Epidemiology
Study Design
and Data Analysis

Third Edition

CHAPMAN & HALL/CRC
Texts in Statistical Science Series

Series Editors
Francesca Dominici, *Harvard School of Public Health, USA*
Julian J. Faraway, *University of Bath, UK*
Martin Tanner, *Northwestern University, USA*
Jim Zidek, *University of British Columbia, Canada*

Texts in Statistical Science

Epidemiology
Study Design
and Data Analysis
Third Edition

Mark Woodward

Professor of Statistics and Epidemiology
University of Oxford, UK

Professor of Biostatistics
The George Institute for Global Health
University of Sydney, Australia

Adjunct Professor of Epidemiology
Johns Hopkins University, USA

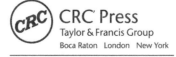

CRC Press
Taylor & Francis Group
Boca Raton   London   New York

CRC Press is an imprint of the
Taylor & Francis Group an **informa** business
A CHAPMAN & HALL BOOK

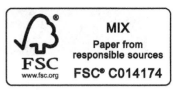

CRC Press
Taylor & Francis Group
6000 Broken Sound Parkway NW, Suite 300
Boca Raton, FL 33487-2742

© 2014 by Taylor & Francis Group, LLC
CRC Press is an imprint of Taylor & Francis Group, an Informa business

No claim to original U.S. Government works

Printed on acid-free paper
Version Date: 20131108

International Standard Book Number-13: 978-1-4398-3970-6 (Hardback)

Visit the Taylor & Francis Web site at
http://www.taylorandfrancis.com

and the CRC Press Web site at
http://www.crcpress.com

To L,
From M

Table of Contents

Preface

This book is about the quantitative aspects of epidemiological research. I have written it with two audiences in mind: the researcher who wishes to understand how statistical principles and techniques may be used to solve epidemiological problems and the applied statistician who wishes to find out how to apply her or his subject in this field. A practical approach is used; although a complete set of formulae are included where hand calculation is viable, mathematical proofs are omitted and statistical nicety has largely been avoided. The techniques described are illustrated by example, and results of the applications of the techniques are interpreted in a practical way. Sometimes hypothetical datasets have been constructed to produce clear examples of epidemiological concepts and methodology. However, the majority of the data used in examples, and exercises, are taken from real epidemiological investigations, drawn from past publications or my own collaborative research. Several substantial datasets are either listed within the book or, more often, made available on the book's web site for the reader to explore using her or his own computer software. SAS and Stata programs for most of the examples, where appropriate, are also provided on this web site. Finally, an extensive list of references is included for further reading.

I have assumed that the reader has some basic knowledge of statistics, such as might be obtained from a medical degree course, or a first-year course in statistics as part of a science degree. Even so, this book is self-contained in that all the standard methods necessary to the rest of the book are reviewed in Chapter 2. From this base, the text goes through analytical methods for general and specific epidemiological study designs, leading on to a practical explanation and development of statistical modelling and then to methods for comparing and summarising the evidence from several studies. Chapters 13 and 14 are new to this edition; they describe some important modern methods in applied statistics. Chapter 13 considers how to translate the results of statistical modelling into clinically useful indices of prognosis, and Chapter 14 shows how to make rational inferences in the absence of complete data or a theoretical formula. As the title suggests, this book is concerned with how to design an epidemiological study, as well as how to analyse the data from such a study. Chapter 1 includes a broad introduction to study design, and later chapters are dedicated to particular types of design: cohort, case-control and intervention studies. Chapter 8 is concerned with the problem of determining the appropriate size for a study.

Some of the material in this book is taken from courses I gave to undergraduate students and students studying the MSc in Biometry at the University of Reading, UK, and to medical and biological students at the Prince Leopold Institute of Tropical Medicine in Antwerp, Belgium. Some of the exercises are based (with permission) on questions that I had previously written for the Medical Statistics examination paper of the Royal Statistical Society.

Outputs in this book were created with:

(1) SAS® software; Copyright 2013, SAS Institute Inc., Cary, NC, USA. All Rights Reserved. Reproduced with permission of SAS Institute Inc., Cary, NC.
(2) Stata Statistical Software; StataCorp. 2013. College Station, TX, USA: Stata-Corp LP.

Neither SAS nor StataCorp is affiliated with Mark Woodward and they have not been asked to endorse this book.

My thanks go to all the authors who gave me permission to present data that they had already published; my apologies to the few authors that I was unable to contact. Thanks also to the following colleagues who allowed me to show data I have been working with, not published elsewhere: Tamakoshi Akiko, John Chalmers, Edel Daly, Dr. Fang, Derrick Heng, Kenneth Hughes, Yutaka Imai, Rod Jackson, Dr. D. J. Jus-sawalla, Matthew Knuiman, Gordon Lowe, Stephen MacMahon, Caroline Morrison, Bruce Neal, Robyn Norton, Saitoh Shigeyuki, Dr. Shimamoto, Piyamitr Sritara, Hugh Tunstall Pedoe, John Whitehead, Professor Wu and B. B. Yeole. I am grateful to Sir Richard Doll for correcting an earlier draft of Table 1.2 and to Julian Higgins and Alex Sutton who provided corrections and insightful comments for Chapter 12.

Thanks for assistance with practical aspects of earlier editions of this book go to Evangelie Barton, Federica Barzi, Alex Owen, Sam Colman and Joan Knock. Thanks to Christine Andreasen for help with proof checking of this edition. I am grateful for the love of my parents, John Woodward and Dorothy Margaret Woodward and my sons, Philip John Woodward and Robert Mark Woodward. Finally, the biggest 'thank you' of all goes to my wife, Lesley Megan Audrey Francis, who was unfailingly sup-portive of my work on this book, and generously understanding when the book took over its author.

M.W.
Baltimore, Maryland, USA
Oxford, England
Sydney, Australia

CHAPTER 1

Fundamental issues

1.1 What is epidemiology?

Epidemiology is the study of the distribution and determinants of disease in human populations. The term derives from the word 'epidemic', which appears to have been derived from *epidemeion*, a word used by Hippocrates when describing a disease that was 'visiting the people'. Modern use of the term (without qualification) retains the restriction to human populations but has broadened the scope to include any type of disease, including those that are far from transient. Thus epidemiologists study chronic (long-duration) diseases, such as asthma, as well as such infectious diseases as cholera that might be inferred from the idea of an 'epidemic'. Chronic diseases (also called non-communicable diseases) are the biggest killers, even in the developing world. Consequently, the majority of epidemiological research addresses chronic diseases and hence most examples is this book are drawn from this field of application.

The **distribution** of disease studied is often a geographical one, but distributions by age, sex, social class, marital status, racial group and occupation (amongst others) are also often of interest. Sometimes the same geographical population is compared at different times to investigate trends in the disease. As an example, consider breast cancer as the disease of interest. This is one of the leading causes of death amongst women in industrialised countries, but epidemiological studies have shown it to be much more common in northern latitudes than in other parts of the world. However, this geographical differential seems to have been decreasing: recent studies suggest a decline in deaths due to breast cancer in industrialised countries, but an increase in Latin America, Africa and some parts of Asia. In general, breast cancer rates have been found to increase with age and to be highest in women of high socioeconomic status who have never married.

The **determinants** of disease are the factors that precipitate disease. Study of the distribution of disease is essentially a descriptive exercise; study of determinants considers the aetiology of the disease. For example, the descriptive finding that women who have never married are more prone to breast cancer leads to investigation of why this should be so. Perhaps the causal factors are features of reproduction, such as a lack of some type of protection that would be conferred by breast feeding. Several studies to address such questions in the epidemiology of breast cancer have been carried out. In general, the factors studied depend upon the particular disease in question and upon prior hypotheses. Typical examples would be exposure to atmospheric pollutants, lifestyle characteristics (such as smoking and diet) and biological characteristics (such as cholesterol and blood pressure). We shall refer to any potential aetiological agent under study as a **risk factor** for the disease of interest; sometimes this term is used in the more restricted sense of being a proven determinant of the disease.

The essential aim of epidemiology is to inform health professionals, and the public at large, in order for improvements in general health status to be made. Both descriptive and aetiological analyses help in this regard. Descriptive analyses give a guide to the optimal allocation of health services and the targeting of health promotion. Aetiological analyses can tell us what to do to lessen our chance of developing the disease in question. Epidemiological data are essential for the planning and evaluation of health services.

Epidemiology is usually regarded as a branch of medicine that deals with populations rather than individuals. Whereas the hospital clinician considers the best treatment and advice to give to each individual patient so as to enable her or him to get better, the epidemiologist considers what advice to give to the general population in order to lessen the overall burden of disease. However, due to its dealings with aggregations (of people), epidemiology is also an applied branch of statistics. Advances in epidemiological research have generally been achieved through interaction of the disciplines of medicine and statistics. Other professions frequently represented in epidemiological research groups are biochemists, sociologists and computing specialists. In specific instances, other professions, such as nutritionists and economists, might be included.

The fascinating history of epidemiology is illustrated by Stolley and Lasky (1995) in their nontechnical account of the subject. Several of the pioneer works are reproduced in Buck *et al.* (1988), which gives a commentary on the development of epidemiological thinking. An alternative (but less comprehensive) annotated collection of key papers is provided by Ashton (1994). See Porta (2008) for a dictionary of terms in common usage by epidemiologists. A superb collection of educational materials relating to epidemiology is available from the University of Pittsburgh 'Supercourse': http://www.pitt.edu/~super1.

1.2   Case studies: the work of Doll and Hill

In this book we shall concentrate on modern applications of epidemiological research. However, as an illustration of the essential ideas, purposes and practice of epidemiology, we shall now consider the innovative work on smoking and lung cancer instigated by Sir Richard Doll and Sir Austin Bradford Hill shortly after the Second World War.

In the period up to 1945 there was a huge increase in the number of deaths due to lung cancer in England and Wales, as well as in other industrialised countries. For instance, the lung cancer death rate amongst men aged 45 and over increased sixfold between 1921–1930 and between 1940–1944 in England and Wales (Doll and Hill, 1950; see also Figure 1.1). This brought attention to a disease that had previously received scant attention in medical journals. A search was on to find the major cause of the disease.

Various factors could have explained the increase, including the possibility that it was an artefact of improved standards of diagnosis. Aetiological explanations put forward included increases in atmospheric pollutants and smoking. Certainly pollution (such as from diesel fuel) and smoking were known to have increased such that the corresponding increase in lung cancer mortality came later — necessary for the relationship to be causal (Section 1.6). Figure 1.1 shows data on lung cancer deaths from 1906 to 1945, taken from government health publications, and industrial records of cigarette sales from 1885 to 1924. Apart from short-term fluctuations in the sales data due to the First World War, a close relationship exists between these variables, but with a time delay. These data come from Peace (1985), who showed that a statistical model assuming a 21-year time lag (consistent with the expected period of growth of a tumour) between the two series was a good fit to these data. Historical evidence of relationships between snuff use and nasal cancer, and between pipe smoking and lip cancer, gave extra credence to the smoking hypothesis.

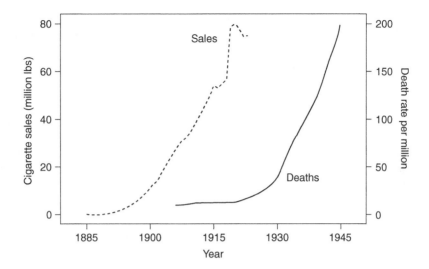

Figure 1.1. Death rate per million population due to lung cancer in England and Wales and cigarette sales in the U.K. over selected time periods.

Example 1.1 By 1948 only very limited evidence, of the kind just related, of a link between smoking and lung cancer was available. Smoking was a commonly enjoyed pastime backed by a lucrative industry, and thus there was reluctance to accept the hypothesis of a link. Consequently, Doll and Hill, a medic and a statistician respectively, instigated a formal scientific study. Between April 1948 and October 1949, they questioned 709 lung cancer patients in 20 hospitals in London (described in Doll and Hill, 1950). These were all the patients admitted to these hospitals with lung cancer, over the period of study, who satisfied certain practical requirements (below 75 years of age, still alive in hospital and able to respond). All cases were asked a set of smoking questions: whether they had smoked at any time; the age at which they started and stopped; the amount they had smoked before the onset of their illness; the main changes in their smoking history; the maximum they had ever smoked; the various proportions smoked in pipes and cigarettes and whether or not they inhaled.

Doll and Hill realized that any results obtained from the lung cancer cases would need to be put into context if they were to provide evidence of causality. For instance, a finding that most of the lung cancer cases smoked would not, by itself, show anything conclusive because it may merely have reflected the norm in general society. Hence, they decided to study a corresponding set of 709 controls. For each case, they sought a noncancer patient, of the same sex and 5-year age group from the same hospital at about the same time, to act as a control. Each control was asked the same questions about smoking habits as was each case.

Table 1.1 gives some basic results from the study (taken from Doll and Hill, 1950). Here 'never-smokers' are people who have never smoked as much as one cigarette each day for as long as a year. The nonzero consumptions show the amount smoked immediately prior to the onset of illness or to quitting smoking altogether. The impact of smoking upon lung cancer may be evaluated by comparing the smoking distributions for cases and controls within each sex group. For men, although the percentage of controls in the 'never' and the 1–4 and 5–14 per day groups exceeds the corresponding percentages of cases, the opposite is true in the higher consumption groups. Thus, cases are more likely to be heavy smokers. A similar pattern is seen for women, although they tended to smoke less and have a more concentrated smoking distribution.

Doll and Hill were aware that their study was not ideal for demonstrating causality. In particular, several potential sources of **bias** — uncontrolled features in the data leading to distorted results and thus, possibly, misleading conclusions — were present. For example, bias could have arisen from inaccuracies in recall of smoking history. It could be that lung cancer patients tended to exaggerate their consumption because they were aware that their illness

Table 1.1. Tobacco consumption[a] by case/control status by sex for patients in London hospitals. Cases are patients with carcinoma of the lung; controls are patients without cancer.

No. of cigarettes/day	Males				Females			
	Cases		Controls		Cases		Controls	
Never-smokers	2	(0%)	27	(4%)	19	(32%)	32	(53%)
1–4	33	(5%)	55	(8%)	7	(12%)	12	(20%)
5–14	250	(39%)	293	(45%)	19	(32%)	10	(17%)
15–24	196	(30%)	190	(29%)	9	(15%)	6	(10%)
25–49	136	(21%)	71	(11%)	6	(10%)	0	
50 or more	32	(5%)	13	(2%)	0		0	
Total	649	(100%)	649	(100%)	60	(100%)	60	(100%)

[a] Ounces of tobacco are expressed in equivalent cigarette numbers; ex-smokers are attributed with the amount they smoked before giving up.

could be related to smoking. A second possibility is that the control group members were not sufficiently compatible with the cases so as to provide a 'fair' comparison. For instance, lung cancer cases were known to arise from a wider catchment area than did the predominantly city-dwelling controls. This could have led to some important differences in lifestyle or environmental exposures, which might have explained the different patterns shown in Table 1.1. In fact, Doll and Hill (1950) provide evidence to show that these particular forms of bias were unlikely to have explained Table 1.1 fully. Nevertheless, other types of bias may not have been recognized. Interestingly, one source of bias, which was not obvious in 1950, will have led to an underestimate of the effect of smoking. This was the use of control patients who had diseases that are now known to be associated with smoking.

Example 1.2 Partially to address concerns regarding their earlier study, Doll and Hill began a much larger study in November 1951. They sent a questionnaire on smoking to all those listed on the British medical register. Altogether there were almost 60 000 on this register; of these, 69% of men and 60% of women responded. These subjects were followed up in succeeding years, leading to a string of published reports from 1954 onwards. This follow-up mainly took the form of recording deaths. Automatic notification was received from death registrations (Section 1.7.2) of anyone who was medically qualified, and obituary notices for the profession were regularly perused. Causes of death were recorded in each case, except in the small number of instances in which this proved impossible to ascertain.

Doll and Hill (1964) report lung cancer rates according to smoking habit over the first 10 years of the study. Table 1.2 gives a small extract from the 10-year results for men (numbers of female

Table 1.2. Lung cancer mortality rates[a] per thousand for male British doctors.

Length of follow-up	Never-smokers	Cigarette smokers (number/day)		
		1–14	5–24	25 or more
10 years[b]	0.07	0.57	1.39	2.27
40 years[c]	0.14	1.05	2.08	3.55

[a] The 10-year data are standardised for age on the England and Wales population. The 40-year data are indirectly standardised from the whole dataset (see Section 4.5 for explanations of terms).
[b] Smoking habit as of 1951 (or last recorded before death).
[c] Smoking habit as of 1990 (or last recorded before death).

smokers were not sufficient to provide a precise picture of the effect of smoking amongst women). Here the definition of a 'never-smoker' is as in Example 1.1. These data provide firm evidence of a relationship between smoking and lung cancer. Not only are never-smokers much less likely to die from lung cancer, but also the chance of death increases as the amount smoked goes up. Heavy (25 or more per day) cigarette smokers have over 30 times the chance of death due to lung cancer compared with never-smokers. This evidence alone does not imply causality; for instance, it could still be that lung cancer symptoms preceded smoking. However, Doll and Hill (1964) were also able to demonstrate a degree of reversibility of effect: those who had given up smoking had a lower lung cancer death rate than continuing smokers, with lower rates for those who had a longer period of abstinence.

The other aspect of the continuing monitoring of the doctors was a succession of mailed questionnaires to produce updated records of smoking habits. Further substantial reports on the progress of male doctors give the results of 20 years (Doll and Peto, 1976), 40 years (Doll *et al.*, 1994) and 50 years (Doll *et al.*, 2004) of follow-up of deaths, related to the updated smoking habits. Table 1.2 gives some results from the 40-year follow-up. At this stage, the 34 339 men recruited in 1951 had been reduced by 20 523 deaths, 2530 migrations abroad and 265 who had been lost to follow-up, leaving 11 121 alive at 1 November 1991. In Table 1.2, the smoking habit shown is that last reported (the last questionnaire had been posted in 1990). Clearly, the relative patterns are the same as in the 10-year results, despite the fact that the percentage who were smoking had reduced from 62% overall in 1951 to 18% in the survivors at 1990.

Since all deaths, due to any cause, were recorded, deaths from diseases other than lung cancer could also be studied and the publications cited look at deaths by cause. Indeed, having already established some evidence of an effect of smoking on lung cancer, one of the original aims of the study was to relate smoking to a range of diseases. Table 1.3 shows some results, within broad disease groupings, from the 40-year analyses; these are taken from Doll *et al.* (1994), which gives much more detailed information. Again, the smoking habit is that reported on the last questionnaire returned: at 1990 or just before death. The relative sizes of the mortality rates for each disease group show the consistency of the effect of smoking. Never-smokers have

Table 1.3. Number of deaths (showing annual mortality rate[a] per 100 000 in parentheses) during 40-years' observation of male British doctors, by cause of death and last reported smoking habit.

| Disease group | Never-smokers | Cigarette smokers (number/day) | | | | Other smokers | |
		Ex	1–14	15–24	25 or more	Ex	Current
Neoplastic	414	885	317	416	406	565	1081
	(305)	(384)	(482)	(645)	(936)	(369)	(474)
Respiratory	131	455	161	170	159	290	392
	(107)	(192)	(237)	(310)	(471)	(176)	(164)
Vascular	1304	2761	1026	1045	799	1878	2896
	(1037)	(1221)	(1447)	(1671)	(1938)	(1226)	(1201)
Other medical	225	458	169	171	149	330	429
	(170)	(202)	(242)	(277)	(382)	(212)	(182)
Trauma and poisoning	114	165	81	80	93	95	196
	(72)	(84)	(103)	(90)	(172)	(79)	(88)
Unknown	27	78	13	13	12	29	45
	(17)	(29)	(33)	(30)	(41)	(16)	(24)
Total	2215	4802	1767	1895	1618	3187	5039
	(1706)	(2113)	(2542)	(3004)	(3928)	(2078)	(2130)

[a] Standardised for age and calendar period.

the lowest death rate (except in the 'unknown' category) and heavy cigarette smokers have the highest rate for each disease group. Former cigarette smokers always have a rate that is intermediate to the never and light (1 to 14 per day) cigarette smokers. Other smokers, a mixed bag, are generally comparable with former cigarette smokers. The overall conclusion is that smoking has an effect detrimental to general health; this effect is partially reversible by quitting.

The results of this, the 'British Doctors Study', could lack general applicability on account of the rather special subject group used. Doctors are certain to be more aware of health issues than are most others and hence may act and be treated rather differently. However, the results are consistent with the very many other studies of smoking and health carried out since the Second World War, including Example 1.1. Coupled with a reasonable biological explanation of the causal pathway (carcinogens in tobacco smoke causing a neoplastic transformation), the epidemiological evidence proves, to any reasonable degree, a causal effect of smoking on the development of lung cancer.

1.3   Populations and samples

1.3.1   Populations

An epidemiological study involves the collection, analysis and interpretation of data from a human population. The population about which we wish to draw conclusions is called the **target population**. In many cases, this is defined according to geographical criteria — for example, all men in Britain. The specific population from which data are collected is called the **study population**. Thus, the British Doctors Study (Example 1.2) has all British doctors in 1951 as the study population. It is a question of judgement whether results for the study population may be used to draw accurate conclusions about the target population; possible problems with making generalisations from the British Doctors Study have already been mentioned. The ultimate target population is all human beings.

Most epidemiological investigations use study populations that are based on geographical, institutional or occupational definitions. Besides questions of generalisation, the study population must also be a suitable base for exploring the hypotheses being studied. For instance, a study of the effects of smoking needs to be set in a study population in which a reasonable number of smokers and nonsmokers can be found. In 1951, this was true amongst British doctors but would not have been true in a manual occupation group in which virtually everyone was a smoker. The optimal study population for comparing smokers and nonsmokers would have equal numbers of each (Section 8.4.3). The British population of doctors was also big enough for any effects to be estimated reliably.

Another way of classifying the study population is by the stage of the disease. We might choose a population that is diseased, disease-free or a mixture. If recommendations for the primary prevention of disease are our ultimate aim, then a study population that is initially disease free would be an ideal choice in a follow-up investigation. Often such a population is impossible or too expensive to identify; for example, the study population in Example 1.2 is a mixture of those with and without existing lung cancer in 1951 (although the seriously ill would not have been able to reply to the questionnaire in any case). If the study population is a set of people with the disease who are then monitored through time, we will be able to study only determinants of progressive (or some entirely different) disease.

If the study population is not readily available, costs will rise and nonresponse may be more likely. Doll and Hill no doubt chose British doctors as their study population in Example 1.2 because they were easily identifiable and likely to be cooperative. However, the issue of availability is often in conflict with that of generalisability.

1.3.2 Samples

If the study requires collection of new data, we shall usually need to sample from our study population. Generalisability is then a two-stage procedure: we want to be able to generalise from the sample to the study population and then from the study population to the target population.

Again, conflict between availability and generalisability (cost and accuracy) at the sampling stage is often present. An extreme example is one in which a volunteer sample is used. Rarely are volunteers typical of the whole. For instance, people who reply to a newspaper advertisement asking them to undergo a physical examination may well differ from the general population in several important ways that could have a bearing upon the results of the epidemiological investigation. They might be predominantly health conscious, so their vital signs are relatively superior. Alternatively, most of them might be out of work (and thus available for daytime mid-week screening) and getting relatively little exercise or eating a relatively poor diet as a consequence. These two scenarios may each produce biased results; if they do, the biases are likely to be in opposite directions. In many instances, we may suspect the direction of bias but have no way of quantifying it. Sampling is most reliable when done randomly, and this will always be the preferred option (Section 1.8.2).

Sometimes epidemiologists use the term 'study population' to refer to the group of people from whom data are collected. The rationale is that this group is the totality of those being studied, perhaps by monitoring for ill health during a follow-up period. However, using the term in this way can be extremely confusing because it conflicts with the general statistical definitions of 'study population' and 'sample' (used here): the epidemiologist's 'study population' is the statistician's 'sample'. A better term for the total group being questioned, examined or followed up would be the 'study group', although 'sample' is often perfectly adequate and technically correct.

1.4 Measuring disease

A typical epidemiological study will require the number of disease outcomes to be counted (as in Example 1.2) or subjects to be selected according to disease status (as in Example 1.1). Thus, we require a definition of what is meant by 'disease' in each specific context. Ideally, we should like to have a clinical definition that can be tested by objective evidence. Frequently, we must rely upon less definitive criteria, if only to keep costs down. Sometimes disease is used in a more general sense than the English language would allow, such as when the disease is a road traffic accident and we are seeking the risk factors that make such accidents more likely. Often epidemiologists are involved in studies of the validity and consistency of diagnostic criteria.

One clear choice in several situations is whether to measure **mortality** (death due to the disease in question) or **morbidity** (being sick with the disease in question). In Example 1.1, lung cancer morbidity was used as a selection criterion and in Example 1.2 lung cancer mortality was used as the primary outcome measure. In general, given two similar studies of the same disease, one of which measures morbidity and the other measures mortality, the determinants of disease identified in one of the studies may differ from those found in the other. This may be a true finding; some factors may cause only relatively minor forms of a disease. Alternatively, the difference may be an artefact of the way in which data were collected. For instance, a survey of post-mortems may find a strong relationship between a particular risk factor and a given disease, but a survey of morbidity amongst live people might find no relationship simply because most of those with the risk factor have already died.

Morbidity may be subdivided into degrees of severity, so comparability of results may still be a problem even within the restricted class of morbidity studies. Often severity is closely linked to the source of information used. Thus, because a family doctor, or general practitioner (GP), will usually refer only her or his most serious cases to a hospital, we can expect disease to mean something rather more serious when we use hospital, rather than GP, records. Sometimes sickness may be identified from self-reports, primarily sickness absence notifications from employees. Generally, only the worst such cases will have seen a GP. There may also be unreported cases of disease, such as those who do not feel ill enough to stay away from work. We might be able to uncover such 'hidden' disease only by screening the general population.

The hierarchy of severity of disease (including death) is sometimes represented by analogy with a partially submerged iceberg. In the situation illustrated by Figure 1.2, data have been derived from death certificates and hospital records; cases of disease that could have been identified by other means (usually only the less severe cases) remain unidentified.

Thus, the decision about how to define disease is bound up with the source of information to be used. Generally, we can expect to find more cases of disease as we move down the disease iceberg. This may seem like a good thing to do, especially when the disease is very rare. However, this will normally correspond with a dilution of the epidemiological essence of the disease, that is, the importance of the condition to the population at large. Mild disease, leading to a quick recovery, or hidden disease, which shows no outward symptoms and has no discernible effect on its host, may have little impact on general health or the use of health services. Furthermore, we risk losing specificity as we broaden our information base; GP diagnoses may lack objective clinical confirmation, and sickness absence reports will be necessarily simplistic and thus relatively vague.

For some diseases, the iceberg of Figure 1.2 has too many layers. Any disease that does not lead to death, or at least not in the normal course of events, will not require the top layer — for example, eczema. Similarly, people with serious accidental injuries will go straight to hospital for attention, missing out the GP stage. Another, less obvious, caveat to the iceberg analogy is that certain types of serious cases of disease may not get routinely reported to any recording system. This would happen if members

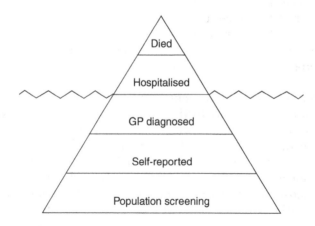

Figure 1.2. The 'disease iceberg'.

of some minority ethnic group were reluctant to use the official health service. Under-reporting of disease, or a biased view of the relationship between disease and some risk factor that is very common (or very unusual) amongst the particular ethnic group, may result. General population screening may be the only answer to this problem.

1.4.1 Incidence and prevalence

As well as deciding how to define disease, we also need to decide how to count it. This leads to consideration of the most important dichotomy in epidemiology: incidence and prevalence of disease. **Incidence** is the number of new cases of the disease within a specified period of time. **Prevalence** is the number of existing cases of disease at a particular point in time. For example, in Table 1.3 we see the incidence of death, overall and by broad cause, over the 40-year period from 1 November 1951. If Doll and Hill had recorded the number of British doctors with lung cancer in 1951, they would have measured the prevalence of this disease. Prevalence is a measure of morbidity, whereas incidence can measure morbidity, mortality or their combination.

Incidence and prevalence are often very different for the same disease in the same population. The prevalence certainly depends upon the incidence, but also depends upon the duration of the disease. A rarely cured chronic disease will have a much greater prevalence than incidence, whereas a disease that leads to death soon after it is diagnosed may have a higher incidence than prevalence. If the incidence and the average duration of the disease are constant over time, then

$$P = ID,$$

where P is prevalence, I is incidence and D is the average duration.

In practice, the assumption of constancy may well be untrue. For many diseases, incidence is not static over successive years. If incidence is dropping, perhaps due to preventive measures consequent to epidemiological research, eventually a very small annual incidence may be observed in a population within which the prevalence is high (principally amongst older adults). This effect will be compounded if the preventive measures also serve to increase the chance of survival for those who already have the disease (here the average duration is also changing).

Normally incidence and prevalence are measured on a relative scale. A simple example is one in which counts of disease are related to the size of the study population (from census results or projections) at the middle of that year. Then we have the following definitions for a specific population and a specific year:

$$\frac{\text{Prevalence rate}}{\text{at mid-year}} = \frac{\text{Number of people with disease at mid-year}}{\text{Mid-year population}}; \qquad (1.1)$$

$$\frac{\text{Incidence rate}}{\text{for the year}} = \frac{\text{Number of new cases of disease in the year}}{\text{Mid-year population}}. \qquad (1.2)$$

In (1.1) and (1.2), the choices of the middle of the year for counting the at-risk population and the prevalence, and the year as the time period for counting the incidence, are arbitrary. Often incidence is averaged over several successive years to obtain an average annual rate. Sometimes the time point used in the numerator and denominator of the prevalence rate are different, although they will usually be in the same calendar year. We shall consider issues of relative measures of incidence and prevalence more fully in Chapter 3. Somewhat confusingly, epidemiologists sometimes refer to the absolute counts of disease and their relative measures, such as (1.1) and (1.2), as prevalence or incidence (as the case may be), although the meaning is usually clear from the context.

As an example of how incidence and prevalence differ, we shall consider *Helicobacter pylori*, a chronic bacterial disease identified in the 1980s. After establishment, the organism responsible generally persists for life unless treatment is given, which is rarely the case at present. Infection seems to be associated with poor social conditions so that, in industrialised countries, many adults will have been infected in childhood, whereas children now (living in better conditions than did their parents) tend to have a low chance of infection. Hence, the overall incidence should be low and the prevalence high. Epidemiological studies in developed countries have shown this to be the case; amongst adults, the incidence rate is estimated to be about 0.5% per year (Parsonnet, 1995) but the prevalence rate is between 37% and 80%, depending upon the ages of the people studied (Pounder and Ng, 1995).

Generally speaking, prevalence measures are better suited to descriptive studies. For instance, comparison of disease prevalence by region suggests how the burden of disease is distributed in a country, which leads to appropriate plans for allocation of resources. Whilst such analyses may *suggest* possible causal factors for the disease, they cannot provide convincing proof. Incidence studies are much better for studying aetiology because they can better establish the sequence of events (Section 1.6 and Section 3.4) and because they are not susceptible to bias by survival. To explain this latter point using an extreme example, suppose that everyone with a certain disease who does not take large daily doses of vitamins dies very quickly. Those who have the disease but do take large daily doses of vitamins survive for several years. Prevalence may then be positively related to vitamin consumption, making it seem as though this is a risky, rather than a healthy, habit.

Most epidemiological investigations are studies of incidence or of prevalence. Lack of identification or consideration of which has been studied is a common source of misconception when interpreting results. In some situations, however, some other way of counting disease is used. One example is when the number of hospital admissions with a particular disease is counted over a period of time. This gives a record of **case incidence**, which will be equal to true incidence only when there are no readmissions of the same patient. Such data may require careful scrutiny and interpretation in any aetiological analysis.

1.5   Measuring the risk factor

Although few general comments can be made about how to measure risk factors, many have the common feature that they can be measured in different ways, and this aspect is worthy of consideration. As an example, consider the risk factor of Section 1.2, tobacco consumption. Doll and Hill asked their subjects to state their smoking habits for themselves. Owing to the possibility of misreporting (most probably under-reporting of smoking consumption in a modern setting), an objective biochemical test may be preferable. Many of these are available, including breath tests and tests on blood, saliva or urine samples, which measure amounts of specific constituents of tobacco smoke (such as nicotine) or their metabolites.

To select a method, the epidemiologist needs to balance the issues of accuracy, cost and intrusion or distress to the subjects. Self-reporting is almost certainly the cheapest option but could give misleading inferences if a particular pattern of misreporting prevails. Tests on blood samples may be most accurate but are invasive and require trained personnel and expensive equipment. Note that a method that causes distress, or is difficult to carry out, may result in several missing values, which will adversely affect the reliability of the results obtained. Sometimes missing values are more likely for certain types of people; for instance, it is more difficult to find a vein in an obese person than in others, so blood samples may be more likely to be absent from the obese. This may lead to biased conclusions (Section 14.9).

Another issue arising in many applications is that of reproducibility. Some risk factors, or sometimes just particular methods for determining them, may be deemed to be unreliable when measured at a single instance, due to variation within the patient over time, between observers or between laboratories. Sometimes this problem may be overcome by taking multiple readings. For instance, duplicate serum cholesterol readings might be taken from any one subject on a single day, and averaged. Often there is long-term within-patient variation, which requires repeat measurement over time to correct atypically high or low values initially recorded, if we wish to quantify the effect of usual values of the risk factor (Section 10.12).

Sometimes the setting within which the risk factor is measured may have an effect. A female subject, for example, may be unwilling to divulge details of her contraceptive practice if the interviewer is male. Similarly, a subject's blood pressure may increase well above its norm when a doctor measures it in a clinic setting (so-called 'white coat hypertension'). These types of problems can lead to bias error and can be avoided only by careful planning.

When we wish to have a historical record of a subject's risk factor status, we generally must rely upon the subject's recall. This issue arose in Doll and Hill's studies (Section 1.2) when they wanted to know previous smoking habits. An exception is when records have been kept automatically, such as records of atmospheric pollution or exposure to hazardous chemicals whilst in employment.

1.6   Causality

Epidemiological research often seeks to identify whether a causal relationship exists between the risk factor and the disease. For instance, we have already considered how far the studies described in Section 1.2 may be interpreted as showing a causal effect of smoking upon lung cancer. As in that example, the first stage in investigating causality is to establish an association; then we go on to consider what the particular association might imply.

1.6.1   Association

A straightforward example of an association between risk factor and disease is one in which a group of people have attended a conference dinner, and a proportion of them become sick overnight. If it happened that everyone who had eaten a particular food became sick, and everyone who avoided that food remained well, then the food would clearly be associated with sickness. Indeed, it would be difficult to argue that it was not causally associated, especially if left-over food were found to be contaminated.

This type of situation is illustrated by the Venn diagram in Figure 1.3(a). In this, and other parts of this figure, the area within the rectangle represents the study population or the sample taken from it. The area within the ellipse containing the letter E represents those exposed to the risk factor (the contaminated food in the example) and the shaded area represents those who have the disease (sickness in the example). In Figure 1.3(a), the exposed and diseased subgroups are conterminous.

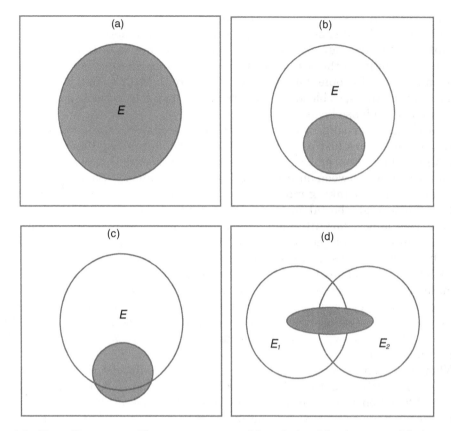

Figure 1.3. Venn diagrams to illustrate some possible relationships between risk factor exposure and disease status.

Most epidemiological problems are not as straightforward. Even when a truly causal factor is investigated, we may well find that not everyone exposed to it becomes diseased. Thus, anecdotal stories of 100-year-old men who have smoked a packet of cigarettes each day since their youth need to be accounted for when discussing the causal effects of smoking. It may be that the situation illustrated by Figure 1.3(b) is encountered: disease occurs only when exposure occurs, but some of those exposed are disease free. An association is still present here: exposure is a necessary but not a sufficient condition for disease. We may be able to build a theory of causation around such an association. Going back to the example of the conference meal, perhaps some people ate too little of the food to experience any discernible reaction, or perhaps some people have a natural immunity.

More complex still is the situation of Figure 1.3(c). Now a proportion of those exposed are diseased, but a proportion of the unexposed are also diseased. Exposure is now neither necessary nor sufficient for disease to occur. Yet an association still exists between risk factor and disease as long as the two proportions just mentioned are very different; in Figure 1.3(c) there is a much higher chance of disease amongst those exposed than amongst those unexposed. Again, we may be able to suggest a causal explanation for the findings. Related to the previous example, some people who did not eat the contaminated food at the dinner may have eaten it the day before, have eaten another contaminated food or have some disease with symptoms similar to the general sickness observed. Most modern-day epidemiological analyses of a single risk factor encounter the situation of Figure 1.3(c).

Figure 1.3(d) illustrates a situation with two risk factors: exposures are now represented as E_1 and E_2. Some people have been exposed to only one, some have been exposed to both and some have been exposed to neither risk factor. It is only in the latter subgroup that disease does not occur. This diagram could be generalised to admit several risk factors, thus having several overlapping ellipses. Any one risk factor is associated with disease if exposure to it coincides with an excess of disease. This is the type of situation for most of the diseases studied by epidemiologists today. For instance, well over 200 risk factors have been suggested for coronary heart disease (CHD). The generalised version of Figure 1.3(d) represents reality; the epidemiologist seeks to fill in the names of the risk factors involved and, ultimately, to provide a causal explanation, where appropriate. In this sense, Figure 1.3(c) could be a special case of Figure 1.3(d) in which two factors are associated with the disease, one of which has not yet been identified. Figure 1.3(b) could be another special case of Figure 1.3(d) where it is only in the presence of both risk factors (one of which is currently unknown) that disease occurs (a rather special example of an **interaction**; see Chapter 4).

1.6.2   Problems with establishing causality

The establishment of an association is a necessary, but certainly not a sufficient, condition to establish causation. For instance, consider a study of dog ownership and blindness. A survey may well find that a greater proportion of blind people own dogs, but it would be bizarre to conclude that dog ownership causes blindness. This example shows that we need to establish which came first. If it could be shown that children born to families with dogs are more likely to go blind in later life, then a basis for a causal relationship exists. We might argue that these children have come into contact with dog faeces and thus contracted toxoplasmosis.

Another problem in establishing causality in epidemiology is that of refuting other plausible explanations of the association observed. This is an inherent problem due to the nature of epidemiological data: observational rather than experimental (Section 1.8). Consider a study that finds CHD to be much more prevalent amongst people with at least one parent who has had CHD (alive or deceased). This is interpreted as showing that a genetic factor must predispose towards CHD. On the face of it, this seems a reasonable interpretation, but are there alternative theories? Those with CHD are probably older than those without, because the disease is progressive and thus age related. Older people will, on the whole, have older parents who thus have an increased chance of CHD. Also, people from the same family tend to have the same lifestyle, for instance in terms of smoking, diet and exercise, each of which is known to have some effect on the chance of CHD. Age and the lifestyle variables may thus explain the link with parental CHD. These variables are then said to be **confounding** factors; the effect of parental history of CHD is *confounded* by these other variables. This important topic is looked at in detail in Chapter 4. One of the greatest challenges in epidemiological research is the unravelling of overlapping associations and causal pathways, made more difficult by the fact that many lifestyle and biological risk factors are strongly interrelated (for example, many people who smoke heavily also have low intakes of vitamins and fibre). Looking at the results of the preceding hypothetical study in another way, they could be said to promote the theory that CHD is an infectious disease. Unless the data are more detailed than we have so far supposed, the only thing against this causal theory is the lack of a convincing biological explanation.

The foregoing gives examples in which data collection and analysis alone are unable to establish causality. We could even adopt the philosophical stance that causality can never be proven absolutely through epidemiological investigation, simply because it is impossible to completely control all the other factors that may be important. Whether or not a causal effect has been established by common consent is a question of the quality of the evidence available. As has already been said in Section 1.2, there is sufficient evidence from many studies to be able to state that smoking causes lung cancer. The jury is still out for many other epidemiological associations.

1.6.3   Principles of causality

A helpful set of principles for judging whether the information available is of sufficient quality to warrant a conclusion of causality were suggested by Sir Austin Bradford Hill. These have been adapted to produce the following seven points. Most of these have already been mentioned or illustrated by example. It is not suggested that any of these principles is necessary or sufficient for causality to be declared, but each will strengthen the evidence in its favour.

1. There should be evidence of a strong association between the risk factor and the disease. Weak relationships may be due to chance occurrence and are more likely to be explainable by confounding.
2. There should be evidence that exposure to the risk factor preceded the onset of disease.
3. There should be a plausible biological explanation.
4. The association should be supported by other investigations in different study settings. This is to protect against chance findings and bias caused by a particular choice of study population or study design.
5. There should be evidence of reversibility of the effect. That is, if the 'cause' is removed, the 'effect' should also disappear, or at least be less likely.
6. There should be evidence of a dose–response effect. That is, the greater the amount of exposure to the risk factor is, the greater is the chance of disease.
7. There should be no convincing alternative explanation. For instance, the association should not be explainable by confounding.

1.7   Studies using routine data

The simplest type of epidemiological study is that which uses routine data, the sources of which will be reviewed in Section 1.7.2 to Section 1.7.4. Routine data are often not suitable for demonstrating causality but are generally useful for descriptive purposes. Often, analyses of such data will suggest hypotheses that more complex studies, using special data collection (Section 1.8), will then address.

The advantages of using routine data are their low cost, ready accessibility and (when official sources are used) authoritative nature. A major disadvantage is that the data are often not adequate for the purposes of the investigation. Several important risk factors may not be included in any routine collection, and the available data may not be sufficiently comprehensive — for example, when they arise from several small-scale samples or relate only to special types of people. It is likely that risk factor and disease data derive from different sources, in which case differences in definition may be a problem. For instance, Figure 1.1 compares risk factor data for the U.K. with disease data from England and Wales and would be misleading if increases in cigarette sales had been restricted to parts of the U.K. outside England and Wales. These problems are made greater when we want to allow for confounding factors because we will need comparable data on these variables also.

1.7.1   Ecological data

Routine data are almost invariably grouped, typically being average values, percentages or totals for geographical regions or for the same region at different times (as in Figure 1.1). Whenever we have grouped (or **ecological**) data, we may encounter the **ecological fallacy**: the assumption that an observed relationship in aggregated data will hold at the individual level. For instance, consider a study using routine data that shows a relationship between the death rate due to AIDS and the percentage who are heavy drinkers for 20 different countries. Drinking is then certainly related to AIDS at the national level, but can we necessarily infer that the relationship will hold amongst individual people? We have no means to answer this question from the aggregate analysis; even a situation in which no person who drinks heavily has AIDS may be compatible with the data.

A classic example of the fallacy is the Durkheim (1951) study of suicides, illustrated by Figure 1.4. Here the suicide rate between 1883 and 1890 is related to the percentage of the population who were Protestant in each of four Prussian provinces. The naïve inference is that those of the Protestant religion are more likely to commit suicide. However, this is not necessarily true. An alternative explanation is that members of minority religious groups were the ones committing suicide, and the more they were in the minority, the greater was the chance of suicide. This is a completely opposite aetiological interpretation of the same data! In fact, Morgenstern (1982) shows that there was still an excess suicide rate amongst Protestants at the individual level, but the relative excess was of the order of 2 rather than the level of 7.6 calculated using the ecological data shown in Figure 1.4.

Ecological analyses may be advantageous when risk factor measurement at the individual level is particularly prone to error. In this situation, we may only be able

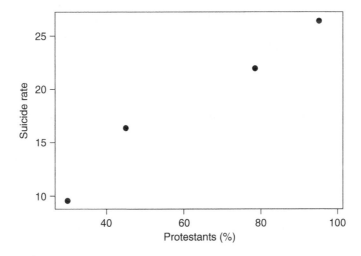

Figure 1.4. Suicide rate per 100 000 population against the percentage who were Protestant in four Prussian provinces, 1883–1890.

to see a true association at the ecological level. For example, it is notoriously difficult to measure the consumption of specific nutrients accurately for any particular individual. This is due to variations in the nutritional content of foods, person-to-person variations in cooking practice and portion size, and day-to-day differences in the eating habits of a given person. When people are grouped, we would expect a reasonably accurate estimate of average consumption to be found, because we would anticipate that under- and overestimation would cancel out. This comment is not restricted to routine data; such a situation may arise with dedicated data collection also.

1.7.2   National sources of data on disease

Routine mortality data derive from the death certificates completed whenever a death occurs. This is usually done by a relative or friend of the deceased at a local registration centre where births and marriages will also be recorded. Information is subsequently compiled at a national registration centre. Registration is thought to be close to 100% complete in most industrialised countries but is very incomplete in many developing countries in which there may be no legal compunction to record deaths; even if there is, compliance may be poor in rural areas.

On the death certificate, demographic characteristics, such as age at death, sex, occupation and place of residence, are recorded along with the cause of death. By convention, causes are specified according to the International Classification of Diseases (ICD): see http:/www.who.int/classifications/icd/en/. This classification is revised periodically. The underlying as well as associated causes of death are recorded. Comparisons of mortality by geographical areas, or over time within the same geographical area, may be compromised by differing diagnostic practices, particularly use of different ICD revisions or different fashions for ascribing precedence when multiple causes are involved.

Routine morbidity data, as shown in Section 1.4, come from different sources. The range available and the degree of comprehensiveness vary from country to country. All over the world, hospitals keep detailed records which, in normal circumstances, are regularly summarised and aggregated for official use. Routine coverage of primary health facilities is much more variable. In countries with a national web of local health centres, data reporting may be as regular as from hospitals. Private health care systems, which are widespread in the U.S. at the primary and hospital levels, usually have complete records. In the U.K., where GPs are effectively self-employed, routine primary care data in a useful form for epidemiological purposes come from occasional national morbidity surveys, regular returns to a national GP study centre from volunteer practices and local initiatives to link computerised databases.

Another common source of data throughout the world is notifications of infectious diseases, such as cholera and typhoid. Such data are useful for studying trends over time as well as for flagging up when and where a new outbreak of disease occurs, often leading to a special epidemiological study to discover the cause. The World Health Organization (WHO) deems certain diseases to be notifiable within all member states, whilst national governments often add other diseases when compiling their national list of notifiable diseases. Health officials will have a statutory responsibility to report each case of a notifiable disease to a local, and thus ultimately a national, registration centre. Some countries have, additionally, disease registers, such as for tuberculosis, cancer or congenital malformations. Sometimes such registration is voluntary.

Other possible sources of routine morbidity data include the sickness benefit forms already mentioned in Section 1.4, school health reports and accident statistics. Records of immunizations and vaccinations can also be relevant.

A further important source of routine data is the population Census, typically carried out every 10 years. This does not usually give data on the number with a disease of interest but does tell us how many are at risk of this disease in the general population. This enables routine disease counts to be put into perspective; see (1.1) and (1.2). Census reports, derived statistics and consequent projections are usually published by the national statistics office of the country concerned.

1.7.3   National sources of data on risk factors

For some risk factors, data can be obtained from official or other routine sources. For instance, Figure 1.1 shows data on cigarette sales from industrial sources. Household, consumer, nutritional and lifestyle surveys are often useful sources of data, particularly on exercise, smoking, drinking and general diet. A prime example is the National Health and Nutrition Examination Survey (NHANES) in the U.S., which has echoes in many countries. Often the surveys that provide risk factor data are carried out by the national statistical office. Risk factors that require invasive measurement are less likely to appear in such compilations, but are sometimes included (such as in NHANES). Otherwise, searches of the epidemiological and medical academic literature may be necessary.

1.7.4   International data

International statistics on population and disease are published regularly by WHO. Subgroups within WHO collate international disease data of specific interest, such as data from dental surveys of children (see, for example, Figure 1.5) and data on cardiovascular disease from the MONICA (multinational MONItoring of trends and determinants in CArdiovascular disease) Project (Tunstall–Pedoe, 2003). International researchers in cancer should be aware of the WHO GLOBOCAN database (http://glob-ocan.iarc.fr/), which includes country-specific data on prevalence, incidence and mortality by site of cancer. Some of these data are estimates used to fill in missing data values, for example in countries where no national cancer registry exists. Risk factor data, at country level, for key chronic disease risk factors are compiled within the WHO Global InfoBase (http://www.who.int/ncd_surveillance/infobase/en/index.html); some of these data are collected using the WHO STEPwise approach to Surveillance (STEPS) methodology (http://www.who.int/chp/steps/en/), which is an excellent model for collecting data on chronic disease risk factors. More useful for other purposes are the national data on development indicators from the United Nations Millennium Development Goals project (http://mdgs.un.org/unsd/mdg/default.aspx). Another useful source of international data for epidemiological purposes arises from the WHO Global Burden of Disease project (http://www.who.int/topics/global_burden_of_disease/en/).

1.8   Study design

An epidemiological study could be designed in several ways so as to collect new data. Two basic principles should always be followed: the study should be comparative and we should seek to avoid all potential causes of bias. As in Example 1.1, where Doll and Hill included controls as well as cases, we will not be able to make judgements about association unless we can make comparisons. Consider also Table 1.3; we would get the completely wrong idea about the effect of smoking from looking at the *numbers* of deaths (which lack the element of comparison to the number at risk) in each smoking category. Bias error, as we have seen by example already, can lead to erroneous conclusions about association and causation.

Two main classes of study type may be identified: observational and interventional. By far the vast majority of epidemiological studies are **observational**, meaning that data are collected simply to see what is happening, as in Example 1.1 and Example 1.2. By contrast, an **intervention** study is an experiment; that is, things are made to happen. We shall start our discussion with intervention studies because these are the gold standard as far as aetiological investigations are concerned. The brief details given here are, where indicated, expanded upon in later chapters. Lengthier discussions on study design appear in Lilienfield and Stolley (1994) and MacMahon and Trichopoulos (1996).

1.8.1   Intervention studies

In Section 1.2 we saw that, in the late 1940s, Doll and Hill and others were interested in the effects of smoking on health. An excellent way of studying this would be to take a large group of people who had never smoked and had no evidence of disease, and to ask a randomly selected half to smoke heavily and the rest to continue to abstain. After several years, the disease experience would be compared between the two halves. Results from such a study would give very strong evidence of a causal effect (or not) of smoking.

This is an example of an intervention study, the essential characteristics of which are that the investigators initially assign the 'treatment' (positive risk factor status) to whomever they wish and then observe what happens prospectively. They can manipulate the allocation so that the groups are comparable, and so avoid any possible problem due to confounding factors. To be more specific, suppose we are studying a certain disease, and its risk factor, both of which are known to be more common amongst old people and amongst men. We could then arrange the intervention study so that the group allocated to be exposed to the risk factor, and the group allocated to be unexposed, have the same age and sex make-up. This way any comparison between the groups using follow-up outcomes cannot be influenced by age or sex differences.

This design seems to be able to remove the problem of confounding that was said to be so important in Section 1.6. So why are most epidemiological studies not done this way? The major reason is an ethical one: it is rarely ethically acceptable to force people to be exposed (or unexposed) to a risk factor. For instance, Doll and Hill would not have found it ethically acceptable to force some people to smoke, especially because they suspected smoking to have a detrimental effect. Other considerations against the intervention approach include the practical impossibility of allocating biological risk factors, such as hypertension, and the difficulty of avoiding 'contamination' during what is usually a long period of follow-up (for example, people allocated to smoke may quit because they are influenced by health education).

We should note that intervention studies can only control potential confounding factors that have been identified and can be measured. However, after allowing for these factors, if the remaining allocation to risk factor groups is performed randomly, then we would expect any other important confounding effects to be averaged out, as long as the sample is large.

Intervention studies in medical research are most commonly encountered as animal experiments or as the clinical trials on patients conducted or financed by pharmaceutical companies. Animal experiments, which are a further topic of ethical debate, are not the subject of this book. Neither are pharmaceutical trials, although a few examples of their practice will be included when the ideas are of use to epidemiologists, or the data illustrate a technical point particularly well. Several specialist books on clinical trials have been published; recommended texts are Pocock (1983) and Piantadosi (2005). In this book, intervention studies are described in Chapter 7.

1.8.2 Observational studies

Because of their predominance in practical epidemiology, observational studies have provided most of the examples used in this book.

The simplest kind of observational study is the epidemiological **survey**, in which a set of people (usually a sample) are observed or questioned to seek information on their risk factor exposure and/or disease status. Epidemiologists often refer to such investigations as **cross-sectional** because they provide a snapshot in time (for example, of the relationship between risk factor and disease). These studies can measure only the prevalence of disease (Section 1.4.1) and must rely upon recall to establish whether risk factor exposure or disease came first. This is frequently unreliable due to a long time-lag and restricted lay knowledge of disease. Consequently, cross-sectional studies are most useful for description. They are better than studies based on routine data because we can collect just what we want and can link the data items person by person.

If sampling is necessary, we prefer a large sample (assuming that bias can be controlled) in order to improve the precision of our estimates. This inevitably pushes up costs, which are of special concern when trained field staff must be utilized. To protect against bias, we should draw the sample randomly from the study population, that is, so that everyone has a known nonzero probability of being sampled. In a **simple random sampling** scheme, everyone has an equal chance of selection.

Often, precision may be improved by **stratification** — that is, drawing separate samples from separate subgroups of the population. For instance, if we believe that the prevalence of the disease in question varies with age and sex, we would be well advised to take separate samples from separate age and sex groups of the study population. Clearly this spreads the sample across the different types of people concerned. In practice, the sample is often drawn in a **clustered** way; for instance we may randomly select a sample of hospitals from which to collect our data on hospital patients. This is done to save costs (for example, travelling expenses) but, unfortunately, tends to decrease the accuracy of estimates made from the data. This happens because the sample is concentrated upon a particular group of people; in the example, we obtain a picture of only the communities served by our chosen hospitals.

The fundamental methodology of surveys is well understood and has wide application. Many excellent books on the topic exist, such as the descriptive text by Moser and Kalton (1971), the predominantly mathematical text by Cochran (1977) and the practical approach of Scheaffer et al. (1995).

A second type of observational study is the **case–control study**. Here the investigators identify a set of people with the disease (the **cases**) and a set without (the **controls**). These two groups are compared with regard to the risk factor. Example 1.1 is an example of a case–control study and Chapter 6 considers the method in detail. Briefly, we note here that these studies are able to study many risk factors (for example, in Example 1.1, Doll and Hill could have asked their subjects about, say, alcohol habits as well as smoking) but cannot study more than one disease. They cannot be used to measure the chance of disease (in terms of incidence or prevalence) because they prespecify that a certain number of diseased and nondiseased people be studied. Also, they are highly susceptible to bias error (see Example 1.1), sources of which are not always obvious. For these reasons, whilst often superior to surveys or routine data examinations, case–control studies are far from ideal for aetiological investigations. Nevertheless, on some occasions they are the best choice in practice, principally when the disease in question is very rare or takes a long time to develop.

The best type of observational study for aetiological purposes is the **cohort study**, in which people are followed through time to record instances of disease (and thus measure incidence). Example 1.2, the British Doctors Study, is an example. Cohort studies' superiority stems from their ability to establish the order of happenings, especially when a disease-free study population is used at the outset. In principle, they can mimic the conditions of an intervention study; for instance, the British Doctors Study could be thought of (in simple terms) as prolonged observation of two groups: smokers and nonsmokers. Smoking then acts like the treatment in an intervention study. However, in the cohort design, people are not assigned to their groups; instead, there is self-selection of risk factor status. Confounding is not controlled and is therefore much more likely to be a problem.

As with intervention studies, cohort studies have the disadvantage that they may require many years of observation, causing considerable expense and probable problems of loss to follow-up. Hence, they are not suitable for diseases with a long latency. They are also not suitable for rare diseases because a large cohort would then be needed in order to obtain a reasonable number of positive disease outcomes to study. Unlike case–control studies, they can study many diseases (see, for example, Table 1.3). Further details are given in Chapter 5.

Perhaps the most famous cohort study is the Framingham Study, a follow-up of 5209 adults resident in Framingham, Massachusetts, begun in 1948. The subjects have been monitored through routine records, surveillance of hospital admissions and a biennial cardiovascular examination. Although primarily designed as a study of the epidemiology of cardiovascular disease, some of the many publications from the study have looked at other diseases. The Framingham Study has shown the great potential of epidemiology; its results have guided public health policy, especially in the U.S. where it is frequently quoted in national statements about cardiovascular disease and how to avoid it.

The foregoing describes the three major types of observational study design used in epidemiological research. Variations on these themes are sometimes used. The use of repeated cross-sectional surveys (for example, when the population census is carried out every 10 years) and specially created disease registers are examples. Both of these methods have been used in the WHO MONICA Project (Tunstall–Pedoe, 2003). Sample surveys were conducted in each study population at various times within the 10-year time span of the study. These surveys give a picture of the changing risk factor profiles (for example, for lipids, blood pressure and smoking) within each geographically defined population. Specimen data from one of the cross-sectional surveys carried out by the Scottish MONICA centre appear in Example 2.13, and elsewhere in this book. Throughout the 10 years, the MONICA centres maintained case registers so as to record every coronary event (morbid and mortal) for every member of the particular study population, thus establishing the overall disease load. Some case register data from the Scottish MONICA centre appear in Table 4.9 and Table 4.10.

1.9   Data analysis

The analytical techniques applied to epidemiological data include general statistical methods, as well as special methods that have been developed to fit the needs of specific epidemiological study designs. Although mathematical formulae, which may be applied without the use of a computer, are supplied for many of the techniques described in this book, even then the size of most epidemiological studies, and the convenience of the medium, make it likely that a computer will be used in practice. Of particular interest to epidemiologists is the excellent Epi Info package, produced by the U.S. Centers for Disease Control and Prevention, which has been written especially for their needs. This may be downloaded from http://www.cdc.gov/epiinfo/downloads.htm.

Unfortunately, this package has limitations; more sophisticated analyses require specialist statistical software. Some such packages include specialised epidemiological tools, including Stata (http://www.stata.com). Although other statistical packages are sometimes mentioned in forthcoming chapters, due to limitations of space, details of use and illustrative outputs are restricted to Stata and SAS (http://www.sas.com). The web site for this book (see Appendix A) contains Stata and SAS programs for many of the examples presented.

As such models are easy to fit using software, epidemiologists frequently use complex statistical models (such as those described in Chapter 9 and thereafter) to analyse their data. Such models provide a general framework within which most of the usual data-based epidemiological questions may be answered, avoiding the need for special formulae (such as several of those given in the early chapters of this book) that are applicable only in specific situations. However, this simplicity of application comes with a price. The epidemiologist may lose the 'feel' for the data, leading to unthinking analyses, which make assumptions about the data, implicit in the statistical model, that are just not true. Hence, associated descriptive procedures and model checking are essential whenever complex models are used.

Exercises

1.1   In a study of risk factors for angina (a chronic condition) subjects were asked the question, 'Do you smoke cigarettes?' Answers were used to classify each respondent as a smoker or nonsmoker. Furthermore, subjects were classified as positive for angina if they had, at some time in the past, been told by a doctor that they had angina.

When the resultant data were analysed, no association was found between cigarette smoking status and angina status.
   (i)   Has the study measured incidence or prevalence of angina?
   (ii)   A considerable body of past evidence suggests that the risk of angina increases with increasing tobacco consumption. Suggest reasons why the study described here failed to find an association.
   (iii) Suggest an alternative design of study that would be more suitable for investigating whether smoking causes angina. Consider the question(s) that you would ask the chosen subjects about their smoking habits.

1.2   A certain general hospital serves a population of half a million people. Over the past 5 years it has treated 20 patients with hairy cell leukaemia. Several of these patients have worked in the petrochemical industry, and hence the hospital physicians wonder if there may be a causal link. In order to explore this possibility, they propose to send a questionnaire to all the survivors from the 20 patients. The questionnaire will ask about lifestyle, including diet and smoking, as well as employment history. Is this a suitable research strategy? If not, suggest an alternative plan.

1.3   A programme is to be developed to study the effects of alcohol consumption on health in a community. The study team in charge of the programme is interested in a number of medical end-points, including coronary heart and liver disease, but results must be obtained within the next year.

Describe a suitable study design for this problem. Give the reasons for your particular choice, and discuss the problems that have led you to reject other possible designs. Your description should include details of the sampling procedure that would be used in the data collection phase. You should also consider the variables about which you would wish to collect data.

1.4   Epidemiological studies of coronary heart disease usually include measurement of each subject's blood pressure. Sometimes this is done by doctors, perhaps in their surgery, and sometimes by nurses, perhaps in the subject's home. It is thought that comparisons of blood pressure between different studies might be compromised by 'white coat hypertension', a temporary rise of blood pressure due to anxiety. The phenomenon is likely to be a greater problem in some settings than in others. How would you design a study to investigate the effect of white coat hypertension in the two settings suggested?

1.5   Figure 1.5 shows the results of an epidemiological investigation into the relationship between the number of decayed, missing and filled teeth (DMFT) and sugar consumption in 29 industrialised nations (Woodward and Walker, 1994). DMFT scores were obtained from WHO's oral health database. These scores are mean values from surveys of 12-year-old children. The surveys were administered within each country, and the results later compiled by WHO. National sugar consumption was estimated from government and/or industrial sources within each country. The horizontal axis on the graph shows the annual consumption divided by the estimated total population of the country (obtained from population census results).

Since the points on the graph show no evidence whatsoever of an increase of DMFT with sugar consumption, the study has been cited (by some people) as evidence that sugar is not harmful to teeth.

(i)   Comment upon any shortcomings that you can see in this investigation, so far as the preceding conclusion is concerned.

(ii)   Given a limited budget and a short time in which to work, how would you design a study to investigate the relationship between sugar consumption and dental health? Describe the data you would record in your study.

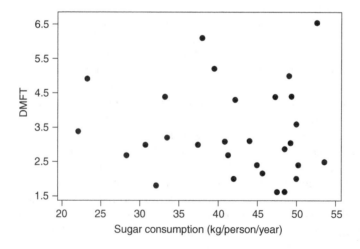

Figure 1.5. Dental health and sugar consumption in 29 industrialised countries.

CHAPTER 2

Basic analytical procedures

2.1 Introduction

The purpose of this chapter is to summarise the most fundamental analytical techniques that are frequently applied to epidemiological data. This is to serve both as a guide to how basic analytical procedures should be used in epidemiology, particularly in written presentations, and as a reference when more advanced, or more subject-specific, techniques are developed in later chapters. Further details on basic statistical procedures may be found in any of the introductory textbooks with medical applications, such as Altman (1991); Armitage *et al.* (2001); Bland (2000); Campbell *et al.* (2007) and Rosner (2010).

In this chapter we discuss both descriptive and inferential techniques, introduced through examples. A **descriptive** analysis is restricted to statements about the data that have been collected (assumed to be a sample from a larger population). **Inferential** analyses go further: they use the observed data to make general statements about the parent population from which the sample data were collected.

2.1.1 *Inferential procedures*

The two major topics in inferential analysis are hypothesis tests and estimation.

A **hypothesis test** seeks to discover whether an assertion about the population appears (on the basis of the sample data) to be unreasonable. Formally, we set up a **null hypothesis** (sometimes denoted by H_0) and seek information (sample data) to try to reject it. If the data do not support rejection, then we say that the null hypothesis fails to be rejected, meaning that it may be true *or* that we just may not have enough data to be able to detect that it is false. The null hypothesis is usually taken to be that of no effect — for example, that a high-fat diet has no effect on the chance of developing breast cancer. Hypothesis tests are first met in Section 2.5.1, where the remaining general definitions are given. Criticisms of hypothesis tests are deferred to Section 3.5.5, where they are developed within a particularly important epidemiological context.

Estimation involves the use of some measure derived from the sample to act as a representative measure for the parent population. For example, the average height of a sample of schoolchildren might be used to estimate the average height of all schoolchildren in the country. Estimation also includes the specification of a **confidence interval**, a range of values which we are fairly confident will contain the true value of the measure of interest in the overall population. Generally, 95% confidence intervals will be specified; we are 95% sure that a 95% confidence interval will contain the true value. To interpret this, we need to imagine that the sampling process is repeated very many times, for instance, 10 000 times. Each time a 95% confidence interval is calculated from the resultant sample data. We then expect that 9500 (that is, 95%) of these intervals will contain the true (population) measure, such as the average height of all schoolchildren. Confidence intervals are first met, and explained by example, in Section 2.5.2.

Generally, estimation is much more useful than hypothesis testing because the estimate gives precise information on the magnitude and direction of an effect. Also, the confidence interval can often be used to make the same decision as would an associated hypothesis test; examples are given in Section 2.5 and Section 2.7.

2.2   Case study

In order to provide a focus, a further epidemiological case study is now introduced. Data from this study are used to illustrate the various techniques presented in this and subsequent chapters.

2.2.1   The Scottish Heart Health Study

Scotland's annual mortality rate from coronary heart disease (CHD) is one of the highest in the world, although the rates vary considerably between regions of the country. Concern about the high overall CHD mortality rate led to the establishment of a Cardiovascular Epidemiology Unit at the University of Dundee, with the remit to undertake a range of epidemiological studies in order to understand the factors associated with CHD prevalence across Scotland.

The Scottish Heart Health Study (SHHS) was one of these epidemiological studies, with the following objectives (Smith *et al.,* 1987):

(a)   To establish the levels of CHD risk factors in a cross-sectional sample of Scottish men and women aged 40 to 59 years drawn from different localities.
(b)   To determine the extent to which the geographical variation in CHD can be explained in terms of the geographical variation in risk factor levels.
(c)   To assess the relative contribution of the established risk factors, as well as some more recently described ones, to the prediction of CHD within a cohort of men and women in Scotland.

Subjects were sampled from 22 of the 56 mainland Scottish local government districts, as defined in the mid-1980s. In each district a number of general practitioners were randomly selected. From their lists of patients, an equal number of people were selected in the four age/sex groups: male, 40 to 49 years old; female, 40 to 49 years old; male, 50 to 59 years old; female, 50 to 59 years old. Each selected subject was sent a questionnaire to complete and an invitation, jointly signed by the general practitioner and the study leader, to attend at a local clinic. The questionnaire included questions on sociodemographic status (age, sex, marital status, employment, etc.), past medical history, exercise, diet, health knowledge and smoking. Also included was the Rose chest pain questionnaire (Rose *et al.,* 1977), which is used in the determination of prevalent CHD.

The subjects took the completed questionnaires with them to the clinic where they were checked. Height, weight and blood pressure were then recorded and a 12-lead electrocardiogram was administered by trained nurses. A blood sample was taken, from which serum total cholesterol, fibrinogen and several other biochemical variables were subsequently measured. From a urine sample, sodium and potassium were evaluated. Clinic sessions were held across the country between 1984 and 1986.

Some selected respondents failed to attend for their clinic appointment. These were invited a second time but, again, not everyone responded. Altogether, information was obtained from 74% of those who received postal questionnaires and invitations, giving a total sample size of 10 359 (5123 men and 5236 women). In very many cases, the information received was not complete; for instance, blood samples were not obtained for 10.6% of the sample.

The resulting dataset comprised 315 variables, representing many aspects of personal circumstances, lifestyle, diet and health that may be related to CHD, and three measures of prevalent CHD (self-reported previous doctor diagnosis, appropriate answers to the self-reported Rose chest pain questionnaire and electrocardiogram indications). Scores of publications were based on this cross-sectional dataset. These were of three major types: descriptions of the state of health of the subjects (e.g., Tunstall–Pedoe et al., 1989); investigations into the relationships between two or more of the variables that are potential risk factors for CHD (e.g., smoking and diet: Woodward et al., 1994); and comparisons of CHD prevalence between specific subgroups (e.g., occupational social class groups: Woodward et al., 1992).

However, as discussed in Chapter 1, prevalence data are not ideal to demonstrate causality. For example, smokers who develop CHD could quit because of their illness so that, by the time they are surveyed, they are recorded as nonsmokers with CHD. Clearly this will tend to produce a misleading inference regarding the smoking–CHD relationship. Consequently, the SHHS was designed as a two-phase study: the cross-sectional 'baseline' study just described, followed by a follow-up cohort study of several years' duration. During this period, a copy of the death registration certificate was collected for any member of the study population who died. Furthermore, Scottish hospital records were examined to identify whenever each of the study population underwent coronary artery surgery (coronary artery bypass graft or percutaneous coronary angioplasty) or was discharged with a coronary diagnosis. After an average of around 8 years' follow-up, this CHD incidence information was collated and a second series of articles began, relating baseline risk factor information to CHD outcome. In these articles, the basic (initial phase) SHHS sample was combined with identical databases from three further Scottish districts collected in 1987, giving a total of 11 718 subjects (see Tunstall–Pedoe et al., 1997). In future years additional baseline surveys were conducted and the length of follow-up was extended.

In Section 2.4 and Section 2.5 we shall consider the subset of 8681 people in the SHHS from whom complete information was received from the original study for all the variables that will be analysed in these sections. For example, anyone who failed to provide a blood sample will not be considered. We will consider these 8681 as a simple random sample (that is, a sample drawn entirely at random, where everyone has an equal chance of selection) of middle-aged Scots. In fact, the sample is not strictly random because of the variable rates of selection by geographical area, age and sex (see Cochran, 1977) and, possibly, because of the missing values, which might be more common in specific types of individuals (see Section 14.9).

In further sections and chapters, other subsets of the SHHS will be analysed. In Section 2.6 a small subset of only 50 people is introduced, in order to provide a tractable example.

2.3   Types of variables

Epidemiological data, such as those collected in the SHHS, consist of a number of observations from different people, on a number of **variables** of interest. Variables are classified into a number of different **types**, and it is of some importance to recognise the type before deciding which analytical methods to apply. The first tier of classification is into the types qualitative and quantitative.

2.3.1 *Qualitative variables*

Qualitative variables are often recorded (like quantitative variables) as a set of numbers, but (unlike quantitative variables) the numbers are merely convenient codes. **Categorical** (or **nominative**) variables are qualitative variables that can take a number of outcomes (or **levels**) that have no intrinsic numerical meaning or order, such as 'cause of death' and 'area of residence'. Numbers might be used to represent each of the levels of such a variable; when there are four areas of residence they might be given codes of 1, 2, 3 and 4 in a database. However such codes are arbitrary; the codes 10, 20, 30, 40 would do equally well, as would 2, 1, 4, 3. All that matters is that we know the key for deciphering the codes. A special, very simple kind of categorical variable is that which can have only two possible outcomes, such as the variable 'sex'. Such variables are called **binary** variables. These arise frequently in epidemiological research, to represent disease outcome (disease/no disease) or survival status (died/survived).

The other type of qualitative variable is the ordinal type. **Ordinal** variables differ from categorical variables by virtue of having a natural order to their outcomes. Common examples are responses recorded as poor/satisfactory/good (or similar), where there is an underlying order in the responses. These are sometimes called **ordered categorical** variables. We might well wish to account for the order when analysing such a variable. Data in the form of ranks, in which items are classified in order of preference or desirability, are a special, and most obvious, case of ordinal data.

Descriptive techniques for qualitative data are described in Section 2.4. Some inferential techniques are described in Section 2.5.

2.3.2 *Quantitative variables*

Quantitative variables are also divided into two subtypes: discrete and continuous variables. **Discrete** variables are those that may increase only in steps, usually of whole numbers. Examples are the number of patients operated upon in a month and the number of births in a year. **Continuous** variables have no such limitation; they may take any value (subject to possible constraints on the minimum and maximum allowable). Most body measurements, such as cholesterol, body mass index and blood pressure, take continuous values. Notice that blood pressure is continuous even though it may have been recorded only as a whole number. This is because it is only the recording convention that has 'chopped off' the decimal places; they are merely hidden, not nonexistent. The essential thing that makes all the variables mentioned in this paragraph quantitative (rather than qualitative) is that the numbers have a unique meaning (subject to the units of measurement adopted). If we were to add, say, one to all the cholesterol measurements this would give rise to totally different conclusions about the hypercholesterolaemic status of the sample.

Descriptive techniques for quantitative data are given in Section 2.6. Some inferential techniques are described in Section 2.7 and Section 2.8.

2.3.3 *The hierarchy of type*

With regard to their use, variable types form a hierarchy in the sense that a variable can always be analysed as if it were of a type further down the hierarchy, but not vice versa:

$$continuous \rightarrow ordinal \rightarrow categorical \rightarrow binary.$$

For instance, we could use the continuous variable 'diastolic blood pressure' to define a new variable, 'hypertension status', which takes value 2 (yes, hypertensive) if diastolic blood pressure is 105 mmHg or greater, and 1 (no) otherwise. We could then analyse this new (binary) representation of diastolic blood pressure. This would not, however, be an efficient use of the data because such grouping must inevitably throw away information. Furthermore, the use of 105 as a cut-point in the example is somewhat arbitrary, and in general we may get totally different conclusions when we vary the definitions of the groups. Hence, use of each variable in its original recorded type is generally to be recommended. Exceptions are in descriptive statistics in which grouping may be acceptable to aid in interpretation and when the assumptions of a statistical method are (possibly) violated unless we 'step down' the hierarchy. The most common example of this latter exception is when **nonparametric** methods, developed for ordinal variables, are used with a continuous outcome variable (Section 2.8.2).

Discrete variables are generally analysed as if they were continuous, possibly after a transformation (Section 2.8.1) or a continuity correction (Section 3.5.3). If a continuous analogue is not acceptable, then methods for ordinal variables would usually be the most appropriate.

2.4   Tables and charts

The major descriptive tools for a single qualitative variable are the **frequency table**, **bar chart** and **pie chart**. These are illustrated by Table 2.1, Figure 2.1 and Figure 2.2, respectively; all show SHHS data on social class. Social class is measured according to occupation, using standard classifications (Office of Population Censuses and Surveys, 1980) to form an ordinal variable.

In the bar chart, the bars are drawn of equal width, but the heights are proportional to the percentages. Other possible scales for the vertical axis are the frequencies or **relative frequencies** (percentages divided by 100), both of which leave the shape of the bar chart unaltered. In a pie chart, the areas of the slices are drawn in proportion to the frequencies by simply dividing the entire 360° of the circle into separate angles of the correct relative size.

Table 2.1, Figure 2.1 and Figure 2.2 all clearly show that there are relatively few in the extreme classification groups, and most in social class IIIm. This gives a useful demographic profile of the sample chosen. Other useful descriptive variables in epidemiological studies are age and sex, although in the case of the SHHS, the distribution by age and sex were determined by the sampling method used. If the SHHS were a true simple random sample — that is, where everyone has equal chance of entering the sample — Table 2.1 would provide an estimated profile by social class of middle-aged

Table 2.1. Occupational social class in the SHHS.

Social class		Number	(%)
I	nonmanual, professional	592	(7)
II	nonmanual, intermediate	2254	(26)
IIIn	nonmanual, skilled	1017	(12)
IIIm	manual, skilled	3150	(36)
IV	manual, partially skilled	1253	(14)
V	manual, unskilled	415	(5)
Total		8681	

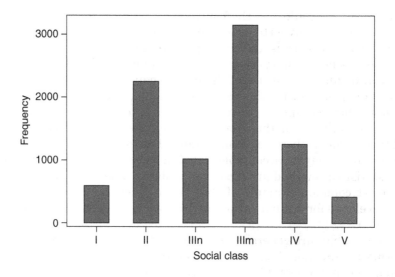

Figure 2.1. Bar chart for occupational social class in the SHHS.

Scots in the 1980s. Percentages are, of course, optional in Table 2.1, but they provide an extremely useful summary.

The table is factually exact, but lacking in visual appeal. Both the pie chart and bar chart look attractive, but the pie chart is harder to interpret because wedge-shaped areas are difficult to compare. Bar charts are also much easier to draw by hand and are far easier to adapt to more complex situations.

The next most complex situation is one in which two qualitative variables are compared. For example, Table 2.2 shows the relationship between social class and

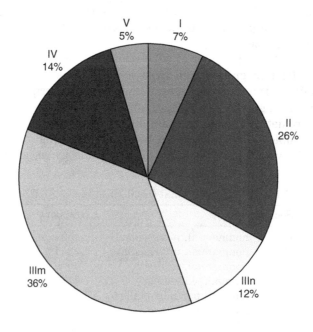

Figure 2.2. Pie chart for occupational social class in the SHHS.

Table 2.2. Social class by prevalent
CHD status in the SHHS.

Social class	Prevalent CHD			
	Yes	(%)	No	Total
I	100	(16.9)	492	592
II	382	(17.0)	1872	2254
IIIn	183	(18.0)	834	1017
IIIm	668	(21.2)	2482	3150
IV	279	(22.3)	974	1253
V	109	(26.3)	306	415
Total	1721	(19.8)	6960	8681

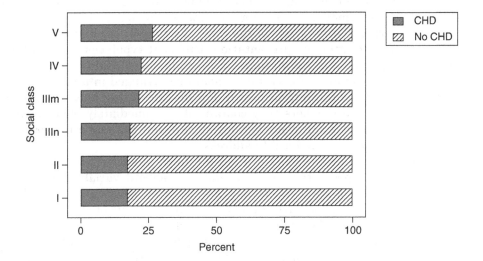

Figure 2.3. Bar chart for occupational social class in the SHHS, showing percentage by CHD status.

prevalent CHD (identified by the three methods described in Section 2.2.1) in the SHHS. Of most interest here is the percentage with CHD in each social class; hence, Table 2.2 gives percentages and Figure 2.3 goes to the extreme of ignoring the actual numbers by fixing each bar to be of the same length. Instead, we could divide each bar in Figure 2.1 into two sections to represent the CHD and no CHD groups, or give separate 'CHD' and 'no CHD' bars grouped together in pairs for each social class. These have the advantage of showing raw numbers, but make relative CHD composition very difficult to judge. From Figure 2.3, we can easily see that CHD is more common as we go up the bars; that is, CHD prevalence is always higher in the more deprived social group. Another element of choice is the orientation, which has been reversed in Figure 2.3 (compared with Figure 2.1).

2.4.1   Tables in reports

Although tables are simple to understand and to produce, careful thought regarding layout is essential to draw attention to the most useful and interesting features of the data. Many epidemiological reports (such as papers submitted for publication) fail to convey their messages due to inadequate attention to such simple descriptive techniques. For ease of reference, recommendations are given here in note form. Tables are also useful to present summary information from quantitative variables. Although discussion of such variables is deferred to Section 2.6, this is the appropriate place to consider the presentation of their tables; consequently, an example is included here (Example 2.1).

1. Each table should be self-explanatory; that is, the reader should be able to understand it without reference to the text in the body of the report. This can be achieved by using complete, meaningful labels for the rows and columns and giving a complete, meaningful title. Footnotes should be used to enhance the explanation.

2. Each table should have an attractive appearance. Sensible use of white space helps enormously; use equal spacing except where large spaces are left to separate distinct parts of the table. Vertical lines should be avoided because these clutter the presentation. Different typefaces (or fonts) may be used to provide discrimination; for example, use of **bold** type or *italics*.

3. The rows and columns of each table should be arranged in a natural order. This is a great help in interpretation. For instance, when rows are ordered by the size of the numbers they contain, it is immediately obvious where relatively big and small contributions come from. Without rank ordering, questions of size may be hard to address.

4. Numbers are easier to compare when the table has a vertical orientation. For example, suppose that we have data on several variables for several hospitals. We then want to compare each variable between hospitals. To achieve this it is best to have rows labelled by the name of the hospital and columns labelled by the subject of the variable. The eye can make comparisons more easily when reading down the page than when reading across. This is especially true when the variables are recorded to varying numbers of significant digits (see Example 2.1). Sometimes vertical orientation may be impossible to achieve because of limitations due to the size of the page. Occasionally such limitations can be overcome by turning the page sideways. Pages written in upright fashion (such as this page) are said to be in portrait format; pages to be read after turning through a right angle are in landscape format. See Table 2.12 for an example.

5. Tables should have consistent appearance throughout the report. Conventions for labelling and ordering rows and columns, for example, should remain the same, as far as possible. This makes the presentation easier to follow, promoting easy comparison of different tables, and reduces the chance of a misinterpretation. A common fault is to interchange the rows and columns of tables within the report; for instance, when one table in the report has sex labelling the rows and age group labelling the columns, whilst another table has sex labelling the columns and age group labelling the rows (see Example 2.2).

Example 2.1 Table 2.3 and Table 2.4 show the same information. Whereas Table 2.3 has the related figures running across the table, Table 2.4 has a vertical orientation. Notice how figures with differing numbers of decimal places are easier to incorporate within a vertical orientation.

Table 2.3. Minimum, median and maximum values for selected variables in developed countries, 1970.

Variable	Minimum	Median	Maximum
Gross national product per person	1949	4236	6652
Population per km^2	1.6	77.2	324.2
Cigarette consumption per person per year	630	2440	3810
Infant mortality per 1000 births	11.0	18.2	29.6

Source: Cochrane, A.L. *et al.* (1978), *J. Epidemiol. Comm. Health*, 32, 200–205.

Table 2.4. Minimum, median and maximum values for selected variables in developed countries, 1970.

	Gross national product per person	Population density per km^2	Cigarette consumption per person/per year	Infant mortality rate per 1000 births
Maximum	6652	324.2	3810	29.6
Median	4236	77.2	2440	18.2
Minimum	1949	1.6	630	11.0

Frequently the first draft of a report will contain many more tables than the final version. Revision will usually result in combining some tables, perhaps because they have common row and column headings, and removing some tables because the information they contain is not necessary to the report, or because the results can be merely included in the written text (usually true only for small tables). On the other hand, revision often increases the size of the tables that remain, by concatenation of two or more of the original tables or because extra information, such as percentages or averages, is added. Tables from the first draft are often replaced by diagrams in the final report, usually because the diagrams are easier for the reader to understand.

Example 2.2 In an investigation of the relationship between smoking habit and CHD in the SHHS, an initial draft publication with seven tables was produced. Two of these are shown as Table 2.5 and Table 2.6. In both tables, the 'diagnosed' are those who have been told that they have CHD by a doctor sometime in the past, whilst the 'undiagnosed' are those who have no previous doctor diagnosis of CHD, but nevertheless appear to have CHD according to medical tests (Rose questionnaire or electrocardiogram). Those without any CHD problems at all are called 'controls'. Table 2.5 describes the CHD status of current smokers and Table 2.6 considers those who currently do not smoke any form of tobacco.

When the investigators carefully considered these two tables, they realized that they were difficult to compare because of inconsistency; whilst Table 2.5 labels 'diagnosis group' across the columns (that is, along the top), Table 2.6 has it across the rows (down the side). More importantly, why do the tables need to be separate? Table 2.7 shows how to combine the two by simply adding the columns of Table 2.6 to the rows of Table 2.5.

Three further modifications were made to produce Table 2.7, which appeared in the subsequent publication. First, it was decided to reverse the percentages. Thus, whereas in Table 2.5 the percentages sum across the rows, in Table 2.7 they sum down the columns. A set of 100% values is shown in Table 2.7 to make it clear to the reader how the percentages were calculated. Of course, there is no 'correct' way to show percentages in a table such as this. What is best depends upon what is important to bring to the reader's attention; in this example, the investigations

Table 2.5. Smoking habit by diagnosis group by sex.

| Sex/smoking habit | CHD diagnosis group | | | |
	Diagnosed	Control	Undiagnosed	Total
Males				
Solely cigarette	125 (8%)	1175 (77%)	226 (15%)	1526
Solely cigar	25 (7%)	313 (83%)	40 (10%)	378
Solely pipe	9 (8%)	80 (72%)	22 (20%)	111
Mixed smokers	39 (8%)	379 (75%)	89 (17%)	507
All smokers	198 (8%)	1947 (77%)	377 (15%)	2522
Females[a]				
Solely cigarette	105 (6%)	1410 (78%)	297 (16%)	1812
Solely cigar	0	12 (100%)	0	12
Mixed smokers	2 (8%)	20 (77%)	4 (15%)	26
All smokers	107 (6%)	1442 (78%)	301 (16%)	1850

[a] No females smoked a pipe.

Table 2.6. Diagnosis group by previous smoking habit by sex for nonsmokers.

| CHD diagnosis group | Males | | Females | |
	Ex-smokers	Never-smokers	Ex-smokers	Never-smokers
Diagnosed	142 (11%)	45 (4%)	58 (6%)	75 (4%)
Control	993 (76%)	888 (83%)	767 (80%)	1581 (78%)
Undiagnosed	164 (13%)	143 (13%)	137 (14%)	375 (18%)

Table 2.7. Men and women classified by self-declared smoking habit and diagnosis group.

| Sex/smoking habit | CHD diagnosis group | | |
	Diagnosed	Undiagnosed	Control
Males			
Solely cigarettes	125 (32%)	226 (33%)	1175 (31%)
Solely cigars	25 (7%)	40 (6%)	313 (8%)
Solely pipes	9 (2%)	22 (3%)	80 (2%)
Mixed smokers	39 (10%)	89 (13%)	379 (10%)
Ex-smokers (of any)	142 (37%)	164 (24%)	993 (26%)
Never-smokers (of any)	45 (12%)	143 (21%)	888 (23%)
Total	385 (100%)	684 (100%)	3828 (100%)
Females			
Solely cigarettes	105 (44%)	297 (37%)	1410 (37%)
Solely cigars	0	0	12 (0%)
Mixed smokers	2 (1%)	4 (0%)	20 (1%)
Ex-smokers (of any)	58 (24%)	137 (17%)	767 (20%)
Never-smokers (of any)	75 (31%)	375 (46%)	1581 (42%)
Total	240 (100%)	813 (100%)	3790 (100%)

Note: Percentages less than 0.5% are given as 0%.

Source: Woodward, M. and Tunstall–Pedoe, H. (1992), *Eur. Heart J.*, 13, 160–165.

changed their initial opinion. It is possible to include both row and column percentages in a table, but the table is then difficult to read and interpret. Since the numbers are given, as well as percentages, the reader can always calculate the row percentages for herself or himself, should this be necessary.

The second major change is that the diagnosis groups are reordered. It was decided to do this because there is a natural order: someone is first disease free (control), then gets the symptoms but is not aware of having CHD (undiagnosed) and then is diagnosed by a doctor. The table is more meaningful when this natural order is used. The third change was to omit the 'total' column from Table 2.5 but include a grand total for each sex, merely to keep the table simple, without detail unnecessary to the essential points.

In the final publication the initial seven draft tables were reduced to four. Despite the reduction in the number of tables, new information was added even as the reduction was made. The compact final report is easier to read and interpret.

2.4.2   Diagrams in reports

Diagrams cannot show numerical information as precisely as tables can, but they may be easier to understand and thus be more powerful as a descriptive tool. Modern computer software makes it easy to produce most standard diagrams, even in a form suitable for publication. Most of the recommendations given for the presentation of tables in Section 2.4.1 are equally suitable for diagrams. In particular, diagrams should be self-explanatory, of an attractive appearance and consistently presented throughout the report. Natural ordering is sometimes possible; for instance, the bars of a bar chart may be arranged according to size.

2.5   Inferential techniques for categorical variables

2.5.1   Contingency tables

When two categorical variables have been recorded, a natural question is whether there is any evidence of an association between the two. For example, Table 2.8 shows the types of tobacco consumed by each sex in the SHHS. This table uses the same SHHS subset (that with no missing values) as in Table 2.1 and Table 2.2. Note that Table 2.7, which considers a similar problem, is taken from a publication that used only the initial (22 districts) phase of the SHHS. A cross-classification table, such as Table 2.8, is known as a **contingency** table.

Does Table 2.8 provide evidence of a sex–tobacco relationship? In other words, are the patterns of tobacco consumption different for men and women? If that were not so, then the percentages within each tobacco group would be the same for men and women. We can see that they are not exactly the same in Table 2.8, where these percentages have been added as an aid to interpretation. However, they may be similar enough for these observed differences to have arisen merely by chance selection of the

Table 2.8. Sex by smoking habit in the SHHS.

Sex	Nonsmoker	Cigarettes	Pipes	Cigars	Mixed	Total
			Smoking habit			
Male	2241 (50%)	1400 (31%)	103 (2%)	352 (8%)	424 (9%)	4520 (100%)
Female	2599 (63%)	1551 (37%)	0 (0%)	9 (0%)	2 (0%)	4161 (100%)
Total	4840	2951	103	361	426	8681

actual sample obtained. What is required is a test of the statistical significance of the relationship: the **chi-square test**.

To compute the chi-square test statistic by hand, we must first calculate the expected frequencies within each cell of the table under the null hypothesis of no association. These are

$$E_{ij} = \frac{R_i C_j}{T}$$

where i denotes the row, j the column, R_i the ith row total, C_j the jth column total and T the grand total. Hence, for Table 2.8, the expected value in, for example, cell $(1, 3)$, the third column in the first row (male pipe smokers), is

$$E_{13} = \frac{4520 \times 103}{8681} = 53 \cdot 6.$$

The complete set of expected values is

$$\begin{array}{ccccc} 2520.1 & 1536.5 & 53.6 & 188.0 & 221.8 \\ 2319.9 & 1414.5 & 49.4 & 173.0 & 204.2 \end{array}.$$

The chi-square test statistic is

$$\sum_i \sum_j \frac{\left(O_{ij} - E_{ij}\right)^2}{E_{ij}}, \tag{2.1}$$

where O_{ij} is the observed value in cell (i, j). In the example, i ranges from 1 to 2 and j from 1 to 5 and the test statistic is

$$\frac{\left(2241 - 2520.1\right)^2}{2520.1} + \cdots + \frac{\left(2 - 204.2\right)^2}{204.2} = 867.8.$$

The test statistic is to be compared with chi-square on $(r - 1)(c - 1)$ degrees of freedom, written $\chi^2_{(r-1)(c-1)}$. The concept of degrees of freedom is discussed in Section 2.6.3.

As with all hypothesis tests (sometimes called **significance tests**), we reject the null hypothesis whenever the test statistic exceeds the cut-point, known as the **critical value**, for a predetermined level of significance. Otherwise, we fail to reject the null hypothesis and conclude that there is insufficient evidence that the null hypothesis is incorrect at this particular level of significance. The critical values can be found from statistical tables such as those in Appendix B, the more complete tables by Fisher and Yates (1963) or from computer packages such as Excel. Table B.3 gives critical values for the chi-square distribution at different degrees of freedom and different levels of significance.

The **significance level** represents the chance that the null hypothesis is rejected when it is actually true. Thus, it represents the chance that a particular kind of error (called **type I error**) occurs, and consequently we wish the significance level to be small. Traditionally, the significance level is given as a percentage and the 5% level of significance is generally accepted to be a reasonable yardstick to use. When a test is significant at the 5% level, the chance of observing a value as extreme as that observed for the test statistic, when the null hypothesis is true, is below 0.05. In, say, 10 000 repetitions of the sampling procedure, we would expect to wrongly reject the null hypothesis 500 times. The argument goes that this is small enough to be an acceptable rate of error.

Although the basic idea of a hypothesis test is to make a decision, results of tests are often given in such a way that the reader can judge the strength of information against the null hypothesis. A simple device is to consider a few different significance levels and report the strongest one at which the test is significant. Most often the following convention is used:

n.s.   not significant at 5%,
*   significant at 5% (but not at 1%),
**   significant at 1% (but not at 0.1%),
***   significant at 0.1%.

The idea is that, because smaller significant levels are more stringent, the number of asterisks defines the strength of evidence against the null hypothesis. Such a demarcation scheme is easy to employ using statistical tables such as Table B.3. For example, the 5%, 1% and 0.1% critical values for χ_4^2 are 9.49, 13.3 and 18.5. If the null hypothesis is true, then there is a 5% chance of observing a chi-square value of 9.49 or above, a 1% chance of 13.3 or above and a 0.1% chance of 18.5 or above. Hence, if the chi-square test statistic, (2.1), is less than 9.49, we fail to reject the null hypothesis at the 5% level of significance; we reject at 5% but not at 1% if it is greater than 9.49 but less than 13.3; we reject at 1% but not at 0.1% if it is greater than 13.3 but less than 18.5; we reject at 0.1% if it is 18.5 or more.

A major drawback with this idea is that, say, significance levels of 4.9% and 1.1% are treated equally. It is preferable to give the exact significance level — the level at which the test is just significant. Traditionally, this is given as a probability, rather than a percentage, and is called the **p value**. The p value is the exact probability of getting a result as extreme as that observed for the test statistic when the null hypothesis is true. Most statistical computer packages will automatically produce p values to several decimal places. We can easily use p values to make decisions at the common significance cut-points; for instance, if p is below 0.05, we reject the null hypothesis at the 5% level of significance. Whenever we reject at the $X\%$ level we automatically reject at the $Y\%$ level for all $Y > X$. If we fail to reject at the $X\%$ level, we automatically fail to reject at the $Y\%$ level for all $Y < X$.

Returning to the example, the test statistic is 867.8, which is to be compared to χ^2 with $(2 - 1)(5 - 1) = 4$ degrees of freedom. Because $\chi_4^2 = 18.5$ at the 0.1% level, we can conclude that the result is significant at the 0.1% level. In fact, because 867.8 is much greater than 18.5, we would certainly be able to reject the null hypothesis, of equal smoking habits for the two sexes, at a much more extreme (smaller) level of significance. Thus there is substantial evidence of a real difference, not explainable by chance variation associated with sampling. From Table 2.8, we can see that men are much more likely to smoke pipes and/or cigars (possibly together with cigarettes).

One word of warning about the chi-square test is appropriate. The test is really only an approximate one (see Section 3.5.3) and the approximation is poor whenever there are small expected (E) values. Small expected values may be avoided by pooling rows or columns, provided that the combined classes make sense. If the table has some kind of natural ordering, then adjacent columns or rows are pooled when necessary. A rule of thumb is that no more than 20% of expected values should be below 5 and none should be below 1. If this cannot be achieved, an exact method, such as is provided by many statistical computer packages, should be used. Section 3.5.4 gives an exact method for a table with two rows and two columns, a 2×2 table. Note that it is small *expected* values that cause problems; small *observed* values, such as in Table 2.8 (female pipes and mixed smoking) are not a problem in themselves, although they are a good indication that small expected values may follow.

2.5.2 Binary variables: proportions and percentages

Binary variables are, as with other categorical variables, generally summarised by proportions or the equivalent percentages, that is, proportions multiplied by 100. For example, consider the binary variable 'smoker' with the outcomes 'yes' and 'no'. Suppose that we are interested in the proportion of female smokers. In Table 2.8 we have details on specific smoking habits. Table 2.9 is a collapsed version of this table. From this, we can easily see that the proportion of female smokers is 1562/4161 = 0.3754; equivalently, the percentage is 37.54%.

With sample data, the proportion found is an estimate of the true proportion in the parent population. Assuming that we have a simple random sample, we can find a 95% confidence interval for this true proportion from

$$p \pm 1.96\sqrt{p(1-p)/n}, \tag{2.2}$$

where p is the sample proportion and n is the sample size. As explained in Section 2.1.1, this gives us limits that we are very confident will contain the true proportion. To be precise, we know that, in the long run, 95% of all such intervals, each calculated from a new simple random sample of the population, will contain the true proportion.

As an example, and taking the female portion of the SHHS as a simple random sample of middle-aged Scotswomen, a 95% confidence interval for the proportion of middle-aged Scotswomen who smoke is

$$0.3754 \pm 1.96\sqrt{\frac{0.3754(1-0.3754)}{4161}},$$

that is,

$$0.3754 \pm 0.0147,$$

Table 2.9. Sex by smoking status in the SHHS.

Sex	Smoking status		
---	Nonsmoker	Smoker	Total
Male	2241	2279	4520
Female	2599	1562	4161
Total	4840	3841	8681

which might otherwise be written as (0.361, 0.390) to three decimal places. We are 95% confident that this interval contains the unknown true proportion of smokers.

The value 1.96 appears in (2.2) because we have chosen 95% confidence and because we have assumed that the distribution of the sample proportion may be approximated by a normal distribution (Section 2.7). For a standard normal distribution (defined in Section 2.7), the middle 95% lies between −1.96 and 1.96 (see Table B.2). Hence, 97.5% of the standard normal lies below 1.96, and 2.5% lies below −1.96, as can be seen, approximately, from Table B.1. The value 1.96 is called the upper 2½% **percentage point** and −1.96 is the lower 2½% percentage point. For the complementary hypothesis test at the $100 - 95 = 5\%$ level of significance (see below), 1.96 is the critical value.

Figure 2.4 illustrates the concept of a 95% confidence interval in the context of the current example, using the general description presented in Section 2.1.1. Should we repeat the sampling process (randomly choosing 4161 Scotswomen) 20 times, we expect to find that 19 of the 20 resultant confidence intervals cover the true percentage of Scotswomen who smoke (since $(95/100) \times 20 = 19$). Of course, our sample could be the odd one out, although we would have to be unlucky for this to have happened. That is the price we pay for sampling and is analogous to the 0.05 probability of finding significance, when the null hypothesis is true, in 5% hypothesis tests. In real life we would never do such repeat sampling — if we did, we would simply combine the samples into one mega sample.

There is no reason to use 95% confidence except that this is most often used in practice, tying in with the common use of the complementary 5% significance level in

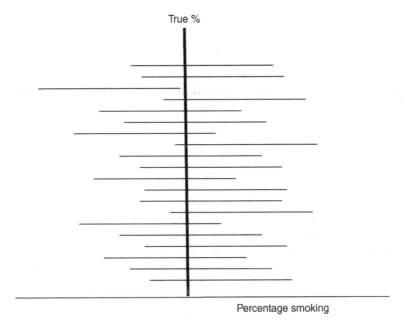

Figure 2.4. Schematic illustration of 95% confidence intervals (shown by horizontal lines) expected from 20 repeat samples of the same number of subjects (Scotswomen, in the example). The vertical line is drawn at the (unknown) percentage of smokers in the population (women in Scotland).

hypothesis tests. Any other high percentage of confidence could be used instead of 95%; Table B.2 gives some useful critical values for confidence intervals and their complementary tests. All that is necessary in order to change the percentage of confidence is to replace 1.96 in (2.2) by the required critical value. Hence, the width (upper minus lower limit) of the confidence interval will be

$$2V\sqrt{p(1-p)/n},\tag{2.3}$$

where V is the critical value. For example, from Table B.2, $V = 1.6449$ for a 90% confidence interval. Table B.2 shows that increasing the percentage of confidence increases V and thus widens the confidence interval (probabilistic limits of error). We can only have greater confidence if we pay the price of having a wider interval of error. Precision would, on the other hand, be improved by increasing n because (2.3) decreases as n increases. So it is a good idea to increase sample size (all else being equal).

The number of female smokers in Scotland is high by international standards, and was much higher still when these data were collected. Suppose that an eminent epidemiologist claimed that the percentage of women who smoke in Scotland was 39%. We could use the sample data to test the null hypothesis that the true proportion of female smokers in Scotland is 39% (at the time of data collection).

The hypothesis test for the null hypothesis that the population proportion is some fixed amount, say Π_0, involves calculation of the test statistic

$$\frac{p - \Pi_0}{\sqrt{\Pi_0(1 - \Pi_0)/n}}\tag{2.4}$$

which is compared to the standard normal distribution (Table B.1 or Table B.2).

For the example quoted, $\Pi_0 = 0.39$ and so the test statistic, (2.4), is

$$\frac{0.3754 - 0.39}{\sqrt{0.39(1 - 0.39)/4161}} = -1.93.$$

As we have already seen, the 5% critical value for the standard normal is 1.96. Because the absolute value of the test statistic, 1.93, is less than 1.96, we fail to reject the null hypothesis (true percentage is 39%), against the alternative that it is some other value, at the 5% level of significance. This is what we might expect, anyway, because $\Pi_0 = 0.39$ is inside the complementary 95% confidence interval found earlier and is, therefore, a reasonably likely value for the true proportion.

This is a particular example of a general procedure; we reject the null hypothesis at the X% level only if the value under the null hypothesis lies outside the $(100 - X)$% confidence interval. In the case of proportions, in contrast to that for means (see Section 2.7), it is just possible, if unlikely, that we get a different result from a hypothesis test compared with using the complementary confidence interval to ascertain significance. This is due to the slightly different approximations used in the two procedures.

One advantage of the test procedure is that it enables us to calculate the p value. From a computer package, $p = 0.054$ for the example. Quoting this figure in a report alerts the reader to the fact that the null hypothesis would, after all, be rejected if a significance level of 5.4%, or some round figure just above it, such as 6%, were used instead of 5%. When we use 5% significance, we shall wrongly reject the null hypothesis one time in 20. Perhaps we are prepared to accept a slightly higher error rate. If we are prepared to be wrong 5.4% of the time (less than one chance in 18), then we could adopt 5.4% significance and thus reject the null hypothesis in the example. If we intend to use the test to make a decision, it is clearly important to fix the significance level *before* data analysis begins.

So far we have not considered the **alternative hypothesis** critically; that is, we have taken it simply to be the negation of the null. In the example used, the alternative hypothesis, denoted H_1, is that the population proportion is not equal to 0.39. This led to a **two-sided test**, in which we reject H_0 if the observed proportion is sufficiently large or sufficiently small. Is this appropriate in the example? Suppose the eminent epidemiologist actually said that *at least* 39% of Scottish women smoke. In this situation, we no longer wish to have a two-sided test; we have the hypotheses

$$H_0 : \Pi = 0.39 \text{ versus } H_1 : \Pi < 0.39,$$

where Π is the population proportion, and we wish to reject the null hypothesis, H_0, in favour of H_1 only when the observed sample proportion is sufficiently *small* (the epidemiologist is only wrong if H_1 is true). Notice that H_0 is as for the two-sided test, only H_1 has changed (previously it was $\Pi \neq 0.39$). We now have a **one-sided** test with a single critical value in the lower tail of the standard normal distribution. Precisely, we have a one-sided 'less than' test. In another situation, H_1 might be formulated as $\Pi > 0.39$; then we have a single critical value in the upper tail. By the symmetry of the normal distribution, this will be the negative of the critical value for the 'less than' test. Since Table B.2 gives two-sided critical values, we shall need to double the required one-sided significance level before using this table for a one-sided test (of either type). Otherwise, we can use Table B.1 more directly.

For a 5% test applied to our example, the critical value is -1.6449 (Table B.1 tells us that it is slightly bigger than -1.65; Table B.2 gives the result to four decimal places when we look up double the required significance level). The test statistic, -1.93, is less than -1.6449, so it is a more extreme value. Hence, we reject H_0 in favour of the one-sided H_1 at the 5% level. Note that this is the opposite decision to that taken after the two-sided test earlier. The p value is 0.027, half of the p value for the earlier two-sided test. Now the epidemiologist's claim is not supported by the data.

This example shows that we should decide not only on the significance level, but also on the alternative hypothesis, before data analysis begins. In most cases, the two-sided alternative is the appropriate one and should be used unless a good reason exists to do otherwise. Consequently, Appendix B gives critical values for the normal (Table B.2) and t (Table B.4) distributions appropriate for two-sided tests.

The chi-square test of Section 2.5.1 requires one-sided critical values of chi-square in order to perform a two-sided test. As observed values move away from expected values in *either* direction, (2.1) will always increase, due to the squaring process in (2.1). Thus, only very large values of (2.1), in the upper tail, are inconsistent with the null hypothesis. Similar comments can be made for the F test from an analysis of variance (Section 9.2.3). Since these are the most common situations in which the distributions are used, Appendix B gives one-sided critical values for the χ^2 and F tests.

2.5.3   Comparing two proportions or percentages

Section 2.5.2 is concerned with the **one-sample** situation, that is, when only one sample of data is analysed. In epidemiological studies, we are more often interested in **two-sample** problems: comparing two samples or one sample split into two subsamples in some meaningful way. For instance, so far we have made inferences about the proportion of female smokers (a one-sample problem), but now we will consider comparing the proportion that smoke between males and females (a two-sample problem).

We obtain a 95% confidence interval for the difference between two population proportions as

$$p_1 - p_2 \pm 1.96\sqrt{\frac{p_1(1-p_1)}{n_1} + \frac{p_2(1-p_2)}{n_2}}, \qquad (2.5)$$

where p_1 is the sample proportion from the first sample (of size n_1) and p_2 and n_2 are the corresponding values for the second sample.

For the difference between male and female smoking proportions, we have, from Table 2.9,

$$p_1 = 2279/4520 = 0.5042, \qquad\qquad p_2 = 0.3754,$$

$$n_1 = 4520, \qquad\qquad n_2 = 4161.$$

Hence, the 95% confidence interval, from (2.5), is

$$0.5042 - 0.3754 \pm 1.96\sqrt{\frac{0.5042(1-0.5042)}{4520} + \frac{0.3754(1-0.3754)}{4161}}$$

which is 0.1288 ± 0.0207 or $(0.108, 0.150)$. We are 95% confident that the male percentage of smokers exceeds the female percentage by between 10.8 and 15.0%. Notice that zero is well outside these limits, suggesting that the male excess has not arisen just by chance. Next we consider how to test this formally.

The test statistic for testing the null hypothesis that the true difference between two population proportions is zero is

$$\frac{p_1 - p_2}{\sqrt{p_c(1-p_c)\left(\dfrac{1}{n_1} + \dfrac{1}{n_2}\right)}}, \qquad (2.6)$$

where

$$p_c = \frac{n_1 p_1 + n_2 p_2}{n_1 + n_2}. \qquad (2.7)$$

We compare (2.6) with the standard normal distribution. In (2.7), p_c is the combined proportion, a weighted average of the two individual sample proportions. An alternative definition is that p_c is the sample proportion for the combined sample, created by pooling samples 1 and 2.

To test the hypothesis that the same percentage of middle-aged Scottish men and women smoke, we first use (2.7),

$$p_c = \frac{(4520)(0.5042) + (4161)(0.3754)}{4520 + 4161} = 0.4425.$$

As noted, we could get this result from Table 2.8 as the proportion of smokers for the sex groups combined. Then, from (2.6), the test statistic is

$$\frac{0.5042 - 0.3754}{\sqrt{0.4425(1 - 0.4425)\left(\dfrac{1}{4520} + \dfrac{1}{4161}\right)}} = 12.07.$$

Since this is above 1.96, we reject the null hypothesis of equal proportions at the 5% level of significance and conclude that the sexes have different proportions of smokers. In fact, we have very strong evidence to reject H_0 because the p value is below 0.0001; that is, we would reject H_0 even if we used a significance level as small as 0.01%. Note that there was no reason to use anything other than the general two-sided alternative hypothesis (proportions unequal) here. Even so, the sample evidence suggests that more men smoke, rather than more women, and our test, like our confidence interval, suggests that this is a 'real' difference.

Another way of looking at the problem of testing the hypothesis that the prevalence of smoking is the same for men and women is to consider the equivalent hypothesis that there is no relationship between smoking and the person's sex. Reference to Section 2.5.1 shows that we test the hypothesis of no relationship through the chi-square test applied to Table 2.9. In fact, this is an equivalent procedure to that used in this section. The only difference when the chi-square test is applied to a 2×2 table is that the test statistic, (2.1), is the square of that introduced here, (2.6). The p value will be exactly the same because the critical values of χ_1^2 are also the squares of those for the standard normal. Further details of how to analyse 2×2 tables are given in Section 3.5.

2.6   Descriptive techniques for quantitative variables

In this section we shall look at two descriptive techniques for epidemiological data on a quantitative variable: numerical summarisation and pictorial shape investigation. In an initial exploration of quantitative data, shape investigation would normally be most important because many analytical techniques are only suitable for data of a certain shape, while summarisation might inadvertently obscure some interesting aspects of the data. In report writing, summarising is generally more important because it is economical in space and easier for the reader to assimilate. It will be convenient to take summarisation first in what follows. The techniques will be illustrated using Scottish Heart Health Study data once again, but for simplicity we shall now take a small subset of these data, for eight variables recorded on 50 subjects (Table 2.10).

Table 2.10. Results for 50 subjects sampled from the Scottish Heart Health Study.

Serum total cholesterol (mmol/l)	Diastolic blood pressure (mmHg)	Systolic blood pressure (mmHg)	Alcohol (g/day)	Cigarettes (no./day)	Carbon monoxide (ppm)	Cotinine (ng/ml)	CHD (1 = yes; 2 = no)
5.75	80	121	5.4	0	6	13	2
6.76	83	139	64.6	0	4	3	2
6.47	76	113	21.5	20	21	284	2
7.11	79	124	8.2	40	57	395	2
5.42	79	127	24.4	20	29	283	2
7.04	100	148	13.6	0	3	0	2
5.75	79	124	54.6	0	3	1	2
7.14	85	127	6.2	0	1	0	2
6.10	76	138	0.0	0	1	3	2
6.55	82	133	2.4	0	2	0	2
6.29	92	141	0.0	0	7	0	2
5.98	100	183	21.5	20	55	245	1
5.71	78	119	50.2	0	14	424	2
6.89	90	143	16.7	0	4	0	1
4.90	85	132	40.6	4	7	82	2
6.23	88	139	16.7	25	24	324	2
7.71	109	154	7.2	1	3	11	1
5.73	93	136	10.8	0	2	0	2
6.54	100	149	26.0	0	3	0	2
7.16	73	107	2.9	25	29	315	1
6.13	92	132	23.9	0	2	2	2
6.25	87	123	31.1	0	7	10	2
5.19	97	141	12.0	0	3	4	1
6.05	74	118	23.9	0	3	0	2
7.12	85	133	24.4	0	2	0	2
5.71	88	121	45.4	0	8	2	2
6.19	69	129	24.8	15	40	367	1
6.73	98	129	52.6	15	21	233	2
5.34	70	123	38.3	1	2	7	2
4.79	82	127	23.9	0	2	1	2
6.78	74	104	4.8	0	4	7	2
6.10	88	123	86.1	0	3	1	1
4.35	88	128	15.5	20	11	554	2
7.10	79	136	7.4	10	9	189	1
5.85	102	150	4.1	0	6	0	2
6.74	68	109	1.2	15	15	230	2
7.55	80	135	92.1	25	29	472	2
7.86	78	131	23.9	6	55	407	1
6.92	101	137	2.5	0	3	0	2
6.64	97	139	119.6	40	16	298	2
6.46	76	142	62.2	40	31	404	1
5.99	73	108	0.0	0	2	4	2
5.39	77	112	11.0	30	11	251	2
6.35	81	133	16.2	0	3	0	2
5.86	88	147	88.5	0	3	0	2
5.64	65	111	0.0	20	16	271	2
6.60	102	149	65.8	0	3	1	2
6.76	75	140	12.4	0	2	0	2
5.51	75	125	0.0	25	16	441	2
7.15	92	131	31.1	20	36	434	1

Note: These data may be downloaded from the book's web site; see Appendix A.

2.6.1   The five-number summary

The basic idea of summarisation is to present a small number of key statistics that may be used to represent the data as a whole. If we want to use only one summary statistic, the obvious choice would be some measure of average. This is usually too great a summarisation, except for very simple uses, because it says nothing about how the data are distributed about the average — that is, how well the average represents the whole. In epidemiological research, we would normally find it much more informative to present the five-number summary given here or the more succinct two-number summary of Section 2.6.3 (or possibly a selection from both).

The five-number summary comprises the following:

- Minimum value
- First quartile, Q_1: 25% of the data are below this and 75% above
- Median (or second quartile), Q_2: 50% of the data are below this and 50% above
- Third quartile, Q_3: 75% of the data are below this and 25% above
- Maximum value

Interpretation (and evaluation) of the extreme values (minimum and maximum) is obvious. The quartiles are the numbers that divide the data into four equal portions. Their derivation is very straightforward when there are, say, nine observations as in the next example.

Example 2.3 To find the five-number summary of the numbers

$$15, 3, 9, 3, 14, 20, 7, 8, 11,$$

first we sort the data, giving:

$$3, 3, 7, 8, 9, 11, 14, 15, 20.$$

The minimum is 3 and the maximum is 20. The median is the middle number (with four below and four above), 9. The first quartile is 7, because this has two below and six above, giving the correct split in the ratio of 1 : 3. Similarly, the third quartile is 14 since three quarters of the remaining data are below, and one-quarter above, this value.

Consider, now, the data on the cholesterol variable in Table 2.10. To apply the same logic, we first need to sort the data. This has been done to produce Table 2.11. From this table, the minimum and maximum are easy enough to find, but an immediate problem occurs when we try to find the median. As there is an even number

Table 2.11. Total serum cholesterol (mmol/l) in rank order.

Rank	Value	Rank	Value	Rank	Value	Rank	Value	Rank	Value
1	4.35	11	5.71	21	6.10	31	6.55	41	7.04
2	4.79	12	5.73	22	6.13	32	6.60	42	7.10
3	4.90	13	5.75	23	6.19	33	6.64	43	7.11
4	5.19	14	5.75	24	6.23	34	6.73	44	7.12
5	5.34	15	5.85	25	6.25	35	6.74	45	7.14
6	5.39	16	5.86	26	6.29	36	6.76	46	7.15
7	5.42	17	5.98	27	6.35	37	6.76	47	7.16
8	5.51	18	5.99	28	6.46	38	6.78	48	7.55
9	5.64	19	6.05	29	6.47	39	6.89	49	7.71
10	5.71	20	6.10	30	6.54	40	6.92	50	7.86

(50) of observations, there is no middle value. It seems reasonable to take the 25th or 26th value, or some summary of the two, as the median, but there is no single right answer. Another problem arises when we try to find Q_1, since no number can possibly have a quarter of the remaining observations (49/4 = 12.25) below it. In fact, because 50/4 = 12.5, the position of Q_1 ought to be 12.5, so it would seem reasonable to take the 12th or 13th value, or some summary of the two.

Unfortunately, there is no universally agreed rule as to which choice to make in these situations. For this reason, different computer packages may give different answers for the quartiles from the same data, although the differences should be small and, usually, unimportant. When the position of a quartile is a whole number, r (say), we shall take the average of the rth and $(r + 1)$th observations in rank order to be the median. For our data, 50/2 = 25, which is a whole number, so we should evaluate the median as half the sum of the 25th and 26th values. On the other hand, if the position of a quartile is not a whole number, we shall take the number in the *next highest* whole number position within the ranked dataset. Since the position for our Q_1 ought to be 12.5, which is not a whole number, we will take the 13th value in rank order to be Q_1. Similarly, Q_3 will be the 38th value. Hence, the five-number summary of the cholesterol data is

$$\begin{array}{ccccc}
4.35 & 5.75 & 6.27 & 6.78 & 7.86 \\
\text{min.} & Q_1 & Q_2 & Q_3 & \text{max.}
\end{array}$$

The intervals between these five numbers are called the **quarters** of the data.

What does the five-number summary tell us about the data? We can see that no one has a cholesterol value of more than 7.86 or less than 4.35 mmol/l; these are important and interesting findings from the epidemiological investigation. Their difference (7.86 − 4.35 = 3.51 mmol/l) is called the **range**, which measures the entire spread (**variation** or **dispersion**) of the data. We can also see the middle value (6.27 mmol/l), which is a measure of **average** for the data. Perhaps not so obvious is the use of Q_1 and Q_3. A small number of unusually low or unusually high values are in many datasets; these are termed **outliers**. Such values may distort the range because they make it much bigger than would be expected if all the data were typical. The range also has an unfortunate tendency to increase as sample size increases; the more people we observe the more chance we have of including the rare 'extreme' person. Certainly the range cannot decrease when we include more observations. The first and third quartiles are not affected by outliers, nor are they sensitive to sample size. Hence, their difference (6.78 − 5.75 = 1.03 mmol/l), called the **interquartile range**, often gives a more representative measure of the dispersion, which may be meaningfully compared with other datasets. Sometimes the semi-interquartile range, or **quartile deviation**, is used instead. This is simply half the interquartile range $(Q_3 − Q_1)/2$.

Example 2.4 Consider Example 2.3 again, but now suppose that the nine numbers are (in rank order)

$$3, 3, 7, 8, 9, 11, 14, 15, 200.$$

That is, as before except that the maximum is now 200 rather than 20. Compared with Example 2.3, the range has increased from 20 − 3 = 17 to 200 − 3 = 197. The interquartile range, however, remains 14 − 7 = 7. Also, the median is unchanged (at the value 9). The number 200 is an outlier because it is more than 10 times larger than any other value. Notice that it could be argued that we cannot claim to know what is typical on the strength of only eight other observations, but the principle behind this simplistic example clearly holds with more appropriate sample sizes.

As well as average and dispersion, the five-number summary gives an impression of the other important feature of observational data, the degree of **symmetry**. Data are symmetrical if each value below the median is perfectly counterbalanced by another value exactly equidistant from, but above, the median (as in a mirror image). We are very unlikely to find such perfect symmetry in observational data, so instead we might look for quartile symmetry, which is where

$$Q_1 - \text{minimum} = \text{maximum} - Q_3$$

and

$$Q_2 - Q_1 = Q_3 - Q_2.$$

For the cholesterol data, these four differences are 1.40, 1.08, 0.52 and 0.51, respectively, showing that almost perfect symmetry exists between the middle quarters of the data, but some lack of symmetry between the outer quarters.

The degree of symmetry is best judged from a diagram of the five-number summary called a **boxplot** (or **box-and-whisker plot**). Figure 2.5 is a boxplot for the cholesterol data. The line in the box marks the median, the edges of the box mark the quartiles, and the arrows (or 'whiskers') go out to the extremes.

The cholesterol data have no obvious outliers, but when outliers are present it is best to isolate them on the boxplot. To do this, we need to impose a definition of an outlier; however, just as with the definition of 'quartile', there is no universally agreed rule, with the consequence that different statistical computer packages may give different results. We will define an outlier in a boxplot by conceptually placing 'fences' at the positions 1½ times the length of the box below Q_1 and above Q_3. The left arrow will then terminate at the smallest observation inside the fences and the right arrow will terminate at the largest observation inside the fences. Any observation outside the fences will be termed an outlier and identified with an asterisk. Figure 2.6 shows a boxplot for alcohol (from Table 2.10) where three outliers are present. When outliers occur, we may prefer to change our five-number summary so that the minimum and maximum are replaced by fairly extreme percentiles, such as the 1st and 99th percentiles (Section 2.6.2).

By eye, from Figure 2.5 and Figure 2.6, we can see that cholesterol is reasonably symmetrical but alcohol is not. Nonsymmetric data are said to be **skewed**. If a bigger

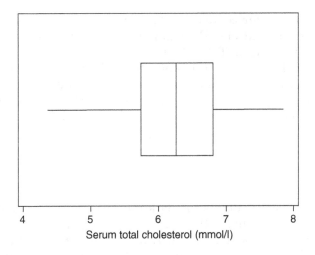

Figure 2.5. Boxplot for cholesterol.

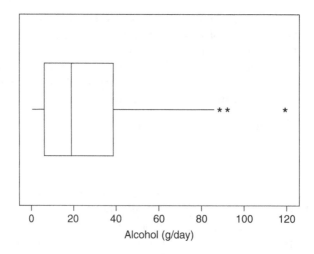

Figure 2.6. Boxplot for alcohol.

portion of the boxplot is to the right of the median, we say that the data are **right-skewed** or **positively skewed**. Otherwise, they are **left-skewed** or **negatively skewed**. Alcohol is right-skewed, from Figure 2.6.

Identification of skew is one of the most important parts of an initial examination of epidemiological data because it points to what is appropriate at further stages of analysis (as we shall see). However, identification of what is *important* skew is not always straightforward since it naturally depends upon what we propose to do with the data. To some extent, it also depends upon the sample size. Although our cholesterol data are not entirely symmetrical, for most practical purposes the slight lack of symmetry is not important. The alcohol data are quite different, with pronounced skew, which must be accounted for in any further analyses. Notice that the symmetry of cholesterol and skewness of alcohol are properties of the *data* rather than the variables. We cannot, for example, be sure that another sample of cholesterol data will not be skewed, although if it were of the same size and taken from a similar parent population, we would anticipate near-symmetry on the basis of our findings.

Boxplots are useful for comparing the same quantitative variable in different populations, or subpopulations. For example, Figure 2.7 shows cholesterol for men with and without CHD, from Table 2.10. Since the same (horizontal) scale has been used, we can see that cholesterol tends to be higher for those with CHD. The dispersion (as measured by the interquartile range) is much the same in each group, although the range is slightly larger for those with CHD. Each distribution shows some evidence of left skew, notably between the first and third quartiles for those with CHD.

2.6.2   Quantiles

Quantiles are values that divide the data into portions of equal size. The quartiles provide an example: they divide the data into four equal parts. Other divisions may be useful to explore how the data are distributed. Tertiles divide into three, quintiles into five, deciles into 10 and percentiles into 100 equal parts, and so on. They may be calculated by extending the methodology used in Section 2.6.1.

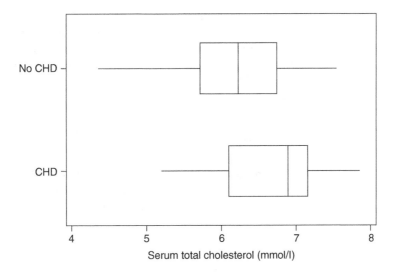

Figure 2.7. Boxplot for cholesterol data by CHD group.

Suppose we want to find the pth q-tile where $0 < p < q$. Let $r = (p/q)n$, let s be the next highest integer above r and denote the ith observation in the dataset, after it has been sorted in ascending order, by $x_{(i)}$. The pth q-tile is then defined to be

$$x_{(s)} \text{ if } r \text{ is not an integer}$$

$$(x_{(r)} + x_{(r+1)})/2 \text{ if } r \text{ is an integer.}$$

In the cholesterol example of Section 2.6.1, n is 50. To find the median, since this is the second quartile, $p = 2$ and $q = 4$. Hence $r = (2/4) \times 50 = 25$. This is an integer, and so the median is $(x_{(25)} + x_{(26)})/2$, i.e., the mean of the 25th and 26th largest cholesterol values, as found before. To find the first quartile, we compute $r = (1/4) \times 50 = 12.5$. Hence the first quartile is $x_{(13)}$, the 13th largest value, as found before.

Example 2.5 Using the data of Example 2.3 (where $n = 9$), the position for the first tertile should be $\frac{1}{3} \times 9 = 3$. As this is a whole number, we take the mean of the third and fourth observations in rank order. Similarly, the second tertile has position $\frac{2}{3} \times 9 = 6$, so that we take the mean of the sixth and seventh observations in rank order. Since the ordered data are

$$3, 3, 7, 8, 9, 11, 14, 15, 20,$$

the first tertile is $(7 + 8)/2 = 7.5$ and the second is $(11 + 14)/2 = 12.5$. Notice that these numbers split the data $3 : 6$ (i.e., $1 : 2$) and $6 : 3$ (i.e., $2 : 1$), respectively, as we would expect of tertiles.

Sometimes a particular quantile is of interest. For instance we may wish to find the 90th percentile of cholesterol from a national population survey such as the SHHS, because this tells us what value we can expect the highest 10% of the national population to exceed. Often the entire set of quantiles (of a particular degree) are required. For example, infant growth curves may have each percentile-for-age of weight marked, these having been calculated from extensive sample data.

When we have data on the same variable from two different sources, a **quantile–quantile plot** is a useful descriptive tool. As the name suggests, this is a plot of the quantiles (for example, deciles) from one source against the same quantiles from the other source. If the two distributions are similar, then we expect to see a straight line on the quantile–quantile plot. This would provide an alternative to the two-sample boxplot (for example, Figure 2.7).

2.6.3   The two-number summary

If the data are reasonably symmetric, then the **mean** (the sum of all the observations divided by the sample size) would often be a better measure of their average than the median. For a sample of size n, the mean is written mathematically as

$$\bar{x} = \frac{1}{n} \sum_{i=1}^{n} x_i \,, \tag{2.8}$$

where x_1, x_2, ..., x_n are the observations.

To calculate the mean for the cholesterol data, we simply sum up the cholesterol values in Table 2.10 and divide by 50. This gives

$$\bar{x} = \frac{1}{50}\left(314.33\right) = 6.287 \; \text{mmol/l.}$$

Similarly, the **standard deviation** is more often used than the interquartile range, or the range, as a measure of spread for symmetric data. This is conceived as a mean of the differences between each observation and their mean; that is, it should tell us the average deviation of the mean from the observations. In fact, we cannot use quite such a simple approach because this mean of differences would always be zero. This is due to the definition of the mean as the arithmetic centre of the data and is easy to prove algebraically. Here, we will simply use an example to illustrate the problem.

Example 2.6 Consider the simple dataset of size 9 from Example 2.3 again. Here the mean is, from (2.8),

$$\bar{x} = \frac{1}{9}\left(15+3+9+3+14+20+7+8+11\right) = \frac{90}{9} = 10.0.$$

The differences from this mean, $x_i - \bar{x}$, are thus

$$5, \; -7, \; -1, \; -7, \; 4, \; 10, \; -3, \; -2, \; 1.$$

The sum of these differences is zero and hence their mean is zero, as stated.

The problem is caused by the positive and negative contributions exactly cancelling each other out. One way of getting over this problem is to square each difference before averaging (because squared values are always positive). This gives rise to the **variance** (denoted s^2), the average of the *squared* differences between each observation and the mean. However, the variance is not very meaningful for practical purposes because it is measured in square units (e.g., squared mmol/l for cholesterol). The standard deviation, s, is hence defined as the square root of the variance.

One final complication is that the averaging process to arrive at the variance should be to add up the squared differences and divide by $n - 1$ rather than the sample size, n. This is necessary to make the variance **unbiased** — that is, to ensure that the mean value of s^2 over many samples equals the true variance. Another explanation is that s^2 uses the divisor $n - 1$ because there are only $n - 1$ independent pieces of information in the data once $\bar{x}$ is known. Look at Example 2.6 again. Once we know $\bar{x}$ and the first eight data items, we automatically know what the ninth item must be. The sum of the first eight numbers is

$$15 + 3 + 9 + 3 + 14 + 20 + 7 + 8 = 79.$$

Since $\bar{x} = 10$, the sum of all nine numbers must be $9 \times 10 = 90$. Hence, the ninth number must be $90 - 79 = 11$, which indeed it is. As in the chi-square test (Section 2.5.1), the term **degrees of freedom** (d.f.) is used to refer to the number of independent pieces of information. Hence, s^2 has $n - 1$ d.f.

When we use a computer package to calculate s^2 (or s), we must check that it has used the $n - 1$ rather than the n divisor (some do not). Division by n is correct only if we have a 100% sample (a **census**) of the population of interest, which is hardly ever the case.

The formula for the variance is thus

$$s^2 = \frac{1}{n-1} S_{xx} \tag{2.9}$$

where

$$S_{xx} = \sum_{i=1}^{n} \left(x_i - \bar{x}\right)^2. \tag{2.10}$$

Example 2.7 Using (2.10) with the data of Example 2.3 gives

$$S_{xx} = 254.$$

Hence, by (2.9), the variance is $s^2 = 254/8 = 31.75$ and the standard deviation is $s = \sqrt{31.75} = 5.63$.

For the cholesterol data of Table 2.10, $S_{xx} = 28.0765$ whence the variance, $s^2 = 0.5730$, and the standard deviation, $s = 0.757$ mmol/l.

With symmetric or near-symmetric data, the mean and standard deviation provide a **two-number summary** of the two major features of the data: their average and their dispersion about this average.

With right-skewed data, the mean will tend to be pulled upwards (above the median) by the few large observations. With left-skewed data, the reverse is true; the mean will be pulled down below the median. Either type of skewness inflates the standard deviation. By contrast, the median and interquartile range are largely unaffected by skewness. We can see this contrast by considering, again, the effect of a single outlier, a particular case of skewness.

Example 2.8 Consider the data of Example 2.3 and Example 2.4 (in rank order):

$$3, 3, 7, 8, 9, 11, 14, 15, 20$$

and

$$3, 3, 7, 8, 9, 11, 14, 15, 200.$$

For the first set of data, $\bar{x} = 10.0$ (as shown in Example 2.6). For the second (with the outlier), it is 30.0. The first mean is a reasonable measure of average for its data; the second certainly is not because it is in no way typical (it is at least twice as big as all but one of the observations). However, in Example 2.3 and Example 2.4 we saw that the median is 9 for both sets of data. Similarly, when 20 is replaced by 200, the standard deviation changes from 5.63 to 63.89, but the interquartile range is unaltered (see Example 2.4).

The mean is thus not a suitable measure of average for highly skewed data, but the question remains as to why we should prefer it to the median for symmetric or near-symmetric data. One reason is that the mean uses every observation in the data; this is not true of the median, which uses only the middle value or values. A second reason is that the mean is what most people think of as 'the average'. Third, the mean has a mathematical expression, (2.8), but the median does not. This allows us to manipulate the mean mathematically and thus enables powerful, more complex methods of analysis to be devised. Thus, we should use the mean if we can, but not when it is unrepresentative of the average, in which case we transform the data (Section 2.8.1) or use the median. The standard deviation should always be used with the mean because it has a similar derivation and its advantages are much the same.

2.6.4   Other summary statistics of spread

Sometimes a quantitative variable is summarised by showing the **standard error** of the mean, rather than the standard deviation, alongside the mean. The standard error of the mean is a measure of the inaccuracy of the sample mean as a representative of the mean of the entire parent population from which the sample was drawn. In fact, it is the standard deviation of the distribution of sample means (the means of repeated samples of the same size from the same population). The standard error of the mean has the value $s/\sqrt{n}$. Notice that this will decrease as the sample size, n, increases. Standard errors may be defined for other summary statistics besides the mean; for instance, the standard error of the difference between two means will be used in Section 2.7.3.

The **coefficient of variation** is defined as the standard deviation divided by the mean. This is a unit-free standardised measure of variation, often used to compare dispersion for variables with different units of measurement. Sometimes it is multiplied by 100 so as to give a percentage measure.

2.6.5   Assessing symmetry

We have already seen how the boxplot may be used to assess symmetry. Here we consider how summary statistics, including those represented on the boxplot, may be used to determine whether a variable is symmetric, or (more likely in practice) reasonably so. This not only determines whether the mean and standard deviation (or standard error) are suitable summary measures but is also a first step in determining whether inferential techniques based upon the normal distribution are appropriate (Section 2.7).

The **coefficient of skewness** is a summary measure of skewness — the opposite of symmetry. It is defined as

$$\frac{k \sum (x - \bar{x})^3}{s^3},$$

where k is some function of the sample size, n. If the distribution of the x variable is perfectly symmetrical, the coefficient of skewness will be zero. Negative values imply left-skewness; positive values imply right-skewness. Different textbooks and computer packages use different forms for k; we shall take $k = n/(n - 1)(n - 2)$. However k is defined, the coefficient of skewness summarises the cubed deviations from the overall mean, standardised by the process of division by the cube of the standard deviation. Due to this standardisation, the coefficient of skewness is, like the coefficient of variation, unit-free.

Unfortunately, the coefficient of skewness has only limited utility for ascertaining symmetry (or lack of it). Besides the issue that k is not uniquely defined, there is no reliable cut-point which could be used to decide which are, and which are not, symmetric data (see also Section 2.7.1). Table 2.12 shows several summary statistics for each of the quantitative variables in Table 2.10. Boxplots of the five variables not presented so far appear in Figure 2.8. The '2' on the boxplot for carbon monoxide indicates two outliers with the same value. In this compound boxplot, each variable has been standardised so as to avoid the gross differences in magnitude that occur when the original variables are plotted on a common scale. For each variable, its median was subtracted from all its values, followed by division by its interquartile range. This standardisation ensures that the boxes are all of equal width and the median line occurs in the same position for all standardised variables. Hence, Figure 2.8 may not be used to compare averages or dispersions; in any case, such comparisons would be meaningless.

From Figure 2.8 diastolic and systolic blood pressure are reasonably symmetrical, although the outlier in systolic blood pressure might usefully be reported separately (without the outlier, the mean becomes 130.2). The other three variables are right-skewed. 'Cigarettes' is so skewed that the minimum, first quartile and median are all equal (to zero). Cotinine is almost as badly skewed; its minimum and first quartile are both zero. Recall that Figure 2.5 and Figure 2.6 show that cholesterol has a slight, but unimportant, left skew and that alcohol is highly right-skewed.

From Table 2.12, notice that the mean is bigger than the median in all four cases in which right-skewness is apparent in the boxplots, as we would expect. In these cases, the relatively few large values distort the mean as a measure of centre of the data. For perfectly symmetric data, the mean and median would be equal since then there is only one 'centre'.

Unless several negative values are present, a variable will usually (although not necessarily) be skewed when the standard deviation is of a similar size to, or exceeds, the mean. This will happen when the coefficient of variation approaches or exceeds 100%, which happens for all four highly skewed variables in Table 2.12. The coefficient

Table 2.12. Summary statistics for variables from Table 2.10.

Summary statistic	Serum total cholesterol (mmol/l)	Diastolic blood pressure (mmHg)	Systolic blood pressure (mmHg)	Alcohol (g/day)	Cigarettes (no./day)	Carbon monoxide (ppm)	Cotinine (ng/ml)
Mean	6.287	84.6	131.3	26.76	8.7	12.8	139.5
Median	6.27	82.5	131.5	19.1	0	6	7
Std deviation	0.757	10.5	14.3	27.75	12.5	14.9	177.3
Std error	0.107	1.5	2.0	3.92	1.8	2.1	25.1
Q_1	5.75	76	123	6.2	0	3	0
Q_3	6.78	92	139	38.3	20	16	284
IQR	1.03	16	16	32.1	20	13	284
Minimum	4.35	65	104	0	0	1	0
Maximum	7.86	109	183	119.6	40	57	554
Range	3.51	44	79	119.6	40	56	554
Skewness	−0.23	0.36	0.69	1.50	1.19	1.68	0.78
CV	12%	12%	11%	104%	143%	117%	127%

Note: IQR = inter-quartile range; CV = coefficient of variation. Sample size, $n = 50$.

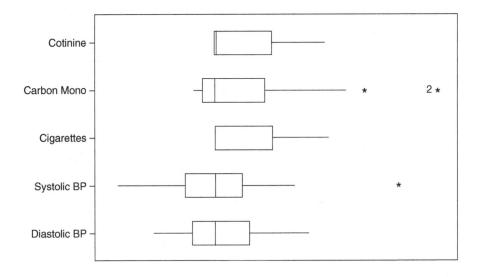

Figure 2.8. Boxplots (using standardised scales) for several variables from Table 2.10.

of skewness is, as anticipated, positive except in the case of the left-skewed variable, cholesterol. Notice how the outlier has inflated the quantitative measure of skewness for systolic blood pressure. Otherwise, the coefficients of skewness tend to follow the relative magnitudes anticipated from the boxplots. Values above about 0.7 seem to be associated with severe positive (right-) skewness.

2.6.6 Investigating shape

The summary statistics shown in Table 2.12 (or some subset of them) provide a short, informative description of the data for a quantitative variable. In some instances, the summary is too extreme and we would wish to show more about the overall shape of the data.

The first step when investigating shape is to create a **grouped frequency table** (or **grouped frequency distribution**), such as Table 2.13, which was created from

Table 2.13. Grouped frequency distribution for total serum cholesterol.

Cholesterol (mmol/l)	Frequency	Percentage	Cumulative percentage
4.0 to less than 4.5	1	2%	2%
4.5 to less than 5.0	2	4%	6%
5.0 to less than 5.5	4	8%	14%
5.5 to less than 6.0	11	22%	36%
6.0 to less than 6.5	11	22%	58%
6.5 to less than 7.0	11	22%	80%
7.0 to less than 7.5	7	14%	94%
7.5 to less than 8.0	3	6%	100%
Total	50	100%	

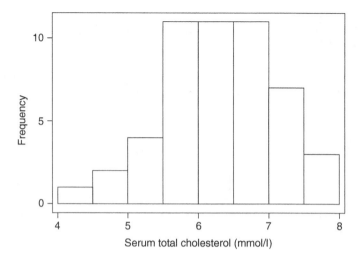

Figure 2.9. Histogram for cholesterol.

the cholesterol data in Table 2.10. As in Table 2.1, the percentages (and cumulative percentages) are optional, but informative.

Figure 2.9 is a **histogram** drawn from Table 2.13; this gives a visual impression of the shape which is apparent, but more difficult to assimilate, from the table. Boxplots also give an impression of some aspects of shape, but histograms show much more; they enable symmetry/skewness to be judged but also show where the 'peaks' and 'troughs' appear (cholesterol clearly peaks in the middle and drops away to either side, but more slowly to the left).

The **class intervals** used in Table 2.13 (i.e., 4.0 to less than 4.5, etc.) and in Figure 2.9 are all of equal size (0.5) and in this situation the histogram is easy to draw; indeed, the histogram is then essentially a bar chart except that the bars have been joined to emphasise the continuous nature of the variable concerned. When the variable concerned is discrete, a continuity correction is applied before the histogram is drawn. This simply joins adjacent classes by starting each bar midway between adjacent class limits (and extending the extreme bars by half a class interval).

It is not essential, nor always very sensible, to maintain equal class sizes, particularly when the data are very bunched in a certain part of the distribution, but very sparse elsewhere. When the class sizes are unequal, we should plot the **frequency density** (relative frequency divided by the class size) on the vertical axis to ensure that the areas of the bars are in the correct relative proportions. Table 2.14 and Figure 2.10 provide an

Table 2.14. Grouped frequency distribution for alcohol.

Alcohol (g/day)	Frequency	Relative frequency	Frequency density
0 but less than 10	16	0.32	0.0320
10 but less than 20	9	0.18	0.0180
20 but less than 30	10	0.20	0.0200
30 but less than 50	5	0.10	0.0050
50 but less than 70	6	0.12	0.0060
70 but less than 120	4	0.08	0.0016
Total	50	1	

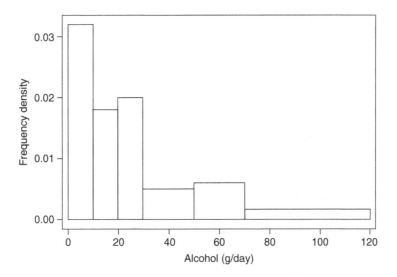

Figure 2.10. Histogram for alcohol.

example; notice how the skew, already apparent from Figure 2.6, is represented. Some computer packages produce histograms as bar charts and hence make no allowance for unequal class sizes. Sometimes histograms are plotted horizontally.

Although the histogram is easy to draw and simple to interpret, its drawbacks are its 'boxy' shape, which seems inappropriate to represent a continuous variable, and its lack of robustness to the choice of the class intervals employed: its overall shape can change greatly when, for instance, the starting point for the first bar is altered. An alternative is a **kernel density plot,** which can be thought of as a continuous analogue to a histogram. These plots would not normally be constructed without access to specialist software, because of the difficulty in drawing them. However, they are aesthetically attractive and give (if appropriately drawn) a direct understanding of the major features of the data. The concept of the kernel density plot, as a development of the histogram, is reasonably straightforward, as will now be explained.

Consider that a histogram is essentially made up of a number of boxes within each group of the frequency distribution. For instance, the bar representing the group 5 to 5.5 mmol/l of cholesterol in Figure 2.9 is essentially constructed by laying, on top of each other, four boxes, one for each of the four values within this range (these values are 5.19, 5.34, 5.39 and 5.42, from Table 2.11). Suppose, instead of taking all four values together, we centred each of these four boxes at its parent value. We then might choose a box width of 0.125 for each box, to mirror the width of the bar, when all four values were taken together, of 5.0 in Figure 2.9. For example, the individual box for the value 5.19 would be centred at 5.19 and would span the range $5.19 - (0.125/2) = 5.1275$ and $5.19 + (0.125/2) = 5.2525$ on the horizontal axis. Each box might be given a height of 1.0, as implied by Figure 2.9, although this is merely a scaling factor which has no bearing on the outline of the plot. Suppose we then piled up the boxes, as in the histogram. More precisely, we would add the heights of the respective boxes together, but now each box would only 'count' within its own range. To explain this, consider the ranges covered by each of the four boxes: Box 1: 5.1275 to 5.2525; Box 2: 5.2775 to 5.4025; Box 3: 5.3275 to 5.4525; Box 4: 5.3575 to 5.4825. Then consider the ranges where they overlap. In the range 5.1275 to 5.2525 only the first box counts; from 5.2525 to 5.2775 there are no boxes that count; from 5.2775 to 5.3275 only box 2 counts; from 5.3275 to 5.3575 boxes 2 and 3 count; from 5.3575 to 5.4025 boxes 2–4 all count; from

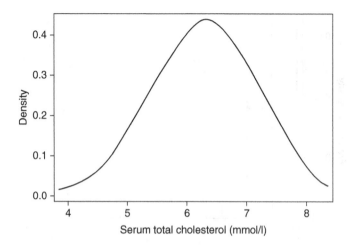

Figure 2.11. Kernel density plot for cholesterol.

5.4025 to 5.4525 boxes 3 and 4 count and from 5.4525 to 5.4825 only box 4 counts. Giving each 'count' a weight of one would produce an outline plot, in the range 5.1275 to 5.4825, with values of 1, 0, 1, 2, 3, 2 and 1 on the vertical scale, sequentially.

The idea of centring individual boxes over each data point and then piling up boxes only when they overlap can be generalised to centring and piling up any kind of shape. In particular, if we choose a smoothed shape that drops away to each side of the centre (i.e., the amount that 'counts' for each data value decreases as we move away from the value), then the addition process can produce an overall smoothed outline. Mathematically, a smaller weight, in the overall plot, is given to each specific point at positions further away from that point. The particular shape chosen is called the **kernel** because it is the basic building block for the plot that results. Figure 2.11 shows the result from using an Epanechnikov kernel applied to the data used in Figure 2.9. This was produced from the KDENSITY command in Stata. Epanechnikov's kernel has a central dome and tapers away equally on each side, like the tip of a missile, and is the default kernel used by Stata. Other kernels are available in Stata and other software.

Whatever the kernel chosen, by narrowing or widening the spread of the kernel the 'total' outline will become less or more smooth, respectively. The width of the kernel, technically the width from the centre to either end-point (e.g., 0.0625 in the demonstration example) is called the **band width**. This should be chosen in relation to the spread of the data and so that all the important features of the data are captured. Figure 2.11 uses a band width of 0.5, which allows us to see the underlying unimodal shape of the data, but hides 'local' peaks and troughs which will appear if a smaller band width is used. Stata chooses a band width that satisfies a certain optimality criterion automatically, but this can be over-ruled, as was done to produce Figure 2.11. Stata's choice of band width, about 0.3, produced a plot with a distinct dimple in the peak which seems most likely to be an artifact of the data (especially as the sample size is small), rather than a true characteristic of cholesterol. In general, the dependence of its shape on the choice of band width is a major drawback of the kernel density plot.

Kernel plots are most useful in comparing two or more distributions of data — for an example, see Figure 10.15 — or for comparing the distribution of a single set

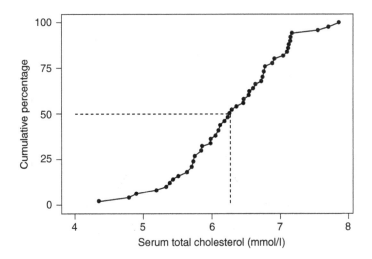

Figure 2.12. Ogive for cholesterol.

of data to some hypothetical distribution — an example is cited in Section 2.7.1. For a comprehensive account of kernel density methodology see Silverman (1998).

Cumulative frequencies (or percentages) may be of more interest than the basic frequencies (percentages) — for example, when we wish to see the percentage of people that have serum total cholesterol less than a certain value. This is easily achieved for our data using Table 2.12, cholesterol values in sorted order. Figure 2.12 plots the percentage of cholesterol values up to and including each successive value in Table 2.11 against the values themselves; for example, 100% is plotted against the maximum value, 7.86. This is called a cumulative (percentage) frequency plot or **ogive**.

The quartiles are easily found (approximately) from an ogive. For example, we find the median by drawing a horizontal line from the 50% position on the vertical scale across to the curve. We drop a vertical line from this point down to the horizontal axis and read off the median. Look at the dotted lines on Figure 2.12 and compare the visual reading with the exact cholesterol median given in Table 2.12.

A less accurate ogive could be drawn from Table 2.13. The right-hand column of this table should be plotted against the upper class limits. For example, 100% is plotted against 8.0. Often the ogive (of either type) is 'smoothed out' to avoid kinks due to sampling variation (such as are apparent in Figure 2.12).

2.7   Inferences about means

When we wish to use quantitative data to make inferences about the wider population from which the sample was drawn, we generally prefer to use the simplest, most useful summary measure for a quantitative variable: the measure of average. As we have seen, the mean is the most useful measure of average if the data are reasonably symmetrical. In this section, we shall take this to be the case and develop confidence intervals and hypothesis tests for means, just as we did earlier for proportions.

In fact, to be more precise, the material in this section assumes that the mean is sampled from a **normal probability distribution**. This should be so if the data have, at least approximately, a normal shape like a long-skirted bell that is symmetric about its middle value (see Figure 2.13). This might be assessed from the histogram. The

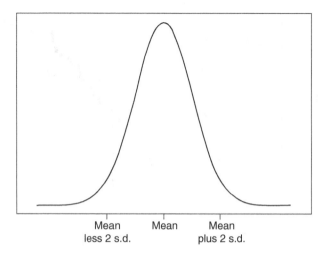

Figure 2.13. The normal curve (s.d. = standard deviation).

approximation must be fairly good for small samples but can be much less exact for large samples. This is because a fundamental theorem of statistics, the **central limit theorem**, says that the sampling distribution of sample means (that is, the means from repeated sampling) will tend to a normal distribution as n tends to infinity. This is the justification for the use of the normal distribution when dealing with proportions in Section 2.5.2 (a proportion is a special type of sample mean). The procedures given there will be justifiable only if n is reasonably big — say, above 100. The distribution of means converges to the normal more quickly when the data have a shape nearer to the normal. In Section 2.8, we shall consider what to do when the data on a quantitative variable do not have a normal distribution, even approximately, so that the central limit theorem cannot be invoked.

The **standard normal distribution** is that normal with mean 0 and standard deviation 1. This is the normal distribution tabulated in Table B.1 and Table B.2. We can change any normal into this standard form by subtracting its mean and dividing by its standard deviation.

2.7.1   Checking normality

Various tests of normality have been suggested (Stephens, 1974), including procedures based upon a measure of skewness (Snedecor and Cochran, 1989). However these are often too sensitive in epidemiological studies where sample sizes are generally large. That is, slight variations from normality cause rejection even when the variations have little effect on the final results of the epidemiological investigation.

Generally descriptive procedures, such as those based on histograms, boxplots and summary statistics are more useful. One disadvantage with these procedures is that they may not be able to distinguish the normal from other symmetric shapes. For example, they may not be able to distinguish a triangular shaped distribution from the normal. Kernel density plots tend to do better in this regard. A descriptive technique that is specific to the normal distribution uses the **normal plot**. This is a plot of the data against their **normal scores**, the expected values *if* the data had a standard normal distribution. If the data do have a normal distribution, the normal plot will produce a straight line.

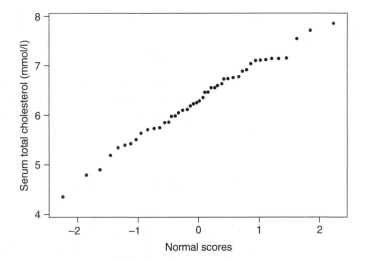

Figure 2.14. Normal plot for cholesterol.

Essentially, normal plots are quantile–quantile plots (Section 2.6.2) where one of the distributions is a theoretical one, and the quantiles plotted are determined by the data.

For example, Figure 2.14 and Figure 2.15 show normal plots for total cholesterol and alcohol, respectively, using the data in Table 2.10. The points in Figure 2.14, but not in Figure 2.15, approximate a straight line fairly well; cholesterol, but not alcohol, is approximately normally distributed. For a test procedure based upon correlations from the normal plot, see Weiss (2001).

Normal scores are available from all the major statistical software packages. To calculate them by hand we would first need to rank the data. For the ith largest data value out of n, we then use Table B.1 to find that value from the standard normal distribution for which $S_i = 100(i/n)\%$ of the standard normal lies below it. For example,

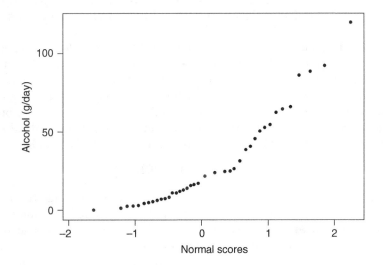

Figure 2.15. Normal plot for alcohol.

Table 2.11 shows that the smallest cholesterol value (with rank = 1) is 4.35. The normal score should correspond to

$$S_1 = 100 \times (1/50) = 2\%.$$

To avoid problems of computation for the highest rank, S_i is often replaced by $100i/(n + 1)$. Further 'corrections' are sometimes made to smooth the results: Figure 2.14 and Figure 2.15 have normal scores computed using $S_i' = 100(i - 0.375)/(n + 0.25)$. This is a commonly used corrected formula for normal scores. For the cholesterol value of 4.35 considered previously,

$$S_1' = 100(1 - 0.375)/(50 + 0.25) = 1.24\%.$$

From Table B.1, the corresponding z value (normal score) is about -2.25 because the chance of a standard normal value below -2.25 is 0.0122, which is as near as this table gets to $1.24/100 = 0.0124$. Thus, 4.12 is plotted against -2.25 in Figure 2.14.

The same technique may be used for probability distributions other than the normal, for instance to check whether the data have a binomial distribution (Clarke and Cooke, 2004).

2.7.2   Inferences for a single mean

A confidence interval for a population mean is given by

$$\bar{x} \pm t_{n-1}\, s/\sqrt{n}, \tag{2.11}$$

where t_{n-1} is the critical value, at some prescribed percentage level, from Student's t distribution on $n - 1$ degrees of freedom (the divisor used to calculate the standard deviation). The t distribution can be thought of as a small-sample analogue of the standard normal distribution (t has a rather wider peak, but otherwise looks much the same). For large n, the standard normal and t are identical, for all practical purposes. Table B.4 gives critical values for t; for example the 5% critical value ranges from 12.7 on 1 d.f. to 1.96 on infinite degrees of freedom. The value 1.96 is also the 5% critical value for the standard normal (see Table B.2), thus demonstrating how t converges to the standard normal.

We can use the cholesterol data in Table 2.10 to find a 95% confidence interval for the mean cholesterol level of all middle-aged Scotsmen, assuming the sample to be a simple random sample of such people. In previous sections, we have seen that these data are quite symmetrical and reasonably near-normal in shape. For these data, $\bar{x} = 6.287$ and standard error = $s/\sqrt{n} = 0.107$. Table B.4 tabulates t at 45 and 50, but not 49 d.f. However, because these are both 2.01 in the 5% column, the 5% critical value for t_{49} must also be 2.01, to two decimal places. Using these results in (2.11) yields

$$6.287 \pm 2.01 \times 0.107,$$

which is 6.287 ± 0.215 mmol/l. Hence, we are 95% confident that the interval (6.07, 6.50) contains the true mean cholesterol level of middle-aged Scotsmen.

The population mean is represented symbolically by μ. A hypothesis test for the null hypothesis $H_0 : \mu = \mu_0$ comes from calculating

$$\frac{\bar{x} - \mu_0}{s/\sqrt{n}} \tag{2.12}$$

and comparing the result with t_{n-1}. This is known as **Student's t test** or simply the **t test**.

Example 2.9 Suppose that we hypothesise that the mean male cholesterol in Scotland is 6.0 mmol/l. We then collect the data shown in Table 2.10. Do these data suggest that our assertion is false?

From (2.12), our test statistic is

$$\frac{6.287 - 6.0}{0.107} = 2.68.$$

As $n - 1 = 49$, we should compare this with t on 49 d.f. The nearest we can get to this using Table B.4 is 50 d.f., showing that this is significant at approximately the 1% level. From a computer package the exact p value was found to be 0.010 — exactly at the 1% level, to three decimal places. Hence, there is strong evidence to suggest that the average cholesterol of Scotsmen (at the time of data collection) is not 6.0; in fact, it seems to be higher.

This result is consistent with the 95% confidence interval we found earlier. As 6.0 is outside the 95% confidence interval, we would expect to reject $H_0 : \mu = 6.0$ at the 5% level of significance. Since 5% is less extreme than 1%, rejection of H_0 at 1% automatically implies rejection at the 5% level. Notice that a two-sided test has been assumed.

2.7.3   Comparing two means

Section 2.7.2 relates to a one-sample problem; that is, the data on cholesterol are taken as a whole. Often we wish to compare mean values of the same variable between two subgroups or between two separate populations. Provided the two samples are drawn independently of each other, we then use the **two-sample t test** and associated confidence interval, which will now be defined.

For example, we saw that serum total cholesterol seems to be different amongst those with and without prevalent CHD in the sample of 50 Scotsmen (see Figure 2.7). Since there is no great skew in these data, we could use the two-sample t test to formally test the null hypothesis that the mean cholesterol is the same in the two groups; that is, the observed difference is simply due to sampling variation.

The general two-sample t test requires calculation of the test statistic,

$$\frac{\bar{x}_1 - \bar{x}_2 - \left(\mu_1 - \mu_2\right)}{\hat{se}}, \tag{2.13}$$

where $\bar{x}_1$ and $\bar{x}_2$ are the two sample means, μ_1 and μ_2 are the corresponding values of the population means under the null hypothesis and $\hat{se}$ is the estimated standard error of the difference between the means (the 'hat' denotes that an estimate is taken). As in the problem we are addressing, often the null hypothesis is $H_0 : \mu_1 = \mu_2$, in which case (2.13) reduces to

$$\frac{\bar{x}_1 - \bar{x}_2}{\hat{se}}. \tag{2.14}$$

We can test H_0 exactly if the two population variances, denoted σ_1^2 and σ_2^2, are equal. In this case,

$$\hat{se} = s_p \sqrt{1/n_1 + 1/n_2}, \tag{2.15}$$

where s_p^2 is the pooled estimate of variance (pooled over the two samples drawn from populations of equal variance) defined by

$$s_p^2 = \frac{\left(n_1 - 1\right)s_1^2 + \left(n_2 - 1\right)s_2^2}{n_1 + n_2 - 2}. \tag{2.16}$$

This is a weighted average of the two sample variances in which the weights are the degrees of freedom. With this value of $\hat{s}e$, we compare (2.13) or (2.14) to t with $n_1 + n_2 - 2$ d.f. The procedure is then called a **pooled t test**.

On the other hand, if we have evidence that σ_1^2 and σ_2^2 are unequal, we have no reason to consider a pooled estimate of variance. Instead, we calculate

$$\hat{s}e = \sqrt{s_1^2 / n_1 + s_2^2 / n_2}. \tag{2.17}$$

Unfortunately, there is no exact test in this circumstance, although various approximate tests have been suggested (see Armitage *et al.*, 2001). One approximation is given by Satterthwaite (1946): compare (2.13) or (2.14), using (2.17), against t with f degrees of freedom where

$$f = \frac{\left[\left(s_1^2 / n_1\right) + \left(s_2^2 / n_2\right)\right]^2}{\left[\left(s_1^2 / n_1\right)^2 \Big/ \left(n_1 - 1\right)\right] + \left[\left(s_2^2 / n_2\right)^2 \Big/ \left(n_2 - 1\right)\right]},$$

rounded to the nearest whole number.

We may calculate a confidence interval for the difference between two population means, $\mu_1 - \mu_2$, as

$$\bar{x}_1 - \bar{x}_2 \pm t\left(\hat{s}e\right), \tag{2.18}$$

where t is the value from the Student's t distribution with the appropriate d.f. for the required percentage confidence. For example, we need the 5% critical value from t on $n_1 + n_2 - 2$ d.f. to obtain a 95% confidence interval when a pooled estimate of variance is used.

Before applying the two-sample t test or computing the associated confidence interval, we clearly need to see whether there is reason to doubt that the two population variances are equal. We can carry out another form of hypothesis test to try to refute this assertion. That is, we test

$$H_0 : \sigma_1^2 = \sigma_2^2 \quad vs \quad H_1 : \sigma_1^2 \neq \sigma_2^2,$$

which is achieved using the test statistic

$$s_1^2 / s_2^2, \tag{2.19}$$

where s_1^2 and s_2^2 are the two sample variances, with $s_1^2 > s_2^2$ (this is *essential*). The test statistic is compared with the F distribution on $(n_1 - 1, n_2 - 1)$ d.f.

Example 2.10 For the SHHS cholesterol values of Table 2.10, split into the two CHD groups, we have the following summary statistics,

$$\text{CHD: } n = 11; \; \bar{x} = 6.708; \; s = 0.803,$$

$$\text{No CHD: } n = 39; \; \bar{x} = 6.168; \; s = 0.709.$$

Since the sample standard deviation is highest in the CHD group, we shall take this group to have subscript '1'. Then the preliminary test of equal population variances, (2.19), gives

$$\frac{\left(0.803\right)^2}{\left(0.709\right)^2} = 1.28.$$

We compare this with $F_{10,38}$. Table B.5 gives one-sided critical values for 10, 5, 2.5, 1 and 0.1%. We have a two-sided test, so these correspond to 20, 10, 5, 2 and 0.2% critical values for our test. $F_{10,38}$ is not given, but $F_{10,35} = 1.79$ and $F_{10,40} = 1.76$ at the 20% level (two-sided) from Table B.5(a). Thus, $F_{10,38}$ must be about 1.77 and we will fail to reject H_0 at the 20% level. From a computer package, the exact p value is 0.552. There is thus no evidence to reject H_0: population variances equal.

Consequently, we may proceed with the pooled t test, that is, with $\hat{s}e$ given by (2.15). From (2.16),

$$s_p^2 = \frac{(10)(0.803)^2 + (38)(0.709)^2}{10+38} = 0.532.$$

Thus, from (2.15),

$$\hat{s}e = \sqrt{0.532}\,\sqrt{1/11 + 1/39} = 0.249,$$

and the test statistic, (2.13), is

$$\frac{6.708 - 6.168}{0.249} = 2.17.$$

This is to be compared with Student's t on $n_1 + n_2 - 2 = 48$ d.f. From Table B.4, 5% critical values are

$$t_{45} = 2.01, \quad t_{50} = 2.01$$

and 2% critical values are

$$t_{45} = 2.41, \quad t_{50} = 2.40.$$

Hence, t_{48} is 2.01 and roughly 2.41 at 5% and 2%, respectively. Thus, we reject H_0 at the 5%, but not at the 2%, level of significance (or at any level below 2%). The exact p value is actually 0.035. We conclude that there is some evidence of a different cholesterol level in the two groups; in fact, it is higher for those with CHD, but the evidence is not strong.

Suppose that we opted to calculate a 99% confidence interval for $\mu_1 - \mu_2$. Since we have accepted a pooled estimate of variance, from (2.18), this is given by

$$6.708 - 6.168 \pm (t_{48})(0.249),$$

where t_{48} is the 1% critical value. Again, Table B.4 does not give the exact value, but a computer package gives it as 2.682. Hence, the 99% confidence interval is 0.540 ± 0.668 mmol/l. That is, we are 99% confident that the average extra amount of serum cholesterol in those with CHD is between -0.13 and 1.21 mmol/l. As would be anticipated, because we have already seen that the hypothesis of no difference was not rejected at the 1% level, this confidence interval contains zero.

2.7.4   Paired data

In Section 2.7.3 we assumed that the two samples are independent. One situation in which this is not the case is that in which the data are **paired**. Pairing means that each individual selected for sample 1 is associated with a like individual, who is then selected for sample 2. For instance, an individual with CHD might be paired with another who is free of CHD, but shares important characteristics, such as being of the same age and sex, that might be expected to influence cholesterol levels and the risk of CHD. Intuitively, this should provide a more reliable picture of how cholesterol levels differ between CHD groups than from purely independent samples (as in Example 2.10). The benefit of pairing — to 'remove' the effect of other variables that may influence the comparison of the two groups (a common goal in epidemiology; see Section 4.2) — is clear by common sense.

One common instance of pairing is when each individual acts as her or his own control, usually encountered where observations are taken before and after some intervention (see Example 2.11). If we can design our comparative study to be paired, this will have the advantage of having less background variation against which to judge observed differences, than in the two-sample case. Smaller variance means tighter confidence limits and a lower p value for any specific difference.

Analysis of paired data must be different from the unpaired case because now the two groups are intrinsically nonindependent. This problem is overcome very easily: we simply subtract one value from the other within each pair. As a result, the paired two-sample problem is reduced to a one-sample problem, to be analysed according to Section 2.7.2. More precisely, let x_{1i} be the first observation from the ith pair, and x_{2i} be the second observation from the same pair (where 'first' and 'second' have some consistent definition from pair to pair). Let $d_i = x_{1i} - x_{2i}$. Then we apply the methods of Section 2.7.2 to the set of differences, $\{d_i\}$.

Let the subscript d denote differenced data. We test $\mu_1 = \mu_2$ by testing for $\mu_d = 0$. From (2.12) the test statistic for $H_0 : \mu_d = 0$ is

$$\frac{\bar{x}_d}{s_d / \sqrt{n}}, \qquad (2.20)$$

which is compared with t_{n-1}. Here, n is the number of *pairs*. Also, from (2.11), a confidence interval for $\mu_1 - \mu_2 = \mu_d$ is

$$\bar{x}_d \pm t_{n-1} s_d / \sqrt{n}. \qquad (2.21)$$

Table 2.15. Total serum cholesterol (mmol/l) at clinic visits 1 and 2
for 44 women in the Alloa Study.

1st Visit	2nd Visit	1st Visit	2nd Visit	1st Visit	2nd Visit
3.795	3.250	7.480	6.955	5.410	5.280
6.225	6.935	4.970	5.100	5.220	5.175
5.210	4.750	6.710	7.480	4.700	4.815
7.040	5.080	4.765	4.530	4.215	3.610
7.550	8.685	6.695	6.160	5.395	5.705
7.715	7.775	4.025	4.160	7.475	6.580
6.555	6.005	5.510	6.010	4.925	5.190
5.360	4.940	5.495	5.010	7.115	6.150
5.285	5.620	5.435	5.975	7.020	6.395
6.230	5.870	5.350	4.705	5.365	5.805
6.475	6.620	5.905	5.465	3.665	3.710
5.680	5.635	6.895	6.925	6.130	5.160
5.490	5.080	4.350	4.260	4.895	5.145
9.865	9.465	5.950	5.325	7.000	7.425
4.625	4.120	5.855	5.505		

Note: Each value shown is the average of two biochemical assays.

Example 2.11 Although the SHHS introduced in this chapter does not involve any paired data directly, the same basic screening protocol was used by the SHHS investigators in the town of Alloa, where a set of individuals were entered into a study to assess the effect of cholesterol screening. A sample of men and women were invited to attend a series of three clinics during which they were given dietary advice to lower their blood cholesterol and a blood sample was taken, from which total cholesterol was subsequently measured and communicated to the subject concerned. Table 2.15 shows the female data collected at the first and second clinics (3 months apart). We can use these data to assess whether this type of cholesterol screening has any short-term effect on blood cholesterol levels.

The data are clearly paired because this is a before and after study of the same individuals. Hence, the first step is to calculate the second clinic minus first clinic differences for each woman. For example, the difference for the first woman is $3.250 - 3.795 = -0.545$. Note that differences may be positive or negative and the sign must be retained. The summary statistics for the differences are

$$\bar{x}_d = -0.1700, \ s_d = 0.5587, \ n = 44.$$

Substituting into (2.21) gives the 95% confidence interval for the true difference as

$$-0.1700 \pm \left(t_{43}\right)\left(0.5587/\sqrt{44}\right).$$

From a computer package, $t_{43} = 2.0167$ at the 5% level. This gives the 95% confidence interval, -0.1700 ± 0.1699, which is the interval from -0.3399 to -0.0001 mmol/l. Because 0 is just outside the 95% confidence interval, we know that the null hypotheses of no difference will be rejected with a p value of just under 0.05. Hence, there is evidence that cholesterol screening has led to a reduction in cholesterol.

It is interesting to compare the results of the valid paired procedure with what we would get if we used the incorrect two-sample approach. Applying (2.18) with either (2.15) or (2.17) to the data in Table 2.15 gives the 95% confidence interval as

-0.17 ± 0.53. This has exactly the same centre as the interval calculated in Example 2.11, as it must because $\bar{x}_d = \bar{x}_1 - \bar{x}_2$ (the mean of the differences is the difference of the means). It is, however, substantially wider than the correct interval, reflecting the fact that here we have failed to take account of the reduction in random variation brought about by pairing. Similarly, the p value from a paired t test (the correct procedure) applied to the data in Table 2.15 is (to two decimal places) 0.05, using (2.20), whereas an incorrect two-sample t test gives a p value of 0.52, using (2.14) with either (2.15) or (2.17).

2.8   Inferential techniques for non-normal data

As explained in Section 2.6.3, the two-number summary is appropriate only when the data are reasonably symmetrical in shape. As explained in Section 2.7, for t tests we require rather more: the data must also be approximately normally distributed. Just what degree of approximation is acceptable cannot be stated in absolute terms. Certainly we require a single-peaked distribution with no great skew, so that the mean is similar to the median. The larger the sample, the less precise the approximation needs to be, although we must be careful whenever analyses by subsets are performed subsequently. Several other statistical procedures common in epidemiological analysis, such as regression and analysis of variance, assume normality (Chapter 9).

As we have already seen, epidemiological data do not always have even an approximately normal shape. Discrete variables, such as counts (for example, the number of cigarettes per day in Table 2.12) rarely have a near-normal shape. Severe skewness is possible even with data on a continuous variable (e.g., cotinine in Table 2.12). As we have seen, medians and allied statistics are more appropriate summaries for such variables. If we wish to consider formal inferential procedures (estimation and testing) with non-normal data, we have two basic choices. We try to **transform** the raw data into a near-normal form or we use **nonparametric** methods of analysis. Both approaches will be described here. Otherwise, we might use complex resampling procedures, as described in Chapter 14.

2.8.1   Transformations

Table 2.16 gives a range of transformations that are often successful with forms of data common in epidemiology. Of all the transformations, the logarithmic (log) is probably the most used. As with all the other transformations, it defines a

Table 2.16. Transformations often successful in removing skew and making data better approximated by the normal curve.

Form of data	Transformation
Slightly right-skewed	Square root
Moderately right-skewed	Logarithmic
Very right-skewed	Reciprocal
Left-skewed	Square
Counts	Square root
Proportions	Arcsine square root

new variable, y (say), from the original observed variable, x (say). In this particular case,

$$y = \log(x),$$

where the base of the logarithm may be anything we choose. Problems in applying this arise when x can take values of zero. In such cases we add a small constant to all the observations. A similar ruse could be used when x can go negative.

Often, proportionate data are reported as percentages, in which case we should divide by 100 before applying the arcsine square root transformation suggested in Table 2.16. This transformation defines

$$y = \sin^{-1}\left(\sqrt{x}\right),$$

where x is a proportion.

The reciprocal transformation,

$$y = 1/x$$

has the unfortunate property of reversing the original ordering of the variables (so that the smallest on the original scale becomes the largest on the transformed scale). To maintain the original order, the negative reciprocal

$$y = -1/x$$

may be used instead.

It is fairly easy to see why the suggested transformations will be useful for skewed data; for example, square roots of small numbers are fairly close to their original numbers (for example, $\sqrt{4} = 2$), whereas taking square roots of large numbers leads to considerable reduction (for example, $\sqrt{144} = 12$). Hence, the upper part of the scale is pulled in. The transformations for counts and proportions arise from theoretical considerations; in the case of proportions, the arcsine square root is strictly justifiable in theory only when all proportions arise from a constant sample size, which is rare in practice.

There is no guarantee that any of the transformations suggested in Table 2.16 will work on any specific set of data. All we can do is to try them out and see what happens. This trial and error approach is not too labour intensive if a statistics or spreadsheet computer package is available.

Some statistical packages implement the Box–Cox (Box and Cox, 1964) method of searching for the most appropriate **power transformation** — that is, a transformation which takes the form

$$y = x^{\theta},$$

for some value of θ. This includes some of the transformations we have already seen; for example, $\theta = -1$ gives the reciprocal transformation.

Theoretical details and recommendations for choosing transformations are given by Snedecor and Cochran (1989). A case study using SHHS data is provided by Millns *et al.* (1995).

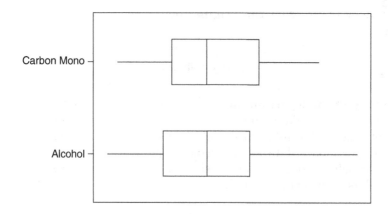

Figure 2.16. Boxplot (using standardised scales) for $\sqrt{\text{alcohol}}$ and $\log_e$(carbon monoxide).

For the highly skewed data in Table 2.10, the square root transformation for alcohol, and log transformation for carbon monoxide, are quite successful in removing skew (see Figure 2.16) and improving approximate normality. Cigarette consumption and cotinine do not seem to be amenable to normalising transformations; certainly none of the basic transformations is at all successful. However, cigarette consumption is really a 'mixture' variable: a mixture of data from nonsmokers (all of whom have a consumption of zero) and smokers. Hence it may be sensible to split the cigarette data by smoking status. In fact, the smokers' data on cigarette consumption (mean = 19.9; median = 20) are very close to perfect quartile symmetry as Figure 2.17 shows. The nonsmokers' data have no variation, so all we can do is to report the proportion (or percentage) of nonsmokers, 28/50 = 0.56 (56%).

Cotinine (which is a biochemical measure of tobacco consumption) could also be split by smoking status, but this may not be appropriate since several nonsmokers have nonzero cotinine values; indeed, one nonsmoker has a cotinine value of 424 ng/ml. This may seem strange, but smoking status in Table 2.10 is self-reported and deception may occur. Small nonzero values of cotinine may also be due to other factors such as passive (secondary) smoking, dietary intake of cotinine and inaccuracies in the assay.

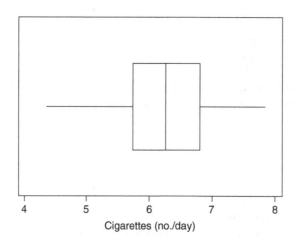

Figure 2.17. Boxplot for cigarette consumption for cigarette smokers only.

Thus, we may decide not to split cotinine data and conclude that we cannot transform to a near-normal shape. In general, we should not expect transformations to be successful whenever the data have more than one peak (unless the data are split), nor when the data are very sparsely distributed.

As well as not always being successful, transformations have the disadvantage that they inevitably produce answers on the transformed scale. For instance, it is perfectly reasonable to use the mean to summarise the square root alcohol data, but the mean (4.42 for the example) is for the square root of daily consumption in $\sqrt{\text{gram}}$ units. Similarly, inferences about differences between means will be valid only on the square root scale. Hence, we get a 95% confidence interval for the difference between mean $\sqrt{\text{alcohol}}$ consumption for smokers and nonsmokers, rather than for the difference between the true mean consumptions.

It may be useful, when presenting results, to back-transform estimates at the last stage of analysis to return to the original scale. For instance, from (2.11), a 95% confidence interval for $\sqrt{\text{alcohol}}$ using the data in Table 2.10 turns out to be 4.417 ± 0.773, that is, (3.644, 5.190). Back-transforming (that is, squaring) the mean and the lower and upper confidence limits gives a back-transformed mean for alcohol of 19.5 g with a 95% confidence interval of (13.3, 26.9) g. Notice that, unlike cases we have seen earlier, the estimate (mean) is not in the middle of this confidence interval.

Back-transformed results should be appropriately labelled so as to avoid ambiguity. For instance, 19.5 g is certainly not an estimate of mean alcohol consumption (see Table 2.12 for a valid estimate). Similarly, the transformed results for the difference in mean $\sqrt{\text{alcohol}}$ between smokers and nonsmokers cannot be squared to define limits for the difference in alcohol because

$$\sqrt{x_1} - \sqrt{x_2} \neq \sqrt{x_1 - x_2}.$$

Due to this issue, transformations are generally more useful in hypothesis testing than in estimation. However, one instance where a back-transformed estimate (and its confidence interval) does have a useful interpretation is where logarithmic transformations are used in a paired sampling problem. Then the back-transformed difference in mean logged values will be the average ratio (see Example 2.13). In general, with non-normal data, the bootstrap resampling procedure (Section 14.2) is recommended when estimation of a mean, or a difference in means, is of interest.

2.8.2 *Nonparametric tests*

When transformations fail, or are thought to be inappropriate, alternative **nonparametric** (or distribution-free) tests may be applied. For example, the **one-sample Wilcoxon test** (or **signed rank sum test**) is a nonparametric analogue sometimes used in place of the one-sample t test. Unlike the t test, which assumes a normal distribution, the Wilcoxon test makes no distributional assumption. Similarly, the **two-sample Wilcoxon test** could replace the two-sample t test.

When we use nonparametric tests in place of parametric ones, we will be treating the variable as of a lower type than it really is (see Section 2.3.3). Thus, some of the information in the data will be ignored; not surprisingly, this makes nonparametric tests rather less powerful than their parametric alternatives ('power' is defined formally in Section 8.2). For instance, we have less chance of rejecting an incorrect null hypothesis using the two-sample Wilcoxon test than using the t test. For this reason, parametric procedures (based, for example, on the normal distribution) are to be preferred when they are possible, even if a prior data transformation is necessary.

Space is insufficient to provide a full account of nonparametric methods here; see Conover (1999) for an extensive exposition. Instead, we shall look at that test most often used in basic epidemiological analysis, the two-sample Wilcoxon test. This treats the data as ordinal; that is, the precise distance between numbers is ignored and only their relative order is used. In some situations, such as clinicians' ranking of severity of disease between patients, the raw data are ordinal and this would be the (two-sample) method of choice at the outset.

The Wilcoxon test procedure begins by ranking the combined dataset from the two samples to be compared. Consider the null hypothesis that the two populations have the same distributions. If H_0 is true, then the ranks for either sample are equally likely to fall anywhere in the list of all possible ranks. Consider now the sum of the ranks for one of the two samples, say, sample 1,

$$T = \sum_{i=1}^{n_1} R_{1i}, \tag{2.22}$$

where R_{11} is the first rank in sample 1, R_{12} is the second rank, etc., and sample 1 has n_1 observations. The idea is then to find all conceivable rank sums should sample 1 take any of the possible n_1 of the combined set of $n_1 + n_2$ ranks. The one-sided p value for the test is then the probability of obtaining a rank sum at least as big as that actually observed, that is, (2.22). This probability is the number of possible rank sums at least as big as that observed, divided by the total number of possible rank sums. Two-sided p values are obtained simply by doubling.

Unfortunately, the process is very cumbersome for hand calculation. Some work can be saved by taking sample 1 in (2.22) to be the smaller of the two samples. Tables of critical values are available, for example, in Conover (1999), but provided either sample size is above 20 a normal approximation may be used. This requires calculation of

$$\frac{T - \dfrac{n_1(n+1)}{2}}{\sqrt{\dfrac{n_1 n_2(n+1)}{12}}}, \tag{2.23}$$

where $n = n_1 + n_2$. To test the null hypothesis, this is compared to the standard normal distribution.

Sometimes there are **tied ranks**, that is, two or more identical numbers in the combined dataset. In this situation, we assign the average rank in the tied range to each member of the tie. For instance, if three values are all equal 10th largest, then the tied range is 10 to 12 and the rank assigned to each is $(10 + 11 + 12)/3 = 11$. The procedure based upon (2.23) works well if there are just a few ties. Otherwise, (2.23) should be replaced by

$$\frac{T - \dfrac{n_1(n+1)}{2}}{\sqrt{\dfrac{n_1 n_2}{n(n-1)} \sum R^2 - \dfrac{(n+1)^2 n_1 n_2}{4(n-1)}}}, \tag{2.24}$$

where $\sum R^2$ is the sum of all the squared ranks.

Table 2.17. Serum total cholesterol (mmol/l) in rank order (with average tied ranks).

Rank	Obs.	Rank	Obs.	Rank	Obs.	Rank	Obs.	Rank	Obs.
1	4.35	10.5	5.71	20.5	6.10*	31	6.55	41	7.04
2	4.79	12	5.73	22	6.13	32	6.60	42	7.10*
3	4.90	13.5	5.75	23	6.19*	33	6.64	43	7.11
4	5.19*	13.5	5.75	24	6.23	34	6.73	44	7.12
5	5.34	15	5.85	25	6.25	35	6.74	45	7.14
6	5.39	16	5.86	26	6.29	36.5	6.76	46	7.15*
7	5.42	17	5.98*	27	6.35	36.5	6.76	47	7.16*
8	5.51	18	5.99	28	6.46*	38	6.78	48	7.55
9	5.64	19	6.05	29	6.47	39	6.89*	49	7.71*
10.5	5.71	20.5	6.10	30	6.54	40	6.92	50	7.86*

Note: An asterisk indicates that the individual concerned has CHD.

Example 2.12 Consider the cholesterol data appearing in Table 2.11 once again. Suppose we wish to consider the null hypothesis that the cholesterol distributions are the same for those with and without CHD.

First we rank the combined data. The result is given as Table 2.17, which differs from Table 2.11 only by the way ties are expressed, and by denoting those with CHD. Here there are four pairs of tied ranks; the average rank is given for each pair.

We will take, for ease of computation, sample 1 to be the smaller group; thus $n_1 = 11$ and $n_2 = 39$, which are big enough for a normal approximation. Using (2.22),

$$T = 4 + 17 + 20.5 + 23 + 28 + 39 + 42 + 46 + 47 + 49 + 50 = 365.5.$$

Hence the test statistic, (2.23), is

$$\frac{365.5 - \dfrac{11 \times 51}{2}}{\sqrt{\dfrac{11 \times 39 \times 51}{12}}} = 1.99.$$

Here, there are few ties, so we should expect (2.23) to be acceptable. To check, we use the more complex formula (2.24). This requires

$$\sum R^2 = \text{sum of squares of all 50 ranks} = 42923.$$

Substituting this into (2.24) gives

$$\frac{365.5 - \dfrac{(11)(51)}{2}}{\sqrt{\dfrac{(11)(39)}{(50)(49)}(42923) - \dfrac{(51)^2 (11)(39)}{(4)(49)}}} = 1.99,$$

which is the same result as from (2.23) to two decimal places.

The 5% two-sided critical value is 1.96 and hence we just reject the null hypothesis at the 5% level (the *p* value is actually 0.048).

Sometimes the Wilcoxon test is said to be a test of the equality of two means or two medians. This will be the case if the two populations differ only in location, not in spread or shape, which would seem to be a reasonable proposition for the cholesterol data according to Figure 2.7. Hence, the similarity between the results of Example 2.10 and Example 2.12 is not unexpected. As discussed already, the distribution of cholesterol approximates a normal curve reasonably well and the sample is moderately big, so Example 2.10 provides the preferred analysis in this case.

Most statistical computer packages will carry out the Wilcoxon test, although some use only the large sample approximation, (2.23). Sometimes the equivalent **Mann–Whitney test** is used instead. See Altman (1991) for comments on the relationship between the Wilcoxon and Mann–Whitney approaches.

2.8.3   Confidence intervals for medians

When the data are certainly not normal, it would be sensible to summarise using medians rather than means (Section 2.6.3). In a two-sample situation, we might find the difference between medians to be useful. Confidence intervals for medians and median differences may be obtained by bootstrapping (Section 14.2).

2.9   Measuring agreement

The chi-square test, two-sample t test and two-sample Wilcoxon test all provide tests of relationships. Sometimes we wish to go further and investigate whether two variables are equivalent. Such a problem arises frequently in laboratory testing. For instance, as mentioned in Section 2.2.1, fibrinogen was measured from blood samples of participants in the SHHS. Since several different fibrinogen assays are available, the question of agreement between pairs of assays is of epidemiological importance, particularly when comparisons between studies that use different methods are envisaged in the future.

2.9.1   Quantitative variables

When the variable is quantitative, as in the preceding fibrinogen example, we should apply each of the two methods to be compared to the same subjects. In our example, the blood plasma from any one individual would be split and a different fibrinogen assay applied to each part. Sometimes the question of agreement in such situations is incorrectly tackled by measuring the correlation (Section 9.3.2) between the two sets of results. This is inappropriate because correlation measures association (in fact, linear association), rather than agreement.

Instead, we should think of the data as paired within individuals and analyse as in Section 2.7.4, unless the normal assumption fails entirely so that the one-sample Wilcoxon test on the differences is necessary. The only difficulty arises when there is evidence that the difference between the paired observations varies with the magnitude of the individual measures, best seen from a plot of the differences against the mean results from the two methods (Bland and Altman, 1986). In practice, it is common for the difference to rise as the mean increases, which suggests that one method's measurement might be a constant multiple of the other's, rather than be a constant amount greater (or less). A convenient approach to this situation is to log transform the data (Section 2.8.1) and to apply the methods of Section 2.7.4; the back-transformed estimate and confidence limits then apply to this multiplicative constant.

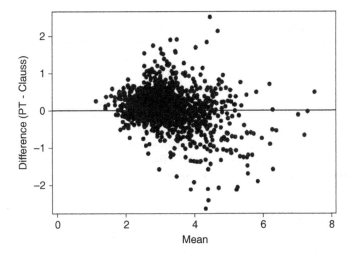

Figure 2.18. Bland–Altman plot for fibrinogen data.

Example 2.13 The web site for this book (see Appendix A) contains data from the fourth MONICA survey in north Glasgow, Scotland. Two measures of fibrinogen, derived using the prothrombin time (PT) and the von Clauss method, were each measured in 1439 men and women. The goal is to see if these methods seem to give the same answers, and to provide a calibration coefficient if they do not.

Figure 2.18 shows the basic Bland–Altman plot of within-subject differences in assay results against within-subject means of assays results. It is clear from this that the discrepancy between the assays increases as the level of fibrinogen increases, because the points show a V-shaped pattern in the horizontal plane. Hence results for both assays were log transformed (to the exponential base, e) and the difference and mean, by subject, were computed for these logged values, and plotted as Figure 2.19. The trend in the difference has now been removed, and we can be confident of making universal conclusions across the range of fibrinogen levels. The mean of the difference in log fibrinogens (PT minus Clauss)

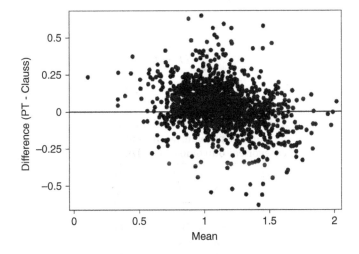

Figure 2.19. Bland–Altman plot for log transformed fibrinogen data.

is 0.038098, with a standard deviation of 0.1484037. A kernel density plot (Section 2.6.6) suggested that the differences in log fibrinogens could be assumed to follow a normal distribution quite closely. Hence, a paired t test (Section 2.7.4) was used to test that the log differences have a mean of zero. This test has a p value < 0.0001, so the null hypothesis was rejected. Using (2.21), a 95% confidence interval for the difference in log fibrinogens was derived as 0.030430 to 0.045765. Taking exponents of the mean and lower and upper confidence limits gives results of 1.039, 1.031 and 1.047, respectively. Hence (Section 2.8.1) the ratio of PT to Clauss results is estimated to be 1.039 with a 95% confidence interval of (1.031, 1.047). Interpreting, for brevity, just the point estimate, we find that PT values are, on average, 3.9% higher than Clauss values; looked at another way, a Clauss value can be recalibrated to a PT value by multiplying by 1.039. See Rumley et al. (2003) for more details of these data and more comprehensive analyses.

2.9.2   Categorical variables

When the variable assessed by the two methods in question is categorical, the data would typically be presented as a square contingency table (see Table 2.18). Perfect agreement would give entries only in the diagonal cells of the table. A common situation in which the issue of agreement arises is when two observers are each asked to assess a subject independently for illness. For instance, two nurses might each be asked to decide whether a person has anaemia based on observation of clinical signs, such as pallor of the eyes and nails. The issue is then one of **interobserver** (or **inter-rater**) **agreement**.

Given a categorical variable with ℓ outcomes (for example, $\ell = 4$ in Table 2.18), we can construct a measure of agreement based upon the difference between the number observed and expected in the ℓ diagonal cells. The numbers expected are the E values in the chi-square test statistic, (2.1). Using the notation of Table 2.18,

$$E_{ii} = \frac{R_i C_i}{n}$$

is the expected value in cell (i, i), the cell that is in both row i and column i.

Hence, agreement may be measured using the observed minus expected differences summed over all the diagonals, that is

$$\sum_{i=1}^{\ell} \left(O_{ii} - E_{ii} \right).$$

Table 2.18. Display of data for an agreement problem with four categorical outcomes (A to D).

Method	Method one				
two	A	B	C	D	Total
A	O_{11}	O_{12}	O_{13}	O_{14}	R_1
B	O_{21}	O_{22}	O_{23}	O_{24}	R_2
C	O_{31}	O_{32}	O_{33}	O_{34}	R_3
D	O_{41}	O_{42}	O_{43}	O_{44}	R_4
Total	C_1	C_2	C_3	C_4	n

If there are just as many observed agreements in classification as would be expected by chance, this sum will be zero. High positive values represent a high degree of agreement.

In this application, it is traditional to compare proportions rather than numbers. The observed proportion that agrees, p_O, is the sum of the observed diagonal elements in the contingency table divided by the number of subjects classified, that is

$$p_O = \left(\sum_{i=1}^{\ell} O_{ii} \right) \Big/ n.$$ (2.25)

The corresponding expected proportion is

$$p_E = \left(\sum_{i=1}^{\ell} E_{ii} \right) \Big/ n = \left(\sum_{i=1}^{\ell} R_i C_i \right) \Big/ n^2.$$ (2.26)

The extent of agreement is now measured by the difference $p_O - p_E$. It is convenient to standardise this difference, and thus use

$$\kappa = \frac{p_O - p_E}{1 - p_E}$$ (2.27)

as the measure of agreement. This is known as **Cohen's kappa** statistic. It takes the value 1 if the agreement is perfect (that is, when $p_O = 1$) and 0 if the amount of agreement is entirely attributable to chance. If $\kappa < 0$, then the amount of agreement is less than would be expected by chance. If $\kappa > 0$, then there is more than chance agreement. Following the suggestions of Fleiss *et al.* (2003), we shall conclude

$$\begin{cases} \text{excellent agreement} & \text{if} \quad \kappa \geq 0.75, \\ \text{fair to good agreement} & \text{if} \quad 0.4 < \kappa < 0.75, \\ \text{poor agreement} & \text{if} \quad \kappa \leq 0.4, \end{cases}$$

although other scoring systems have been suggested. Fleiss *et al.* (2003) also suggest an approximate objective test of randomness, that is, a test of kappa = 0. This requires calculation of

$$\left(\frac{\kappa}{\hat{se}(\kappa)} \right)^2,$$ (2.28)

which is compared to chi-square with 1 d.f. In (2.28), the estimated standard error of κ is

$$\hat{se}(\kappa) = \sqrt{\frac{1}{(1 - p_E)^2 n} \left\{ p_E^2 + p_E - \sum_{i=1}^{\ell} \frac{R_i C_i}{n^3} \left(R_i + C_i \right) \right\}}.$$ (2.29)

As we are usually interested only in agreement that is better than chance, a one-sided test is often used in this application.

An approximate 95% confidence interval for the true measure of agreement is

$$\kappa \pm 1.96\,\hat{se}(\kappa). \qquad (2.30)$$

This uses a normal approximation; as usual, the values $\pm$ 1.96 are derived from Table B.2 as the cut-points within which 95% of the standard normal lies. For other percentages of confidence, we replace 1.96 by the corresponding critical value from the normal distribution.

Example 2.14 In Table 2.1, and elsewhere in this chapter, we have seen the occupational social class distribution of the SHHS subjects. In keeping with the decision made by the study investigators, married women were classified according to their husbands' occupations. It is of interest to compare the social classification by this method and when all women are classified according to their own occupation. Table 2.19 gives the data from the same selection criteria that gave rise to Table 2.1, showing all women for whom a classification could be made by both methods.

In this case, the number of categories, $\ell = 6$. From (2.25),

$$p_O = (22 + 471 + 379 + 197 + 266 + 97)/3334 = 0.4295.$$

From (2.26),

$$\begin{aligned} p_E = (&36 \times 194 + 841 \times 826 + 1137 \times 507 + 308 \times 1097 \\ &+ 668 \times 525 + 344 \times 185)/3334^2 \\ =\ &0.1827. \end{aligned}$$

Hence, from (2.27),

$$\kappa = \frac{0.4295 - 0.1827}{1 - 0.1827} = 0.302.$$

Also, using (2.29), the estimated standard error of kappa turns out to be $\hat{se}(\kappa) = 0.0078$.

Here the degree of agreement is poor. Notice that this does not imply that either way of classifying a woman's social class is in any way 'wrong', but does signify that we might anticipate different results in epidemiological analyses that use the different methods.

Table 2.19. Social class for women in the SHHS according to husband's and own occupations.

Husband's occupation	Own occupation						
	I	II	IIIn	IIIm	IV	V	Total
I	22	80	73	6	9	4	194
II	11	471	241	31	60	12	826
IIIn	3	61	379	20	29	15	507
IIIm	0	159	326	197	263	152	1097
IV	0	60	92	43	266	64	525
V	0	10	26	11	41	97	185
Total	36	841	1137	308	668	344	3334

2.9.3   *Ordered categorical variables*

In many instances, the outcomes of the categorical variable have a rank order. For instance, the classification of anaemia in the example of Section 2.9.2 might be unlikely/possible/probable/definite, rather than just no/yes. In this situation, a worse discrepancy occurs when the two methods give results two ordinal categories apart than when they are only one apart, etc.

To allow for such problems, Cohen (1968) suggested a weighted version of the kappa statistic. The **weighted kappa** statistic is given by (2.27) again, but with (2.25) and (2.26) replaced by

$$p_O = \left(\sum_{i=1}^{\ell} \sum_{j=1}^{\ell} w_{ij} O_{ij} \right) \bigg/ n \tag{2.31}$$

$$p_E = \left(\sum_{i=1}^{\ell} \sum_{j=1}^{\ell} w_{ij} R_i C_j \right) \bigg/ n^2, \tag{2.32}$$

where the weight for cell (i, j) is

$$w_{ij} = 1 - \frac{|i - j|}{\ell - 1}, \tag{2.33}$$

in which $|i - j|$ means the absolute value (with sign ignored) of $(i - j)$. The test for weighted kappa = 0 and 95% confidence interval follow from (2.28) and (2.30) as before, but now using the estimated standard error of weighted kappa, which is

$$\hat{se}(\kappa_w) = \sqrt{ \frac{1}{(1 - p_E)^2 n} \left\{ \sum_{i=1}^{\ell} \sum_{j=1}^{\ell} \frac{R_i C_j}{n^2} \left(w_{ij} - w_i - w_j' \right)^2 - p_E^2 \right\} }, \tag{2.34}$$

where

$$w_i = \sum_{j=1}^{\ell} \frac{C_j w_{ij}}{n} \tag{2.35}$$

and

$$w_j' = \sum_{i=1}^{\ell} \frac{R_i w_{ij}}{n}. \tag{2.36}$$

Example 2.15 In the problem of Example 2.14 social class is graded, and a discrepancy of several social classifications is more important than one of only a few. Hence, it seems reasonable to weight the measure of concordance. The weights given by (2.33) are shown in Table 2.20; as required, we weight (for agreement) more strongly as we approach the diagonals.

From (2.31), Table 2.19 and Table 2.20,

$$p_O = (1 \times 22 + 0.8 \times 80 + \cdots + 1 \times 97)/3334 = 0.8263.$$

Table 2.20. Weights for Example 2.15.

Husband's occupation	Own occupation					
	I	II	IIIn	IIIm	IV	V
I	1	0.8	0.6	0.4	0.2	0
II	0.8	1	0.8	0.6	0.4	0.2
IIIn	0.6	0.8	1	0.8	0.6	0.4
IIIm	0.4	0.6	0.8	1	0.8	0.6
IV	0.2	0.4	0.6	0.8	1	0.8
V	0	0.2	0.4	0.6	0.8	1

From (2.32), Table 2.19 and Table 2.20,

$$p_E = (1 \times 194 \times 36 + 0.8 \times 194 \times 841 + \cdots + 1 \times 185 \times 344)/3334^2$$

$$= 0.6962.$$

Hence, by (2.27), the weighted kappa is

$$\kappa_w = \frac{0.8263 - 0.6962}{1 - 0.6962} = 0.428.$$

This is now just inside the good agreement range. Inspection of Table 2.19 shows why the weighted kappa is larger than the unweighted: the discrepancies that do occur tend not to be extreme.

We can obtain the estimated standard error of the weighted kappa using (2.34). This requires prior evaluation of the six equations specified by (2.35) and the six equations specified by (2.36). For illustration, one of each of these will be evaluated.

From (2.35) when $i = 3$,

$$w_3 = (36 \times 0.6 + 841 \times 0.8 + \cdots + 344 \times 0.4)/3334 = 0.7847.$$

From (2.36), when $j = 5$,

$$w_5' = (194 \times 0.2 + 826 \times 0.4 + \cdots + 185 \times 0.8)/3334 = 0.6671.$$

Substituting these, together with other components, into (2.34) gives $\hat{se}(\kappa) = 0.0110$. From (2.30) a 95% confidence interval for the true weighted kappa, relating self to husband's occupational social classification for middle-aged Scotswomen, is $0.428 \pm 1.96 \times 0.0110$; that is, (0.41, 0.45).

Stata has several commands for computing kappa and weighted kappa statistics, the most useful of which is KAP. In SAS, PROC FREQ should be used with the AGREE option to the TABLES statement.

2.9.4   Internal consistency

Sometimes there is no single variable that captures the concept that we wish to analyse, yet there are several individual aspects of this concept that we can score. For example, functional independence, for instance in the elderly, can cover several aspects such as bladder control and ability to climb stairs. In these situations it is common to question people on each item separately, score each item on a pre-defined scale and then sum to get an overall score. For example, the modified Barthel score (Mahoney and Barthel, 1965) uses a 10-item questionnaire to record aspects of functional independence, to be completed by subjects or their carers. We may then wish to know whether there is agreement between items; that is whether individual items might reasonably be considered to be measures of a single, underlying, construct, often known as **internal consistency**. This may be investigated through the use of **Cronbach's alpha**, defined as

$$\alpha = \frac{k}{k-1}\left(1 - \frac{\sum s_i^2}{s_T^2}\right),$$

where k is the number of items, s_i is the standard deviation of scores on the ith item (for $i = 1,...,k$) and s_T is the standard deviation of the total score. If the items are independent, $\alpha = 0$; if they are all measuring exactly the same thing, $\alpha = 1$. Conventionally, values of $\alpha > 0.7$ are taken to mean that internal consistency is acceptable; values below 0.5 signify that it is unacceptable and the scoring system requires modification.

See Bland and Altman (1997) for a simple numerical example using Cronbach's alpha, as well as more insight into its derivation. The Stata command ALPHA, and the SAS option ALPHA used with the PROC CORR procedure, produces this statistic.

2.10   Assessing diagnostic tests

Epidemiological investigations often require classification of each individual studied according to some binary outcome variable, the most important example of which is disease status (yes/no). These classification procedures will be called **diagnostic tests**. In some situations, the accuracy of the diagnosis will not be in question, most obviously when the 'disease' is death from any cause.

Sometimes the state of affairs may be less certain. In particular, clinical and laboratory procedures are often used for diagnosis. Examples include cancer screening clinics and analysis of blood samples for signs of an illness. Such tests may not be 100% reliable, and it is of interest to quantify just how reliable any particular test really is. This may be achieved by applying the test to a number of individuals whose true disease status is known and interpreting the results. Notice the contrast to the situation of Section 2.9.2: here we will also be comparing two sets of results, but now one set of results provides the standard. The problem is one of calibration rather than investigating equivalence.

Two types of error can occur during diagnostic testing. Consider the problem of classifying disease status once more. First, the test could wrongly decide that a person with the disease does not have it. Second, the test could wrongly decide that a person without the disease does have it. Clearly, we would wish for the probabilities of each type of error to be small.

Consider data from a test of n subjects presented in the form of Table 2.21, showing the test decision (the rows) and the true state of affairs (the columns). Notice that this assumes that we are testing for the presence of disease; in some applications, 'disease' would not be the appropriate label for the columns (for example, when assessing preparatory pregnancy testing kits). Nevertheless, we shall continue to assume this situation for simplicity.

Table 2.21. Display of data from a
diagnostic test.

| Test | True disease status | | |
result	Positive	Negative	Total
Positive	a	b	$a + b$
Negative	c	d	$c + d$
Total	$a + c$	$b + d$	n

From Table 2.21, we can see that the (estimated) probabilities of the two wrong
decisions are

1. For false negatives, $c/(a + c)$.
2. For false positives, $b/(b + d)$.

In fact, the complementary probabilities are more often quoted — that is, the probability of making the right decision whenever a person has the disease, called the **sensitivity** of the test, and the probability of making the right decision whenever a person
does not have the disease, called the **specificity** of the test. These are thus estimated as

1. Sensitivity $= a/(a + c)$.
2. Specificity $= d/(b + d)$.   (2.37)

Notice that these are, respectively, the relative frequency of correct decisions amongst true
positives and true negatives. They may be calculated using the two columns of the table.

Sometimes we may also wish to consider the probability that someone really does
have the disease, once the test has given a positive result, called the **predictive value
of a positive test**. Also, we may consider the probability that someone really does
not have the disease once the test has given a negative result, called the **predictive
value of a negative test**. From Table 2.21, estimated predictive values are

1. For a positive test, $a/(a + b)$.
2. For a negative test, $d/(c + d)$.   (2.38)

Notice that these two calculations use the two rows of the table.

Because all the measures in (2.37) and (2.38) are proportions, we can use the
material of Section 2.5.2 to make inferences; for instance, (2.3) may be used to attach
confidence intervals to any of the results.

Although sensitivity, specificity and predictive values are defined for the case in
which true disease outcome is known, they are frequently used, in practice, to compare
a test against some standard test that is generally assumed to be correct. Notice that
this is, strictly speaking, only *relative* sensitivity, etc.

Example 2.16 Ditchburn and Ditchburn (1990) describe a number of tests for the rapid diagnosis
of urinary tract infections (UTIs). They took urine samples from over 200 patients with symptoms of UTI; these were sent to a hospital microbiology laboratory for a culture test. This test
is taken to be the standard against which all other tests are to be compared. All the other tests
were much more immediate and thus suitable for use in general practice. We will consider only
one of the rapid tests here, a dipstick test to detect pyuria (by leucocyte–esterase estimation).
The results are given in Table 2.22.
From (2.37) and (2.38),

Sensitivity = 84/94 = 0.894.
Specificity = 92/135 = 0.681.
Predictive value of a positive test = 84/127 = 0.661.
Predictive value of a negative test = 92/102 = 0.902.

Table 2.22. Results of a dipstick test
for pyuria.

Dipstick test	Culture test (standard)		
	Positive	Negative	Total
Positive	84	43	127
Negative	10	92	102
Total	94	135	229

Thus, assuming the culture test to be the truth, the pyuria test is rather better at diagnosing UTI than diagnosing absence of UTI (sensitivity greater than specificity). Also, more of the apparent UTI cases than apparent UTI noncases (according to the pyuria test) will have been incorrectly diagnosed (predictive value greatest for the negative test).

It would be incorrect to conclude that predictive values give no useful information once sensitivity and specificity are known. Predictive values depend upon the relative numbers of true positives and negatives that have been tested. For instance, suppose the methodology described in Example 2.16 was repeated in a different population and produced the results shown in Table 2.23. Sensitivity and specificity are just as before ($252/282 = 0.894$ and $92/135 = 0.681$, respectively). The predictive values are now $252/295 = 0.854$ (positive test) and $92/122 = 0.754$ (negative test), which are not only different in magnitude from before, but also in reverse order (positive test now bigger). This is because the sample in Table 2.23 has more true (culture) positives than negatives, whereas in Table 2.22 the opposite is true.

2.10.1 Accounting for sensitivity and specificity

Sometimes there are several tests to compare. For example, Ditchburn and Ditchburn (1990) also give the results of another dipstick test, this time for nitrate. This test has a sensitivity of 0.57 — below that for the pyuria test, but a specificity of 0.96 — higher than that for the pyuria test. If we needed to choose one of the two tests, which should we choose?

One often used criterion is the **likelihood ratio**, defined to be

$$\frac{s}{1-p}, \tag{2.39}$$

where s is sensitivity, and p is specificity, for the different tests. This will increase if sensitivity or specificity increases with the other remaining constant, or if both sensitivity and specificity increase. Thus, the largest values of (2.39) are considered best. However, (2.39) may go up or down if sensitivity and specificity move in

Table 2.23. Alternative (hypothetical)
results of a dipstick test for pyuria.

Dipstick test	Culture test (standard)		
	Positive	Negative	Total
Positive	252	43	295
Negative	30	92	122
Total	282	135	417

opposite directions, as in the dipstick tests example. Consequently, the likelihood ratio criterion has limited utility.

In general, we need to consider the relative importance, or 'weight', that we will give to sensitivity and specificity. For instance, if the disease in question is likely to lead to death and the preferred treatment (subsequent to a positive diagnosis) has few side-effects, then it will be more important to make sensitivity as large as possible. On the other hand, if the disease is not too serious and no known treatment is completely free of unpleasant side-effects, then more weight might be given to specificity. The cost of the treatment given to those with positive test results could also come into consideration. If the weight, however decided, given to sensitivity is w (and the weight given to specificity is thus $1 - w$), then we would seek to maximise

$$M = ws + (1 - w)p \tag{2.40}$$

where s is sensitivity and p is specificity, as before.

In many situations, the primary aim will be to maximise the total number of correct decisions made by the test. Here we should make a distinction between correct decisions used during the test (that is, on the sample of people tested) and when the test is later applied to the whole population. These may not be the same; in particular, the sample chosen for testing may have been selected to give a particular ratio of true positives and negatives. If we take the 'sample' criteria, then we maximise the number of correct decisions by taking

$$w = \frac{\text{no. of positive samples}}{\text{total no. of samples}}.$$

Applied to Example 2.16, $w = 94/229$ and so $1 - w = 1 - 94/229 = 135/229$, the number of negative samples divided by the total number of samples. Hence, from (2.40),

$$M = \frac{94}{229} \times \frac{84}{94} + \frac{135}{229} \times \frac{92}{135} = \frac{84 + 92}{229},$$

which is the overall proportion of correct test results, as we would expect. On the other hand, if we take the 'population' criterion, then we maximise the number of correct decisions by taking

$$w = \frac{\text{no. of people with disease in the population}}{\text{total population size}},$$

that is, the disease prevalence in the population. Often this is not known exactly and must be estimated. Another possibility is to give equal weight to sensitivity and specificity (Youden, 1950), in which case, $w = 0.5$. The choice of which particular value to use for w may be crucial in comparative diagnostic testing.

Example 2.17 Carbon monoxide in expired air (CO) is often used to validate self-reported smoking habits. Consider the problem of determining the cut-point for CO, which best discriminates between nonsmokers and smokers. For instance, if the CO cut-point used is 6 ppm, then everyone with a value of CO above 6 ppm will test positive and anyone else will test negative for being a smoker. Such a test is useful in epidemiological research when there is reason to believe that self-reported smoking may be inaccurate. However, how should the best cut-point be decided?

This question was addressed by Ruth and Neaton (1991). They recorded the CO of 5621 smokers and 3274 nonsmokers in the Multiple Risk Factor Intervention Trial conducted in the U.S. These

Table 2.24. Results of a test for smoking status in the Multiple Risk Factor Intervention Trial.

CO value (ppm)	No. of smokers above this value	No. of nonsmokers at or below this value	Sensitivity (s)	Specificity (p)	0.5s + 0.5p
LOW-1	5621	0	1.000	0.000	0.500
5	5460	817	0.971	0.250	0.610
6	5331	1403	0.948	0.429	0.688
7	5200	1914	0.925	0.585	0.755
8	5057	2360	0.900	0.721	0.810
9	4932	2696	0.877	0.823	0.850
10	4818	2972	0.857	0.908	0.882
20	3499	3266	0.622	0.998	0.810
30	1984	3273	0.353	1.000	0.676
40	874	3273	0.155	1.000	0.578
HIGH	0	3274	0.000	1.000	0.500

Note: LOW is the smallest CO value observed and HIGH is the largest CO value observed; these are not specified in the source paper.

Source: Ruth, K.J. and Neaton, J.D. (1991), *Prev. Med.*, 20, 574–579.

values are summarised in Table 2.24. The table also gives the results of calculations of sensitivity and specificity, calculated from (2.37) repeatedly, using each possible cut-point. These are combined using (2.40) with Youden's equal weighting; the best cut-point is CO = 10 ppm.

Different weightings of sensitivity and specificity would give different results. In the extreme case in which only sensitivity is important (so that $w = 1$), the optimum cut-point will be zero — that is, everyone is designated a smoker. Clearly, we can never miss a smoker using this rule, although the test is unlikely to be acceptable in practice! At the opposite extreme, suppose that only specificity is important ($w = 0$). Then, we should simply designate everyone as a nonsmoker. Again, it is difficult to envisage a situation in which this would be a useful procedure. These extreme situations illustrate the importance of considering both sensitivity and specificity.

Interpretation of the performance of different cut-points is enhanced by diagrams, such as a plot of sensitivity, specificity and their sum against the cut-point used (see Figure 2.20). A common plot in this context is that of sensitivity against (1 − specificity), called the **receiver operating characteristic (ROC) plot**. This is particularly helpful when we wish to compare two (or more) diagnostic tests. For instance, Ruth and Neaton (1991) also give data on a second objective test for smoking status, the level of thiocyanate (SCN) in each subject's blood. These data, together with CO data, were used to produce a simple combination test of smoking status: anyone with levels of SCN and CO below or at each cut-point was designated a nonsmoker, and all others were designated smokers. The ROC curves for the CO test (from Table 2.24) and the combined (SCN + CO) test are shown in Figure 2.21.

A test that produces a diagonal line for its ROC plot (each sensitivity matched by an equal lack of specificity) is undiscriminating in that the chance of a right decision when someone has the disease is equal to the chance of a wrong decision when someone does not. A perfect test would always have perfect sensitivity or specificity, and hence its ROC curve would go straight up the vertical axis to a sensitivity of 1 and then straight across, parallel to the horizontal axis. A test nearer this ideal, that is, with a larger area under the ROC curve, is the better. Thus, in Figure 2.21 the combined (SCN + CO) test is best, although only marginally. There is no question but that the

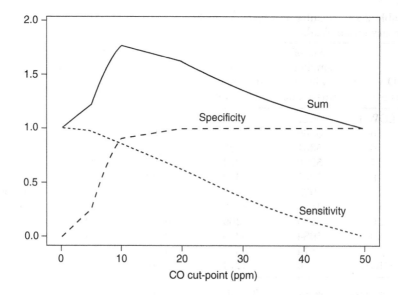

Figure 2.20. Sensitivity, specificity and their sum (solid line) against the cut-point used to distinguish smokers from nonsmokers for the data in Table 2.24. Here it is assumed that LOW = 1 and HIGH = 50.

combined test has the larger area under the curve here; for any given false positive rate, it always has at least as high a true positive rate as does the CO test.

The procedure used to combine SCN and CO information for Figure 2.21 is crude. Ruth and Neaton (1991) included a better method, based on logistic regression modelling (Chapter 10). For an example that is very similar to Example 2.17 but using the SHHS data referred to repeatedly in this chapter, see Woodward and Tunstall–Pedoe (1992b).

ROC analyses are conveniently carried out using Stata, which includes procedures for calculating sensitivity, specificity and area under the curve (the ROCTAB procedure); plotting (ROCPLOT); and comparing areas (ROCCOMP). The SAS package procedure PROC LOGISTIC may also be used. For more details on ROC curves, see Hanley and

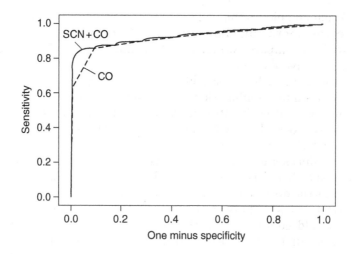

Figure 2.21. Receiver operating characteristic plot for two tests designed to distinguish smokers from nonsmokers: the CO test (dashed line) and the SCN + CO test (solid line).

McNeil (1982) and Zweig and Campbell (1993). Chapter 13 considers the use of sensitivity, specificity and ROC curves in prognosis and extends the methodology introduced here.

Exercises

2.1   Mason *et al.* (1997) studied the habit of illicit drug taking by remand prisoners at the time of their arrival at Durham jail. The following table shows the number of types of illicit drugs used in the past year by the unconvicted prisoners studied.
      (i)   Construct a suitable diagram and calculate a suitable summary measure of average for these data.
      (ii) Estimate the proportion of new remand prisoners in the jail who have taken illicit drugs in the year prior to entry. Calculate a 95% confidence interval for this proportion.

No. of drugs	No. of subjects
0	236
1	108
2	96
3	55
4	27
5	17
6	8
7	1

2.2   The web site for this book (see Appendix A) contains data from the Bombay (now Mumbai) lung cancer registry. This registry obtained data from all cancer patients registered in the 168 government and private hospitals and nursing homes in Bombay, and from death records maintained by the Bombay Municipal Corporation. The survival times of each subject ($n = 682$) with lung cancer from time of first diagnosis to death (or censoring) were recorded over the period 1 January 1989 to 31 December 1991.
      (i)   Construct a table to show the distribution of lung cancer patients by sex, education and marital status.
      (ii) The table of sex by tumour type turns out to be:

Sex	Type of tumour		
	Local	Regional	Advanced
Male	165	169	229
Female	37	39	43

Test the null hypothesis that the distribution of tumour types is the same for men and women. Find a 95% confidence interval for the percentage of advanced tumours (both sexes combined).

2.3   For the Scottish Heart Health Study data on carbon monoxide in Table 2.10, draw a histogram and ogive and construct a normal plot. Compare these with results for carbon monoxide given in Table 2.12 and Figure 2.8. How would you describe the distribution of carbon monoxide?

2.4   Refer to the third Glasgow MONICA data available from the web site for this book (see Appendix A). The MONICA Study is an international collaborative investigation into cardiovascular disease. Data from a random sample of 40 of the subjects in the third MONICA survey in north Glasgow are provided. The variables selected here are the subject's age and alcohol consumption in the past week, ascertained by questionnaire, and protein C and protein S measurements from blood samples. Alcohol consumption was classified using standard alcohol grades. See Lowe *et al.* (1997) for analysis of the full dataset involving 1564 people.

(i)   Draw histograms for protein C and protein S.

(ii)   Find the five-number summaries of the protein C and protein S data. Draw boxplots for each variable.

(iii)   Find the two-number summaries of the protein C and protein S data.

(iv)   Find the coefficients of skewness of the protein C and protein S data.

(v)   Are data for either of the variables highly skewed? If so, try suitable transformations to obtain a reasonably symmetric form, repeating the operations in (i) through (iv), as necessary, on the transformed data.

(vi)   Produce normal plots for protein C and protein S in their raw state and in whatever transformed state was decided upon in (v). Do these plots confirm your findings in (v)?

(vii)   Find a 95% confidence interval for the mean protein C and another for the mean protein S. Use back-transformations where necessary.

(viii) Divide the subjects into two groups: those who drank alcohol in the past week (alcohol status = 1 or 2) and those who did not (alcohol status = 3, 4 or 5). Find a 95% confidence interval for the proportion who have drunk in the past week.

(ix)   An interesting question is whether protein S varies with drinking in the past week. Construct a pair of boxplots, on the same scale, to compare drinkers and nondrinkers (in the past week).

(x)   Test whether mean protein S is the same for drinkers in the past week and nondrinkers using a *t* test. Note that a preliminary test of the equality of variances is required.

(xi)   Use a Wilcoxon test to compare the distributions of protein S for drinkers and nondrinkers (in the past week).

(xii)   Repeat (ix) to (xi) for protein C, using an appropriate transformation when required.

(xiii) Summarise your findings from (ix) to (xii), in words.

(xiv)   Find a 95% confidence interval for the difference in mean protein S for drinkers compared with nondrinkers. Does this agree with your result in (x)?

(xv)   For the full dataset, the mean protein S is 108.9. Test the null hypothesis that the mean of the subset of 40 observations used in this exercise is 108.9 against the two-sided alternative that it is not.

2.5   Oats are an important source of fibre and nutrients but are often avoided by people with coeliac disease. Srinivasan *et al.* (1996) gave 10 patients with the disease an 'oats challenge': 50 g of oats per day for 12 weeks. Results for enterocyte height (μm) before and after the challenge were:

Patient	1	2	3	4	5	6	7	8	9	10
Before	36.3	36.0	40.8	44.9	32.8	28.8	38.4	31.1	29.8	30.2
After	35.3	38.3	37.9	37.6	28.8	27.1	42.6	34.7	30.6	36.8

    (i)   Test the null hypothesis that the oats challenge had no effect on entero-cyte heights.

    (ii)   Find a 90% confidence interval for the difference in mean values after and before the challenge.

    (iii) What conclusion do you draw?

2.6   Sugar derived from the diet is classified into three types:

- Extrinsic sugar — derived from sweets, puddings, etc.
- Intrinsic sugar — naturally occurring in fresh fruit, vegetables and grain.
- Lactose sugar — derived from milk.

Bolton–Smith and Woodward (1995) compared the dietary intake (expressed as a percentage of total dietary consumption of energy from all foods) of each sugar type to the body mass index (BMI) for subjects in the Scottish Heart Health Study and the first Scottish MONICA survey. Results from the study follow.

Draw a diagram, or diagrams, to illustrate these data, so as to show comparisons between BMI groups for each specific sugar type. Comment on the major features of the data.

BMI group (kg/m²)	Type of sugar			
	Extrinsic	Intrinsic	Lactose	Total
Males				
<20	14.2	1.5	3.3	19.0
20–25	12.5	1.9	3.3	17.6
25–30	10.4	2.1	3.4	15.9
>30	8.8	2.2	3.4	14.4
Females				
<20	12.2	2.8	4.0	19.1
20–25	9.4	3.2	4.2	16.8
25–30	8.0	3.3	4.2	15.4
>30	7.5	3.4	4.0	14.8

2.7   McKinney et al. (1991) compared mothers' reports of childhood vaccinations with the records of the children's general practitioners. For the first whooping cough vaccination, the concordance between the two sources of data (neither of which can be considered to represent the truth) can be judged from the following table. Use this table to estimate the kappa statistic, together with an approximate 95% confidence interval.

GP's record	Mother's report		
	No vaccination	Vaccination	Total
No vaccination	79	37	116
Vaccination	11	167	178
Total	90	204	294

2.8 In the study of Mason *et al.* (1997) used in Exercise 2.1, all unconvicted men remanded into custody in Durham jail from 1 October 1995 to 30 April 1996 were given a detailed interview. From this, the researchers were able to ascertain who did and did not take drugs at the time of incarceration. The following table shows the research findings for cannabis, showing also whether the prison's reception screening programme had detected cannabis use.

Screening finding	Research finding	
	User	Nonuser
User	49	6
Nonuser	201	118

Treating the research finding as the truth, estimate (i) the sensitivity; (ii) the specificity and the predictive values of (iii) a positive test and (iv) a negative test. Give confidence intervals corresponding to each estimate. Interpret your findings.

2.9 The following table shows the results of the thiocyanate (SCN) test for smoking reported by Ruth and Neaton (1991). Find the sensitivity and specificity for each SCN cut-point. Find the optimum cut-point according to each of the following criteria:

(i) Youden's equal weighting of sensitivity and specificity.
(ii) To maximise the number of correct decisions for the sample data.
(iii) To maximise the number of correct decisions in a population in which 25% of people smoke.

SCN value	No. of smokers above this value	No. of nonsmokers below or at this value
LOW-1	5621	0
20	5602	149
40	5502	1279
60	5294	2271
80	5030	2806
100	4750	3057
120	4315	3185
140	3741	3240
160	2993	3259
180	2166	3268
200	1417	3271
220	823	3274
HIGH	0	3274

Note: LOW is the smallest observed SCN value; HIGH is the largest observed SCN value.

2.10 Suppose that you were asked to write a report on the studies of Doll and Hill described in Section 1.2. Assuming that you could obtain access to the raw data, how (if at all) would you redesign Tables 1.1 to 1.3 for inclusion in your report?

CHAPTER 3

Assessing risk factors

3.1 Risk and relative risk

In epidemiology, we are often interested in evaluating the chance that an individual who possesses a certain attribute also has a specific disease. The most basic epidemiological measure is the probability of an individual becoming newly diseased given that the individual has the particular attribute under consideration. This is called the **risk** of disease; as defined in Section 1.1, the attribute considered is called the **risk factor**. Hence, risk measures the probability of disease incidence.

Although risk is a useful summary of the relationship between risk factor and disease, it is not sufficient by itself for assessing the importance of the risk factor to disease outcome. For instance, we may find that 30% of a sample of women who use a particular type of contraceptive pill develop breast cancer, so the risk of breast cancer is 0.3 for pill users. This would seem impressive evidence implicating the pill, unless it transpired that a similar percentage of nonpill users have also developed breast cancer. As in most procedures in epidemiology, a comparison group is required; the simplest one to take here is the group without the risk factor. This leads to the definition of the **relative risk** (or **risk ratio**) as the ratio of the risk of disease for those with the risk factor to the risk of disease for those without the risk factor. If the relative risk is above 1, the factor under investigation increases risk; if less than 1, it reduces risk. A factor with a relative risk less than 1 is sometimes referred to as a **protective factor**. In most cases, we shall use the general term 'risk factor' without specifying the direction of its effect. Sometimes (somewhat unnecessarily) risk is called **absolute risk**, to distinguish it from relative risk.

Computation of the risk and relative risk is particularly simple from a 2 × 2 table (two rows by two columns) of risk factor status against disease status, designated algebraically by Table 3.1. This represents data from n subjects free from disease at the outset of the study (the **baseline**). Each individual's risk factor status at baseline was recorded, as was whether she or he went on to develop the disease during the study.

From Table 3.1, we see that, for example, the number of people with the risk factor but without the disease is b. Note that $n = a + b + c + d$. In general,

$$\text{Risk} = \frac{\text{number of cases of disease}}{\text{number of people at risk}}. \tag{3.1}$$

From Table 3.1, the exposure-specific risks are, for those with the risk factor, $a/(a + b)$; and for those without the risk factor, $c/(c + d)$. The relative risk (denoted λ) for those with the risk factor, compared with those without, is estimated by

$$\hat{\lambda} = \frac{a/(a+b)}{c/(c+d)} = \frac{a(c+d)}{c(a+b)}. \tag{3.2}$$

Table 3.1. Display of data from an incidence study.

Risk factor status	Disease status		
	Disease	No disease	Total
Exposed	a	b	$a + b$
Not exposed	c	d	$c + d$
Total	$a + c$	$b + d$	n

In most real-life situations, the data collected in an epidemiological study will be a sample of data on the subject of interest. Hence, the risk and relative risk calculated from the data are estimates for the equivalent entities in the population as a whole — for instance, all premenopausal women in the earlier example relating to use of the pill. In fact, we shall see in Section 6.2 that the sample values are not appropriate estimates for the population equivalents for case–control studies. As a consequence, risk and relative risk should *not* be calculated from case–control studies.

We should specify the sampling error inherent in our sample-based estimates of the true (population) risk and relative risk. As in other cases, this is best done by specifying the standard error (sample-to-sample variation in the value of the estimate) or a confidence interval. We shall use the symbol R to represent the population risk and r to represent the sample risk.

By definition, the population risk is simply a probability, and the standard error is estimated by

$$\hat{\mathrm{se}}(r) = \sqrt{r(1 - r)/n}\,. \tag{3.3}$$

Using a normal approximation, as was used to define (2.2), the 95% confidence interval for R is

$$r \pm 1.96\hat{\mathrm{se}}(r)\,. \tag{3.4}$$

The value 1.96 appears because this is the 5% critical value for the normal distribution. As usual, if we require a different percentage confidence interval, we simply alter this value; see (2.3). As with (3.1), we could use (3.3) and (3.4) for the risk amongst those exposed or amongst those unexposed or, indeed, for everyone (both groups combined).

The confidence interval for the relative risk is slightly more difficult to compute. The distribution of the sample relative risk is skewed and a log transformation is necessary to ensure approximate normality (Section 2.8.1). Katz *et al.* (1978) showed that, in the notation of Table 3.1,

$$\hat{\mathrm{se}}(\log_e \hat{\lambda}) = \sqrt{\frac{1}{a} - \frac{1}{a + b} + \frac{1}{c} - \frac{1}{c + d}}\,, \tag{3.5}$$

where λ is the population relative risk and $\hat{\lambda}$ is its estimate in the sample, defined by (3.2). Hence, the 95% confidence interval for $\log_e \lambda$ is

$$\log_e \hat{\lambda} \pm 1.96\hat{\mathrm{se}}(\log_e \hat{\lambda})\,,$$

with lower and upper limits of

$$L_{\log} = \log_e \hat{\lambda} - 1.96\hat{se}(\log_e \hat{\lambda}),$$
$$U_{\log} = \log_e \hat{\lambda} + 1.96\hat{se}(\log_e \hat{\lambda}). \tag{3.6}$$

We really want a 95% confidence interval for λ. This is obtained by raising the two limits in (3.6) to the power e. That is, the lower and upper limits in the 95% confidence interval for the relative risk, λ, are

$$L = \exp(L_{\log}),$$
$$U = \exp(U_{\log}). \tag{3.7}$$

Example 3.1 In 1985, employees of the Electricity Generating Authority of Thailand (EGAT) aged 35 to 54 years old were asked to complete a questionnaire that asked, amongst other things, whether they currently smoked. Vital status (alive/dead) was ascertained 12 years later in 3315 employees or ex-employees who could still be traced; these were 95% of those who had answered the question on smoking (Sritara *et al.*, 2003). Table 3.2 enumerates those who died due to cardiovascular disease (CVD) over the period 1985 to 1997 against smoking status in 1985.

From (3.1), overall risk of death due to CVD is 46/3315 = 0.013876. The risk for smokers is 31/1417 = 0.021877, whilst for nonsmokers it is 15/1898 = 0.007903. From (3.2), the relative risk is 0.021877/0.007903 = 2.7682. From (3.4), the 95% confidence interval for the risk of a cardiovascular death for smokers is

$$0.021877 \pm 1.96\sqrt{0.021877(1 - 0.021877)/1417};$$

that is, 0.021877 ± 0.007617 or (0.01426, 0.02949). From (3.5), the estimated standard error of the log of the relative risk is

$$\sqrt{\frac{1}{31} - \frac{1}{1417} + \frac{1}{15} - \frac{1}{1898}} = 0.31256.$$

From (3.6), 95% confidence limits for the log of the relative risk are then

$$L_{\log} = \log_e(2.7682) - 1.96 \times 0.31256 = 0.40558,$$

$$U_{\log} = \log_e(2.7682) + 1.96 \times 0.31256 = 1.63081.$$

Table 3.2. Smoking and cardiovascular deaths in the EGAT study.

Smoker at entry?	Cardiovascular death during follow-up?		
	Yes	No	Total
Yes	31	1386	1417
No	15	1883	1898
Total	46	3269	3315

From (3.7), 95% confidence limits for the relative risk of a cardiovascular death for smokers compared with nonsmokers are then

$$L = \exp(0.40558) = 1.500,$$

$$U = \exp(1.63081) = 5.108.$$

Hence (with appropriate rounding), we estimate that the risk of a cardiovascular death for smokers is 0.022, and we are 95% sure that the interval (0.014, 0.029) contains the true population risk. The estimated relative risk of a cardiovascular death for smokers compared with nonsmokers is 2.77, and we are 95% sure that the interval (1.50, 5.11) contains the true population relative risk. Note that numbers were originally calculated to several decimal places, because several results are subsequently used to derive other results and because we will wish to make comparisons with other analytical methods later. Two decimal places (or two significant digits — those following any leading zeros) are usually sufficient in a presentation. In brief, we conclude that about 2% of smokers experience a cardiovascular death — almost 2.8 times as many as nonsmokers. That is, we estimate that smoking elevates risk by almost 180%.

Notice that (3.3) could be applied to calculate a confidence interval for the overall risk (pooled over smoking status) or the risk for nonsmokers, if either were required. Also, there is no theoretical necessity to calculate relative risk as smokers' risk over nonsmokers' risk in Example 3.1. Instead, the inverse, nonsmokers' risk over smokers' risk, could be calculated in a similar way, if this is of practical interest. In fact, it is simply the reciprocal of the relative risk found already: $1/2.768 = 0.36$. Similarly, the 95% confidence limits for the relative risk of a cardiovascular death for nonsmokers compared with smokers are found as the reciprocals of the limits found already, except that the order of the two limits is reversed; that is, the lower limit is $1/5.108 = 0.20$ and the upper limit is $1/1.500 = 0.67$. There is no advantage in stating both sets of results, but this example shows that it is important to specify clearly what is being related (in the numerator) to what (in the denominator). The outcome used to define the denominator in the relative risk is called the **base** or **reference**. Generally, the base is taken as absence of the risk factor in a situation akin to Example 3.1.

When relative risk is quoted for a protective factor, it may be convenient to express it as a percentage risk reduction defined as $100(1 - \lambda)$. For example, if the relative risk for stomach cancer for a diet high in whole-grain cereals compared with other diets is 0.4, then the whole-grain cereal diet is associated with a 60% risk reduction.

3.2   Odds and odds ratio

As we have seen, the risk is a probability. Whenever a probability is calculated, it would also be possible to calculate an alternative specification of chance called the **odds**. Whereas the probability measures the number of times the outcome of interest (for example, disease) occurs relative to the total number of observations (that is, the sample size), the odds measures the number of times the outcome occurs relative to the number of times it does not. The odds can be calculated for different groups; here we would be interested in the odds for those exposed to the risk factor and the odds for those unexposed. The ratio of these two is called the **odds ratio**. Similar to the relative risk, an odds ratio above 1 implies that exposure to the factor under investigation increases the odds of disease, whilst a value below 1 means the factor reduces the odds of disease. In general,

$$\text{Odds} = \frac{\text{number of cases of disease}}{\text{number of noncases of disease}}. \tag{3.8}$$

From Table 3.1, the exposure-specific odds are, for those with the risk factor, a/b; and for those without the risk factor, c/d. The odds ratio for those with the risk factor, compared to those without, is given by

$$\hat{\psi} = \frac{a/b}{c/d} = \frac{ad}{bc}. \tag{3.9}$$

The Greek letter ψ (psi) is commonly used (as here) to represent the population odds ratio. In (3.9), the hat, once again, denotes a sample value that is an estimate of its population equivalent.

Another way of deriving the odds is as the ratio of the risk to its complement; for example, the odds for those with the risk factor are given by $r/(1 - r)$. This can easily be seen from (3.1) and (3.8). In everyday life, odds are most often heard about in gambling situations, such as the odds of a horse winning a race. Epidemiologists take 'odds' and 'odds ratio' to refer to the chance of a disease *incidence*, just as they do 'risk' and 'relative risk'. In practice, the odds are rarely of interest, and the odds ratio is generally quoted alone (Section 3.3).

As with the relative risk, the distribution of the odds ratio is better approximated by a normal distribution if a log transformation is applied. Woolf (1955) showed that

$$\hat{se}(\log_e \hat{\psi}) = \sqrt{\frac{1}{a} + \frac{1}{b} + \frac{1}{c} + \frac{1}{d}}, \tag{3.10}$$

and hence 95% confidence limits for $\log_e \psi$ are

$$\begin{aligned} L_{\log} &= \log_e \hat{\psi} - 1.96\hat{se}(\log_e \hat{\psi}), \\ U_{\log} &= \log_e \hat{\psi} + 1.96\hat{se}(\log_e \hat{\psi}); \end{aligned} \tag{3.11}$$

and the 95% confidence limits for ψ are

$$\begin{aligned} L &= \exp\left(L_{\log}\right), \\ U &= \exp\left(U_{\log}\right). \end{aligned} \tag{3.12}$$

Example 3.2 For the EGAT study, Table 3.2 gives the following results. From (3.8), the overall odds of a cardiovascular death are $46/3269 = 0.014072$; the odds of a cardiovascular death for smokers are $31/1386 = 0.022367$, whilst for nonsmokers they are $15/1883 = 0.007966$. From (3.9), the odds ratio for a cardiovascular death, comparing smokers to nonsmokers, is

$$\frac{0.022367}{0.007966} = \frac{31 \times 1883}{1386 \times 15} = 2.8077.$$

From (3.10), the estimated standard error of the log of the odds ratio is

$$\sqrt{\frac{1}{31} + \frac{1}{1386} + \frac{1}{15} + \frac{1}{1883}} = 0.31651.$$

From (3.11), 95% confidence limits for the log of the odds ratio are then

$$L_{log} = \log_e(2.8077) - 1.96 \times 0.31651 = 0.41201 \ ,$$

$$U_{log} = \log_e(2.8077) + 1.96 \times 0.31651 = 1.65273 \ .$$

From (3.12), 95% confidence limits for the odds ratio for a cardiovascular death comparing smokers to nonsmokers are then

$$L = \exp(0.41201) = 1.510,$$

$$U = \exp(1.65273) = 5.221.$$

The odds of a cardiovascular death are estimated to be 2.81 times greater for smokers as for nonsmokers, and we are 95% sure that the interval (1.51, 5.22) contains the true odds ratio. In brief, smoking is estimated to elevate the odds of a cardiovascular death by 181%.

Although it would be unusual to want to do so, it is possible to compute the odds ratio and its confidence interval for nonsmokers compared with smokers. As in the case of the relative risk (Section 3.1), we can do this from the results of Example 3.2 without recourse to the data. We simply take the reciprocal of the original odds ratio and its confidence limits, with order reversed: 0.36 (0.19, 0.66). As with the relative risk, it is important to specify what is being compared with what, whenever an odds ratio is stated.

Note that the formulae for the limits of confidence intervals given in this section and Section 3.1 are really only approximations. For example, (3.4) uses a normal approximation to the true binomial distribution of the number who are cases out of the number at risk. See Clarke and Cooke (2004) for an introduction to the binomial distribution and Conover (1999) for details on exact binomial procedures and the normal approximation. Modern computer packages, including Stata (Section 3.10), will provide more accurate results, based on exact theory. Other approximate formulae for confidence intervals commonly used are due to Cornfield (1956), for the odds ratio, and Greenland and Robins (1985), for the relative risk. Generally, results will be virtually the same by the alternative approaches whenever sample sizes are large.

3.3   Relative risk or odds ratio?

As we have seen, risk and odds measure the chance of disease incidence in some way, and thus the relative risk and odds ratio measure comparative chance. Risk is the preferred measure because it is a probability and probabilities are well understood as long-run versions of proportions. Odds are less well understood.

So, why consider odds at all? The answer is that, in practice, the odds ratio is often a good approximation to the relative risk, and in some cases the odds ratio is all that we can estimate (the situation in case–control studies; see Chapter 6) or is the most convenient to calculate (in logistic regression analysis; see Chapter 10).

The odds ratio will be a good approximation to the relative risk whenever the disease in question is rare. Referring to Table 3.1, when the disease is rare, it must be that

$$a + b \simeq b,$$
$$c + d \simeq d,$$

$$(3.13)$$

where $\simeq$ means 'approximately equal to'. Hence, from (3.2), (3.9) and (3.13),

$$\hat{\psi} = \frac{ad}{bc} \simeq \frac{a(c+d)}{(a+b)c} = \hat{\lambda}.$$

A little algebra will show that

$$\frac{\hat{\psi}}{\hat{\lambda}} = \frac{1-r_{\bar{E}}}{1-r_E},$$

where r_E is the risk of disease amongst those exposed to the risk factor and $r_{\bar{E}}$ is the risk amongst those unexposed. From this we can see that $\hat{\psi}/\hat{\lambda}$ will be more than one whenever the relative risk $(r_E/r_{\bar{E}})$ is more than one. That is, the odds ratio will always be bigger than the relative risk whenever the relative risk is more than one. Conversely, the odds ratio will always be smaller than the relative risk whenever the relative risk is less than one. Taking these conclusions together, the odds ratio is always more extreme than the relative risk (except when the relative risk is one, in which case the odds ratio will also be one).

Comparison of Example 3.1 and Example 3.2 shows that the relative risk (2.77) and odds ratio (2.81) for a cardiovascular death, comparing smokers to nonsmokers, are very similar for the EGAT study. Cardiovascular deaths are quite unusual, despite being the leading cause of death amongst middle-aged Thais. Many other diseases will have lower overall incidence rates, suggesting even better agreement. However, the approximation is only good if incidence is relatively low amongst *both* those with and those without the risk factor. For example, if few nonsmokers have a cardiovascular death, but virtually all smokers do, then the odds ratio would be substantially larger than the relative risk. Another way of looking at this is that the approximation will be good whenever both the risk in the unexposed group and the relative risk are low.

Example 3.3 Consider the hypothetical results of Table 3.3. An extra column of risks has been added to enhance interpretation; this is often useful in written reports. In this case, the disease is rare overall (only about 1 person in 100 has it) and yet the relative risk is

$$\hat{\lambda} = \frac{0.5}{0.00102} = 490,$$

whereas the odds ratio is

$$\hat{\psi} = \frac{9 \times 981}{1 \times 9} = 981,$$

just over twice as big. Thus, the odds ratio does not provide a good approximation to the relative risk in this case.

Table 3.3. Hypothetical data from an incidence study.

Risk factor status	Disease status			
	Disease	No disease	Total	Risk
Exposed	9	9	18	0.5
Not exposed	1	981	982	0.00102
Total	10	990	1000	0.01010

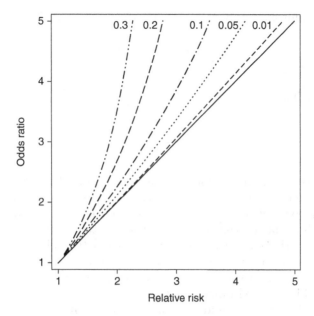

Figure 3.1. The odds ratio against the relative risk. The fanned lines are each drawn at a specific value (as so labelled) of the risk of disease in subjects who are unexposed to the risk factor. The diagonal solid line is the line of equality between the odds ratio and the relative risk.

Situations akin to Table 3.3, in which the risk factor is virtually the sole causal agent for the disease, arise infrequently in practical epidemiological research, as do odds ratios/relative risks in the hundreds or more. Table 3.3 shows a very extreme example of how the odds ratio can overestimate the relative risk and it could be argued that exact values matter little when the direction of effect is so obvious. However, because the relative risk and odds ratio are not the same, it is appropriate to specify which of the two is being reported. Many epidemiological publications have been in error in this regard, usually by wrongly calling an odds ratio a relative risk. It would be possible to compute both in any follow-up investigation, as in Example 3.1 and Example 3.2, although not in a case–control study. However, we would normally only want to report one.

To give a more complete picture of the relationship between the odds ratio and relative risk for common values of the relative risk, Figure 3.1 plots one against the other for relative risks in the range 1 to 5. Results are shown at selected levels of the risk of disease for those unexposed to the risk factor. Notice how, as expected, the odds ratio is never smaller than the relative risk, and how it moves further away from equality (represented by the diagonal solid line) as either the relative risk or the unexposed risk increases. When the unexposed risk is 0.01, the approximation is good at all levels of the relative risk. When it is 0.05, the difference is great enough once the relative risk is as high as four that we likely would not be prepared to accept the odds ratio as a good approximation (the odds ratio is 4.75 when the relative risk is 4.0). Once the unexposed risk gets as high as 0.30 the odds ratio is a poor approximation to the relative risk except at very low values of the relative risk greater than one. For relative risks below one (not illustrated) the odds ratio will always be smaller than the relative risk and the two measures will diverge as the relative risk decreases and as the risk for unexposed subjects increases.

3.4 Prevalence studies

In the preceding sections, risk, relative risk, odds and odds ratio have been defined as measures of chance in incidence studies. Technically, there is no reason why the same definitions could not be used in prevalence studies; (3.1) to (3.13) could be defined quite properly in a mathematical sense. Unlike general English usage, epidemiologists reserve all these key terms to refer to incidence. However, this is really rather unfortunate because it is perfectly natural to want to talk about risk in relation to prevalence data such as those in Table 2.2. To overcome this difficulty, the prefix 'prevalence' should be used; for example, the coronary heart disease (CHD) **prevalence odds ratio** for manual (classes IIIm, IV and V) compared with nonmanual (classes I, II and IIIn) workers can be calculated from Table 2.2 as

$$\frac{(668 + 279 + 109)/(2482 + 974 + 306)}{(100 + 382 + 183)/(492 + 1872 + 834)} = 1.35.$$

Thus, manual workers have 35% higher odds of having CHD than do nonmanual workers. If one is prepared to be less pedantic, a more elegant name for the measure in this example is the odds ratio for prevalent CHD.

Example 3.4 Smith *et al.* (1991) give the results of a cross-sectional study of peripheral vascular disease (PVD) in Scotland. Table 3.4 shows prevalent cases and noncases of the disease classified by cigarette smoking status for men. Hence,

Overall prevalence risk of PVD = 56/4956 = 0.0113

Prevalence risk of PVD for cigarette smokers = 15/1727 = 0.00869

Prevalence risk of PVD for non-cigarette smokers = 41/3229 = 0.0127

Prevalence relative risk = 0.00869/0.0127 = 0.68

Prevalence odds of PVD for cigarette smokers = 15/1712 = 0.00876

Prevalence odds of PVD for non-cigarette smokers = 41/3188 = 0.0129

Prevalence odds ratio = 0.00876/0.0129 = 0.68

Notice that the prevalence relative risk and odds ratio are the same (to two decimal places), as would be expected for a disease as rare as peripheral vascular disease.

Table 3.4. Cigarette smoking and peripheral vascular disease in a sample of Scottish men.

Cigarette smoker?	Peripheral vascular disease?		
	Yes	No	Total
Yes	15	1712	1727
No	41	3188	3229
Total	56	4900	4956

Table 3.5. Cigarette smoking and peripheral vascular disease in a sample of Scottish men.

| Cigarette smoking status | Peripheral vascular disease? | | | Prevalence |
	Yes	No	Total	
Current smoker	15	1712	1727	0.0087
Ex-smoker	33	1897	1930	0.0171
Never smoked	8	1291	1299	0.0062
Total	56	4900	4956	0.0113

The results of Example 3.4 seem to go against expectation: cigarette smoking appears to be protective (relative risk below 1). This illustrates one great drawback with prevalence studies: individuals with pre-existing disease may have altered their lifestyle, possibly due to medical advice, so that they are now no longer exposed to the risk factor. In the example, a smoker may quit once he has experienced PVD or other cardiovascular symptoms.

Example 3.5 The original article that gave rise to Example 3.4 distinguished between ex-smokers and never-smokers when considering the nonsmoking group. Table 3.5 shows the results when this more extensive classification is used. As we expect, those who have never smoked have the lowest prevalence; ex-smokers have the highest prevalence, with current smokers somewhere between the two.

In other situations, we may not be able to identify those previously exposed to whatever risk factor is of interest. The results may then be biased in favour of the risk factor, as in Example 3.4. Of course, even in Example 3.5, there is no guarantee that disease has caused people to give up or, indeed, that disease has even preceded giving up. We can infer that this is likely, but it is not proven unless we can ascertain the sequence of events for each current nonsmoker.

Other problems with prevalence studies are mentioned in Section 1.4.1. All these problems show that if we wish to demonstrate direct causality from risk factor to disease, we would be wise to use incidence, rather than prevalence, data.

3.5   Testing association

We have seen that the relative risk and odds ratio are meaningful measures of association between risk factor and disease. Both measure the relative chance of disease with the risk factor compared to without. If the risk factor has no effect, the relative risk and odds ratio should turn out to be around unity. In practice, we take a sample of data and measure the sample relative risk or odds ratio; we could then consider whether this sample result provides evidence that the equivalent population value is different from unity. If not, then we would conclude that no evidence of an association between the risk factor and the disease in question exists. Such a result would cast doubt upon the theory that the (supposed) risk factor causes the disease.

Considering the display of Table 3.1, it is clear that a test of no association between risk factor and disease is achieved by the chi-square test (Section 2.5.1). From Table 3.1, the expected (E) values when the null hypothesis of no association (equivalent to $H_0 : \lambda = 1$ or $H_0 : \psi = 1$) is true are

$$(a + b)(a + c)/n \quad (a + b)(b + d)/n$$

$$(c + d)(a + c)/n \quad (c + d)(b + d)/n.$$

Using (2.1), a little algebraic manipulation produces the specific form of the chi-square test statistic for a 2×2 table:

$$\frac{n(ad - bc)^2}{(a + b)(c + d)(a + c)(b + d)} . \tag{3.14}$$

As there are two rows and two columns, the degrees of freedom associated with this chi-square statistic are $(2 - 1)(2 - 1) = 1$. Hence, we compare (3.14) with χ_1^2.

Example 3.6 Consider the EGAT data of Table 3.2 once again. By (3.14), the chi-square test statistic is

$$\frac{3315(31 \times 1883 - 1386 \times 15)^2}{(1417 \times 1898 \times 46 \times 3269)} = 11.58.$$

From Table B.3, $\chi_1^2 = 10.8$ at the 0.1% level and hence the result is significant at this level. The exact p value is 0.0007, found from a computer package. We conclude that there is strong evidence of an association between smoking and cardiovascular death. The relative risk and odds ratio are significantly different from 1 at the conventional 5% level of significance.

One thing to note about the preceding result is that we cannot use it to conclude that smoking causes cardiovascular disease. Although the result certainly does not refute the idea of a causal link, the association *could* be the result of external forces. For instance, it could be that smokers are mainly older people and it is older people who experience cardiovascular deaths. Smoking and cardiovascular disease are then, perhaps, only associated because of their common causal link with age. This issue is considered further in Chapter 4.

The chi-square test is a two-sided test, so the conclusion in Example 3.6 was that $\lambda \neq 1$, or $\psi \neq 1$. To ascertain the direction of the link between risk factor and disease, we simply look at the estimate of λ, or ψ. From Example 3.1 and Example 3.2, we see that the estimated values, $\hat{\lambda} = 2.77$ and $\hat{\psi} = 2.81$, are greater than 1. Hence, we conclude that smokers are more likely to have a cardiovascular death, and we have evidence that the observed association is not simply due to chance.

We can also tie up the results of Example 3.1 and Example 3.2 with Example 3.6 where, because the result was significant at $p = 0.0007$, it must also be significant at the less extreme $p = 0.05$. The 95% confidence intervals for λ and ψ were (1.50, 5.11) and (1.51, 5.22), respectively. Both exclude unity, which agrees with the result $\lambda \neq 1$ or $\psi \neq 1$, at the 5% level of significance.

3.5.1 Equivalent tests

As already described in Section 2.5.1, the chi-square test of no association in a 2×2 table is entirely equivalent to the test of equality of two proportions. In the current context, this implies that we can equally well test the null hypothesis of no association between risk factor and disease, $\lambda = 1$ or $\psi = 1$, by testing whether the same proportion have the disease in the risk factor-positive and risk factor-negative groups. In some contexts, the chi-square approach is somewhat easier; in others, the test of equal proportions will seem more natural. As noted in Section 2.5.3, the only difference is that everything is squared in the chi-square formulation.

Example 3.7 For the EGAT study, the proportions who died from CVD in the sample were 0.021877, for smokers, and 0.007903, for nonsmokers (Example 3.1). The proportion for smokers and nonsmokers combined may be obtained from (2.7) as

$$p_c = \frac{1417 \times 0.021877 + 1898 \times 0.007903}{1417 + 1898} = 0.013876,$$

as already derived, more directly, in Example 3.1. Then, from (2.6), the test statistic for testing whether the population proportions dying from CVD are the same for smokers and nonsmokers is

$$\frac{0.021877 - 0.007903}{\sqrt{0.013876(1 - 0.013876)\left(\dfrac{1}{1417} + \dfrac{1}{1898}\right)}} = 3.403.$$

This result is to be compared with the standard normal distribution (Table B.2). A computer package was used to obtain the exact p value as 0.0007 for a two-sided test (that is, when the alternative hypothesis is that the two proportions are unequal). This is the same result as that obtained in Example 3.6. Notice that the square of the test statistic in this example equals the test statistic in Example 3.6 ($3.403^2 = 11.58$), as it should.

Another equivalent test is less interesting to the epidemiologist, but perfectly acceptable. This is a test of whether the same proportion have the risk factor in the diseased and nondiseased groups. In the EGAT example, this compares the proportion smoking: 31/46 for those who die from CVD and 1386/3269 for those who do not die from CVD. The test statistic, (2.6), for this comparison is exactly the same as in Example 3.7.

One word of caution: these tests on proportions will make practical sense only if the entire data are drawn as a random sample. For instance, if those diseased and undiseased are sampled independently, as in a case–control study, then a test that compares proportions with disease (similar to Example 3.7) would not be suitably formulated (although it would be mathematically correct). The chi-square test considered as a test of no association does not have this practical difficulty.

3.5.2   One-sided tests

In most cases, we will wish to perform two-sided tests of no association between risk factor and disease, simply because we will still wish to identify situations in which the risk factor is actually protective against the disease. To take the EGAT example, we certainly do not expect smoking to prevent CVD, but we would not want to miss discovering such a relationship if the data suggest it.

If we decide that a one-sided test is appropriate in the situation in which (say) only an increased risk in the presence of the risk factor ($\lambda > 1$) is of interest, the procedure is straightforward if we use the normal test of Section 3.5.1. We read off one-sided p values directly from Table B.1 or an equivalent table with greater coverage. Due to the symmetry of the normal distribution, the p value for a one-sided test is always half of that for the equivalent two-sided test. Hence, if a one-sided alternative were sensible in Example 3.7, the p value for the test of equality of risk would be $0.0007/2 = 0.00035$. We can obtain this result only approximately from Table B.1; it tells us that the proportion of the standard normal below 3.50 is 0.99977 and hence the probability of a value of 3.50 or more, when the null hypothesis is true, is just above $1 - 0.99977 = 0.00033$. We really need the probability of 3.403 or more (the value of the test statistic in Example 3.7), which is slightly less than 3.5, so the probability required will be slightly more than 0.00033.

When the chi-square test is adopted, the one-sided procedure is not as obvious. This is because the chi-square test is a test of the null hypothesis of no association against the alternative of *some* association; in the current context, it is always two-sided. Consequently, Table B.3 gives two-sided p values. However, because we have already seen that the two tests are equivalent when applied to a 2×2 table, the solution is very obvious: we simply halve the chi-square p value whenever a one-sided test is required. The same procedure is possible whenever a chi-square test with one degree of freedom is concerned. In most other situations in which chi-square tests are used (see Section 2.5.1), the concept of a one-sided test will not be meaningful and the problem does not arise.

3.5.3 Continuity corrections

The chi-square test and the equivalent normal test just described are really only approximate tests. An exact test is possible and will be described in Section 3.5.4. One aspect of the approximation is that the data in a 2×2 table of risk factor status against disease outcome must be discrete and yet the probability distribution (chi-square or normal) used to test the data is continuous. In order to improve this continuous approximation to a discrete distribution, a **continuity correction** is sometimes used. The correction generally used is **Yates's correction**, which reduces the absolute difference between the observed and (under the null hypothesis) expected numbers in the chi-square test statistic, (2.1), by a half. That is, (2.1) becomes

$$\sum_i \sum_j \frac{\left(\left|O_{ij} - E_{ij}\right| - \frac{1}{2}\right)^2}{E_{ij}} \tag{3.15}$$

which, for a 2×2 table, becomes

$$\frac{n\left(\left|ad - bc\right| - \frac{1}{2}n\right)^2}{(a + b)(c + d)(a + c)(b + d)}, \tag{3.16}$$

replacing (3.14). In (3.15), $\left|O_{ij} - E_{ij}\right|$ denotes the absolute value (that is, negative outcomes are treated as positive) of $O_{ij} - E_{ij}$. Similarly for $\left|ad - bc\right|$ in (3.16). Using Yates's correction in the test for equality of two proportions alters (2.6) to give

$$\frac{\left|p_1 - p_2\right| - \frac{1}{2}\left(\frac{1}{n_1} + \frac{1}{n_2}\right)}{\sqrt{p_c(1 - p_c)\left(\frac{1}{n_1} + \frac{1}{n_2}\right)}}. \tag{3.17}$$

Example 3.8 Reworking Example 3.6 using (3.16) rather than (3.14) gives the test statistic

$$\frac{3315\left(\left|31 \times 1883 - 1386 \times 15\right| - 3315/2\right)^2}{1417 \times 1898 \times 46 \times 3269} = 10.58.$$

This is smaller by one than the result when Yates's correction is not used (Example 3.6). The p value for this test turns out to be 0.0011, slightly larger than the 0.0007 found earlier. Hence, the continuity correction has made only a slight difference to the result and leaves the conclusion unchanged: there is strong evidence that smoking is associated with cardiovascular death.

This example could be based upon the normal test. Once again, this gives an entirely equivalent result. Using (3.17) on the EGAT data gives a test statistic of 3.253, the square root of the 10.58 found here.

There is an ongoing debate as to whether Yates's correction is worthwhile. In its favour, it gives a better approximation to the exact result (see Example 3.9 and the discussion in Mantel and Greenhouse, 1968). Against Yates's correction is the argument that it is more complex to understand and calculate (Kleinbaum *et al.*, 1982). As long as absolute faith is not attached to significance level cut-points (see Section 2.5.2), the distinction should not be important unless the numbers are small. Given its extra complexity, the continuity correction is worthwhile only when numbers are fairly small. However, if at least one of the expected numbers is very small, an exact test should always be used; the continuity correction is then not sufficient.

3.5.4   Fisher's exact test

As already mentioned, the chi-square test is an approximate test. An exact procedure, at least under the assumption that the row and column totals (called the **marginal totals**) are fixed, is given here. This is typically used whenever any expected value in a 2×2 table is below 5.

Attributed to Sir Ronald Fisher, the procedure works by first using probability theory to calculate the probability of the observed table, given fixed marginal totals. Referring to Table 3.1, the probability of the observed outcomes a, b, c and d, with the marginal totals $(a + c)$, $(b + d)$, $(a + b)$ and $(c + d)$ fixed, may be shown (Mood *et al.*, 1974) to be

$$\frac{(a + c)!(b + d)!(a + b)!(c + d)!}{n!a!b!c!d!}, \tag{3.18}$$

where, for example, $n!$ is read as 'n factorial' and is defined as the product of all integers up to and including n. Hence,

$$n! = n(n - 1)(n - 2) \ldots (2)(1).$$

By definition, $0! = 1$.

Fisher's procedure requires the probability of the observed and all more extreme tables to be computed, using (3.18) repeatedly. The sum of all these probabilities is the p value for the test. 'More extreme' here means all tables that provide more evidence of an association. Thinking in terms of relative risks, if the observed relative risk is larger than 1, then all more extreme tables give relative risks even larger than 1. On the other hand, if the relative risk from the observed table is below 1, more extreme tables have even smaller relative risks. Due to this, Fisher's exact test, unlike the chi-square test, is fundamentally *one-sided*. However, it is possible to formulate a two-sided version; see Fleiss *et al.* (2003) for details.

Example 3.9 illustrates how Fisher's exact test works. In fact, the exact test may not be necessary in this example because there are no expected frequencies below 5. The example has been deliberately chosen to show the effect of the continuity correction in a situation in which the chi-square test is acceptable, yet the numbers concerned are small enough to allow the exact test to be conducted easily.

Table 3.6. Results of a study of women
pregnant with twins in Zimbabwe.

Activity	Hypertension status		Total	Risk
	Yes	No		
Best rest	3	55	58	0.0517
Normal	9	51	60	0.1500
Total	12	106	118	

Example 3.9 Crowther *et al.* (1990) describe a comparative study of hospitalisation for bed rest against normal activity for 118 Zimbabwean women who were expecting twins. Around half of the women were allocated to each of the two activity regimens. Table 3.6 gives measurements of hypertension status (where hypertension is defined as a blood pressure $\geq$ 140/90 mmHg) for the mothers at the time of their deliveries. This table can be used to test the null hypothesis: pregnant women (with twins) are no more likely to develop maternal hypertension than those left to get on with normal daily living.

Clearly bed rest tends to reduce the chance of hypertension compared with normal activity; the estimated relative risk is 0.0517/0.1500 = 0.345. The one-sided alternative is H_1 : bed rest reduces hypertension. Using (3.18), we can calculate the probability of the observed outcomes 3, 55, 9, 51 in Table 3.6 as

$$\frac{(12!)(106!)(58!)(60!)}{(118!)(3!)(55!)(9!)(51!)} = 0.0535.$$

Now we must identify all the more extreme tables. The easiest way to do this is to consider the smallest observed frequency, 3. If this were to decrease, then the risk for the bed rest group would also decrease. At the same time, this would automatically cause the risk in the normal activity group to increase because the marginal totals are fixed; thus, any decrease from the value 3 in Table 3.6 is balanced by an equal increase from the value 9, and so on. When the risk in the bed rest group increases and that in the normal activity group decreases, the relative risk becomes even smaller than it was originally. Hence, decreasing the value 3 in Table 3.6 produces more extreme tables. As frequencies cannot be negative, there are three more extreme tables. These are given in outline below, with the consequent relative risk (given in brackets) and probability, calculated from (3.18), shown underneath.

2 56	1 57	0 58
10 50	11 49	12 48
(0.179)	(0.078)	(0)
0.0146	0.0023	0.0002

The *p* value for the test is the sum of the four probabilities:

$$0.0535 + 0.0146 + 0.0023 + 0.0002 = 0.071.$$

Hence, we marginally fail to reject the null hypothesis at the 5% level of significance. Evidence is insufficient to conclude that bed rest has a real effect on the chance of a pregnant woman developing maternal hypertension. However, the *p* value is small enough to suggest that a rather larger study would be worthwhile.

As pointed out earlier, all expected values are greater than 5 in this example; hence, the chi-square test might be used, rather than the exact test, because it is easier to compute. Without the continuity correction, (3.14) gives the test statistic as 3.12. With the continuity correction, (3.16) gives the test statistic as 2.13. These results correspond to *p* values of 0.0774 and 0.1440, respectively. Because the chi-square test is two-sided, we must halve these (Section 3.5.2) to obtain results comparable with the one-sided Fisher's exact test. Thus, the uncorrected chi-square test gives a p value of 0.039 and the continuity-corrected chi-square test has $p = 0.072$. The latter is very close to the exact result.

A more rigorous account of Fisher's exact test, and when it should be used, is given by Campbell (2007). In general, if the chi-square, continuity-corrected chi-square and Fisher tests give different inferences, the latter should be used.

3.5.5 Limitations of tests

In most epidemiological analyses, hypothesis tests are less useful than estimation procedures (see Altman *et al.*, 2000, for a general discussion). Specific problems include the arbitrary nature of the cut-point used to define 'significance' (for example, $p < 0.05$) and the dependence of the conclusion upon the sample size. The observed value of the test statistic, and hence the p value, depend upon both the magnitude of the effect measured and the amount of information available to estimate the effect. For this reason, some researchers suggest reporting, rather than the p value, the size of the effect divided by its standard deviation (see Section 13.4.4).

Example 3.10 Table 3.7 shows hypothetical data from two studies of the same relationship between risk factor and disease. In both studies, the risk, relative risk, odds and odds ratio are the same, so the estimated effect of the risk factor is the same. This should be so because study B simply has all cell contents twice as large as in study A. However, a significant relationship exists between risk factor and disease in study B but not in study A, at least using the conventional 5% level of significance.

No matter how small the effect, it is always possible to find it significant if a large enough sample is used. This is true even when we choose to take a very extreme significance level, such as $p < 0.0001$. As epidemiological studies frequently involve several thousand subjects, this issue is of real concern. The epidemiologist must consider clinical, as well as statistical, significance.

Arguably, we have already seen an instance of this issue in Example 2.13. Although the prothrombin time method produced highly significantly ($p < 0.0001$) different estimates of fibrinogen compared with the von Clauss method, the actual excess was only, on average, about 4%. Since fibrinogen values, in this example, rarely exceed 6 and never exceed 8, this may not be a clinically important difference.

Table 3.7. Results from two hypothetical incidence studies.

Risk factor status	Study A			Study B		
	Disease	No disease	Risk[a]	Disease	No disease	Risk[a]
Exposed	10	15	0.40	20	30	0.40
Not exposed	5	20	0.20	10	40	0.20
Relative risk[b]			2.00			2.00
Odds ratio[c]			2.67			2.67
p value[d]			0.12			0.03
n			50			100

[a] Using (3.1).
[b] Using (3.2).
[c] Using (3.9).
[d] Using (3.14).

Table 3.8. Results from a hypothetical large incidence study.

Risk factor status	Disease status		Risk[a]
	Disease	No disease	
Exposed	4140	5860	0.414
Not exposed	4000	6000	0.400
Relative risk[b]			1.03
Odds ratio[c]			1.06
p value[d]			0.04
n			20 000

[a] Using (3.1).
[b] Using (3.2).
[c] Using (3.9).
[d] Using (3.14).

Example 3.11 Table 3.8 shows further hypothetical data wherein the relative risk is only 1.03 (the odds ratio is 1.06), suggestive of an effect that has little or no medical importance. However, the result is statistically significant at the conventional 5% level. Conclusions based solely on the hypothesis test would be misleading. The large sample size (20 000) has caused the test to be extremely sensitive to small effects. Note that this order of magnitude for the sample size is not unusual in certain types of epidemiological studies.

In conclusion, whilst hypothesis tests are useful to check whether results are attributable to chance, estimates of effects should be considered before conclusions are drawn. In many cases, the confidence intervals for the estimates will encompass all the useful information of the hypothesis test. For instance, we can see that the result is (at least approximately) significant at the 5% level if the value of the effect under the null hypothesis is outside the 95% confidence interval for the effect.

3.6 Risk factors measured at several levels

Up to now we have assumed that the risk factor is measured only at two levels: exposed and unexposed. Often the risk factor will, instead, have many levels; for example, Table 2.2 shows social class, measured on an ordered six-point scale, against prevalent CHD. We may extend the ideas of relative risks and odds ratios from 2×2 tables, such as Table 3.2, to $\ell \times 2$ tables (for $\ell > 2$), such as Table 2.2 where $\ell = 6$, very easily. A convenient approach is to choose one level of the risk factor to be the base (reference) level and compare all other levels to this base. For example, in Table 2.2, we could choose social class I to be the base. We can find the prevalence relative risk, for example, of social class II relative to social class I, by thinking of the two corresponding rows of Table 2.2 as the *only* rows. Ignoring all other rows leaves Table 2.2 in the form of a 2×2 table, as shown in Table 3.9.

Then, from (3.2), the relative risk of prevalent CHD for social class II compared with I is

$$\hat{\lambda}_{\mathrm{II}} = \frac{382/2254}{100/592} = 1.003.$$

Confidence intervals and tests for relative risks, odds ratios, etc. all follow as previously described.

Table 3.9. A portion of Table 2.1.

Social class	Prevalent CHD		
	Yes	No	Total
II	382	1872	2254
I	100	492	592
Total	482	2364	2846

Notice that we must be careful how we lay out the subtable so as to correspond with Table 3.1: the base must be the bottom row and positive disease must be the left-hand column. Similar tables to Table 3.9 can be drawn up for the other **contrasts** with social class I; for example, the relative risk for social class V compared with social class I is

$$\hat{\lambda}_V = \frac{109/415}{100/592} = 1.55.$$

Thus, all five contrasts with social class I may be obtained.

It should be apparent that it is not necessary to formally draw out the five subtables, of which Table 3.9 is the first. Calculations may be done straight from the 6×2 table, Table 2.2, by ignoring all but the relevant rows for each contrast. Indeed the prevalence relative risks, apart from rounding error, can be found very easily as quotients of the percentage prevalences already given (in parentheses) in Table 2.2. For example,

$$\hat{\lambda}_V = \frac{26.3}{16.9} = 1.56,$$

which is only in error due to the rounding of percentages in Table 2.2.

As ever, choice of the base level is arbitrary. There is a sound statistical argument that the base level should be chosen as that level with risk, or odds, that has the smallest standard error. In practice, the base is usually taken to be the level with the lowest risk (or odds) or, if the levels have some natural order (as in Table 2.2), the lowest level.

It is possible to have a moving base; for instance, we could compare social class II with I, then III with II, etc., but this is more difficult to interpret. In fact, we can easily construct relative risks or odds ratios for other comparisons as quotients of the basic contrasts already derived. For instance, the relative risk for social class V relative to social class II is

$$\hat{\lambda}_V / \hat{\lambda}_{II} = 1.55/1.003 = 1.55.$$

This works because the risk for social class I in the denominator of $\hat{\lambda}_V$ and $\hat{\lambda}_{II}$ simply cancels out:

$$\frac{\text{risk}_V}{\text{risk}_I} \div \frac{\text{risk}_{II}}{\text{risk}_I} = \frac{\text{risk}_V}{\text{risk}_{II}}.$$

To test for a significant overall effect of the risk factor on disease, we apply the chi-square test, (2.1), with $\ell - 1$ d.f. to the $\ell \times 2$ table.

3.6.1   Continuous risk factors

The ideas of relative risk and odds ratio are so attractive that it is natural to want to specify one or the other for all the risk factors in an epidemiological study. Whenever the relationship between risk factor and the disease is shown in a table, this is straightforward. If the data are continuous (or discrete with several outcomes), tables are not feasible for the raw data. Instead, tables of manageable size may be derived by grouping the continuous risk factor. Relative risks or odds ratios may then be derived from the grouped table.

The grouping has drawbacks. Inevitably, considerable information on the risk factor is lost; for example, we do not know how risk varies within each group. Also, different ways of grouping can produce quite different results and inferences. This phenomenon may easily be seen from a simple artificial example.

Example 3.12 Table 3.10 shows a risk factor with three levels, 1, 2 and 3, representing increasing doses. Suppose that we decide to group the three levels into two. If we combine 1 and 2 as 'low dose', leaving 3 as 'high dose', then the relative risk (high compared with low dose) is, from (3.2),

$$\frac{189/200}{197/210} = 1.01.$$

We conclude that the dose has little effect; high dose increases risk by a negligible amount.

On the other hand, if 1 is low dose and 2 and 3 are combined to define high dose, then the relative risk becomes

$$\frac{385/400}{1/10} = 9.6,$$

which is almost 10 times as big as before; we now conclude that high dose increases risk. Obviously, the choice of cut-off for high dose has made a considerable difference. Even though this is an extreme example, the problem could arise whenever grouping is performed.

A similar problem occurs when hypothesis tests are used; one grouping system may produce a significant effect, say at the 5% level of significance, whereas another does not. In fact, this happens in Example 3.12, using the chi-square test with Yates's correction and Fisher's exact test as appropriate.

So as to avoid the possibility of a biased selection (a choice that leads to a desired result), an objective method of grouping is preferable. In some situations, we may be able to use some pre-existing standard system of grouping; for example, there is a standard international classification system for body mass index (weight divided by the square of height), a measure of excess body fat (World Health Organization, 1995).

Table 3.10. Hypothetical results of a study of risk factor dose.

Risk factor	Disease status		
dose	Disease	No disease	Total
1	1	9	10
2	196	4	200
3	189	11	200
Total	386	24	410

Another objective way of grouping is to divide the data into groups of equal size. This has the statistical advantage of providing maximum power when one group is compared with another. This might be achieved by simply dividing the range of values taken by the risk factor into equal parts. In practice, this rarely gives groups of even approximately equal size because of nonuniformity in distribution of the risk factor. Instead, the quantiles of the risk factor are found and used as the cut-points that define the groups. For example, the three quartiles define four equal groups, called the **fourths** or **quarters.** Unfortunately, modern practice has often been to use the term 'quartiles' to represent both the cut-points and the groups they define. This confusing double meaning is avoided in this book.

A further question then arises: how many groups should be used? There is no simple answer. Taking few groups means that much information is lost; for instance, we cannot possibly discover any evidence of curvature in the relationship between risk factor and disease if we take only two groups. On the other hand, many groups will be hard to interpret and will inevitably result in wide overlapping confidence intervals (for risk, etc.), unless the sample size is large. In practical epidemiological research, it is rare to find more than five groups used.

Example 3.13 Table 3.11 shows data from the follow-up (cohort) phase of the Scottish Heart Health Study (SHHS) (Tunstall–Pedoe *et al.,* 1997). Here, the 4095 men who had their cholesterol measured and were free of CHD at baseline are classified by cholesterol and CHD status, whether or not they developed CHD in the 6 years after their cholesterol was measured. The continuous variable cholesterol has been grouped into its fifths; the quintiles that define the limits of these fifths are 5.40, 6.00, 6.55 and 7.27 mmol/l. Notice that the fifths are not quite the same size due to multiple values at the quintiles.

Here the first fifth has been taken as the base group (relative risk = 1) and all other fifths are compared with this using (3.2), (3.5), (3.6) and (3.7) repeatedly. Risk clearly increases with increasing cholesterol. At the 5% level, no significant difference (in risk) can be seen between the second and first or between the third and first fifths, but a significant difference exists between the fourth and first and between the fifth and first fifths.

3.6.2   A test for linear trend

When the risk factor is defined at ℓ levels, we have seen that the chi-square test, (2.1), can be used to test association. Essentially, this is a test of the null hypothesis

$$H_0 : R_1 = R_2 = R_3 = ... = R_\ell$$

against H_1: they are not all equal, where the R values represent the risks at each of the ℓ levels. An equivalent formulation may be made in terms of odds. Under H_0 all ℓ

Table 3.11.   Total serum cholesterol and CHD status from the SHHS follow-up.

Cholesterol fifth	Disease status CHD	No CHD	Total	Relative risk (95% CI)
1	15 (1.85%)	798	813	1
2	20 (2.46%)	794	814	1.33 (0.69, 2.58)
3	26 (3.18%)	791	817	1.72 (0.92, 3.23)
4	41 (4.96%)	785	826	2.69 (1.50, 4.82)
5	48 (5.82%)	777	825	3.15 (1.78, 5.59)
Total	150 (3.66%)	3945	4095	

Note: CI = confidence interval.

risks are equivalent to some overall average risk. In epidemiology, we are often interested in **dose–response effects** — that is, situations in which an increased value of the risk factor means a greater likelihood of disease. As discussed in Section 1.6.3, this would provide meaningful evidence of a causal relationship.

It is possible to use the chi-square approach to test for a dose–response trend whenever the ℓ levels of the risk factor are graded (that is, the risk factor is ordinal, or at least treated as such). The theory behind the procedure is based upon the ideas of simple linear regression (Section 9.3.1). Consequently, we should denote the result as a test of *linear* trend. See Armitage (1955) for details of the theory and Maclure and Greenland (1992) for a general discussion of the methodology. Although the previous paragraph talked about increasing risk, the direction of trend could be positive or negative. Negative trend means an increasing protective effect of the risk factor; for instance, increasing blood levels of vitamin D have been hypothesised to give increased protection against certain diseases.

To apply the test, we need, first, to assign representative scores for each level of the risk factor. These should reflect the rank ordering; for example, the social class groupings in Table 2.2 could be labelled from 1 (class I) to 6 (class V). Table 3.12 displays the theoretical form of the data.

The test statistic, for the test of linear trend, is

$$X^2_{(L)} = \left\{ T_1 - \left(n_1 T_2 / n \right) \right\}^2 \Big/ V, \tag{3.19}$$

where

$$T_1 = \sum_1^{\ell} a_i x_i \quad T_2 = \sum_1^{\ell} m_i x_i \quad T_3 = \sum_1^{\ell} m_i x_i^2 \tag{3.20}$$

and

$$V = n_1 n_2 \left(n T_3 - T_2^2 \right) \Big/ n^2 (n-1) \tag{3.21}$$

and the remaining variables are defined by Table 3.12. We compare $X^2_{(L)}$ against chi-square with 1 d.f.

Table 3.12. Display of data from a dose–response study.

Risk factor level (score)	Disease status Disease	No disease	Total
x_1	a_1	b_1	m_1
x_2	a_2	b_2	m_2
.	.	.	.
.	.	.	.
.	.	.	.
x_ℓ	a_ℓ	b_ℓ	m_ℓ
Total	n_1	n_2	n

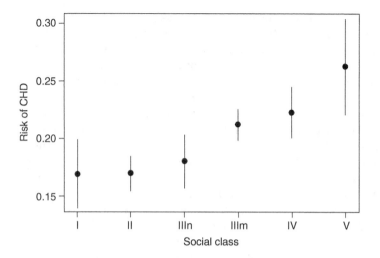

Figure 3.2. Prevalence risks (with 95% confidence intervals) for CHD by social class; SHHS.

Example 3.14 Figure 3.2 shows the risks for prevalent CHD (with confidence intervals), calculated from (3.1) and (3.3), for the SHHS social class data of Table 2.2. There is clear indication of a trend here (see also the related Figure 2.3). Scoring social class from 1 to 6, we have, from (3.20),

$$T_1 = 100 \times 1 + 382 \times 2 + 183 \times 3 + 668 \times 4 + 279 \times 5 + 109 \times 6$$

$$= 6134$$

$$T_2 = 592 \times 1 + 2254 \times 2 + 1017 \times 3 + 3150 \times 4 + 1253 \times 5 + 415 \times 6$$

$$= 29506$$

$$T_3 = 592 \times 1 \times 1 + 2254 \times 2 \times 2 + 1017 \times 3 \times 3 + 3150 \times 4 \times 4$$

$$+ 1253 \times 5 \times 5 + 415 \times 6 \times 6 = 115426.$$

Then, from (3.21),

$$V = \frac{1721 \times 6960 \left(8681 \times 115426 - 29506^2 \right)}{8681^2 \times 8680} = 2406.3357.$$

Hence, (3.19) gives

$$X^2_{(L)} = \frac{\left(6134 - 1721 \times 29506 / 8681 \right)^2}{2406.3357} = 33.63.$$

From Table B.3, $\chi^2_1 = 10.8$ at the 0.1% level. Hence, the test is highly significant: there is evidence of a linear trend.

When the levels are defined by groups, as in Example 3.13, the conventional epidemiological approach is to use the rank scores 1, 2, 3, ..., just as in Example 3.14. The trend in question then represents a consistent rise in risk from group to successive group (fifth to successive fifth in Example 3.13). A more meaningful test may be to test for a consistent rise across the range of the risk factor. In this case we should use a numerical summary score that represents the location of each group. The median value of the risk factor within the group is a sensible choice.

The overall chi-square test (with $\ell - 1$ d.f.) and that for linear trend (with 1 d.f.) may well give opposite results. For instance, the overall test may not be significant ($p > 0.05$), but the linear test highly significant ($p < 0.001$). This means that, although the risks in the ℓ groups are never very different from their overall average, they do tend to systematically increase (or decrease). Evidence of a trend is a more powerful indication of causality than is evidence of an association.

3.6.3 A test for nonlinearity

Sometimes the relationship between the risk factor and disease is nonlinear. For example, it could be that low and high doses of the risk factor are harmful compared with average doses. Such a U-shaped relationship has been found by several authors who have investigated the relationship between alcohol consumption and death from any cause (see, for example, Duffy, 1995).

To test for a nonlinear relationship, we calculate the difference between the overall chi-square test statistic, (2.1), and the trend test statistic, (3.19). This difference is compared against chi-square with d.f. given by the difference in the d.f. of these two components, $(\ell - 1) - 1 = \ell - 2$ d.f. This gives a test for *any* nonlinear relationship. In Section 9.3.3 and Section 10.7.4, we shall consider some specific nonlinear relationships within the context of statistical modelling.

Example 3.15 The chi-square test statistic, (2.1), for the data in Table 2.2 turns out to be 36.40. In Example 3.14, we found the test statistic for linear trend, $X^2_{(L)} = 33.63$. Hence, the test statistic for nonlinear trend is $36.40 - 33.63 = 2.77$. Compared against chi-square on $6 - 2 = 4$ d.f., this is not significant ($p = 0.60$). Hence, we have found no evidence that the risk of prevalent CHD rises in anything but a linear fashion as we go down the social scale, from highly advantaged to highly disadvantaged.

3.7 Attributable risk

Although the relative risk is very useful as a measure of the relative importance to the disease of the risk factor, it does not tell us the overall importance of that risk factor. For instance, Kahn and Sempos (1989) report results from the Framingham study that show the relative risk of coronary heart disease to be 2.8 for those with systolic blood pressure of 180 mmHg or more compared with others, whereas the relative risk for cigarette smoking is only 1.9. Hence, it might appear that it would be more important to target health education measures to reduce hypertension than to reduce smoking.

This is not necessarily true because we must also take account of the prevalence of the risk factors. In a population in which hypertension is very rare but smoking is common, the overall impact on heart disease of reducing the prevalence of high blood pressure will be minimal, although it would be extremely important to reduce smoking (we will address this comparison in Example 3.17). What is required is a measure that combines relative risk and the prevalence of the risk factor: the **attributable risk** or **aetiologic fraction**. This will measure the proportion of cases of disease attributable to the risk factor.

As with the relative risk, epidemiologists generally reserve the term 'attributable risk' to refer to disease incidence. Consider, then, Table 3.1 as the results of an incidence study; suppose that the n individuals are a random sample from the background population who are followed up over time to record cases of disease. If exposure to the risk factor were removed, then everyone would experience the risk of the nonexposed group, which is $c/(c + d)$. Hence, we would expect to have an overall proportion of $c/(c + d)$ cases of disease; that is, we would expect $nc/(c + d)$ cases of disease amongst the n people. In fact, we have $a + c$ cases, so the excess number of cases attributable to the risk factor is

$$(a + c) - \frac{nc}{c + d}. \tag{3.22}$$

The attributable risk (denoted θ) is then estimated by

$$\hat{\theta} = \frac{1}{a + c}\left\{(a + c) - \frac{nc}{c + d}\right\} = \frac{r - r_{\bar{E}}}{r}. \tag{3.23}$$

Here r is the overall risk of disease and $r_{\bar{E}}$ is the risk in the unexposed group for the sample data. Both are calculated by (3.1); that is, $r = (a + c)/n$ and $r_{\bar{E}} = c/(c + d)$.

Approximate 95% confidence limits for the attributable risk are given by

$$\frac{(ad - bc)\exp(\pm u)}{nc + (ad - bc)\exp(\pm u)}, \tag{3.24}$$

where $\pm$ is replaced by a minus sign for the lower limit and a plus sign for the upper limit, and

$$u = \frac{1.96(a + c)(c + d)}{ad - bc}\sqrt{\frac{ad(n - c) + c^2b}{nc(a + c)(c + d)}}. \tag{3.25}$$

As usual, we replace 1.96 by the appropriate critical value from the normal distribution in (3.25) whenever we wish to derive confidence intervals for some percentage other than 95%. As with the odds ratio and relative risk, other methods for calculating approximate confidence limits have been developed. The limits in (3.24) were suggested by Leung and Kupper (1981). They have been found to produce shorter confidence limits than other simple methods across the majority of likely values for θ (see Whittemore, 1983).

Example 3.16 In Example 3.1, $r = 0.013876$ and $r_{\bar{E}} = 0.007903$. The attributable risk of a cardiovascular death for smoking is thus estimated to be, from (3.23),

$$\hat{\theta} = \frac{0.013876 - 0.007903}{0.013876} = 0.430.$$

Thus, 43% of the risk of a cardiovascular death is estimated to be attributable to smoking.

From (3.25) and by reference to Table 3.1 and Table 3.2,

$$u = \frac{1.96 \times 46 \times 1898}{31 \times 1883 - 1386 \times 15} \sqrt{\frac{31 \times 1883(3315 - 15) + 15^2 \times 1386}{3315 \times 15 \times 46 \times 1898}}$$

$$= 0.95988.$$

Then, from (3.24), approximate 95% confidence limits for the attributable risk are

$$\frac{\{31 \times 1883 - 1386 \times 15\} \exp(\pm\, 0.95988)}{3315 \times 15 + \{31 \times 1883 - 1386 \times 15\} \exp(\pm\, 0.95988)},$$

giving the 95% confidence interval (0.224, 0.664) or, in percentage terms, 22 to 66%.

Notice that (3.22) is the excess number of cases in the *sample*; if we require an estimate of the excess number of cases in the *population*, we should multiply $\hat{\theta}$ and its confidence limits by the total number of cases of disease in the population. Most often we would do this for a national population for which the number of cases would be recorded in official routine statistics.

As the derivation of (3.23) suggests, the *population* (as opposed to the sample) attributable risk is

$$\theta = \frac{R - R_{\bar{E}}}{R}, \tag{3.26}$$

where R and $R_{\bar{E}}$ are the population equivalents of the sample values of r and $r_{\bar{E}}$, respectively. An alternative definition, derived from (3.26) using probability theory, is

$$\theta = \frac{p_E(\lambda - 1)}{1 + p_E(\lambda - 1)}, \tag{3.27}$$

where p_E is the probability of exposure to the risk factor and λ is, as usual, the relative risk (exposed versus unexposed). This definition shows explicitly how the attributable risk combines the relative risk and the prevalence of the risk factor. When we have sample data, we substitute sample estimates of p_E and λ into (3.27), as usual.

Note that θ is defined only when $\lambda > 1$. Although we can always invert the numerator and denominator risks making up λ to ensure that $\lambda > 1$, we may wish to see how many, or what proportion of, cases of disease are prevented by a protective risk factor. Kleinbaum *et al.* (1982) describe the appropriate methodology for this situation.

Table 3.13 illustrates how θ depends upon p_E and λ, using (3.27) repeatedly. If the risk factor is rare and has little relative effect on the disease, then the attributable risk is low. If the risk factor is common and has a large relative risk, then the attributable risk is high. Within these extremes, a considerable attributable risk can occur when the relative risk is low, provided the risk factor is common, or when the risk factor is fairly rare, provided the relative risk is high.

Often, (3.27) is used to produce an estimated θ when the procedure represented by (3.23) cannot be applied. This includes the situation in which a case–control study

Table 3.13. Attributable risk[a] for various values of the relative risk and prevalence[a] of the risk factor.

Prevalence (%)	Relative risk							
	1.5	2	2.5	3	4	5	10	15
1	0.5	1.0	1.5	2.0	2.9	3.8	8.3	12.3
5	2.4	4.8	7.0	9.1	13.0	16.7	31.0	41.2
10	4.8	9.1	13.0	16.7	23.1	28.6	47.4	58.3
20	9.1	16.7	23.1	28.6	37.5	44.4	64.3	73.7
30	13.0	23.1	31.0	37.5	47.4	54.5	73.0	80.8
40	16.7	28.6	37.5	44.4	54.5	61.5	78.3	84.8
50	20.0	33.3	42.9	50.0	60.0	66.7	81.8	87.5
60	23.1	37.5	47.4	54.5	64.3	70.6	84.4	89.4
70	25.9	41.2	51.2	58.3	67.7	73.7	86.3	90.7
80	28.6	44.4	54.5	61.5	70.6	76.2	87.8	91.8
90	31.0	47.4	57.4	64.3	73.0	78.3	89.0	92.6
95	32.2	48.7	58.8	65.5	74.0	79.2	89.5	93.0
99	33.1	49.7	59.8	66.4	74.8	79.8	89.9	93.3

[a] Expressed as a percentage.

has been carried out (Section 6.2.4). Occasionally, we might combine data from other studies to estimate θ. For instance, if we wished to estimate the national attributable risk for cardiovascular death due to smoking in Thailand, we might use the estimate of λ from Example 3.1 (the Thai EGAT study) and combine this with an estimate of p_E (here, the proportion of smokers) from a national smoking survey. This would be necessary because, although the relative risk, λ, from the EGAT occupational study might well be a good estimate of the national relative risk (Section 5.1.4), the proportion of smokers amongst EGAT workers (a relatively affluent and well-educated group) is almost certainly not a good estimate of the national Thai equivalent. The confidence limits given in (3.24) would, however, no longer be valid (see Leung and Kupper, 1981).

The next example shows how prevalence data from the cross-sectional (baseline) phase of the SHHS can be combined with pre-existing data to estimate the attributable risks for high blood pressure and smoking used as examples earlier. Of course, once follow-up data from the SHHS (as described in Section 5.2) are available, the SHHS can be used to estimate incidence rates and θ without regard to other studies. This example supposes that an estimate of θ is required at the time of the cross-sectional study when only prevalence risks may be estimated from the SHHS data.

Example 3.17 Shewry *et al.* (1992) used data from the initial phase (22 districts) of the SHHS to estimate the prevalence of cigarette smoking amongst middle-aged Scotsmen to be 0.392. At the time of this publication, no incidence data were available from the study. Table 3.14 shows corresponding data on systolic blood pressure. From this, the prevalence of high blood pressure

Table 3.14. Systolic blood pressure in the initial phase of the SHHS.

Systolic blood pressure	Number
Low (under 180 mmHg)	4920
High (180 mmHg or more)	124
Total	5084

(as defined here) is estimated to be 124/5084 = 0.024. If we suppose that the CHD relative risks of 2.8 for high blood pressure and 1.9 for cigarette smoking from the Framingham study (as stated in Kahn and Sempos, 1989) are appropriate to middle-aged Scottish men, then (3.27) allows the attributable risks in Scotland to be estimated.

The results are, for high blood pressure,

$$\frac{0.024(2.8-1)}{1 + 0.024(2.8-1)} = 0.04;$$

for cigarette smoking,

$$\frac{0.392(1.9-1)}{1 + 0.392(1.9-1)} = 0.26.$$

Thus, we estimate that 26% of the male cases of CHD in Scotland are attributable to cigarette smoking, but only 4% to high (systolic) blood pressure. Notice that this contrast is despite high blood pressure's higher relative risk.

Unfortunately, the term 'attributable risk' does not have a standard meaning. For example, Schlesselman (1982), amongst others, defines it to be the difference between the risks in the exposed and unexposed groups. Hence, caution is required when interpreting published results. Frequently, it is useful to define a second type of attributable risk, which relates only to those exposed to the risk factor. By the same argument as used earlier, the attributable risk amongst only those exposed to the risk factor in the population is

$$\frac{R_E - R_{\bar{E}}}{R_E} = \frac{\lambda - 1}{\lambda},$$

where R_E is the risk in the exposed group, estimated by $a/(a + b)$.

Although the attributable risk is conventionally computed by assuming that the exposure is binary (i.e. yes/no), many risk factors have, at least approximately, a linear relationship with risk, usually on the logarithmic scale. For example, the threshold of 180 mmHg used in Example 3.17 for SBP is really an arbitrary one, and, indeed, is far higher than would be used in modern definitions of 'hypertension' (these definitions, themselves, differ across jurisdictions). The relationship between SBP and CHD has been shown to be log-linear in that the relative risk comparing two SBP levels the same distance apart is the same) from SBP levels at least as low as 115 mmHg upwards. In such cases, it can make more sense to consider the attributable risk, in any specific setting (say a country), by reference to how much greater the mean level of the risk factor is to that setting (country) with the lowest mean value, i.e., by comparison to what is known as the **theoretical-minimum-risk exposure**. Details are beyond the scope of this book: see Lopez *et al.* (2006).

Finally, notice that attribution does not necessarily imply causation, even though θ will often be interpreted in this way. For instance, we might use Example 3.17 to conclude that 26% of coronary cases would be avoided if cigarette smoking were to cease. If, however, a third factor is involved, which causes smoking and CHD, then the conclusion will be overoptimistic. Similarly, another risk factor (such as stress) may become more important as smoking is removed, again causing the conclusion to be overoptimistic. In general, this is a problem of confounding (Chapter 4); see Benichou (2001), Gefeller (1992) and Whittemore (1983) for discussions of this issue and solutions. A further issue is that the effect of smoking is not instantly reversible; even if someone stops smoking now, a residual ill effect may persist for several years. In some situations, the risk effect may not be at all reversible in the current population.

3.8   Rate and relative rate

Our definition of risk in Section 3.1 uses the proportion who have disease among so many individuals at risk. In some situations, we know the number who have disease but do not know the exact number at risk; that is, we know the numerator but not the denominator required to find the risk. Instead, we may have an estimate of the number at risk, typically the mid-year population of the at-risk group. This gives rise to the estimate of a disease **rate**,

$$\hat{\rho} = e/p, \qquad\qquad (3.28)$$

where e is the number of events (a count of the number of cases of disease) and p is the mid-year population. This equation generalises the definition of the prevalence rate given by (1.1), when the disease count is at a particular time, and of the incidence rate given by (1.2), when the disease count is the number of new cases within a particular time period. In general, the rate and the risk will be different, although if events are unusual, one will be a good approximation of the other.

Example 3.18 Table 3.15 gives data on the male population of Scotland in 1995. These data come from routine sources, including death registrations and the Census. The final two columns are calculated using (3.28), giving a cause-specific and overall mortality rate, respectively, for each 5-year age group. The mid-year population acts as the denominator for both of these incidence rates.

   If the disease events occur randomly and independently, a reasonable assumption is that their number follows a Poisson distribution (Clarke and Cooke, 2004). Assuming that the denominator is a fixed known quantity, the estimated standard error of the disease rate is then

$$\hat{se}(\hat{\rho}) = e/\sqrt{p}.$$

Table 3.15. Demographic data and derived mortality rates for Scotsmen in 1995.

Age group (years)	Number of deaths CHD	Number of deaths Total	Mid-year population	Mortality rate (per thousand) CHD	Mortality rate (per thousand) Total
40–44	81	419	166 582	0.5	2.5
45–49	190	736	173 587	1.1	4.2
50–54	294	1010	141 048	2.1	7.2
55–59	515	1613	131 738	3.9	12.2
60–64	823	2531	121 420	6.8	20.8
65–69	1222	3724	108 649	11.2	34.3

Source: General Register Office for Scotland (Crown Copyright).

We can find approximate 95% confidence limits for the number of events, (e_L, e_U), from

$$e_L = \left(\frac{1.96}{2} - \sqrt{e} \right)^2,$$

$$e_U = \left(\frac{1.96}{2} + \sqrt{e+1} \right)^2,$$

(3.29)

giving 95% confidence limits for the disease rate of (ρ_L, ρ_U) where

$$\rho_L = e_L/p,$$

$$\rho_U = e_U/p.$$

(3.30)

This uses a normal approximation, which works well for $e > 100$. Different percentage confidence limits are, as usual, obtained by replacing 1.96 by the appropriate percentage point in (3.29). Exact values of (e_L, e_U) come from tables of the Poisson distribution: see Altman *et al.* (2000).

Suppose that we have data from two groups. For example, group 1 might be those exposed, and group 2 those unexposed, to some risk factor. In group 1, there are e_1 events, the mid-year population is p_1 and the estimated disease rate is thus $\hat{\rho}_1 = e_1/p_1$ and similarly for group 2 with '2' subscripts. The estimated **relative rate**, group 2 compared with group 1, is then

$$\hat{\omega} = \frac{\hat{\rho}_2}{\hat{\rho}_1} = \left(\frac{p_1}{p_2} \right) \left(\frac{e_2}{e_1} \right).$$

(3.31)

Consider the probability that, when an event occurs, it occurs in group 2. Call this quantity π. From sample data, it is estimated by

$$\hat{\pi} = e_2/(e_1 + e_2).$$

(3.32)

An approximate 95% confidence interval for π comes from (2.2). Let the 95% confidence limits be (π_L, π_U). Comparing (3.31) and (3.32) shows that

$$\hat{\omega} = \left(\frac{p_1}{p_2} \right) \left(\frac{\hat{\pi}}{1 - \hat{\pi}} \right).$$

Thus, the 95% confidence limits (ω_L, ω_U) for the relative rate are

$$\omega_L = \left(\frac{p_1}{p_2} \right) \left(\frac{\pi_L}{1 - \pi_L} \right),$$

$$\omega_U = \left(\frac{p_1}{p_2} \right) \left(\frac{\pi_U}{1 - \pi_U} \right).$$

(3.33)

Table 3.16. Demographic data for Scots aged
40–59 years in 1995.

	CHD deaths	Mid-year population
Women	306	634 103
Men	1080	612 955

Source: General Register Office for Scotland (Crown
Copyright).

Example 3.19 Suppose that we wished to compare national male and female coronary death
rates amongst 40- to 59-year-olds in Scotland. Table 3.16 gives relevant data (the male data
may also be derived from Table 3.15).

Considering 1995 as a sample year, we can estimate coronary death rates by sex group and
the relative rate of coronary death. From (3.28), the rate for men is 1080/612955 = 1.76 per
thousand. From (3.29), the 95% confidence limit for the number of male deaths is (e_L, e_U) where

$$e_L = \left(\frac{1.96}{2} - \sqrt{1080} \right)^2 = 1016.548,$$

$$e_U = \left(\frac{1.96}{2} + \sqrt{1081} \right)^2 = 1146.402.$$

Hence, using (3.30), the 95% confidence interval for the male coronary death rate is obtained
by dividing each of the preceding by 612 955 — that is, (1.66, 1.87) per thousand. Similar
calculations give the estimated female coronary rate (with 95% confidence interval) as 0.483
(0.430, 0.540) per thousand.

The estimated coronary death relative rate for men compared with women is, from (3.31),

$$\hat{\omega} = \frac{634103}{612955} \times \frac{1080}{306} = 3.65.$$

As expected, except for rounding error, this is equal to the ratio of the male and female rates
(that is, 1.76/0.483). Middle-aged men are thus 3.65 times as likely to die from a coronary attack
as are women, in Scotland.

The estimated proportion of coronary deaths that are male is $\hat{\pi} = 1080/(1080 + 306) = 0.77922$,
from (3.32). An approximate 95% confidence interval (π_L, π_U) for the proportion of deaths that
are male comes from (2.2):

$$\pi_L = 0.77922 - 1.96\sqrt{0.77922(1 - 0.77922)/1386}$$

$$= 0.77922 - 0.02184 = 0.75738;$$

and so

$$\pi_U = 0.77922 + 0.02184 = 0.80106.$$

From (3.33), the 95% confidence interval for the coronary death relative rate, comparing men to women, is (ω_L, ω_U) where

$$\omega_L = \frac{634103}{612955} \times \frac{0.75738}{1 - 0.75738} = 3.23,$$

$$\omega_U = \frac{634103}{612955} \times \frac{0.80106}{1 - 0.80106} = 4.17.$$

In many cases, a reasonable assumption is that the relative rate is a good approximation to the relative risk. Then, by analogy with (3.27), an attributable risk might be estimated from data on disease rates as

$$\frac{\hat{p}_E(\hat{\omega} - 1)}{1 + \hat{p}_E(\hat{\omega} - 1)}.$$

3.8.1   *The general epidemiological rate*

So far we have looked at rates in which the denominator is the population at risk. More generally, an epidemiological rate is any quotient where the denominator is assumed to be fixed and the numerator is a count of the number of events, this being a random variable. The estimated rate compares the observed value of the numerator to this fixed denominator. The denominator does not need to be in the same units of measurement as the numerator, although the comparison achieved must have some physical interpretation to be useful. In Section 5.6, we shall see another kind of epidemiological rate in which the denominator is the number of person-years of observation.

3.9   Measures of difference

The relative risk, odds ratio and relative rate are *proportionate* comparative measures of chance. Such measures seem the most natural because chance itself is conventionally measured proportionately. However, difference measures may also be used; indeed, some epidemiologists argue that these are preferable (see Poole, 2010). The **risk difference** (sometimes called the **absolute risk difference**) for cardiovascular death in Example 3.1, smokers compared with nonsmokers, is $0.021877 - 0.007903 = 0.013974$. The risk of a cardiovascular death is thus around 0.014 (that is, 14 chances in 1000) higher for smokers compared with nonsmokers. Sometimes, this is phrased from the viewpoint of prevention and termed the **absolute risk reduction** — here, abstinence from smoking leads to an absolute risk reduction of 0.014. A 95% confidence interval for the risk difference may be calculated using (2.5).

When relative risk and risk difference are compared between populations or subgroups of a single population, we can get completely different inferences. Whenever 'background' risk is larger, any specific absolute increase will be associated with a smaller proportionate increase. Take a simple situation in which a study population has exposed and unexposed groups of the same size: 100. Suppose the risk of disease in the unexposed group is low, say 1 in 100; then two extra deaths in the exposed group make the relative risk, $(3/100)/(1/100) = 3$ and the risk difference, $(3/100) - (1/100) = 2/100$, or 2 per hundred. Consider another study population that also has 100 in each group, but a higher rate of disease, say 1 in 10, in the unexposed group.

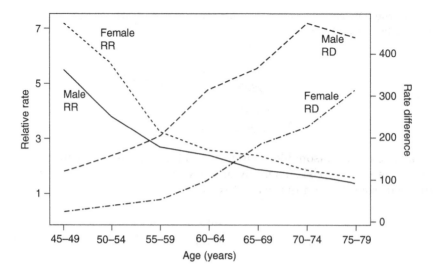

Figure 3.3. Relative rate (RR) and rate difference (RD) (per 100 000 per year) for coronary heart disease by age group (45- to 79-year-olds) and sex, comparing current smokers to never-smokers; American Cancer Prevention Study II.

Two extra deaths in the exposed group make the relative risk 1.2, much smaller than before, but leave the risk difference unchanged at 2 per 100.

Figure 3.3 shows a more extreme example, this time using rates from real data on current cigarette smokers and lifetime never-smokers in the American Cancer Society's Second Cancer Prevention Study (National Cancer Institute, 1997). From this figure, we see that if we choose relative rate as our epidemiological measure of excess risk, we conclude that women, at all ages shown, have higher excess risk of heart disease from smoking than men, and that this excess risk decreases with age. On the other hand, if we use the rate difference, we get completely the opposite conclusions for the sex and age comparisons.

It is important to understand why the patterns in Figure 3.3 have occurred and thereby to understand the difference between relative and absolute measures. The difference between the rates for smokers and never-smokers is small amongst young women, presumably because the smokers have a short history of smoking and so have been exposed to a minor cumulative dose. However, the rates are low amongst young women because it happens that heart disease is not very prevalent amongst this group. The result is that the small absolute extra risk for smokers creates a large relative risk amongst young women. The reverse is true for old men.

When we wish to make comparisons between groups for which the background risk varies appreciably, it may be best to calculate an absolute and a relative measure of excess chance of disease. These measures could be based on risks, rates, odds or similar metrics.

3.10   EPITAB commands in Stata

Stata has a suite of so-called EPITAB commands that carry out most of the standard epidemiological procedures covered in this chapter, as well as some of those in Chapter 4 to Chapter 6 (see also Section 4.10). The CS command will produce risks, relative risks, risk differences, odds ratios, attributable risks (overall and amongst those exposed) and *p* values from chi-square or Fisher's exact tests. An 'immediate'

Output 3.1. Results from CSI in Stata for the data of Table 3.2.

	Exposed	Unexposed	Total
Cases	31	15	46
Noncases	1386	1883	3269
Total	1417	1898	3315
Risk	.0218772	.0079031	.0138763

	Point estimate	[95% Conf. Interval]
Risk difference	.0139741	.0053788 .0225695
Risk ratio	2.768196	1.500194 5.107944
Attr. frac. ex.	.6387539	.3334196 .8042265
Attr. frac. pop	.4304646	
Odds ratio	2.807744	1.50989 5.221191(Woolf)

chi2(1) = 11.58 Pr>chi2 = 0.0007

form of this, CSI, will even allow the four numbers in the basic epidemiological table, Table 3.1, to be entered as part of the command rather than requiring a dataset to be 'opened'. Output 3.1 shows the results from using CSI applied to the data in Table 3.2. From this we can see several results already reported in Section 3.1, Section 3.5, Section 3.7 and Section 3.9. The commands used to create Output 3.1 are included on the web site for this book.

Some other commands in this suite are the IR (with immediate form IRI) command, which deals with rates (Section 3.8), whilst the CC (and CCI) command is similar to CS (and CSI) but is suitable for unmatched case–control studies and the MCC (and MCCI) command is suitable for matched case–control studies (Chapter 6). In some cases the computations of confidence limits improve on the approximate equations, which are more suitable for hand computation, provided in this book.

Exercises

3.1 The following table shows data from a random sample of middle-aged men taken in Kuopio, Finland (Kauhanen *et al.*, 1997). A beer binger is defined as someone who usually drinks six or more bottles of beer per drinking session. This was recorded at the outset of the study; mortality was recorded from death certificates over an average of 7.7 years' follow-up.

Beer binger?	Cardiovascular death?		
	Yes	No	Total
Yes	7	63	70
No	52	1519	1571
Total	59	1582	1641

(i)   Estimate the risks of cardiovascular death for bingers and for nonbingers, together with 95% confidence intervals.

(ii)   Estimate the relative risk of cardiovascular death for bingers compared with nonbingers, together with a 95% confidence interval.

(iii)   Estimate the odds of cardiovascular death for bingers and for nonbingers.

(vi)   Estimate the odds ratio for cardiovascular death for bingers compared with nonbingers, together with a 95% confidence interval.

(v)   Test the null hypothesis that beer binging has no relationship with cardiovascular death.

(vi)   Estimate the attributable risk of cardiovascular death for beer binging, together with a 95% confidence interval.

3.2   From an investigation into asthma in seven primary schools in the South of England, Storr et al. (1987) reported data on 55 pupils with asthma. Twenty of these pupils lost 10 days or more of schooling over the previous year. Of these 20, 8 had parents who provided adequate medication. A further 35 pupils with asthma lost less than 10 days of schooling; 4 of these had parents who provided adequate medication. Use Fisher's exact test to see whether the time lost from school is unrelated to the provision of adequate medication. Interpret your result.

3.3   In a Danish study of healthy mothers (Tetzchner et al., 1997), urinary incontinence and pudendal nerve terminal motor latency (PNTML) were recorded 12 weeks after delivery. PNTML was recorded as high if it was in excess of the normal range for the relevant laboratory; otherwise, it was low. Of the 17 women with high PNTML, 6 were incontinent; of the women with low PNTML, 19 were incontinent and 110 were not.

(i)   Estimate the relative risk for incontinence, comparing high against low PNTML, and find the associated 95% confidence interval for the true relative risk.

(ii)   Estimate the odds ratio for incontinence, comparing high against low PNTML, and find the associated 95% confidence interval for the true odds ratio.

(iii)   Test the null hypothesis that PNTML has no effect on incontinence.

(iv)   Estimate the attributable risk for incontinence ascribable to high PNTML, and compute the associated 95% confidence interval.

3.4   Refer to the total columns of Table C.1 in Appendix C, which contains summary data from the third Glasgow MONICA survey.

(i)   Estimate the prevalence risks of cardiovascular disease (CVD) by factor IX status for each sex.

(ii)   Estimate the prevalence relative risk for high compared with low factor IX, together with 95% confidence limits for each sex.

(iii)   Repeat (i), but for odds.

(iv)   Repeat (ii), but for the odds ratio.

(v)   Test whether factor IX has an effect on CVD for men and women separately.

(vi)   Interpret all your results.

3.5   Wilson and McClure (1996) give the data shown in the following table on the number of babies of extremely low birthweight (less than 1000 g) admitted to a regional neonatal intensive care unit on the first day of life. 'Survival' means that the baby was discharged alive; gestational age was estimated from the date of the last menstrual period, fetal ultrasonography and physical examination of the baby.

Calculate the chi-square test statistics for effect of gestational age:
(i)   Overall
(ii)   Linear trend
(iii)   Nonlinear
Interpret your results. (*Hint*: In calculating (ii) use x values of 0, 1, 2, 3, 4, 5 and 8 to ease computation.)

Gestational age (weeks)	Number of babies	Number of survivors
23	4	0
24	12	5
25	16	9
26	17	10
27	13	12
28	5	4
29–33	10	10

3.6 In the second Cancer Prevention Study in the U.S., 578 027 adult women with complete reproductive histories were followed up for 7 years (Calle *et al.*, 1995). Of 425 599 women without a history of spontaneous abortions, 951 died from breast cancer. For women who had experienced one spontaneous abortion, 208 out of 101 773 died from breast cancer; for two spontaneous abortions, 54/32 887 died from breast cancer; for three or more spontaneous abortions, 34/17 768 died from breast cancer.
(i)   Estimate the risk of death from breast cancer for women who have had at least one spontaneous abortion, and compute the associated 99% confidence interval.
(ii)   Estimate the relative risk for those who have had at least one, compared with those who have had no, spontaneous abortions, and compute the associated 99% confidence interval.
(iii)   Test for a significant linear trend in the percentage dying from breast cancer. To do this, you need to assume some average in the 'three or more' group. In order to provide a verifiable calculation, you may take this to be four.

3.7 Pearson *et al.* (1991) studied the uptake of well-woman clinics in Liverpool. The following table shows the number of attendees in 1986, together with the estimated 1986 mid-year population of Liverpool (provided by the City Council), by 10-year age groups.

Age group (years)	Clinic attendees	Liverpool population
15–24	36	40 941
25–34	88	33 350
35–44	95	29 014
45–54	47	25 381
55–64	27	28 382
65–74	4	25 750

(i)   Find the age-specific attendance rates per thousand population.
(ii)   Find a 95% confidence interval for the rate per thousand in the 35- to 44-year age group.
(iii) Find the relative rates for each of the other age groups compared with the 15- to 24-year group.
(iv)   Find a 95% confidence interval for the relative rate comparing women aged 35 to 44 years with women aged 15 to 24 years.

CHAPTER 4

Confounding and interaction

4.1 Introduction

In the last chapter we were concerned with only two variables: the risk factor and the disease status. Often a third factor may have an important influence on the apparent relationship between these two variables. If the third factor can explain (at least partially) this relationship, then **confounding** is present. For instance, a relationship between the number of children and prevalent breast cancer for a sample of mothers may be explained by the ages of the mothers: older mothers tend to have more children and also have a greater chance of having contracted breast cancer. Age is then the third factor that explains the observed relationship between number of children and breast cancer. The effect (upon breast cancer) of multiple childbearing is confounded with the effect of age.

If, instead, the third factor modifies the relationship between risk factor and the disease, then **interaction** is present. For instance, suppose that the relationship between salt consumption and cerebrovascular disease (stroke) is quite different for men and women; perhaps women with relatively high salt intakes have a moderately elevated risk of stroke compared to other women, whereas men with high salt intake have substantially greater risk than do other men. Sex would then be the third factor that modifies the relationship between salt and stroke. Sex would be said to interact with salt consumption in determining the risk of a stroke.

The issues of confounding and interaction need to be considered whenever an epidemiological study is designed or analysed. Consideration of likely confounding and interaction effects is necessary even before a study is begun because analytical methods to deal with confounding or interaction can only be applied if data on the specific third factor are collected. In most cases, there will not be a single potential confounding variable or a single potential interaction variable. Thus, the term 'third factor' could refer to a set of factors.

Although confounding and interaction are very different phenomena, they are often confused. Part of the reason for this is that we may be unsure, at the stage of designing a study, whether a particular variable that we decide to record has a confounding or interactive effect on the specific relationship that we wish to study. Indeed, we may have several risk factors that we decide to measure, and part of the study aims is to decide which risk factors are confounded and which interact with others in regard to the disease outcome of interest. Methods for detecting and dealing with confounding and interaction are described in Section 4.2 to Section 4.6; interaction is considered in Section 4.7 to Section 4.9.

4.2   The concept of confounding

A confounding variable, or **confounder**, is an extraneous factor that wholly or partially accounts for the observed effect of the risk factor on disease status. The 'effect' here could be an apparent relationship or an apparent lack of relationship. In the first case, the confounder is causing the relationship to appear; in the second, the confounder is masking a true relationship. Two hypothetical examples will illustrate how these situations could arise.

Example 4.1 Table 4.1 shows the cross-tabulation of risk factor status (exposure/no exposure in these examples) and disease outcome for a hypothetical prospective study of 320 subjects. Using the methodology of the previous chapter and, specifically, (3.1) and (3.2), we find that the relative risk of disease (exposure versus not) is 5.52. This is formally significant ($p < 0.0001$), from (3.15). Hence, we conclude that the risk factor does, indeed, have an effect on disease.

However, suppose that we also have data on a third variable, a potential confounding factor denoted by C. Again, suppose we simply recorded whether C was present or absent for each subject. Table 4.2 shows the relationship between the risk factor and disease separately for those individuals with C present and those with C absent. In the former case, both those exposed and unexposed to the risk factor have a risk of disease of 0.1 and hence the relative risk is 1. In the latter case, the two risks are 0.8 and hence the relative risk is also 1. When considered within levels of C, the supposed risk factor has absolutely no effect on the disease. The apparent relationship, seen in Table 4.1, is entirely explained by confounding with C.

Careful inspection of the tables shows why the confounding occurs: presence/absence of the confounder and the risk factor tend to go together. C is, itself, a risk factor for the disease with a relative risk (for presence versus absence) of

$$\frac{\left(80 + 8\right)\big/\left(80 + 8 + 20 + 2\right)}{\left(1 + 20\right)\big/\left(1 + 20 + 9 + 180\right)} = 8.$$

When we think that we are seeing the effect of the risk factor, we may really be seeing the effect of C.

Table 4.1. Risk factor status by disease status in Example 4.1.

Risk factor status	Disease status		
	Disease	No disease	Risk
Exposed	81	29	0.7364
Not exposed	28	182	0.1333
Relative risk			5.52

Table 4.2. Risk factor status by disease status by confounder (C) status in Example 4.1.

Risk factor status	Confounder absent			Confounder present		
	Disease	No disease	Risk	Disease	No disease	Risk
Exposed	1	9	0.1000	80	20	0.8000
Not exposed	20	180	0.1000	8	2	0.8000
Relative risk			1.00			1.00

Table 4.3. Risk factor status by disease status in Example 4.2.

Risk factor status	Disease status		
	Disease	No disease	Risk
Exposed	240	420	0.3636
Not exposed	200	350	0.3636
Relative risk			1.00

Table 4.4. Risk factor status by disease status by confounder (C) status in Example 4.2.

Risk factor status	Confounder absent			Confounder present		
	Disease	No disease	Risk	Disease	No disease	Risk
Exposed	135	415	0.2455	105	5	0.9545
Not exposed	5	45	0.1000	195	305	0.3900
Relative risk			2.45			2.45

Example 4.2 Table 4.3 shows results from another hypothetical prospective study. This time, before we consider the confounder, the potential risk factor has absolutely no effect: the risk is the same whether it is present or absent. In Table 4.4, the three-way cross-classification identifies that, on the contrary, exposure to the risk factor is more likely to lead to disease: in fact, 2.45 times as likely. Indeed, if we apply formal hypothesis tests, using (3.15), to either of the subtables of Table 4.4, the relative risk is significantly different from unity ($p = 0.03$ and $p < 0.0001$, respectively). This relationship is entirely masked by the confounder, C, in the simple analysis of Table 4.3.

In this example, the presence of the confounder tends to go with the absence of the risk factor whilst the absence of the confounder tends to go with the presence of the risk factor. As in Example 4.1, C is, itself, a risk factor for the disease. The relative risk, C present versus C absent, is

$$\frac{\left(105 + 195\right)/\left(105 + 195 + 5 + 305\right)}{\left(135 + 5\right)/\left(135 + 5 + 415 + 45\right)} = 2.11.$$

In Table 4.3, exposure to the risk factor and C are effectively cancelling each other out.

When there is **perfect confounding**, the relative risks (or other estimates of relative chance of disease) for the various levels (there need not be only two) of the confounder are the same, and this common value is different from the relative risk when the confounding variable is ignored. Example 4.1 and Example 4.2 illustrate perfect confounding. Indeed, they are quite extreme examples of perfect confounding because, in each case, there appears to be no effect of the risk factor (relative risk of 1) or a substantial effect, depending on the analysis. Generally, confounding is more likely to lead to underestimation or overestimation of an effect, unless it is controlled for (as in the next example).

Perfect confounding is extremely unlikely in real-life epidemiological data. Furthermore, approximations to perfect confounding are neither necessary nor sufficient for confounding to be present. The degree of confounding may be much more marginal

Table 4.5. Housing tenure by CHD outcome after 6 years; SHHS men.

| | CHD? | | |
Housing tenure	Yes	No	Risk
Rented	85	1821	0.0446
Owner-occupied	77	2400	0.0311
Relative risk			1.43

Table 4.6. Housing tenure by CHD outcome after 6 years by cigarette smoking; SHHS men.

| | Nonsmokers | | | Smokers | | |
Housing tenure	CHD	No CHD	Risk	CHD	No CHD	Risk
Rented	33	923	0.0345	52	898	0.0547
Owner-occupied	48	1722	0.0271	29	678	0.0410
Relative risk			1.27			1.33

or less consistent across the subtables. We can be sure, however, that confounding is not an important issue whenever the estimates in the different levels, or **strata**, of the confounder are all very similar and are also not very different from the overall estimate. As we shall discover in Section 4.7, if the estimates differ substantially by strata and no stratum has a small sample size, then interaction is present and should be allowed for.

Example 4.3 Table 4.5 shows data from 6 years' follow-up of men in the Scottish Heart Health Study (SHHS). These data are for those with no symptoms of coronary heart disease (CHD) at the beginning of the study. The variable 'housing tenure' records whether they rent or own their accommodation. As can be seen, the chance of a CHD event is substantially higher amongst the renters.

When this study began, housing rental in Scotland was predominantly a feature of the more disadvantaged social groups. The more disadvantaged tend to have a less healthy lifestyle, and hence the question arises as to whether the risk of renting is explained by confounding with lifestyle. In particular, 57% of the renters but only 35% of the owner–occupiers smoke cigarettes, and cigarette smoking is a well-established risk factor for CHD.

Table 4.6 shows Table 4.5 split by cigarette smoking status. As before, living in rented housing seems to be a risk factor. However, its effect has been reduced (because of the smaller relative risks), once we account for smoking. Certainly, confounding is present here because a similar reduction has occurred in each stratum. Since the reductions are minor, we can conclude that the degree of confounding is small.

Confounding can arise in real-life data because of an interrelationship between the variables in general or because of the way in which the data were collected. For instance, if (antisocial) drug taking and heavy (alcoholic) drinking tend to go together, then the effects of drug taking on any alcohol-related disease are sure to be confounded by the effects of heavy drinking. This is an example of a general relationship leading to confounding.

On the other hand, consider an intervention study of the effect of an active prophylactic drug compared with placebo. Suppose that the patients selected to receive the active drug, by chance, turned out to be predominantly male; patients on the placebo, by contrast, are predominantly female. Suppose that the disease is more likely in men.

Then we should expect to find that the drug does not perform as well as it should because its effect is confounded with that of sex. Notice that we would not have expected this type of confounding if there had not been the sex bias in drug allocation; hence, this is confounding by design. In the extreme case in which everyone in one treatment group is male and everyone in the other is female, the effects of drug and sex are indistinguishable, or **aliased**. Clearly, this would be a very poor study design.

4.3   Identification of confounders

In our discussion so far, we have looked at only the basic concepts and some possible consequences of confounding. Here we shall consider what conditions are necessary before a variable may be considered a confounder. Let us denote the disease by D, the risk factor by F and the third variable by C. If C is to be a confounder it must:

- Be related to the disease, but not be a consequence of the disease.
- Be related to the risk factor, but not be a consequence of the risk factor.

After Schlesselman (1982), path diagrams will be used to illustrate situations in which C is and is not a confounder of the F–D relationship. The arrows show relationships that exist regardless of all other relationships inherent in the path diagram. Double-sided arrows are used to denote noncausal relationships; single-sided arrows show the direction of causality.

Figure 4.1 shows three of the possible situations wherein C is a confounder, and Figure 4.2 gives particular examples. Figure 4.2(a) is an oft-quoted example of confounding. Grey hair tends to be related to any disease, such as stroke, that is age related. However, this does not mean that grey hair is a risk factor for such diseases; it is simply caused by the ageing process. The other two examples in Figure 4.2 were introduced earlier. In Figure 4.2(c), it is supposed that house renting is not causally related to CHD, but rather that other causal factors besides smoking are present that are also confounded with renting. If it is, indeed, the fact of renting that is causal, then the F–D arrow should be single-sided, pointing at CHD. There would still be confounding with smoking.

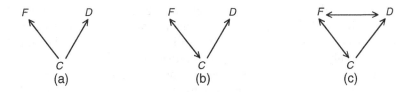

Figure 4.1. Some situations in which C is a confounder for the F–D relationship.

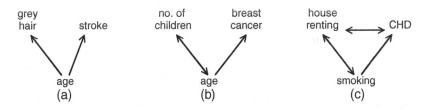

Figure 4.2. Some examples that may fit the situations in Figure 4.1.

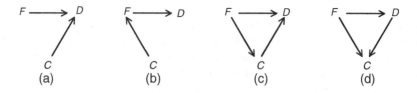

Figure 4.3. Some situations in which C is not a confounder for the F–D relationship.

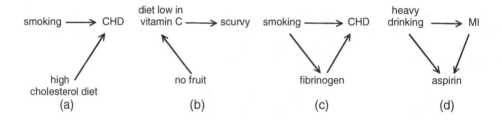

Figure 4.4. Some examples that may fit the situations in Figure 4.3.

The example of the prophylactic intervention study in Section 4.2 is of type (c), whilst the example relating antisocial drugs and alcohol is of type (b) or type (c). In two of the three examples in Figure 4.2, the confounder is age, which is the most common confounding variable in epidemiological investigations.

Figure 4.3 illustrates four possible situations in which C is *not* a confounder; Figure 4.4 gives a potential example for each case. To see why C is not a confounder, it is useful to consider the consequence of controlling (adjusting) the F–D relationship for C. In Section 4.4 to Section 4.6, we shall see how to carry out adjustments; the technical details are not important at this stage.

The most straightforward situation is (a), where F and C act independently. It would not be incorrect to control for C here, but it would serve no purpose. The example given supposes that the effects of smoking and a diet rich in cholesterol are independent with regard to CHD. In (b), C causes D only through the intermediate agent, F. Not eating fruit causes a low intake of vitamin C, which causes scurvy. In (c) and (d), F causes C. Thus, in (c), smoking and fibrinogen are both risk factors for CHD, but smoking promotes increased fibrinogen. Controlling smoking for fibrinogen would not be sensible because this would, effectively, mean controlling the effect of smoking for part of itself. In (d), the added feature is that D causes C. People who have had myocardial infarction (MI) are routinely advised to take aspirins to help avoid a recurrence. Controlling any risk factor (such as heavy drinking) associated, causally or noncausally, with aspirin-taking would not be sensible because this is, effectively, controlling the effect on disease for a consequence of the disease itself. Hence, (d) fails on two counts.

4.3.1   A strategy for selection

As the foregoing has shown, what makes something a confounder depends upon data-based observed relationships and *a priori* knowledge of the supposed biological processes at work. In order to decide which variables are potential confounders, path diagrams need to be considered for all candidate variables. Figure 4.5 summarises the necessary conditions; Figure 4.1 and Figure 4.3 are special cases.

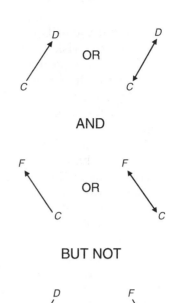

Figure 4.5. Conditions for C to be a confounder for the F–D relationship.

Any variable that satisfies the conditions in Figure 4.5 should be considered as a confounder. If we are not sure about the positive aspects, but know that the negative ones are false, then nothing is wrong with proceeding as if confounding occurs and subsequently assessing whether this was really worthwhile (using the methods presented in Section 4.4). For this reason, all known risk factors for the specific disease are potential confounders; this should be borne in mind at the stage of study design. Similarly, age and sex are always worth considering, when appropriate.

4.4   Assessing confounding

Once the data have been collected, we can use analytical methods to assess the effect of any variable that is a potential confounder. As in other problems, we can choose to use analytical techniques based upon estimation or hypothesis tests. The former is preferable because it is the most straightforward and the most meaningful.

4.4.1   Using estimation

We can assess confounding by estimating the effect of the risk factor with and without allowing for confounding. For instance, in Example 4.3 the relative risk of renting is 1.43 unadjusted, and around 1.30 (the average over the two strata) after adjustment for smoking. We would then estimate the effect of confounding as E_C/E, where E is the unadjusted, and E_C is the adjusted, estimate. In the example, this is $1.30/1.43 = 0.91$; adjustment has reduced the relative risk by 9%

One problem with this approach is that the answer will depend upon the measure of comparative chance of disease (exposed versus not exposed) that is used. An extensive description of this issue is given by Miettinen and Cook (1981). For example, consider the use of odds ratios, rather than relative risks, as the measure of comparative chance of disease in Example 4.2. The unadjusted odds ratio is 1.00, the same as the relative risk, but the odds ratios by strata are 2.93 and 32.85, which are very different from the relative risks and from each other. On the other hand, the assessment of confounding by comparing relative risks and by comparing odds ratios will be similar whenever the disease is rare (see Section 3.3). Thus, in Example 4.3, the odds ratios are 1.45 (unadjusted) and 1.28 and 1.35 in the smoking groups. Because these are very similar to the relative risks, the value of E_C/E will be much the same by both criteria.

The method of stratification, used in Example 4.1 to Example 4.3, provides separate estimates (of whatever parameter is used to represent the relative chance of disease) by strata. The arithmetic mean, over the strata, may be used to represent E_C, but there are several better ways of deriving an adjusted estimate. In Section 4.5 and Section 4.6, we shall discuss methods of adjustment based on tables (non-parametric methods); in Chapter 9 to Chapter 11, we shall see how to use statistical models for adjustment.

For simplicity, all the examples so far have considered binary confounding and risk factor variables. The methods of adjustment presented in this chapter will handle confounding variables with many levels; the modelling methods of later chapters will also cope with continuous variables. However, when the risk factor has more than two levels, there is no single measure of confounding E_C/E because this will vary by the levels being compared. The best strategy is to present sets of estimates, unadjusted (or, perhaps, adjusted only for nonmodifiable risk factors, such as age) and adjusted, side by side. The reader can then judge the effects of confounding. Of course, if confounding has little effect, then one set of estimates will suffice.

Example 4.4 Table 4.7 presents unadjusted and age-adjusted coronary event rates and risks of death subsequent to a coronary event, for men in north Glasgow, 1991, by socioeconomic (deprivation) group. These data will be described and the numerical results derived in Example 4.6 and Example 4.8.

Coronary event rates not only change quite considerably after adjustment, but also change in rank order (group IV is highest after adjustment; group III was highest before). Hence, adjustment has had an important effect here, and it is useful to present the unadjusted and adjusted values (see also Figure 4.6). The risks of coronary death, on the other hand, remain much the same and retain the same overall pattern after adjustment. In this case, there is little point in presenting both sets of values; adjustment has clearly had virtually no effect. We conclude that age is a confounder for the deprivation-event, but not the deprivation-death, relationship.

4.4.2   Using hypothesis tests

As in other situations (see Section 3.5.5), hypothesis tests by themselves are of limited use. The situation is worse here because no direct test for successful confounding is available.

Table 4.7. Coronary event rates and risk of death by deprivation group; north Glasgow men in 1991.

Deprivation group	Coronary event rate (per thousand)		Risk of coronary death	
	Unadjusted	Age adjusted	Unadjusted	Age adjusted
I (most advantaged)	2.95	3.28	0.57	0.59
II	4.32	4.20	0.50	0.50
III	6.15	5.30	0.51	0.52
IV (least advantaged)	5.90	5.75	0.56	0.56

What we can do is test whether F and D are related after the adjustment for C has been made; that is, we can test for an adjusted relationship between F and D, often interpreted as an **adjusted effect** of F on D. We might compare the result to a similar test before adjustment has been made. If, for example, F is highly significantly related to D before adjustment ($p < 0.001$), but not after adjustment (say, $p > 0.1$), then the evidence is that the confounder has really had an effect. Conversely, when there is still a significant effect of F on D after adjustment for C, we may infer that F has an effect on D over and above any effect of C. Such a significant adjusted effect is often called an **independent effect** by epidemiologists, especially when the effect of F has been adjusted for all (other) known risk factors for D simultaneously (Section 4.4.3). Note that this is not the same as **statistical independence**, which signifies that the risk of disease given exposure to F is exactly the same whether or not a person has also been exposed to C.

The word of caution expressed in Section 3.5.5 needs reiterating: the results of hypothesis tests depend upon sample size. Thus, a significant adjusted effect could be simply a reflection of a large study sample. The very act of allowing for the confounder has an effect on the overall estimate of unexplained (background) variation, and thus the effective sample size is different before and after adjustment. If the confounder has several missing values, we may even have used different actual sample sizes for the unadjusted and adjusted tests and hence will not even be comparing like with like when we compare the tests.

4.4.3 Dealing with several confounding variables

For simplicity, the foregoing examples have taken the situation in which only one confounding variable is present; in practice there could be several. The analytical methods for dealing with one confounder may easily be extended to the case of several confounders: for example, stratification (as used in Example 4.1 to Example 4.3) would use all the confounders simultaneously. Thus, if we consider smoking (yes/no) and exercise (coded as seldom/sometimes/often/very often) as confounders for the relationship between housing tenure and CHD in Example 4.3, we would define $2 \times 4 = 8$ strata and corresponding subtables (see also Example 4.12).

The interpretation of the effect of several confounders is much less straightforward. The effect of any one confounder may be quite different when a second confounder is also considered. For instance, it might be that coffee drinking is a confounder for the relationship between smoking and some specific type of cancer. However, perhaps controlling for coffee drinking has no effect when the smoking–cancer relationship has already been controlled for alcohol consumption. This may be because coffee and alcohol are related. On the other hand, if the smoking–cancer relationship is adjusted for, say, coffee and tea drinking simultaneously, it could be that there is no (joint) confounding effect. Coffee may be a confounder, but not in conjunction with tea, possibly because coffee and tea drinking are inversely related.

In essence, the problem here is that of confounding (or interaction) of confounders, and the causes may be more subtle than the simple examples given previously may suggest. In general, we cannot necessarily predict what the joint or adjusted effects of two confounders will be simply from observing their relationship to each other and their individual relationships to the disease. It is how they affect the relationship between risk factor and disease that is crucial.

As with the effect of any one confounder, the best way to assess joint confounding is to compare unadjusted and adjusted estimates. 'Adjusted' here could encompass adjustments for each single confounder, all possible pairs, all possible triples, etc. In practice, this will often be too unwieldy, especially for presentation purposes. Often the most useful adjustment will be that for all the potential confounders simultaneously: for

Table 4.8. Odds ratios (95% confidence intervals) for myocardial infarction by cigarette smoking habit amongst men aged 30 to 54 living in the northeast U.S.

Smoking habit	Unadjusted	Age adjusted	Multiple adjusted[a]
Never smoked	1	1	1
Ex-smoker	1.5 (1.0, 2.2)	1.1 (0.7, 1.7)	1.2 (0.8, 1.9)
<25 per day	2.1 (1.4, 3.2)	2.1 (1.4, 3.1)	2.5 (1.6, 3.9)
25–34 per day	2.5 (1.6, 3.8)	2.4 (1.5, 3.7)	2.9 (1.8, 4.7)
35–44 per day	4.1 (2.7, 6.4)	3.9 (2.5, 5.9)	4.4 (2.8, 7.1)
≥45 per day	4.4 (2.8, 7.0)	4.0 (2.5, 6.4)	5.0 (3.1, 8.3)

[a] Adjusted for age; geographic region; drug treatment for hypertension; history of elevated cholesterol; drug treatment for diabetes mellitus; family history of myocardial infarction or stroke; personality score; alcohol consumption; religion and marital status.

example, all previously well-established risk factors for the disease. However, we should be aware that this may include some redundant confounders and may hide some interesting and useful facts about interrelationships.

Example 4.5 Kaufman *et al.* (1983) describe a case–control study of cigarette smoking as a risk factor for MI, which was carried out in parts of Connecticut, Massachusetts, New York and Rhode Island. Table 4.8 gives their results for different levels of smoking; these are as reported, except that the unadjusted results have been calculated from figures supplied in their article, using (3.9) and (3.12). This table gives data for 501 cases of MI and 827 controls (subjects with no MI).

Adjustment for age reduces the effect of smoking, but adjustment for the complete set of potential confounders identified by Kaufman *et al.,* increases the effect (except amongst ex-smokers). The downward effect of age as a confounder is swamped by the upward effect of one or more of the other confounders. With the information available, we cannot investigate this further. Clearly we can say that current smoking has a real effect on MI, regardless of the effect of age or of the other potential confounders taken together. Kaufman and colleagues sensibly include a test of dose–response amongst current smokers. This is reported as statistically significant ($p < 0.001$) after both age and multiple adjustment.

Whenever several variables are recorded in addition to disease status, it may be that each in turn will be considered as *the* risk factor with all the remaining variables as confounders. In different situations, any specific variable may act as the risk factor or as one of the confounders (perhaps the only one).

4.5   Standardisation

The method of *standardisation* deals with confounding by choosing a **standard population**, with a known distribution of the confounding variable, and evaluating the theoretical effect of the risk factor, as observed in the study population, on the standard population. In this way, the effect of the particular distribution of the confounding variable in the study population is removed.

The vast majority of practical applications of standardisation occur when the confounding variable is age, leading to **age standardisation**. Sometimes sex standardisation is employed concurrently, leading to **age/sex standardisation**. This is a standard tool in demography (see Pollard *et al.,* 1990), for example, when comparing death rates between communities. The classic example of the need for age standardisation in demographic analyses is the comparison of mortality rates between a seaside resort and an industrialised town. The former tends to have higher death rates despite its healthier environment; the explanation is that elderly people tend to retire to the seaside. Age standardisation tends to reverse the ranking of these two death rates.

In epidemiology, standardisation is often used in a very similar way. As in the preceding example, it is generally used to facilitate meaningful comparisons between two or more groups. Instead of all-causes death rates, cause-specific death rates, morbidity rates, hospitalisation rates, referral rates, etc. may be standardised. Although age standardisation is most usual, standardisation for any variable is possible as long as the distribution of this variable is known.

This leads to consideration of what population to choose as the standard. The choice is essentially arbitrary, as long as the standard can be considered typical of the type of population(s) under study. Various artificial standard populations have been constructed including Segi's synthetic World Standard Population; see the discussion at http://www3.who.int/whosis/discussion_papers/pdf/paper31.pdf.

Otherwise, the standard population is usually chosen to be a superset of the study populations to be compared or one of the study populations. Hence, if we wished to compare cancer rates by towns in the U.S., we might choose the entire population of the U.S. as the standard, or we might take one of the study towns as the standard. Unfortunately, the choice of the standard can affect the results considerably, so using a superpopulation or universal standard is preferable because they are more objective.

For simplicity, the remainder of this section will deal with standardisation for age. Other variables would be handled similarly. Standardisation may be applied to event rates or risks. Rates are dealt with in Section 4.5.1 and Section 4.5.2; risks are discussed in Section 4.5.3. Throughout, we shall assume that the effect on disease of whatever risk factor is investigated is reasonably homogeneous across age groups. If not, interaction will occur between the risk factor and age (see Section 4.7) and standardisation is inappropriate.

4.5.1   Direct standardisation of event rates

The **direct standardised event rate** is the number of events (for example, deaths) that would be expected in the standard population if the age-specific event rates in the study population prevailed, divided by the size of the standard population. To avoid small numbers, this is usually multiplied by 1000.

Let the superscript s denote the standard population. Suppose that the study and standard populations have been subdivided into the same set of age groups (say, 0 to 9, 10 to 19, 20 to 29 years, etc.). Let e_i be the number of events in the ith age group of the study population; p_i be the size of the ith age group of the study population; $p_i^{(s)}$ be the size of the ith age group of the standard population and $p^{(s)} = \sum p_i^{(s)}$ be the total size of the standard population. Then, the direct age standardised event rate per thousand is

$$\mathrm{dsr} = \frac{1000}{p^{(s)}} \sum \left(\frac{e_i}{p_i} \right) p_i^{(s)}. \tag{4.1}$$

If we assume that the observed number of events, e_i, has a Poisson distribution, then the standard error of the direct standardised rate is

$$\mathrm{se(dsr)} = \frac{1000}{p^{(s)}} \left\{ \sqrt{\sum e_i \left(\frac{p_i^{(s)}}{p_i} \right)^2} \right\}. \tag{4.2}$$

An approximate 95% confidence interval for the direct standardised rate is

$$\text{dsr} \pm 1.96\text{se(dsr)}.$$

An exact method for obtaining a confidence interval is given by Dobson *et al.* (1991).

Example 4.6 Morrison *et al.* (1997) describe an investigation into the variation of CHD rates by social class groups in north Glasgow using data collected as part of the World Health Organization MONICA Study (Tunstall–Pedoe, 2003). All north Glasgow residents aged 25 to 64 years were included in the investigation; here we will consider only men and only one of the years covered by the study. That part of Glasgow north of the River Clyde was divided into four areas of differing degrees of deprivation but roughly equal population size. The level of deprivation was determined from 1991 census data on key neighbourhood characteristics (McLoone, 1994).

Table 4.9 shows the number of coronary events and population size (from the population census) by age and ranked deprivation group (I = least disadvantaged; IV = most) in 1991. Also shown is Segi's World Standard Population for this age range. This will be used as the standard population here; reasonable alternatives would be the Scottish male population at the 1991 Census or the total male population of north Glasgow.

Table 4.9 also shows the crude event rate (the total number of events divided by the total population size) per thousand in each deprivation group. There is an increase from groups I to II to III but a drop from III to IV. It may be that this break in the pattern is due to age differences within the deprivation groups. Group III has a relatively older age structure (see Table 4.9) and CHD rates are well known to increase with age. Hence, it seems sensible to remove the age effect by standardising each of the four rates for age, so as to produce a more meaningful comparison.

This is simple, but tedious, to achieve using (4.1). Spreadsheet packages can handle such repeated calculations very efficiently. For illustration, consider the direct age standardised rate per thousand for deprivation group III. From (4.1) this is

$$\frac{1000}{45}\left(\frac{0}{4351} \times 8 + \frac{0}{3232} \times 6 + \frac{1}{2438} \times 6 + \frac{9}{2241} \times 6 \right.$$

$$\left. + \frac{17}{2360} \times 6 + \frac{19}{2708} \times 5 + \frac{43}{2968} \times 4 + \frac{53}{2802} \times 4 \right) = 5.30.$$

Similar calculations give the set of standardised rates, by increasing rank of deprivation group, of 3.28, 4.20, 5.30 and 5.75 per thousand. These increase with rank, so we can conclude that the chance of a male CHD event increases with worsening deprivation, once age differences are taken account of.

From (4.2), the standard error of the standardised rate for deprivation group III is

$$\frac{1000}{45}\left\{ \sqrt{0\left(\frac{8}{4351}\right)^2 + 0\left(\frac{6}{3232}\right)^2 + 1\left(\frac{6}{2436}\right)^2 + 9\left(\frac{6}{2241}\right)^2 + 17\left(\frac{6}{2360}\right)^2} \right.$$

$$\left. + 19\left(\frac{5}{2708}\right)^2 + 43\left(\frac{4}{2968}\right)^2 + 53\left(\frac{4}{2802}\right)^2 \right\} = \frac{1000}{45} \times 0.02077 = 0.462.$$

Similarly, the other standard errors are (I) 0.399, (II) 0.451 and (IV) 0.493.

Table 4.9. Coronary events and population by age and deprivation group; north Glasgow men in 1991 and Segi's World Standard Population aged 25–64.

Age group (years)	Deprivation group								World standard popn
	I		II		III		IV		
	Events	Popn	Events	Popn	Events	Popn	Events	Popn	
25–29	0	4 784	0	4 972	0	4 351	0	4 440	8
30–34	0	4 210	0	4 045	0	3 232	1	3 685	6
35–39	1	3 396	4	3 094	1	2 438	5	2 966	6
40–44	6	3 226	7	2 655	9	2 241	10	2 763	6
45–49	7	2 391	13	2 343	17	2 360	15	2 388	6
50–54	16	2 156	11	2 394	19	2 708	24	2 566	5
55–59	17	2 182	28	2 597	43	2 968	28	2 387	4
60–64	25	2 054	44	2 667	53	2 802	56	2 380	4
Total	72	24 399	107	24 767	142	23 100	139	23 575	45
Rate (per thousand)	2.95		4.32		6.15		5.90		

By using (4.1) directly, our solution to Example 4.6 has bypassed a stage that is sometimes useful. As already noted, direct standardisation is the application of **age-specific rates** (that is, rates for each age group) in the study population to the age structure of the standard population. Sometimes the age-specific rates are of interest in their own right and are thus calculated as an intermediate stage. From (3.28), the age-specific rate in age group i is $\hat{\rho}_i = e_i/p_i$. In Example 4.6, we obtain age-specific rates for the four deprivation groups by dividing adjacent columns in Table 4.9. Given the set of age-specific rates for a particular study population, (4.1) becomes

$$\mathrm{dsr} = \frac{1000}{p^{(\mathrm{s})}} \sum \hat{\rho}_i p_i^{(\mathrm{s})},$$

and (4.2) becomes

$$\mathrm{se(dsr)} = \frac{1000}{p^{(\mathrm{s})}} \left\{ \sqrt{ \sum \frac{\hat{\rho}_i}{p_i} (p_i^{(\mathrm{s})})^2 } \right\}.$$

4.5.2   Indirect standardisation of event rates

Indirect standardisation is a two-stage process. First, in contrast to the direct method, the age-specific event rates in the standard population are applied to the study population. This produces the **expected number** of events in the study population. When the observed number of events is divided by this expected number, the result is called the **standardised event ratio** (SER). When events are deaths, this becomes the **standardised mortality ratio** or SMR. Often the SMR is multiplied by 100 for presentation purposes. An SMR below 100 indicates a study population with a mortality rate that is less than the standard, having allowed for age differentials; above 100 means above the standard. This procedure is particularly useful when the standard is the national population and SMRs are calculated for several towns or other geographical areas.

The second stage in calculation of the indirect standardised rate is to multiply the SER by the crude (that is, total) event rate in the standard population. Consequently, the standard rate is adjusted up or down accordingly.

Adding to the notation introduced in Section 4.5.1, let $e = \sum e_i$ be the total number of events in the study population (the observed number of events); $e_i^{(\mathrm{s})}$ be the number of events in the ith age group of the standard population; $e^{(\mathrm{s})} = \sum e_i^{(\mathrm{s})}$ be the total number of events in the standard population; $\rho_i^{(\mathrm{s})} = e_i^{(\mathrm{s})}/p_i^{(\mathrm{s})}$ be the event rate in the ith age group for the standard population; and $\rho^{(\mathrm{s})} = e^{(\mathrm{s})}/p^{(\mathrm{s})}$ be the overall event rate in the standard population. Then, the expected number of events in the study population is

$$E = \sum \rho_i^{(\mathrm{s})} p_i = \sum \left(\frac{e_i^{(\mathrm{s})}}{p_i^{(\mathrm{s})}} \right) p_i. \tag{4.3}$$

By definition,

$$\mathrm{SER} = \frac{\text{observed number of events}}{\text{expected number of events}} = \frac{e}{E}. \tag{4.4}$$

Assuming a Poisson distribution for the observed number of events, e, the standard error of the indirect standardised rate is

$$se(SER) = \frac{\sqrt{e}}{E}. \tag{4.5}$$

If results are to be expressed in percentage form, (4.4) and (4.5) should be multiplied by 100.

As with the direct standardised rate, the indirect rate is often expressed per thousand people. It is then

$$isr = 1000 \times SER \times \rho^{(s)} = 1000 \times SER \times \frac{e^{(s)}}{p^{(s)}}, \tag{4.6}$$

with standard error

$$se(isr) = 1000\rho^{(s)}se(SER) = 1000\rho^{(s)} \frac{\sqrt{e}}{E} = \frac{1000\,e^{(s)}\sqrt{e}}{p^{(s)}E}. \tag{4.7}$$

Note that the SER should not be premultiplied by 100 when using (4.6) and (4.7). See Section 5.7.2 and Section 5.7.3 for more details of SERs.

Example 4.7 The indirect method of standardisation may be applied to the problem of Example 4.6. However, age-specific coronary event rates are not available for the idealised World Standard Population, so a different standard population must be chosen. This time, we shall use an internal standard: the total population over the four deprivation groups. The necessary data, obtained from Table 4.9, are given in Table 4.10.

Table 4.10. Population by age and deprivation group and total number of coronary events by deprivation group; north Glasgow men in 1991.

Age group	Deprivation group populations				Total		
(years)	I	II	III	IV	Events	Pop.	Rate/1000
25–29	4 784	4 972	4 351	4 440	0	18 547	0
30–34	4 210	4 045	3 232	3 685	1	15 172	0.0659
35–39	3 396	3 094	2 438	2 966	11	11 894	0.9248
40–44	3 226	2 655	2 241	2 763	32	10 885	2.9398
45–49	2 391	2 343	2 360	2 388	52	9 482	5.4841
50–54	2 156	2 394	2 708	2 566	70	9 824	7.1254
55–59	2 182	2 597	2 968	2 387	116	10 134	11.4466
60–64	2 054	2 667	2 802	2 380	178	9 903	17.9744
Total	24 399	24 767	23 100	23 575		95 841	
No. of events	72	107	142	139	460		
Rate/1000	2.95	4.32	6.15	5.90			4.7996

Consider calculation of the expected number of events for deprivation group I. By (4.3), this requires multiplication of the right-hand column by the group I population column of Table 4.10. That is, the expected number per thousand is

$$0 \times 4784 + 0.0659 \times 4210 + 0.9248 \times 3396 + 2.9398 \times 3226$$

$$+ 5.4841 \times 2391 + 7.1254 \times 2156 + 11.4466 \times 2182$$

$$+ 17.9744 \times 2054 = 103273,$$

and thus $E = 103.273$. Then, from (4.4) and (4.5), the standardised event ratio is $72/103.273 = 0.6972$ with standard error $\sqrt{72}/103.272 = 0.0822$. Hence, the first deprivation group (the least deprived) has coronary events at around 70% of the rate that is the local norm. Applying (4.6) converts the SER into the indirect standardised event rate,

$$0.6972 \times 4.7996 = 3.35.$$

Notice that we did not need to multiply by a thousand here because $\rho^{(s)} = 4.7996$ is already expressed per thousand (see Table 4.10). By (4.7), the standard error of the indirect standardised rate is $4.7996\sqrt{72}/103.273 = 0.394$.

Similar calculations can be made for the other deprivation groups. The four expected numbers of events are, by increasing rank, 103.273, 118.505, 125.632 and 112.590. The standardised event ratios (with standard errors) are 69.72 (8.216), 90.29 (8.729), 113.03 (9.485) and 123.46 (10.471). The indirect standardised rates (and standard errors) are a constant multiple of the preceding. These are 3.35 (0.394), 4.33 (0.419), 5.42 (0.455) and 5.93 (0.503).

From Example 4.6, the direct standardised equivalents are 3.28 (0.399), 4.20 (0.450), 5.30 (0.462) and 5.75 (0.493), which are very similar but always slightly smaller. Because we have used a different standard population here, we would not expect identical results. In any case, the methods of computation have clear differences.

One useful way of comparing the raw (unadjusted), direct and indirect standardised rates is through the relative rates that they define. For example, choosing deprivation group I to be the 'base' group, we obtain relative indirect standardised rates of 1, 1.29, 1.62, 1.77, by increasing deprivation rank. Figure 4.6 plots the three sets

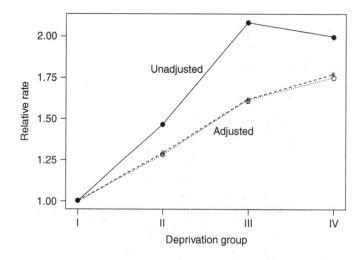

Figure 4.6. Unadjusted (raw) and age-adjusted coronary event relative rates for north Glasgow men in 1991. The dotted line shows adjustment by direct standardisation and the dashed line shows adjustment by indirect standardisation.

of relative rates: the two adjusted sets are virtually indistinguishable. Because deprivation group I (the base group) has the youngest age structure in north Glasgow, failure to account for age differences has exaggerated the relative rates, particularly in deprivation group III.

Although the data used in Example 4.6 and Example 4.7 have permitted direct and indirect standardisation, in some situations the available data may allow only one method to be used. For instance, we may not know the age-specific numbers of events for the desired standard population (in which case the direct method is necessary) or we may not know them for the study population. The latter case sometimes occurs with demographic data from developing countries, when the number of deaths by age is not known very accurately and yet the total number of deaths is known to a reasonable degree of certainty. Only the indirect method, using some suitable standard population with known or assumed age-specific death rates, can be used in this context.

4.5.3   Standardisation of risks

Theoretically, risks could be directly or indirectly standardised, but direct standardisation will be the only method described here. Essentially, the methodology is identical to that already used for rates except that the binomial probability distribution is appropriate rather than the Poisson. As in Section 4.5.1, age-specific values in the study population will be applied to the standard population. Hence, if e_i, $p_i^{(s)}$ and $p^{(s)}$ are as in Section 4.5.1, n_i is the number at risk in the ith age group of the study population and $r_i = e_i/n_i$ is the risk in the ith age group of the study population, then the age-standardised risk is

$$\text{sr} = \frac{1}{p^{(s)}} \sum \left(\frac{e_i}{n_i} \right) p_i^{(s)} = \frac{1}{p^{(s)}} \sum r_i p_i^{(s)}. \tag{4.8}$$

If we assume that the number of events, e_i, out of the number at risk, n_i, has a binomial distribution, then the standard error of the standardised risk is

$$\text{se(sr)} = \frac{1}{p^{(s)}} \left\{ \sqrt{\sum \frac{(p_i^{(s)})^2}{n_i^3} e_i (n_i - e_i)} \right\} \tag{4.9}$$

$$= \frac{1}{p^{(s)}} \left\{ \sqrt{\sum \frac{r_i(1-r_i)}{n_i} (p_i^{(s)})^2} \right\}.$$

If we wish to express the results in percentage form, (4.8) and (4.9) should be multiplied by 100.

Example 4.8 The study of Morrison *et al.* (1997), described in Example 4.6, recorded whether or not each coronary event led to death within 28 days. Table 4.11 shows the numbers of deaths and coronary events within each age and deprivation group. The number of coronary events are shown in Table 4.9. Since only one event was aged below 35, Table 4.11 does not include the 25- to 34-year-olds. To avoid confusion, 'events' are called 'coronaries' in Table 4.11. In this context, the outcome is death. Table 4.11 also shows the crude risks (total number of deaths divided by the total number of men experiencing a coronary attack) in each deprivation group. These show no obvious pattern by deprivation group; is this lack of effect due to confounding by age?

Table 4.11. Number of coronaries and number of coronaries leading to death within 28 days, by age and deprivation group; north Glasgow men in 1991.

Age group (years)	Deprivation group								Total coronaries
	I		II		III		IV		
	Deaths	Coronaries	Deaths	Coronaries	Deaths	Coronaries	Deaths	Coronaries	
35–39	1	1	0	4	1	1	2	5	11
40–44	3	6	4	7	4	9	5	10	32
45–49	4	7	8	13	7	17	6	15	52
50–54	7	16	5	11	10	19	11	24	70
55–59	10	17	12	28	19	43	15	28	116
60–64	16	25	24	44	31	53	38	56	178
Total	41	72	53	107	72	142	77	138	459
Risk	0.569		0.495		0.507		0.558		

To answer this question, we shall calculate age-standardised risks. For example, let us take deprivation group II. From (4.8), the standardised risk for this group is

$$\frac{1}{459}\left(\frac{0}{4} \times 11 + \frac{4}{7} \times 32 + \frac{8}{13} \times 52 + \frac{5}{11} \times 70 + \frac{12}{28} \times 116 + \frac{24}{44} \times 178\right)$$

$$= \frac{228.9091}{459} = 0.499.$$

From (4.9) the standard error of this is

$$\frac{1}{459}\left\{\sqrt{\frac{11^2}{4^3}0(4-0) + \frac{32^2}{7^3}4(7-4) + \frac{52^2}{13^3}8(13-8) + \frac{70^2}{11^3}5(11-5)}\right.$$

$$\left. + \frac{116^2}{28^3}12(28-12) + \frac{178^2}{44^3}24(44-24)\right\} = \sqrt{491.7250}\Big/459 = 0.04831.$$

Similar calculations for the other three groups lead to the full set of standardised risks (and standard errors) by increasing deprivation rank: 0.587 (0.0575), 0.499 (0.0483), 0.520 (0.0409) and 0.558 (0.0418). The age-standardised risks are clearly very similar to the crude risks, so age appears to have a minimal effect (that is, no confounding). The four standardised risks are quite similar, with no gradient by increasing deprivation. Hence, having controlled for age, we can conclude that deprivation seems to have no systematic effect on the chance of survival after a coronary attack. Deprivation seems to be a factor that affects the chance of a coronary event (see Example 4.6 or Example 4.7) but does not affect the subsequent survival.

4.6   Mantel–Haenszel methods

In Example 4.1 to Example 4.3, we considered stratifying the risk factor versus disease table by the levels of the confounding variable. Mantel and Haenszel (1959) took this approach and then considered how best to calculate a summary measure of the odds ratio across the strata. The method they used assumes a common true odds ratio for each stratum; differences in observed odds ratios are purely due to chance variation. Their estimate is now known as the **Mantel–Haenszel estimate** (of the odds ratio).

Consider the subtable for any individual stratum. Table 4.12 introduces the notation that will be used here; the i subscript denotes stratum i. We shall denote

Table 4.12. Display of data for stratum i of the confounding variable.

Risk factor status	Disease status		
	Disease	No disease	Total
Exposed	a_i	b_i	E_i
Not exposed	c_i	d_i	$\bar{E}_i$
Total	D_i	$\bar{D}_i$	n_i

the row totals by E_i (for exposure) and $\bar{E}_i$ (for nonexposure), and the column totals by D_i (for disease positive) and $\bar{D}_i$ (for no disease). Other notation follows the style of Table 3.1.

The Mantel–Haenszel estimate is a weighted average of the odds ratios in the individual strata. The weight for any one stratum is chosen to be equal to the precision, measured as the inverse of the estimated variance, of the odds ratio for that stratum. In this way, the most precise stratum-specific odds ratio gets the largest weight; generally this will tend to give greater weight to the bigger strata, that is the strata with larger n_i.

It turns out (Mantel and Haenszel, 1959) that this results in an estimate of the common odds ratio,

$$\hat{\psi}_{\text{MH}} = \left(\sum \frac{a_i d_i}{n_i}\right) \bigg/ \left(\sum \frac{b_i c_i}{n_i}\right), \tag{4.10}$$

where both summations go over all strata.

In order to derive a confidence interval for this estimate, we need to consider its standard error. Instead, we will consider the standard error of the natural logarithm of $\hat{\psi}_{\text{MH}}$ because this quantity has a more symmetrical distribution that is much better approximated by a normal distribution (just as for the odds ratio in a single stratum; see Section 3.2). Various estimators for the standard error of $\log_e \hat{\psi}_{\text{MH}}$ have been suggested. Robins *et al.* (1986b) show that the following estimator has useful properties:

$$\hat{\text{se}}\left(\log_e \hat{\psi}_{\text{MH}}\right) = \sqrt{\frac{\sum P_i R_i}{2\left(\sum R_i\right)^2} + \frac{\sum P_i S_i + \sum Q_i R_i}{2\sum R_i \sum S_i} + \frac{\sum Q_i S_i}{2\left(\sum S_i\right)^2}}, \tag{4.11}$$

where, for stratum i,

$$\begin{aligned} P_i &= (a_i + d_i)/n_i, & Q_i &= (b_i + c_i)/n_i, \\ R_i &= a_i d_i/n_i, & S_i &= b_i c_i/n_i. \end{aligned} \tag{4.12}$$

The 95% confidence limits for $\log_e \hat{\psi}_{\text{MH}}$ are then

$$\begin{aligned} L_{\log} &= \log_e \hat{\psi}_{\text{MH}} - 1.96\,\hat{\text{se}}\left(\log_e \hat{\psi}_{\text{MH}}\right), \\ U_{\log} &= \log_e \hat{\psi}_{\text{MH}} + 1.96\,\hat{\text{se}}\left(\log_e \hat{\psi}_{\text{MH}}\right); \end{aligned} \tag{4.13}$$

and the 95% confidence limits for $\hat{\psi}_{\text{MH}}$ are thus

$$\begin{aligned} L &= \exp\left(L_{\log}\right), \\ U &= \exp\left(U_{\log}\right). \end{aligned} \tag{4.14}$$

Example 4.9 The data in Table 4.6 involve two strata for the confounder 'smoking status'. For convenience, the data are presented again in Table 4.13 with totals included. Each stratum is now in the form of Table 4.12.

Table 4.13. Data from Table 4.6, with totals.

Housing tenure	Nonsmokers			Smokers		
	CHD	No CHD	Total	CHD	No CHD	Total
Rented	33	923	956	52	898	950
Owner-occupied	48	1722	1770	29	678	707
Total	81	2645	2726	81	1576	1657

Using (4.10), the common odds ratio is estimated by

$$\hat{\psi}_{MH} = \frac{\left(\dfrac{33 \times 1722}{2726}\right) + \left(\dfrac{52 \times 678}{1657}\right)}{\left(\dfrac{923 \times 48}{2726}\right) + \left(\dfrac{898 \times 29}{1657}\right)} = \frac{42.123}{31.969} = 1.32.$$

If we consider the strata individually, we can find the odds ratios from (3.9) as 1.28 (nonsmokers) and 1.35 (smokers). As we would expect, the Mantel–Haenszel summary is somewhere between the two separate estimates; in fact, it is just about in the middle in this example, although this will not always happen.

We can attach confidence limits to $\hat{\psi}_{MH}$ using (4.11) to (4.14). First, we use (4.12) to find

$$P_1 = \frac{33 + 1722}{2726} = 0.6438, \qquad P_2 = \frac{52 + 678}{1657} = 0.4406,$$

$$Q_1 = \frac{923 + 48}{2726} = 0.3562, \qquad Q_2 = \frac{898 + 29}{1657} = 0.5594,$$

$$R_1 = \frac{33 \times 1722}{2726} = 20.85, \qquad R_2 = \frac{52 \times 678}{1657} = 21.28,$$

$$S_1 = \frac{923 \times 48}{2726} = 16.25, \qquad S_2 = \frac{898 \times 29}{1657} = 15.72.$$

Thus

$$\sum P_i R_i = 0.6438 \times 20.85 + 0.4406 \times 21.28 = 22.80,$$

$$\sum P_i S_i = 0.6438 \times 16.25 + 0.4406 \times 15.72 = 17.39,$$

$$\sum Q_i R_i = 0.3562 \times 20.85 + 0.5594 \times 21.28 = 19.33,$$

$$\sum Q_i S_i = 0.3562 \times 16.25 + 0.5594 \times 15.72 = 14.58,$$

$$\sum R_i = 20.85 + 21.28 = 42.13,$$

$$\sum S_i = 16.25 + 15.72 = 31.97.$$

In (4.11), these give

$$\hat{se}(\log_e \hat{\psi}_{MH}) = \sqrt{\frac{22.80}{2 \times 42.13^2} + \frac{17.39 + 19.33}{2 \times 42.13 \times 31.97} + \frac{14.58}{2 \times 31.97^2}} = 0.1649.$$

Then, by (4.13) and (4.14), the confidence interval for $\hat{\psi}_{MH}$ is

$$\exp(\log_e(1.32) \pm 1.96 \times 0.1649);$$

that is, (0.95, 1.82). The smoking-adjusted estimate of the odds ratio for CHD, comparing renters to owner–occupiers, is 1.32 with 95% confidence interval (0.95, 1.82).

4.6.1   The Mantel–Haenszel relative risk

Although Mantel and Haenszel sought to produce only a summary estimate of the common odds ratio over strata, the same basic technique can be used to derive a summary estimate of the common relative risk, assuming that the relative risk is constant across the strata (Tarone, 1981). The formulae that follow are taken from Greenland and Robins (1985).

The Mantel–Haenszel estimate of relative risk is

$$\hat{\lambda}_{MH} = \frac{\sum \left(a_i \bar{E}_i / n_i \right)}{\sum \left(c_i E_i / n_i \right)}. \tag{4.15}$$

The estimated standard error of the logarithm of this is

$$\hat{se}\left(\log_e \hat{\lambda}_{MH}\right) = \sqrt{\frac{\sum \left(E_i \bar{E}_i D_i - a_i c_i n_i \right) / n_i^2}{\left(\sum \left(a_i \bar{E}_i / n_i \right) \right) \left(\sum \left(c_i E_i / n_i \right) \right)}}; \tag{4.16}$$

hence, 95% confidence limits $(L_{\log}, U_{\log})$ for $\log_e \lambda_{MH}$ are

$$
\begin{aligned}
L_{\log} &= \log_e \hat{\lambda}_{MH} - 1.96\ \hat{se}\left(\log_e \hat{\lambda}_{MH}\right), \\
U_{\log} &= \log_e \hat{\lambda}_{MH} + 1.96\ \hat{se}\left(\log_e \hat{\lambda}_{MH}\right),
\end{aligned}
\tag{4.17}
$$

and the 95% confidence limits (L, U) for $\hat{\lambda}_{MH}$ are

$$
\begin{aligned}
L &= \exp\left(L_{\log}\right), \\
U &= \exp\left(U_{\log}\right).
\end{aligned}
\tag{4.18}
$$

Example 4.10 Consider, again, the data in Table 4.13. This time we shall seek to estimate the common relative risk. From (4.15), the Mantel–Haenszel estimate is

$$\hat{\lambda}_{MH} = \frac{(33 \times 1770/2726) + (52 \times 707/1657)}{(48 \times 956/2726) + (29 \times 950/1657)} = \frac{43.614}{33.460} = 1.30.$$

From (4.16), the standard error of the log of λ_{MH} is estimated by $\sqrt{T/B}$, where

$$T = \left(956 \times 1770 \times 81 - 33 \times 48 \times 2726\right)\big/2726^2$$
$$+ \left(950 \times 707 \times 81 - 52 \times 29 \times 1657\right)\big/1657^2$$
$$B = \left(33 \times 1770/2726 + 52 \times 707/1657\right)\left(48 \times 956/2726 + 29 \times 950/1657\right).$$

Hence,

$$\text{standard error} = \sqrt{\frac{17.863 + 18.904}{43.614 \times 33.460}} = 0.1587.$$

Then, by (4.17) and (4.18), the confidence interval for λ_{MH} is

$$\exp(\log_e(1.30) \pm 1.96 \times 0.1587);$$

that is, $(0.95, 1.78)$. The smoking-adjusted estimate of the relative risk of CHD for renters compared with owner–occupiers is 1.30, with 95% confidence interval $(0.95, 1.78)$. Note that, in this case, the Mantel–Haenszel estimate is the same as the arithmetic mean over the strata (Example 4.3). As with the Mantel–Haenszel odds ratio, this will not always be the case and is unlikely to be even approximately true when the sample sizes, n_i, differ substantially across the strata.

4.6.2 The Cochran–Mantel–Haenszel test

Whether odds ratios or relative risks are used to estimate relative propensity for disease, the association between the risk factor and the disease, controlling for the confounder, can be tested using a test attributed to Cochran as well as Mantel and Haenszel.

Within any stratum, when row and column totals are known, knowledge of any one cell in the 2×2 contingency table automatically fixes the other three cells. Hence, the test for no association can be based upon a test of the values in, say, the top left-hand cell of each stratum. Recall that the observed value in this cell is a_i for stratum i. This will be a value from a hypergeometric distribution with expected (that is, mean) value $E(a_i)$ and variance $V(a_i)$ where

$$E(a_i) = \frac{D_i E_i}{n_i}, \qquad V(a_i) = \frac{D_i \bar{D}_i E_i \bar{E}_i}{n_i^2 (n_i - 1)}. \tag{4.19}$$

Notice that the expected value is just what we would compute in the standard chi-square test of no association (Section 2.5.1). If the distribution from which each a_i is derived is not very skewed, we expect the distribution of

$$\frac{\left(\sum a_i - \sum E(a_i)\right)^2}{\sum V(a_i)} \tag{4.20}$$

to be approximately chi-square on one degree of freedom. Here the summations each run over all the strata. We might, instead, use a continuity-corrected (Section 3.5.3) version of (4.20),

$$\frac{\left(\left|\sum a_i - \sum E(a_i)\right| - \frac{1}{2}\right)^2}{\sum V(a_i)}. \tag{4.21}$$

Hence, the test for no residual association between risk factor and disease, after accounting for confounding, is to compare (4.20) or (4.21) with χ_1^2.

Example 4.11 Once more, consider the data in Table 4.13. Here we have, using (4.19),

$$a_1 = 33, \qquad\qquad a_2 = 52,$$

$$E(a_1) = \frac{81 \times 956}{2726} = 28.406, \qquad\qquad E(a_2) = \frac{81 \times 950}{1657} = 46.439,$$

$$V(a_1) = \frac{81 \times 2645 \times 956 \times 1770}{2726^2 \times 2725} = 17.903, \qquad V(a_2) = \frac{81 \times 1576 \times 950 \times 707}{1657^2 \times 1656} = 18.857.$$

Then, using (4.21), the continuity-corrected test statistic is

$$\frac{\left(\left|(33 + 52) - (28.406 + 46.439)\right| - 0.5\right)^2}{17.903 + 18.857} = 2.54.$$

Comparing with Table B.3, we see that this is not significant even at the 10% level. Hence, we conclude that there is no evidence of an association between housing tenure and CHD, after allowing for cigarette smoking status. There is no evidence to refute the hypothesis that the adjusted odds ratio equals 1 (or that the adjusted relative risk is 1).

4.6.3 Further comments

The Mantel–Haenszel approach is based upon an assumption that the parameter representing the comparative chance of disease does not vary by levels of the confounding variable. See Section 4.8 for tests of this assumption.

The confidence interval formulae for Mantel–Haenszel odds ratios and relative risks given here behave well in a range of circumstances; however, other procedures have been suggested that may have the advantage of simplicity or may be more appropriate in a specific situation. A discussion is given by Robins *et al.* (1986b). In particular, when the sample size is small, an exact method of analysis, not employing the normal distribution approximation, will be advisable; see Thomas (1975) and Mehta *et al.* (1985).

The Mantel–Haenszel approach is used in various other contexts in epidemiology; for example, in the log-rank test for survival data (Section 5.5.1); in person-years analysis (Section 5.7.4); in matched case–control studies (Section 6.6.2) and in meta-analysis (Section 12.5.2). It has been generalised in various ways, including situations in which the risk factor is measured at several (more than two) levels (see Yanagawa *et al.*, 1994).

To conclude the discussion of this topic here, the data analysed in the original Mantel and Haenszel (1959) paper are presented and analysed.

Example 4.12 Table 4.14 shows the results of a case–control study of epidermoid and undifferentiated pulmonary carcinoma. The issue of interest is whether, having accounted for occupation and age, smoking is a risk factor for this disease. Mantel and Haenszel (1959) give data for only nonsmokers and heavy (one pack or more per day) smokers.

Table 4.14. Cases of epidermoid and undifferentiated pulmonary carcinoma and controls classified by occupation, age and smoking habit.

Occupation	Age (years)	Cases (diseased)		Controls (no disease)	
		Nonsmokers	≥1 Pack/day	Nonsmokers	≥1 Pack/day
Housewives	<45	2	0	7	0
	45–54	5	2	24	1
	55–64	6	3	49	0
	≥65	11	0	42	0
White-collar	<45	0	3	6	2
workers	45–54	2	2	18	2
	55–64	4	2	23	2
	≥65	6	0	11	1
Other	<45	0	1	10	3
occupations	45–54	1	4	12	1
	55–64	6	0	19	1
	≥65	3	1	15	0

Table 4.15. Strata derived from Table 4.14, expressed in the form of Table 4.12 with smoking as the risk factor.

0	0	0		2	1	3		3	0	3		0	0	0
2	7	9		5	24	29		6	49	55		11	42	53
2	7	9		7	25	32		9	49	58		11	42	53

3	2	5		2	2	4		2	2	4		0	1	1
0	6	6		2	18	20		4	23	27		6	11	17
3	8	11		4	20	24		6	25	31		6	12	18

1	3	4		4	1	5		0	1	1		1	0	1
0	10	10		1	12	13		6	19	25		3	15	18
1	13	14		5	13	18		6	20	26		4	15	19

Notice that, in contrast to Example 4.9 to Example 4.11, smoking is now the risk factor rather than the confounder. As stated in Section 4.4.3, the status of any variable depends upon the question(s) to be answered. Here there are two confounding variables: employment, with three levels, and age with four. There are thus $3 \times 4 = 12$ strata for the confounding variables. The resultant subtables, one for each stratum, are given as Table 4.15.

Since this is a case–control study, it is not appropriate to estimate the relative risk. Instead, we can use (4.10) to (4.14) to find the Mantel–Haenszel odds ratio (with 95% confidence interval) as 10.68 (4.47, 39.26). Applying the Cochran–Mantel–Haenszel test with the continuity correction, (4.21), gives a test statistic of 30.66, which is extremely significant ($p < 0.0001$). Hence, there is strong evidence that smoking is associated with the disease after allowing for employment and age; heavy smokers are estimated to have over 10 times the odds of disease compared with nonsmokers of the same age and occupation group.

4.7   The concept of interaction

Interaction occurs between two risk factors when the effect of one risk factor upon disease is different at (at least some) different levels (outcomes, strata) of the second risk factor. Hence, the equivalent term, **effect modification**. When no interaction occurs, the effects of each of the risk factors are consistent (**homogeneous**) across the levels of the other risk factor.

An example of an interaction occurs in the cohort study of elderly people by Fransen *et al.* (2002), in which the chance of death or institutionalisation within 2 years was much higher for those who had previously suffered a hip fracture at the start of these 2 years, but the excess risk associated with a hip fracture was significantly higher for men than women. This is an interaction between hip fracture status (yes/no) and sex. Another example is given by Barbash *et al.* (1993) who found that nonsmokers had a higher short-term chance of death after a first MI than smokers. Since smoking is known to cause premature death in general populations — most of whom have not had an MI — an interaction between MI status (yes/no) and smoking is thus suggested (we shall explore this suggestion subsequently).

Just as with confounding, the analysis of interaction may produce different results depending upon how the comparative chance of disease is measured. In Section 4.8, we shall see how to deal with the relative risk, odds ratio and risk difference. Until then, we shall continue to leave the choice of measurement unspecified.

For simplicity, let us assume (for now) that both of the risk factors have only two outcomes: call these exposure and nonexposure. Then, interaction occurs when the comparative effect of exposure compared with nonexposure for one risk factor is different for the subgroup who are, and the subgroup who are not, exposed to the second risk factor.

Figure 4.7 gives a set of **interaction diagrams** that illustrate three ways in which interaction could happen, as well as the situation of no interaction. **Antagonism** is when the effect of risk factor *A* works in the opposite direction when acting in the

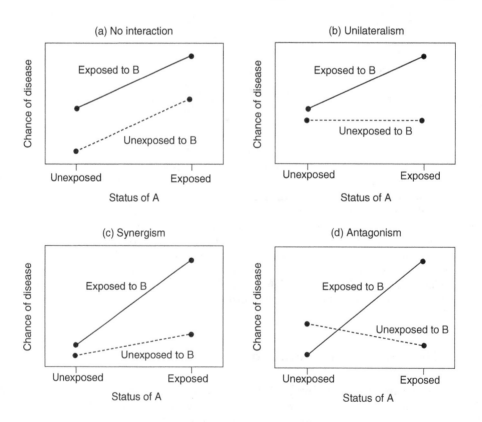

Figure 4.7. Interaction diagrams illustrating four different situations for risk factors *A* and *B*.

presence of exposure, to the direction in which it acts in the absence of exposure, to risk factor B. This is the strongest type of interaction because it represents a reversal of effect (a qualitative difference). **Synergism** is when the effect of A is in the same direction, but stronger in the presence of B. **Unilateralism** is when A has no effect in the absence of B, but a considerable effect when B is present. In fact, presence and absence of exposure are interchangeable in these definitions. Figure 4.7 illustrates the situations in which A and B (themselves interchangeable) are risk factors, rather than protective factors, for the disease. Unilaterism could, alternatively, appear as a sideways 'V', that is, with both lines emanating from the same point. To see this, consider how Figure 4.7(b) would look if B, rather than A, were 'plotted' on the horizontal axis.

As Figure 4.7(a) shows, lack of interaction does not mean that the chance of disease (however measured) after exposure to A is the same regardless of the exposure status of B. When the chance of disease is measured by risk, this would be the situation of statistical independence. This would appear as a *single* line, rather than the parallel lines for no interaction. Lack of interaction means that the *comparative* chance is constant.

In practice, we are hardly likely to find exact agreements in comparative chance — that is, exactly parallel lines on the interaction diagram. Chance sampling variation may explain slight, or even (with small samples) fairly large, differences. Conversely, sampling variation may explain crossing of lines on the interaction diagram when no true interaction occurs in the population. Thus, it is reasonable to carry out tests of interaction so as to sift out the 'real' effects. These will be described in Section 4.8. As in other applications, these tests should be combined with consideration of estimates, for instance, through interaction diagrams.

A quite common, although not generally appropriate, method of testing for an interaction is through separate tests in each stratum of the second risk factor. For instance, the interaction between smoking and MI status, suggested earlier, might be investigated by testing the effect of smoking for those who have had an MI and then repeating the procedure for those who have not. Then the respective p values are compared and the lowest taken to signify the greatest effect. However, one subgroup may be small, leading to a high p value (nonsignificance) even for a large effect, but the other subgroup may be large, leading to a small p value (significance) when the size of the effect is similar to that in the other subgroup. Unilateralism is then incorrectly inferred from this separate testing method. As explained in Section 3.5.5, the p value depends upon sample size as well as the magnitude of the effect. Notice that the absurdity of this inference would be obvious if an interaction diagram were inspected. The only situation in which this approach could have any meaning is that in which the sample sizes in the subgroups are equal, although, even then, what follows in Section 4.8 is recommended.

4.8 Testing for interaction

In this section, we shall consider tests for interaction, sometimes also called **tests of homogeneity**. Since, as already noted, a different conclusion may arise when different basic measures of excess risk are used, we shall consider relative risk, odds ratio and risk difference separately.

4.8.1 Using the relative risk

For simplicity, as before, we shall suppose that two risk factors (A and B) are being studied, each of which is measured at two levels (exposed to the risk factor and unexposed). When relative risks are used to measure the relative chance of disease, we shall say no interaction occurs when

$$\frac{R_{11}}{R_{01}} = \frac{R_{10}}{R_{00}}, \tag{4.22}$$

where R_{11} is the risk for those exposed to A and to B; R_{10} is the risk for those exposed only to A; R_{01} is the risk for those exposed only to B; and R_{00} is the risk for those exposed neither to A or B. That is, there is no interaction if the relative risk for exposure : no exposure to A is the same in both strata of B. Multiplying both sides of (4.22) by R_{01}/R_{10} shows that A and B are interchangeable in this definition (at least when both risk factors have only two levels).

When B has several ℓ strata, 'no interaction' means that there is a constant relative risk across all the strata. A test of the null hypothesis of no interaction is thus derived by considering the situation in which the table of risk factor versus disease for one variable (say, A) is split into subtables by the ℓ strata of the second risk factor, B. This is as in Table 4.12, except that the confounding variable has now become risk factor B. Because the Mantel–Haenszel summary measure of relative risk is only appropriate when there is a constant relative risk across the strata (Section 4.6.1), a test of the null hypothesis of no interaction is also a test of the suitability of application of the Mantel–Haenszel technique (assuming other requirements for confounding are met). Thus, whenever we seek to apply the Mantel–Haenszel procedure, we should first apply a test for interaction.

A test for a common relative risk, λ_0, across all strata is given by comparing

$$\sum \frac{\left(a_i - E\left(a_i\right)\right)^2}{V\left(a_i\right)} \tag{4.23}$$

to chi-square on $\ell - 1$ d.f. Here the summation runs over all the ℓ strata and a_i is (as usual) the observed value in the top left-hand cell of the 2×2 table for stratum i. Also

$$E\left(a_i\right) = \frac{E_i D_i \lambda_0}{\bar{E}_i + E_i \lambda_0} \tag{4.24}$$

and

$$V\left(a_i\right) = \left(\frac{1}{E\left(a_i\right)} + \frac{1}{E\left(b_i\right)} + \frac{1}{E\left(c_i\right)} + \frac{1}{E\left(d_i\right)}\right)^{-1}, \tag{4.25}$$

such that

$$E\left(b_i\right) = E_i - E\left(a_i\right),$$

$$E\left(c_i\right) = D_i - E\left(a_i\right), \tag{4.26}$$

$$E\left(d_i\right) = n_i - E\left(a_i\right) - E\left(b_i\right) - E\left(c_i\right),$$

using notation from Table 4.12.

To be able to evaluate (4.24) and thus, ultimately, (4.23), we need to fix a value for λ_0. One way to do this, which works reasonably well in practice, is to use the Mantel–Haenszel estimate, $\hat{\lambda}_{\mathrm{MH}}$, as defined by (4.15).

Returning to the simple situation in which each risk factor has two levels (that is $\ell = 2$), another way of looking at the definition of 'no interaction' with relative risks comes from multiplying both sides of (4.22) by R_{01}/R_{00}, which gives

$$\frac{R_{11}}{R_{00}} = \frac{R_{10}}{R_{00}} \times \frac{R_{01}}{R_{00}}. \tag{4.27}$$

If we think of the four groups defined by joint exposure/no exposure to A and B, three relative risks can be defined relative to the base level 'no exposure to A or B': λ_{AB} for the group 'exposure to both'; $\lambda_{A\bar{B}}$ for 'exposure to A alone'; and $\lambda_{\bar{A}B}$ for 'exposure to B alone'. Thus (4.27) becomes

$$\lambda_{AB} = \lambda_{A\bar{B}} \lambda_{\bar{A}B}, \tag{4.28}$$

which is a multiplicative relationship. For this reason, the model for interaction assumed here is called a **multiplicative model**.

Notice also that taking logarithms of both sides of (4.22) gives

$$\log R_{11} - \log R_{01} = \log R_{10} - \log R_{00}.$$

That is, the differences in log(risk) in the two strata defined by exposure and nonexposure to B must be equal for there to be no interaction. This suggests that the most useful interaction diagram in this situation is one in which log(risk) is plotted on the vertical axis (see Figure 4.8 and Figure 4.9). This is because it is easier to interpret absolute, rather than relative, differences pictorially.

The interaction effect across the two levels of B might be summarised as a ratio of relative risks. Thus, if λ_1 and λ_2 are the two relative risks comparing the levels of A (e.g., exposure versus no exposure), we might take the ratio λ_1/λ_2 which has a 95% confidence interval of

$$\exp\left(\log_e \hat{\lambda}_1 - \log_e \hat{\lambda}_2 \pm 1.96 \sqrt{\left(\hat{\mathrm{se}}\left(\log_e \hat{\lambda}_1\right)\right)^2 + \left(\hat{\mathrm{se}}\left(\log_e \hat{\lambda}_2\right)\right)^2} \right),$$

where the estimated standard errors are given by (3.5).

Example 4.13 In Section 4.7, it was reported that smoking may have a different effect on the risk of premature death after an MI occurs. Here we shall explore this suggestion using data from the 6-year follow-up of the SHHS to see whether an interaction is present between smoking and previous MI status in the prediction of CHD. Table 4.16 shows cigarette smoking status at the start of the SHHS against whether or not a CHD event (nonfatal MI or coronary death) occurred in the following 6 years, separately for those who had and had not already suffered an MI when the study began. On this occasion, SHHS data are shown for women only; also, women with unknown smoking or previous MI status have been excluded.

Interaction is clearly suggested because smokers have a higher risk amongst those without a previous MI and a lower risk amongst those with a previous MI. This suggests that antagonism may occur.

The relative risks are, from (3.2) or directly (as here): for no previous MI, 3.15/1.31 = 2.40; for previous MI, 13.56/21.15 = 0.64. Figure 4.8 gives a suitable interaction diagram for this problem. There is clear crossing of lines.

Table 4.16. Smoking status by CHD outcome by previous MI status; SHHS women.

Smoking	No previous MI			Previous MI		
status	CHD	No CHD	Total	CHD	No CHD	Total
Smoker	67 (3.15%)	2061	2128	8 (13.56%)	51	59
Nonsmoker	46 (1.31%)	3454	3500	11 (21.15%)	41	52
Total	113	5515	5628	19	92	111

To test the null hypothesis of no interaction, we first calculate the value of $\hat{\lambda}_{MH}$. From (4.15), this is

$$\hat{\lambda}_{MH} = \frac{\left(67 \times 3500/5628\right) + \left(8 \times 52/111\right)}{\left(46 \times 2128/5628\right) + \left(11 \times 59/111\right)} = 1.954.$$

Taking this to be the λ_0 in (4.24) gives, for stratum 1 (no previous MI),

$$E\left(a_1\right) = \frac{2128 \times 113 \times 1.954}{3500 + 2128 \times 1.954} = 61.355.$$

Using this to complete the expected table for the first stratum gives, as expressed by (4.26),

$$E(b_1) = 2128 - 61.355 = 2066.645,$$

$$E(c_1) = 113 - 61.355 = 51.645,$$

$$E(d_1) = 5628 - 61.355 - 2066.645 - 51.645 = 3448.355.$$

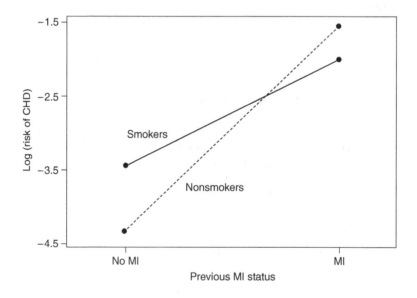

Figure 4.8. Logarithm of risk of CHD by smoking status and previous MI status; SHHS women.

Then, in (4.25),

$$V(a_1) = \left(\frac{1}{61.355} + \frac{1}{2066.645} + \frac{1}{51.645} + \frac{1}{3448.355} \right)^{-1} = 27.446.$$

Similar calculations for stratum 2 (those with previous MI) give

$$E\left(a_2\right) = 13.094, \qquad V(a_2) = 3.458.$$

Substituting into (4.23) gives the test statistic

$$\frac{(67 - 61.355)^2}{27.446} + \frac{(8 - 13.094)^2}{3.458} = 8.67.$$

This is to be compared with χ^2 on $\ell - 1 = 2 - 1 = 1$ d.f. From Table B.3, $0.005 > p > 0.001$ and hence we have strong evidence to reject the null hypothesis; that is, we conclude that interaction between smoking and previous MI status occurs.

Example 4.14 In Example 4.10, we assumed that the two strata defined by smoking status in Table 4.13 had a common relative risk and used the Mantel–Haenszel relative risk of 1.30 to estimate it. We can now test whether this assumption was reasonable. Figure 4.9 is an interaction diagram for this problem; as in Example 4.13, we will be testing whether the lines are parallel.

From (4.24) through (4.26):

$$E\left(a_1\right) = 33.41, \qquad E\left(a_2\right) = 51.51,$$

$$V\left(a_1\right) = 19.01, \qquad V\left(a_2\right) = 17.89,$$

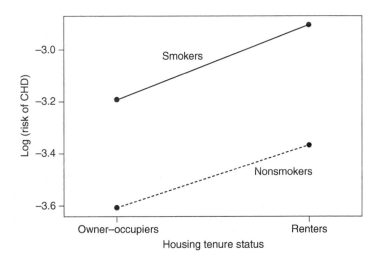

Figure 4.9. Logarithm of risk of CHD by smoking status and housing tenure status; SHHS men.

and (4.23) then takes a value of 0.02, which is clearly not significant at any sensible significance level. Hence, no interaction occurs here (as Figure 4.9 suggests); we are justified in using the summary relative risk.

4.8.2   Using the odds ratio

When the odds ratio is used (as it must be in case–control studies) in place of the relative risk, theoretical details follow in very much the same way as in Section 4.8.1. As with relative risks, no interaction means that there is a constant odds ratio for exposure, compared with no exposure, to A across the strata of B (or vice versa), giving a multiplicative model of interaction. This would be a preliminary test for the adoption of the Mantel–Haenszel odds ratio, (4.10).

A test for a constant odds ratio across the strata, as represented by Table 4.12 for stratum i of risk factor B, uses (4.23) again. All calculations are just as in Section 4.8.1 except that (4.24) is replaced by

$$E(a_i) = \frac{P_i \pm \sqrt{P_i^2 - 4\psi_0(\psi_0 - 1)E_i D_i}}{2(\psi_0 - 1)}, \tag{4.29}$$

where

$$P_i = (\psi_0 - 1)(E_i + D_i) + n_i \tag{4.30}$$

and ψ_0 is some estimate of the common odds ratio under the null hypothesis, such as the Mantel–Haenszel estimate. Although (4.29) will yield two outcomes, we require only the outcome that gives positive values for all the expected cell values. We shall need to use (4.29) to calculate the result of (4.25) via (4.26) for each stratum and thus produce the test statistic, (4.23).

Similar to the relative risk, when A and B each have two strata the interaction effect might be summarised as ψ_1/ψ_2, the ratio of the two odds ratios comparing the levels of A (one at each level of B). This has 95% confidence interval

$$\exp\left(\log_e \hat{\psi}_1 - \log_e \hat{\psi}_2 \pm 1.96\sqrt{\left(\hat{\text{se}}\left(\log_e \hat{\psi}_1\right)\right)^2 + \left(\hat{\text{se}}\left(\log_e \hat{\psi}_2\right)\right)^2} \right),$$

where the estimated standard errors are given by (3.10).

Example 4.15 Consider the problem of Example 4.13 again, but this time suppose that we choose to measure comparative chance by odds ratios. From (3.9), the odds ratios are 2.44 (no previous MI) and 0.58 (previous MI). As these are substantially different and very similar to the corresponding relative risks, we shall anticipate rejecting the null hypothesis of no interaction.

The first step in carrying out the formal test is to calculate $\hat{\psi}_{\text{MH}}$ from (4.10). This is

$$\hat{\psi}_{\text{MH}} = \frac{\left(67 \times 3454/5628\right) + \left(8 \times 41/111\right)}{\left(2061 \times 46/5628\right) + \left(51 \times 11/111\right)} = 2.013.$$

Then, for stratum 1 (no previous MI), when $\hat{\psi}_{MH}$ is used for the common (over all strata) value of ψ_0, (4.30) becomes

$$P_1 = (2.013 - 1)(2128 + 113) + 5628 = 7898.133.$$

Using (4.29), we find

$$E\left(a_1\right) = \frac{7898.133 \pm \sqrt{7898.133^2 - 4 \times 2.013 \times 1.013 \times 2128 \times 113}}{2 \times 1.013}$$

$$= \frac{7898.133 \pm 7772.973}{2.026}$$

$$= 61.777 \text{ or } 7734.998.$$

Of these, only the smaller will give positive expected values for all the remaining cells of the first stratum; thus, $E(a_1) = 61.777$ and then, by (4.26),

$$E(b_1) = 2128 - 61.777 = 2066.223,$$

$$E(c_1) = 113 - 61.777 = 51.223,$$

$$E(d_1) = 5628 - 61.777 - 2066.223 - 51.223 = 3448.777.$$

From (4.25),

$$V(a_1) = \left(\frac{1}{61.777} + \frac{1}{2066.223} + \frac{1}{51.223} + \frac{1}{3448.777}\right)^{-1} = 27.410.$$

Similar calculations for the second stratum (previous MI) give

$$E(a_2) = 12.741, \quad V(a_2) = 3.549.$$

Substituting into (4.23) gives the test statistic

$$\frac{(67 - 61.777)^2}{27.410} + \frac{(8 - 12.741)^2}{3.549} = 7.33.$$

When compared with χ^2 on $\ell - 1 = 1$ d.f. (Table B.3), we find $0.01 > p > 0.005$. There is strong evidence to reject the null hypothesis; we conclude that interaction, measured through odds ratios, occurs between smoking and previous MI status in the 6-year prediction of coronary events in the SHHS.

As we would expect for a (reasonably) rare disease, the numerical results in Example 4.13 and Example 4.15 are very similar. If we apply the test for a common odds ratio to the data of Table 4.13, we can expect similar results to those in Example 4.14.

The tests defined here and in Section 4.8.1 involve various approximations, such as a chi-square distribution for the test statistic. These approximations will be acceptable whenever the cell numbers are large in each stratum's 2×2 table. As with single tables (see Section 2.5.1), we can expect problems whenever several expected numbers are less than about five. This suggests that the number of strata may need to be restricted, perhaps by combining strata in some sensible way. For instance, application of the test for a common odds ratio given here should not be applied to the set of stratified tables given as Table 4.15. Indeed, it cannot be applied because some of the expected cell values will be zero, which leads to a requirement for division by zero in (4.25). This may be avoided by combining adjacent age groups in the original table, Table 4.14. More accurate procedures for testing for a common summary parameter over stratified tables are given by Breslow and Day (1993, 1994).

4.8.3   Using the risk difference

When the risk difference is used to measure excess risk, no interaction means a constant risk difference for exposure, compared with no exposure, to A across all the strata of B. That is,

$$R_{11} - R_{01} = R_{10} - R_{00} \qquad (4.31)$$

when A and B each have two levels. Let Δ_{AB} be the risk difference for the group 'exposure to A and B'; $\Delta_{A\bar{B}}$ be the risk difference for 'exposure to A alone'; $\Delta_{\bar{A}B}$ be the risk difference for 'exposure to B alone'; all compared with the base group 'unexposed to A and B'. Add $R_{01} - R_{00}$ to both sides of (4.31) to get

$$R_{11} - R_{00} = (R_{10} - R_{00}) + (R_{01} - R_{00}), \qquad (4.32)$$

$$\text{i.e., } \Delta_{AB} = \Delta_{A\bar{B}} + \Delta_{\bar{A}B},$$

which is an additive relationship. Hence, the model for interaction assumed here is called an **additive model**. One advantage of this additive formulation is that risk can be plotted on the interaction diagram, allowing a more direct interpretation than for relative risks or odds ratios.

   When there are two levels for both risk factors, an approximate test (using a normal approximation) for an interaction using risk differences is to compare

$$\frac{\left(\left(r_{11} - r_{01}\right) - \left(r_{10} - r_{00}\right)\right)^2}{\mathrm{v\hat{a}r}\left(r_{11}\right) + \mathrm{v\hat{a}r}\left(r_{01}\right) + \mathrm{v\hat{a}r}\left(r_{10}\right) + \mathrm{v\hat{a}r}\left(r_{00}\right)} \qquad (4.33)$$

with chi-square on one d.f. In (4.33) each r is the sample value of the corresponding R and each variance estimate, $\mathrm{v\hat{a}r}(r_{ij})$, is obtained, by reference to Section 2.5.3, as

$$\mathrm{v\hat{a}r}\left(r_{ij}\right) = r_{ij}\left(1 - r_{ij}\right)/n_{ij}, \qquad (4.34)$$

where n_{ij} is the sample size (denominator) for r_{ij} and i and j take the values 0 and 1. A 95% confidence interval for the difference in risk differences is

$$\left(r_{11} - r_{01}\right) - \left(r_{10} - r_{00}\right) \pm 1.96\sqrt{\mathrm{v\hat{a}r}\left(r_{11}\right) + \mathrm{v\hat{a}r}\left(r_{01}\right) + \mathrm{v\hat{a}r}\left(r_{10}\right) + \mathrm{v\hat{a}r}\left(r_{00}\right)}.$$

Example 4.16 Once again, consider the data of Table 4.16. Here $r_{11} = 8/59 = 0.13559$; $r_{01} = 11/52 = 0.21154$; $r_{10} = 67/2128 = 0.03148$; $r_{00} = 46/3500 = 0.01314$, where smoking has been taken (without loss of generality) as risk factor A. The risk differences for smoking compared with not smoking are thus

$$r_{11} - r_{01} = -0.07595 \text{ for those with a previous MI}$$

$$r_{10} - r_{00} = 0.01834 \text{ for those without a previous MI}$$

and thus the difference in risk differences is $-0.07595 - 0.01834 = -0.09429$. From (4.34), $\hat{\mathrm{var}}(r_{11})$ $= (8/59)(51/59)/59 = 0.001987$. Continuing for the other estimated variances gives a result for (4.33) of $(-0.09429)^2/0.005212 = 1.71$. From a computer package, $p = 0.19$. We conclude that no interaction takes place between smoking and previous MI status.

4.8.4   Which type of interaction to use?

As we have seen, we can adopt multiplicative or additive models of interaction. Examination of the results of Example 4.13 and Example 4.16 (which gave opposite conclusions) will show that it is crucial to make it clear which type of interaction is being used. It is easy to see that additive and multiplicative models for interactions with risks will almost always give different indications of when there is no interaction from (4.32) which becomes, on division throughout by R_{00},

$$\lambda_{AB} - 1 = \lambda_{A\bar{B}} - 1 + \lambda_{\bar{A}B} - 1$$

$$\text{i.e., } \lambda_{AB} = \lambda_{A\bar{B}} + \lambda_{\bar{A}B} - 1.$$

This will be the same condition as (4.28) only if $\lambda_{A\bar{B}} = 1$ or $\lambda_{\bar{A}B} = 1$, both of which are highly unlikely. This suggests it would be better to talk of 'modification of relative risk effects' or 'heterogeneity of relative risks' rather than 'interaction' when dealing with relative risks, etc.

The approach of equating interaction with heterogeneity used here leads to what is sometimes called 'statistical interaction' to distinguish it from other approaches (discussed by Rothman and Greenland, 1998). The same approach is taken, at least from standard usage, by statistical computer packages. Of the models that will be introduced in later chapters, logistic, Cox and Poisson regression all assume multiplicative models for interaction. By contrast, the general linear model (standard regression and analysis of variance) assumes an additive model. For example, analysis of variance compares means. Since, unlike risks, means are not proportionate, the additive scale is the natural choice; we compare means through their difference (Section 2.7.3), rather than their ratio.

4.8.5   Which interactions to test?

In the face of a large dataset, including several potential risk factors, many interactions could be investigated. This could include high-order interactions (three-way or above), although these are worth considering only if the number of observations is extremely large and there is some prior reason for expecting such a complex interaction. With small datasets, the chance of detecting a high-order interaction is minimal, even when it exists. On the other hand, we must beware of false positives when many hypothesis tests are carried out in order to trawl for interactions; with 5% significance tests, we expect to reject the null hypothesis of no interaction wrongly five times in a hundred. Furthermore, high-order interactions are difficult to interpret. Hence, it is often reasonable to restrict to investigating two-way interactions.

When there are several variables, the false positives problem is also relevant for two-way interactions. Furthermore, an unreasonable amount of work may be concerned with testing two-way interactions for all variables. Consequently, the approach sometimes taken in epidemiological data analysis is to test only for two-way interactions between those variables that have already been identified as true risk (or protective) factors or confounders. With this approach, we must accept that we would miss identifying an important interaction that involves two risk factors that are, by themselves, not associated with disease or death. On some occasions, this could be a real problem. To take an extreme example, two drugs may each be beneficial in treating a disease with no side effects when used alone, but in combination they might cause death.

4.9   Dealing with interaction

Whenever we have detected interaction between two risk factors, it will *not* be appropriate to consider the effects of each independently of the other. Thus, when A and B interact in determining the chance of disease, as measured through the relative risk, we should not quote the relative risk for A or the relative risk for B (the so-called **main effects** of A and B, respectively). To do so would give a misleading result.

This is most obvious when evidence of antagonism exists. For instance, the relative risk of CHD for smoking (main effect, ignoring previous MI status) from Table 4.16 is

$$\frac{75/2187}{57/3552} = 2.14.$$

Taking this as the estimate of relative risk for all people is clearly inappropriate when applied to someone with a previous history of MI, because it goes in the wrong direction (increased rather than decreased risk). Another incorrect approach is to take the average of the two relative risks, by strata of previous MI status, as a measure of overall risk. The answer would then be (from Example 4.13),

$$(2.40 + 0.64)/2 = 1.52,$$

which is very misleading when used for either previous MI group. It badly underestimates the relative risk for one subgroup and is in the wrong direction for the other.

Instead of giving main effects, we should state the estimates of effect for one risk factor separately for each stratum of the second. Hence, it is appropriate to carry out separate analyses for those with and without previous MI from Table 4.16. The relative risks, with 95% confidence intervals from (3.5) through (3.7) in parentheses, for smoking compared with nonsmoking are for no previous MI, 2.40 (1.65, 3.47); for previous MI, 0.64 (0.28, 1.47).

Because unity is in the second, but not the first, confidence interval, we would conclude that smoking certainly seems to be a risk factor for a first MI, but the evidence for a protective effect after an initial MI is inconclusive. That is, there could be unilateralism rather than antagonism.

Output 4.1. Results from CS in Stata for the data of Table 4.6.

```
(i)  Odds ratio
        smoker  |      OR      [95% Conf. Interval]   M-H Weight

             0  | 1.282638    .8203543   2.005522    16.25238 (Cornfield)
             1  | 1.353813    .8533568   2.147543    15.71635 (Cornfield)

         Crude  | 1.454888    1.063705   1.989923
  M-H combined  | 1.317629    .9537528   1.820331

Test of homogeneity (M-H)      chi2(1)  =  0.027  Pr>chi2 =  0.8701

                Test that combined OR = 1:
                           Mantel-Haenszel chi2(1) =      2.80
                                       Pr>chi2 =    0.0940
(ii)  Relative risk

        smoker  |      RR      [95% Conf. Interval]   M-H Weight

             0  | 1.272882    .8229229   1.96887     16.83346
             1  | 1.334446    .8562663   2.079665    16.62643

         Crude  | 1.434602    1.060108   1.94139
  M-H combined  | 1.303474    .9549737   1.779152

Test of homogeneity (M-H)      chi2(1)  =  0.022  Pr>chi2 =  0.8817
```

This is not the appropriate place to investigate the (apparently bizarre) change in effect of smoking. One obvious possibility is that some change takes place in the smoking habit subsequent to an MI, but before smoking habits are ascertained. The great weakness in the analysis here, chosen for its simplicity rather than its scientific completeness, is the absence of any consideration of lifetime tobacco consumption.

4.10   EPITAB commands in Stata

Stata's CS command, part of the EPITAB suite (Section 3.10), can be used to find strata-specific odds ratios or relative risks, combine them using the Mantel–Haenszel method (or other weighting methods) and carry out both the tests for homogeneity and for a null effect after adjustment. Output 4.1 shows the results from running the CS command twice (once for the adjusted odds ratio and once for the adjusted relative risk), applied to the housing tenure data (Table 4.6). The results are comparable with the corresponding results in Example 4.9 to Example 4.11 and Example 4.14. The commands used are included on the web site for this book.

Exercises

4.1   The age-standardised mortality ratios for male doctors in England and Wales in 1982 to 1983 were 57 for lung cancer, 115 for hepatic cirrhosis (a rough measure of alcohol abuse) and 172 for suicide (Rawnsley, 1991). These results take the national population as the standard (SMR = 100). Interpret these results and speculate as to their causes; consider why it was thought necessary to standardise for age.

4.2   In each of the following situations, F is the risk factor, D is the study disease and C is a third variable. In which cases could C possibly be a confounder?
       (i) F = regular use of mouthwashes; D = oral cancer; C = smoking.
       (ii) F = smoking; D = lung cancer; C = yellow staining on teeth.
       (iii) F = dental disease; D = cardiovascular disease; C = smoking.
       In the cases in which C could be a confounder, what prior evidence would convince you that C really is worth considering as a likely confounder when designing a study to relate F to D? Search the literature to locate previous publications that contain such evidence.

4.3   In a study of risk factors for a certain disease, smoking status and average daily fat consumption were recorded. Suppose that the relative risks for the combinations of smoking status and level of fat consumption (never smoker, low fat consumers = 1) were:

| Fat consumption | Smoking status | | | |
	Never	Ex	Light	Heavy
Low	1	1.5	2.0	3.0
Medium	1.2	1.8	2.4	3.6
High	1.5	2.3	3.0	4.5
Very high	2.0	3.5	4.0	6.0

       Risk is clearly accentuated by having a relatively high value of the second risk factor, whatever the value of the first, so that those who are both very high fat consumers and heavy smokers are at most risk. Does the table suggest that one of the two variables might be confounded with the other? Does it suggest that fat consumption and smoking interact in their effect upon the disease?

4.4   Refer to the following table of demographic data from Romania in 1993 (United Nations, 1996).

| Age group (years) | Population | | Deaths | |
	Urban	Rural	Urban	Rural
0–9	1 800 680	1 359 501	3 526	4 997
10–19	2 128 150	1 642 941	1 010	1 049
20–29	1 967 110	1 450 550	1 599	1 977
30–39	2 118 205	1 019 015	4 333	3 300
40–49	1 691 033	1 139 065	8 312	6 903
50–59	1 200 412	1 396 080	14 896	16 739
60–69	921 072	1 380 709	24 191	32 443
70–79	404 304	670 133	23 706	38 872
80 and above	175 238	291 062	25 909	49 561

       (i)   Find the crude death rates (per thousand) in urban and rural areas.
       (ii)   Using the overall population as the standard, find the age-standardised death rates (per thousand) for both the rural and the urban areas, using the direct method.
       (iii) Using the overall population as the standard, find the standardised mortality ratios for urban and rural areas. Use these to find the indirect standardised death rates (per thousand).
       (iv)   Interpret your results.

4.5 Cole and MacMahon (1971) present the following data from a case–control study of bladder cancer:

High-risk occupation?	High cigarette consumption?	No. of cases	No. of controls
No	No	43	94
No	Yes	173	189
Yes	No	26	20
Yes	Yes	111	72

(i) Estimate the odds ratio for bladder cancer comparing high-risk to other occupations (ignoring cigarette consumption).

(ii) Test the null hypothesis that the odds ratio is the same for those who work in high-risk and in other occupations.

(iii) Calculate the Mantel–Haenszel odds ratio for high-risk versus other occupations, adjusted for cigarette consumption.

(iv) Test the null hypothesis that the smoking-adjusted odds ratio is one.

(v) Interpret your results.

4.6 Refer to the following table, which gives summary results derived from the north Glasgow male coronary event registration data presented in Table 4.11.

Age group (years)	Deprivation group			
	I & II		III & IV	
	Deaths	Coronaries	Deaths	Coronaries
35–44	8	18	12	25
45–54	24	47	34	75
55–64	62	114	103	180

(i) Find the age-specific risks of death for coronary cases from the two deprivation groups. Find their logarithms and plot them on a graph. Does the graph suggest a possible effect of age or deprivation group or any interaction between age and deprivation group?

(ii) Find the relative risk (ignoring age) of a death for coronary cases in deprivation groups III and IV compared with I and II, together with the corresponding 95% confidence interval.

(iii) Find the Mantel–Haenszel age-adjusted relative risk and confidence interval corresponding to (ii).

(iv) Test whether the effect of age on the relative risk of death differs between deprivation groups (that is, test for an age–deprivation group interaction using relative risks).

(v) Repeat (ii) replacing relative risk by odds ratio.

(vi) Repeat (iii) replacing relative risk by odds ratio.

(vii) Repeat (iv) replacing risk by odds and relative risks by odds ratios.

(viii) Test for an effect of deprivation on the chance of death, ignoring age.

(ix) Test for an effect of deprivation on the chance of death, adjusting for age.

(x) Interpret your results.

4.7 Refer to the MONICA data of Table C.1 in Appendix C.

(i) Estimate the prevalence relative risk for high versus low factor IX.

(ii) Find the Mantel–Haenszel sex-adjusted estimate of the prevalence relative risk (high versus low).

(iii) Find the Mantel–Haenszel age-adjusted estimate of the prevalence relative risk (high versus low).

(iv) Find the Mantel–Haenszel age/sex-adjusted estimate of the prevalence relative risk (high versus low). This requires taking the 10 age/sex groups as strata.

(v) Test whether the relative risks by factor IX status are the same for both sexes.

(vi) Test whether the relative risks by factor IX status are the same for all age groups.

(vii) Test whether the relative risks by factor IX status are the same for all 10 age/sex groups.

(viii)–(xi) Repeat (i) to (iv) replacing relative risk by odds ratio.

(xii)–(xiv) Repeat (v) to (vii) replacing relative risks by odds ratios.

(xv) Interpret your results and summarise your conclusion about the effect of factor IX on prevalent CVD.

CHAPTER 5

Cohort studies

5.1   Design considerations

A **cohort**, or **prospective**, study is one in which individuals are followed over time
to monitor their health outcomes. The simplest approach is to select two groups of
people at the start of the study, the **baseline**. One group consists of people who possess
some special attribute thought to be a possible risk factor for a disease of interest,
whilst the other group does not. Both groups are followed over time and the incidence
of disease compared between the groups. Hence, in a study of the hazards of working
in the coal industry, a group of coal miners and a second group of employees in other
heavy industries might be selected at baseline. Both groups would then be monitored
for (say) 10 years, after which time the incidence of (say) bronchitis is compared
between the groups. The nonfactor group (other heavy industries in the example) is
included to act as a control group for purposes of comparison — that is, to enable the
excess morbidity associated with the risk factor (coal mining) to be found. Figure 5.1
gives a schematic representation of this type of cohort study.

Sometimes we may be able to study the entire population exposed to the risk factor,
such as every person who was present in a factory at the time of a radiation leakage.
Most often, both groups will need to be sampled. When sampling, as always, we prefer
to take random samples in order to avoid possible bias (Section 5.1.4).

Ideally, everyone who enters the study should be free of the disease being studied.
Thus, in the coal mining example, only people without symptoms of bronchitis would be
included at baseline. In this situation, we may show that the hypothesised cause does
indeed precede the effect. During the follow-up, we shall be recording disease *incidence*.

5.1.1   Advantages

1. Cohort studies give direct information on the sequence of happenings. This
   is ideal for demonstrating causality.
2. Many diseases can be studied simultaneously. We do this by ensuring that
   we record all episodes of all the required diseases during the follow-up.

5.1.2   Disadvantages

1. Cohort studies are often very expensive and time-consuming. This is because
   they typically require monitoring of a large set of subjects over a long time
   period.
2. They are not suitable for diseases with a long latency because the time period
   for the study would then become unacceptably long. If, for example, young

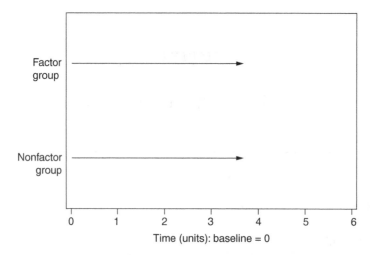

Figure 5.1. Schematic representation of a cohort study.

disease-free cigarette smokers and nonsmokers were followed up to investigate lung cancer, we might need to plan for at least a 20-year time horizon,
in order to give the tumours time to grow and be identified (Section 1.2).

3. Cohort studies are not suitable for rare diseases. If the disease is rare, then
we would either need to take an enormous baseline sample or to monitor for
a very long time, both of which may be unacceptable. For instance, consider
a disease that has an incidence rate of 5 cases per 100 000 per year. Suppose
we decide that we need around 100 cases before we can make any meaningful
evaluation of the risk profile for the disease. We would then expect to need,
for example, an initial cohort of 200 000 subjects if we wished to finish after
10 years. Alternatively, given an initial cohort of 40 000 subjects, we would
expect to continue monitoring for 50 years!

4. There may be study effects; that is, someone may act differently simply by
virtue of being studied. For instance, some people may alter their dietary
habits once they are entered into a study of smoking as a risk factor for
coronary heart disease (CHD) because they become more aware of current
'healthy eating' advice. They would then be expected to have a lower incidence
of CHD than other smokers. This problem is much reduced by the inclusion
of a nonfactor group, as is recommended, because this group would experience
the same influences during observation.

5. Exposure to the factor of interest may change, especially when the time horizon
is long, for reasons unconnected with the investigation. The result is that
someone initially classified to the factor group might have the attributes necessary to the nonfactor group before the study is over. For instance, a smoker
may quit within a few weeks of the baseline study and yet continue to be
counted amongst the smokers in subsequent analyses. When risk factors are
repeatedly remeasured during follow-up, the cohort study is usually called a
longitudinal study. Provided that changes to risk factors are monitored, along
with disease outcome, this can be accounted for in the analysis by various
methods, such as the person-years approach (Section 5.7) and generalised
estimating equations (Section 9.11).

6. Withdrawals may occur. Provided that withdrawals are made for reasons unconnected with disease, they may be accounted for using appropriate methods of analysis. Withdrawal and consequent loss to follow-up may, however, be a direct or indirect consequence of disease. Thus coal miners with bronchitis may emigrate to a warmer climate in order to avoid further distress, or a smoker with lung cancer might commit suicide because of depression caused by the disease. In both examples, the result would be to bias the conclusions in favour of the supposed risk factor; that is, it seems to have less effect on disease than it actually has.

5.1.3   *Alternative designs with economic advantages*

As well as the basic design (Figure 5.1), many alternative types of cohort study exist, any of which may be preferable in a given situation. Those listed next have advantages in saving costs and/or time.

1. Omission of the nonfactor group. This is not recommended because, without parallel study of a control group, we cannot judge whether any effects seen are due to the factor, study effects or simply 'background' effects, such as air pollution.
2. Use of an external comparison group rather than a nonfactor group. This has the advantage of studies of type 1, that only one group must be monitored, whilst maintaining a comparative aspect. The external group is often the national population. For example, in a study of workers exposed to styrene in the reinforced plastics and composites industry, Wong (1990) calculated cause-specific death rates for a cohort of workers and compared these with routine statistics for the U.S. The major difficulty with this approach is the possibility of bias. Routine statistics may not be complete (even in the U.S.) and are unlikely to be as detailed as the information collected on the cohort. Study effects could also cause differential bias. One important difference with this design is that *rates*, rather than risks, are generally the basic unit of measurement. As such, it requires a special approach to analysis; we defer discussion of this until Section 5.7.
3. Mortality, rather than morbidity, is the outcome recorded. As already mentioned, this was the method used by Wong (1990), whose major aim was to study the relationship between exposure to styrene and cancer. Death is a sensible outcome measure here, but would not be if diseases that rarely lead to death, such as skin disorders, were of major interest. The disadvantage of recording only deaths is that the number of positive outcomes found is smaller (or at least, no bigger) than when episodes of sickness are used. This means that a larger cohort or a longer time horizon needs to be used to identify the same number of positive outcomes. Clearly there could also be important differences between relationships of risk factors with morbidity and mortality, because the latter represents the extreme. In the Scottish Heart Health Study (SHHS) (Section 2.2.1), both types of outcome were recorded.
4. Event notification arises from routine statistics, rather than special observation. As mentioned for studies of type 2, routine statistics (such as death registrations, hospital patient administration systems and disease registers) may be incomplete or insufficiently detailed. There may also be substantial

loss to follow-up through migration. Even so, this is likely to be the only viable method of monitoring in a large study. Provided that the factor and nonfactor groups experience equal problems, this method is sound. In the SHHS, the cohort was monitored by having each member flagged by the Registrar General for Scotland. Whenever any member died, the death certificate was copied and sent to the study team for analysis. The cohort was also followed up for coronary morbidity by linking hospital in-patient records, for patients with chosen diagnoses, to the SHHS database, linking by name, age, sex and address (Tunstall–Pedoe et al., 1997).

5. Retrospective cohort studies. Sometimes it is possible to trace the cohort backwards in time to ascertain risk factor status some years before. This method is attractive because it does not involve waiting for years before the study is complete. It is, however, essential to have complete and accurate records for the method to give unbiased results. For example, it would not be sensible to study the hazards of smoking by asking a sample of people to recall their smoking habits 10 years ago and then comparing morbidity between people who were smokers and nonsmokers at that time. Besides problems of accurate recall, we would expect that a greater proportion of those who smoked 10 years ago will have already died. Retrospective cohort studies are frequently used in studies of occupational mortality, including the study by Wong (1990) already cited and in studies using routinely collected health data, such as medical insurance databases.

5.1.4   Studies with a single baseline sample

A very common cohort study design is to take a single baseline sample and identify the factor and nonfactor groups of Figure 5.1 from the sample data. This approach has the great advantage that information on the variable used to stratify the risk factor groups is not required beforehand. A disadvantage, when there is a single risk factor of key interest, is that the distribution of this risk factor cannot be controlled; we may end up with a disparate number in the factor and nonfactor groups, which is statistically inefficient (Section 8.4.3).

The single baseline sample design would be the obvious approach when several risk factors are of interest. For example, as explained in Section 2.2.1, in the baseline survey for the SHHS, a random sample of Scottish men and women were sampled and invited to complete a questionnaire and attend a screening clinic. Consequently, information on several possible risk factors for coronary heart disease was obtained which could then be used to subdivide the sample in several ways — for example, by baseline smoking status (current smoker/nonsmoker) and parental history of coronary heart disease (yes/no). When the cohort was followed up over time, relative risks, etc. were calculated for each individual risk factor (as well as combinations), as already seen in several examples in Chapter 4. More examples follow in this and later chapters.

An extra advantage of this design is that, provided the sample is randomly selected, an unbiased estimate of the prevalence of the risk factor may be obtained (for example, the percentage of people who are current smokers at baseline). This is necessary in order to obtain a direct estimate of the attributable risk (Section 3.7). Also, although the basic two-group cohort design exemplified by Figure 5.1 is easily extended to categorical risk factors with more than two levels (e.g., smoking status: never/ex/current smokers), unlike the single baseline design, it cannot allow for measurement of a risk factor in continuous form. As discussed in Section 3.6.1, this allows for a richer range of analyses.

One common misconception is that the single baseline sample must be a random sample of the general population. Although this is preferable because it allows reliable estimation of population prevalence and attributable risk, it is generally unnecessary if the sole purpose is to estimate relative chance of disease (e.g., a relative risk). Then, nonrandom samples are problematic only if we have reason to believe that the factor making the sample nonrandom (or an associated factor) acts as an effect modifier (see Section 4.7).

For instance, many cohort studies are carried out within occupational workforces; these are convenient study populations because they are relatively cheap and easy to follow. In these studies, unlike that of Wong (1990) mentioned earlier, we are not interested in studying the risks conferred by employment. Instead we study risk factors amongst study populations who happen to have this employment. For example, the study enumerated in Example 3.1 is a cohort study of cardiovascular risk factors conducted amongst employees of the Electricity Generating Authority of Thailand (EGAT). Although it would have been particularly difficult to follow up a random population sample of Thais, due to migration and underdeveloped administrative systems, EGAT has its own detailed recording systems. Thus, it was relatively straightforward for the EGAT investigators to follow up, for example, those who did and did not smoke at study baseline and compute the relative chance of cardiovascular death 12 years later (Table 3.2). It could not be expected that the risk of cardiovascular death would be the same in EGAT as in the general Thai population, because those in employment will be relatively more healthy (otherwise they would not be fit for continuing employment). Epidemiologists call this the 'healthy worker effect'. Similarly, the prevalence of smoking at baseline in EGAT may well be different from that of all Thais of a similar age at the same time (Section 3.7). However, unless we feel that some aspect associated with their employment will interact with smoking in influencing cardiovascular risk, we have no reason to suppose that the EGAT relative risks, comparing those with and without smoking, will be any different from what would be found in the general population.

Example 5.1 The Avon Longitudinal Study of Pregnancy and Childhood (ALSPAC) is a birth cohort study of all pregnancies amongst women resident in three English health districts with expected delivery dates between 1 April 1991 and 31 December 1992. The study recruited 14 893 pregnancies, leading to 14 210 surviving children. This builds on previous national studies (of 1946, 1958 and 1970 birth cohorts) and is part of a European network of similar studies. The study aims to follow each child through to adulthood. Initial information before, at and after birth was gathered from a number of sources, including self-completion questionnaires given to mothers and fathers, hospital and other health records and biological samples from mother and/or child (urine, blood, teeth, hair, nails and placenta). Reports on various factors that may be associated with the development of children and the well-being of parents and their offspring have been published. These include the effects of maternal smoking on birthweight (Passaro *et al.,* 1996) and light drinking in pregnancy related to mental health and academic outcomes of offspring at 11 years of age (Sayal *et al.,* 2013). For further information see http://www.bristol.ac.uk/alspac/.

5.2 Analytical considerations

5.2.1 Concurrent follow-up

If everyone in the cohort starts at the same time and is followed up for the same length of time (or, at least, until the event of interest, such as death, occurs), then analysis may proceed as in Chapter 3, taking account of confounding and interaction as necessary, as explained in Chapter 4. This is the **fixed cohort** situation and is relatively easy to deal with. Section 5.2.2 to Section 5.6 will consider situations in which the opposite, the **variable cohort** situation, occurs. This is when the set of individuals at risk changes during the study for reasons other than loss due to the event of interest.

Even with a fixed cohort, the simple analyses of risk based, for example, on relative risks have the disadvantage that they cannot differentiate between short- and long-term effects. This would be a problem, for instance, if a high blood pressure at age 50 is a risk factor for all-causes mortality (death from any cause) in the first few years, but not a noticeable risk in the review made after 30 years of follow-up. Of course, everyone must die eventually, so relative risks for death must inevitably tend to unity as follow-up time increases.

An alternative approach is to carry out a **survival analysis**, which is a simultaneous analysis of progress for different durations of follow-up; the times of events are analysed rather than the mere fact of the events. Survival analysis is ideal for the variable cohort situation. Note that the word 'survival' here does not necessarily relate to lack of death; it could mean failure to become diseased. In general, 'survival' means lack of experience of the event of interest. We shall develop the basic ideas of survival analysis in Section 5.3. A further alternative, based upon the person-years of experience of the cohort, is described in Section 5.7.

5.2.2   Moving baseline dates

Sometimes recruitment into a study is not simultaneous, but happens over a period of time. For instance, in the SHHS, follow-up was recorded from the day that the individual attended a clinic, where blood pressure, height, weight, etc. were recorded (Section 2.2.1). The nurses who administered these clinics had to travel to different parts of Scotland; hence, subjects from different parts of the country had different baseline dates. Indeed, 35 months passed between the first and last clinic sessions.

The usual way to deal with this problem is simply to ignore it; follow-up is measured as elapsed time since baseline, using a different starting point for each subject. This assumes that any effects are homogeneous (unchanged) with respect to calendar time. Provided that the baseline dates do not vary greatly, this is usually a reasonable assumption; see Section 5.8 for further discussion.

5.2.3   Varying follow-up durations

As just noted, baseline calendar times may vary. Conversely, the calendar time at which evaluation of effects is made will generally be the same for each member of the cohort. Therefore, lengths of follow-up may vary. For example, the paper by Tunstall–Pedoe et al. (1997), which is the source of information about the follow-up in the SHHS used here, described coronary events (hospital diagnosis of myocardial infarction, coronary artery surgery or death) for every member of the SHHS cohort up to the last day of 1993. At this date, elapsed follow-up time since baseline varied from 9.1 years for the earliest recruits (November 1984 to December 1993) to 6.2 years for the last recruits (October 1987 to December 1993). The mean elapsed time was 7.7 years. Notice that elapsed time here is *potential* follow-up time; some individuals will have early termination, for example, due to coronary death.

Treating the study as if it were a fixed cohort, we could seek to use the simple risk analyses of Chapter 3 in this situation in three different ways. The first is to analyse only those with complete (potential) follow-up. This is wasteful of information and not acceptable unless the wastage is only marginal.

The second is to perform a simple risk analysis for all events up to, but not exceeding, the minimum elapsed time. In the SHHS, this is 6.2 years. For ease of interpretation, this might be rounded down to some convenient value. Thus, Example 3.13, Example 4.3 and Example 4.13 (and their extensions) all used the first 6 years of observation in the SHHS. This approach is fine for providing simple examples that are easy to interpret, but is unsatisfactory as a definitive analysis of risk — again, because it wastes information. For instance, people known to have their first coronary event in their seventh, eighth or ninth year of study would, nevertheless, be counted as disease free in the 6-year follow-up analysis.

The third method uses this extra information by simply ignoring the variation in follow-up durations. That is, we record each individual as disease positive or negative during her or his follow-up and proceed as in Chapter 3. Of course, this means that some people will have had rather longer to experience an event; thus, all else being equal, they have more chance of an event than those with shorter follow-ups. This should not cause a problem as long as the time homogeneity assumption is satisfied (which generally requires the variation in follow-up to be small) and the length of follow-up is not related to the risk factor being studied.

As an example of where a problem could occur, consider the analysis of coronary risk by housing tenure status (owner–occupiers versus renters) in the SHHS. As explained in Section 5.2.2, the date of entry into the SHHS varies with the location of the local clinic. Consequently, the elapsed follow-up time, up to the end of 1993, varies by the area of residence of the subject. Suppose that, by chance, early recruitment was made in areas where rented accommodation is far more common than is the norm in Scotland. Renters will then tend to have been observed for longer periods of follow-up and thus have more chance of an event, all else being equal. The analysis, based upon the assumption of a fixed cohort, would then be biased against renters.

In fact, no such problems of bias have been noted in the SHHS data. Consequently, analysis of varying follow-up periods will be used for these data as illustrations in Chapter 10, in which statistical models for the situations of Chapter 3 are presented. Nevertheless, this is not the preferred method of dealing with varying follow-ups; survival analysis is better because it removes the chance of bias. Published accounts of the SHHS follow-up use survival analysis for this and other reasons.

Since survival analysis considers risk during successive duration intervals, it can easily deal with varying follow-ups. For instance, someone who joins a study only 2 years before its closure can provide information for risk calculation in the first and second, but not in subsequent, years. Separating out the years in this way makes it unimportant that the number at risk (the denominator in the risk calculation) varies by year.

Anyone who has not yet experienced an event but has a shorter follow-up time than the maximum possible is said to be **censored**; the data supplied by such a person are **censored data**. Thus, in a 20-year study of the risk of working in the coal-mining industry that finishes today, someone who started work 10 years ago and is still in good health has been censored. Notice that censoring can occur only for people who have yet to experience the event of interest. Even someone recruited only a few days before the study ends will be uncensored should she or he have had an event, the illness or cause of death under study, in the few available days. When the study is effectively open-ended, so that maximum follow-up time is not predetermined, all subjects who have no recorded event at the time of review are censored. This is so in the SHHS; live subjects continued to be followed up after the review date of 31 December 1993 (used in Tunstall–Pedoe *et al.* (1997) and in this chapter), for future analyses. In later chapters some data from follow-up beyond 1993 will be analysed.

5.2.4   *Withdrawals*

As noted in Section 5.1.2, **withdrawals** are a possible complication. Withdrawals are people who are lost to follow-up before experiencing an event. Their duration of study (length of time when they were at risk of an event) will be less than the difference between the dates of the end of the study and their entry. We cannot know whether they would have had an event if they had lasted for their complete possible follow-up duration.

For example, in the SHHS, withdrawals occur when a study member leaves the United Kingdom. Figure 5.2 illustrates the progress of SHHS subjects from their baseline (in 1984, 1985, 1986 or 1987) to the closing date of 31 December 1993. For any year of entry, some individuals will experience an event before the closing date, some will be event-free survivors at the closing date (censored) and some will have left the U.K. before the closing date (withdrawn). Each line represents a representative subject from a specific year of entry and, for simplicity, each representative is shown as entering in mid-year.

Let us suppose that the withdrawal happened for reasons not associated with the disease of interest — for instance, a subject who left the study environment in order to take up a promotion at work. If we choose to analyse the cohort data using simple risk analyses, as in Chapter 3, in the presence of withdrawals, we clearly cannot treat the withdrawals as event positive. We have two choices: ignore the withdrawals altogether or include them amongst those negative for the event. In the former case, we will ignore the known information that they survived for some time without an event, and thus tend to overestimate the risk. In the latter, we ignore the fact that they could have gone on to experience an event had they been fully followed up, and thus tend to underestimate the risk. Thus, neither choice is ideal. Simple risk analysis will be acceptable only if the number of withdrawals is small — for instance, in the SHHS, where only 14 of the 11 629 subjects were withdrawals.

Assuming that the reason for withdrawal is unimportant, the problem of withdrawals is very similar to that of variable follow-up durations. Hence, withdrawals may be treated as censored subjects in a survival analysis, as we shall do for data

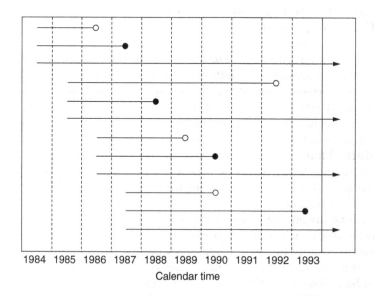

1984 1985 1986 1987 1988 1989 1990 1991 1992 1993
Calendar time

Figure 5.2. Follow-up periods in the SHHS. Solid dots denote events (e.g., deaths); open dots denote withdrawals; and arrows denote event-free survivors at the closing date for analyses.

from the SHHS. If withdrawal should occur for some reason connected with the outcome of interest, as in the bronchitis example in Section 5.1.2 (migration due to illness), then withdrawal should be counted as a positive event.

If withdrawal is related to the risk factor but not the outcome variable, it does not invalidate the analysis but may suggest that the outcome measure is insubstantial. For instance, if many people leave the coal mining industry, but not other industries, due to heart disease, then the study of bronchitis introduced in Section 5.1, which treats such withdrawals as censored, would still be valid but might not be the most useful study of occupational risk for miners. See also Section 5.6.

5.3   Cohort life tables

A **cohort life table**, which will simply be called a life table here, is a tabular presentation of the progress of a cohort through time. To construct the life table, the first step is to divide the entire follow-up period into consecutive intervals of time. Then calculate the following quantities: n_t the number of survivors at time t; e_t the number of events in the study interval that begins at time t; p_t the estimated probability of surviving the entire study interval that begins at t; q_t the estimated probability of an event (or **failure**) during the study interval that begins at t; and s_t the estimated probability of surviving from baseline to the end of the study interval that begins at t. Taking baseline to be time 0, then n_0 will be the total number of subjects in the study. As explained in Section 5.2.1, 'survival' is a general term meaning absence of experience of the event of interest. When the event of interest is death from any cause, survival will have the most straightforward interpretation. Notice that the intervals of time need not be equal in length, although they will be in the next few examples.

All the n and e results come from observation. The q values are risks and so, by (3.1) or simple logic,

$$q_t = e_t/n_t. \tag{5.1}$$

Since surviving is the complement to experiencing an event,

$$p_t = 1 - q_t. \tag{5.2}$$

Finally, because each p value gives the estimated probability of survival during a particular interval (indexed by t), the estimated probability of complete, or **cumulative**, survival from baseline to the end of a given interval will be the product of all p values up to and including that for the given interval. That is,

$$s_t = p_0 p_1 p_2 \cdots p_{t-1}. \tag{5.3}$$

When the event of interest is an attack of the disease that is not necessarily fatal, it will be possible for any one individual to suffer more than one event during follow-up. Then the word 'event' in all the preceding will be taken to refer to the first event. Once an individual has an event, she or he is immediately treated as a nonsurvivor. For example, when analysing coronary events in the SHHS, someone who has a hospital diagnosis of myocardial infarction after 26 months' follow-up, but dies of a subsequent heart attack some months later, would nevertheless have a completed survival time of 26 months.

Table 5.1. Life table for a hypothetical cohort.

Time (t)	No. free of disease (n)	No. of events (e)	Interval risk (q)	Interval survival (p)	Cumulative survival (s)
0	1000	5	0.0050	0.9950	0.9950
1	995	10	0.0100	0.9899	0.9850
2	985	20	0.0203	0.9797	0.9650
3	965	35	0.0363	0.9637	0.9300
4	930	50	0.0538	0.9462	0.8800
5	880				

Example 5.2 A cohort of 1000 men at high risk of disease, but currently disease free, is recruited. In the first year of study, 5 of the men are newly diagnosed with the disease. In the second year, a further 10; in the third year, 20; in the fourth year, 35; and in the fifth year 50 new cases are identified. The resultant life table, employing (5.1) through (5.3), is Table 5.1.

From this table, we see that the estimated probability of survival for 5 years is 0.88. This could well be the most useful single outcome measure for the study. Notice that we could get this in a straightforward manner from the n column: 880 survivors at time 5 compared with 1000 at time 0 gives an estimated 5-year survival probability of 880/1000 = 0.88.

Figure 5.3 shows the estimated cumulative survival probability, s_t, for the data in Table 5.1 plotted against time: a graph of the estimated **survival function**, or a **survival plot**. This is a **step function**; that is, it moves in discrete steps rather than in a smooth curve. As a consequence, the chance of survival to a point intermediate to those enumerated in the life table will be estimated to be equal to that chance evaluated at the previous life table time cut-point. Thus, the estimated chance of survival for 2.5 years is taken as equal to the estimated chance of survival for 2 years: 0.9850. The steps in a survival plot must always be in a downward direction because the chance of survival cannot increase with time. By definition, the probability of survival to time 0 is unity.

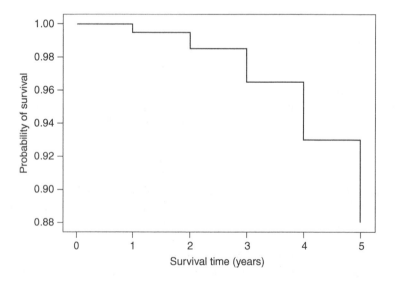

Figure 5.3. Estimated cumulative survival probabilities against time from Table 5.1.

5.3.1   *Allowing for sampling variation*

We can estimate the standard error of the interval-specific risks by using (3.3):

$$\hat{\text{se}}\left(p_t\right) = \sqrt{p_t\left(1 - p_t\right)/n_t}.$$

Similarly,

$$\hat{\text{se}}\left(q_t\right) = \sqrt{q_t\left(1 - q_t\right)/n_t}.$$

Further inferences on these interval-specific probabilities follow from Section 2.5.2.

We can estimate the standard error of the cumulative survival probability (Greenwood, 1926) as

$$\hat{\text{se}}\left(s_t\right) = s_t\sqrt{\sum_{i=0}^{t-1}\frac{q_i}{n_i - e_i}}\,, \tag{5.4}$$

from which an approximate 95% confidence interval (using a normal approximation) for cumulative survival from baseline to the end of the interval that begins at time t is

$$s_t \pm 1.96\,\hat{\text{se}}\left(s_t\right). \tag{5.5}$$

Example 5.3 The estimated standard error of the estimated 5-year survival probability in Example 5.2 is, from (5.4),

$$\hat{\text{se}}\left(s_5\right) = s_5\sqrt{\sum_{i=0}^{4}\frac{q_i}{n_i - e_i}}$$

$$= 0.88\sqrt{\frac{0.0050}{995} + \frac{0.0100}{985} + \frac{0.0203}{965} + \frac{0.0363}{930} + \frac{0.0538}{880}}$$

$$= 0.01028.$$

Hence, from (5.5) and Table 5.1, the approximate 95% confidence interval for survival up to 5 years is

$$0.8800 \pm 1.96 \times 0.01028,$$

that is, 0.8800 ± 0.0201 or $(0.8599, 0.9001)$. We are 95% sure that the interval from 0.86 to 0.90 contains the true probability of surviving for 5 years.

An approximate test of the null hypothesis that the cumulative survival probability is s, where s is some preconceived value, comes from comparing

$$\left\{\frac{s_t - s}{\hat{\text{se}}(s_t)}\right\}^2, \tag{5.6}$$

to chi-square with 1 d.f.

Table 5.2. Number of men experiencing a CHD
event or being censored by period of observation;
SHHS selected subset.

Period of follow-up (years)	Censored	Events	Total
0 but less than 1	7	17	24
1 but less than 2	12	22	34
2 but less than 3	24	26	50
3 but less than 4	19	23	42
4 but less than 5	21	37	58
5 but less than 6	15	38	53
6 but less than 7	501	31	532
7 but less than 8	2143	20	2163
8 but less than 9	1375	5	1380
9 but less than 10	66	0	66
Total	4183	219	4402

5.3.2 Allowing for censoring

As explained in Section 5.2, subjects may be lost to follow-up for various reasons.
Here we shall not distinguish between these causes but will take them all into the
single category of censored individuals. For instance, Table 5.2 shows the results of
follow-up for a selected subset of men in the SHHS. This subset consists of men who
were free of coronary disease and had a known category of housing tenure at baseline;
housing tenure will be used to define subgroups in subsequent examples. Follow-up
has been subdivided into whole-year intervals from baseline. As Figure 5.2 shows,
the calendar date of baseline varies by individual and the maximum possible completed follow-up time, from baseline to study end at 31 December 1993, is less than
10 years.

The basic life table approach can be adapted in several ways to allow for withdrawals. Consider the first interval in Table 5.2. The seven men censored before a
single completed year of follow-up could have all been lost at the beginning. Because
4402 men were recruited in all, this would lead to an estimated failure probability of
$17/(4402 - 7) = 0.003868$ in this year, using (5.1). If, instead, the seven men were lost
at the end of the first year, the appropriate estimated failure probability would be
$17/4402 = 0.003862$. Clearly, the truth lies somewhere between these two extremes.
A reasonable approximation is to subtract half the number censored from the raw
denominator, 4402. That is, we take the estimated failure probability to be
$17/(4402 - 3.5) = 0.003865$.

A general formula for this censoring-adjusted estimated failure probability is

$$q_t = e_t / n_t^*$$

(5.7)

where

$$n_t^* = n_t - \frac{1}{2}c_t$$

(5.8)

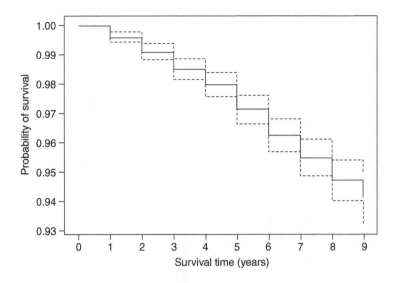

Figure 5.4. Actuarial estimates and 95% confidence intervals for cumulative survival probabilities of coronary events; selected subset of SHHS men.

and c_t is the number censored during the interval which begins at time t. Use of (5.8) is called the **actuarial method** for analysing survival data. Using (5.7), the procedures described by (5.2) and (5.3) are still valid for this new situation; (5.4) becomes

$$\hat{se}\left(s_t\right) = s_t \sqrt{\sum_{i=0}^{t-1} \frac{q_t}{n_t^* - e_t}} \tag{5.9}$$

and (5.5) and (5.6) are still valid.

Example 5.4 Table 5.3 is the life table for SHHS men using the data in Table 5.2 and, consecutively, (5.8), (5.7), (5.2), (5.3) and (5.9). The n_t^* values are given in the 'adjusted number' column. Figure 5.4 shows the estimated cumulative survival probabilities from Table 5.3, together with 95% confidence intervals calculated from (5.5).

As in Example 5.2, a useful summary measure for the life table is the longest possible survival probability; here, the probability of survival for 9 years is estimated as 0.941081. Notice that this is not the same as the total number of men who have not experienced an event divided by the total number studied, 4183/4402 = 0.950250, because the latter takes no account of loss to follow-up. Unlike Example 5.2, the intermediate life table values *are* required to produce an appropriate measure of overall survival.

5.3.3   Comparison of two life tables

As discussed in Section 5.1, cohort studies are much more useful if they involve an element of comparison. Life tables can be constructed for each subgroup of the cohort and the survival experiences compared by graphical, or more formal, methods. In Section 5.5, we shall develop a global test for the comparison of survival; here, we shall restrict ourselves to comparing two specific survival probabilities, one from each of the two subgroups.

Table 5.3. Life table for coronary events; selected subset of SHHS men.

Time (years)	Number	Censored	Events	Adjusted number	Interval risk	Interval survival	Cumulative survival probability	
							Estimate	Standard error
0	4402	7	17	4398.5	0.003865	0.996135	0.996135	0.0009356
1	4378	12	22	4372.0	0.005032	0.994968	0.991122	0.0014152
2	4344	24	26	4332.0	0.006002	0.993998	0.985174	0.0018253
3	4294	19	23	4284.5	0.005368	0.994632	0.979885	0.0021226
4	4252	21	37	4241.5	0.008723	0.991277	0.971337	0.0025268
5	4194	15	38	4186.5	0.009077	0.990923	0.962521	0.0028804
6	4141	501	31	3890.5	0.007968	0.992032	0.954851	0.0031697
7	3609	2143	20	2537.5	0.007882	0.992118	0.947325	0.0035636
8	1446	1375	5	758.5	0.006592	0.993408	0.941081	0.0045033
9	66	66	0					

Table 5.4. Extract from life tables for SHSS men living in owner-occupied and rented accommodations.

	Owner-occupiers					Renters				
				Cumulative survival probability					Cumulative survival probability	
Time (years)	Number	Censored	Events	Estimate	Standard error	Number	Censored	Events	Estimate	Standard error
0	2482	2	8	0.996776	0.0011382	1920	5	9	0.995306	0.0015609
1	2472	5	12	0.991932	0.0017968	1906	7	10	0.990075	0.0022657
2	2455	10	11	0.987478	0.0022349	1889	14	15	0.982184	0.0030282
3	2434	9	8	0.984227	0.0025058	1860	10	15	0.974241	0.0036323
4	2417	12	17	0.977287	0.0030006	1835	9	20	0.963597	0.0043024
5	2388	4	21	0.968686	0.0035126	1806	11	17	0.954499	0.0047943
6	2363	247	15	0.962197	0.0038679	1778	254	16	0.945249	0.0052762
7	2101	1286	9	0.956258	0.0043212	1508	857	11	0.935617	0.0059684
8	806	755	3	0.949563	0.0057661	640	620	2	0.929946	0.0071534
9	48	48	0			18	18	0		

The standard error of the difference between two cumulative survival probabilities, $s_t^{(1)}$ and $s_t^{(2)}$, is estimated as

$$\hat{se}\left(s_t^{(1)} - s_t^{(2)}\right) = \sqrt{\hat{se}\left(s_t^{(1)}\right)^2 + \hat{se}\left(s_t^{(2)}\right)^2}, \qquad (5.10)$$

leading to an approximate 95% confidence interval for the true difference of

$$s_t^{(1)} - s_t^{(2)} \pm 1.96\, \hat{se}\left(s_t^{(1)} - s_t^{(2)}\right). \qquad (5.11)$$

An approximate test of the null hypothesis that the two survival probabilities are equal is given by comparing

$$\left\{ \frac{s_t^{(1)} - s_t^{(2)}}{\hat{se}\left(s_t^{(1)} - s_t^{(2)}\right)} \right\}^2 \qquad (5.12)$$

to chi-square with 1 d.f.

Example 5.5 The data of Table 5.2 were disaggregated by housing tenure status and separate life tables were constructed for owner–occupiers and renters. The essential results are shown in Table 5.4, from which Figure 5.5 was drawn to compare the two survival functions pictorially. The chance of survival without a coronary event is greatest in the owner–occupier groups at all times. This agrees with, but adds to, the finding of Example 4.3: those who live in rented accommodation (predominantly those of lower social status in 1980s Scotland) are more likely to experience CHD.

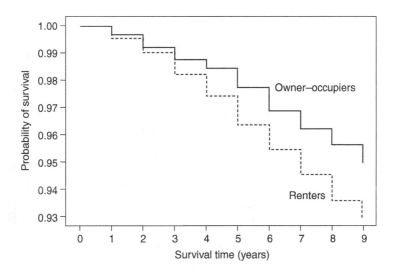

Figure 5.5. Estimated cumulative survival probabilities for coronary events comparing owner–occupiers (solid line) and renters (dashed line); SHHS men.

We might wish to compare 9-year survival to see whether the observed difference is statistically significant. Using (5.10), the test statistic, (5.12), becomes

$$\frac{(0.949563 - 0.929946)^2}{0.0057661^2 + 0.0071534^2} = 4.56.$$

From Table B.3, this result is significant at the 5% level of significance ($0.05 > p > 0.025$). Hence, there is evidence of a real difference.

Suppose that, for some reason, 5-year survival was of key interest. An approximate 95% confidence interval for the difference in the probability of survival for 5 years for owner–occupiers compared with renters is, from (5.10) and (5.11),

$$0.977287 - 0.963597 \pm 1.96\sqrt{0.0030006^2 + 0.0043024^2};$$

that is, 0.01369 ± 0.01028 or $(0.00341, 0.02397)$.

Figure 5.6 shows the difference in estimated survival probabilities up to each whole number of years of survival. In this instance, 99% confidence intervals for this difference are shown. Recall that, as in other cases based upon the normal distribution, we can make the formula for a 95% confidence interval into one for an alternative percentage of confidence by replacing the two-sided 5% critical value, 1.96, by the appropriate alternative: here, 2.5758, the 1% critical value (see Table B.2).

The difference in survival always favours owner–occupiers and tends to increase with time. Confidence limits also get wider with time. As there are few events and many censored at that time, we should expect the considerable lack of precision in the final year that the figure shows.

5.3.4   Limitations

We have already noted that the life table approach produces a step function, leading to consequent overestimation of survival probabilities at points intermediate to the cut-points that define the life table intervals. This suggests that it will be better to choose small intervals whenever several specific probabilities are likely to be of interest.

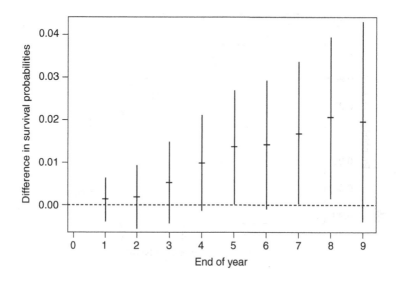

Figure 5.6. Difference between estimated survival probabilities for owner–occupiers and renters by year of follow-up; SHHS men. Bars show 99% confidence intervals.

For each interval in the life table, the actuarial method, defined by (5.8), assumes that the number of events amongst $n_t - c_t$ people who are at risk for the entire interval and c_t people who are at risk for part of the interval is equal to the expected number of events from $n_t - \frac{1}{2}c_t$ people who are at risk for the entire interval. This will be accurate if the average time to censoring is half the length of the interval, which would be true if censoring occurs uniformly within the interval, and if the risk of an event in any small time period is constant throughout the interval.

In some situations, the approximation is not reasonable because either or both of these conditions are known to be violated. It may be that the average time to censoring is not halfway through the interval. Perhaps, for example, it is two-thirds of the way through. In this case, we adjust (5.8) accordingly to

$$n_t^* = n_t - \tfrac{1}{3}c_t.$$

In general, we might prefer to use

$$n_t^* = n_t - (1 - a_t)c_t, \tag{5.13}$$

where a_t is the average proportion of the interval that is survived before censoring occurs, for the interval that begins at time t. Sometimes a_t will be unknown and a value of 0.5, leading to (5.8), will be the best 'guess'. If the interval is small, the number censored, c_t, is unlikely to be large and hence the choice of value for a_t in the general expression, (5.13), is unlikely to be important. Notice that this is certainly not the case in Example 5.4 and Example 5.5 in which hundreds are censored in the seventh, eighth and ninth years of follow-up.

Alternatively, it may be that the risk of an event in, say, any single day increases (or decreases) as a person progresses through an interval defined in the life table. Consider a whole human life span represented by 10-year intervals in a life table for a birth cohort study. During the first 10 years, the instantaneous risk of death decreases rapidly, particularly during the first year as the baby develops in strength. A child leaving the study, say, halfway through the initial 10-year interval from birth will have already experienced the most vulnerable period. Using (5.7) with (5.8) will then overestimate the risk of death. Similarly, during the last 10 years of life, the instantaneous risk of death will increase as the elderly person grows frailer, so we can expect underestimates when censoring occurs in the final 10-year interval.

To avoid such problems, small intervals are recommended (again). Then the exact time at which withdrawals occur will not be crucial to the approximation, and instantaneous risk is unlikely to vary substantially within any of the intervals. Small intervals may only be required at survival durations in which censoring is common or risk is known to be changing rapidly.

5.4   Kaplan–Meier estimation

The **Kaplan–Meier** (KM) or **product-limit** approach to estimating the survival function (Kaplan and Meier, 1958) provides a response to the limitations of the standard life table identified in Section 5.3.4. In the KM approach, the observed event times for the cohort studied define the values of t at which s_t is evaluated; in the life table approach these values are round numbers, usually set in advance of data collection. The KM approach leads to a life table with the smallest possible intervals. This uses the maximum amount of information in the data, ensuring that the steps in s_t are as small as possible. Furthermore, the possible problems concerned with withdrawals are minimised. The only disadvantages are that the KM approach requires more (usually much more) computation and produces a less useful tabular display.

Essentially, KM estimation is life table estimation with the life table times (cut-points used to define the intervals) taken to be equal to the times of events in the cohort. Thus, with no censoring, (5.1) through (5.6) are still valid. However, in the presence of censoring, (5.1) and (5.4) are used rather than (5.7) and (5.9), or any other adjusted formula. As already mentioned, the choice of approximation used to deal with censoring is unlikely to be important when the intervals in the equivalent life table are small. The procedures for comparing cumulative survival probabilities given in Section 5.3.3 are also applicable, including (5.10) through (5.12).

Applying the KM methodology to the SHHS data analysed in Example 5.4 leads to a presentational problem: the resultant life table will be huge because there are hundreds of events. Instead, for illustrative purposes, we shall go through the calculations for the first year of follow-up (up to 365 days from a subject's baseline) only.

Example 5.6 During the first year of follow-up in the SHHS, the completed survival times (in days) for the male subset defined in Section 5.3.2 were:

$$1, 46, 91^*, 101, 101, 103, 119, 133^*, 137, 145^*, 156, 186^*,$$

$$208, 215, 235, 242, 251, 294, 299, 300, 309^*, 312, 336^*, 357^*.$$

Here, * denotes a censored observation (others are event times). A schematic representation of the loss to follow-up in year 1 is given by Figure 5.7. Note the double event at time 101.

The KM estimates of the survival function and their estimated standard errors are given in Table 5.5 (from Table 5.3, we already know that there were 4402 men at baseline). Seventeen coronary events occurred during the year, two of which occurred on the same day of follow-up. Hence, excluding the start and end rows, Table 5.5 has 16 rows. The seven censoring times do not define a row of the table, but the loss due to censoring must be accounted for when determining the number who survive to each specified time. For example, because 4401 survived to 46 days, then one man experienced a coronary event on this day and then another man was censored at 91 days, the number surviving to 101 days is $4401 - 1 - 1 = 4399$. At 365 days there were $4402 - 17 - 7 = 4378$ still under study and event free. The number at risk in the KM life table is that just *before* the time of the event (or events) occurring on that day.

5.4.1   An empirical comparison

It is of interest to compare KM results with the actuarial results (from Section 5.3). The probability of survival to 1 year in Table 5.5 is 0.996136, compared with 0.996135 in Table 5.3. These are in excellent agreement; this magnitude of difference is no more than might be expected from rounding error. This is not always so. When KM estimation was used for the entire 9 years of SHHS data, the end-of-year estimates were as shown

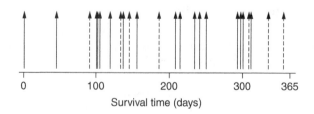

Figure 5.7. Loss to follow-up during the first year of study; selected subset of SHHS men. Solid arrows denote coronary events; dashed arrows denote censoring.

Table 5.5. Data and Kaplan–Meier estimation of the
survival function; year 1 of follow-up for the selected subset
of SHHS men.

| Time | Number | | Survival probability | |
(days)	at risk	Events	Estimate	Standard error
0	4402		1	
1	4402	1	0.999773	0.0002271
46	4401	1	0.999546	0.0003212
101	4399	2	0.999091	0.0004542
103	4397	1	0.998864	0.0005077
119	4396	1	0.998637	0.0005561
137	4394	1	0.998410	0.0006007
156	4392	1	0.998182	0.0006421
208	4390	1	0.997954	0.0006810
215	4389	1	0.997727	0.0007178
235	4388	1	0.997500	0.0007528
242	4387	1	0.997273	0.0007862
251	4386	1	0.997045	0.0008183
294	4385	1	0.996818	0.0008491
299	4384	1	0.996591	0.0008788
300	4383	1	0.996363	0.0009075
312	4381	1	0.996136	0.0009354
365	4378			

in Table 5.6, which also gives the actuarial results reproduced from Table 5.3 for ease
of comparison. The agreement in the estimates of survival probabilities, as well as their
standard errors, is very good until the last 3 years, when they begin to drift apart. This
is not surprising because this is the period when there are several hundred censored
and relatively few events. As noted already, the study described here could not be
expected to produce accurate results for these later years.

When there are many events, published tabular displays of KM analyses will generally be extracts from the whole life table, such as are given in Table 5.6. Graphical
displays are more straightforward: Figure 5.8 gives KM estimates (and 95% confidence
intervals) for the entire follow-up of the SHHS cohort. This is the direct equivalent of
Figure 5.4; notice that the steps in the KM survival function are much less pronounced
than in the actuarial function, leading to a smoother display.

Table 5.6. Comparison of actuarial and Kaplan–Meier (KM)
results for the survivor function; SHHS selected subset.

| Time | Estimate | | Standard error ($\times 10\,000$) | |
(years)	Actuarial	KM	Actuarial	KM
1	0.996135	0.996136	9.356	9.354
2	0.991122	0.991125	14.152	14.148
3	0.985174	0.985177	18.253	18.249
4	0.979885	0.979885	21.226	21.226
5	0.971337	0.971339	25.268	25.267
6	0.962521	0.962525	28.804	28.800
7	0.954851	0.954982	31.697	31.607
8	0.947325	0.947144	35.636	36.308
9	0.941081	0.936608	45.033	70.003

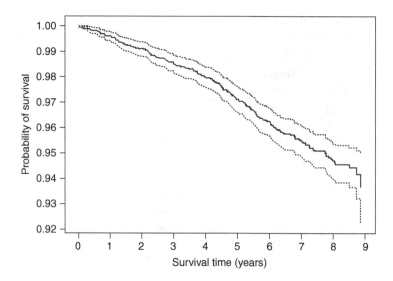

Figure 5.8. Kaplan–Meier estimates and 95% confidence intervals for cumulative survival probabilities for coronary events; selected subset of SHHS men.

Kaplan–Meier plots may be produced from the STS command in Stata or PROC LIFETEST in SAS, as well as from other standard statistical software.

5.5   Comparison of two sets of survival probabilities

In Section 5.3.3, we saw how to use Greenwood's formula, (5.4), to construct a test for equality and confidence interval for the difference between two cumulative survival probabilities, one from each of two cohorts (or two subgroups of a single cohort). Here we consider the more general problem of comparing two complete sets of such probabilities; that is, we seek summary measures of comparative survival across the entire period of follow-up.

5.5.1   Mantel–Haenszel methods

Suppose that the follow-up times for both the cohorts to be compared are divided into the same consecutive intervals, just as in Table 5.4. Consider the number surviving to the start of each interval and the number of events in each interval, just as we have done before. Table 5.7 shows the relevant values extracted from Table 5.4.

Consider the first interval (0 to 1 year of follow-up). We can write the survival experience of the two groups during this interval as a 2×2 table (Table 5.8). We could then use the methods of Chapter 3 to compare the survival experiences within this first year, although this would take no account of those censored. Of more interest here is the fact that tables akin to Table 5.8 may be constructed for each interval in Table 5.7: nine tables in all. We seek a summary measure of the chance of an event or, conversely, of survival, across the nine intervals: a situation analogous to that of Section 4.6, in which Mantel–Haenszel methodology was used to produce summaries over strata defined by a confounding variable. Now the strata are the intervals of time, but otherwise the methodology transfers.

Example 5.7 Mantel–Haenszel methods will now be used to summarise survival in the SHHS example. Table 5.9 gives the set of 2×2 tables produced from Table 5.7 (the first of which is

Table 5.7. SHHS coronary survival data for men living in owner-occupied and rented accommodations.

Interval (years)	Owner–occupiers		Renters	
	Number[a]	Events	Number[a]	Events
0 but less than 1	2482	8	1920	9
1 but less than 2	2472	12	1906	10
2 but less than 3	2455	11	1889	15
3 but less than 4	2434	8	1860	15
4 but less than 5	2417	17	1835	20
5 but less than 6	2388	21	1806	17
6 but less than 7	2363	15	1778	16
7 but less than 8	2101	9	1508	11
8 but less than 9	806	3	640	2

[a] Number at the beginning of the interval.

Table 5.8. Survival experience by housing tenure status during the first year of follow-up; SHHS men.

Housing tenure	Event	No event	Total
Renters	9	1911	1920
Owner–occupiers	8	2474	2482
Total	17	4385	4402

Table 5.9. Survival experience by housing tenure status for each interval defined in Table 5.7.[a]

9	1911	1920		10	1896	1906		15	1874	1889
8	2474	2482		12	2460	2472		11	2444	2455
17	4385	4402		22	4356	4378		26	4318	4344

$E(a_1) = 7.415$ $\quad\quad\quad E(a_2) = 9.578$ $\quad\quad\quad E(a_3) = 11.306$

$V(a_1) = 4.166$ $\quad\quad\quad V(a_2) = 5.382$ $\quad\quad\quad V(a_3) = 6.353$

15	1845	1860		20	1815	1835		17	1789	1806
8	2426	2434		17	2400	2417		21	2367	2388
23	4271	4294		37	4215	4252		38	4156	4194

$E(a_4) = 9.963$ $\quad\quad\quad E(a_5) = 15.968$ $\quad\quad\quad E(a_6) = 16.364$

$V(a_4) = 5.618$ $\quad\quad\quad V(a_5) = 9.000$ $\quad\quad\quad V(a_6) = 9.235$

16	1762	1778		11	1497	1508		2	638	640
15	2348	2363		9	2092	2101		3	803	806
31	4110	4141		20	3589	3609		5	1441	1446

$E(a_7) = 13.310$ $\quad\quad\quad E(a_8) = 8.357$ $\quad\quad\quad E(a_9) = 2.213$

$V(a_7) = 7.540$ $\quad\quad\quad V(a_8) = 4.839$ $\quad\quad\quad V(a_9) = 1.230$

[a] See Table 5.8 for labels.

Table 5.8). Underneath each table $E(a_i)$ and $V(a_i)$ are given ($i = 1, 2, ..., 9$), the mean and variance of each top left-hand cell value (see Table 4.12). These are calculated from (4.19).

From (4.21), the continuity-corrected Cochran–Mantel–Haenszel test statistic for the null hypothesis of no overall difference in survival experience between the housing tenure groups is

$$\frac{\left(\left|\sum a_i - \sum E(a_i)\right| - \frac{1}{2}\right)^2}{\sum V(a_i)} = \frac{\left(\left|115 - 94.474\right| - 0.5\right)^2}{53.363} = 7.52.$$

From Table B.3, for 1 d.f., this is significant at the 0.1% level (the exact p value is 0.006). Hence, there is evidence of a difference in the overall chance of survival. As the sum of observed values ($\sum a_i$) is greater than the sum of expected ($\sum E(a_i)$) for those who experience an event amongst renters, we can conclude that renters are the more likely to have a coronary attack.

We can use (4.10) or (4.15) to estimate the common odds ratio or relative risk across the intervals. Both turn out to be 1.46. Hence, we estimate that renters are almost half as likely again to experience a coronary event within any one year of the nine. This may be compared with Example 4.3, in which the relative risk for an event within 6 years was found to be about 1.3, when no account was taken of those censored. The difference is explained by reference to Table 5.4: a disproportionate number of renters were censored (mainly due to death from other causes) in the earlier years of follow-up.

5.5.2   The log-rank test

In Section 5.5.1 the treatment of censored individuals was rather crude. For instance, it may be that one of the two cohorts (subgroups) loses several subjects during an interval whilst the other does not. The analysis would then be biased against the cohort with no censoring. As in Section 5.4, we can minimise the chance of such a problem by taking the intervals to be as small as possible. In the current situation, we choose the intervals between successive events for the two subgroups *combined*.

When the Cochran–Mantel–Haenszel test of Section 4.6.2 is applied to survival data using KM intervals, it is called the **log-rank test**. In Example 5.8, we apply this test to data from the first year of the SHHS. As with KM estimation, the log-rank test is computationally intensive and it would be impractical to provide a detailed numerical example of its application to the entire 9 years of the SHHS. In practice, a computer package would be used.

The name 'log-rank test' (or 'logrank test') is sometimes applied to other, similar test procedures. These include the procedures given in Section 5.5.3 and the test used by Peto *et al.* (1977). This is unfortunate because it may lead to confusion. An alternative derivation of the log-rank test, as defined here, is given by Cox and Oakes (1984).

Example 5.8 During the first year of follow-up in the SHHS, the completed survival times (in days) for the men in owner–occupied accommodation were:

46, 101, 103, 119, 208, 215, 235, 299, 309*, 336*.

For those in rented accommodation, they were:

1, 91*, 101, 133*, 137, 145*, 156, 186*, 242, 251, 294, 300, 312, 357*.

As before, * denotes a censored observation. We could proceed, as in Example 5.7, to list the set of 16 2 × 2 tables of tenure by survivorship (one for each interval between events). However, this is not necessary in order to apply (4.21), the continuity-corrected log-rank test statistic. A table

Table 5.10. SHHS coronary survival data during the first year of follow-up for men living in owner–occupied and rented accommodations.

Interval (days)	Owner–occupiers $\bar{E}_i$	c_i	Renters E_i	a_i	Expectation $E(a_i)$	Variance $V(a_i)$
1 to less than 46	2482	0	1920	1	0.4362	0.2459
46 to less than 101	2482	1	1919	0	0.4361	0.2459
101 to less than 103	2481	1	1918	1	0.8720	0.4917
103 to less than 119	2480	1	1917	0	0.4360	0.2459
119 to less than 137	2479	1	1917	0	0.4361	0.2459
137 to less than 156	2478	0	1916	1	0.4360	0.2459
156 to less than 208	2478	0	1914	1	0.4358	0.2459
208 to less than 215	2478	1	1912	0	0.4355	0.2458
215 to less than 235	2477	1	1912	0	0.4356	0.2459
235 to less than 242	2476	1	1912	0	0.4357	0.2459
242 to less than 251	2475	0	1912	1	0.4358	0.2459
251 to less than 294	2475	0	1911	1	0.4357	0.2459
294 to less than 299	2475	0	1910	1	0.4356	0.2459
299 to less than 300	2475	1	1909	0	0.4354	0.2458
300 to less than 312	2474	0	1909	1	0.4355	0.2458
312 to 365	2473	0	1908	1	0.4355	0.2458
Total		8		9	7.4086	4.1798

in the format of Table 5.7 has all the necessary information, from which (4.21) can be applied repeatedly by interpreting the items in each row in terms of the 2×2 table that they define. This shorthand approach has been used in Table 5.10 (from Table 5.4, we already know that there were 2482 owner–occupiers and 1920 renters at baseline). The columns labelled $\bar{E}_i$ and E_i are the number of survivors (after events and censoring have been accounted for) at the start of interval i and c_i and a_i are the numbers of events within interval i for owner–occupiers and renters, respectively. This notation is derived from Table 4.12.

As an example of the calculations required to obtain the final two columns, consider the first row of Table 5.10. By reference to Table 4.12 and analogy with Example 5.7, (4.19) gives

$$E\left(a_1\right) = \frac{\left(1 + 0\right) \times 1920}{1920 + 2482} = 0.4362,$$

$$V\left(a_1\right) = \frac{\left(1 + 0\right)\left(\left(1920 - 1\right) + \left(2482 - 0\right)\right) \times 1920 \times 2482}{\left(1920 + 2482\right)^2 \left(1920 + 2482 - 1\right)} = 0.2459.$$

Notice that the expected number of events in the renters group, under the null hypothesis of no difference (in survival) between the groups, is equal to the risk of an event in the combined cohort times the number at risk in the renters group. This seems intuitively reasonable.

From (4.21), the continuity-corrected log-rank test statistic is

$$\frac{\left(\left|9 - 7.4086\right| - 0.5\right)^2}{4.1798} = 0.2850.$$

This is to be compared with χ_1^2 but is clearly not significant at any reasonable significance level. We conclude that there is no evidence of a difference between coronary survival probabilities in the first year of follow-up.

Just as the choice of which group to place in the first row of Table 5.8 and Table 5.9 is arbitrary, we could choose to swap the owner–occupiers and renters data, keeping the labels for $\bar{E}_i$, etc. fixed, in Table 5.10. We would then find that $\sum(a_i) - \sum E(a_i)$ has the same magnitude but opposite sign to that found previously. $\sum V(a_i)$ would remain the same. As a consequence, the value of the log-rank test statistic would stay the same.

5.5.3 Weighted log-rank tests

A class of alternative tests to the log-rank test are the **weighted log-rank tests**. These are generally derived from the log-rank statistic without continuity correction (4.20), which may be written as

$$L = E^2/V, \tag{5.14}$$

where

$$E = \sum\left(a_i - E\left(a_i\right)\right), \qquad V = \sum V\left(a_i\right) \tag{5.15}$$

and the summations run over all time intervals. Weighted log-rank test statistics are of the form

$$L_w = E_w^2/V_w, \tag{5.16}$$

where

$$E_w = \sum w_i\left(a_i - E\left(a_i\right)\right), \quad V_w = \sum w_i^2 V\left(a_i\right) \tag{5.17}$$

and the $\{w_i\}$ are a set of weights, one for each time interval. The log-rank test is a special case in which $w_i = 1$ for all i. Weighted log-rank test statistics are each compared to chi-square with 1 d.f.

The most common weighted log-rank test takes $w_i = n_i$, the number at risk at the start of time interval i. This test is variously known as the **Breslow, Gehan** or **(generalised) Wilcoxon test**. It gives greatest weight to the time intervals with the greatest numbers at risk; inevitably, these are the earliest time intervals. Most other weighting schemes take w_i to be some function of n_i; for example $w_i = \sqrt{n_i}$ leads to the **Tarone–Ware test**.

Example 5.9 Figure 5.9 shows the KM estimates of the survivor function for coronary events by housing tenure status for the entire 9 years of the SHHS data. Once more we see that owner–occupiers have the best outcomes at all times. The complete set of data (as used here in its entirety, and earlier in summary or extract) may be downloaded; see Appendix A.

The application of the log-rank test to the entire dataset is a straightforward extension of Example 5.8. It turns out that $E = 20.435$ and $V = 53.7180$, using (5.15). The continuity-corrected log-rank statistic is then, from (4.21) and (5.14),

$$(20.435 - 0.5)^2/53.7180 = 7.40,$$

whilst the uncorrected form, (5.14), is

$$20.435/53.7180 = 7.77.$$

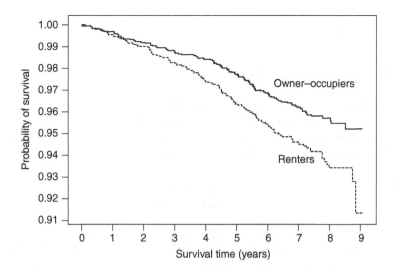

Figure 5.9. Kaplan–Meier estimates of the cumulative survival probability for owner–occupiers (solid line) and renters (dashed line); SHHS men.

As we saw earlier, the SHHS results are unreliable in the final couple of years due to the large number censored and the small number of events. Hence, there is a case for weighting the test procedure in favour of the earlier intervals. The generalised Wilcoxon test was applied to the data and gave $E_w = 78\,493$ and $V_w = 8.866 \times 10^8$ using (5.17). From (5.16), the test statistic is

$$78493^2 \big/ \left(8.866 \times 10^8\right) = 6.95.$$

Neither the continuity correction nor the Wilcoxon weighting has had a large effect upon the result in this example. When each of these three test statistics is compared with χ^2_1, the p value is below 0.01 (see Table B.3). Hence, we can conclude that there is evidence of a real difference; the benefit of being an owner–occupier does not seem to be simply due to chance. Compare this conclusion with that of Example 5.8; Figure 5.9 shows little difference between the tenure groups in the first year, but a widening gap thereafter.

In Section 4.6.3 we noted that the Cochran–Mantel–Haenszel test assumes that the comparative chance of an event does not vary by level of the confounding factor. Translated into the current application, the log-rank test assumes that the comparative chance of an event does not vary by the time intervals between events. This is widely known as the **proportional hazards** assumption. We shall consider this assumption more fully in Chapter 11. For now, it is sufficient to note that it is an assumption of time homogeneity: the chances of an event in the two groups are assumed to be in constant proportion over time.

The null hypothesis for the log-rank test is that the constant proportion is unity (that is, no difference). The alternative hypothesis is that this constant proportion is something other than unity. Under conditions of proportional hazards, the log-rank test is the most powerful test available (see Section 8.2 for a formal definition of 'power'). Otherwise, a weighted test will be preferable. Hence, we require a method of testing for proportional hazards, an issue discussed in Section 11.8. In most applications, the log-rank test is used rather than any kind of weighted test unless the proportional hazards assumption is clearly false.

The log-rank test may be applied using the STS TEST command in Stata or PROC LIFETEST in SAS.

5.5.4 Allowing for confounding variables

The log-rank test may easily be extended to allow adjustment for confounding variables. We split the data into strata defined by the levels of the confounder. Then we find the E and V statistics of (5.15) for each stratum: call these E_j and V_j for the jth stratum. The **stratified log-rank test statistic** is then

$$L_s = \sum E_j^2 \Big/ \sum V_j,$$

where the summations run over all strata. This is, once more, compared against chi-square with 1 d.f. Similar stratified tests may be constructed for weighted log-rank tests. An alternative way of dealing with confounding is through a statistical model for survival analysis; see Chapter 11.

5.5.5 Comparing three or more groups

The log-rank test and its associates may be extended to deal with the problem of comparing three or more sets of survival functions; see Collett (2003). In practice, such situations are more commonly dealt with using the statistical models of Chapter 11.

5.6   Competing risk

Although the study may be designed to study only one disease, for example heart disease, follow-up may be terminated due to death from some other disease, such as cancer. In a sense, heart disease and death from cancer are then **competing risks**. The simplest way to deal with a competing cause is to treat it as a type of censoring mechanism. This may be acceptable if the second type of event is independent of the event we are interested in, for example having a benign skin tumour may well not affect the future chance of having a heart attack. When having the second event does affect the chance of a future event of the type that we wish to study, we should consider taking this into account. Dying from cancer, or any other non-coronary cause, clearly makes the chance of a future heart attack zero, and thus provides an example where competing risk should be considered.

Treating the competing risk as a form of censoring gives us estimated probabilities of an event on the assumption that the competing cause does not occur. Another way of looking at this is that predicted probabilities will be for the hypothetical universe where the competing cause does not exist. Consider the data of Example 5.6. Some of the men who were censored had non-coronary deaths, so that we should consider the results in the 'estimate' column of Table 5.5 as the time-specific probabilities of survival from CHD when death (other than a coronary death) is assumed not to intervene. So we estimate that a middle-aged man in Scotland has (at the time of study) 99.6% chance of being free from CHD within 12 months' time, assuming that he does not die from other causes in this period. In fact, in competing risk (CR) analysis the language concerning survival becomes awkward and hence it is more usual to talk about the chance of failure than the chance of survival. Using KM the change is straightforward using (5.2). So the man in our example has a 0.4% chance of a coronary event within 12 months, if he does not die from another cause first.

If, instead, we wish to make a probabilistic statement based upon his complete chance of being CHD-free, allowing for his overall chance of death, then we need a different approach to estimation than KM, although we shall still use the KM construct wherein the times of events define the study intervals in our life table. Our competing risk analysis will estimate the time-specific probability of a coronary event allowing for the fact that death from another cause may occur first. We will develop this using a hypothetical example based on the real data of Example 5.6, but where events occur in clusters, rather than (apart from the double event at 101 days) singularly. This will be assumed purely for demonstration purposes — to ensure that the probabilities derived using KM and CR differ to a noticeable degree. Precisely, our artificial example will have all the single CHD events in Example 5.6 involve 50 people; and all the censored events involve 100 people, 60 of whom have a non-CHD death and 40 of whom are lost to follow-up due to emigration. The first five columns of Table 5.11 show all the assumed numbers, from which we shall derive CR estimates for CHD incidence.

Although several approaches to CR analysis have been suggested, for simplicity here we shall only look at the most commonly used method that does not involve statistical modelling: **cause-specific estimation**. In Example 11.9 a second method will be used, that being the method most commonly used in modelling. The cause-specific approach argues that, if we want to allow for competing risks, we should consider the risk of an index event (that is, the event of interest) in each study interval only for those people who have survived to the start of the interval free of both the index and the competing event. In this way, we explicitly allow for occurrences of the competing event when estimating survival.

Suppose we generalise the notation used earlier in this chapter so that the joint risk of an event (the index event or the competing event) during the interval t is $q_t^{(J)}$ and the corresponding chance of joint survival in the interval is $p_t^{(J)}$. Then, by analogy to (5.1),

$$q_t^{(J)} = \left(e_t^{(1)} + e_t^{(2)} \right) \Big/ n_t,$$

where e and n are as defined in Section 5.3 and the '(1)' and '(2)' superscripts denote the index and competing event, respectively. When censoring is present, n will deflate due both to events (of either type) and censoring. By analogy to (5.2) and (5.3):

$$p_t^{(J)} = 1 - q_t^{(J)}$$

and

$$s_t^{(J)} = p_0^{(J)} p_1^{(J)} p_2^{(J)} \ldots p_t^{(J)}.$$

Once someone has reached the start of interval t, from (5.1) again, they have a probability

$$q_t^{(1)} = e_t^{(1)} \Big/ n_t$$

of having the index event in that interval. Hence the probability of both surviving, free of both events, to the start of interval t and then failing (i.e., having the index event) in that interval is the conditional probability,

$$d_t^{(1)} = s_{t-1}^{(J)} q_t^{(1)}.$$

Table 5.11. Computations of cause-specific CHD incidence allowing for competing risk due to non-CHD death: numerically scaled up hypothetical version of the data used in Example 5.6 (surv. = survival and cond. = conditional). The final column (in italics) shows the estimated cumulative failure from CHD when competing risk is ignored (i.e., treated as censored).

Time	Number at risk	CHD	Died	Censored	Interval joint risk $(q^{(J)})$	Interval joint surv. $(p^{(J)})$	Cumulative joint surv. $(s^{(J)})$	Interval risk $(q^{(1)})$	Interval cond. risk $(d^{(1)})$	Cumulative failure $(f^{(1)})$	Kaplan-Meier failure
0	4402						1				
1	4402	50	0	0	0.011358	0.988642	0.988642	0.011358	0.011358	0.011358	0.011358
46	4352	50	0	0	0.011489	0.988511	0.977283	0.011489	0.011358	0.022717	0.022717
91	4302	0	60	40	0.013947	0.986053	0.963653	0	0	0.022717	0.022717
101	4202	100	0	0	0.023798	0.976202	0.940720	0.023798	0.022933	0.045650	0.045975
103	4102	50	0	0	0.012189	0.987811	0.929253	0.012189	0.011467	0.057117	0.057603
119	4052	50	0	0	0.012340	0.987660	0.917786	0.012340	0.011467	0.068583	0.069232
133	4002	0	60	40	0.014993	0.985007	0.904027	0	0	0.068583	0.069232
137	3902	50	0	0	0.012814	0.987186	0.892442	0.012814	0.011584	0.080167	0.081159
145	3852	0	60	40	0.015576	0.984424	0.878541	0	0	0.080167	0.081159
156	3752	50	0	0	0.013326	0.986674	0.866834	0.013326	0.011708	0.091875	0.093404
186	3702	0	60	40	0.016207	0.983793	0.852785	0	0	0.091875	0.093404
208	3602	50	0	0	0.013881	0.986119	0.840947	0.013881	0.011838	0.103713	0.105988
215	3552	50	0	0	0.014077	0.985923	0.829109	0.014077	0.011838	0.115550	0.118573
235	3502	50	0	0	0.014278	0.985722	0.817272	0.014278	0.011838	0.127388	0.131157
242	3452	50	0	0	0.014484	0.985516	0.805434	0.014484	0.011838	0.139226	0.143742
251	3402	50	0	0	0.014697	0.985303	0.793596	0.014697	0.011838	0.151063	0.156327
294	3352	50	0	0	0.014916	0.985084	0.781759	0.014916	0.011838	0.162901	0.168911
299	3302	50	0	0	0.015142	0.984858	0.769921	0.015142	0.011838	0.174739	0.181496
300	3252	50	0	0	0.015375	0.984625	0.758083	0.015375	0.011838	0.186576	0.194081
309	3202	0	60	40	0.018738	0.981262	0.743878	0	0	0.186576	0.194081
312	3102	50	0	0	0.016119	0.983881	0.731888	0.016119	0.011990	0.198567	0.207071
336	3052	0	60	40	0.019659	0.980341	0.717500	0	0	0.198567	0.207071
357	2952	0	60	40	0.020325	0.979675	0.702916	0	0	0.198567	0.207071
365	2852										

To obtain the cumulative probability of failure from the index event, allowing for the competing risk, we then sum all the conditional probabilities up to and including the current interval to give

$$f_t^{(1)} = d_1^{(1)} + d_2^{(1)} + d_3^{(1)} + \cdots + d_t^{(1)}.$$

In columns 6–11 of Table 5.11 these equations are applied to the hypothetical scaling up of Example 5.6.

In order to demonstrate the differences between the KM and CR approaches, KM estimation was used for the same hypothetical data. As already explained, KM lumps those who have died into the group of censored subjects, for each time interval. The final column of Table 5.11 was thus produced using the methods of Section 5.4. Notice that the CR failure estimates are never greater than the KM estimates. This makes sense because only the CR estimates take account of death as an event that might preclude CHD. With these hypothetical data, the chance of a coronary event *per se* is 20.7% whereas the chance of a coronary event, if death from smoking does not occur first, is 19.9%. Some researchers considering these results would consider that only the CR estimates are valid, since the competing event of death is always possible in real life whilst the KM estimates are only interpretable in the hypothetical universe where they are excluded. They would regard the KM estimates of failure as biased upwards.

Notice that it is only competing events that occur before the event of interest that are at issue. For instance, once someone has CHD she or he automatically 'leaves' the life table; that person may die from some non-coronary cause later, but this is irrelevant to our current purpose. Another point to note is that there may be several competing events, but they can (again, for the current purpose) all be taken together. For example, in the CR analyses of CHD we took all non-coronary causes of death as a single competing event.

Choudhury (2002) constructs confidence intervals for cause-specific estimation and Gray (1988) develops a parallel test to the log-rank test which allows for competing risk. Cause-specific incidence probabilities, with confidence intervals, can be obtained from the user-supplied STCOMPET routine in Stata, whilst Lin *et al.* (2012) describe SAS macros for handling CR analyses.

5.7   The person-years method

An alternative to the life table method of analysis for cohort data is the person-years method. The person-years is computed as time followed-up multiplied by the number of people. For instance, four people followed-up for ten years gives 40 person-years; three people followed-up for ten years and one followed-up for five years gives 35 person-years.

The person-years incidence rate is estimated to be

$$\hat{\rho} = e/y, \qquad (5.18)$$

where e is the number of events (just as in earlier sections) and y is the number of person-years of follow-up. To calculate y, we must sum all the follow-up periods of the study subjects. Once someone is censored or has an event, that person's follow-up is terminated. This gives an alternative way of dealing with censoring. Sometimes (5.18)

Table 5.12. Data from a hypothetical chemical company.

Individual no.	Date entered	Date left	Years studied	Death?
1	5 Oct 1962	1 Dec 1999	37y, 2m	yes
2	10 Oct 1975	31 Dec 2003	28y, 3m	no
3	10 Jun 1985	31 Dec 2003	18y, 7m	no
4	30 Aug 1990	28 Sep 2000	10y, 1m	no
5	8 May 1968	8 Jul 1997	29y, 2m	yes
6	1 Nov 1972	10 May 1985	12y, 6m	yes
7	21 Mar 1960	30 Jun 1997	37y, 3m	no
8	8 Jun 1967	29 Jul 1971	4y, 2m	yes
		Total	177y, 2m	yes = 4
				no = 4

is called an **incidence density** to distinguish it from a rate when the denominator is a number of people, as in (3.28).

The only difference between (3.28) and (5.18) lies in the denominator. We develop inferential procedures for each rate assuming that its denominator is a fixed quantity; the only variable quantity is the numerator, which is the number of events in each case. Hence, the confidence intervals and tests given in Section 3.8 are applicable in the current context; we simply replace the number, n, by the person-years, y, in each formula (where necessary).

Example 5.10 Suppose that the eight male employees who work in a high-exposure (to potential toxic substances) department of a chemical company are investigated in an all-causes mortality study. Table 5.12 shows the dates when each man joined the study (that is, began employment in the high-exposure department) and the dates of leaving the study (through death, leaving for another job, retirement or end of study).

Notice that years studied have been calculated to the nearest month. It would be possible to calculate more accurately by counting individual days. If we further approximate 1 month = $1/12 = 0.0833$ years, we get $y = 177.1667$ years. From (5.18), the mortality rate is then $e/y = 4/177.1667 = 0.0226$ or 22.6 per thousand per year.

Users of Stata will find the STPTIME command useful for person-years analyses and other computations covered in this section.

5.7.1   Age-specific rates

Since age is often a basic determinant of propensity for disease, person-years analyses usually take account of age. This is achieved by dividing the time spent in the study into periods spent within distinct age groups, separately for each subject. Of course, during follow-up each individual could pass through several age groups. If e_i is the number of events that occurred whilst subjects were in age group i and y_i is the number of years in total spent in the study whilst in age group i (the person-years at age i) then the person-years incidence rate for age group i is estimated, using (5.18), as

$$\hat{\rho}_i = e_i / y_i. \qquad (5.19)$$

Calculation of the component of y_i attributable to any particular individual is somewhat tricky and would normally be done by computer for any large cohort. Figure 5.10 is a flow-chart specifying a general method for calculating y_i for a single person within

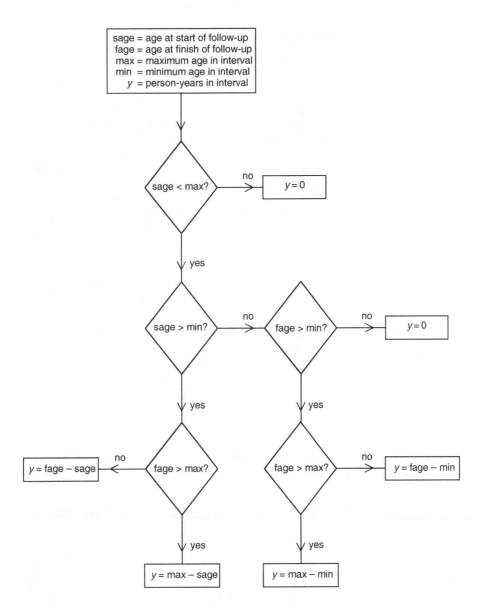

Figure 5.10. Flow-chart for the calculation of age-specific person-years for a single individual and a single age group.

a single age interval denoted by i. The results from all individuals will be summed to give the value of y_i in (5.19) for each i.

Example 5.11 Consider Example 5.10 again, but now include information on date of birth (see Table 5.13). This enables the total employment experience of each person to be divided up by the time spent at different ages. Three age groups are used here; notice that they do not need to span an equal number of years. All durations are rounded to the nearest month, as before.

Ages at start and end have been calculated using the start and end dates from Table 5.11. For example, consider individual number 1:

Age at entry = (5 Oct 1962) − (31 Jul 1935) = 27 years, 2 months,

Age at leaving = (1 Dec 1999) − (31 Jul 1935) = 64 years, 4 months.

Table 5.13. Further data from a hypothetical chemical company (+ denotes a death).

Individual number	Date of birth	Age at start	Age at finish	Experience when aged (years)		
				<40	40–54	55 & over
1	21 Jul 1935	27y, 2m	64y, 4m	12y, 10m	15y, 0m	9y, 4m+
2	1 Aug 1939	36y, 2m	64y, 5m	3y, 10m	15y, 0m	9y, 5m
3	8 Jun 1957	28y, 0m	46y, 7m	12y, 0m	6y, 7m	—
4	17 Jun 1950	40y, 2m	50y, 3m	—	10y, 1m	—
5	3 Jan 1937	31y, 4m	60y, 6m	8y, 8m	15y, 0m	5y, 6m+
6	14 May 1942	30y, 6m	43y, 0m	9y, 6m	3y, 0m+	—
7	30 Jun 1932	27y, 9m	65y, 0m	12y, 3m	15y, 0m	10y, 0m
8	10 Aug 1932	34y, 10m	39y, 0m	4y, 2m+	—	—
			Total	63y, 3m	79y, 8m	34y, 3m
			e_i	1	1	2
			y_i	63.250	79.667	34.250
			$\hat{p}_i$	0.01581	0.01255	0.05839

The components of y_i for each i ($i = 1, 2, 3$) were calculated using Figure 5.10. When $i = 1$, min = 0 and max = 40. When $i = 2$, min = 40 and max = 55. When $i = 3$, min = 55 and max = ∞. Consider, again, the first individual. For him, sage = 27.167 and fage = 64.333. Following the flow-chart through for age group 1, we obtain

$$y = \text{max} - \text{sage} = 40 - 27.167 = 12.667 \text{ years (or 12 years, 10 months)}.$$

For age group 2, we obtain

$$y = \text{max} - \text{min} = 55 - 40 = 15 \text{ years}.$$

For age group 3, we obtain

$$y = \text{fage} - \text{min} = 64.333 - 55 = 9.333 \text{ years (or 9 years, 4 months)}.$$

5.7.2 Summarisation of rates

The set of age-specific estimated rates $\{\hat{p}_i\}$ is generally summarised using the standardised event ratio (SER), as defined by (4.4). This requires some suitable standard population as a basis for comparison. This will often be the national population of which the cohort followed is a subset.

Example 5.12 Suppose that the national statistical digest for the country from which data were collected in Example 5.10 and Example 5.11 reported average annual male death rates (per thousand) of 1.8 for 25- to 39-year-olds; 9.0 for 40- to 54-year-olds and 19.2 for 55- to 64-year-olds. The expected number of deaths in the chemical company department during the course of the cohort study is then, from (4.3),

$$E = 1.8 \times 63.250 + 9.0 \times 79.667 + 19.2 \times 34.250 = 1488.453$$

per thousand. Hence, we would expect to see 1.488 deaths if the chemical company employees had the same chance of death as all males in the country. From (4.4) the standardised mortality ratio (SMR: the SER when the events are all deaths) is 4/1.488 = 2.69, or 269%. Hence, the high-exposure department of the chemical factory is apparently a dangerous place to work, with a death rate 2.69 times the national average (age-standardised).

If the population from which the cohort was selected has the same chance of an event as does the standard population, after age adjustment, then observed and expected numbers of events should be very similar. We can test for equality (that is, study population SER = 1) by calculating

$$\frac{\left(\left|e - E\right| - \frac{1}{2}\right)^2}{E},$$ (5.20)

which is compared against chi-square with 1 d.f. Note that the $\frac{1}{2}$ is a continuity correction, which is appropriate here because e comes from a Poisson distribution and can only take integer values.

Approximate 95% confidence intervals for the SER may be obtained from the approximate result that $\sqrt{e}$ has a normal distribution with variance $\frac{1}{4}$ (Snedecor and Cochran, 1989). This leads to the limits for the study population SER of

$$\mathrm{SER}\left(1 \pm \frac{1.96}{2\sqrt{e}}\right)^2.$$ (5.21)

Unfortunately, (5.20) and (5.21) are inaccurate when e is small. When e is below 20, exact procedures are recommended; see Breslow and Day (1994) and Altman *et al.* (2000). Neither (5.20) nor (5.21) would be suitable for the hypothetical data of Example 5.11, but they could be used for each deprivation group in Example 4.7. The methods of this (and the next) section may be applied equally well to data from other types of studies that are summarised as SERs or indirect standardised rates.

5.7.3 Comparison of two SERs

The methodology of Section 5.7.1 and Section 5.7.2 would be applicable when a single cohort is followed. When two (or more) cohorts or subcohorts are observed, we would normally seek to compare them. We can do this directly, using an extension of the Mantel–Haenszel procedure (see Section 5.7.4), or indirectly by comparing SERs. The latter comparison is indirect because an SER is already a comparative measure where the base is the standard population. If we take the same standard population for each SER, we have a logical framework for comparison.

By analogy with the idea of a relative risk, we can calculate the **relative SER**,

$$\omega_S = \frac{\mathrm{SER}_2}{\mathrm{SER}_1},$$ (5.22)

to compare two standardised event rates, SER_2 relative to SER_1. Since, by (4.6), the indirect standardised rate is a constant times the SER, ω_S may also be called a **standardised relative rate.**

From Breslow and Day (1994), 95% confidence limits for ω_S are given by (ω_L, ω_U), where

$$\omega_L = \frac{E_1 e_2}{E_2 F_L (e_1 + 1)}, \qquad \omega_U = \frac{E_1 F_U (e_2 + 1)}{E_2 e_1}.$$ (5.23)

Here e_1 and E_1 are, respectively, the observed and expected number of events in cohort 1; similarly for cohort 2. F_L is the upper $2\frac{1}{2}\%$ point of the F distribution on $(2e_1 + 2, 2e_2)$ d.f. and F_U is the upper $2\frac{1}{2}\%$ point of the F distribution with $(2e_2 + 2, 2e_1)$ d.f.; see Table B.5(c).

Breslow and Day (1994) also derive an approximate test of the null hypothesis that two SERs are equal. This requires calculation of the test statistic (with continuity correction),

$$\frac{\left(\left|e_1 - E_1^*\right| - \frac{1}{2}\right)^2}{E_1^*} + \frac{\left(\left|e_2 - E_2^*\right| - \frac{1}{2}\right)^2}{E_2^*}, \tag{5.24}$$

which is to be compared against chi-square with 1 d.f. In (5.24),

$$E_i^* = (\text{SER})E_i, \tag{5.25}$$

for $i = 1, 2$, where SER is the overall standardised event ratio for the two cohorts combined. Since (5.24) is only an approximation, it will not necessarily agree with the result from (5.23). When the results are in conflict, it will be better to base the test on inclusion (fail to reject H_0) or exclusion (reject H_0) of unity within the confidence interval. Breslow and Day (1994) also give an exact test that requires evaluating probabilities from the binomial distribution.

Example 5.13 In addition to the chemical company that was the subject of the last three examples, another (much larger) chemical company in the same country also has employees working in similar high-exposure conditions. In the period 1960 to 2003, 43 deaths occurred amongst this company's high-exposure workforce. This compares with 38.755 that were expected according to national statistics.

Clearly, both workforces have higher than expected numbers of deaths when compared with the experiences of the country as a whole. We shall now compare the second workforce with the first.

Letting subscript '1' denote the original chemical company, we have from the preceding and Example 5.10 and Example 5.12,

$$e_1 = 4, \ e_2 = 43,$$

$$E_1 = 1.488, \quad E_2 = 38.755.$$

Hence, the estimated relative SMR, from (4.4) and (5.22), is

$$\hat{\omega}_S = \frac{43 / 38.755}{4 / 1.488} = 0.413.$$

Thus, the second workforce has less than half the (indirectly standardised) rate of the first.

To obtain 95% confidence limits for ω_S, we first find the upper $2\frac{1}{2}\%$ point of F with $(2 \times 4 + 2, 2 \times 43) = (10, 86)$ and $(2 \times 43 + 2, 2 \times 4) = (88, 8)$ d.f. From a statistical computer package, these were found to be 2.201 and 3.749, respectively. Using these, (5.23) gives the lower and upper confidence limits as

$$\frac{1.488 \times 43}{38.755 \times 2.201 \times (4 + 1)} = 0.150 \ \text{and} \ \frac{1.488 \times 3.749 \times (43 + 1)}{38.755 \times 4} = 1.583.$$

Thus, the 95% confidence limits are (0.150, 1.583); there is quite a wide range of error, including a relative age-standardised mortality rate of unity.

We can go on (if we wish) to test the hypothesis that the relative SMR is unity using (5.24). First, we find the overall SMR, which is, from (4.4),

$$\frac{4+43}{1.488+38.755} = 1.168.$$

Using this in (5.25) gives

$$E_1^* = 1.168 \times 1.488 = 1.738,$$

$$E_2^* = 1.168 \times 38.755 = 45.266.$$

Substituting into (5.24) gives the test statistic

$$\frac{\left(\left|4 - 1.738\right| - 0.5\right)^2}{1.738} + \frac{\left(\left|43 - 45.266\right| - 0.5\right)^2}{45.266} = 1.855.$$

This value is well below the 10% critical value from χ_1^2, so the null hypothesis fails to be rejected. No conclusive evidence exists that either company is worse than the other, after allowing for age differentials.

5.7.4   Mantel–Haenszel methods

In Section 5.7.2 and Section 5.7.3, we have seen how to use standardisation to control for variation in age (the confounding variable) and then how to compare two cohorts (or subgroups of a single cohort) using the standard population as an intermediate reference. A more direct way of comparing two cohorts is to use a Mantel–Haenszel (MH) procedure.

As in Section 4.6, the MH approach requires the data for the two cohorts to be subdivided by the strata of the confounding variable(s). As in Section 5.7.1 to Section 5.7.3, we will take age to be the sole confounder (although this is not necessary). Suppose that membership of one cohort denotes exposure, whilst membership of the other is no exposure: for example, smokers versus nonsmokers. Then we record e_{1i} events in the ith age group of cohort 1 (unexposed) and y_{1i} person-years in the ith age group of cohort 1. Here, i ranges over all the age groups used. Similar variables e_{2i} and y_{2i} are defined for cohort 2 (exposed).

It is useful to compare these definitions with those given by Table 4.12 for the fixed cohort problem (where no individual is censored). Two of the terms are identical: $a_i = e_{2i}$ and $c_i = e_{1i}$, but y_{1i} takes the place of $\overline{E}_i$ whilst y_{2i} takes the place of E_i. These latter two relationships are not equalities because, although the Es are real numbers of people, the ys are accumulated durations. Nevertheless, the MH estimate of the age-adjusted **relative rate**, $\hat{\omega}_{\text{MH}}$, turns out to be remarkably similar to the MH estimate of the age-adjusted relative risk, $\hat{\lambda}_{\text{MH}}$, given by (4.15). The estimate is

$$\hat{\omega}_{\text{MH}} = \frac{\sum e_{2i} y_{1i}/y_i}{\sum e_{1i} y_{2i}/y_i}, \tag{5.26}$$

where $y_i = y_{1i} + y_{2i}$ is the total number of person-years at age i (which takes the place of n_i in (4.15)) and the summations run over all age groups. As person-years are used, (5.26) could also be called an age-adjusted **incidence density ratio**. Note that (5.26) compares the exposed to the unexposed. See Rothman and Boice (1979) for a derivation of this MH estimator and Greenland and Robins (1985) for further comment. Breslow (1984) suggests the following estimate for the standard error of the log of the MH estimate:

$$\hat{se}\left(\log_e \hat{\omega}_{MH}\right) = \sqrt{\sum\left(y_{1i}y_{2i}e_i/y_i^2\right)}\Big/\left(\left(\sqrt{\hat{\omega}_{MH}}\right)\left(\sum\left(y_{1i}y_{2i}e_i\Big/y_i\left(y_{1i} + \hat{\omega}_{MH}y_{2i}\right)\right)\right)\right), \tag{5.27}$$

where $e_i = e_{1i} + e_{2i}$ is the total number of events at age i, and the summations run over all age groups.

From (5.27), we get approximate 95% confidence limits $(L_{\log}, U_{\log})$ for $\log_e\omega_{MH}$ of

$$L_{\log} = \log_e\hat{\omega}_{MH} - 1.96\hat{se}\left(\log_e \hat{\omega}_{MH}\right)$$
$$U_{\log} = \log_e\hat{\omega}_{MH} + 1.96\hat{se}\left(\log_e \hat{\omega}_{MH}\right) \tag{5.28}$$

and hence approximate 95% confidence limits (L, U) for ω_{MH} are

$$L = \exp\left(L_{\log}\right),$$
$$U = \exp\left(U_{\log}\right). \tag{5.29}$$

Breslow and Day (1994) provide the following test statistic of the null hypothesis $\omega_{MH} = 1$, that is, no association between exposure and disease after allowing for age differences:

$$\frac{\left(\left|e_2 - \sum\left(y_{2i}e_i/y_i\right)\right| - \frac{1}{2}\right)^2}{\sum\left(y_{1i}y_{2i}e_i/y_i^2\right)}. \tag{5.30}$$

This is compared against chi-square with 1 d.f. Here $e_2 = \sum e_{2i}$ is the total number of events in the exposed group. Once again, the summations run over all age groups and the $\frac{1}{2}$ is a continuity correction.

Finally, recall that MH summarisation is appropriate only if there is homogeneity of exposure-disease association across the age strata (Section 4.6.3). A test of the null hypothesis that the relative rate is homogeneous across age groups is given by comparing

$$\sum\frac{\left(e_{1i} - \hat{e}_{1i}\right)^2}{\hat{e}_{1i}} + \sum\frac{\left(e_{2i} - \hat{e}_{2i}\right)^2}{\hat{e}_{2i}} \tag{5.31}$$

against chi-square with $\ell - 1$ d.f., where ℓ is the number of age groups (the number of items in each summation) and

$$\hat{e}_{1i} = \frac{e_i y_{1i}}{y_{1i} + \hat{\omega}_{MH}y_{2i}},$$
$$\hat{e}_{2i} = \frac{e_i y_{2i}\hat{\omega}_{MH}}{y_{1i} + \hat{\omega}_{MH}y_{2i}}. \tag{5.32}$$

This result is derived by Breslow and Day (1994), although they also suggest an improved, but more complex, procedure requiring the use of an alternative estimator for ω to the MH estimator used in (5.32).

Table 5.14. Number of coronary events and person-years by age group and housing tenure; SHHS men.

Age group (years)	Housing tenure	Coronary events	Person-years	Coronary rate (per thousand)	Relative rate
40–44	renters	2	1107.447	1.806	0.97
	owners	3	1619.328	1.853	
45–49	renters	24	3058.986	7.846	1.88
	owners	19	4550.166	4.176	
50–54	renters	31	3506.530	8.841	1.72
	owners	25	4857.904	5.146	
55–59	renters	28	3756.650	7.453	1.25
	owners	27	4536.832	5.951	
60–64	renters	28	2419.622	11.572	1.19
	owners	26	2680.843	9.698	
65–69	renters	2	351.710	5.687	0.51
	owners	4	356.394	11.224	
Total	renters	115	14 200.945	8.098	1.45
	owners	104	18 601.467	5.591	

Example 5.14 We now return to the example from the SHHS used in earlier sections. Using the algorithm of Figure 5.10, the person-years of follow-up were calculated, by 5-year age group, for men who rent as well as men who occupy their own accommodations. Furthermore, all coronary events were also grouped by the same 5-year age groups. Results are given in Table 5.14. For completeness, age-specific coronary event rates and the relative rate (renters versus owner–occupiers), calculated from (5.18) and (3.31), are included. As the SHHS studied 40- to 59-year-olds, and the maximum follow-up time is less than 10 years, there are no person-years of observation at ages above 69 years.

The age-specific relative rates range from 0.51 to 1.88. We can summarise these by the MH estimate, (5.26),

$$\hat{\omega}_{MH} =$$

$$\frac{(2 \times 1619.328)/(1619.328 + 1107.447) + \cdots + (2 \times 356.394)/(356.394 + 351.710)}{(3 \times 1107.447)/(1619.328 + 1107.447) + \cdots + (4 \times 351.710)/(356.394 + 351.710)}$$

$$= \frac{64.584}{45.888} = 1.407,$$

which is, as expected, different from the unadjusted relative rate, 1.45 (seen in the 'total' line in Table 5.14).

Notice that, because renters provide the numerator for the relative rate, they take the place of the exposed group, with subscript '2' in (5.26) to (5.32). $\hat{\omega}_{MH}$ can be used, in (5.32) and then (5.31), to test whether the relative rate is homogeneous across the age strata. We require all six values of $\hat{e}_{1i}$ and $\hat{e}_{2i}$ from (5.32). For example, when $i = 1$ (age group 40 to 44 years),

$$\hat{e}_{11} = \frac{(3 + 2) \times 1619.328}{1619.328 + 1.407 \times 1107.447} = 2.548,$$

$$\hat{e}_{21} = \frac{(3 + 2) \times 1107.447 \times 1.407}{1619.328 + 1.407 \times 1107.447} = 2.452.$$

When all such terms are calculated, (5.31) becomes $1.981 + 1.699 = 3.68$. This is to be compared against chi-square with $(6 - 1) = 5$ d.f. and is not significant ($p > 0.5$). Hence, we conclude that the difference in observed relative rates by age group was consistent with random error.

We have now established that it is sensible to use a summary measure of the relative rate and shall go on to consider the accuracy of our chosen measure, $\hat{\omega}_{MH}$. From (5.27),

$$\hat{se}\left(\log_e \hat{\omega}_{MH}\right) = \left(\sqrt{\sum T_i}\right) \bigg/ \left(\left(\sqrt{\hat{\omega}_{MH}}\right)\left(\sum B_i\right)\right)$$

where, for example,

$$T_1 = \left(1619.328 \times 1107.447 \times 5\right) \big/ \left(1619.328 + 1107.447\right)^2.$$

$\hat{\omega}_{MH} = 1.407$ and $B_1 =$

$$\left(1619.328 \times 1107.447 \times 5\right) \big/ \left(\left(1619.328 + 1107.447\right)\left(1619.328 + 1.407 \times 1107.447\right)\right).$$

Hence, $\hat{se}\left(\log_e \hat{\omega}_{MH}\right) = \dfrac{\sqrt{53.771}}{\sqrt{1.407} \times 45.599} = 0.1356.$

This leads to 95% confidence limits for $\log_e \omega_{MH}$ of $\log_e(1.407) \pm 1.96 \times 0.1356$, that is, 0.3415 ± 0.2658, using (5.28). Raising the two limits to the power e gives the 95% confidence interval for ω_{MH}, $(1.08, 1.84)$, as specified by (5.29).

Finally we can test whether the common relative rate is significantly different from unity by computing (5.30), which turns out to be

$$\frac{\left(\left|115 - 96.304\right| - 0.5\right)^2}{53.771} = 6.16.$$

This is compared with χ_1^2. From Table B.3, $0.025 > p > 0.01$; hence, we conclude there is evidence that renters have higher coronary rates than do owner–occupiers, after correcting for age.

5.7.5   Further comments

Although the person-years method has been described so that adjustment is made for age, it is frequently used to adjust simultaneously for calendar period. This means extending the algorithm of Figure 5.10 to subdivide follow-up by calendar time as well as age.

Sometimes the exposure to the risk factor may alter during follow-up; for example, a smoker may quit smoking during the study. The individual person-years of follow-up for any exposure level accumulate only the years when the individual was at that particular exposure level. For example, if someone dies whilst exposed, she or he will still have made a contribution to the person-years for nonexposure if her or his exposure started after the study began. More details of this specific point, and of person-years methodology in general, are given by Breslow and Day (1994). This includes extensions to the situation of only two exposure levels, although this generalisation is often achieved in practice through the Poisson regression model described in Section 11.10. See also Section 11.6.1 and Section 11.11.

As was seen directly in Example 5.14, the use of Mantel–Haenszel methods with person-years data provides an alternative to the survival analysis methods of Section 5.3 to Section 5.5. Kahn and Sempos (1989) compare the two methods and conclude that there is little to choose between them in terms of the assumptions needed for validity; for example, both assume lack of bias caused by withdrawals. However, the person-years method often requires a considerable amount of work to produce the basic data — via Figure 5.10, for example. Also, observing how survival probability alters with follow-up duration has an advantage, which is a direct result of survival analysis.

Person-years analysis is the method of choice when there is no control group, other than some standard population that has not been followed up for the purposes of the study (study type 2 in Section 5.1.3).

5.8   Period-cohort analysis

In this chapter, we have assumed that any effects that are investigated are homogeneous over calendar time so that subjects with different baseline times may be taken together (Section 5.2.2). In this final section, we briefly review the case in which this assumption is invalid.

We will expect lack of homogeneity (a **period-cohort effect**) due to such things as changes in general health care or natural fluctuations in disease, whenever baseline dates vary over several years. As an example, Table 5.15 shows some data from the Connecticut Tumor Registry that are presented and analysed by Campbell *et al.* (1994). The table shows breast cancer incidence data for the years 1938 to 1982, by 5-year intervals.

The year-of-birth groups define birth cohorts (at least approximately, because migration into and out of Connecticut will have occurred). The baseline dates (years of birth) range over more than 60 years, so we should consider the possibility of period-cohort effects. If there is time homogeneity, the age-specific rates should be reasonably constant over the cohorts. They are clearly not, from inspection of any column in Table 5.15 or from Figure 5.11, which illustrates rates for selected cohorts from Table 5.15.

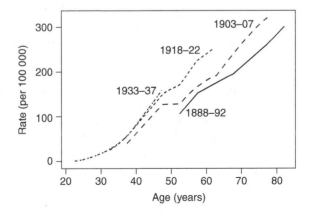

Figure 5.11. Breast cancer rates by age group for selected birth cohorts in Connecticut.

Another example in which it will be advisable to consider time-specific cohorts is an occupational health study in which important recent improvements in safety precautions are known to have been implemented.

The simplest analysis, when time homogeneity fails, will be to analyse the cohorts separately. However, this results in small numbers and incomplete estimation in most cohorts (see the gaps in Table 5.15) and may not ultimately be necessary if the sole object is to compare survival or person-years rates between levels of a risk factor. In the latter case, cohort amalgamation may still be acceptable if no *interaction* is associated with the risk factor. For instance, the roughly parallel curves in Figure 5.11 suggest that the risk factor, age, may act in the same relative way throughout (see the comments in Section 4.7). Hence, for analyses of the effect of age, the whole dataset might still be considered as one. Campbell *et al.* (1994) fit a statistical model to the complete dataset in Table 5.15, using both period and cohort information.

Methods for dealing with time-specific cohorts, allowing for interactions with age, are discussed by Kupper *et al.* (1985). A thorough treatment of the modelling issues is given by Clayton and Schifflers (1987a, b).

5.8.1   Period-specific rates

Finally, we consider a topic that, although closely allied to the material of this chapter, is actually a technique for use with cross-sectional data. This is the use of rates calculated from data collected in a single time period (for instance, over the past year) to produce a view of how a population would be expected to progress if it always experienced these rates.

For example, the breast cancer rates by age group in Connecticut during 1978 to 1982 (the most recent 5-year period covered by the data) may be extracted from Table 5.15 by considering how old each birth cohort would be once it reaches the period 1978 to 1982. It turns out that the appropriate rates are those along the bottom diagonal: that is, from 25.9 (for 30- to 34-year-olds) to 320.2 (for 80- to 84-year-olds), as plotted in Figure 5.12 (solid line).

Period-specific rates have the advantage of being relatively quick to calculate; to determine the solid line in Figure 5.12, we need data only on population size and breast cancer incidence in 1978 to 1982, rather than any protracted follow-up. They are also up to date; we would need to go back to the 1898 to 1902 cohort in Table 5.15 to obtain cohort-specific data on 80- to 84-year-olds, although then data from this cohort give an analysis of, say, 40- to 44-year-olds that is of considerable vintage. Often, period-specific rates are calculated from readily available data such as national demographic publications, which give mid-year population estimates and deaths in the past 12 months (such as appear in Table 3.15).

Unfortunately, period-specific rates are misleading whenever there is an important period-cohort effect. For example, Figure 5.12 (solid line) shows a slight fall in the rate of breast cancer at around age 80. This suggests that the oldest women alive may have some protection conferred by their age. This is seen to be misleading when we consider the first three birth cohorts (1888 to 1902) in Table 5.15. For each of these cohorts, the rates continue to increase with age. The dip in the solid line of Figure 5.12 arises because the 80- to 84-year-olds alive in 1978 to 1982 lived through the time of least overall risk from breast cancer (over all the time studied); we can see this from the general tendency for rates to increase as we go down the columns of Table 5.15, starting at the third row. As a consequence, they have accumulated less risk than the 75- to 79-year-olds alive in 1978 to 1982. Two risk processes are influencing the results: an increase of risk with age and an increase of risk with calendar time (possibly caused by changes in lifestyle or environmental pollution).

Table 5.15. Breast cancer rates[a] 1938–1982 by age group and year of birth; Connecticut.

Year of birth	Age group (years)												
	20–24	25–29	30–34	35–39	40–44	45–49	50–54	55–59	60–64	65–69	70–74	75–79	80–84
1888–1892							106.8	152.7	174.5	193.9	228.1	263.0	302.2
1893–1897						91.8	102.5	156.5	170.8	211.1	235.4	275.0	317.7
1898–1902					85.8	104.3	117.6	150.9	168.3	213.6	257.5	318.8	320.2
1903–1907				39.8	84.8	126.9	129.1	170.2	189.7	237.8	285.8	321.7	
1908–1912			19.7	48.3	97.6	127.2	154.3	183.6	214.5	263.5	303.8		
1913–1917		5.9	15.8	53.4	100.0	138.6	147.6	184.5	229.0	271.8			
1918–1922	1.5	8.2	26.2	56.2	102.9	150.1	171.6	226.9	254.4				
1923–1927	1.5	6.3	24.5	57.5	114.1	168.3	195.9	214.1					
1928–1932	3.5	9.0	27.5	59.5	127.4	183.9	174.4						
1933–1937	0.4	9.6	25.0	55.6	106.9	160.8							
1938–1942	0.8	9.1	24.1	55.8	95.3								
1943–1947	0.2	8.3	26.0	58.8									
1948–1952	1.8	8.0	25.9										

[a] Cases per 100 000 woman-years.

Source: Data prepared by the National Cancer Institute.

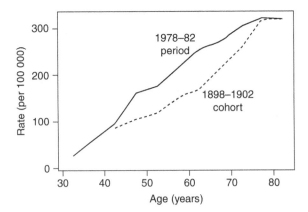

Figure 5.12. Breast cancer rates in Connecticut by age. The solid line shows the rates recorded during the most recent period of observation (1978–1982). The dashed line shows the rates experienced by the 1898–1902 birth cohort as it passed through successive time periods from age 40–44 years onwards.

The same phenomenon may lead to underestimation of relative rates by age group, which could be constructed from Figure 5.12 (solid line) or (more accurately) from the bottom diagonal of Table 5.15. For example, the relative rate comparing 75- to 79-year-olds to 50- to 54-year-olds using 1978 to 1982 data (from the diagonal in Table 5.15) is 321.7/174.4 = 1.84. For each of the four cohorts within which this calculation is possible in Table 5.15 (the 1888 to 1907 birth cohorts), the same relative rate varies between 2.46 and 2.71. To illustrate the underestimation of relative rates, the data from one of the birth cohorts (1898 to 1902) have been added to Figure 5.12 (as a dashed line). The dashed line gives much lower rates in the earlier years of life, producing a greater contrast with the later years than does the solid line. Such problems are always possible with cross-sectional data but are not always acknowledged.

Period-specific rates by age may be used to construct a period-specific life table, usually called a **current life table**. This is the type of life table found in demographic yearbooks and publications of national statistical services. The layout of a current life table is similar to that of a cohort life table, although extra functions are often added. Several examples of their use are given by Pollard *et al.* (1990); fine details of their construction are given by Shryock *et al.* (1976).

Exercises

5.1 Shaper *et al.* (1988) describe a cohort study of a random sample of 7729 middle-aged British men. Each man was asked, at baseline, his current alcohol consumption (amongst other things). During the next 7.5 years, death certificates were collected for any of the cohort who died. The following table was compiled:

Number of	None	Occasional	Light	Moderate	Heavy
Subjects	466	1845	2544	2042	832
Deaths	41	142	143	116	62

with header spanning "Alcohol consumption group" over None, Occasional, Light, Moderate, Heavy.

(i) Calculate the risk and the relative risk (using the nondrinkers as the base group) of death for each alcohol consumption group. Calculate 95% confidence intervals for each risk and relative risk. Plot a graph of the relative risks, showing the confidence limits. What do the results appear to show about the health effects of drinking?

(ii) Why might the conclusions based on the preceding table alone be misleading? Given adequate funding, describe how you would go about answering the question of how alcohol consumption is related to middle-aged mortality. State the data collection method you would employ and which variables you would record.

5.2 Refer to the brain metastases data of Table C.2 (in Appendix C), treating anyone who did not die from a tumour as censored.

(i) Construct a life table using intervals of 6 months (so that the cut-points are 0, 6, 12, etc.) using the actuarial method. Include 95% confidence intervals for the survival probabilities.

(ii) Find the Kaplan–Meier estimates of the survivor function, together with 95% confidence intervals.

(iii) Produce a diagram to compare your estimates in (i) and (ii).

(iv) Construct separate life tables with intervals of 6 months (using the actuarial method) for those who have and have not received prior treatment. Use these to compare survival probabilities at 12 months for those who have and have not received prior treatment, giving a 95% confidence interval for the difference.

(v) Use the Mantel–Haenszel test on the life table results to compare survival experiences for those who have and have not received prior treatment.

(vi) Find Kaplan–Meier survival estimates for the two prior treatment groups. Then use the log-rank test to compare survival experiences for those who have and have not received prior treatment.

(vii) Use the generalised Wilcoxon test to repeat (vi). Compare the two results with that of (v).

5.3 Refer to the lung cancer data of Exercise 2.2.

(i) Find the Kaplan–Meier estimates of survival function for literate and illiterate people separately.

(ii) Plot these estimates on a single graph.

(iii) Compare the two one-year survival probabilities, giving a 99% confidence interval for each and for their difference.

(iv) Use the log-rank test to compare survival experience between literate and illiterate people.

5.4 An investigation has been carried out to explore the relationship between industrial exposure to hydrogen cyanide and coronary heart disease. The investigation studied men employed in a variety of factories, all of whom were regularly exposed to hydrogen cyanide at work. Over a 10-year period, 280 men died from coronary heart disease. In all, 15 000 man-years of follow-up were observed.

(i) If the national annual death rate from coronary heart disease amongst the male working population is 182 per 100 000, calculate the relative rate for those exposed to industrial hydrogen cyanide using the national working population as the base. Does this suggest that industrial exposure to hydrogen cyanide is an important risk factor for coronary heart disease?

(ii)   Discuss the shortcomings of this investigation. Suggest ways in which the study design could be improved so as to provide better insight into the relationship of interest.

5.5   Liddell *et al.* (1977) describe an occupational cohort study of all 10 951 men born between 1891 and 1920 who worked for at least 1 month in the chrysotile mining and milling industry in Quebec. The paper, from which data are given below, describes 20 years' follow-up for each man until the end of 1973. From estimates of the concentration of airborne respirable dust, year by year, for each specific job within the industry and using full employment records, the investigators calculated the overall dust exposure for each man. The number of lung cancer deaths was presented within a number of dust exposure groups and compared with the expected number based on the complete cohort.

Total dust exposure	Lung cancer deaths	
$(pf^{-3}y \times 10^6)$	Observed	Expected
Less than 3	28	31.93
3–10	11	19.09
10–30	17	18.76
30–100	37	40.08
100–300	34	45.02
300–600	43	31.04
600 or greater	28	12.13

Calculate the SMR for each dust exposure group, together with its 95% confidence interval. Plot the results on a graph and describe the effect of dust exposure in words.

5.6   Kitange *et al.* (1996) studied adult mortality in Tanzania, where no accurate death registration system existed. During the period from 1 June 1992 to 31 May 1995, adult deaths were recorded in three areas of the country through a system of field reports and 'verbal autopsies'. A population census was also carried out for each area. The areas chosen were within the urban centre of Dar es Salaam and the rural areas of Hai and Morogoro. The following table gives observed and expected numbers of deaths for women in each area (expected numbers have been estimated from other statistics given in the source paper and cannot accurately be quoted with more significant digits). The standard population used by the authors was the female population of England and Wales in 1991.

Deaths	Dar es Salaam	Hai	Morogoro
Observed	615	693	1070
Expected	69.4	153	111

(i)   Estimate the standardised mortality ratios (SMRs), together with 95% confidence intervals, within each area.

(ii)   Compare the SMR for women in Hai to that in Dar es Salaam by calculating the relative SMR and its 95% confidence interval.

(iii) Repeat (ii) comparing Morogoro to Dar es Salaam.

(iv)   Interpret your results.

5.7   In a cohort study of 34 387 menopausal women in Iowa, intakes of certain
       vitamins were assessed in 1986 (Kushi *et al.*, 1996). In the period up to the
       end of 1992, 879 of these women were newly diagnosed with breast cancer.
       The following table shows data for two vitamins, classified according to
       ranked categories of intake.

| Category | Vitamin C | | Vitamin E | |
of intake	Events	PY[a]	Events	PY[a]
1 (low)	507	124 373	570	143 117
2	217	57 268	129	33 950
3	76	19 357	71	19 536
4	55	17 013	28	6 942
5 (high)	24	7 711	81	22 176

[a] PY = woman-years (as reported: note that their sum unex-
     pectedly differs by one between vitamins).

       For each vitamin, calculate the relative rates (with 95% confidence intervals)
       taking the low-consumption group as base. Do your results suggest any
       beneficial (or otherwise) effect of additional vitamin C or E intake?

5.8   Refer to the smelter workers data in Table C.3.
       (i)   Find the overall relative rate of death, high versus low arsenic expo-
              sure, together with a 95% confidence interval.
       (ii)   Find the Mantel–Haenszel relative rate corresponding to (i), adjusting
              for age group and calendar period simultaneously. Give the corresponding
              95% confidence interval.
       (iii) Test whether exposure has an effect, adjusting for age group and cal-
              endar period.
       (iv)   Carry out a test of the assumption necessary for the application of the
              Mantel–Haenszel method.

CHAPTER 6

Case–control studies

6.1 Basic design concepts

The first step in a **case–control**, **case-referent** or **retrospective** study is to detect a number of people with the disease under study: the **cases**. We then select a number of people who are free of the disease: the **controls**. The cases and controls are then investigated to see which risk factors differ between them.

Example 6.1 Autier *et al.* (1996) describe a study of cutaneous melanoma in which 420 adult cases (selected from five hospitals in Belgium, France and Germany) were compared with 447 adult controls (selected from the local communities served by the hospitals). Of the cases, 75% reported that they had not been protected against sunlight (for instance, by wearing a hat or applying sunblock) during their childhood. This exceeds the corresponding percentage, 69%, amongst controls. Hence, to be a case is more closely associated with lack of childhood protection than to be a control, and exposure to sunlight in childhood may thus be a risk factor for melanoma.

The clear difference between a case–control and a cohort study is that here we select by disease status and look back to see what, in the past, might have caused the disease. By contrast, in a cohort study, we wait to see whether disease develops. Diagrammatically, the comparison may be made between Figure 6.1 and Figure 5.1.

6.1.1 Advantages

1. Case–control studies are quicker and cheaper than follow-up studies because no waiting time is involved. This makes them particularly suitable for diseases with a long latency.
2. Many risk factors can be studied simultaneously. For example, the cases and controls may be asked a series of questions on aspects of their lifestyles.
3. Case–control studies are particularly well suited to investigations of risk factors for rare diseases, where, otherwise, there may well be problems in generating a sufficient number of diseased people to produce accurate results.
4. Case–control studies usually require much smaller sample sizes than do equivalent cohort studies. Sample size calculation is the topic of Chapter 8; case–control and cohort study sample sizes are compared in Section 8.7.3.
5. Case–control studies are generally able to evaluate confounding and interaction rather more precisely for the same overall sample size than are cohort studies. This is because case–control studies are usually more equally balanced.
6. Transient risk factors, such as contaminated food and pollution caused through industrial accidents are ideally studied through the case–control approach.

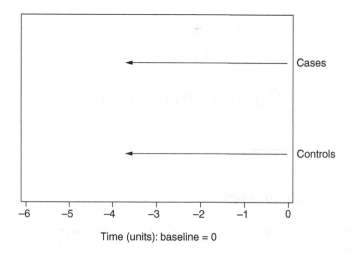

Figure 6.1. Schematic representation of a case–control study.

6.1.2 Disadvantages

1. Case–control studies do not involve a time sequence and so are not able to demonstrate causality. For example, when more of the cases are heavy drinkers, how do we know that drinking preceded the disease? Perhaps the disease led to heavy drinking as a source of comfort. Sometimes it will be possible to question the time sequence of risk factor exposure and disease, but there are frequently problems with the accuracy of recall.

2. Being a case might reflect survival rather than morbidity. For instance, suppose that heavy smokers who have a heart attack tend to die immediately, before they reach hospital. A case–control study of heavy smoking and myocardial infarction (MI), which selects both cases and controls from hospital, will then find rather fewer heavy smokers amongst the cases than the controls. This may even suggest that heavy smoking is protective against MI.

3. Case–control studies can investigate only one disease outcome. This is because sampling is carried out separately within the study groups (case and control), which are defined according to the disease outcome. Other diseases would produce different study groups.

4. Case–control studies cannot provide valid estimates of risk or odds and can provide only approximate estimates of relative risk, which are inaccurate in certain circumstances (Section 3.3 and Section 6.2).

5. Case–control studies are very likely to suffer from bias error. In many instances, problems arise from the way controls are sampled (Section 6.4). Another source of bias is differential quality of information. Since they are more interesting in a medical sense, cases may be researched more thoroughly. The very fact that someone has a disease may mean that she or he has been subjected to a more rigorous investigation, perhaps x-ray screening, blood testing and the like. Also, when asked to provide information, the cases may well be more likely to be accurate than the controls, simply because they have personal interest in the results of the research (see Example 6.2). In most such instances, a case is more likely to be correctly recorded as having been exposed to a particular risk factor. By contrast, in a comparison of recall

of mothers from a case–control study of sudden infant death syndrome, Drews *et al.* (1990) found that mothers of cases were more likely to report false prior medical events. Either way, there is bias against the misreported variable when it is considered as a risk factor.

Disadvantage 5 is the one most often quoted in the criticism of the case–control approach. Together with disadvantage 1, this places case–control studies below cohort studies in the hierarchy of study validity when the purpose is to investigate cause and effect. As this is such a common goal in epidemiological investigations, this is a serious drawback.

Case–control studies are often used for pragmatic reasons (for example, to save cost or time), rather than for considerations of validity. As a consequence, case–control studies need to be conducted very carefully, with full regard to possible sources of bias. To be persuasive, they need to be reported with evidence of avoidance or minimisation of bias. Steps to avoid bias include blindness of the analyst to the case or control status of any one individual (Section 7.3.2) and careful selection of cases and controls (Section 6.3 and Section 6.4).

Where possible, checks for bias should be carried out. For example, consider Example 1.1. Subsequent to their initial work, Doll and Hill (1952) were able to identify a number of lung cancer 'cases' who were wrongly diagnosed — that is, they were treated as cases in the analysis but should have been treated as controls (or, perhaps, ignored altogether). They found no difference between the smoking habits (as ascertained during the case–control study) of this misclassified set and the controls, although the true cases had much higher levels of tobacco consumption. Hence, there was no evidence of a bias in risk factor assessment.

Although bias error might occur, it is unlikely fully to explain large estimates of association between risk factor and disease, such as odds ratios that exceed 3. Furthermore, we can be more confident that bias has had no important effect whenever a dose–response effect (greater odds ratio, compared with the base level, at higher levels of the risk factor) is found.

Example 6.2 During January 1984, six cases of Legionnaires' disease were reported to the health authority in Reading, U.K., all of whom became ill between 15 and 19 December 1983 (Anderson *et al.,* 1985). This cluster suggested a point source outbreak. A local search was then conducted to discover whether there had been any other Legionnaires' disease cases with onsets within the same 5 days. General practitioners and hospital physicians were asked to consider recent referrals and report any possible cases for further investigation, whilst hospital discharge and autopsy records were reviewed and outpatient x-rays were checked for possible cases, so far undiagnosed. The result was that 13 cases were detected in all. The cases had no obvious factor in common, such as all working in the same place, so that no clear source of the legionella bacterium (an aquatic organism) was apparent. However, all cases had visited Reading town centre just before their illness.

A case–control study was mounted to compare exposure between the cases and a selected set of 36 people without the disease (the controls). Cases and controls were compared by the number who had visited each of six designated parts of Reading town centre, just prior to the outbreak. Results are given in Table 6.1.

Frequency of visiting most parts of Reading was high amongst both groups, which is not surprising as the period covered was just before Christmas. However, most of the cases, but rather fewer controls, visited the Butts Centre shopping mall. This suggests that the Butts Centre might be a source of the legionella bacterium. A formal analysis is given by Example 6.10.

Subsequently, a water sample from a cooling tower in one of the buildings in the Butts Centre was found to have the legionella species, *Legionella pneumophila*. It was concluded that the disease may have been spread by atmospheric drift of contaminated water droplets from this tower.

Table 6.1. Number of people visiting parts of Reading town centre in the 2 weeks preceding onset of Legionnaires' disease.

Area of Reading	Cases	Controls
Abbey Square	9	19
Butts Centre	12	21
Forbury Gardens	3	6
Minster Street	9	21
South Street	4	9
Train station	3	9
Overall	13	36

In this investigation, the case–control approach is the only one possible because of the transient nature of the risk factor and because speed of hypothesis testing was of paramount importance to avoid further infections, which could lead to deaths. Cohort studies of Legionnaires' disease will, in any case, be impractical because of the rare nature of the disease (only 558 cases were reported in England and Wales in the 4 years preceding the Reading outbreak), despite the common presence of the bacterium in many natural and artificial water supplies. Hence, extremely large samples would be required.

One possible bias in the Reading study is differential quality of reporting. Cases are likely to have given careful thought to what they did just before becoming ill. On the other hand, controls, with no personal interest in the disease, may well have been rather less precise in their recall. For example, some controls may have forgotten a trip that they made, several weeks before being questioned, to the shops in the Butts Centre. Hence, the observed case–control differential may be due to bias error. This type of bias is sometimes called **anamnestic bias**.

6.2   Basic methods of analysis

6.2.1   Dichotomous exposure

Consider, first, the simple situation in which exposure to the risk factor is dichotomous. Without loss of generality, we shall (as usual) refer to the two outcomes as 'yes' or 'no' to exposure. Data from the study then appear as a 2×2 table in the form of Table 3.1. For example, Table 6.2 gives the data reported by Autier *et al.* (1996) described in Example 6.1. No data were available for 43 subjects whose childhood protection against the sun could not be ascertained.

As in Example 6.1, it is straightforward to compare the proportion (or percentage) of cases and controls with (or without) sun protection. However, this is not the most

Table 6.2. Sun protection during childhood by case–control status for cutaneous melanoma in Belgium, France and Germany.

Sun protection?	Cases	Controls	Total
Yes	99	132	231
No	303	290	593
Total	402	422	824

useful comparison. The epidemiologist would really like to compare the chance of disease for those who have, and those who have not, been protected from the sun.

Because Table 6.2 is in the form of Table 3.1, the temptation is to calculate any of the summary estimates of association given in Chapter 3, including the risk and relative risk. This would be incorrect, because we do not have a single random sample when a case–control study is undertaken. Instead we have a sample of cases and a separate sample of controls: a sample that is **stratified** by case–control status. This means that our overall sample would not necessarily contain anything like the same proportion of diseased subjects as are in the population within which the study is based. Since cases are generally rare and controls are plentiful, the proportion of diseased individuals in the sample will usually be much higher. For instance, the proportion of melanoma cases in the sample presented in Table 6.2 is $402/824 = 0.49$. Considerably fewer than 49% of adults have cutaneous melanoma; the annual incidence rate is approximately 1 per 10 000 and the lifetime risk is about 1 in 200 (Boyle *et al.*, 1995).

To understand what we can estimate using case–control data, it is useful to consider the distribution of diseased and undiseased people by risk factor exposure status in the population: see Table 6.3(a). After Schlesselman (1982), let us suppose that the case–control study samples a fraction f_1 of those diseased and a fraction f_2 of those without the disease. That is, we sample from the *columns* of Table 6.3(a). The result is Table 6.3(b).

The risk in the population is, from (3.1), $A/(A+B)$ for those exposed to the risk factor and $C/(C+D)$ for those unexposed; the relative risk is, from (3.2),

$$\frac{A(C + D)}{C(A + B)},$$

comparing the exposed to the unexposed. The expected values of these quantities in the case–control sample are, for those exposed to the risk factor:

$$f_1 A \big/ \big(f_1 A + f_2 B\big) \neq A \big/ \big(A + B\big);$$

for those unexposed:

$$f_1 C \big/ \big(f_1 C + f_2 D\big) \neq C \big/ \big(C + D\big);$$

and for the relative risk:

$$\frac{f_1 A \big(f_1 C + f_2 D\big)}{f_1 C \big(f_1 A + f_2 B\big)} \neq \frac{A\big(C + D\big)}{C\big(A + B\big)}.$$

Table 6.3. Risk factor status by (a) disease status in the population and (b) case–control status in the sample (showing expected values).

Risk factor status	(a) Population values			(b) Expected values in the sample		
	Diseased	Not diseased	Total	Cases	Controls	Total
Exposed	A	B	$A + B$	$f_1 A$	$f_2 B$	$f_1 A + f_2 B$
Not exposed	C	D	$C + D$	$f_1 C$	$f_2 D$	$f_1 C + f_2 D$
Total	$A + C$	$B + D$	N	$f_1(A + C)$	$f_2(B + D)$	n

This demonstrates that the sample risk and the sample relative risk are not valid estimates of their population equivalents in a case–control study.

A similar problem arises for the odds. In the population, the odds of disease are, from (3.8), A/B for those exposed to the risk factor and C/D for those unexposed. The expected values of the odds in the case–control sample are

$$f_1 A / f_2 B \neq A/B$$

for those exposed and

$$f_1 C / f_2 D \neq C/D$$

for those unexposed. However, for the odds ratio, the sampling fractions f_1 and f_2 cancel out. That is, using (3.9), the expected sample value is

$$\frac{(f_1 A)(f_2 D)}{(f_2 B)(f_1 C)} = \frac{AD}{BC} = \psi,$$

where ψ (as usual) is the odds ratio in the population. Hence, we can use a case–control study to estimate the odds ratio, but not the risk, relative risk or odds.

The only exception to the preceding statement would be when $f_1 = f_2$. However, as already indicated, this is very unlikely in practice. The fraction of the diseased sampled, f_1, will tend to be much closer to unity than will the fraction of the nondiseased sampled, f_2.

Lack of ability to estimate the relative risk directly is not too much of a disadvantage if the disease is rare amongst both those with and without the risk factor, which is very often the situation when a case–control study is undertaken. In this situation, the odds ratio is a good approximation to the relative risk (Section 3.3.1). Indeed, many authors use the term relative risk to refer to the odds ratio from a case–control study. As this is confusing and inexact, the distinction will be maintained here.

Although there are restrictions on the range of estimation available from a case–control study, the chi-square test of Section 3.5 is applicable without modification. Similarly, Fisher's exact test (Section 3.5.4) may be used, where necessary.

Example 6.3 From the data in Table 6.2, we estimate the odds ratio for melanoma (sun protection versus no sun protection) to be

$$\frac{99 \times 290}{132 \times 303} = 0.72,$$

using (3.9). The approximate standard error of the log of this odds ratio is calculated from (3.10) to be

$$\sqrt{\frac{1}{99} + \frac{1}{132} + \frac{1}{303} + \frac{1}{290}} = 0.1563.$$

From (3.11) and (3.12), approximate 95% confidence limits for the odds ratio are thus

$$\exp\left\{\log_e(0.72) \pm 1.96 \times 0.1563\right\},$$

that is, (0.53, 0.98). Hence, sun protection in childhood reduces the risk of melanoma by a factor of around 0.72 (those protected have 72% of the risk of the unprotected). We are 95% sure that the interval from 0.53 to 0.98 contains the true odds ratio (approximate relative risk). If we prefer to write conclusions in terms of the elevated risk from lack of protection, we could say that the odds ratio (95% confidence interval) for lack of protection versus protection is 1/0.72 (1/0.98, 1/0.53); that is, 1.39 (1.02, 1.89).

To test the null hypothesis of no association between exposure and case–control status, we use (3.16). The observed value of this is

$$\frac{824\left\{\left|99 \times 290 - 132 \times 303\right| - 824/2\right\}^2}{231 \times 593 \times 402 \times 422} = 4.19.$$

From Table B.3, this is significant at the 5% level (the exact p value is 0.04). Hence, there is evidence that lack of sun protection in childhood is associated with melanoma in adulthood. Note that this conclusion is consistent with unity lying just outside the 95% confidence interval.

In a cohort study (with a fixed cohort), the estimation problems described here do not arise, even when stratified sampling is used. This is because the sampling will be from those with and without the risk factor: the rows of Table 6.3(a). A little algebra will show that sampling fractions will always cancel out, whatever measure of chance, or comparative chance, of disease is used in a cohort study.

6.2.2   Polytomous exposure

When exposure to the risk factor is measured at several levels, we proceed as in Section 3.6. That is, we choose a base level and compare all other levels to this base.

Example 6.4 Table 6.4 gives results from a case–control study of *Escherichia coli* by Fihn *et al.* (1996). Cases were women aged 18 to 40 years selected from the records of a health maintenance organisation in Washington state. Controls were randomly sampled from the same database, chosen from those women without *E. coli* infections within the same age structure as the cases. Table 6.4 gives odds ratios for ethnicity relative to the chosen base group. Caucasians were chosen as the base because they are the largest group in number and thus most accurately measured.

There is some evidence of a relationship between ethnicity and case–control status; the chi-square statistic, (2.1), is 11.10 ($p = 0.03$). Those with *E. coli* seem more likely to be Hispanics and Asians and less likely to be 'Others'. However, only 'Others' seem to be significantly different from the Caucasians at the 5% level, because unity is inside all the other 95% confidence intervals for the odds ratios.

Table 6.4. Ethnicity by case–control status in a study of *E. coli* in Washington state.

Ethnicity	Cases	Controls	Odds ratio (95% confidence interval)
Caucasian	514	541	1
African American	25	25	1.05 (0.60, 1.86)
Hispanic	13	5	2.74 (0.97, 7.73)
Asian	32	21	1.60 (0.91, 2.82)
Other	20	37	0.57 (0.33, 0.99)
Total	604	629	

When the levels are ordinal, we would normally wish to consider a trend in the odds ratios. This cannot be achieved by the method of Section 3.6.2 because that uses risks that are nonestimable here. A method for analysing trend in odds ratios is given in Section 10.4.4.

6.2.3 Confounding and interaction

Just as with any kind of epidemiological study, the results obtained for a single risk factor may be compromised by confounding or interaction with other variables. The Mantel–Haenszel method of Section 4.6 may be applied to deal with confounding. Indeed, the source paper (Mantel and Haenszel, 1959) analysed a case–control study; see Example 4.12. Unfortunately, confounding may arise through the selection process in a case–control study; we should then adjust only if the confounder has a known association with disease in the parent population (see Day *et al.*, 1980). Interaction in case–control studies may be analysed as described in Section 4.8.2. Alternatively, virtually all of Chapter 10 is appropriate to case–control studies; statistical models are used there to adjust for confounding or to deal with interaction.

6.2.4 Attributable risk

In Section 3.7, attributable risk, θ, was defined as the proportion of cases of disease that were apparently due to the risk factor. We can estimate θ from a case–control study as long as:

1. The odds ratio is a good approximation to the relative risk.
2. The prevalence of the risk factor amongst controls is a good approximation to the prevalence in the entire population.

The rare disease assumption, previously used only to justify proposition 1, makes these reasonable propositions as long as controls are sampled randomly from amongst those without the disease (see Cole and MacMahon, 1971).

In symbols, using the notation of Section 3.7,

1. ad/bc is an approximate estimate of λ.
2. $b/(b + d)$ is an approximate estimate of p_E.

Hence, after some algebraic manipulation, (3.27) gives

$$\tilde{\theta} = \frac{ad - bc}{d(a + c)} \, , \tag{6.1}$$

where $\tilde{\theta}$ is the estimated attributable risk from a case–control study.

Assuming that the disease is rare, we can obtain approximate 95% confidence limits for the attributable risk in a case–control study as

$$\left\{ 1 + \frac{1 - \tilde{\theta}}{\tilde{\theta}} \exp(\pm u) \right\}^{-1} , \tag{6.2}$$

where

$$u = \frac{1.96d(b+d)}{a(b+d) - b(a+c)} \sqrt{\frac{a}{c(a+c)} + \frac{b}{d(b+d)}} \,. \tag{6.3}$$

These limits were suggested by Leung and Kupper (1981), using the same method that gave rise to (3.24). A logistic regression modelling approach to adjust the attributable risk for confounders is described by Benichou and Gail (1990); a SAS macro to carry out their computations is given by Mezzetti *et al.* (1996). Other methods are reviewed by Benichou (1991) and Coughlin *et al.* (1994).

Example 6.5 In a case–control study of paternal smoking and birth defects in Shanghai, China, 1012 cases with nonsmoking mothers were identified during the period from 1 October 1986 to 30 September 1987. An equal number of controls with nonsmoking mothers were selected from problem-free births during the same period (Zhang *et al.*, 1992). Results are given in Table 6.5.
 From Table 6.5, we can estimate the odds ratio for a birth defect, comparing babies whose fathers smoke to those whose fathers do not, to be

$$\hat{\psi} = \frac{639 \times 419}{593 \times 373} = 1.21.$$

To be able to go on to calculate attributable risk, we need to ascertain that birth defects are rare and that the controls are a fair sample from the population of babies. During the year of monitoring of births in this study, 75 756 newborns were recorded, of whom 1013 (less than 2%) had defects. Note that only one of these had to be excluded from the case definition used for Table 6.5 due to maternal smoking. Although case and control selection was based on hospital records, the controls should be a random selection from the community at large because all deliveries in Shanghai are made in hospital. Hence, we can estimate attributable risk from these data.
 From (6.1), the estimated attributable risk is

$$\hat{\theta} = \frac{639 \times 419 - 593 \times 373}{419 \times 1012} = 0.10979.$$

To calculate the corresponding 95% confidence interval, we first use (6.3) to find

$$u = \frac{1.96 \times 419 \times 1012}{639 \times 1012 - 593 \times 1012} \sqrt{\frac{639}{373 \times 1012} + \frac{593}{419 \times 1012}} = 0.99262.$$

Table 6.5. Paternal smoking by case–control status for birth defects in Shanghai.

Paternal smoking?	Cases	Controls
Yes	639	593
No	373	419
Total	1012	1012

Then, from (6.2), the 95% confidence limits are

$$\left\{1 + \frac{1 - 0.10979}{0.10979}\exp(\pm0.99262)\right\}^{-1} = (0.0437, 0.2497).$$

Hence, we estimate that 11.0% of birth defects are attributable to paternal smoking, and we are 95% sure that the interval from 4.4 to 25.0% contains the true attributable percentage.

6.3   Selection of cases

Thus far the issues of subject selection have been deliberately skimmed over, so as to provide a simplified introductory account. This complex issue in the design of a case–control study will now be addressed. Case selection is considered here; control selection and its relation with case selection is the subject of Section 6.4.

6.3.1   Definition

Before cases can be selected, a precise definition of the disease to be studied must be formulated. If this is not precise, there will be a danger of misclassification of potential cases and controls. If the definition is too broad, then the case–control study may be futile. For instance, the definition, 'mental illness' will encompass a range of conditions with very different aetiology. Even if certain clinical conditions are strongly associated with specific risk factors, the complete set of cases may have no, or only a minimal, excess of these risk factors compared with controls.

When the disease is very rare, the temptation is to broaden the definition so as to capture extra cases. Thus, in some analyses of the Legionnaires' disease study (Example 6.2), people diagnosed with primary pneumonia were included together with proven Legionnaires' disease sufferers because the two are difficult to distinguish. The danger is that this dilutes the true effect of exposure on the real disease. The Legionnaires' disease study considered several different definitions and thus had several different, but overlapping, case series. However, this type of approach might lead to bias if only the best results are presented.

6.3.2   Inclusion and exclusion criteria

Sometimes subjects with the disease are considered eligible to be cases only if they satisfy certain inclusion and exclusion criteria. These may be chosen so as to improve the validity of the study — for example, when subjects with co-existing diseases or well-established risk factors are excluded. Thus, babies with mothers who smoke were excluded from the cases in Example 6.5. It may be desirable to restrict selection to cases with an onset of disease within a limited time period and in a specific place. This is so whenever a **point source** of disease (in time and space) is sought, for example, during an outbreak of food poisoning and in the Legionnaires' disease study of Example 6.2. Some restrictions on time and place are, in any case, necessary for practical reasons in all case–control studies.

Sometimes diseased people are excluded from the case series because they have no, or very little, chance of exposure to the risk factor. Thus, in a study of oral contraceptives as a risk factor for breast cancer, we should exclude postmenopausal women; including them would be a waste of resources. Exclusions on grounds of efficiency often utilise age and sex criteria.

6.3.3   Incident or prevalent?

Incident disease is a better criterion for case selection. Prevalent cases introduce a greater element of ambiguity in the time sequence, as discussed in Section 1.4.1 and Section 3.4. For instance, alcohol consumption may be associated with the absence of diabetes simply because many of those with diabetes have been told to stop drinking by their doctor.

The great advantage with prevalent cases is their ready availability in large numbers for certain conditions. This would represent a distinct saving in time and effort when studying a rare, but nonfatal, chronic condition. When prevalent cases are used, steps should be taken to minimise the chance of error; for example, lifetime histories of exposures might be sought.

6.3.4   Source

Cases are usually selected from medical information systems. The most common source is hospital admission records, but operating theatre or pathology department records, sickness absence forms and disease registers are other potential sources. Further possibilities are given in Example 6.2. As in the study described there, several sources may be utilised so as to broaden the search, when necessary.

6.3.5   Consideration of bias

Case selection will be biased if the chance of having the risk factor, for those from whom the cases are drawn, is different from the chance of having the risk factor for all of those who have the disease (that is, in the parent population). If we let p_{case} be the probability of exposure (assumed, for simplicity, to be dichotomous) amongst cases and p_{disease} be the corresponding probability for all those with the disease, then we have bias if

$$p_{\text{case}} \neq p_{\text{disease}}.$$

Such bias will occur whenever the chance of becoming a case depends, in some way, on the fact of exposure to the risk factor.

An example arises in which hormone replacement therapy (HRT) is considered as a risk factor for cervical cancer. Women patients registered with a particular health centre who take HRT daily are required to attend at an annual HRT clinic, held at the health centre, as a condition of renewal of their prescription. At the clinic, they undergo a cervical smear. Although other female patients will routinely be given notice that they are due for a smear, this is done only at intervals of several years and many will not attend for the screening test. Hence, undetected cervical cancer is more likely amongst those who are not receiving HRT and

$$p_{\text{case}} > p_{\text{disease}}.$$

In this example, the potential problem might be removed if only advanced stages of the disease are considered. Then it may well be that all the diseased will have been detected, whatever the subject's history.

A second example shows bias in the opposite direction. Pearl (1929) studied data from autopsies and found that cancer and tuberculosis (TB) were rarely found together. He thus suggested that cancer patients might be treated with tuberculin (the protein of the TB bacterium). Hence, (lack of) TB is supposed to be a risk factor for cancer. However, not all deaths were equally likely to be autopsied. It happened that people who died from cancer and TB were less likely to be autopsied than those who died from cancer alone. Hence,

$$p_{\text{case}} < p_{\text{disease}}.$$

In this case, the bias arises specifically because of the source (autopsies) used. This type of bias is known as **Berkson's bias,** as reviewed by Walter (1980a) and Feinstein *et al.* (1986). More examples appear in Section 6.4.

Although we should be concerned whenever the case selection is biased, this may not, in itself, invalidate the case–control analysis. As seen in Section 6.2, the analysis will be based on a comparison of cases and controls. Consequently, the result (that is, the odds ratio for exposure versus no exposure) will be biased only if there is *differential* bias in case and control selection. Further details appear in Section 6.4.2.

6.4   Selection of controls

Controls should be a representative subgroup of members of the same base group that gave rise to cases, who have the particular characteristic that they have not (yet) developed the disease. With all else equal (specifically, exposure to the risk factor of interest), a case and a control should have had the same chance of becoming classified as a case, if they had become diseased. In practice, such comparability is often difficult to achieve, making this the most challenging aspect of case–control study design. A thorough exposition of principles and practice is given by Wacholder *et al.* (1992) and several numerical examples are given by Sackett (1979). A more concise account is provided in this section.

6.4.1   General principles

Four general principles involved in control selection may be identified. The first two of these derive from the general requirement of comparability given previously. The other two are concerned with efficiency and validity of attribution of effect of the particular risk factor.

1. Controls should be drawn from amongst those who are free of the disease being studied. Usually, we would exempt anyone who, although disease free now, has had the disease in the past.
2. Controls should be drawn from the same general population as gave rise to the cases. This is necessary to protect (as far as possible) against the possible distorting effects of unknown, or unmeasured, confounders and effect modifiers. The same inclusion/exclusion criteria used for cases (Section 6.3.2) should be applied, as far as is appropriate, without introducing any new criteria. Thus, in Example 6.5, controls were drawn from nonsmoking mothers because the decision had been made to exclude cases whose mothers smoked.

3. The source from which controls are selected should not give rise to bias error. By analogy with Section 6.3.5, bias in inferences drawn specifically about controls arises when

$$p_{\text{control}} \neq p_{\text{undiseased}}$$

where p denotes the chance of exposure. We shall see examples of this problem in Section 6.4.2.

4. Controls should have some potential for the disease. For instance, women who have had their womb removed should not be considered as controls in a study of endometrial cancer. If they were, some of those without a womb but with the risk factor would be expected to have become cases if they had retained their womb. Consequently, the comparison between cases and controls would underestimate the effect of the risk factor, assuming that no equal (or greater) bias is associated with the cases.

Notice that there is not, as sometimes stated, any reason to exclude a control purely because she or he has no potential for exposure to the risk factor. Besides the issues raised in 1 through 4 above, we are interested in comparing all those who have no exposure. See Poole (1986) for a discussion of this issue.

Controls are generally drawn from the same source (such as the same hospital) as cases, or from the community served by the same medical services. Hospital controls are considered in Section 6.4.2, community controls in Section 6.4.3 and other types of control in Section 6.4.4. When possible, more than one type of control group might be used. In this situation, comparison of the control groups may highlight problems. If the groups are the same (in terms of risk factor profiles), then no particular problem is found and the control groups should be combined. This does not rule out bias caused by selection of controls, but makes it less likely. If the control groups are different in some important way, bias may well be associated with at least one of them and further investigation is necessary. This may result in ignoring one (or more) of the control groups subsequently. Drawbacks are that it may not be easy to reconcile differences, and the whole process will be demanding in resources. When the disease is particularly rare, the make-up of the control group may be checked against the make-up (say, by age, sex and race) of the national population as a whole.

Example 6.6 Moritz *et al.* (1997) describe a comparison of hospital and community controls when female cases of hip fracture aged 45 years or more were selected from hospitals in New York City and Philadelphia. They found that the estimates of effect for some risk factors differed greatly when the different control groups were used separately in the analysis. Table 6.6 shows a selection of their results.

Table 6.6. Odds ratios (with 95% confidence intervals)[a] in a study of hip fracture using two different control groups.

Risk factor	Hospital controls	Community controls
Fall in past 6 months	1.08 (0.71, 1.53)	1.70 (1.22, 2.35)
Current (vs. never) smoking	1.30 (0.85, 1.98)	2.49 (1.61, 3.83)
Stroke	1.36 (0.87, 2.11)	2.51 (1.60, 3.94)
Poor vision	2.62 (1.27, 5.37)	1.42 (0.81, 2.48)

[a] Adjusted for several potential confounding variables.

When community controls (a sample of women living in the communities in which the cases lived) were used, falling during the past 6 months, smoking and stroke were much more important risk factors than when hospital controls (sampled from the same hospitals as the cases) were used. On the other hand, the use of hospital controls (women sampled from surgical, orthopaedic or medical wards) suggested a stronger effect of poor vision on the risk of a hip fracture.

The explanation for the difference is likely to be that hospital controls tend to be less healthy in a general sense (although apparently not in terms of eyesight). The authors of the source paper suggest that community controls may be better for studying frail, elderly individuals.

6.4.2   Hospital controls

Hospitals are a convenient and cheap source of controls, especially in situations when a clinical procedure, such as a blood sample, is required to measure the risk factor. They have the advantage that their medical data are likely to be of comparable quality to those from the cases and may have been collected prior to classification as controls (removing the possibility of observer bias). There is a good chance that their quality of recall will also be similar to that for cases (reducing the chance of anamnestic bias) because they are in the same environment. As with the cases, they are likely to be thinking about the antecedents of their illness and they are likely to be co-operative, especially because they have time to spare.

One disadvantage is that the risk factor for the study disease may also be a risk factor for the condition that a particular control has, which is the cause of her or his hospitalisation. For example, in the study of lung cancer and smoking by Doll and Hill (Example 1.1), the controls were to be noncancer patients selected from the same hospitals as the cases. As mentioned in Section 1.2, several of the controls had been hospitalised for diseases that we now know to be related to smoking. Hence,

$$p_{\text{control}} > p_{\text{undiseased}},$$

and there was thus a bias in favour of the risk factor in the analysis that compares lung cancer cases and controls. Exactly the same kind of bias appears to have operated when hospital controls were used in the study reported in Example 6.6 (a large effect of smoking was found only when community controls were used).

The reverse situation could occur if we studied aspirin and MI. We would expect lack of aspirin taking to be likely to lead to hospitalisation for MI because of aspirin's platelet-inhibiting property. However, if our controls contain, for example, large numbers who suffer from arthritis, then we should expect many of these to be taking aspirin to alleviate pain. Hence, when we consider lack of aspirin as the risk factor for MI,

$$p_{\text{control}} < p_{\text{undiseased}}$$

and we have bias in the direction contrary to the risk factor — that is, we have a reduced estimate of the benefit of aspirin for avoiding an MI (heart attack).

To reduce such problems, it is best to choose controls from a range of conditions, exempting any disease that is likely to be related to exposure (as discussed by Wacholder and Silverman, 1990). In order to ensure comparability with cases, conditions for which the hospital (of the cases) is a regional specialty might be excluded. Otherwise, the controls may have, for example, a much wider socioeconomic profile because they are drawn from a wider catchment population. If the hospital is a regional

Table 6.7. Risk factor by disease[a]
status for hospital patients.

| Risk factor | Disease status | |
status	Disease	No disease
Exposed	$f_1 A$	$f_2 B$
Unexposed	$f_3 C$	$f_4 D$

[a] 'Disease' refers to the specific disease
   being studied.

specialty for the disease under study (that is, the condition suffered by the cases), then a number of local hospitals might be used to provide controls.

The second major disadvantage is the possibility of Berkson's bias — differential rates of hospitalisation. To see how this arises, consider the distribution of exposure and disease in the population, Table 6.3(a), once again. Suppose that fractions f_1 of those exposed and diseased, f_2 of those exposed and not diseased, f_3 of those unexposed and diseased and f_4 of those unexposed and not diseased are hospitalised. The result is Table 6.7, showing the hospital population distribution.

If all those hospitalised were studied in the case–control study, then the odds ratio is

$$\psi_H = \frac{f_1 A f_4 D}{f_2 B f_3 C} = \left(\frac{f_1 f_4}{f_2 f_3}\right)\frac{AD}{BC} = \left(\frac{f_1 f_4}{f_2 f_3}\right)\psi. \tag{6.4}$$

If the hospitalisation fractions (the fs) are different, then $\psi_H \neq \psi$, the true odds ratio for the entire population. When a random sample is drawn from amongst those in hospital with the study disease and/or (more likely) those in hospital without this disease, ψ_H is the expected value, and the same problem arises. Differential hospitalisation rates might be caused by the influence of a second disease.

Example 6.7 Sackett (1979) reports a study of 2784 individuals sampled from the community. Of these, 257 had been hospitalised during the previous 6 months. Data from the whole and for the hospitalised subset only are given in Table 6.8. Both data displays show the presence or absence of respiratory disease and the presence or absence of diseases of the bones and organs of movement (labelled 'bone disease').

If we were to consider bone disease as a risk factor for respiratory disease, we would find a large effect if we drew our case–control sample from hospital (25 versus 8%). However, there is really almost no effect (8 versus 7%) in the entire population.

Table 6.8. Bone disease by respiratory
disease status in (a) the general population
and (b) hospitalised subjects.

| | Respiratory disease in | | | |
| Bone | (a) Population | | (b) Hospital | |
disease?	Yes	No	Yes	No
Yes	17	184	5	18
No	207	2376	15	219
% Yes	8%	7%	25%	8%

More particularly,

$$\hat{\psi}_H = \frac{5 \times 219}{18 \times 15} = 4.06,$$

whereas

$$\hat{\psi} = \frac{17 \times 2376}{1840 \times 207} = 1.06.$$

Hence, hospital subjects would give a misleading picture of association. Comparing the two parts of Table 6.8, we can see that hospitalisation rates are much higher when someone has both diseases ($f_1 = 5/17 = 0.29$) than when she or he has only one disease ($f_2 = 0.10$, $f_3 = 0.07$) or neither disease ($f_4 = 0.09$). This causes the bias in the hospitalised odds ratio.

In general, we might expect higher hospitalisation rates when someone has multiple illnesses (as in Example 6.7) because then she or he is rather more ill than when suffering from only one condition. This can cause a bias even when the 'second' condition is not a subject of study, because the risk factors for this second condition will then be over-represented amongst cases of the condition of interest. For instance, suppose lack of vitamin K is a risk factor for bone disease. Hospital cases of respiratory disease will, on the basis of Example 6.7, be more likely to have low levels of vitamin K than the controls, even though vitamin K consumption has no effect on respiratory disease.

One point to emphasise about Berkson's bias is that (in this context) it requires *differential* hospitalisation rates between cases and controls. For instance, we would not expect this kind of bias should there be (as often happens) lower rates of hospitalisation amongst those of lower social class or amongst ethnic minority groups, provided that the effect of class or ethnicity is the same for those diseased and undiseased. We can see this from (6.4). Suppose that exposure to the risk factor multiplies the chance of hospitalisation by a factor of e, regardless of the health problem. For example, the most deprived members of society might have 80% of the chance of hospitalisation that others have, whenever they become sick (that is, $e = 0.8$). Then,

$$f_1 = f_3 e \quad \text{and} \quad f_2 = f_4 e$$

so that (6.4) becomes

$$\psi_H = \frac{(f_3 e)f_4}{(f_4 e)f_3} \psi = \psi.$$

For this and other potential sources of bias, we will not have bias in the overall measure of comparison, ψ, when there is equal bias in case and control selection. Of course, in practice, we may often suspect that bias occurs without having the means to quantify it and thereby see whether it is equally distributed.

6.4.3   Community controls

Controls taken from the community have the great advantage of being drawn directly from the true population of those without the disease. Assuming that they are drawn randomly, they provide a valid basis for the estimation of the attributable risk when the disease is rare (Section 6.2.4). They would almost certainly be the ideal source when cases are also identified in the community because of the complete generalisability in this situation. Even when cases are detected in hospital, community controls should not have the problem of selection bias that is due to their exposure status.

The disadvantages with random community controls are that they are inconvenient to capture and their data are often of inferior quality. Interviews will often need to be carried out, and medical investigations may be required, which will necessitate personal contact. Locating and visiting a random selection of controls at home may be expensive and time consuming. Subjects may be unwilling to co-operate, especially when asked to attend a clinic and/or to submit to invasive procedures. Convenient sampling frames, such as local taxation or voting registers, may introduce a selection bias (for example, a socioeconomic bias). Indeed, all the types of bias generally associated with sample surveys, such as bias caused by nonresponse and poor-quality fieldwork, may occur. Such problems may not arise for cases, especially when they are drawn from hospitals, and hence there could be an important differential bias.

Another possible problem is that a bias in case selection might well 'cancel' out if hospital controls were used and becomes important only when community controls are employed. For instance, those with the disease might be more likely to be hospitalised if they are of high socioeconomic status, particularly if the disease is not generally fatal (for example, conditions related to fertility). Controls (for instance, parents identified from school records) will presumably have a complete social mix. The effect of factors associated with social status will then be judged in a biased way. Thus, if the well-off eat a diet relatively high in protein, then

$$p_{case} > p_{disease}$$

where p is the probability of a high protein diet. Assuming controls are sampled randomly, no equivalent bias occurs in controls. The study might thus find an erroneous link between dietary protein and infertility.

6.4.4   Other sources

Other sources for controls are medical systems other than hospitals (as in Example 6.4) and special groups in the community who have some relation to the cases (such as friends, neighbours and relatives). Usually the medical systems used to locate controls are those that give rise to the cases (as in Example 6.4). The issues will be similar to those discussed in Section 6.4.2. Relative controls should be particularly useful when genetic factors are possible confounders.

Special community controls are generally used only in **matched** case–control studies. In the simplest kind of matched study, each case is individually paired with a control who is (say) a near neighbour. The idea is that this should ensure that such factors as exposure to air pollution, socioeconomic status and access to medical care are balanced between cases and controls, thus removing any confounding effect. A full description of matched studies appears in Section 6.5 and Section 6.6; the question of whether to match is a further issue in the selection of controls.

Special community controls have the advantage of not requiring a sampling frame, although neighbourhood controls may be difficult to obtain due to nonresponse within a limited population. For example, the Legionnaires' disease study of Example 6.2

used neighbourhood controls; this led to many revisions of the control selection due to failure to locate co-operative neighbours who satisfied other inclusion criteria (see Example 6.10).

Friends and relatives are unlikely to refuse to co-operate and so are easy and cheap to identify and recruit. However, other types of bias are often a problem, particularly because the sample is necessarily nonrandom. For instance, lonely people will be missed out of friend control groups and small households are relatively unlikely to yield neighbourhood controls, if only because the chance of an empty house when a call is made is greater. In both cases, a consequent bias against social activities, such as smoking and drinking, might be present in the final analysis. An example is given by Siemiatychi (1989). On the other hand, special controls are often too similar to the cases, meaning that the risk factor tends to be rather more common in controls than it would otherwise be, leading to bias in the other direction. This problem is known as **overmatching** (discussed further in Section 6.5.2).

6.4.5   How many?

Sometimes the number of cases is fixed because we can detect no more. This was certainly true in the Legionnaires' disease outbreak in Reading (Example 6.2) where case searching was intense and thus probably all-inclusive. On the other hand, the number of available controls is usually very large, indeed virtually unlimited in some situations. A naïve approach would be to choose just as many controls as there are cases; however, when it is possible to choose more, should we do so? The statistical answer to this question is 'yes', because there will then be greater precision in estimates and tests. However, economic and time considerations may also come into play, especially as the extra precision will be subject to the 'law of diminishing returns'. As a consequence, rarely will it be worth having a case : control ratio above 1 : 4.

One measure of precision is the power of the test for an exposure–disease relationship (see Section 8.2 for a definition of 'power'). Figure 6.2 shows how power increases as the number of controls increases, when the number of cases is fixed. The

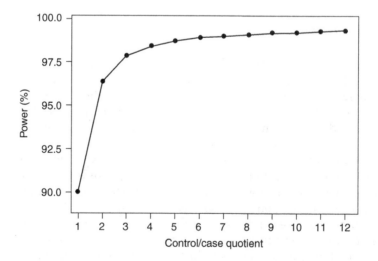

Figure 6.2. Power against control/case quotient. This shows the power to detect an approximate relative risk of 2 when the risk factor has a prevalence of 30%, a two-sided 5% significance test is to be used and 188 cases are available.

points on this figure correspond to situations in which the number of controls is an integer multiple of the number of cases (between 1 and 12). Of course, this multiple could be fractional; consideration of fractional multiples would produce a smooth curve for the figure.

Notice how much better a 1 : 2 study is than a 1 : 1 study, showing that it is worthwhile to double the number of controls. The extra power soon becomes less important as the control/case quotient increases; above 4 (a case : control ratio of 1 : 4), little improvement occurs when the control/case quotient is increased.

The theory required to produce Figure 6.2 is given in Section 8.7; in particular, (8.22) defines the power. Figure 6.2 illustrates a special situation suggested by Example 8.18, but the concept is a general one.

6.5   Matching

In Chapter 4, we have seen how to adjust for confounding during the analysis stage of an epidemiological investigation. Such adjustment may, instead, be made at the design stage by the process of **matching**. The simplest type of matching is one in which each case is matched with a single control (**1 : 1 matching** or **pair matching**), so that the control has identical (or at least very similar) values of the confounding variables. In this design, the case and control groups are identically balanced, so any difference between them cannot be due to the confounders.

Common matching variables are age and sex. In particular circumstances, race, marital status, hospital, time of admission to hospital, neighbourhood, parity, blood group and social class (amongst others) may be sensible matching criteria. Continuous variables, such as age, are matched within a prespecified range. Sometimes this is done by grouping the variables; for example, age might be categorised into 5-year age groups and the control must be within the same 5-year age group as the case. A better technique is to insist that the control is aged within so many years either side of the case's age — for example, no more than 2½ years younger or older. The finer the groupings are, the more effective the matching is.

6.5.1   Advantages

1. There is direct control of the confounders. This means that the 'adjustment' of the relationship between risk factor and disease is achieved automatically and intuitively, leading to a clear interpretation. This is the most common reason for matching.
2. Matching ensures that adjustment is possible. In exceptional circumstances, there might be no overlap between the cases and a randomly sampled set of controls. For instance, all the cases may be elderly, but the controls include no elderly people. Adjusting for age, using the Mantel–Haenszel (Section 4.6) or some other procedure, would not then be possible.
3. Under certain conditions, matching improves the efficiency of the investigation. For instance, a smaller sample size could be used, or the effect of the risk factor could be estimated with a narrower confidence interval. Many studies of the relative efficiency of matched and unmatched case–control studies have been carried out: for example, McKinlay (1977), Kupper et al. (1981), Thompson et al. (1982) and Thomas and Greenland (1983). The comparison is complex because relative efficiency depends upon several factors, many of which may be difficult

to quantify in advance of data collection. In summary, the matched design is more efficient only if the matching variable is a true confounder (that is, related to the disease and to the risk factor), and if only a moderate number of recruited controls must be rejected because they cannot be matched to a case.

6.5.2   Disadvantages

1. Data collection is more complex. It may be difficult to find a suitable match, especially when there are several matching variables. For example, we may need to locate a disease-free Afro-Caribbean woman in her fifth pregnancy from a neighbourhood that is predominantly Caucasian. This may make the investigation more expensive than the corresponding unmatched study, especially when the potential controls must be questioned before a decision can be reached as to whether they should be accepted or discarded (McKinlay, 1977). Of course, we can always relax the matching criteria, perhaps by eliminating a matching factor or widening the groups for a continuous variable, but this inevitably reduces the fundamental benefit of matching.

2. Data analysis must take account of the matching. A matched study requires a matched analysis, which is often considerably more complex to understand and compute (Section 6.6).

3. The effect (on disease) of the matching variable cannot be estimated. By design, we know that the probability of being a case, given a certain level of exposure to the matching variable, in a paired study is ½. Thus, we cannot take account of the matching variable as a risk factor in its own right. We can, however, analyse the interaction between the risk factor and the matching variable (Thomas and Greenland, 1985).

4. Adjustment cannot be removed. We cannot estimate the effect of the risk factor without adjustment for the matching variable. Sometimes the contrast between unadjusted and adjusted odds ratios is an important component of the interpretation of the epidemiological data.

5. There may be overmatching. This occurs when the matching has been done incorrectly or unnecessarily. That is, the matching variable has some relationship with the risk factor or disease, but it is not a true confounder or is so highly correlated with other matching variables as to be superfluous. This may simply result in loss of efficiency, but may also cause biased results. MacMahon and Trichopoulos (1996) suggest an example of overmatching in which the consequent odds ratio is correct, but the procedure is inefficient because many data items are redundant. This is where matching is done on religion in a study of oral contraceptive risk. Assuming religion is unrelated to disease, matching on religion may well produce many case–control pairs who have no chance of exposure to oral contraceptives because of their religious beliefs. They can provide no information about risk (see Section 6.6.2 for a proof).

As the preceding suggests, whether or not to match is not an easy question to answer. The precise comparison between the efficiency of matched and unmatched designs depends upon several factors, including the strengths of relationships, the way confounding is addressed in the analysis of the unmatched design and the type of matching used. When there is a large pool of controls, from which information on risk factor and confounder exposure may be obtained cheaply, it is unlikely that a

Table 6.9. Relative efficiencies for number of matched controls
per case.

Number of controls	Relative efficiency compared with one less	Relative efficiency compared with pairing
2	1.333	1.333
3	1.125	1.500
4	1.067	1.600
5	1.042	1.667
6	1.029	1.714
7	1.021	1.750
8	1.016	1.778
9	1.013	1.800
10	1.010	1.818

pair matched study will be a worthwhile alternative to the unmatched design. See
Thompson *et al.* (1982) and Thomas and Greenland (1983) for detailed discussions.

6.5.3   One-to-many matching

Since it is highly likely that many more controls are available than cases, we can often
contemplate matching each case with several controls, so as to improve efficiency (for
example, precision of estimates). We shall refer to this as $1 : c$ matching, meaning that
one case is matched to c controls. As c increases, more and more of the 'spare' controls
will be used up, provided they can be matched with cases. This increases overall sample
size and hence gives more precise estimation.

The relative precision of matching, say, r, rather than s controls to each case was
studied by Ury (1975). For large samples, he showed that the relative efficiency is $r(s +
1)/s(r +1)$. Using this formula, Table 6.9 has been constructed to show the relative
efficiency for a range of numbers of controls compared both to pairing and to one less
control (for each case). Clearly, pairing is inefficient; even $1 : 2$ matching is a third again
as efficient. In agreement with the comments made for unmatched studies (in Section
6.4.5), there is little to gain from having more than four matched controls per case (for
example using five controls is only 4% more efficient than using four).

6.5.4   Matching in other study designs

Although matching is given here as a methodology for case–control studies, it could also
be applied to cohort or intervention studies (Section 10.17.8). There we would match
across risk factor states, rather than disease states. For example, we might match a
smoker to a nonsmoker of the same sex and age in a cohort study of lung cancer. As
Kleinbaum *et al.* (1982) show, matching has theoretical attractions for such follow-up
designs.

6.6   The analysis of matched studies

When a case–control study (or, indeed, any other type of study) is matched, the
analysis *must* take account of the matching. If, instead, the standard unmatched
analysis is used, the odds ratio will tend to be closer to unity; hence, we are liable

Table 6.10. Results from a paired case–control study.

Case exposed to	Control exposed to the risk factor?	
the risk factor?	Yes	No
Yes	c_1	d_1
No	d_2	c_2

to miss detecting the effect of a true risk factor. This is because the cases and controls will be more similar to each other than they would have been, if independent sampling had taken place. The appropriate analysis for matched studies turns out to be very simple for $1:1$ matching (Section 6.6.1), but more complex in the general case (Section 6.6.2 to Section 6.6.4). In this section, we restrict to analyses based on 2×2 tables, or combinations of such tables.

6.6.1 $1 : 1$ Matching

The results of a paired study, with subjects classified by exposure/no exposure to the risk factor of interest, should be presented in terms of the study pairs. In particular, the format of Table 6.10 is appropriate to display the data, rather than that of Table 3.1. Table 6.10 displays information about the case–control pairs observed. Each member of the pair is either exposed or unexposed to the risk factor and is (of course) either a case or a control, giving the four possible outcomes shown in the table.

Pairs with the same exposure status for both case and control are called **concordant** pairs; the total number of concordant pairs is $c_1 + c_2$. Pairs with different exposures are called **discordant**; there are $d_1 + d_2 = d$ discordant pairs.

Let ϕ be the probability that a discordant pair has an exposed case. Then, from Table 6.10, ϕ is estimated by the proportion

$$\hat{\phi} = d_1 / (d_1 + d_2) = d_1 / d. \tag{6.5}$$

Under the usual null hypothesis that no association exists between the risk factor and disease, each discordant pair is just as likely to have the case exposed as to have the control exposed. Thus, the null hypothesis can be written as

$$H_0 : \phi = \tfrac{1}{2}.$$

This is a test of the value of a proportion. Adopting a normal approximation, the general case of this is considered in Section 2.5.2. From (2.4), a test of no association in a paired study has the test statistic

$$\frac{\hat{\phi} - 0.5}{\sqrt{0.5(1 - 0.5)/d}} = \frac{2d_1 - d}{\sqrt{d}}. \tag{6.6}$$

We compare (6.6) to the standard normal distribution (Table B.1 or B.2). Alternatively, we could square (6.6) to give

$$\frac{(2d_1 - d)^2}{d}, \tag{6.7}$$

which we compare to chi-square on 1 d.f. (Table B.3). As usual (Section 3.5.3), a continuity correction might be applied to (6.6) or (6.7). For instance, (6.8) is the continuity-corrected chi-square statistic

$$\frac{\left(\left|2d_1 - d\right| - 1\right)^2}{d} . \tag{6.8}$$

The test based on any of (6.6) through (6.8) is referred to as **McNemar's test** — the test for no association in a paired study of proportions. It is a direct analogue of the paired t test for a quantitative variable (Section 2.7.4).

To obtain an estimate of the odds ratio, ψ, we may use the following relationship between ϕ and ψ:

$$\psi = \phi/(1 - \phi) , \tag{6.9}$$

which is easy to prove from basic rules of probability (Cox, 1958). Taking (6.5) and (6.9) together gives an estimate for ψ of

$$\hat{\psi} = d_1/d_2. \tag{6.10}$$

Note that (6.9) shows that when $\phi = \frac{1}{2}$, the value of the odds ratio, ψ, is 1. Hence, (6.6) through (6.8) give tests of $\psi = 1$, as we would anticipate.

When d is large, we can use (2.2) to get 95% confidence limits for ϕ by a normal approximation, thus leading to confidence limits for ψ using (6.9). However, d is often fairly small in paired case–control studies and it is then necessary to use exact limits for ψ. Breslow and Day (1993) give these limits as (ψ_L, ψ_U), where

$$\psi_L = d_1 / \left\{ \left(d_2 + 1 \right) F_L \right\}$$
$$\psi_U = \left(d_1 + 1 \right) F_U / d_2 \tag{6.11}$$

in which F_L and F_U are the upper 2½% points of F on $(2(d_2 + 1), 2d_1)$ and $(2(d_1 + 1), 2d_2)$ d.f., respectively.

Because McNemar's test is an approximate one, when numbers are small a preferable testing procedure (for $H_0 : \psi = 1$) at the 5% level is to calculate the 95% confidence interval for ψ from (6.11) and reject H_0 if unity is outside it. A more direct method is given by Liddell (1980).

Example 6.8 A case–control study of presenile dementia by Forster *et al.* (1995) identified 109 clinically diagnosed patients aged below 65 years from hospital records. Each case was individually paired with a community control of the same sex and age, having taken steps to ascertain that the control did not suffer from dementia.

Table 6.11 shows the status of the 109 pairs for one of the risk factors explored in the study: family history of dementia. Information on the relationship between family history of dementia and disease comes from the 37 discordant pairs, 25 of which had an exposed case. The 66 pairs in which neither person had a relative with dementia, and 6 pairs in which both had a relative with dementia, yield no information about this relationship.

Using (6.8), McNemar's continuity-corrected test statistic is

$$\frac{\left(\left|2 \times 25 - 37\right| - 1\right)^2}{37} = 3.89.$$

Table 6.11. Family history of dementia and case–control status in a paired study of presenile dementia.

Case has a relative with dementia?	Control has a relative with dementia?	
	Yes	No
Yes	6	25
No	12	66

Compared with χ^2_1, using Table B.3, this is just significant at the 5% level. Hence, there is evidence of an effect of family history on dementia.

From (6.10), the odds ratio is estimated to be

$$25/12 = 2.08,$$

so that a family history of dementia roughly doubles an individual's chance of presenile dementia.

The 95% confidence limits for the odds ratio are, from (6.11),

$$\psi_L = 25/13F_L$$

$$\psi_U = 26F_U/12$$

where F_L and F_U are the upper 2½% points of F on $(2 \times 13, 2 \times 25) = (26, 50)$ and $(2 \times 26, 2 \times 12) = (52, 24)$ d.f., respectively. From using the F.INV.RT function in Excel, these were found to be 1.9066 and 2.1006, respectively. Hence, the 95% confidence interval for the odds ratio is

$$(25/(13 \times 1.9066), 26 \times 2.1066/12) = (1.01, 4.55).$$

6.6.2   1 : c Matching

When each case is matched to c controls, a test statistic that generalises McNemar's test may be derived using the same methodology as that used in Section 6.6.1. Alternatively, the Mantel–Haenszel (MH) approach may be used. Both approaches give the same results, as shown by Pike and Morrow (1970). We will consider the MH derivation only. Derivations of formulae will be provided, using the results of Section 4.6. Details may be omitted without loss of ability to use the consequent formulae.

In order to apply the MH methodology, we must first define the strata. In Section 4.6, the strata were the groups defined by the confounding variable; here, each case–control matched set is a distinct stratum.

1 : 1 Matching revisited

To fix ideas, consider, again, 1 : 1 matching, where each set (stratum) is of size 2. Given n case–control pairs, we have n strata, but the strata can be of only four types. Table 6.12 shows these four possibilities. Each of the constituent tables is of the form of Table 3.1; notice that it is correct to consider the data *within* a matched set in this format. For convenience, Table 6.12 is divided into three sections, each classified by the number exposed within the pair. When there is one exposure there are two possible tables (case exposed or control exposed). Each table naturally has an overall total of 2, because all sets are of this size.

The Cochran–Mantel–Haenszel (CMH) test statistic, (4.21), requires calculation of the expectation and variance of the top-left cell of each table. The expectation, from (4.19), is the product of the 'cases' total and the 'exposed' total divided by n, the grand total (which is always 2). For a 'no exposures' table, this is $1 \times 0/2 = 0$; for a 'one exposure' table, it is $1 \times 1/2 = 1/2$ and for a 'two exposures' table, it is $1 \times 2/2 = 1$.

Table 6.12. Types of tables (showing risk factor exposure status by case–control status) possible for each pair in a paired case–control study.

No exposures

	Cases	Controls	Total
Exposed	0	0	0
Unexposed	1	1	2
Total	1	1	2

One exposure

	Cases	Controls	Total
Exposed	1	0	1
Unexposed	0	1	1
Total	1	1	2

	Cases	Controls	Total
Exposed	0	1	1
Unexposed	1	0	1
Total	1	1	2

Two exposures

	Cases	Controls	Total
Exposed	1	1	2
Unexposed	0	0	0
Total	1	1	2

The variance, from (4.19), is the product of the four marginal totals divided by $n^2 (n - 1) = 2 \times 2 \times 1 = 4$. For a 'no exposures' table, this is $1 \times 1 \times 0 \times 1/4 = 0$; for a 'one exposure' table, it is $1 \times 1 \times 1 \times 1/4 = 1/4$; and for a 'two exposures' table, it is $1 \times 1 \times 2 \times 0/4 = 0$. Notice that the 'no exposures' and 'two exposures' tables have no variance and thus provide no information. We can exclude them from further consideration on these grounds, but we shall retain them for now to see what happens.

In order to compute the CMH test statistic, we need to sum the elements in the top-left cell of each table making up the whole dataset, to sum the expectations and sum the variances. Hence, we need to know how many there are of each kind of table. As usual, let a denote the observed number in this top-left cell for some arbitrary case–control set. Also, let t_i be the number of sets with i exposures and m_i the number of the t_i in which the case is exposed. Then, the four 2×2 tables making up Table 6.12 have, reading downwards and left to right, t_0, m_1, $t_1 - m_1$ and t_2 occurrences, respectively, in the observed data. These tables have, respectively, $a = 0$, $a = 1$, $a = 0$ and $a = 1$ and thus

$$\sum a = t_0 \times 0 + m_1 \times 1 + (t_1 - m_1) \times 0 + t_2 \times 1 = m_1 + t_2.$$

Using E and V to denote the corresponding expectations and variances gives

$$\sum E = t_0 \times 0 + t_1 \times \tfrac{1}{2} + t_2 \times 1 = \tfrac{1}{2} t_1 + t_2,$$

$$\sum V = t_0 \times 0 + t_1 \times \tfrac{1}{4} + t_2 \times 0 = \tfrac{1}{4} t_1.$$

Notice that, when calculating $\sum E$ and $\sum V$ (but not $\sum a$), we do not need to distinguish the two types of table with one exposure. Note also that $m_0 = 0$ and $m_2 = t_2$.

The continuity-corrected CMH test statistic, (4.21), is

$$\frac{\left(\left|\sum a - \sum E\right| - \frac{1}{2}\right)^2}{\sum V} = \frac{\left(\left|\left(m_1 + t_2\right) - \left(\frac{1}{2}t_1 + t_2\right)\right| - \frac{1}{2}\right)^2}{\frac{1}{4}t_1}$$

$$= \frac{\left(\left|2m_1 - t_1\right| - 1\right)^2}{t_1}. \tag{6.12}$$

Now t_1 is the number of pairs with one exposure — that is, the number of discordant pairs. In Section 6.6.1, we called this quantity d. Similarly, $m_1 = d_1$ in the notation of Section 6.6.1. With these substitutions, (6.12) reduces to the McNemar test statistic, (6.8).

Thinking, once more, of each case–control set (pair, in the 1 : 1 situation) as a stratum, a MH estimate of the odds ratio, $\hat{\psi}_{\text{MH}}$, may be obtained similarly from (4.10). There is a simplification here that $n = 2$ in every stratum. The odds ratio turns out to be the sum of the products of diagonals in each stratum's 2×2 table, divided by the sum of the products of the off-diagonals. For each of the tables making up Table 6.12, the diagonal products are, respectively, 0×1, 1×1, 0×0 and 1×0. Hence, the numerator for $\hat{\psi}_{\text{MH}}$ is

$$t_0 \times 0 + m_1 \times 1 + \left(t_1 - m_1\right) \times 0 + t_2 \times 0 = m_1.$$

The corresponding off-diagonal products are 0×1, 0×0, 1×1 and 1×0, giving a denominator for $\hat{\psi}_{\text{MH}}$ of

$$t_0 \times 0 + m_1 \times 0 + \left(t_1 - m_1\right) \times 1 + t_2 \times 0 = t_1 - m_1.$$

Thus,

$$\hat{\psi}_{\text{MH}} = m_1 / \left(t_1 - m_1\right), \tag{6.13}$$

which reduces to the estimate of the odds ratio given in Section 6.6.1, (6.10), when we substitute $d = t_1$ and $d_1 = m_1$.

Notice, finally, that neither (6.12) nor (6.13) contains any contribution from the 'no exposures' or 'two exposures' tables. The terms from either type of concordant pair have been zero or have cancelled out. In general, it does no harm to include concordant sets in calculations because they will make no overall contribution. However, excluding them simplifies the arithmetic.

1 : 2 Matching

So far the MH approach has provided no new results, but the notation and methodology for $c = 1$ is easily extended to $c > 1$. Now there will be $2(c + 1)$ different types of 2×2 tables to consider, each table representing a type of matched set. One further example will be given before the general results are stated. This is the situation in which $c = 2$;

all strata now are of size 3 (one case and two controls in each set). The $2(c + 1) = 6$ different 2×2 tables and appropriate calculations for each type of table are given as Table 6.13.

Using Table 6.13, with (4.21), the CMH test statistic is thus

$$\frac{\left(\left|\sum a - \sum E\right| - \frac{1}{2}\right)^2}{\sum V} = \frac{\left(\left|m_1 + m_2 - \frac{1}{3}t_1 - \frac{2}{3}t_2\right| - \frac{1}{2}\right)^2}{\frac{2}{9}(t_1 + t_2)}. \tag{6.14}$$

Table 6.13. Types of tables (showing risk factor exposure status by case–control status) possible for each set in a 1 : 2 case–control study. (DP = diagonal product; OP = off-diagonal product)

No exposures

0	0	0
1	2	3
1	2	3

$E = \dfrac{1 \times 0}{3} = 0$

$V = \dfrac{1 \times 2 \times 0 \times 3}{3^2 \times 2} = 0$

No. of tables: t_0
$a = 0$; DP = 0; OP = 0.

One exposure

1	0	1
0	2	2
1	2	3

0	1	1
1	1	2
1	2	3

$E = \dfrac{1 \times 1}{3} = \dfrac{1}{3}$

$V = \dfrac{1 \times 2 \times 1 \times 2}{3^2 \times 2} = \dfrac{2}{9}$

No. of tables: m_1 No. of tables: $t_1 - m_1$
$a = 1$; DP = 2; OP = 0. $a = 0$; DP = 0; OP = 1.

Two exposures

1	1	2
0	1	1
1	2	3

0	2	2
1	0	1
1	2	3

$E = \dfrac{1 \times 2}{3} = \dfrac{2}{3}$

$V = \dfrac{1 \times 2 \times 2 \times 1}{3^2 \times 2} = \dfrac{2}{9}$

No. of tables: m_2 No. of tables: $t_2 - m_2$
$a = 1$; DP = 1; OP = 0. $a = 0$; DP = 0; OP = 2.

Three exposures

1	2	3
0	0	0
1	2	3

$E = \dfrac{1 \times 3}{3} = 1$

$V = \dfrac{1 \times 2 \times 3 \times 0}{3^2 \times 2} = 0$

No. of tables: t_3
$a = 1$; DP = 0; OP = 0.

Note: Row and column labels as in Table 6.12.

Also, from (4.10),

$$\hat{\psi}_{MH} = \frac{2m_1 + m_2}{\left(t_1 - m_1\right) + 2\left(t_2 - m_2\right)}. \tag{6.15}$$

Thus we have the appropriate calculations for a $1:2$ matched study. Note, again, that concordant sets provide no contibution to the final equations (that is, none of m_0, t_0, m_3 or t_3 appear in (6.14) or (6.15)).

General $1:c$ matching

General results for $1:c$ matching are obtained from the same approach. The CMH test statistic for testing the null hypothesis of no association between case–control status and exposure status is

$$\left(\left|\sum_{i=1}^{c} m_i - \sum_{i=1}^{c}\left(\frac{i}{c+1}\right)t_i\right| - \frac{1}{2}\right)^2 \Bigg/ \sum_{i=1}^{c}\left\{\frac{i(c+1-i)}{(c+1)^2}\right\}t_i .$$

This may be rewritten as

$$\left(\left|(c+1)\sum_{i=1}^{c} m_i - \sum_{i=1}^{c} it_i\right| - (c+1)/2\right)^2 \Bigg/ \sum_{i=1}^{c} i(c+1-i)t_i. \tag{6.16}$$

We compare (6.16) with chi-square on 1 d.f.
    The MH estimate of the odds ratio is

$$\hat{\psi}_{MH} = \frac{\displaystyle\sum_{i=1}^{c}\left(c+1-i\right)m_i}{\displaystyle\sum_{i=1}^{c} i\left(t_i - m_i\right)}. \tag{6.17}$$

When $c = 1$, (6.16) and (6.17) reduce to (6.12) and (6.13), respectively; when $c = 2$, they reduce to (6.14) and (6.15).
    Miettinen (1970) gives an approximate formula for the standard error of $\log_e \hat{\psi}$:

$$se\left(\log_e \hat{\psi}\right) = \left[\psi\sum_{i=1}^{c} \frac{i\left(c+1-i\right)t_i}{\left(i\psi + c + 1 - i\right)^2}\right]^{-0.5} . \tag{6.18}$$

We can substitute $\hat{\psi}_{MH}$ for ψ in (6.18) to obtain an estimated result, $\hat{se}(\log_e \hat{\psi})$. An approximate 95% confidence interval for $\log_e \psi$ is then (L_{log}, U_{log}), given by

$$\log_e \hat{\psi}_{MH} \pm 1.96\hat{se}\left(\log_e \hat{\psi}\right), \tag{6.19}$$

Table 6.14. Exposure amongst matched sets showing number of cases and matched controls with a history of BCG vaccination.

Case with BCG?	Number of controls with BCG						Total no. of sets
	0	1	2	3	4	5	
Yes	1	5	1	3	20	27	57
No	11	15	11	5	7	5	54

leading to approximate 95% confidence limits for ψ of

$$\left(\exp\{L_{\log}\}, \ \exp\{U_{\log}\}\right). \tag{6.20}$$

Although the preceding formulae are complex, they are easily implemented using a spreadsheet package, as the tabular approach taken in the next example shows. Alternatively, the method of Robins *et al.* (1986b), given by (4.11) through (4.14), could be applied to the individual case–control sets.

Example 6.9 Rodrigues *et al.* (1991) describe a study of the protection against tuberculosis conferred by BCG vaccination amongst children of Indian ethnic origin born in England. Cases were selected from lists of notifications of the disease, picking out names associated with the Indian subcontinent. Controls were selected from district child health registry or school health records, again picking out Indian names only.

Five controls were matched to each case on the basis of sex and date of birth. BCG vaccination history was determined from historical records for both cases and controls. Results are given in Table 6.14, which is in a compact form, suitable for publication. Using the notation introduced earlier, the first three columns of Table 6.15 re-express the data. The remaining columns of Table 6.15 give the components of (6.16) and (6.17), which are then summed. Notice that $c + 1 = 6$ here.

For example, Table 6.14 shows three matched sets with the case and three controls exposed, and seven matched sets with the case unexposed but four controls exposed. There are thus 10 sets with four exposures, of which three have the case exposed (shown in the row labelled '$i = 4$' in Table 6.15). The t_i values come from adding successive diagonals across Table 6.14 (i.e., $1 + 15$, $5 + 11$, $1 + 5$, etc.), and the m_i values are the numbers in the 'Yes' row of Table 6.14. Concordant sets (the bottom-left and top-right cells of Table 6.14) do not contribute to inferences and hence are ignored in Table 6.15. If they were included in the table, results would stay the same.

Table 6.15. Calculations for Example 6.9 where $i =$ number of exposures, $t_i =$ total number of sets with i exposures and $m_i =$ number of t_i in which the case is exposed.

i	m_i	t_i	it_i	$i(6-i)t_i$	$(6-i)m_i$	$i(t_i - m_i)$
1	1	16	16	80	5	15
2	5	16	32	128	20	22
3	1	6	18	54	3	15
4	3	10	40	80	6	28
5	20	25	125	125	20	25
Total	30		231	467	54	105

Table 6.16. Extra calculations (for a confidence interval) for Example 6.9.[a]

i	t_i	$H = i(6 - i)t_i$	$J = (i\psi + 6 - i)^2$	H/J
1	16	80	30.4073	2.6309
2	16	128	25.2865	5.0620
3	6	54	20.6376	2.6166
4	10	80	16.4604	4.8601
5	25	125	12.7551	9.8000
			Total	24.9696

[a] Notation as in Table 6.15.

From (6.16) and the first three totals in Table 6.15, we have the test statistic

$$\left(\left|6 \times 30 - 231\right| - 6/2\right)^2 \big/ 467 = 4.93.$$

Compared with χ_1^2, this is significant at the 5% level; from Table B.3, $0.05 > p > 0.025$.

From (6.17) and the final two totals in Table 6.15, the odds ratio for BCG versus no BCG is estimated to be $54/105 = 0.51$. Hence, BCG vaccination seems approximately to halve the chance of tuberculosis amongst Indian children born in England.

In order to calculate $\hat{se}(\log_e \hat{\psi})$, Table 6.16 was constructed. Here the first three columns are all copied from Table 6.15; ψ is estimated as $54/105$, the MH estimate just derived. When the total given in Table 6.16 is substituted into (6.18), we obtain,

$$\hat{se}(\log_e \hat{\psi}) = \left[\frac{54}{105} \times 24.9696\right]^{-0.5} = 1/\sqrt{12.8415} = 0.2791.$$

From (6.19), approximate 95% confidence limits for $\log_e \psi$ are

$$\log_e\left(\frac{54}{105}\right) \pm 1.96 \times 0.2791,$$

that is, $(-1.2120, -0.1179)$. Exponentiating both limits gives approximate 95% confidence limits for ψ of $(0.30, 0.89)$, as stated by (6.20).

6.6.3   1 : Variable matching

On occasion, a study may plan to match each case with c controls (where $c > 1$), but the data that eventually arrive for analysis have some incomplete sets. This may be because of failure to locate c controls with all the matching criteria, due to drop-outs or as a consequence of missing values (failure to ascertain the exposure status of some controls). In such situations, we have a 1 : variable matched study. Although conceptually more difficult, these studies are straightforward to deal with using the methodology of Section 6.6.2.

Suppose that we let j denote the number of controls that are matched with any one case, where $j = 1, 2, ..., c$. We can derive a test of $H_0 : \psi = 1$ by calculating the Es and Vs according to (4.19) for each value of i within each value of j in the observed data.

Using a superscript (j) to denote the matching ratio, we obtain

$$E_i^{(j)} = \left(\frac{i}{j+1}\right) t_i^{(j)}$$

$$V_i^{(j)} = \left\{\frac{i(j+1-i)}{(j+1)^2}\right\} t_i^{(j)}$$

(6.21)

for $i = 1, 2, \ldots, j$ within each value of j. Substituting into (4.21) gives the CMH test statistic

$$\left(\left|\sum_{j=1}^{c}\sum_{i=1}^{j} m_i^{(j)} - \sum_{j=1}^{c}\sum_{i=1}^{j} E_i^{(j)}\right| - \tfrac{1}{2}\right)^2 \bigg/ \left(\sum_{j=1}^{c}\sum_{i=1}^{j} V_i^{(j)}\right),$$

(6.22)

which is to be compared with χ_1^2.

A similar method gives rise to an estimate of the odds ratio,

$$\hat{\psi}_{MH} = \sum_{j=1}^{c}\sum_{i=1}^{j} T_i^{(j)} \bigg/ \sum_{j=1}^{c}\sum_{i=1}^{j} B_i^{(j)},$$

(6.23)

where

$$T_i^{(j)} = \left(j+1-i\right) m_i^{(j)} \big/ \left(j+1\right)$$

$$B_i^{(j)} = i\left(t_i^{(j)} - m_i^{(j)}\right) \big/ \left(j+1\right).$$

(6.24)

Similarly, (6.18) may be generalised to give a standard error for $\log_e \hat{\psi}$ of

$$\left[\psi \sum_{j=1}^{c}\sum_{i=1}^{j} \frac{i(j+1-i) t_i^{(j)}}{(i\psi + j+1-i)^2}\right]^{-0.5},$$

from which a 95% confidence interval for ψ follows using (6.19) and (6.20).

Example 6.10 In the study of Legionnaires' disease in Reading (Example 6.2), each person with the disease was supposed to be matched by three controls. The matching criteria were age (within 10 years), sex, neighbourhood of residence and mobility (ability to move around). Due to the combination of the factors, only one control could be found for one of the cases and only two controls for one of the others. The remaining 11 cases all received three matched controls. Tables of exposure status against case–control status were drawn up for each designated area in Reading. Table 6.17 gives the table for 'exposure' to the Butts Centre.

Calculation of the test statistic and estimate of the odds ratio is illustrated by Table 6.18. Substituting the totals from this table into (6.22) gives the test statistic

$$\frac{(|7 - 3.9167| - 0.5)^2}{1.6597} = 4.02,$$

Table 6.17. Exposure amongst matched sets, showing the number of cases and matched controls who visited Reading's Butts Centre in the 2 weeks preceding the case's onset of illness.

Matching ratio	Case visited Butts Centre?	Number of controls visiting Butts Centre			
		0	1	2	3
1 : 1	Yes	0	1		
	No	0	0		
1 : 2	Yes	0	1	0	
	No	0	0	0	
1 : 3	Yes	**2**	**2**	**2**	**4**
	No	0	**1**	0	0

Note: Discordant sets are marked in bold.

Table 6.18. Calculations for Example 6.10, where j = number of controls matched to a case; i = number of exposures; $t_i^{(j)}$ = total number of sets of size $j + 1$ with i exposures; $m_i^{(j)}$ = number of the $t_i^{(j)}$ in which the case is exposed; $E_i^{(j)}$ and $V_i^{(j)}$ are defined by (6.21) and $T_i^{(j)}$ and $B_i^{(j)}$ are defined by (6.24).

j	i	$m_i^{(j)}$	$t_i^{(j)}$	$E_i^{(j)}$	$V_i^{(j)}$	$T_i^{(j)}$	$B_i^{(j)}$
2	2	1	1	0.6667	0.2222	0.3333	0
3	1	2	3	0.7500	0.5625	1.5000	0.2500
	2	2	2	1.0000	0.5000	1.0000	0
	3	2	2	1.5000	0.3750	0.5000	0
Total		7		3.9167	1.6597	3.3333	0.2500

which is significant at the 5% level (see Table B.3). The odds ratio for visiting the Butts Centre, compared with not visiting it, is, from (6.23),

$$\frac{3.3333}{0.2500} = 13.33.$$

Hence, there is a strong indication that the Butts Centre was a source of the legionella bacterium.

6.6.4   Many : many matching

A major disadvantage with 1 : 1 (paired) matching is that if the matched control is 'lost' (for example, due to a failed blood analysis), then the corresponding case is inevitably also lost. This not only reduces accuracy in the final results, but also means that time and resources (for example, in laboratory testing of this case's blood) will have been wasted. The adoption of a 1 : many matching scheme, with the fall-back of a 1 : variable scheme if necessary, protects against this problem. With this scheme, however, if the *case* is lost, the corresponding matched controls will also be lost. To protect against this (opposite) problem, a many : many matched scheme may be possible in special circumstances.

A many : many matching scheme also arises when the goal of matching is simply to ensure that the control sample has a similar overall make-up to the case sample, in terms of potential confounding variables. Hence, if the cases consist of 100 young men, 50 old men, 25 young women and 25 old women, then the control sample will be made the same. Here, matching is done at a group level rather than at an individual level, as we have supposed up to now. Effectively this combines, into a single group, cases that match with each other and their corresponding controls. When the matched groups have an equal number of cases and controls (as in the preceding example), this is sometimes called **frequency matching**.

As McKinlay (1977) and Kleinbaum *et al.* (1982) point out, pairing is often arbitrary in that a case could have been matched with another case's control when two or more cases have common matching variable values. When an arbitrary number of controls is selected to match any group of cases, a **category matching** scheme has been used. When controls are plentiful, this would usually be a better choice than frequency matching; controls would outnumber cases, typically chosen to be in the same ratio, in each matched group. In practice, even when desired, frequency matching may be achieved only approximately due to drop-outs or failure to locate the total number required. Note that matching within groups requires the distribution of cases to be known, which is not possible if cases are identified sequentially as the study progresses. One instance in which the case distribution will be known is in a nested case–control study (Section 6.7).

The MH methodology of Section 4.6 can be applied directly to the matched sets of a many : many scheme. However, if there are many sets, this may require extensive computation. Alternatively (and completely equivalently), the approach of Section 6.6.2 and Section 6.6.3 may be extended to the many : many situation. Practical situations generally will have variable numbers of both cases and controls (that is, variable case : control ratios). Consequently, this is the situation that we will consider. Of course, this is the most general situation, from which the fixed ratio situation may be derived as a special case.

Suppose that $m_{ik}^{(rs)}$ is the number of matched sets with r cases and s controls in which there are i exposures to the risk factor, k of which are exposed cases. The test statistic for testing no association ($\psi = 1$) is

$$\left(\left| \sum k m_{ik}^{(rs)} - \sum E_{ik}^{(rs)} \right| - \tfrac{1}{2} \right)^2 \Big/ \left(\sum V_{ik}^{(rs)} \right), \tag{6.25}$$

where

$$E_{ik}^{(rs)} = \left(\frac{ir}{r+s} \right) m_{ik}^{(rs)},$$

$$V_{ik}^{(rs)} = \left\{ \frac{i(r+s-i)rs}{(r+s)^2(r+s-1)} \right\} m_{ik}^{(rs)}. \tag{6.26}$$

The estimated odds ratio (exposure versus no exposure) is

$$\hat{\psi}_{\mathrm{MH}} = \left(\sum T_{ik}^{(rs)} \right) \Big/ \left(\sum B_{ik}^{(rs)} \right), \tag{6.27}$$

where

$$T_{ik}^{(rs)} = k(s - i + k) m_{ik}^{(rs)} \big/ (r+s),$$

$$B_{ik}^{(rs)} = (i - k)(r - k) m_{ik}^{(rs)} \big/ (r+s). \tag{6.28}$$

In (6.25) and (6.27), the summations are quadruple summations over r, s, i and k. The procedure required is to calculate the value $km_{ik}^{(rs)}$ and the four quantities in (6.26) and (6.28), for each observed combination of r, s, i and k. Each of the five sets of quantities is then summed and the sums are substituted into (6.25) and (6.27). To save unnecessary work, all concordant sets may be discarded at the outset (as usual).

Example 6.11 Table 6.19 shows an excerpt from an unpublished many : many matched case–control study of D-dimer and MI carried out by Professor G.D.O. Lowe (this study was nested within the Scottish Heart Health Study; see Section 6.7). Here, we take 'exposure' to D-dimer to be a high value, above a threshold. Table 6.19 has data for 28 cases and 107 controls. Two of the sets (2 and 4), involving 2 cases and 6 controls, are concordant and can be discarded. Using (6.26) and (6.28), calculations on the remaining 18 sets are presented in Table 6.20. In order to clarify the calculations, each set is taken separately in Table 6.20, rather than grouping together sets with common values of r, s, i and k (that is, sets 5, 6 and 7 and sets 10 and 11). As a consequence, $m_{ik}^{(rs)} = 1$ in each row of the table, so we can use each of (6.25), (6.26) and (6.28) with the $m_{ik}^{(rs)}$ term deleted.

From substituting the totals from Table 6.20 into (6.25), the test statistic is

$$\left(\left|14 - 12.8047\right| - 0.5\right)^2 \Big/ 5.2230 = 0.09,$$

which is clearly not significant at any reasonable significance level. The estimated odds ratio is, from (6.27) and the totals of the final two columns in Table 6.20,

$$\hat{\psi}_{MH} = 5.7111 / 4.5158 = 1.26.$$

Table 6.19. Results from a matched case–control study of D-dimer and myocardial infarction.

Set number	Matching ratio	Number of exposed[a]	
		Cases	Controls
1	1 : 2	0	1
2	1 : 3	0	0
3	1 : 3	1	1
4	1 : 3	1	3
5	1 : 4	0	1
6	1 : 4	0	1
7	1 : 4	0	1
8	1 : 4	0	2
9	1 : 4	0	3
10	1 : 4	1	1
11	1 : 4	1	1
12	1 : 4	1	2
13	1 : 4	1	3
14	1 : 7	1	3
15	2 : 7	1	2
16	2 : 7	1	5
17	2 : 8	1	7
18	2 : 8	2	3
19	3 : 11	1	4
20	3 : 12	2	8

Note: Discordant sets have their set numbers in bold.

[a] Exposure = high D-dimer.

Table 6.20. Calculations for Example 6.11 on a set-by-set basis so that $m_{ik}^{(rs)} = 1$.

Set no.	Cases r	Controls s	Exposures i	Cases exp. k	$E_{ik}^{(rs)}$	$V_{ik}^{(rs)}$	$T_{ik}^{(rs)}$	$B_{ik}^{(rs)}$
1	1	2	1	0	0.3333	0.2222	0	0.3333
3	1	3	2	1	0.5000	0.2500	0.5000	0
5	1	4	1	0	0.2000	0.1600	0	0.2000
6	1	4	1	0	0.2000	0.1600	0	0.2000
7	1	4	1	0	0.2000	0.1600	0	0.2000
8	1	4	2	0	0.4000	0.2400	0	0.4000
9	1	4	3	0	0.6000	0.2400	0	0.6000
10	1	4	2	1	0.4000	0.2400	0.6000	0
11	1	4	2	1	0.4000	0.2400	0.6000	0
12	1	4	3	1	0.6000	0.2400	0.4000	0
13	1	4	4	1	0.8000	0.1600	0.2000	0
14	1	7	4	1	0.5000	0.2500	0.5000	0
15	2	7	3	1	0.6667	0.3889	0.5556	0.2222
16	2	7	6	1	1.3333	0.3889	0.2222	0.5556
17	2	8	8	1	1.6000	0.2844	0.1000	0.7000
18	2	8	5	2	1.0000	0.4444	1.0000	0
19	3	11	5	1	1.0714	0.5828	0.5000	0.5714
20	3	12	10	2	2.0000	0.5714	0.5333	0.5333
Total				14	12.8047	5.2230	5.7111	4.5158

Note: E, V, T and B variables are defined by (6.26) and (6.28).

Hence, those with high D-dimer have approximately 1.26 times the risk of MI compared with those with low D-dimer, but this contrast is not significant. A confidence interval for ψ_{MH} may be found from (4.11) to (4.14), using the 20 sets as 20 strata. This gives a 95% confidence interval of (0.53, 3.02). Applying (4.10) and (4.21) to the same 20 strata gives the same results for the test statistic and estimate, as it must.

6.6.5   A modelling approach

An alternative method for analysing matched case–control studies is through a conditional logistic regression model (Section 10.13.2). This approach can conveniently extend the range of analyses presented here to deal with multiple exposure levels, confounding variables not included in the matching criteria and interaction.

6.7   Nested case–control studies

A **nested case–control study** is a case–control study set within a cohort (or, possibly, an intervention) study. Taking a cohort study that has run for some time, the cases are identified as those in the cohort study who have developed the disease of interest. For each case, a random selection of corresponding controls is drawn from amongst all those in the cohort who have not experienced the disease at the time when the case gets the disease. These controls may get the disease later and may also act as controls for other cases.

Figure 6.3 illustrates the mechanism for a simple (if unrealistic) cohort of eight men and women. When subject A gets the disease (that is, when his event occurs),

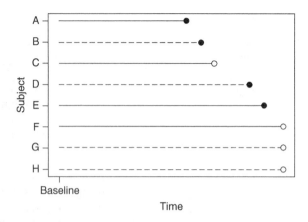

Figure 6.3. Hypothetical cohort study involving eight men and women (solid lines for men; dashed lines for women) showing outcomes as solid dots, denoting events (incident disease), or open dots, denoting censoring (end of follow-up; no event recorded). Subjects are ordered by finish times and given arbitrary labels.

all other subjects are at risk and thus eligible to be selected as controls for A. We call the set of subjects at risk at this time the **risk set** for A, which will be denoted as {A; B, C, D, E, F, G, H}, where the subject to the left of the semicolon is the case. As four subjects in the cohort study get the disease before follow-up is terminated, there are four risk sets; the remaining three are {B; C, D, E, F, G, H}, {D; E, F, G, H} and {E; F, G, H}. From each risk set, we draw a random sample of the controls. Often the same number of controls is drawn from each risk set. For instance, when two controls were randomly selected from each of the four preceding sets, the resulting sampled risk sets were: {A; C, H}, {B; D, G}, {D; F, H} and {E; F, G}, and these would constitute the data elements for the nested case–control study. Notice that D is a control for B even though she later becomes a case, and that F, G and H all act as controls for two cases. Thinking of time as a matching variable, these four sampled risk sets would then be the sets in a 1 : 2 matched case–control study, just as described in Section 6.6.2.

Nested case–control studies may be mounted when, some time after the cohort study has begun, it is decided that further risk factors or confounding variables, not measured when the cohort was recruited, should be analysed. Of course, these extra variables need only be measured on those subjects who appear in the sampled risk sets. This new information might be obtained by recalling the sampled subjects, but this is likely to lead to recall error. A better approach is to use materials taken at the time when the individuals entered the cohort study, such as blood and urine samples or detailed dietary and medication histories, from which the new variables may be measured. Since the nested case–control study will not require every member of the cohort to be measured, there will be savings, which may be important when measurements are expensive or intricate. Furthermore, as the cohort follow-up proceeds, new hypotheses may arise, for example, concerning risk factors recently suggested and/or biochemical assays just invented. Wise designers of cohort studies will, wherever possible, have banked resources, such as blood samples, that can be used to address such issues.

Example 6.12 In a cohort study of risk factors for cancer, Lin *et al.* (1995) recruited 9775 men. Blood samples were taken and frozen at recruitment into the cohort study. Over a follow-up of around 7 years, 29 incident cases of gastric cancer were identified. By this time, a number of authors had published studies suggesting that *Helicobacter pylori* might be a risk factor for gastric cancer. Since *H. pylori* can be ascertained through an assay on blood samples, Lin and colleagues decided to exploit their stored samples to test this emerging theory through a nested case–control study. Between five and eight controls were sampled for each case, giving 220 controls altogether. Laboratory work was much reduced compared with analysing the entire cohort: 249 assays rather than 9775 (less some with missing samples) were required.

The great advantage of a nested study, over a standard case–control design, is that cases and controls come from the same population, avoiding the issues of selection bias discussed in Section 6.3 and Section 6.4. If exposure status (that is, the risk factor) is measured on materials sampled at cohort baseline, bias due to differential quality of information between cases and controls is also much less likely, particularly if the person doing the measurements is blinded (Section 7.3.2) to case–control status. As already indicated, relative to the parent cohort study, and assuming the disease under study is rare, nested case–control studies save numbers, and thus expense, due to sampling of controls within the risk sets. In practice, the nested study typically uses less than 20% of the parent cohort. However, this loss of numbers does make the design less statistically efficient than the cohort study; with very large numbers, for a $1 : c$ nested case–control study, the power (Section 8.2) for unadjusted analyses is $c/(c + 1)$ times that of the cohort study (Langholz and Clayton, 1994). For a moderate value of c, this loss of efficiency is relatively small compared with the savings in cost, e.g., when $c = 5$ the loss of efficiency is only a sixth.

Ernster (1994) and Wacholder (1991) give details and examples of nested case–control studies. Variations on the sampling method described here appear in Robins *et al.* (1986a). As already noted, nested case–control studies may also be set within intervention studies (Chapter 7). This presents no extra complications, although it would then be sensible to match by treatment group. For an example, see Woodward *et al.* (2005).

6.7.1   Matched studies

In most situations, the nested case–control study is matched not only on follow-up time, as explained previously (which is essential), but also on important confounding variables that were measured in the cohort study. Just as with any case-control study, this matching provides a direct way of dealing with confounding. The added bonus here is that no further work is required to obtain the values of these confounders. In the gastric cancer study of Example 6.12, matching was done on age, sex and residence, all of which were recorded in the baseline questionnaire for the parent cohort study.

With Figure 6.3 as an example, suppose we decide to match by sex. The consequence is that the risk sets are smaller because only people of the same sex are allowed to share any risk set. They are: {A; C, E, F}, {B; D, G, H}, {D; G, H} and {E; F}. As before, we would sample from the controls within any set and analyse as for a matched study. Notice that, if we tried to do a 1 : 2 matched study as before, we would not be able to draw two controls to match with E, leaving us with 1 : variable matching (easily dealt with; see Section 6.6.3). In practice, cohort studies are likely to have thousands of subjects, rather than eight, but a similar issue can arise when there are several matching variables. As ever, we should beware of overmatching (Section 6.5.2). Variable matching may also occur because of missing values — for instance, when certain frozen stored blood samples are found to be unusable, perhaps due to prior accidental thawing.

6.7.2   Counter-matched studies

In certain situations, a better alternative to matching is **counter-matching**. Whereas matching is used to control for confounding, counter-matching is used to maximise the variation in exposure to the risk factor. Thus, matched studies match according to levels of the confounding factor, and counter-matched studies match according to levels of the risk factor, or some proxy. This approach would be ideal when a cohort study has been completed that shows a significant, and medically important, association between a risk factor and a disease, but there is a remaining question whether a confounder that was not measured in the cohort study might explain the observed association. If this confounder could be retrospectively measured, a counter-matched (on risk factor exposure) nested case–control study would be expected to be more efficient than an unmatched (except for time) nested case–control study (Langholz and Clayton, 1994).

Given any risk set, counter-matching requires stratifying the members of that risk set according to levels of the counter-matching variable and selecting a random sample from each stratum (thus spreading the exposure) to make up the controls in the sampled risk set, within the constraint that the desired matching ratio is maintained in all sampled risk sets. For 1 : 1 matching with a binary exposure, we sample purely from within the opposite stratum to that occupied by the case, giving rise to the term 'counter-matching'. Consider Figure 6.3: a 1 : 1 counter-matched design for sex would require, for instance within the risk set for the female subject B, random sampling of one from the three male subjects C, E and F. The sampled risk set might be {B; F}. Similarly, we might obtain, by suitable random sampling, the other three sampled risk sets {A; H}, {D; E} and {E; H}.

Analysis of counter-matched studies requires weighted analyses, beyond our present scope. See Langholz and Clayton (1994) for a concise account.

6.8   Case–cohort studies

A **case–cohort study** is, like the nested case–control study, set within a parent cohort study. Both designs take the cases identified from the cohort study in the same way, but the case–cohort study, rather than adding matched controls, adds a random subset of the initial cohort, called the **subcohort**. No matching is involved. The case–cohort study thus consists of all the members of the subcohort plus all those who were identified as having got the disease during follow-up (the cases), with some overlap between these two sources. As with nested studies, case–cohort studies use fewer subjects than the full cohort. Table 6.21 shows that the expected number in the case–cohort study is $D + \pi(N - D)$, where N is the number in the cohort study, D is the number of incident cases

Table 6.21. Expected numbers (shown in bold) in a case–cohort study according to source (where π = proportion sampled for the subcohort).

Baseline categorisation	Follow-up outcome		
	Disease	No disease	Total
Subcohort	πD	$\pi(N - D)$	πN
Not	$(1 - \pi)D$	$(1 - \pi)(N - D)$	$(1 - \pi)N$
Total	D	$N - D$	N

of disease during follow-up and π is the fraction sampled for the subcohort. In Example 6.12, 29 cases were found in a cohort of size 9775. If, instead of a nested design, a case–cohort design had been chosen, with the subcohort being 5% of the cohort, the expected number of subjects would have been $29 + 0.05 \times (9775 - 29) = 516$.

Case–cohort studies are often used when nested case–control studies could be used, sharing the advantages of being less liable to bias error and saving cost. Various comparisons of the two designs have been made (for example, Barlow *et al.*, 1999; Ernster, 1994; Langholz and Thomas, 1990; and Wacholder, 1991). These are inconclusive regarding statistical efficiency but lead to the conclusion that the case–cohort design is more flexible, yet may be more prone to bias error, compared with the nested design.

Taking the relative advantages of the case–cohort design first, the most important is that the subcohort can be used for any outcome of interest. That is, if we wish to study two diseases, the subcohort, of size πN, can contribute to the case–cohort study of both diseases. The second disease merely requires the addition of the expected $(1 - \pi)D$ nonsubcohort cases for that disease, and subsequent measurement of the risk factor. As the nested study involves matching, it would require a (virtually) complete new set of measurements. So, if we require analyses of the same risk factor on several diseases, the case–cohort design is a better choice.

Another advantage is that analyses may be made according to any time scale, unlike under the nested design in which the initial time matching precludes such flexibility. Examples of alternative time scales, which may be useful in certain circumstances, are age and time since a significant event (such as the menopause) occurred. Unlike nested studies, case–cohort studies can spread the extra measurements (those not taken for all the parent cohort study) over time. The subcohort can be identified as the cohort is recruited, and the extra measurements can thus start immediately. In a nested study, the best that can be done is to start the measurements once the first incident case is identified. Repeat measurements can be done on the subcohort, leading to a direct correction for regression dilution bias (Section 10.12). Finally, the subcohort can directly serve as any other cohort might do; for example, as a basis for computing risk scores (Chapter 13) and for making comparisons with external populations (Wacholder and Boivin, 1987).

The chance of bias is higher in case–cohort, compared with nested, studies, when the subcohort is selected at baseline, since then the nonsubcohort members may not be followed up as carefully as the subcohort members (by definition, these are somewhat 'special'). Since the majority of cases are likely to come from outside the subcohort, this could lead to underestimation of the association between the risk factor and the disease, or incomplete adjustment for confounding. If the extra (noncohort) measurements are taken from blood (or other) samples, in a fresh state for the subcohort and after storage for the nonsubcohort cases, the earlier and later values may not be comparable due to deterioration of the samples — again leading to bias. Should the subcohort be selected after follow-up is completed (similar to a nested case–control study), the case–cohort study would avoid these issues of bias.

Analysis of case–cohort studies may be undertaken with the Stata routine STSEL-PRE, the SAS macros available from http://lib.stat.cmu. edu/general/robphreg or other specialist software. These programs use weighted Cox proportional hazards regression models (Section 11.6); see Barlow *et al.* (1999) for a description of popular weighting methods and the SAS macros mentioned previously. Another method of analysis is described by Breslow *et al.* (2009) and Ganna *et al.* (2012). A further Stata procedure, STCASCOH, may be useful for creating the case–cohort dataset.

6.9   Case–crossover studies

Sometimes the risk factor of interest is transient but repeatable, for example, the use of mobile telephones by drivers of cars (which may lead to a crash), bouts of anger (which may lead to a heart attack) and contaminants in the air (which may lead to respiratory disease). For such risk factors, a special type of matched study can be very useful — the **case–crossover study**, in which each case acts as her or his own control.

The basic method is to identify a set of cases (here called 'subjects') and decide upon a time window preceding onset of the condition (the **case window**) wherein exposure to the risk factor will be evaluated for each subject. For instance, we might take all drivers hospitalised after a nonfatal car crash and ascertain, by interview, whether each used a mobile phone in the 5 minutes preceding the crash. Then, for each subject, a second, nonoverlapping, time window (the **control window**) of the same length, during which the subject did not experience the condition being researched, is chosen. Exposure to the risk factor in the control window is also ascertained. For example, each person who crashed their car might be asked whether they used their mobile phone during the same 5 minutes on the previous occasion when they drove their car, at roughly the same time of the day, before the trip that included their crash. As in the basic case–control approach, the effect of the risk factor is estimated through comparison of exposures in the case and control windows, over all subjects. This is achieved by analysing the data as a 1 : 1 matched case–control study, just as in Section 6.6.

Example 6.13 In an Italian case–crossover study of sleep disturbance and injury amongst children (Valent *et al.*, 2001), each child was asked about her or his sleep in the 24 hours before the injury occurred (the case window) and in the 24 hours before that (the control window). Amongst 181 boys, 40 had less than 10 hours sleep on both the days concerned; 111 had less than 10 hours sleep on neither day; 21 had less than 10 hours sleep only on the day before the injury; and 9 had less than 10 hours sleep only on the penultimate day before the injury. Using (6.10) and (6.11), the odds ratio (95% confidence interval) for injury, comparing days without and with 10 hours or more sleep, is 2.33 (1.02, 5.79).

The case–crossover approach is suitable for studying the transient effects of an intermittent exposure of a rare, acute condition. When it is suitable, it provides an optimal approach to controlling for any confounder that is not transient, because of the self-matching. As it does not require controls, clear cost savings are realised compared with case–control designs (matched or otherwise). Indeed, because case–crossover data are analysed as for matched studies, in which concordant pairs (or sets) give no information, case–crossover studies require only subjects with some exposure to be recruited. Thus, this design might be used when the only data are reports on people exposed to the risk factor, such as health records of intermittent drug users. The basic design is easily extended by picking several control windows per subject, leading to analysis as for one to many matched case–control studies (Section 6.6.2, Section 6.6.3 and Section 6.6.5).

Unfortunately, the design is susceptible to bias error. Recall bias is quite likely, in much the same way as for a case–control design (Section 6.1.2). In some situations, this may be overcome by choosing a control window after the case window. Obviously, this is not always possible, for example, when deaths are studied or when exposure changes due to becoming a case.

The biggest problems are concerned with the choices of the window(s). Choice of the length of the case window depends upon how the risk factor is hypothesised to work; for example, mobile phone use that ceased 30 minutes ago is highly unlikely to be risk-forming for drivers, whereas pollution outbreaks several days ago could still affect respiration. Sometimes different window lengths are tried, but the resultant odds ratios may differ in an unexpected way, presenting difficulties in interpretation.

Control windows must be chosen extremely carefully, ensuring that the subject had equal chance of exposure to the risk factor in their case and control windows. Also, any systematic differences over time need to be controlled. For instance, traffic levels differ by time, day and place; ideally, we would like a control window that reproduces all these, compared with the case window, in any study of car drivers. Such control may, however, be possible only at the expense of recall error. To avoid carry-over effects, it may be sensible to allow a **wash-out** period (i.e., a period of time not selected into a window) between the case and control windows. In Example 6.13, no such wash-out period was included, which would have led to underestimation of the odds ratio if it were generally true that a day with many hours of sleep is generally preceded by a day with few hours of sleep, amongst children. Sensitivity analyses are often undertaken to compare the results from different choices for control windows.

Further details about case–crossover design strategies are given in Mittleman *et al.* (1995) and Maclure and Mittleman (2000). An example of the use of a case–crossover study to examine the association between mobile phone use and car crashes is given by McEvoy *et al.* (2005).

Exercises

6.1 In a case–control study of the use of oral contraceptives (OCs) and breast cancer in New Zealand, Paul *et al.* (1986) identified cases over a 2-year period from the National Cancer Registry and controls by random selection from electoral rolls. The following data were compiled.

Used OCs?	Cases	Controls
Yes	310	708
No	123	189
Total	433	897

(i) Estimate the odds ratio for breast cancer, OC users versus nonusers. Specify a 95% confidence interval for the true odds ratio.

(ii) Test whether OC use appears to be associated with breast cancer.

6.2 Morrison (1992) carried out a case–control study of risk factors for prostatic hypertrophy in Rhode Island. Cases were all men who had a first experience of prostatic surgery, but who did not have prostatic or bladder cancer, during the period from November 1985 to October 1987. Random population controls were selected from administrative lists, filtering out by telephone interview those with a history of prostatic surgery or prostatic or bladder cancer. Of 873 cases, 48 reported that they were Jewish. Of 1934 controls, 64 were Jewish.

(i) Calculate the odds ratio (with a 95% confidence interval) for prostatic surgery for Jews compared with non-Jews.

(ii) Test for the significance of a relationship between being of the Jewish religion and undergoing prostatic surgery.

6.3   In September 1993 only the second outbreak of *Salmonella enteritidis* phage
       type 4 (SE) occurred in the U.S. (Boyce *et al.*, 1996). As with the first, the
       infection occurred amongst people who had eaten at a certain Chinese fast-
       food restaurant in El Paso, Texas. To investigate the second outbreak, a
       case–control study was instigated. Cases were people with diarrhoea or
       culture-confirmed SE that occurred after the patient ate at the restaurant
       between 27 August and 15 September 1995. Controls were well meal com-
       panions of the cases or persons subsequently identified as having eaten at
       the restaurant, without undue effects, during the outbreak. The following table
       shows the number of cases and controls who reported eating each of four
       menu items from the restaurant.

Food item	Cases ($n = 19$)	Controls ($n = 17$)
Breaded chicken	14	11
Any chicken	16	16
Egg rolls	14	3
Fried rice	14	9

       Which food item do you suspect is the source of SE? Provide suitable ana-
       lytical evidence to support your assertion.

6.4   Scragg *et al.* (1993) report a study of bed sharing and sudden infant death
       syndrome (SIDS). Cases of SIDS were compared with a random sample of
       controls selected from lists of births. Of the 393 cases, 248 usually shared a
       bed, whereas of the 1591 controls, 708 usually shared a bed. Estimate the
       attributable risk of SIDS for bed sharing, together with a 95% confidence
       interval.

6.5   Horwitz and Feinstein (1978) report that a side-effect of exogenous oestrogen
       use is vaginal bleeding. Vaginal bleeding is a potential sign of endometrial
       cancer amongst postmenopausal women. Consider the implications of these
       observations in the design of a case–control study of oestrogen intake and
       endometrial cancer.

6.6   In a case–control study of risk factors for dental caries, McMahon *et al.* (1993)
       present the following data relating to age of child, age of mother and whether
       the child has dental caries. Caries is defined here as a minimum of four
       decayed, missing or filled teeth.

Age of mother (years)	Age of child (months)					
	<36		36–47		≥48	
	Caries	Control	Caries	Control	Caries	Control
<25	1	1	1	5	8	9
25–34	4	16	18	67	46	113
≥35	1	2	3	14	10	35

       Find (i) unadjusted (raw) and (ii) Mantel–Haenszel adjusted (for child age)
       odds ratios for dental caries by age of mother, taking the oldest women as
       the reference group. Give 95% confidence intervals in each case. (iii) Interpret
       your results.

6.7   For Example 6.8, Example 6.9 and Example 6.10, find the odds ratio of each, *ignoring* matching. What effect has ignoring matching had on each odds ratio?

6.8   A case–control study of acute lymphoblastic leukaemia amongst Spanish children found 128 cases aged below 15 years from hospital records (Infante–Rivard *et al.*, 1991). Each case was matched by year of birth, sex and municipality to a single control. Community controls were randomly selected using Census lists. The following table shows an analysis of the mothers' exposure to dust from cotton, wool or synthetic fibres during pregnancy. Exposure was established by interview at home or in hospital.

Case exposed to dust?	Control exposed to dust?	
	Yes	No
Yes	1	11
No	2	114

   (i)   Find the estimated odds ratio for exposure compared with nonexposure, together with a 95% confidence interval.
   (ii)   Test the null hypothesis that exposure to dust is not associated with acute lymphoblastic leukaemia.

6.9   In a study of the relationship between criminality and injury, cases were selected from English-speaking men with acute, traumatic spinal cord injuries admitted to hospital in Louisiana between 1 January 1965 and 31 December 1984 who were still alive at the time of study and could be contacted by telephone (Mawson *et al.*, 1996). Controls were selected from holders of Louisiana driver's licences, matched with individual cases on age, sex, race, ZIP code of residence and educational attainment. Subjects were asked if they had ever been arrested, convicted of a crime or placed in a correctional institution before the date of their spinal injury. Controls were asked the same questions, with the relevant date being that of the spinal injury of the case to whom they had been matched. Results for arrests before the age of 17 years for case–control pairs are:

Case arrested?	Control arrested?	
	Yes	No
Yes	7	33
No	16	83

   (i)   Calculate the odds ratio for spinal cord injury, comparing those with a history of criminal arrests to those without. Give a 95% confidence interval for your estimate.
   (ii)   Test the null hypothesis that criminality is not associated with spinal injury.
   (iii) Which issues concerned with the design and analysis of this study (as presented here) might temper the conclusion that criminality is related to spinal injury?

6.10 Miller *et al.* (1978) identified 136 cases of bladder cancer at Ottowa Civic
Hospital, Canada. Each case was matched by two controls for sex and 10-year
age group; controls were largely recruited from the same hospital as the cases.
The following table gives a classification of the number of heavy smokers (20
or more cigarettes per day) within each of the case–control triples.

Number of exposures in the triple	Number of triples	Number of triples with an exposed case
0	12	0
1	40	17
2	53	42
3	31	31

   (i)   Estimate the odds ratio for bladder cancer, heavy smokers versus not.
         Give a 95% confidence interval for the true odds ratio.
   (ii) Test whether heavy smoking is associated with bladder cancer.

6.11 Pike *et al.* (1970) give the results of a matched case–control study of children
with microscopically proven Burkitt's lymphoma at Mulago Hospital,
Uganda. Patients were individually matched with one or two unrelated persons of the same age, sex, tribe and place of residence. The method used was
to visit homes near the home of the patient until one or two suitable subjects
were found. Individuals were then characterised as haemoglobin AA or AS
to test the hypothesis that haemoglobin AA is a risk factor for Burkitt's
lymphoma. The following table reproduces the way in which results are given
in the source paper.

Burkitt's tumour patient	Matched controls				
	Single controls		Two controls		
	AA	AS	AA, AA	AA, AS	AS, AS
AA	13	6	7	3	1
AS	2	1	1	2	0

   (i)   Test the hypothesis of no association against the one-sided alternative
         that children with haemoglobin AA are more susceptible to the lym-
         phoma.
   (ii) Estimate the corresponding odds ratio and compute the associated 99%
         confidence interval.
   (iii) Interpret your results.

6.12 In a matched case–control study of venous thromboembolism (VTE) and use
of hormone replacement therapy (HRT), Daly *et al.* (1996) screened women
aged 45–64 years admitted to hospitals in the Oxford Regional Health Authority (UK) with a suspected diagnosis of VTE. From these, 103 cases of idiopathic
VTE were recruited. Each case was individually matched with up to two
hospital controls with diagnoses judged to be unrelated to HRT use, such as
diseases of the eyes, ears or skin. Matching criteria were 5-year age group,
district of admission and date of admission (between 2 weeks before and 4
months after the admission date of the corresponding case). Altogether there
were 178 controls. The data are available from the web site for this book
(Appendix A).

Confirm the following summary table:

Matching ratio	Case uses HRT?	Number of controls using HRT		
		0	1	2
1 : 1	yes	7	3	
	no	17	1	
1 : 2	yes	15	15	4
	no	27	11	3

Using this summary table,
(i)   Test for no association between hormone replacement therapy (HRT) use and venous thromboembolism.
(ii) Estimate the odds ratio, and find the associated 95% confidence interval, for HRT users versus nonusers.

6.13 A medical investigator plans to carry out a case–control study of risk factors for asthma amongst infants. Cases are to be identified from referrals to the paediatric department of a certain hospital. Each case will be matched by two controls selected from the hospital records; matching being on the basis of whether the baby was born in a high-level care department of a hospital (such as an intensive care unit). Is this a sensible matching criterion? Suggest other possible matching criteria and identify how you would select your controls.

6.14 For the case–crossover study of Example 6.13,
(i)   Apply the general formulae for one to many case–control studies, (6.16) through (6.20), where $c = 1$, to obtain a test statistic and odds ratio with its 95% confidence limits. Show that the odds ratio is the same as that given in the text but that the confidence interval is slightly narrower (reflecting the approximation used in (6.18)).
(ii) Show that the same odds ratio and confidence interval as in (i) is obtained from applying the general MH formulae, (4.10) through (4.14), to the 'one exposure' subtables of Table 6.12 for these data.

CHAPTER 7

Intervention studies

7.1 Introduction

An **intervention study**, or **clinical trial**, is an experiment applied to existing patients, in order to decide upon an appropriate therapy, or to those presently free of symptoms, in order to decide upon an appropriate preventive strategy. These experiments involve giving **treatments** to the subjects in the study. For example, to test the efficacy of a novel drug formulation in the treatment of a specific disease, some patients with the disease are given the new drug and some are given an established drug. The two groups are then compared prospectively for incidence of the disease and other outcomes of interest, known collectively as **end-points**. Other examples of intervention studies are comparisons of hospital procedures (e.g., day care against overnight stay or medical against surgical treatment for patients with similar complaints), field trials of vaccines and evaluation of contraceptive practices. Thus, here the term 'treatment' has a very general meaning.

The essential feature of an intervention study is that the allocation of subject to treatment is *planned*; that is, the investigators decide who should receive which treatment (usually using some probabilistic mechanism). Contrast this with cross-sectional surveys, cohort and case-control studies wherein, for example, there is no control over who is and who is not a cigarette smoker.

Example 7.1 Crombie *et al.* (1990) describe an intervention study of vitamin and mineral supplementation to improve verbal and nonverbal reasoning of schoolchildren, which was carried out in Dundee, Scotland. Various reasoning (IQ) tests were applied to two groups of schoolchildren aged between 11 and 13 years old. One group (of size 42) then received vitamin and mineral supplements. The other group (of size 44) received a **placebo** treatment — inactive tablets that were indistinguishable from the active tablets. The tablets were taken for 7 months, after which time the IQ tests were repeated. Table 7.1 gives the baseline and final values for two of the tests administered.

Since important differences could exist between the two groups before treatment began, it is most meaningful to compare the differences in IQ scores — that is, final minus initial score — between the two groups. Such differences are sometimes called **deltas**. Summary statistics and the results of *t* tests, using (2.14) through (2.16), are given for deltas from both IQ tests in Table 7.2. Although those on active treatment show the greatest improvement (on average), no significant difference is found between the supplement and placebo groups, for either test. We conclude that there is no evidence of an effect upon IQ of supplementation. More complete analyses are given in the source paper.

Table 7.1. Initial and final values of IQ scores for 86 children in Dundee.

Placebo group ($n = 44$)				Active group ($n = 42$)			
Nonverbal test		Verbal test		Nonverbal test		Verbal test	
Initial	Final	Initial	Final	Initial	Final	Initial	Final
89	83	87	84	70	87	57	63
82	97	73	87	91	91	68	75
107	107	59	72	106	104	78	89
95	101	105	108	92	87	86	84
110	100	97	105	103	114	81	93
106	97	75	84	105	115	85	89
114	112	113	118	106	106	85	86
97	96	86	89	82	78	80	82
103	103	95	97	101	98	86	84
109	122	101	94	86	106	76	86
97	80	84	89	101	102	99	97
93	103	93	93	97	97	100	93
107	110	96	94	84	85	76	85
84	102	73	86	90	100	87	97
69	79	70	80	88	90	77	85
109	100	97	95	121	106	95	92
98	101	77	76	101	110	82	89
72	78	86	87	100	97	91	89
70	78	82	87	116	126	108	110
99	122	79	79	108	121	98	111
105	118	96	104	127	125	94	98
133	133	130	126	95	100	88	88
87	93	84	82	90	91	83	92
104	120	101	89	112	117	101	93
118	112	98	95	115	119	98	109
113	121	105	118	112	111	80	87
89	99	90	92	104	108	99	107
101	97	76	79	107	98	88	88
95	95	82	83	137	131	109	109
103	101	98	100	109	115	91	99
99	107	90	96	99	116	82	85
101	111	89	89	80	82	84	90
118	104	106	104	105	112	90	99
114	115	103	100	99	104	82	84
111	105	87	89	78	85	70	77
81	75	78	64	70	98	92	89
90	74	89	77	135	135	117	116
104	87	75	74	117	129	108	104
83	91	69	79	84	88	91	80
101	98	79	86	103	104	87	88
113	98	78	98	108	112	85	87
97	101	83	92	130	128	102	100
93	92	84	89				
119	130	121	126				

Note: These data may be downloaded; see Appendix A.

Table 7.2. Mean differences (with standard errors in parentheses) in IQ score deltas, together with tests of no difference between treatments.

IQ test	Placebo group	Active group	t test Statistic	p value
Nonverbal	1.50 (1.49)	3.90 (1.24)	1.24	0.22
Verbal	2.64 (1.06)	3.14 (0.90)	0.36	0.72

7.1.1   Advantages

Intervention studies are most efficient for investigating possible causal relationships between risk factors and disease because:

1. We can ensure that the 'cause' precedes the 'effect'.
2. We can ensure that possible confounding factors do not confuse the results because we can allocate subjects to treatment in any way we choose. For instance, consider a comparative trial of two treatments for a chronic condition that inevitably worsens with age. We can allocate each treatment to patient groups with the same (or very similar) age distribution, thus avoiding any age differences in the subsequent group comparisons.
3. We can ensure that treatments are compared efficiently. This means using our control over allocation to spread the sample over the treatment groups so as to achieve maximum power in statistical tests such as the t test of Example 7.1. This may simply require allocating an equal number of subjects to each treatment group (Section 8.4.3). We may also wish to look for effects of combinations of treatments or interactions between treatments and personal characteristics. Then we can arrange so that we obtain sufficient numbers of observations of each distinct type, in order to evaluate such effects efficiently.

7.1.2   Disadvantages

1. Since intervention studies involve the prospective collection of data, they may share many of the disadvantages of cohort studies listed in Section 5.1.2.
2. Ethical problems are associated with giving experimental treatments. These are considered in more detail in Section 7.2, but note that such considerations often rule out the use of intervention studies in epidemiological investigations. For example, it is unethical to force chosen individuals to smoke or drink heavily merely for experimental purposes, because smoking and heavy drinking have known undesirable effects.
3. In many instances, intervention studies screen out 'problem' subjects, such as the very young, the elderly and pregnant women, who may have a special (possibly adverse) reaction to treatment. This may restrict the generalisability of results.

7.2   Ethical considerations

Although ethical issues are crucial in any epidemiological investigation, they are inevitably most important in experimental situations (Pocock, 1983) and thus are most conveniently addressed here. Ethical requirements of medical studies are defined in the Declaration of

Helsinki, see http://www.wma.net/en/30publications/10policies/b3/index.html. These requirements are primarily concerned with individual rights; for instance, each subject should receive an explanation of the study and her or his consent should be obtained. In addition to such issues, steps should be taken to avoid bias (Section 7.3) and an adequate sample size should be used (Chapter 8) or else the study will be unethical in the sense of being misleading or wasteful of resources.

7.2.1   The protocol

One of the principles of the Declaration of Helsinki is that the study should have a protocol. The protocol serves three main purposes. First, it is a justification for the study, which will be scrutinized by ethical committees and, possibly, funding agencies. Second, it is a reference manual for use by all those involved in the administration and analysis of the study. Third, it specifies the analytic methods to be used before the data are collected, thus avoiding bias through 'cherry-picking' of results. Although no list can possibly cover the needs of all protocols, the following is a specimen list of section headings suitable for intervention studies. Several of the items will be appropriate for protocols in observational studies also. Further details on protocol design are provided by Sylvester *et al.* (1982) and in the SPIRIT checklist (Chan *et al.*, 2013).

1. Rationale: The background to the study. When a novel treatment is involved, this might include an explanation of how it is thought to work against the disease in question and why it might be an improvement on existing treatment. References to previous literature on the subject would normally be included.
2. Aims of study: What, exactly, does the study seek to discover? For instance, the aims may be to compare efficacy (suitably defined) and side-effects of a new treatment against an existing treatment.
3. Design of study: A specification of the basic design used (Sections 7.4 to 7.6) and how the measures to avoid bias (Section 7.3) will be implemented.
4. Selection of subjects: This should include the number to be assigned to each treatment group, as well as inclusion and exclusion criteria. Inclusion criteria usually contain the precise definition of disease to be used (for example, the symptoms that must be exhibited) and appropriate age limits (if any) for entry to the study. Exclusion criteria often include other medical conditions that may cause complications and pregnancy. Subjects may also be excluded because they have received treatment that may affect their responses in the current investigation.
5. Drugs and dosages: A list of the medications (or alternatives) to be taken by the subjects, the dosage(s) to be used and the form of the medication (tablets, injections, inhalers, etc.). If appropriate, the drug supplier is mentioned here, if not specified elsewhere.
6. Assessments: What the study will measure. This is likely to include measures of efficacy (blood pressure, lung function etc.), records of adverse events (headaches, nausea etc.) plus records of adherence (how many tablets were actually taken each day) and concurrent medication (or other form of treatment) received. Adherence gives important information on tolerance of treatment and treatment administration. Records of concurrent medication may be used in two main ways. If this medication is something that alleviates the symptoms of the very disease being studied, then its consumption is evidence of lack of efficacy of the treatment allocated. If the medication is normally taken for

other complaints, then its consumption might indicate a side-effect of the treatment allocated. Furthermore, in the event that many subjects take the same concurrent medication, we may wish to look at the effect of taking a combination of the study treatment and the concurrent medication.

7. Documentation: A list of the forms for recording information. This may include physicians' record cards to be completed during clinic visits and daily record cards to be completed by the subject. The latter would typically record compliance and side-effects, plus self-assessments of well-being (particularly in studies of chronic conditions).

8. Procedure: Usually the longest part of the protocol, this specifies what should be done, and by whom, at each stage of the study. Many intervention studies involve several clinic visits, and here we should state, for example, what measurements will be taken at each particular visit, including the precise methodology to use (for example, 'diastolic blood pressure by sphygmomanometer taking the fifth Korotkoff sound'). Instructions for the doctor to give to her or his patients would also be included (such as how many tablets should be taken per day and how the daily record card should be completed).

9. Withdrawals: Subjects may withdraw or may be removed from the study by the investigating physician (or others), possibly for medical reasons or because of serious protocol deviations. This section of the protocol specifies how the reasons for withdrawal should be recorded (often on a special form) and describes any other consequent administrative procedures. Reasons for withdrawal may, of course, provide evidence of side-effects.

10. Adverse events: As for withdrawals. Severe adverse events would often lead to withdrawal in any case.

11. Consent: A statement that subject consent (or a proxy, if necessary) will be sought and how this will be obtained.

12. Ethics: A statement that the appropriate ethical committee will be, or has already been, consulted. A copy of the ethical guidelines to be adopted, such as the Declaration of Helsinki, is sometimes included as an appendix.

13. Analysis: Details of the statistical methods to be used upon the subsequent dataset. If there are special features of the required analysis, such as separate subgroup analyses (for example, by age group), these should be given here.

14. Data discharge: Details of data confidentiality and the rules governing disclosure.

15. Investigators' statement: A declaration that the protocol will be followed, which the principal investigators (and others) will sign.

7.3   Avoidance of bias

Just as in any other exercise in data collection, intervention studies may suffer from bias error if not conducted in an appropriate fashion. In this section, we will consider five principles that should be followed in order to reduce the chance of a biased conclusion. See also Section 7.4 for some examples of the application of these principles.

7.3.1   Use of a control group

Just as for cohort studies, intervention studies should be *comparative* — that is, a control group should be researched alongside a treated group. Here we assume, as we will subsequently in this chapter, that only two groups are involved, but in general several treatment groups could be involved. The control group may be treated with a placebo (as in Example 7.1) or another active treatment, such as the existing standard therapy.

If there had been no placebo group in the Dundee vitamin study, the only data would be the right-hand portion of Table 7.1. Then the appropriate procedure (for each IQ test) would be to use a paired t test (Section 2.7.4). The t statistics are 3.16 and 3.50, leading to p values of 0.003 and 0.001, for nonverbal and verbal tests, respectively. Thus, without the control group, we would conclude that vitamin supplementation *does* improve IQ — the opposite to the conclusion in Example 7.1. One contributory factor to the result here may be the increased experience of the children between testing dates; some improvement in certain aspects of IQ might be expected regardless of treatment.

If we fail to use a control group, we can never be sure that our results are not, at least in part, due to background causes. One possible background influence is the psychological boost of treatment, which may cause an improvement in patient health by itself. This is demonstrated in the following example, which is described in greater detail by Miao (1977) and Freedman *et al.* (1997).

Example 7.2 In 1962, gastric freezing was introduced as an innovative treatment for duodenal ulcers on the evidence of an uncontrolled trial (that is, with no control group) of 24 patients, all of whom had relief of symptoms when the trial concluded after 6 weeks (Wangensteen *et al.*, 1962). The standard treatment in nonsevere cases was not curative and, in severe cases, involved surgery that sometimes failed and sometimes was fatal, so this new treatment soon became popular. Seven years later a controlled trial of gastric freezing was published using 82 patients in the treated (gastric freeze) group and 78 in the control (pretend freeze) group. When the trial was evaluated after 6 weeks both groups tended to show an improvement; after 2 years, however, both groups tended to become clinically worse. There was no significant difference between the two groups at any time. This is suggestive of a short-term psychological boost after treatment, which disappeared in the long term; gastric freezing appears to have no real effect. Partially as a result of the second, properly conducted trial, gastric freezing was abandoned as a treatment for duodenal ulcers.

7.3.2   Blindness

In intervention studies, blindness is the policy of keeping someone unaware of which treatment has been given. Studies are said to be **single-blind** if the subject does not know which treatment she or he has received. This is desirable to avoid psychological boosts that may affect the results. For instance, those who know that they have received a placebo are unlikely to receive the same lift as those who know their treatment is active. For this reason, the controlled gastric freezing trial (Example 7.2) used a pretend freeze, identical to the actual freeze in all observable aspects, for the control group.

Intervention studies are **double-blind** if the doctor, nurse or whoever is assessing the outcomes (subject response, physical measurements, laboratory tests, etc.), as well as the subject, is unaware of the treatment received. This avoids **observer bias** — that is, situations in which the observer 'sees' an imaginary benefit (such as an improved state of health or fewer side-effects) for those subjects treated with the observer's preferred treatment. However subconscious the observer's prejudice may be, the results would be biased in favour of any preconceived preference. Sometimes the person interpreting the set of results, possibly a statistician, is also kept blind for similar reasons. The study would then be **triple-blind**.

Although blindness is desirable, it is not always possible. An obvious example is when a radiation treatment is compared with a surgical treatment for breast cancer. In drug trials, blindness is usually easy to achieve by the use of dummy tablets, such as used in the Dundee vitamin study (Example 7.1). On the other hand, it is essential that the treatment allocation is coded and that someone is able to break the code in times of medical problems during the study and when final results are required.

7.3.3   Randomisation

Subjects should be allocated to treatment group according to some chance mechanism (Section 7.7). When this is done, the study is called a **randomised controlled trial** (RCT). Randomisation is necessary to avoid systematic bias; the following example provides a cautionary tale of what can happen without randomisation.

Example 7.3 Gore and Altman (1982) describe a controlled trial of free milk supplementation to improve growth amongst schoolchildren in Lanarkshire, Scotland, in 1930. Ten thousand children were allocated to the treated group, who received the milk, and a similar number to the control group, who received no supplementation. Well-intentioned teachers decided that the poorest children should be given priority for free milk, rather than using strictly randomised allocation. The consequence was that the effects of milk supplementation were indistinguishable from (that is, confounded with) the effects of poverty. Since the poorer children were lighter at baseline, this could bias in favour of milk 'treatment' because the lightest children had more potential to grow. Furthermore, the study began in winter and ended in summer and, at both times, the children were weighed fully clothed. This is likely to have led to an underestimation of weight gain in both groups, but less so in the poorer (milk supplementation) group because their warm winter clothes were sure to have been lighter. Again, there is a bias towards better results in the group given free milk. Of course, other potential effects are associated with poverty. Quite how much, and even in what direction overall, the nonrandomised allocation procedure affected the results is unclear. Firm conclusions about the benefit or otherwise of milk supplementation cannot be drawn from this study.

Randomisation can be expected to reduce the chance of bias caused by imbalance between the treatment groups in confounding variables at baseline. The degree of benefit can be expected to increase as the number of subjects in the trial increases, provided an appropriate randomisation scheme (Section 7.7) is used. For example, the ADVANCE RCT (Patel *et al.*, 2008), of intensive versus standard glycaemic control amongst 11 140 patients with diabetes, reported 21 independent comparisons, between treatment groups, of binary variables (such as the percentage of women and the percentage taking aspirin) at baseline. The largest difference between the treatments groups was 1.2%, whilst one-third of the 21 comparisons showed a difference, between groups, of 0.1% or less. Similarly, of 16 comparisons of quantitative variables (such as age and systolic blood pressure), the biggest difference was 1 unit, with three-quarters of the comparisons showing differences of 0.1 units or less (however, such comparisons of continuous variables depend on the measurement scales used, so their interpretation is not straightforward).

Chance imbalances can, nevertheless, occur even in large trials. Just as in observational studies, variables that are unbalanced between treatments, and are associated with the disease, can confound the result of the RCT. Hence it would be prudent to compare treatments after adjusting for such potential confounding variables. Since we can only do this if these variables have been recorded, it is always sensible to include the measurement of key prognostic variables for the disease(s) under study in the protocol for the trial. Adjustments for any variables used to stratify randomisation (Section 7.7.2) should also be allowed for in the analyses (Kahan and Morris, 2012). In practice, RCTs are often analysed without adjustment, often because such results are thought to be more acceptable to clinical scrutiny. Even if these are presented as the headline results, comparative sensitivity analyses with adjustments should be carried out.

When considering how well balanced the trial is across important prognostic factors, it is not correct to use a hypothesis test (Altman, 1985). By definition, in an RCT, subjects in the two groups are 'the same' in the population at large, and the test will thus only be of the efficacy of the randomisation process used. Furthermore, as commented upon elsewhere in this book, the larger the sample size (Section 3.5.5) and the greater the number of comparisons made (Section 9.2.5), the more likely we are to get at least one positive result, all else being equal. Hence the same degree of difference can lead to a different conclusion in different trials. Rather, our concern is whether there are important differences in the *sample* we have obtained. A convenient measure of 'closeness' in this context is the standardised mean effect size (SMES), which is the difference in means divided by its standard deviation (SD) (Section 13.4.4). Note that this quantity is independent of the units of measurement (solving the issue with continuous variables raised earlier). Assuming that the sample sizes in the two arms of the trial are similar, the square root of the mean variance in each arm can be used as the SD in computing the SMES for a continuous variable (if sample sizes are not similar a weighted mean would be more sensible). For example, in ADVANCE, the published paper (Patel *et al.*, 2008) states that the mean (SD) creatinine in the intervention group is 86 (24) μmol/l, and in the standard control group is 87 (27) μmol/l. This is the continuous variable with the greatest difference at baseline, as reported in the paper. The SMES is thus

$(86 - 87)/\sqrt{((24 \times 24) + (27 \times 27))/2} = -0.033$. For a binary variable we can take the standard deviation in the SMES to be the square root of the mean of $p(1 - p)$ from each group, where p is the proportion with positive outcomes. In Patel *et al.* (2008), the binary variable with the greatest contrast, at baseline, was use of acarbose, reported to occur in 9.2% of the intervention group and 8.0% of the standard group.

The SMES is thus $(0.092 - 0.080)/\sqrt{((0.092 \times 0.908) + (0.08 \times 0.92))/2} = 0.043$. Generally percentage SMES values are easier to understand and compare: 3.3% and 4.3% in the examples here. An obvious question, then, is how large should the percentage SMES be before we conclude that imbalance is important? The answer depends upon clinical, as well as statistical, judgement. Certainly the variable concerned has to be a prognostic factor for the outcome(s) used in the RCT, otherwise imbalance is a moot point. In ADVANCE the combined primary outcome was macrovascular or microvascular disease. Since acarbose is only one of several drugs that are taken for glycaemic control, it is unlikely to be a crucial prognostic factor, but creatinine is a key factor in defining renal disease (one component of microvascular disease) and so this is a key prognostic variable in ADVANCE. A potential statistical threshold for important imbalance is 10%, suggested by research in propensity scoring (Section 10.17.7). If this is adopted, both the variables in ADVANCE cited here would be considered to be balanced between the treatment groups.

7.3.4   Consent before randomisation

To avoid bias in the eventual composition of the treatment groups, subjects should be checked for consent (and eligibility) for each treatment before being randomly allocated to a treatment group (Kramer and Shapiro, 1984). It is usually more attractive to a physician to randomize first because then she or he will need to explain only one treatment to any one subject. As well as being easier, this avoids possible loss of trust when the doctor must admit uncertainty about which of the treatments is best in this individual case. However, there is always the chance that a specific treatment will be rejected by a specific type of person, leading to potential bias. For example, in a comparison of drug and homeopathic treatments for a severe chronic condition, it may well be that those who agree to participate after being allocated to homeopathic treatment are predominantly people who have been failed by 'normal' treatments and hence are inherently rather more sick. Bias is then against the homeopathic treatment.

7.3.5   Analysis by intention-to-treat

During the intervention study, subjects may stop or modify their allocated treatment for many reasons, including illness, toxicity, migration or simply in error. Treatment efficacy is normally analysed according to treatment allocated rather than treatment actually received, ignoring any information on adherence — the principle of analysis by **intention-to-treat**. This protects against bias because someone who stops or even crosses to the other treatment (e.g., the well-established control drug) may well have done so because of an adverse effect of the treatment. Also, it should reflect practice in the real world rather more accurately. The disadvantage is that this will not measure the true relative effectiveness of the treatments as administered (Sheiner and Rubin, 1995); in general, we would expect underestimation of the administered treatment difference.

In some circumstances, a complete intention-to-treat analysis will be impossible or at least would require some imputation (Section 14.9) or use of a surrogate endpoint. This would be an issue when we are recording change in physical parameters, such as cartilage thickness for old people with osteoarthritis, where a substantial number of subjects are likely to die before the study ends. Thus, the decision regarding adoption of the intention-to-treat principle should be based on careful consideration of the goals of the intervention study. At the very least, when the standard intention-to-treat analysis is not straightforward, alternative analyses should be carried out as part of a sensitivity analysis.

7.4   Parallel group studies

All of the intervention studies described so far are of the simplest design wherein subjects are allocated into two (or more) treatment groups and everyone within a group receives the same treatment, which is different from the treatment given to other group(s). Furthermore, the number of subjects to be allocated to each group (notwithstanding withdrawals) is fixed in advance. Such studies are called **parallel group studies**; Section 7.5 and Section 7.6 consider two alternative study designs for intervention studies. Guidelines for reporting parallel group studies are given at http://www.consort-statement.org/. The same web site has links to other useful material for the design and reporting of intervention studies.

Although the design is very different, the analysis of a parallel group intervention study proceeds exactly as for an equivalent cohort study. Here we shall look at two further examples of parallel group studies, so as to reinforce the basic ideas and provide illustrations of how the principles of Section 7.3 are put into practice. More complex examples may involve issues such as censoring and thus require the analytical methods introduced in Chapter 5 and developed in Chapter 11.

Example 7.4 Several accounts have been given of the large-scale field trial of the Salk polio vaccine carried out in the U.S. in 1954, including those by Snedecor and Cochran (1989) and Pocock (1983). The description here draws mainly on the account by Freedman *et al.* (1997).

Although the first outbreak of poliomyelitis did not happen until 1916, by 1954 hundreds of thousands of Americans, particularly children, had contracted the disease. The vaccine of Jonas Salk was just one of many proposed, but it had already proved successful at generating antibodies to polio during laboratory tests. A field trial of the vaccine amongst children was deemed appropriate. As the annual incidence rate of polio was, thankfully, only about 1 in 2000, several thousand subjects were needed (Chapter 8).

There were ethical objections to the use of a placebo control group in the field trial, given the nature of the disease, but this was overruled because polio tends to occur in epidemics. The number of cases in the U.S. in 1953, for instance, was about half of that in 1952, so that a drop during 1954 might have been attributable to a natural lull in the disease, had an uncontrolled experiment been used.

Two different approaches to allocating children to treatment (vaccination or control) group were used. The National Foundation for Infantile Paralysis (NFIP) suggested vaccinating all children in the second grade whose parents gave consent. First- and third-grade children were to act as controls (without seeking parental consent). This approach has two serious flaws. First, it is likely that a greater proportion of consenting parents would be from advantaged social classes than we would expect to find in the general population. This is primarily because the more advantaged are usually better educated. Schoolchildren from high social class families are more likely to contract polio because they live in more hygienic accommodation and so are less likely to have already contracted a mild form of the disease in early life, when protected by maternal antibodies. Hence, to confine vaccination to children whose parents gave consent is to bias against the vaccine. The error is that of seeking consent after allocation (Section 7.3.4). The second problem with the NFIP method is that, because of the contagious nature of polio, a clustering effect is highly likely. Hence, just by chance, a relatively high (or low) incidence could have occurred amongst second-grade children in 1954, even if the trial had never occurred.

The second design used was an RCT that included all children whose parents consented to their entering the trial. These children were subsequently randomly assigned to the vaccinated or control group within each participating school. Randomisation was carried out within schools so as to balance out any geographic variations (for example, some schools may have been in particularly high-risk areas).

The RCT was double-blind. Children and their families were kept blind to treatment allocation by the use of saline fluid injections for the control group which mimicked the active vaccinations. The evaluating physicians were also kept blind because some forms of polio were difficult to diagnose, and it was thought likely that a sick child who was known to be unvaccinated was more likely to receive a positive diagnosis for polio than a child known to be vaccinated. Since the merits of the Salk vaccine were still being debated, subconscious bias during evaluation was very possible.

Some schools used the NFIP method whilst others adopted the RCT. Table 7.3 gives rounded figures to summarise the results. In this table, results from those children without parental consent have been omitted, but these were also recorded.

There is a clear benefit of vaccine in both trials, with either 29 or 43 fewer cases of polio per 100 000 children after vaccination. Formal significance tests could be carried out for each trial using the methods of Section 3.5 to compare two proportions on the exact source data. In fact it is clear, even from the rounded figures, that both trials produced extremely significant results (given the enormous sample sizes). However, Table 7.3 also shows a clear difference between

Table 7.3. Polio incidence rates per 100 000 (with sample size, in thousands, in parentheses) in the two Salk vaccine trials.

Group	NFIP	RCT
Vaccinated	25 (225)	28 (200)
Control	54 (725)	71 (200)
Difference	−29	−43

the two trials, with the RCT predicting a much greater effect of vaccination. This demonstrates the bias, as expected, from the NFIP method; in fact, it underestimates the effect of the vaccine by $43 - 29 = 14$ cases per 100 000. The evidence of this RCT played an important part in the subsequent decision to put the Salk vaccine into widespread use.

Example 7.5 The study of Crowther *et al.* (1990), already met in Example 3.9, was a parallel group study of the benefits of hospitalisation for bed rest (from 28 to 30 weeks' gestation until delivery) in twin pregnancies. Subjects were women attending a special multiple pregnancy antenatal clinic. Women with cervical sutures, hypertension, a Caesarean section scar, an anteparteum haemorrhage or uncertain gestational age were excluded. Subjects were randomly allocated to the treated (hospitalised bed rest) group or control (no hospitalisation, normal routine) group. Consent was obtained before randomisation and ethical approval was granted by the local University Research Board. Although it was clearly not possible to make the subjects blind, the neonatalogist who made gestational age assessments was unaware of the treatment given.

Randomisation achieved two groups of women that were fairly similar in all important aspects (average height, weight, gestational age etc.). There were no withdrawals or loss to follow-up. However, of the 58 women in the treated group, 4 did not attend for hospitalisation and a further 11 required leave of absence from hospital for domestic reasons. Of the 60 women in the control group, 22 required antenatal admission to hospital because complications developed. Rather than treat these as protocol deviations to be excluded, they were retained in the analysis according to the principle of analysis by intention-to-treat. Crowther *et al.* (1990) conclude that the study is thus truly a comparison of a policy of recommended routine hospitalisation in uncomplicated twin pregnancy against a policy of advising hospitalisation only if complications supervened.

Various end-points of the trial were analysed. Mean values (for example, mean gestational age at delivery) were compared using t tests, and proportions (for example, the proportion who underwent a Caesarean section) were compared by using odds ratios (Section 3.2). In Example 7.1, we saw an example of the analysis of means. To illustrate an analysis of data in the form of proportions, consider Table 7.4, which gives data on delivery time from the study of Crowther *et al.* (1990). From this, it is easy to calculate the odds ratio for bed rest versus no bed rest, from (3.9), as

$$\hat{\psi} = \frac{36 \times 20}{22 \times 40} = 0.82.$$

The 95% confidence limits for this odds ratio are easily derived from (3.12) to be (0.39, 1.74). Because unity lies well within this interval, we conclude that hospitalisation for bed rest has no significant effect upon the odds of a delivery before 37 weeks. A chi-square test (with and without a continuity correction, as explained in Section 3.5.3) gives a p value of 0.60. Notice that the analysis of Table 7.4 might have been better based on the relative risk rather than the odds ratio (Section 3.3).

No significant differences were found in any measure of pregnancy outcome, but twins in the treated group were significantly heavier and less likely to be small for gestational age or stillbirths (although the analysis used ignores any correlation between siblings). Hence, the

Table 7.4. Treatment group by gestational age at delivery for the bed rest study.

Treatment group	Gestational age (weeks)		
	Below 37	37 or more	Total
Bed rest	36	22	58
Control	40	20	60
Total	76	42	118

study suggests that recommended bed rest may enhance fetal growth, but provides no evidence of any effect on aspects of the pregnancy itself.

7.4.1   Number needed to treat

Besides the usual measures of relative chance of disease, such as the relative risk or odds ratio, binary outcomes of controlled intervention studies are often quantified by stating the expected **number needed to treat** (NNT) with the intervention to avoid one outcome. This number is easy to derive given the risks of the outcome: r_c in the control group and r_g in the intervention group. When n people are exposed to the control, the expected number of events is

$$E_c = r_c\, n.$$

Similarly, for n people exposed to the intervention, the corresponding expected number is

$$E_g = r_g\, n.$$

Thus, if intervention is to lead to one less outcome,

$$1 = r_c\, n - r_g\, n$$

and n will then be the NNT. Hence,

$$\text{NNT} = 1/(r_c - r_g), \tag{7.1}$$

that is, the reciprocal of the risk difference. An approximate 95% confidence interval for NNT can be derived by taking reciprocals of the confidence limits for the risk difference, computed using (2.5).

    The NNT will be negative whenever the risk difference is negative, which means that the intervention is harmful rather than protective. When the risks are not significantly different, we expect the confidence interval for the risk difference to include zero (see comment in Section 2.5.2); thus, one of the confidence limits will be negative and the other positive. The corresponding confidence interval for NNT will then be of a very different form to other confidence intervals in this book because the reciprocal of zero is infinity. They will be comprised of two distinct parts: (1) an interval from minus infinity to the reciprocal of the negative risk difference limit; and (2) an interval from the reciprocal of the positive risk difference limit to plus infinity (Altman, 1998).

    In a general context, the NNT resulting from (7.1) should be interpreted as the expected number needed to be exposed to the intervention, rather than the control, for a time equal to the duration of the study from which data were derived, to prevent one outcome. We might prefer to specify the NNT for a single year, because this is easier to understand. To do this, we may use the definition of cumulative survival probability, (5.3), to estimate r_c and r_g per year, assuming constant risk per year. Hence, if the risk per year in the control group is r_{c1} and the study lasted for y years, (5.3) gives

$$1 - r_c = (1 - r_{c1})^y.$$

Hence,

$$r_{c1} = 1 - (1 - r_c)^{1/y}. \tag{7.2}$$

An identical computation leads to an estimated 1-year risk for those exposed to the intervention. The two 1-year risks are substituted into (7.1) and we then proceed just as before. If we decide to specify the NNT for any other time period, we can use much the same procedure to estimate risks over the required period. The z-year risk in the control group, for instance, is

$$r_{cz} = 1 - (1 - r_{c1})^z. \tag{7.3}$$

Example 7.6 Ohkubo *et al.* (2004) describe a parallel group study comparing an ACE-inhibitor with placebo for patients who had previously suffered a stroke. The median follow-up for those who continued until the end of the study was 4.2 years. Of Asian participants in the study, 26 out of 1176 treated with the intervention experienced pneumonia, compared with 48 out of 1176 in the control group.

Here, $r_c = 48/1176 = 0.040816$ and $r_g = 26/1176 = 0.022109$ and hence, from (7.1),

$$NNT = 1/(0.040816 - 0.022109) = 1/0.018707 = 53.5.$$

We thus expect to save one case of pneumonia by treating 53 patients with the ACE-inhibitor for 4.2 years. As this is somewhat difficult to interpret, we might, instead, give an NNT for 5 years. To get this, first compute r_{c1} and r_{g1}. From (7.2),

$$r_{c1} = 1 - (1 - 0.040816)^{1/4.2} = 0.009873.$$

Similar computations give $r_{g1} = 0.005309$. Then, by (7.3),

$$r_{c5} = 1 - (1 - 0.009873)^5 = 0.048400,$$

and, again, the same computations for the other group give $r_{g5} = 0.026265$. Hence, using (7.1) again,

$$NNT_5 = 1/(0.048400 - 0.026265) = 1/0.022135 = 45.2,$$

where the subscript '5' is used to differentiate this from the earlier NNT, which is appropriate for the duration of the study. We need to treat 45 patients with ACE-inhibitors for 5 years to avoid one case of pneumonia.

To illustrate computations of confidence intervals, we shall take the 5-year problem only. From (2.5), the approriate confidence interval for the risk difference is

$$0.22135 \pm 1.96 \sqrt{\frac{0.048400 \times 0.951600}{1176} + \frac{0.026265 \times 0.973735}{1176}},$$

i.e., 0.022135 ± 0.015297 or $(0.006838, 0.037432)$. Taking reciprocals of both limits (and reversing the order) gives the 95% confidence interval for NNT_5 of $(26.7, 146.2)$.

If we are not prepared to assume constant risks per year, in order to interpolate NNT, we will require complete information on follow-up, year-by-year, such as that presented in Table 5.1. We then use (5.2), as previously, allowing risk to vary by year (or some other time period). This issue is discussed by Altman and Andersen (1999), who also show how to use results from Cox models (see Section 11.6) in NNT estimation.

Although the concept of NNT was developed for intervention studies, it may also be applied, without mathematical revision, to cohort studies, although then it is better to use a name such as 'number needed to avoid the risk factor'. For instance, in

Example 3.1, the number needed to avoid smoking to save one cardiovascular death is $1/(0.021877 - 0.007903) = 71.6$ in a 12-year period. Naturally, the interpretation will be somewhat different from when a treatment is assessed. In this example, the effect of smoking does not instantly disappear and it might be more appropriate to think of the number of people needed to have never begun smoking to avoid one death in 12 years. To account for confounding, the 'number needed to avoid' might be calculated from adjusted relative risks or odds ratios (Bender and Blettner, 2002).

7.4.2   Cluster randomised trials

Sometimes the subjects in an intervention study naturally occur in separate groups (called clusters in the current context; see Section 1.8.2) and, rather than randomise individuals to treatment, we randomize the clusters. The result is known as a **cluster randomised trial** (Donner and Klar, 2000). Almost always, cluster randomisation is used for convenience or out of necessity. For instance, suppose the object is to compare two methods of general public health education: intensive and control. Communities randomised to the intensive regimen are offered such things as free smoking cessation clinics and exercise classes and are the targets of billboard and postal advertising relating to healthy lifestyle advice. None of these activities is provided in control communities. Another example would be when we wish to compare two different training programmes given to doctors, to see which is most effective in practice. In both examples, although we will measure outcomes, such as lung function or blood pressure, on individual people, their treatment was decided according to their cluster (i.e., where they live or who their doctor is).

Besides ease of implementation, cluster randomised trials are less likely than others to be subject to treatment contamination, that is, when subjects take the alternative treatment (assuming two treatments only). Typically, this works through control subjects being influenced to follow the intensive regimen. An example would be when underweight, frail elderly people living in nursing homes are to be allocated a supplementary or a normal diet. If individuals are randomly allocated to a diet, the carers may well be tempted to start giving the supplementary diet to an individual in the control group who has lost weight during the trial. Such treatment contamination is less likely in a trial in which nursing homes are randomised to diet, because everyone in any one home has the same diet. Indeed, adherence to treatment in general would be expected to be better when everyone in the same nursing home gets the same diet.

The cluster randomised approach has two important drawbacks compared to individual randomisation. First, considerably more individuals need to be recruited so as to obtain the same level of precision in the results (see Section 8.8). Second, the resulting data are considerably more complex to analyse because we can no longer reasonably assume that all observations are independent of each other (within the same cluster, they will certainly not be), as is assumed in basic statistical procedures. Consequently, more sophisticated analysis techniques are required. Specifically, we need to use methods that allow for clustering such as PROC SURVEYMEANS in the SAS package or the complex survey ('SVY') routines in the Stata package, or more general statistical models that allow for nonindependent correlation structures (see Section 9.11 and Section 10.15).

7.4.3   Stepped wedge trials

In a **stepped wedge trial**, assuming the standard situation wherein an intervention is to be compared with a control, each individual, or more typically each cluster, starts

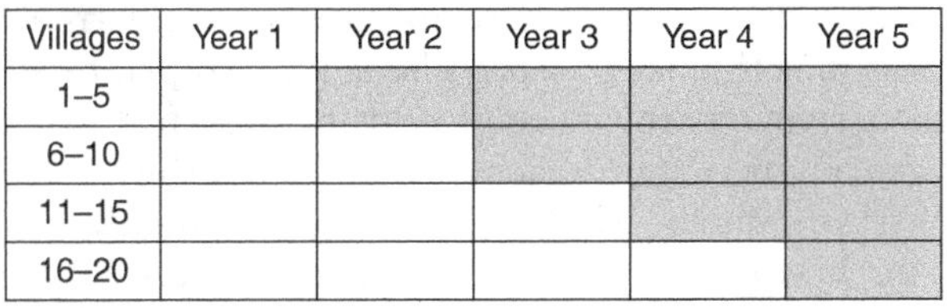

Villages	Year 1	Year 2	Year 3	Year 4	Year 5
1–5		▓	▓	▓	▓
6–10			▓	▓	▓
11–15				▓	▓
16–20					▓

Figure 7.1. Schematic representation of a stepped wedge trial: Example 7.7. Villages receive the intervention only in the years represented by shaded cells.

out on the control and each is progressively switched — in random order — to the intervention over successive periods. By the end of the trial, all are on the intervention. Measures of efficacy are taken during each study period. Such a design is useful when the intervention is fairly certain to be effective, usually because of past scientific evidence, but the magnitude of its effectiveness is not certain in the current context. In such cases it may be considered unethical to withhold the treatment from anyone, in the medium term.

Example 7.7 Suppose that a novel system of cardiovascular (CV) health promotion and surveillance, using local health workers, is to be implemented in an African province as a model for future roll-out to other provinces, and other countries in the region. The researchers are confident that the system will have advantages for health, based on the experience of Western nations and the known high levels of blood pressure in the study area. However, whether the intervention would be cost-effective is unclear. The prospective funders of the study, reasonably, insist that every person to be included in the trial must have a share of the benefits. Hence a parallel group study, of intervention versus control, is untenable. A before-and-after study design is rejected on the usual grounds of lacking a control — knowledge of CV risk factors may well increase with time, regardless of the novel intervention, due to improving communication with the outside world. A crossover trial would not be very useful because of the carry-over effects of new knowledge. Hence the researchers opt for a stepped wedge design. This is to last for five years and will involve twenty villages (i.e., clusters). In year one, all twenty villages are studied without the intervention (baseline and 12-monthly surveys of CV risk factors are conducted). In year two, villagers in a further random five villages receive the novel health system; in year three, another random five villages; in year four, another random five villages; in year five, the final five villages. Once a village starts receiving the intervention, it never stops (at least until the study ends): see Figure 7.1. The effectiveness (and cost) of the intervention can then be evaluated both overall and as it accumulates over time.

The main disadvantages of stepped wedge trials are that, like cross-over trials (Section 7.5), they inevitably require a long period of observation and are relatively complex to analyse. Lack of space precludes further discussion here: see Hussey and Hughes (2007) for details of the design and analysis of stepped wedge trials.

7.4.4 Non-inferiority trials

In a standard clinical trial comparing two treatments, the null and alternative hypotheses are

$$H_0 : e_1 - e_2 = 0 \quad \text{versus } H_1 : e_1 - e_2 \neq 0,$$

where e_1 and e_2 are the effect sizes under the two treatments being compared. For example, e might be the delta mean (as in Example 7.1) or the log odds (as in

Example 7.5). This design is ideal when an experimental treatment is compared with a placebo. Sometimes the use of a placebo is inappropriate, generally for ethical reasons, and so an active control is used as the reference. An example of this is where the control treatment is standard care, such as in the ADVANCE trial (Section 7.3.3). In such cases it may be that the new, experimental, treatment is being considered primarily because it has advantages besides efficacy, such as being cheaper, less invasive or derived synthetically rather than from animal products. Then the new treatment may be suitable for wide-scale adoption even if it is marginally inferior to the active treatment currently in common use, taken as the reference in the current context. Suppose that we can express the margin of difference, M, beyond which we will decide that the new treatment (call this N) will be considered inferior to the currently used reference treatment (call this R). The trial should then be designed with hypotheses:

$$H_0 : e_R - e_N \geq M \text{ versus } H_1 : e_R - e_N < M,$$

and we then have a **non-inferiority trial**. Here we assume that $M > 0$ and that a larger e represents relatively more benefit. In the first of the two examples for e given earlier, this would be true when a larger delta mean is advantageous. In the second example, where the basic metric used in the trial is an odds ratio, we could take the log inverse odds for e since an odds conventionally measures harm. The null hypothesis represents the *status quo*: N is at least marginally worse than R, which should remain the mainstay of treatment. The alternative hypothesis represents at least non-inferiority: we could advise that N be adopted. We can test H_0 versus H_1 using a one-sided test, but it is conventional to construct a 95% confidence interval for $e_R - e_N$ and reject H_0 in favour of H_1 at the 2.5% level whenever the upper limit falls below M.

Example 7.8 Kim *et al.* (2013) describe a non-inferiority trial of same-day discharge from hospital following percutaneous coronary intervention. Same-day discharge was compared with the standard policy of next-day discharge (i.e., staying overnight) for a range of outcomes, the primary outcome being the patient's self-reported ability to cope well during the 7 days following discharge. The investigators pre-specified that same-day discharge (with much reduced costs) would be considered non-inferior provided coping was less than 12 percentage points lower following same-day, compared to following next-day, discharge (i.e., the effect size, e, is the percentage coping and $M = 12\%$).

The study protocol called for a sample size of 600, to be randomly allocated, in equal numbers, to same- or next-day discharge. Due to lack of funding, only 298 actually entered the trial. Amongst this 298, 77% of the 148 randomised to next-day discharge, and 79% of the 150 randomised to same-day discharge, coped well. This led to a conclusion of non-inferiority.

The authors considered what conclusions might have been made, should the trial have involved the full target of 600 people. Assuming that the percentage coping under next-day discharge was as observed (77%), Figure 7.2 shows the different conclusions that would have been drawn under a selection of possible outcomes for the percentage coping after same-day discharge (Kim *et al.* (2013) produced a similar figure). Confidence intervals were calculated using (2.5). We see that, when patients leave hospital on the day of their surgery, if 55% cope well (scenario A) this discharge policy is inferior (fail to reject H_0) to the next-day discharge policy. If the percentage is 69% (scenario B) the evidence is inconclusive since the confidence interval straddles the edge of the zone of non-inferiority (same-day is worse but not significantly so at the 2.5% level). Scenarios C–E all lead to (at least) a conclusion of non-inferiority because all the confidence intervals lie completely within the zone of non-inferiority. In scenario C (same-day coping = 75%) same-day is expected to be worse, and in scenario D

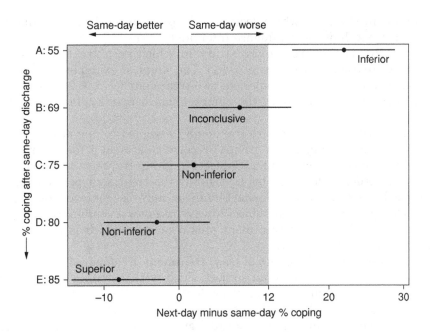

Figure 7.2. Schematic diagram of a non-inferiority trial under five scenarios with the percentage coping after next-day discharge fixed at 77%: Example 7.8. Conclusions drawn relate to the same-day discharge policy. Note that the vertical labels are not drawn on a proper arithmetic scale.

(same-day coping = 80%) better, than next-day, but this does not lead to different conclusions for the test. In scenario E (same-day coping = 85%) the entire confidence interval is below zero and we can thus go further and conclude that same-day is the superior discharge policy. Further calculations shown that same-day discharge will be considered inferior, under the hypothetical conditions, whenever it is associated with lower than 58% coping, and superior whenever it is associated with greater than 83% coping.

One of the main difficulties in non-inferiority trials is to fix the non-inferiority margin, M. D'Agostino et al. (2003) give some guidance and suggest that the decision should be made jointly in relation to statistical and clinical considerations. Often past evidence of feasible differences (for example, comparing the reference treatment to a placebo) can help. Piaggio et al. (2012) give sound advice on the design, analysis and reporting of a non-inferiority trial, as well as a related trial design, the **equivalence trial**. Such a trial has equivalence margins at $-M$ as well as M, and equivalence is concluded if the whole of the confidence interval lies between $\pm M$.

7.5 Cross-over studies

The most important drawback of a parallel group study is that any differences between the two (or more) treatment groups will affect the results. Although randomisation will prevent any systematic differences occurring, chance imbalances in such things as age, sex, height and weight between groups are possible, especially if the size of the study is fairly small. Even if the between-group differences in these so-called **prognostic factors** (which would be called confounding variables at the analysis stage) are not significant, such person-to-person differences cause extra variation in the measurements obtained, which decreases the precision of the results (for example, it increases the width of the confidence intervals).

An alternative is the **cross-over study** in which each treatment is given, at different times, to each subject (Senn, 2002). The simplest example, and the only one we will consider here, is the two-period, two-treatment (or 2 × 2) cross-over. More complex designs are discussed in the comprehensive text by Jones and Kenward (2003).

In the 2 × 2 design, subjects are (randomly) assigned to one of two groups; call them groups A and B. Subjects in group A receive treatment 1 for a suitable length of time and then receive treatment 2. Subjects in group B receive the two treatments in the opposite order (2 followed by 1). Usually the treatment periods are of equal length, typically a few weeks. Single blindness may be achieved by the **double dummy** technique wherein each subject always receives a combination of two treatments, the appropriate active treatment plus a placebo which is indistinguishable from the other active treatment.

In a cross-over study, the effect of (say) treatment 1 compared with treatment 2 may be assessed for each individual subject. Such **within-subject differences** are then summarised to obtain an overall evaluation of efficacy. Since within-subject variation is almost certainly less than between-subject variation, a cross-over should produce more precise results than a parallel group study of the same size. Alternatively, this advantage of cross-overs could be viewed as a saving in sample size: a cross-over should obtain the same precision as a parallel group study without using as many subjects. This saving of resources is the most common justification for using a cross-over design.

Unfortunately, cross-overs have several disadvantages that restrict their application. These are:

1. Justification: The advantage of more precision, or fewer subjects, is valid only when within-subject variation is less than between-subject variation. Although this does generally happen in practice, there is no theoretical reason why it should always be so.

2. Suitability: Cross-over studies are suitable only for long-term conditions for which treatment provides only short-term relief (and certainly not a cure). Otherwise, no justification could be offered for the second treatment period. Examples of use include studies of bronchitis, angina, migraine, 'jet lag', colostomy appliances and contraceptive devices.

3. Duration: Each subject must spend a long time in the trial, possibly twice as long as in the comparable parallel group study. This may lead to several withdrawals, and lack of adherence to treatment, because of fatigue. With extremely long trials, problems of cost and changes in the condition of the illness may also occur.

4. Carry-over effects: It is possible that, when given first, one treatment has a residual effect in the second period, called a **carry-over effect**. An obvious case in which this is likely is when treatment 1 is active and treatment 2 is a placebo. Subjects in group A may still have some benefit from treatment 1 even after they have crossed over to the placebo. A straightforward comparison of within-subject differences would then be biased against the active treatment because some (group A) placebo results are better than they should be. To protect against carry-overs, many cross-over trials include a **washout** period between the two treatment periods (similar to that used in case–crossover studies; Section 6.9). Sometimes a

placebo is applied during this period, or sometimes the second period treatment is applied early — that is, before the start of the second treatment period proper. In either case, the washout period is ignored in the analyses. As in other types of intervention study, cross-over studies may have a **run-in** period before the first treatment period proper begins, so as to wash out any residual effects of previous medications. The run-in period also allows subjects to become acclimatised to trial conditions, which may also be an important advantage in parallel group trials.

A differential carry-over effect is one of several possible causes of a **treatment by period interaction** — that is, a differential effect of treatment in different periods. A test for the presence of such an interaction may be constructed (as we shall see later) but, unfortunately, this test usually has low power, by which we mean that there is a good chance of failing to detect an interaction (caused by carry-over or otherwise) even when it is medically important (see Section 8.2 for technical details). The reason for this is that this particular test is based upon between-subject differences and the sample size is usually small. Note that the treatment by period interaction is indistinguishable from (aliased with) an effect of treatment group in a two-treatment, two-period cross-over.

5. Complexity: Cross-overs are more complex to analyse than parallel group studies.

7.5.1   Graphical analysis

As in many other situations, the first step in analysing cross-over data should be to plot the data. Various different plots have their use in 2×2 cross-overs (as discussed by Hills and Armitage, 1979). Consider, first, graphs of mean response against period, labelled by treatment received. Figure 7.3 illustrates possible forms for such a graph for a trial of treatments R and S. In each case, the responses under the same treatment have been joined by a line. This should not be interpreted as subjects' progress through the trial; remember that someone who takes R in period 1 will take S in period 2 and vice versa. The lines emphasise treatment by period interactions, when they occur, because these are manifested as nonparallel lines. In extreme cases of interaction (Section 4.7), the lines will cross. A case study example of the type of plot given in Figure 7.3 is included as Figure 7.4.

For other useful plots, see the figures, like Figure 7.4, associated with Example 7.9. Figure 7.5 shows response against period for each subject separately for each treatment group. Here the lines *do* represent subjects' progress (the left-hand side marks the response in period 1 and the right the response in period 2, for a given subject). These plots are able to show up atypical subjects, such as those whose trial progress goes in the opposite direction to others, or who have very small or very large effects. Such subjects require further scrutiny; for instance, they may be protocol violations.

Scatterplots (Section 9.3.1) may also be useful in this respect. Figure 7.6 shows a scatterplot of results in period 2 against results in period 1, labelled by treatment group. A treatment effect would show as a clustering of symbols either side of the diagonal line. A similar scatterplot, but showing results when using the different treatments, rather than in different periods, could be used to detect period effects. Period effects are probably not of direct interest; the study aims to explore treatment effects. They may, however, be of secondary interest. For instance, Figure 7.3(b) and Figure 7.3(c) are cases in which response has increased over time for each treatment group (that is, regardless of order), which suggests a benefit of longer term treatment. Figure 7.3(a) suggests no such effect.

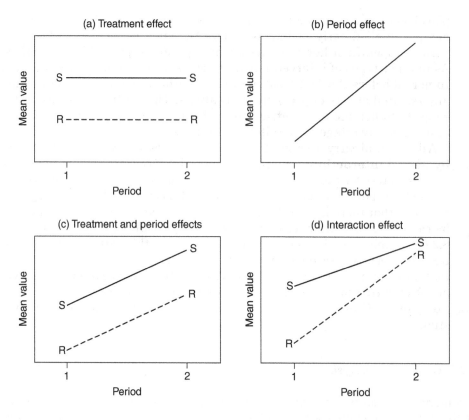

Figure 7.3. Plots of mean response against treatment period with interpretation of result: 'R' denotes that treatment R was used, 'S' denotes that treatment S was used (points are coincident in (b)).

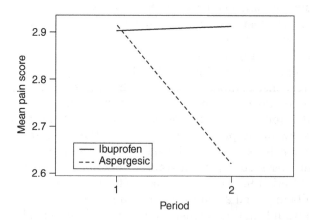

Figure 7.4. Mean pain score (over all subjects) when using a particular treatment against treatment period; arthritis study, Example 7.9.

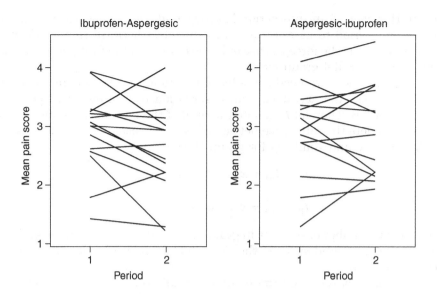

Figure 7.5. Mean pain score (over a 2-week period) against treatment period classified by treatment group; arthritis study, Example 7.9.

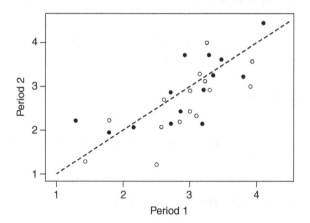

Figure 7.6. Mean pain score (over a 2-week period) in the second period against the same quantity (for the same subject) in the first period of treatment; arthritis study, Example 7.9. Open circles represent the ibuprofen–Aspergesic group; closed circles represent the Aspergesic–ibuprofen group.

7.5.2 Comparing means

The plots of Figure 7.3 are somewhat idealised because exactly parallel lines are unlikely in practice. Furthermore, we would like to be able to quantify what is a small and what is a large difference. Hence, we continue by assessing the statistical significance of the various possible effects.

Before we can test for a treatment (or period) effect, we should first test for a treatment by period interaction. If no evidence for such an interaction is found, then we may go ahead and test for treatment (and period) effects using the cross-over data (see below). However, if an interaction is discovered, we cannot use the information from the second period to assess the treatment effect because this would introduce bias. Instead, we would be forced to use only the data from the first period of treatment and analyse as a parallel group study.

To develop the tests, we need some basic notation. Let x_{A1} denote an observation from group A in period 1; x_{A2} denote an observation from group A in period 2; and similarly for group B. Then let t_A denote the total of the two observations for a subject in group A; d_A denote the difference between first- and second-period observations for subjects in group A; and similarly for group B. Hence,

$$t_A = x_{A1} + x_{A2}, \quad d_A = x_{A1} - x_{A2},$$

$$t_B = x_{B1} + x_{B2}, \quad d_B = x_{B1} - x_{B2}.$$

Also, let n_A be the number of subjects in group A; $\bar{t}_A$ and $s(t)_A$ be the mean and standard deviation of the t_A; $\bar{d}_A$ and $s(d)_A$ be the mean and standard deviation of the d_A; and similarly for group B.

Analyses will be based upon these sums and differences across periods. We shall assume that the data obtained approximate to a normal distribution reasonably well, so that t tests may be used. Otherwise, transformations (Section 2.8.1) should be tried and, if these fail to induce normality, nonparametric alternatives may be used (Section 2.8.2). We shall also assume that the pooled estimate of variance, (2.16), is appropriate to use. In the case of totals this will be

$$s(t)_p^2 = \frac{(n_A - 1)s(t)_A^2 + (n_B - 1)s(t)_B^2}{n_A + n_B - 2}, \tag{7.4}$$

and, in the case of differences,

$$s(d)_p^2 = \frac{(n_A - 1)s(d)_A^2 + (n_B - 1)s(d)_B^2}{n_A + n_B - 2}. \tag{7.5}$$

Three tests are possible, for the effects now listed.

1. **Treatment by period interaction.** If no such interaction occurs, then the means of the two totals (t_A and t_B) should be equal. This is tested formally by applying (2.14) to the data on totals for the separate groups; that is, we compare

$$\frac{\bar{t}_A - \bar{t}_B}{\sqrt{s(t)_p^2 \left[\dfrac{1}{n_A} + \dfrac{1}{n_B} \right]}} \tag{7.6}$$

with $t_{n_A + n_B - 2}$ using some appropriate significance level. If this test is significant, then, unless we have some way of accounting for the interaction from other data, we should abandon the cross-over analysis, as already explained. Given that an alternative analysis is still available, many investigators choose to protect against the low power of this test for interaction by using it with a higher significance level than that planned for the test of treatment difference. Typically, when a 5% test is used to compare treatments, a 10% test is used to test for the treatment by period interaction (although there is no statistical basis for this amount of 'correction').

2. **Treatment difference.** Cross-over data are paired data, and hence the paired t test (Section 2.7.4) could be applied to the entire set of treatment differences (that is, d_A and $-d_B$ combined), which would be compared with zero. The weakness of this test is that it ignores the period effect and, in the presence of an important period effect, it may give misleading results. A rather safer procedure, which is not affected by period differences, is the two-sample t test to compare the means of the d_A and d_B. Here, $\bar{d}_A$ estimates $\mu_R - \mu_S$, where μ_R and μ_S are the true mean effects of treatments R and S, respectively, where R is the treatment taken in the first period by subjects in group A, and S the other treatment. $\bar{d}_B$ will estimate $\mu_S - \mu_R$. A test of $\mu_R - \mu_S = 0$ (no treatment effect) can be made by comparing $\bar{d}_A - \bar{d}_B$ with zero. Hence, the test statistic

$$\frac{\bar{d}_A - \bar{d}_B}{\sqrt{s(d)_p^2 \left[\dfrac{1}{n_A} + \dfrac{1}{n_B} \right]}} \qquad (7.7)$$

is compared with $t_{n_A + n_B - 2}$. An unbiased estimate for $\mu_R - \mu_S$ is given by $\frac{1}{2}(\bar{d}_A - \bar{d}_B)$. The associated confidence interval, derived from (2.18), also includes the factor $\frac{1}{2}$. It is

$$\frac{1}{2}\left(\bar{d}_A - \bar{d}_B\right) \pm \frac{1}{2}\left(t_{n_A + n_B - 2}\right)\sqrt{s(d)_p^2 \left[\dfrac{1}{n_A} + \dfrac{1}{n_B} \right]}. \qquad (7.8)$$

3. **Period difference.** If it is interesting, this may be tested (regardless of any treatment effect) by comparing the average of the d_A against the average of the *negative* values of d_B. This follows from the method used to compare treatments. In the calculations, the only change now is that we must replace $-\bar{d}_B$ by $+\bar{d}_B$ in (7.7) and (7.8).

The procedures given here may easily be implemented using standard software that applies the pooled t test and associated confidence interval. Generalisations of the approach, using statistical modelling, are given by Barker *et al.* (1982) and Jones and Kenward (2003). See also Section 9.11 and Section 10.15.

Example 7.9 Hill *et al.* (1990) describe a 2×2 cross-over trial to compare lysine acetyl salicylate (Aspergesic) with ibuprofen in the treatment of rheumatoid arthritis. Here, ibuprofen was the usual prescribed treatment; there was interest in whether a cheap, over-the-counter medicine might work equally well. Thirty-six patients were randomly assigned to the two treatment order groups at entry (half to each). After 2 weeks on their first treatment, patients crossed over to the opposite treatment. A further 2 weeks later, the trial ended. There was no run-in or washout period, but the trial was double-blind (including use of the double dummy procedure).

At baseline, a general medical examination was carried out, and the recorded baseline values of the two treatment groups were found to be similar (in summary terms), as expected.

Table 7.5. Average pain scores from the rheumatoid arthritis study, showing sums and differences across treatment periods.

Ibuprofen–Aspergesic group ($n = 15$)				Aspergesic–ibuprofen group ($n = 14$)			
Period 1	Period 2	Sum	Diff.	Period 1	Period 2	Sum	Diff.
3.143	3.286	6.429	−0.143	1.286	2.214	3.500	−0.928
3.000	2.429	5.429	0.571	4.100	4.444	8.544	−0.344
3.071	2.357	5.428	0.714	3.357	3.267	6.624	0.090
3.286	2.929	6.215	0.357	3.214	2.929	6.143	0.285
2.846	2.200	5.046	0.646	3.286	3.714	7.000	−0.428
2.571	2.071	4.642	0.500	3.800	3.231	7.031	0.569
3.214	3.143	6.357	0.071	3.143	2.214	5.357	0.929
3.929	3.571	7.500	0.358	3.467	3.615	7.082	−0.148
3.909	3.000	6.909	0.909	2.714	2.154	4.868	0.560
2.615	2.692	5.307	−0.077	1.786	1.929	3.715	−0.143
1.786	2.214	4.000	−0.428	2.714	2.857	5.571	−0.143
1.429	1.286	2.715	0.143	2.930	3.710	6.640	−0.780
3.000	2.929	5.929	0.071	2.143	2.071	4.214	0.072
3.250	4.000	7.250	−0.750	2.860	2.430	5.290	0.430
2.500	1.214	3.714	1.286				
	Total	82.87	4.228		Total	81.58	0.021
	Mean	5.52	0.282		Mean	5.83	0.0015
	Std. dev.	1.35	0.524		Std. dev.	1.45	0.527

At the two subsequent clinic visits (at the half-way point and the end), patient and investigator assessments of progress were recorded and several measurements (grip strength, blood pressure, haematology, etc.) were taken. Between the clinic visits (that is, whilst on treatment), diary cards were completed each day by the patients. The data recorded included a pain assessment score on a 1 to 5 scale (1 = no pain; 2 = mild pain; 3 = moderate pain; 4 = severe pain; 5 = unbearable pain). These data are summarised in Table 7.5, which shows the average (mean) pain score for each patient in each treatment period (plus other statistics). As in the source publication, Table 7.5 only represents 29 of the original 36 patients. Five withdrew from the trial, one was considered noncompliant because of the vast quantities of study medication that he returned unused, and one patient failed to return his second diary card.

Graphical analyses of these data are given by Figure 7.4 to Figure 7.6. Figure 7.5 and Figure 7.6 suggest there is little treatment effect, because several of the lines on each side of Figure 7.5 go up and several go down and the points in Figure 7.6 are near to the diagonal and do not cluster by type of symbol (representing group membership). Figure 7.4 suggests that there could be a treatment by period interaction because the lines (just) cross. Mean pain scores are virtually identical, except when Aspergesic is taken in the second period, in which case they are lower. This agrees with Figure 7.5 and Table 7.5 in which we note that 11/15 do better with Aspergesic when it is used in the second period compared with half (7/14) when it is used first. Thus, perhaps Aspergesic works better when taken *after* ibuprofen, which would imply a treatment by period interaction, perhaps caused by a differential carry-over of ibuprofen (although other explanations are possible). Other diagrams (boxplots and histograms not shown here) suggest that the pain scores in Table 7.5 have a distribution reasonably close to the normal distribution (for instance, no severe skew). Hence, t tests are acceptable.

A test for treatment by period interaction involves computing

$$s(t)^2_p = \frac{14 \times 1.35^2 + 13 \times 1.45^2}{15 + 14 - 2} = 1.96$$

from (7.4). Substituting this into (7.6) gives

$$\frac{5.52 - 5.83}{\sqrt{1.96\left(\dfrac{1}{15} + \dfrac{1}{14}\right)}} = -0.60,$$

which is not significant when compared to t on 27 d.f. ($p > 0.5$ from Table B.4). Despite our earlier concern, no evidence of an interaction is found and hence the lack of parallel lines seen in Figure 7.4 is attributable to chance variation. We can thus go on to use the full cross-over to test for treatment and period effects. We need to calculate first

$$s(d)_p^2 = \frac{14 \times 0.524^2 + 13 \times 0.527^2}{15 + 14 - 2} = 0.276$$

from (7.5). Substituting this into (7.7) gives the test for treatment effect,

$$\frac{0.282 - 0.0015}{\sqrt{0.276\left(\dfrac{1}{15} + \dfrac{1}{14}\right)}} = 1.44,$$

which is not significant when compared against t with 27 d.f. ($p > 0.2$ from Table B.2). A similar test for a period effect requires comparison of

$$\frac{0.282 + 0.0015}{\sqrt{0.276\left(\dfrac{1}{15} + \dfrac{1}{14}\right)}} = 1.45$$

with the same t value. Again, this is not significant. Hence, we conclude that there is no significant effect of treatment or period of treatment. We have no evidence that Aspergesic is better or worse than ibuprofen.

Using (7.8), we can quantify the difference in pain score when using Aspergesic compared with ibuprofen. This gives the 95% confidence interval as

$$\frac{1}{2}(0.282 - 0.0015) \pm \frac{1}{2} \times 2.052 \times \sqrt{0.276\left(\frac{1}{15} + \frac{1}{14}\right)},$$

that is, 0.14 ± 0.20. In this calculation, 2.052 is t_{27} at the two-sided 5% level, obtained from using the T.INV.2T function in Excel. As the hypothesis test has already suggested, the interval contains 0. We expect Aspergesic to produce an average of 0.14 more 'units of pain' than ibuprofen, but this is not significantly different from 'no difference' in mean pain score. The 95% confidence interval for period difference is unlikely to be required here, but for completeness it is

$$\frac{1}{2}(0.282 + 0.0015) \pm 0.20,$$

or 0.14 ± 0.20. This is the extra mean pain score in period 1 compared to period 2. Notice that, to two decimal places, it is the same as the treatment difference. This is not, of course, generally so. This has happened here because $\bar{d}_B$ is so small.

One final point about the analysis is that Figure 7.5 shows the possible existence of an outlier. One patient in the ibuprofen–Aspergesic group has a very large decrease in pain between periods 1 and 2 (this is the last patient in this group in Table 7.5). Reference to this patient's other data from the trial gave no reason to suspect an error in these results. To be safe, the data were reanalysed omitting this patient; the conclusions from the hypothesis tests were not altered.

7.5.3   Analysing preferences

At the end of a cross-over trial, subjects are sometimes asked to state which treatment period they preferred. This may be a general question such as, 'During which period did you feel better?' or a more particular question such as, 'In which period did you experience the fewest problems?' Sometimes the investigating physician may also be asked to state the treatment period in which she or he thought the subject's health was better. We wish to analyse such data to discover which (if any) treatment is preferred. This can be achieved using **Prescott's test** (Prescott, 1981), which is a test for linear trend in a contingency table of treatment group against preference stated. The general layout of such a table is shown in Table 7.6.

Prescott's test statistic may be derived directly from (3.19). However, because the numbers in cross-over trials are usually quite small, it is advisable to use a continuity correction. This means subtracting $\frac{1}{2}n$ from the numerator of (3.19). The result is

$$\frac{n\left(n\left(n_{A3} - n_{A1}\right) - n_A\left(n_3 - n_1\right) - \frac{1}{2}n\right)^2}{n_A n_B\left(n\left(n_3 + n_1\right) - \left(n_3 - n_1\right)^2\right)}, \tag{7.9}$$

which should be compared against chi-square with 1 d.f.

The drawback with this procedure is that the approximation to chi-square will be in doubt if some of the expected frequencies are very small. In this event, we would be forced to use the exact form of Prescott's test, which is akin to Fisher's exact test (Section 3.5.4) but computationally more demanding. An alternative, but less sensitive, test that is easier to compute in the exact form is **Gart's test** (Gart, 1969), sometimes known as the **Mainland–Gart test**. This is based upon the 2×2 contingency table formed by deleting the 'no preference' column from Table 7.6. Now Fisher's exact test may be applied, if necessary.

Treatment effect is usually estimated by the odds ratio,

$$\hat{\psi} = \frac{n_{A1}/n_{A3}}{n_{B1}/n_{B3}}, \tag{7.10}$$

Table 7.6. Display of preference data.

Treatment group	Prefer 1st period treatment	No preference	Prefer 2nd period treatment	Total
A	n_{A1}	n_{A2}	n_{A3}	n_A
B	n_{B1}	n_{B2}	n_{B3}	n_B
Total	n_1	n_2	n_3	n

Table 7.7. Preference data relating to pain assessment from the Aspergesic trial.

Treatment group	Prefer 1st period treatment	No preference	Prefer 2nd period treatment	Total
Ibuprofen–Aspergesic	6	3	8	17
Aspergesic–ibuprofen	7	3	3	13
Total	13	6	11	30

which gives the relative odds in favour of a preference for treatment R, *given that a preference is stated.* As in Section 7.5.2, R is the treatment given in period 1 to subjects in group A.

The procedures described so far are all for treatment effects. Just as in Section 7.5.2, we can also look at period effects; as before this is achieved by a minor change to the equations for treatment effects. Here we simply interchange n_{B1} and n_{B3} in Table 7.6. This causes changes in n_1 and n_3 (and the corresponding headings should now be 'prefer treatment R' and 'prefer treatment S', where S is the treatment given in period 2 to subjects in group A), but all else is unchanged. We can then apply Prescott's (or Gart's) test to this new table or, equivalently, simply make the necessary changes to (7.9) and (7.10). The latter becomes the odds in favour of a preference for period 1, given that a preference is stated.

Example 7.10 In the trial described in Example 7.9, one of the questions at the end of the trial was, 'Compared to the last visit [to the clinic] is your pain worse/the same/better?' In our terminology, these translate to: worse = treatment given in period 1 preferred; same = no preference; better = treatment given in period 2 preferred. There were 30 responses to this question (no missing values). The results are given in Table 7.7.

The numbers here are quite small, but we would expect the chi-square test with a continuity correction to be reasonably accurate. Using (7.9), the test statistic is

$$\frac{30(30(8-6)-17(11-13)-15)^2}{17 \times 13(30(11+13)+(11-13)^2)} = 1.18.$$

By Table B.3, this is not significant ($p > 0.1$).

To test for a period effect using the χ_1^2 statistic for Prescott's test, we apply (7.9) to the table

6	3	8	17
3	3	7	13
9	6	15	30

which results in the test statistic

$$\frac{30(30(8-6)-17(15-9)-15)^2}{17 \times 13(30(15+9)-(15-9)^2)} = 0.64.$$

This is clearly not significant at any reasonable significance level.

7.5.4 Analysing binary data

Another type of data that may arise from a cross-over study is the binary form — for example, the answer to the question, 'Did you feel any chest pain since the last clinic visit?' in an angina study. Binary data may be analysed in exactly the same fashion as preference data. This is achieved by taking a subject who has success in period 1 but failure in period 2 as a 'period 1 preference'; similarly, a subject who has success in period 2 but failure in period 1 is a 'period 2 preference'. All others have 'no preference'. We would then analyse as in Section 7.5.3.

7.6   Sequential studies

In many intervention studies, subjects are recruited at different times. For instance, a general practitioner (GP) may enter each new patient that arrives for consultation with a specific disorder into the study; unless the disorder is particularly common, this may require recruitment over several weeks, or even months. Consequently, results for particular patients, such as response to a 2-week exposure to treatment, may well be available serially in time. Suppose, then, that the benefits of one treatment over another are clear from the early results. Is there any point in continuing the experiment under these circumstances? Indeed, is it ethically acceptable to continue to allocate a treatment once it is known to be inferior?

To avoid this ethical dilemma, some intervention studies use a **sequential** design. This means that the number of subjects studied is not fixed in advance but is allowed to vary depending upon the clarity of the information received. Hence, if early observations show an obvious treatment difference, then the study will stop early. If not, it continues. Such a design is suitable only when data do arrive serially in time. As well as the ethical consideration, a sequential study (suitably designed and analysed) can be expected to finish before the conventional fixed-sample parallel group study would do so. This not only reduces costs for the current study but also should be of benefit to future subjects, because the results will be available rather earlier than they would otherwise have been.

The practical disadvantages are that the required quantities of the treatment, human resources and equipment are unknown in advance and that data must be compiled and calculations made at regular intervals (these are sometimes called **interim analyses**). Sequential data are also more difficult to analyse. Space is insufficient to describe the methods of analysis here; see Whitehead (1997) for a thorough exposition. A simple picture will describe the essential idea (Figure 7.7). This shows the stopping boundaries for a particular sequential test called the **triangular test**. A suitable test statistic, the formula for which is determined by statistical theory, is calculated at each interim analysis, assumed here to happen when each single new result is obtained (this assumption is not necessary and may well be inconvenient in practice). Progress during the study, as results accumulate, is shown as a 'walk' across the plot from left to right. The walk begins within the 'no decision yet' zone and continues until the 'reject null hypothesis' or 'fail to reject' boundary is crossed. In the hypothetical example illustrated, the rejection boundary was crossed and the study terminated once the 20th subject's result was available. The conclusion was that the null hypothesis should be rejected.

In many situations, it is appropriate to plot some function of the accumulated sample size, rather than the sample size itself, on the horizontal axis. The triangular test is only one of a number of sequential test designs available; see Whitehead (1997) for a general discussion and Jennison and Turnbull (1990) for a comparison of some of the more popular designs.

An example of a sequential intervention study is described by Moss *et al.* (1996). This was a comparison of prophylactic therapy with an implanted cardioverter-defibrillator and conventional medicine in the treatment of subjects with specific severe coronary

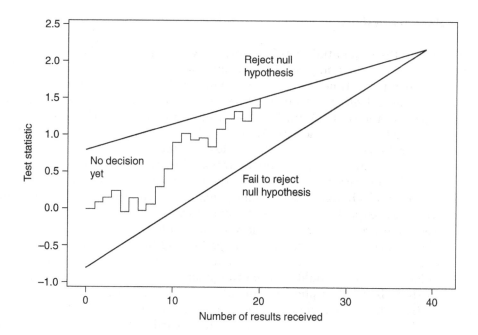

Figure 7.7. A triangular sequential test: the null hypothesis is that the mean subject response takes some predetermined value against a one-sided alternative.

symptoms. The end-point recorded was death from any cause. A two-sided sequential triangular test was adopted; the test statistic used to formulate the stopping boundaries was the log-rank test (Section 5.5.2). Data were analysed weekly from the point when 10 deaths had been reported. By the time the study was terminated, the first of the 192 patients recruited had been followed up for 61 months and the last for 1 month (the average duration of follow-up was 27 months). The conclusion reached was that the treatments had a different effect ($p = 0.009$); the implant appeared to reduce mortality. Early stopping, compared with a fixed-sample design, meant that the results could be published and acted upon more quickly.

7.6.1   The Haybittle–Peto stopping rule

Many parallel group RCTs are designed to have a few pre-planned interim analyses, usually for the purpose of stopping early when the outcome is already clear. Although these are really sequential trials, the complexities of the general sequential trial are often avoided by adopting the **Haybittle–Peto rule**. This states that we should stop the trial at any interim analysis where the absolute value of the estimated treatment effect (e.g., the log relative risk or the difference between the treatment means) is bigger than three times its standard error. With this rule, the p values and confidence intervals derived at the end of the trial do not need correcting for bias caused by the interim analyses (DeMets and Lan, 1994). This is an approximate result, based on an assumption of a normal distribution for the treatment effect (which explains the use of the log transformation for relative risk above — see Section 3.1). Jennison and Turnbull (1990) give a precise algorithm which requires slight changes to the p value used at the end of the trial, but this is unnecessary in the vast majority of practical applications.

7.6.2   Adaptive designs

An extension of the sequential trial is an **adaptive design**. This is a trial in which accumulating study data, and possibly data sourced externally, are used to modify the study design at interim times without undermining the validity and integrity of the trial. At the interim looks the trial could be stopped for efficacy (the intervention is clearly superior to the control), futility (the trial is unlikely to find the intervention to be superior) or for safety concerns. Alternatively, the trial could be continued, with or without alterations to the design. Examples of alterations include increasing the rate of recruitment, altering the relative rates of recruitment into the treatment groups, decreasing or increasing the dose of the intervention treatment, adding extra treatment arms and changing the primary endpoint. Information from variables related to the disease (particularly those thought to be surrogate outcomes), compared between treatment groups in interim analyses, may allow an informed re-evaluation of the chance of a conclusive outcome, perhaps leading to early stopping. Data from other recent studies, trials or otherwise, may be used to help the re-evaluation. Although adaptive designs could be used in epidemiological investigations, they are far more likely to be used in pharmaceutical trials and thus beyond the main scope of this book. Good accounts of adaptive designs include Berry (2011), with applications in oncology, Mehta *et al.* (2009), with applications in cardiovascular disease and Bretz *et al.* (2009), with a statistical focus.

7.7   Allocation to treatment group

Whatever the design, any comparative intervention study should have a set of rules for allocating subjects to treatment groups. Earlier we have seen the benefit of randomisation, which is to protect against systematic bias, so we will certainly want rules involving a chance mechanism. We will assume that subjects will be allocated to either of two treatment groups — call them A and B — and that an equal number are required in each. Generalisations from these restrictions are not difficult. We will also assume that subjects arrive one at a time for recruitment by the investigator (assumed to be a physician, perhaps at a GP clinic or hospital). Consent should have been obtained before allocation begins (Section 7.3.4).

The allocation schemes described fall into two types: those using global (unstratified) randomisation (Section 7.7.1) and those stratifying randomisation so as to achieve balance between the groups in terms of key prognostic factors (such as age and sex), which are thought to have an important effect on the outcome of the intervention study (Section 7.7.2).

In the examples that follow, we shall use a random number table, Table B.6. To make things easier to follow, we will always begin drawing random numbers at the top left-hand position and move left to right across the table. In general, a random starting point within the table should be chosen as well, perhaps, as a random direction.

7.7.1   Global randomisation

Here, subjects will be allocated to treatment groups A or B using randomisation rules that are unrestricted with regard to prognostic factors. We shall look at four alternative schemes.

In **complete randomisation**, each subject is allocated to group A or B using a fair coin (for example, heads = A; tails = B) or some equivalent mechanism, such as

Table B.6. To use a random number table, we assign an equal number of random digits to each group; for example, we could allocate 0 to 4 to A and 5 to 9 to B. Then, because the first 10 random numbers in Table B.6 are

$$1, 4, 7, 2, 6, 0, 9, 2, 7, 2,$$

the allocations for the first 10 subjects are

$$\text{A, A, B, A, B, A, B, A, B, A.}$$

This simple scheme has two drawbacks: overall imbalance between the groups is fairly likely (in the example, there are six As and only four Bs) and prognostic factors may not be balanced (for example, all the As could, by chance, be men and all the Bs could be women). These problems are unlikely to be important for very large studies, in which case this may be the preferred allocation scheme because of its simplicity.

In the **alternation** scheme, the first subject is allocated as before and thereafter the assignments alternate. Hence, using Table B.6, we draw the first random number, 1, which corresponds to allocation A (by the rules used previously). The sequence of allocations thus is

$$\text{A, B, A, B, A, B, A, B, A, B, ...}$$

This scheme ensures equal allocation (obviously this is exactly true only if the overall sample size is even). It still does not guarantee balance in prognostic factors and, furthermore, has the disadvantage of predictability. Once the investigating physician has discovered the pattern, she or he may defer or refuse recruitment because the next allocation is known in advance. This will lead to bias in many cases. Clearly, the problem is not as bad in double-blind studies, but it is not impossible for a few subjects' codes to be broken, inadvertently or due to medical necessity. The investigator may then be able to guess the pattern.

An improvement on alternation is a block allocation scheme, **random permuted blocks**, which is much less predictable. We will look at the specific example of blocks of size 4. Consider all the different possible sequences of allocations of four successive subjects containing two As and two Bs. These are the permuted blocks:

1. A, A, B, B
2. A, B, A, B
3. A, B, B, A
4. B, A, A, B
5. B, A, B, A
6. B, B, A, A.

Blocks are then chosen at random by selecting random numbers between 1 and 6. This could be done (for example) with a fair die or by using Table B.6 (ignoring the numbers 7, 8, 9 and 0). Hence, the first five numbers obtained from Table B.6 are

$$1, 4, 2, 6, 2$$

Referring back to the previous numbering scheme gives the allocation of the first 20 subjects as

$$\text{A, A, B, B, B, A, A, B, A, B, A, B, B, B, A, A, A, B, A, B}$$

(split the letters into groups of four to see the relationship with the list of permuted blocks).

This scheme may not be entirely unpredictable because, in single-blind studies, an investigator who discovers the block size will then know at least every last assignment in the block in advance, assuming that she or he is devious enough to keep a record of past assignments. This problem is unlikely to occur when the block size is large (say, 10 or more), but it may be worthwhile varying the block size as allocation proceeds.

The **biased coin** method is akin to complete randomization except that, at each allocation, we evaluate the correspondence in treatment group size up to that point and allocate to the group currently undersized with a probability of more than 1/2. The probabilities used are commonly 3/5, 2/3 or 3/4. We will take 2/3 as an example. To apply the scheme, we will take the random numbers 1, 2, 3, 4, 5, 6 for the smallest group, and 7, 8, 9 for the largest group. In the case of a tie in sample size, we simply allocate to each group with probability 1/2, exactly as for the complete randomisation scheme (0 to 4 = A; 5 to 9 = B).

The first 11 numbers obtained from Table B.6 are now written with the consequent allocation according to the preceding rules; the lower-case letters in-between describe the relative sample sizes *before* the present allocation is made (a = A larger, b = B larger, t = tie):

1,	4,	7,	2,	6,	0,	9,	2,	7,	2,	9
t	a	t	b	t	b	b	b	b	b	b
A,	B,	B,	A,	B,		B,	A,	B,	A,	B

Note that the zero has been rejected.

This scheme is not guaranteed to provide a balance in numbers (indeed the sample sizes are 6 : 4 in favour of B in the example), but the degree of inequality is unlikely to be important except in very small studies. Prognostic factors may be unbalanced.

7.7.2   Stratified randomization

Here we shall assume that a number of prognostic factors are known to have an important influence on the outcome to be used in the study. We shall look at two allocation schemes that seek to remove the differential effect of such prognostic factors by balancing their contribution to the two treatment groups. For example, we might wish to allocate as many men to group A as to group B, thus achieving balance with regard to sex.

Such balancing is not essential. For one thing, randomisation should achieve at least an approximate balance in the long run (that is, big samples) because it is a fair allocation scheme. The problem is that studies may be fairly small in relation to the number of prognostic factors and the degree of balance that is required. As discussed in Section 7.3.3, lack of balance may be allowed for at the analysis stage using methods designed to control for confounding (Chapter 4). Balance is, however, desirable on the grounds that the results are then more obvious and more likely to be convincing. It is also statistically more efficient. Hence, as long as important prognostic factors are known and the sample size overall is not big, restricted randomisation is to be preferred. On the other hand, it is pointless to try to balance for a factor unless we are very confident that it has a real effect. Restricted randomisation is more complex and more prone to error in application. Rarely will it be worthwhile balancing on more than three prognostic factors.

In what follows, as an example, we shall assume that we wish to balance on three factors: age, sex and severity of illness. Age is to be balanced at three levels (below 30, 30 to 49 and 50 years or more) and severity at two levels (severe, not severe).

In the **stratified random permuted blocks** scheme, subjects are grouped into cross-classified strata defined by the prognostic factors. Our example has 12 such strata ($3 \times 2 \times 2$). A random permuted block scheme is used within each stratum using random numbers, just as in the unstratified scheme. The only difference now is that we shall have several (12 in the example) parallel sequences of random numbers, and thus blocks. Such a process has little chance of predictability by the investigator, and blocks of size 2 (A, B and B, A only) may well be acceptable.

The drawback with this scheme is that it does not guarantee equality in total group size or in the relative numbers for individual prognostic factors between treatment groups. Either or both may have serious discrepancies. For our example, suppose that 100 subjects are recruited to the study and that the number in each cross-class is as shown in Table 7.8. Suppose that random permuted blocks of size 2 are used within each stratum, and the resulting allocation is as shown in Table 7.9. This splits each individual number in Table 7.8 into two components and, because blocks of size 2 are used, the difference is never more than 1 between the left and right halves of Table 7.9.

The sex ratio in group A is 29 : 22 in favour of women but in group B is 25 : 24 in favour of men. If the disease affects women more seriously than men, this imbalance would lead to bias (against the treatment given to group A in a parallel group study), unless the analysis takes it into account. In this example, there are also slight imbalances in overall sample size (51 : 49 in favour of A), age and severity of illness. Examples with serious imbalances in any of these are not difficult to construct. Therefore, although the cross-classes are almost exactly balanced, the totals for any individual prognostic factor may be quite dissimilar.

In general, the problems illustrated by the example will tend to worsen as overall sample size decreases, block size increases and the number of cross-classes (that is, number of prognostic factors or levels used within factors) increases. Hence, small block sizes are preferable, but even then if subjects or resources are scarce and there are several important prognostic factors, the scheme may not be suitable.

Table 7.8. Cross-classification of 100 subjects by sex, severity of illness and age group.

Sex	Severity of illness	Age (years)		
		Below 30	30–49	50 and over
Men	severe	5	11	9
	not severe	9	13	0
Women	severe	3	13	15
	not severe	7	15	0

Table 7.9. Result of stratified random permuted block (of size 2) allocation for the data in Table 7.8.

Allocation to A			Allocation to B		
2	5	4	3	6	5
4	7	0	5	6	0
2	7	8	1	6	7
4	8	0	3	7	0

Note: Labels as in Table 7.8 for each treatment group.

Minimisation is a generalisation of the biased coin method, by means of which we seek to balance the individual (marginal) totals of the prognostic factors. The basic idea is that when a new subject arrives for allocation, we should calculate a score for each treatment group that reflects how similar the current allocation outcome is, in overall terms, to the characteristics of this new subject. The subject is then allocated to the group with lowest score using a probability greater than 1/2. As with the simple biased coin method, the probability taken is often 3/5, 2/3 or 3/4. Tied scores require the use of a probability of 1/2.

The simplest method of scoring is to count the number with each individual prognostic factor in common with the new subject and sum over all the factors. For example, suppose the result of current allocations is given by Table 7.10. The next subject is a woman aged 26 without a severe case of the illness. To decide the treatment group into which she should go, we add up the numbers for the levels of Table 7.10 which have matching characteristics. These are: for A, $22 + 12 + 21 = 55$; for B : $25 + 11 + 22 = 58$. Hence, we allocate her to group A with a probability of, say, 2/3. Notice that this particular outcome would be expected to improve the balance for overall group sizes, sex and severity of illness but actually increase the imbalance for age.

This scheme is not guaranteed to produce exactly equal numbers (as is clear from the example), but the degree of imbalance is unlikely to be important except in very small studies. Notice that minimisation does not even try to balance out numbers in the cross-classes, such as those shown in Table 7.8. Balance may be perfect for each prognostic factor when taken alone, but serious imbalance may be present across some cross-classes. For instance, groups A and B may have the same number of men and women and the same number of severe and nonsevere cases, yet all the men in group A might be severe, and all the men in B nonsevere, cases. This, of course, is the opposite problem to that encountered with stratified random permuted blocks. If we really would like balance across cross-classes with the minimisation scheme, we should take each cross-class as a separate classification contributing to the score. However, this is likely to be tedious to implement.

Sometimes minimisation is applied using an allocation probability of unity for the group with the smallest score. This is undesirable because the process is now no longer random, but it may be justifiable on pragmatic grounds in multicentre studies and when there are several prognostic factors. Other rules for scoring, to be contrasted with the simple totalling method suggested here, are described by Whitehead (1997). A comprehensive account of randomisation schemes in general, covering more complex allocation schemes to those considered here, is given by Rosenberger and Lachin (2002).

Table 7.10. Result of current allocations (within each sex, age and severity group separately) when the next subject arrives.

Factor	Level	A	B
Sex	men	27	25
	women	22	25
Age (years)	below 30	12	11
	30–49	25	27
	50 and over	12	12
Severity of illness	severe	28	28
	not severe	21	22

7.7.3   Implementation

Rather than having an investigator spin a coin, toss a die, consult random number tables or use some equivalent device for randomisation during subject contact, randomisation is often done externally, such as through a web site where subject details are entered on-line; treatment allocation is returned automatically (possibly blinded). Alternatively, randomisation lists may be prepared in advance and distributed to investigators. Often this list is transferred to a sequence of cards, which are then placed in numbered, opaque, sealed envelopes. As each subject arrives, the next envelope is opened to reveal the A or B allocation. Pocock (1983) cautions that doctors have been known to open and then reseal envelopes to discover forthcoming allocations in advance; subjects may then be rejected or deferred because the particular treatment is thought to be unsuitable for them, giving rise to bias.

Biased coin and minimisation schemes require three sets of sealed envelopes: one for the situation in which B is in the ascendancy (for example, with cards in the ratio 2 : 1 in favour of A), one for a tie (1 : 1) and one for A in the ascendancy (1 : 2). They also require that a careful check on past allocations be maintained. The stratified random permuted block scheme requires a set of envelopes for each stratum. Further details about allocation of subjects to treatment are given by Pocock (1979). Similar material is included in Pocock (1983).

7.8   Trials as cohorts

Intervention studies routinely record variables at baseline that are thought to be related to disease, if only to check their balance between the treatment groups. If we ignore the fact that treatments were administered, the clinical trial has the form of a cohort study. Hence we can analyse the trial data as we would data from a cohort study. For instance, blood pressure is routinely recorded at baseline in clinical trials of blood pressure lowering medications. Suppose that such a trial records stroke outcomes during follow-up. The consequent study can be viewed, forgetting about treatment, as a cohort study of the effects of blood pressure on stroke, and the data analysed accordingly.

Whether such an analysis is sensible requires careful consideration. A good plan would be to run analyses separately by treatment arm and to test for a treatment by risk factor interaction. If these analyses suggest that the treatment has had an effect on the risk factor–disease association then we might decide to only make use of the results from the control arm, especially if the trial was placebo-controlled. Otherwise, all data could be analysed together, with adjustment for the treatment allocation.

The main advantage in using trial data to estimate aetiological effects is that the data are likely to be of relatively high quality compared to standard cohort studies. For instance, follow-up data are likely to be comprehensive and outcomes may be adjudicated by clinical committees. The main disadvantage is that results from trial data may not be generalisable.

Exercises

7.1   In the Lifestyle Heart Trial, subjects with angiographically documented coronary heart disease were randomly assigned to an experimental or a usual-care group (Ornish *et al.,* 1990). Experimental subjects were prescribed a low-fat vegetarian diet, moderate aerobic exercise, stress management training, smoking and group support. The usual-care subjects were not asked to change their lifestyle. Progression or regression of coronary artery lesions was assessed in both groups by angiography at baseline and after about a year. Regression was observed in 18 of the 22 experimental subjects and 10 of the 19 control subjects.

    (i)   Is this evidence of a significant effect of the lifestyle change regimen? Calculate suitable summary statistics to represent the effect.

    (ii)   Discuss the potential problems of this intervention study and suggest moves that might be made to control these problems in similar studies.

7.2   In a study of four treatments for eradication of *H. pylori*, Tham *et al.* (1996) report the following eradication results (expressed as ratios of eradications to number treated):

- Omeprazole + amoxycillin + metronidazole: 6/20.
- Ranitidine + amoxycillin + metronidazole: 8/20.
- Omeprazole + placebo: 0/20.
- Omeprazole + clarithromycin: 4/20.

Test whether a significant difference exists between:

    (i)   The first two treatments in this list.

    (ii)   The third treatment (the only one not involving an antibiotic) and all the rest combined.

7.3   Refer to the cerebral palsy data of Table C.4 (in Appendix C).

    (i)   Test whether the addition of rhizotomy has a significant effect on motor function.

    (ii)   Summarise the effect of adding rhizotomy, giving a 95% confidence interval for your summary statistic.

7.4   Dorman *et al.* (1997) describe a randomised controlled comparison of a brief and a long questionnaire to ascertain quality of life for stroke survivors. Although the short questionnaire solicits less information, it may be worth adopting, in the future, if it leads to a higher response rate. The study involved 2253 survivors from the U.K. centres of the International Stroke Trial: 1125 received the short form and 1128 the long form; both were sent out by post. After two mailings, 905 short and 849 long questionnaires had been returned.

    (i)   Carry out a suitable test to ascertain whether the short questionnaire is worth considering further.

    (ii)   Find a 99% confidence interval for the difference in response rates.

    (iii) If the short questionnaire, rather than the long one, were to be used in a study of 25 000 stroke survivors, how many extra respondents would you expect? Give a 99% confidence interval for this result.

7.5   Refer to the Norwegian Multicentre Study data of Table C.5.

    (i)   Construct a separate actuarial life table for each treatment group. Include a standard error for each cumulative survival probability using Greenwood's formula.

    (ii)   Plot the estimates of cumulative survival probability on a graph and interpret the presentation.

    (iii) Use a Cochran–Mantel–Haenszel test to compare overall survival between the Blocadren and placebo groups.

7.6   The following gives a series of objectives that have arisen, each of which suggests the use of an intervention study. State which kind of study design — parallel group, cluster randomised, cross-over or sequential — you would suggest.

    (i)   Comparison of two types of inhaler that are to be used to provide fixed amounts of salbutamol to patients with asthma. Lung function before and immediately after inhaler use will be compared.

(ii)   Comparison of the use and absence of use of antiarrhythmic drugs as an adjunct to electric shock treatment during episodes of ventricular fibrillation. The outcome measured will be survival for 1 hour.

(iii)   Comparison of two diets that may cause reductions in blood cholesterol. Subjects will be healthy volunteers and the outcome measure will be change in serum total cholesterol after 4 weeks on the diet.

(iv)   Comparison of a new and an existing treatment for a rare, fatal disease. Outcome will be survival time.

(v)   Comparison of two hospital care management systems. The primary outcome will be patient satisfaction with the care received.

(vi)   Investigation of dental hygiene practices and blood coagulation. Volunteer subjects will be asked to brush teeth twice a day or to refrain from tooth brushing. Changes in blood coagulation measures will be assessed after 2 weeks.

7.7   For the rheumatoid arthritis data of Table C.6, draw suitable diagrams to assess the treatment and period effects. Test for (i) a treatment by period interaction, (ii) a treatment effect and (iii) a period effect. Interpret your results.

7.8   Whitehead (1997) describes a sequential test, called a sequential probability ratio test, for the comparison of two proportions. This requires plotting Z against V at each time of observation, where

$$Z = \frac{nS - mT}{m + n}$$

$$V = \frac{mn(S + T)\left[(m - S) + (n - T)\right]}{(m + n)^3}.$$

Here m and n are, respectively, the number of patients in groups 1 and 2; and S and T are, respectively, the number of treatment successes in groups 1 and 2.

Du Mond (1992) describes a sequential study in which this test was used to compare ganciclovir against placebo in the prevention of pneumonia following bone marrow transplantation. The upper and lower stopping boundaries for this test, for which results appear in Table C.7, turn out to be $Z = 2.58 + 0.675V$ and $Z = -2.58 + 0.675V$, respectively. Taking the ganciclovir group as group 1 and the placebo group as group 2, we conclude that ganciclovir is effective if we hit the upper boundary and we conclude 'no difference' if we hit the lower boundary.

(i)   Using the data given in Table C.7, mark the preceding boundaries and the results on a plot of Z against V. What decision is made at the termination of the study?

(ii)   Compare the boundaries for this test with those for the triangular test shown in Figure 7.7. Is there any particular disadvantage with the boundaries used in this test?

7.9   A study is planned to assess the desirability, and overall impact on the health services, of day surgery (hospital patients sent home after surgery without overnight stay). Several hospitals agree to take part in the study. At each hospital, some surgical patients will be given day surgery and others will be kept as in-patients for at least one night. The two groups will be compared using various subjective criteria (including self-assessed health during the weeks following surgery) and factual criteria (such as the number of calls made to community and primary health care services during the weeks following surgery).

Describe a suitable method for allocating hospital patients to intervention groups. You may assume that a list of suitable surgical procedures for day surgery has already been established. Consider how you would put your allocation scheme into practice.

CHAPTER 8

Sample size determination

8.1 Introduction

Whenever an epidemiological study is being planned, the question always arises of how many subjects to include — that is, what sample size to use. This is clearly a vital question and would constitute a crucial part of any research proposal. Too large a sample means wasted resources; the result may be statistically significant but have no practical significance, as when a very small relative risk, say below 1.05, turns out to be statistically significant. Rarely will such a small increase in risk be biologically or medically important. This issue was discussed in Section 3.5.5. On the other hand, too small a sample leads to lack of precision in the results. This may render the entire study worthless: a result that would have medical significance has little chance of being found statistically significant when it is true. For instance, when Frieman *et al.* (1978) investigated 71 intervention studies that reported absence of an effect when comparing two treatments, it transpired that about two-thirds of these studies had a chance of 70% or less of detecting a true improvement of one treatment over the other of 50%. Seldom, if ever, would a 50% improvement be of no medical importance and hence such studies run a high risk of missing vital information.

The essential problem is to decide upon a value for the sample size, n, which is just sufficient to provide the required precision of results. The first consideration in calculating n is the method of analysis that will subsequently be used on the data after collection. As we have seen in earlier chapters, this may well depend upon the type of data involved. Each different method of analysis will have an associated method for calculating sample size. This makes the entire subject too extensive, and often too complex, to cover fully here. Instead, we shall restrict our description to the situation most commonly assumed when determining sample size in epidemiological research: carrying out a hypothesis test using a normal assumption or approximation. This leads to sample size formulae that are reasonably easy to compute by hand. Exact methods require the use of commercial software packages, although the error when using the approximate formulae is rarely important, especially given that some of the parameters that are used in the computations are themselves necessarily approximate, as we shall see. Both of the packages that this book concentrates upon, SAS and Stata, have facilities to deal with sample size design. Programs using PROC POWER in SAS to solve some of the examples in this chapter are included on the web site for this book (see Appendix A). Stata includes a suite of commands which have the POWER prefix. Specialist software includes nQuery Adviser (http://www.statistical-solutions-software.com/nquery-advisor-nterim/) and PASS (http://www.ncss.com/software/pass/)

We shall look at four particular cases: tests for a single mean; comparison of two means; a single proportion; and comparison of two proportions. Sample size requirements when a more complex statistical analysis is planned, such as survival analysis, are covered in technical journal articles. For example, Freedman (1982) gives tables of sample sizes for use with the log-rank test; Julious (2004) and Julious and Campbell (2012) give details of sample size requirements across a wide range of clinical trial designs; Hsieh (1989) gives sample sizes for use in logistic regression analysis (Chapter 10); and Hsieh and Lavori (2000) consider sample sizes for the proportional hazards model (Chapter 11). The book of sample size tables by Machin *et al.* (2009) may also be useful. Specific sample size problems, beyond our current scope, can, of course, sometimes be addressed by using the software packages already mentioned.

So, rather than attempting to give exact formulae or a truly comprehensive account of the subject, this chapter aims to introduce the essential ideas and issues relating to sample size, common to all epidemiological study design issues, and to produce and interpret indicative results based upon relatively simple formulae. Excel programs that carry out the computations for the formulae given in this chapter have been packaged and are available from the web site for this book.

The approach of calculating n for hypothesis tests is sometimes called the **power calculation method**. The application of this method in epidemiological research is generally straightforward as long as the sampling scheme to be used is simple random sampling. More complex sampling methods are considered briefly in Section 8.8. Note that case–control studies require a slightly different approach to determining n compared with other types of study, and hence they are considered separately in Section 8.7. An alternative approach to the power calculation method is to determine n so as to ensure that the resultant 95% (or other) confidence interval is of a specified maximum width. This method, which has much to commend it, is described by Bristol (1989). PROC POWER in SAS implements this method as an alternative to its default power calculations.

Sometimes it may be useful to look at the sample size problem the other way around — that is, to ask, given a particular value of n (perhaps the most that can be afforded), what precision we might expect to get in the results. Here 'precision' might be the power (defined in the next section) or, say, the minimum relative risk that we can expect to find. This important problem will be addressed here along with direct computations of n.

8.2 Power

The **power** of a hypothesis test is the probability that the null hypothesis is rejected when it is false. Often this is represented as a percentage rather than a probability. The distinction will not be crucial in our account because it will be made clear which definition is being used.

In this section we shall consider, through examples, what determines the power of a hypothesis test. To simplify the explanation, we shall consider one particular hypothesis test: the test for a mean value, as outlined in Section 2.7.2. Suppose that we wish to carry out a one-sided test so that the two hypotheses under consideration are

$$H_0 : \mu = \mu_0$$

$$H_1 : \mu > \mu_0.$$

Furthermore, suppose that we plan to use a 5% significance test. For this test, we know that we should reject H_0 whenever T is greater than the upper 5% (one-sided) t value on $n - 1$ d.f., where T is the test statistic, (2.12),

$$T = \frac{\bar{x} - \mu_0}{s / \sqrt{n}}$$

for sample size n. The trouble with using this formula in any discussion of sample size is that the standard deviation, s, will be unknown before the sample is drawn. To simplify matters, and consequently derive an approximate result for the sample size, we will assume that the population standard deviation, denoted σ, is known. In this situation, we replace (2.12) by

$$T = \frac{\bar{x} - \mu_0}{\sigma/\sqrt{n}}$$

and compare T with the standard normal, rather than Student's t, distribution. Then we should reject H_0 in favour of H_1 whenever $T > 1.6449$. Note that 1.6449 is the critical value for a two-sided 10% test and thus a one-sided 5% test (see Table B.2). Hence, by definition,

$$\text{Power} = p\bigl(T > 1.6449 \big| H_1 \text{ true}\bigr),$$

where the vertical line denotes 'given'. In words, the power for a 5% test is the probability that the test statistic, T, exceeds 1.6449 given that the alternative hypothesis, H_1, is true.

It will be of interest to evaluate this equation for specific outcomes under the alternative hypothesis, H_1. That is, suppose we rewrite H_1 as

$$H_1 : \mu = \mu_1,$$

where $\mu_1 > \mu_0$. Then the power for the specific alternative $\mu = \mu_1$ becomes

$$\text{Power} = p\bigl(T > 1.6449 \big| \mu = \mu_1\bigr).$$

When $\mu = \mu_1$, the standardisation process of taking away the mean and dividing by the standard error (Section 2.7) changes this to

$$\text{Power} = p\left(Z > 1.6449 + \frac{\mu_0 - \mu_1}{\sigma/\sqrt{n}} \right),$$

where Z is a standard normal random variable (as tabulated in Table B.1 and Table B.2). By the symmetry of the normal distribution, for any value z, $p(Z > z) = p(Z < -z)$. Hence,

$$\text{Power} = p\left(Z < \frac{\mu_1 - \mu_0}{\sigma/\sqrt{n}} - 1.6449 \right). \tag{8.1}$$

We can evaluate the right-hand side of (8.1) and find an answer (at least approximately) from Table B.1. Alternatively, as noted in earlier chapters, exact values for the standard normal distribution can be obtained from Excel, or other computer packages. We shall quote exact figures from the latter method here; the results can be checked approximately with Table B.1.

Example 8.1 The male population of an area within a developing country is known to have had a mean serum total cholesterol value of 5.5 mmol/l 10 years ago. In recent years, many Western foodstuffs have been imported into the country as part of a rapid move towards a market economy. It is believed that this will have caused an increase in cholesterol levels. A sample survey involving 50 men is planned to test the hypothesis that the mean cholesterol value is still 5.5 against the alternative that it has increased, at the 5% level of significance. From the evidence of several studies, it may be assumed that the standard deviation of serum total cholesterol is 1.4 mmol/l. The epidemiologist in charge of the project considers that an increase in cholesterol up to 6.0 mmol/l would be extremely important in a medical sense. What is the chance that the planned test will detect such an increase when it really has occurred?

Here $\mu_0 = 5.5$, $\mu_1 = 6.0$, $\sigma = 1.4$ and $n = 50$. Substituting these into (8.1) gives the result,

$$\text{Power} = p\left(Z < \frac{6.0 - 5.5}{1.4/\sqrt{50}} - 1.6449\right)$$

$$= p\left(Z < 0.8805\right) = 0.8107.$$

Hence, the chance of finding a significant result, when the mean really is 6.0, is about 81%.

The determination of power for Example 8.1 is shown diagrammatically by Figure 8.1. The **rejection region** (or **critical region**) for the test is the area to the right of $T = 1.6449$. This is determined so as to contain 5% of the distribution of T when the null hypothesis $\mu = 5.5$ is true (shaded). When the alternative hypothesis, $\mu = 6.0$, is true, the test statistic, T, no longer has mean zero; its mean is now

$$\frac{\mu_1 - \mu_0}{\sigma/\sqrt{n}} = \frac{6.0 - 5.5}{1.4/\sqrt{50}} = 2.5254.$$

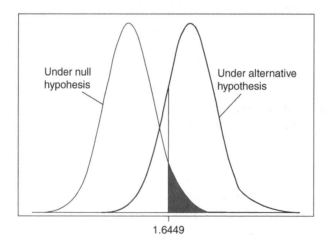

Figure 8.1. Distribution of the test statistic, T, when H_0 is true and when H_1 is true for Example 8.1.

This causes the entire distribution of T to be shifted 2.5254 units to the right. The area to the right of 1.6449 is now well over 5%; indeed, it is clearly over 50% of the whole. As we have seen, it is actually 81%.

In Example 8.1, a difference of 0.5 mmol/l in mean cholesterol was thought to be medically important. Suppose that this was reconsidered and, instead, a difference of 0.6 was sought, that is, $\mu_1 = 6.1$. Using this new value for μ_1 in (8.1) gives the result,

$$\text{Power} = p(Z < 1.3856) = 0.9171.$$

That is, the power has increased from a little over 81% when seeking to detect a true mean of 6.0 to a little under 92% for a true mean of 6.1 mmol/l. We can see that an increase should be expected from Figure 8.1, because the right-hand normal curve would be moved further to the right if the mean under the alternative hypothesis was increased. There would then be a larger area to the right of the 1.6449 cut-point under the right-hand curve.

It may be useful to consider the power for a whole range of values for μ_1. For Example 8.1, this simply means substituting repeatedly for μ_1 in the equation

$$\text{Power} = p\left(Z < \frac{\mu_1 - 5.5}{1.4/\sqrt{50}} - 1.6449 \right),$$

which is derived from (8.1). The results may be displayed in a graph called a **power curve**. A power curve for Example 8.1 is shown as Figure 8.2. Notice that power increases, up to its maximum of 100%, as the value for the alternative hypothesis, H_1, moves away from the H_0 value (5.5 mmol/l). This makes intuitive sense: bigger differences should be far more obvious and thus more likely to be detected. Notice that the significance level of the test (5% in Example 8.1) is obtained as the 'power' when $\mu_1 = \mu_0 = 5.5$ in Figure 8.2.

The power and significance level, when expressed as probabilities, are (respectively) analogous to the sensitivity and (1 − specificity) for diagnostic tests (Section 2.10). Instead of the power, some analysts prefer to consider the complementary probability, (1 − power). This is known as the probability of **type II** error, the error

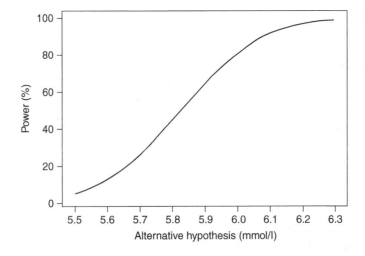

Figure 8.2. A power curve for Example 8.1 (one-sided test, $n = 50$).

of failing to reject H_0 when it is false. This is generally given the symbol β. Contrast this with type I error, α, the error of rejecting H_0 when it is true (defined in Section 2.5.1), which is just the significance level expressed as a probability. In Example 8.1, $\alpha = 0.05$ and $\beta = 1 - 0.8107 = 0.1893$.

In (8.1), we assumed that a 5% test was to be used. This will not always be true. In general, if we plan to carry out a test at the $100\alpha\%$ level then we simply need to replace 1.6449 with z_α in (8.1), where

$$p(Z < z_\alpha) = 1 - \alpha.$$

For some specific values of α we can find z_α directly from Table B.1 or indirectly from Table B.2. The equation for power for a $100\alpha\%$ test then becomes

$$\text{Power} = p\left(Z < \frac{\mu_1 - \mu_0}{\sigma/\sqrt{n}} - z_\alpha\right). \tag{8.2}$$

We are now in a position to specify what determines the power of a test. From (8.2), we can see that power will increase as

$$\frac{\mu_1 - \mu_0}{\sigma/\sqrt{n}} - z_\alpha$$

increases. In particular, therefore, power increases as

- σ decreases.
- μ_1 moves away from μ_0.
- z_α decreases, i.e., α increases (becomes less extreme).
- n increases.

Generally, we can do nothing to change σ because it is an inherent property of the material at our disposal (in Example 8.1, we cannot change the person-to-person variability in cholesterol). We can alter the value of μ_1 at which we evaluate power, but this will not change the essential characteristics of the test. We can alter α, but an increased α means a greater chance of type I error. We can, however, increase n so as to improve the test globally (albeit at extra cost). Intuitively, this makes perfect sense: the larger the value of n is, the more information we have available and thus the more precise our results (notwithstanding possible bias error).

Figure 8.3 shows the power curves for the situation of Example 8.1, but where $n = 100$ and $n = 200$, superimposed over Figure 8.2 (where $n = 50$). When $n = 200$, the power reaches 100% (to three decimal places) for any alternative hypothesis value of 6.047 mmol/l or greater. This shows the pivotal role of sample size in hypothesis testing, tying in with the material of Section 3.5.5.

8.2.1   Choice of alternative hypothesis

Up to now we have considered only one-sided 'greater than' alternatives. In Example 8.1, we expect cholesterol to increase because of a move towards a Western diet. Suppose that a similar survey were planned in the United States, where we might expect cholesterol to have decreased over the last 10 years due to greater public awareness of the risks associated with elevated cholesterol levels. In this situation,

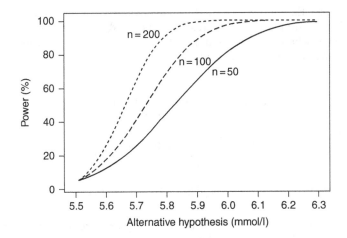

Figure 8.3. Power curves for Example 8.1 (one-sided test) when $n = 50$ (solid line), $n = 100$ (dashed line) and $n = 200$ (dotted line).

we might decide that a one-sided test with a 'less than' alternative is appropriate. Due to the symmetry of the normal distribution, the only change to what went before is that we now reject H_0 whenever T is less than -1.6449, rather than greater than 1.6449, for a 5% test. The equation for power now becomes

$$\text{Power} = p\left(Z < \frac{\mu_0 - \mu_1}{\sigma/\sqrt{n}} - 1.6449 \right). \tag{8.3}$$

This is exactly the same as (8.1) except that $\mu_0 - \mu_1$ has replaced $\mu_1 - \mu_0$. Consequently, the new power curve is simply the mirror image of the old. For example, there must be an 81% chance of detecting a *reduction* of 0.5 mmol/l in mean serum total cholesterol according to the result of Example 8.1 (assuming $n = 50$ and $\sigma = 1.4$, as before) when a 5% test against a 'less than' alternative is used.

When the alternative hypothesis is two-sided (as is most usual in practice) the hypotheses become

$$H_0 : \mu = \mu_0$$

$$H_1 : \mu = \mu_1$$

where $\mu_1 \neq \mu_0$, such that μ_1 can lie either side of μ_0. The test statistic, T, is the same as for the one-sided case, but the critical value is now 1.96 because 5% of the standard normal distribution is either less than -1.9600 or greater than 1.9600 (see Table B.2). Proceeding as in the one-sided situation, we can show (Woodward, 1992) that an approximate result for a 5% significance test is

$$\text{Power} = \begin{cases} p\left(Z < \dfrac{\mu_1 - \mu_0}{\sigma/\sqrt{n}} - 1.96 \right) & \text{for } \mu_1 > \mu_0 \\[4mm] p\left(Z < \dfrac{\mu_0 - \mu_1}{\sigma/\sqrt{n}} - 1.96 \right) & \text{for } \mu_1 < \mu_0. \end{cases} \tag{8.4}$$

Example 8.2 Consider Example 8.1 again, but where we wish to test for a cholesterol difference in either direction, so that a two-sided test is to be used. What is the chance of detecting a significant difference when the true mean is 6.0 mmol/l, and when the true mean is 5.0 mmol/l?

When the true mean is 6.0, $\mu_1 > \mu_0$ and, by (8.4),

$$\text{Power} = p\left(Z < \frac{\mu_1 - \mu_0}{\sigma/\sqrt{n}} - 1.96 \right)$$

$$= p\left(Z < \frac{6.0 - 5.5}{1.4/\sqrt{50}} - 1.96 \right)$$

$$= p\left(Z < 0.5654 \right) = 0.7141.$$

When the true mean is 5.0, $\mu_1 < \mu_0$ and, by (8.4) or by symmetry, the result is the same, 0.7141. Hence, there is about a 71% chance of detecting an increase or decrease of 0.5 mmol/l using a two-sided test.

The general formula for power with a $100\alpha\%$ two-sided test is

$$\text{Power} = \begin{cases} p\left(Z < \dfrac{\mu_1 - \mu_0}{\sigma/\sqrt{n}} - z_{\alpha/2} \right) & \text{for } \mu_1 > \mu_0 \\[3mm] p\left(Z < \dfrac{\mu_0 - \mu_1}{\sigma/\sqrt{n}} - z_{\alpha/2} \right) & \text{for } \mu_1 < \mu_0, \end{cases} \tag{8.5}$$

where $p(Z < z_{\alpha/2}) = 1 - (\alpha/2)$. For some values of α, $z_{\alpha/2}$ can be read directly from Table B.2 where (using notation in this table) $P = 100\alpha\%$. With all else equal, the power is always lower using a two-sided test because $z_{\alpha/2}$ replaces z_α in the basic formulae (see also Example 8.1 and Example 8.2). Just as before, power increases as n increases, σ decreases, α increases or μ_1 moves away from μ_0. The latter is illustrated by Figure 8.4, a power curve for the situation of Example 8.2. Notice the

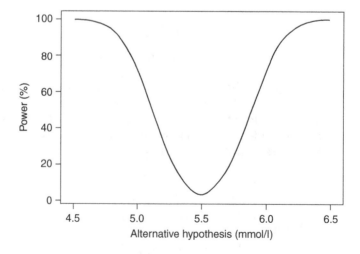

Figure 8.4. A power curve for Example 8.2 (two-sided test when $n = 50$).

symmetry of such a two-sided power curve. As in Figure 8.2 and Figure 8.3, the significance level of the test is given by the 'power' in the case where $\mu_1 = \mu_0 = 5.5$.

8.3 Testing a mean value

The theory of Section 8.2 is directly applicable to the problem of determining sample size when the subsequent data will be used to test a hypothesis about the mean of the parent population. This problem often arises in cross-sectional epidemiological sample surveys. We will develop the methodology by changing the terms of reference in our earlier example.

Example 8.3 Consider the problem of Example 8.1 again. The epidemiologist decides that an increase in mean total serum cholesterol up to 6.0 mmol/l from the known previous value of 5.5 mmol/l is so important that he would wish to be 90% sure of detecting it. Assuming that a one-sided 5% test is to be carried out and that the standard deviation, σ, is known to be 1.4 mmol/l, as before, what sample size should be used?

Notice that the problem of Example 8.1 has now been turned around: power is known to be 0.90, but n is now to be determined. The problem is solved by turning (8.1) around in a similar fashion. When the numerical values are substituted, (8.1) becomes

$$0.90 = p\left(Z < \frac{6.0 - 5.5}{1.4/\sqrt{n}} - 1.6449 \right).$$

Now, from Table B.2, $p(Z < 1.2816) = 0.90$ because the table shows us that 10% of the standard normal is above 1.2816. Hence,

$$\frac{6.0 - 5.5}{1.4/\sqrt{n}} - 1.6449 = 1.2816;$$

when rearranged, this gives the formula

$$n = \frac{\left(1.6449 + 1.2816\right)^2 (1.4)^2}{(6.0 - 5.5)^2} = 67.14.$$

In practice, this will need to be rounded upwards, to be safe, so that 68 subjects should be sampled. In Example 8.1, we saw that the suggested sample size of 50 would give a test with 81% power, thus leaving a chance of almost 1 in 5 that the important difference would fail to be detected. This example shows that 18 further subjects are needed to increase power to the required level of 90%.

Consideration of Example 8.3 shows that the general formula for sample size for a one-sided test may be obtained from (8.2) as

$$n = \frac{\left(z_\alpha + z_\beta\right)^2 \sigma^2}{\left(\mu_1 - \mu_0\right)^2} \tag{8.6}$$

where $100\alpha\%$ is the significance level for the test, $100(1 - \beta)\%$ is the predetermined power of detecting when the true mean is μ_1 and, as usual,

$$p\left(Z < z_\alpha\right) = 1 - \alpha$$

and also, by analogy,

$$p\left(Z < z_\beta\right) = 1 - \beta.$$

Example 8.4 Consider Example 8.3 again, but suppose that the epidemiologist has decided to change his requirements. He now wishes to be 95% sure of detecting when the true mean is 6.1 mmol/l (with all else as before).

This time, $1 - \beta = 0.95$, and from Table B.2, as seen already,

$$p(Z < 1.6449) = 0.95,$$

so that $z_\beta = 1.6449$. If $\alpha = 0.05$ (as before), then z_α is also 1.6449. Substituting the numerical values into (8.6) gives

$$n = \frac{(1.6449 + 1.6449)^2 (1.4)^2}{(6.1 - 5.5)^2} = 58.92,$$

so that 59 subjects will be needed.

Next, we should consider other alternative hypotheses. As we have seen in Section 8.2.1, one-sided 'less than' alternatives simply involve swapping $\mu_1 - \mu_0$ for $\mu_0 - \mu_1$ in the formula for power, as with (8.1) and (8.3). Since $\mu_1 - \mu_0$ is squared in the formula for n, this formula, (8.6), is valid for both types of one-sided alternatives. Two-sided alternatives are, by a similar argument that led to (8.4), dealt with simply by substituting $\alpha/2$ for α in (8.6); that is,

$$n = \frac{\left(z_{\alpha/2} + z_\beta\right)^2 \sigma^2}{\left(\mu_1 - \mu_0\right)^2} \tag{8.7}$$

for a two-sided test with significance level $100\alpha\%$.

Inspection of (8.6) and (8.7) shows that the sample size requirement increases as

- σ increases.
- μ_1 moves towards μ_0.
- z_α or $z_{\alpha/2}$ increases, i.e., α decreases.
- z_β increases, i.e., β decreases, i.e., power increases.

As discussed in Section 8.2, the standard deviation, σ, is a property of the material sampled and is not ours to vary. Intuitively, it makes sense that a larger sample would be needed when the person-to-person variability is greater, because then we would expect to have to sample more widely to obtain an accurate overall picture. Sample size requirements should increase as μ_1 moves towards μ_0 because then we are trying to differentiate between hypotheses that are more similar, which inevitably requires more information. Since α and β are probabilities of error, it seems reasonable that more information is required to reduce either of them.

Table 8.1. Values of z_α or $z_{\alpha/2}$ for common values of the significance level and of z_β (in bold) for common values of power.

One-sided			Two-sided			Power	
5%	1%	0.1%	5%	1%	0.1%	90%	95%
1.6449	2.3263	3.0902	1.9600	2.5758	3.2905	**1.2816**	**1.6449**

(Significance level spans the One-sided and Two-sided groups.)

8.3.1 Common choices for power and significance level

As we saw in Section 2.5.1, the significance level for a test is generally chosen to be 5, 1 or 0.1% (that is, $\alpha = 0.05$, 0.01 or 0.001). Power (as a percentage) is often chosen to be 80, 90 or 95%. As discussed in Example 8.3, 80% power is really too small for comfort, despite its common use in medical grant applications; 90% power (i.e., $\beta = 0.1$) is acceptable for most purposes. For easy reference, Table 8.1 shows the values of z_α (or $z_{\alpha/2}$) and z_β, which correspond to useful common choices (derived from Table B.2).

Other values for the significance level and percentage power may well be more appropriate in certain circumstances (Table B.1 or a computer package would then need to be used). Usually the power and alternative hypothesis are determined jointly because $1 - \beta$ is the probability of detecting when the true mean really is μ_1.

8.3.2 Using a table of sample sizes

Table 8.1 merely provides values of z_α (or $z_{\alpha/2}$) and z_β for substitution into (8.6) or (8.7). Table B.7 in Appendix B goes further and gives the values of n. However, to make Table B.7 of manageable size, it is necessary to introduce a new parameter, S, which is the standardised difference between the two hypothesised values for the mean, using the standard deviation as the standardising factor. That is,

$$S = \frac{\mu_1 - \mu_0}{\sigma}. \tag{8.8}$$

When μ_1 is less than μ_0, the negative sign for S should be ignored.

The values in Table B.7 have been calculated using six decimal places for the standard normal percentage points and have been rounded to avoid trailing decimals. Consequently, the answers given might disagree slightly with values calculated from (8.6) or (8.7) using Table 8.1, due to rounding error. Table B.7 gives values for n appropriate to one-sided tests directly. For two-sided tests, we should use the column of the table corresponding to half the significance level required (equivalent to using $z_{\alpha/2}$ rather than z_α). Similar comments hold for Table B.8 to Table B.10.

Example 8.5 An intervention study is planned to compare drug treatment with alternative medicine in the treatment of a specific medical condition. The drug is to be stockpiled in a health centre ready for distribution. The drug is supplied in sachets, which are supposed to contain exactly 2 mg of the drug. It is thought that supplies may have been overfull, which could compromise the results of the study (although posing no danger to the subjects treated). Consequently, a number of sachets will be sampled and their mean content tested against the null hypothesis that the mean really is 2.0. A 1% significance test will be used because the health centre wishes to be very sure that the sachets are overweight before complaining to the supplier. The standard deviation of sachet contents is known, from past experience, to be 0.2 mg. The health centre decides that it is important to be 95% sure of detecting when the true mean content is 2.1 mg. How many sachets should be sampled?

Since the concern here is about overfilling, a one-sided test will be used. Now $\mu_0 = 2.0$; $\mu_1 = 2.1$; $\sigma = 0.2$ and, from Table 8.1, $z_\alpha = 2.3263$ and $z_\beta = 1.6449$. Using (8.6) we obtain

$$n = \frac{(2.3263 + 1.6449)^2 (0.2)^2}{(2.1 - 2.0)^2} = 63.08,$$

which would be rounded up to 64. Alternatively, we could use Table B.7. Then, we need only to calculate S from (8.8),

$$S = \frac{2.1 - 2.0}{0.2} = 0.5.$$

When $S = 0.5$, the significance level is 1% and power 95%, Table B.7 gives the answer 64, just as before.

Example 8.6 Take the situation of Example 8.5 again, but now suppose that there is also concern in case the sachets are underweight. This, too, is a potential source of bias in the study. A two-sided test would now be appropriate.

Assuming all else is unchanged, Table 8.1 gives $z_{\alpha/2} = 2.5758$ and $z_\beta = 1.6449$ and thus, by (8.7),

$$n = \frac{(2.5758 + 1.6449)^2 (0.2)^2}{(2.1 - 2.0)^2} = 71.26,$$

which rounds up to 72. Alternatively, to use Table B.7, we must look up the significance level of 0.5% because our test is two-sided. As before, $S = 0.5$ and power is 95%. Table B.7 also gives the answer 72. Notice that a larger sample size is needed for this two-sided test compared with the one-sided equivalent in Example 8.5. This reflects the power differential between these two types of test, commented upon earlier.

Table B.7 cannot possibly include every value of S (or significance level, or power). Thus the value of S in Example 8.3 is $(6.0 - 5.5)/1.4 = 0.3571$, which does not appear in Table B.7. In these situations, we can get a rough idea of sample size by taking the nearest figure for S. In the example, the nearest tabulated figure is 0.35, which has $n = 70$ (for one-sided 5% significance and 90% power). This is only slightly above the true value of 68 for $S = 0.3571$, given in Example 8.3. However, this process can lead to considerable error when S is small, so it is preferable to use the formula, (8.6).

8.3.3   The minimum detectable difference

Sometimes we have budgetary or other restrictions that cause the maximum possible value for n to be determined by other than statistical considerations. In this case, we may use (8.2) or (8.5) to determine the power with which we can expect to detect when the alternative hypothesis is true.

Alternatively, we might like to consider what is the difference from the null hypothesis, $d = \mu_1 - \mu_0$, that we can expect just to be able to detect with specified power. This is called the **minimum detectable difference**: we will be able to detect this, or any larger difference, with the given n and specified power. By inverting (8.6), we get the result that

$$d = \frac{\sigma}{\sqrt{n}} (z_\alpha + z_\beta) \tag{8.9}$$

for a one-sided test. Replace z_α by $z_{\alpha/2}$ for a two-sided test, as usual.

Example 8.7 Suppose that, in the problem of Example 8.3, only one nurse is presently available to take the necessary blood samples. Due to time constraints, it is estimated that she will be able to take blood from only 50 patients. How small an increase in cholesterol from the known value of 5.5 mmol/l of 10 years ago can we expect to detect now, using a 5% test with 90% power?

Substituting the numerical values from Example 8.3 into (8.9) gives

$$d = \frac{1.4}{\sqrt{50}}(1.6449 + 1.2816) = 0.579 \text{ mmol/l}.$$

Thus, we are 90% certain of detecting when the true mean cholesterol is 5.5 + 0.579 = 6.079 mmol/l. The investigators now must decide whether this is good enough (probably not, because the minimum detectable difference of 0.579 is bigger than the difference of 0.5, which is considered medically important; see Example 8.3), or whether a second nurse should be employed so as to enable n to be increased.

8.3.4   *The assumption of known standard deviation*

Notice that we have assumed throughout that the standard deviation, σ, is known. In practice this is rarely true and we will, instead, need to rely upon an estimate, usually obtained from past experience. An alternative approach based on Student's t-distribution, which does not assume that σ is known, is applied by PROC POWER in SAS and other software. Theoretically, this is preferable, but for good estimates of σ and moderately large n, the results should be similar to those obtained from the equations given here.

8.4   Testing a difference between means

So far we have been concerned solely with one-sample situations in which we wish to test a hypothesis about a mean. This is the simplest situation from which to introduce the methodology. Most often epidemiological investigations are comparative; in this section we will extend our discussion to the problem of testing for the equality of two means. This situation is most likely to arise in a cross-sectional or intervention study. A similar problem could also arise in a cohort study with a fixed cohort, but in these studies the usual end-point of interest is a disease incidence, which is a proportion rather than a mean (Section 8.6).

Our new problem is a two-sample one. Although we still wish to know how many subjects we should select altogether, now an extra factor must be considered: how to distribute the entire sample size between the two groups. Although equal sample sizes are often used, this is by no means always the case. Thus, in an experimental study of a new procedure against an existing standard, giving the new treatment to more than half of the patients might be worthwhile simply in order to obtain more information about its performance (presumably the performance of the standard procedure is already well known). In a cohort study, if we take a single random sample (rather than a separate one from those with and without the risk factor), we expect the sample distribution by risk factor status to be as in the parent population and thus not necessarily 1 : 1 (Example 8.14). Economic considerations may also have an effect. For instance, one of the two treatments in an intervention study may be extremely expensive and this might cause us to prefer to allocate fewer to this treatment. In a case–control study, the number of cases might be necessarily fixed, but the number of controls practically unlimited (Section 6.4.5).

We will assume, for simplicity, that the standard deviations are the same in each group. As before, we will assume that this common standard deviation, σ, is known. Let the sample sizes (to be determined) in the two groups be n_1 and n_2. Define the allocation ratio r to be n_1/n_2 and let the overall sample size be n. That is,

$$n = n_1 + n_2 = (r+1)n_2.$$

Consider a test of the null hypothesis that the group means are equal against the alternative that their difference is δ. Using the notation μ_1 and μ_2 for the two population means, the hypotheses are thus

$$H_0 : \mu_1 = \mu_2$$

$$H_1 : \mu_1 - \mu_2 = \delta,$$

where $\delta < 0$ or $\delta > 0$ for the two possible one-sided tests and $\delta \neq 0$ for a two-sided test. Sample size is to be determined as to achieve a power of $1 - \beta$ of detecting when the true difference is δ. The theory outlined in Section 8.2 and Section 8.3 may be extended to show that

$$n = \frac{(r+1)^2 \left(z_\alpha + z_\beta\right)^2 \sigma^2}{\delta^2 r} \tag{8.10}$$

for a one-sided test (of either type). For a two-sided test, the same formula is used except that z_α is replaced by $z_{\alpha/2}$.

Example 8.8 In Example 8.1 and its extensions, we assumed that the mean value of serum total cholesterol 10 years ago was known and only the present-day value needed to be tested. Consider, now, the problem of deciding how many to sample in two surveys separated in time by 10 years. Suppose that we wish to test, at the 5% level of significance, the hypothesis that the cholesterol means are equal in the 2 years against the one-sided alternative that the mean is higher in the second of the 2 years. Suppose that equal-sized samples are to be taken in each year, but that these will not be the same individuals — that is, the two samples are independent (see Example 8.11 for the paired situation). Our test is to have a power of 95% for detecting when the later mean exceeds the earlier mean by 0.5 mmol/l. The standard deviation is assumed to be 1.4 mmol/l each time.

Here $\sigma = 1.4$, $\delta = 0.5$, $r = 1$ (because $n_1 = n_2$) and $z_\alpha = z_\beta = 1.6449$ (from Table 8.1). Hence, by (8.10),

$$n = \frac{(1+1)^2(1.6449 + 1.6449)^2(1.4)^2}{(0.5)^2 \times 1} = 339.40.$$

To satisfy the set conditions, this would need to be rounded up to the next highest *even* number, 340. Hence, we should sample 170 individuals in the first year and a further 170 in the second year.

8.4.1   Using a table of sample sizes

Notice that (8.10) is closely related to (8.6). If we consider that both δ and $\mu_1 - \mu_0$ are a difference between two means, then the relationship between the two equations is that (8.6) must be multiplied by $(r + 1)^2/r$ to arrive at (8.10). Hence, Table B.7 may be used in the two-sample situation. All that is necessary is to multiply each entry in the table by $(r + 1)^2/r$. When $r = 1$ (i.e., 1 : 1 allocation), this multiplier becomes 4. Hence, for Example 8.8, we get the standardised difference, $S = 0.5/1.4 = 0.3571$. As we have seen already, the nearest tabulated value to this is 0.35. With 5% significance and 95% power, Table B.7 gives $n = 89$. Multiplying by 4 gives a value of 356 when $S = 0.35$, which is roughly comparable with the true answer of 340 when $S = 0.3571$.

Example 8.9 Undernourished women taking oral contraceptives sometimes experience anaemia due to increased iron absorption. A study is planned to compare regular intake of iron tablets against a course of placebos. Oral contraceptive users are to be randomly allocated to the two treatment groups and the mean serum iron concentrations compared after 6 months. It is thought, from earlier studies, that the standard deviation of the increase in serum iron concentration is 4 μg% over a 6-month period. The average increase in serum iron concentration without iron supplements is also 4 μg%. The investigators wish to be 90% sure of detecting when the iron supplement doubles the serum iron concentration using a two-sided 5% significance test. It has been decided that four times as many women should be allocated to the iron tablet treatment so as to obtain a better idea of its effect, because there is little chance of any side-effects and this treatment is very cheap.

Here the difference to be detected is $8 - 4 = 4$ μg% and, because $\sigma = 4$ μg%, $S = 1$. Table B.7 gives a starting value for n of 11, which needs to be multiplied by $(r + 1)^2/r = (4 + 1)^2/4 = 6.25$. Hence the overall sample size required is 68.75, which needs to be rounded up to the nearest multiple of 5, that is, 70. We should allocate $70/5 = 14$ women to the placebo treatment and four times as many (56) to the iron tablet treatment. (8.10) gives exactly the same answer after rounding up.

Due to rounding error, Table B.7 can give different results to (8.10), but the difference is likely to be important only in extreme cases (very large or very small values for r).

Figure 8.5 shows how the sample size requirement decreases as the standardised difference, S, increases from 0.5 to 2.0 for Example 8.9. This emphasises what should already be apparent from the use of S in Table B.7: the sample size depends on the size of the difference to be tested *relative* to the standard deviation of the material in question. Figure 8.5 is a typical sample size curve and shows that we should be prepared for large samples if we wish to detect, with a high probability, a difference between

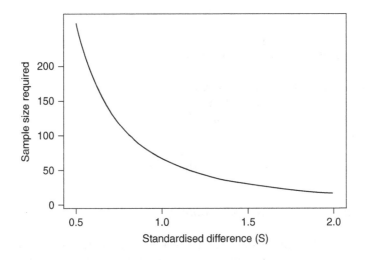

Figure 8.5. Sample size against standardised difference for Example 8.9.

means that is less than the standard deviation ($S < 1$). Note that Figure 8.5 gives results straight from (8.10) — that is, without rounding up to the nearest multiple of five.

8.4.2   Power and minimum detectable difference

It is a simple matter to turn (8.10) around to obtain expressions for the power, given the sample size (and the difference to be detected), and for the minimum detectable difference, given the sample size (and the power). These are, respectively,

$$z_\beta = \frac{\delta\sqrt{nr}}{(r+1)\sigma} - z_\alpha \qquad (8.11)$$

and

$$\delta = \frac{(r+1)(z_\alpha + z_\beta)\sigma}{\sqrt{nr}}. \qquad (8.12)$$

In fact, (8.11) gives an expression for z_β that would need to be converted into an expression for power $(1 - \beta)$ using the usual equation,

$$p(Z < z_\beta) = 1 - \beta.$$

As always, replace z_α by $z_{\alpha/2}$ in (8.11) and (8.12) for a two-sided test.

Example 8.10 Consider Example 8.8 again. Suppose that, because of human resource constraints, only 50 people may be sampled for blood in the first year, whilst it is anticipated that it will be possible to sample 100 in the second year. What is the minimum increase in cholesterol that can be detected with 95% power when a 5% significance test is used?

Here, $n = n_1 + n_2 = 150$ and $r = n_1/n_2 = 2$. From Example 8.8, $\sigma = 1.4$ and $z_\alpha = z_\beta = 1.6449$. Hence, from (8.12),

$$\delta = \frac{(2+1)(1.6449+1.6449)(1.4)}{\sqrt{(150)(2)}} = 0.80 \text{ mmol/l}.$$

So, with the human resources available, the investigators can expect to find, with 95% power, an increase of as little as 0.80 mmol/l in cholesterol.

Notice that Example 8.10 takes sample 2 to be the sample in the earlier year, because the increase is the second minus the first value. If, instead, sample 1 were taken as the earlier sample, we would have $r = n_1/n_2 = 0.5$. When substituted into (8.12), this gives exactly the same answer as before, but now we would interpret δ as a decrease over time. Strictly speaking, (8.12) gives a result for $\pm\delta$, but we can always choose to take sample 1 to be that with the highest mean and so force δ to be positive.

8.4.3   Optimum distribution of the sample

Given a fixed overall sample size, n, the optimum allocation of this between the two groups is an equal allocation; that is, $n_1 = n_2$ or $r = 1$. This can be proven from (8.11) using differential calculus. Hence, if there are no strong reasons to do otherwise, we should allocate the sample equally between the two groups.

8.4.4 Paired data

So far, we have assumed that the two samples are independent. If they are, instead, paired (such as measurements before and after some medical intervention; see Section 2.7.4), then (8.10) is inappropriate. We should then apply (8.6) or (8.7) to the differenced data, where δ takes the place of $\mu_1 - \mu_0$. We now need to be careful that the variance, σ^2, is correct for the differenced data (i.e., the deltas).

Example 8.11 Take the situation of Example 8.8 again, but this time suppose that the *same* individuals are to be sampled in the two years. The data are now paired and we should apply (8.6). Suppose that the standard deviation of the *increase* in cholesterol is known to be 1.0 mmol/l. Then, taking all else as in Example 8.8, (8.6) gives

$$n = \frac{(1.6449 + 1.6449)^2 (1.0)^2}{(0.5)^2} = 43.29,$$

which is rounded up to 44. Here, $S = 0.5/1.0 = 0.5$ and the answer may be obtained directly from Table B.7.

Notice that the sample size requirement of 44 in Example 8.11 is well below that of 170 (per sample) in the unpaired case (Example 8.8). Provided that the correlation between the 'before' and 'after' measurements is high and positive (as is likely in practice), pairing will give a considerable saving in sample numbers. However, there may be costs elsewhere. In Example 8.11, it may be difficult to keep track of the 44 individuals over the 10-year period. Furthermore, bias error may also be present because the individuals concerned may be more health conscious simply by virtue of being studied. This may lead them to (say) consume less saturated fat than other members of the population.

In the paired situation, (8.2) or (8.9) may be used to find power or minimum detectable difference, correcting for two-sided tests (when necessary) as usual.

Sometimes no data can be found from which to calculate the standard deviation of the differences, and so (8.2), (8.6), (8.7) and (8.9) cannot be used. However, in these cases it may be possible to find, from past publications in medical journals, estimates of the standard deviation in each arm of the paired comparison and the correlation (Section 9.3.2) between the values in each arm. An alternative approach to sample size issues with paired means, implemented by PROC POWER in SAS, uses such data.

8.5 Testing a proportion

All of our discussion about sample size requirements so far has been concerned with mean values. Similar formulae may be derived to deal with hypothesis tests for proportions by using a normal approximation to the binomial distribution that naturally arises, assuming independent outcomes. In this section, we will consider the one-sample situation.

Here the problem is to test the hypotheses

$$H_0 : \pi = \pi_0$$

$$H_1 : \pi = \pi_1 = \pi_0 + d,$$

where π is the true proportion; π_0 is some specified value for this proportion for which we wish to test; and π_1 (which differs from π_0 by an amount d) is the alternative value, which we would like to identify correctly with a probability (power) of $1 - \beta$. For one-sided tests, $\pi_1 < \pi_0$ or $\pi_1 > \pi_0$ ($d < 0$ or $d > 0$) and for two-sided tests $\pi_1 \neq \pi_0$ ($d \neq 0$). Applying the power calculation method outlined in Section 8.2 and Section 8.3 gives the result (assuming a $100\alpha\%$ significance test is used):

$$n = \frac{1}{d^2} \left(z_\alpha \sqrt{\pi_0(1-\pi_0)} + z_\beta \sqrt{\pi_1(1-\pi_1)} \right)^2 \tag{8.13}$$

for a one-sided test. Replace z_α by $z_{\alpha/2}$ for a two-sided test. Power can be derived from

$$z_\beta = \frac{d\sqrt{n} - z_\alpha \sqrt{\pi_0(1-\pi_0)}}{\sqrt{\pi_1(1-\pi_1)}}.$$

Example 8.12 Suppose that, in a country where male smoking has been extremely common in recent years, a government target has been to reduce the prevalence of male smoking to, at most, 30%. A sample survey is planned to test, at the 5% level, the hypothesis that the proportion of smokers in the male population is 0.3 against the one-sided alternative that it is greater. The test should be able to find a prevalence of 32%, when it is true, with 90% power.

In this problem, $\pi_0 = 0.30$ and $\pi_1 = 0.32$; hence, $d = 0.02$. For 5% significance (in a one-sided test) and 90% power, $z_\alpha = 1.6449$ and $z_\beta = 1.2816$ from Table 8.1. Hence, by (8.13),

$$n = \frac{1}{(0.02)^2} \left\{ 1.6449\sqrt{(0.3)(0.7)} + 1.2816\sqrt{(0.32)(0.68)} \right\}^2 = 4567.2.$$

Thus, with rounding, 4568 should be sampled.

Notice that the sample size required in the last example is in the thousands. This is not uncommon in problems concerned with proportions, which typically require much larger sample sizes than problems concerned with means.

8.5.1   Using a table of sample sizes

Example 8.12 could also be solved using Table B.8(a). In this table, the answer 4567 appears in the fourth column of the second row. The difference (of one) is due to rounding error. Notice, from this table, that the values for n increase as π_0 (the null hypothesis value) approaches 0.5 from either side. Also, as in Table B.7, n increases as the difference to be detected, d, decreases.

8.6   Testing a relative risk

Consider, now, a two-sample problem in which the outcomes to be compared are proportions. The hypotheses to be tested may be written as

$$H_0 : \pi_1 = \pi_2$$

$$H_1 : \pi_1 - \pi_2 = \delta$$

for some specified δ, where π_1 and π_2 are the two population proportions. As in Section 3.1, it is usually more convenient to consider the relative risk, the ratio of π_1 to π_2, rather than the difference $\pi_1 - \pi_2$. Hence, we will consider instead,

$$H_0 : \pi_1 = \pi_2$$

$$H_1 : \pi_1/\pi_2 = \lambda.$$

Here, group 2 will be the reference group because it is the denominator for the relative risk. For one-sided tests, $\lambda < 1$ or $\lambda > 1$ and for two-sided tests, $\lambda \neq 1$. Notice that, should we prefer to formulate the alternative hypothesis as a difference rather than a ratio (Section 3.9), we can easily calculate λ as $\lambda = 1 + (\delta/\pi_2)$ and then proceed as below.

Problems of comparing proportions may arise in cohort studies, cross-sectional surveys and intervention studies. The methods discussed in this section are applicable in all such studies. Although a case-control study would also normally seek to compare two proportions, the equations given in this section would not be appropriate because of the special sampling design used (Section 8.7).

Using the power calculation method and adopting the notation of previous sections (including $r = n_1/n_2$), the total sample size requirement ($n_1 + n_2$) for a one-sided test turns out to be

$$n = \frac{r+1}{r(\lambda-1)^2 \pi^2} \left[z_\alpha \sqrt{(r+1)p_c(1-p_c)} + z_\beta \sqrt{\lambda\pi(1-\lambda\pi) + r\pi(1-\pi)} \right]^2, \qquad (8.14)$$

where $\pi = \pi_2$ is the proportion in the reference group and p_c is the common proportion over the two groups, which is estimated from (2.7) as

$$p_c = \frac{\pi(r\lambda+1)}{r+1}. \qquad (8.15)$$

When $r = 1$ (equal-sized groups), (8.15) reduces to

$$p_c = \frac{\pi(\lambda+1)}{2} = \frac{\pi_1 + \pi_2}{2},$$

the arithmetic mean of the two separate proportions (under H_1). Replace z_α by $z_{\alpha/2}$ for a two-sided test.

Notice that n depends upon $\pi = \pi_2$, the true proportion in the reference group. In general, this will not be known but will be estimated from past experience.

Example 8.13 A cohort study of smoking and coronary heart disease (CHD) amongst middle-aged men is planned. A sample of men will be selected at random from the population and asked to complete a questionnaire. Subsequently, they will be monitored to record ill health and death. The investigators wish to submit their results for publication after 5 years, at which point they would like to be 90% sure of being able to detect when the relative risk for CHD is 1.4 (smoking : not), using a one-sided 5% significance test. Previous evidence (Doll and Peto, 1976) suggests that non-smokers have an average annual death rate from CHD of 413 per 100 000 per year. Assuming that equal numbers of smokers and nonsmokers are to be sampled, how many should be sampled overall?

Over a 5-year period the estimated chance of death is $5 \times 413/100000 = 0.02065$. This gives the value for π. The relative risk to be detected, λ, is 1.4, $z_\alpha = 1.6449$ and $z_\beta = 1.2816$ (from Table 8.1). We are assuming that the sample ratio, r, is unity. Then we must first use (8.15) to obtain

$$p_c = \frac{(0.02065)(2.4)}{2} = 0.02478.$$

Notice here that $\lambda\pi = 0.02891$ and that p_c is the arithmetic mean of π and $\lambda\pi$ as it should be, because $r = 1$. Then by (8.14),

$$n = \frac{2}{0.4^2 \times 0.02065^2}\left[1.6449\sqrt{2 \times 0.02478 \times 0.97522}\right.$$
$$\left. + 1.2816\sqrt{0.02891 \times 0.97109 + 0.02065 \times 0.97935}\right]^2 = 12130.16.$$

Thus, rounding up to the next highest even number, 12 132 men should be sampled (6066 smokers and 6066 nonsmokers).

In practice, the procedure assumed in the last example would be difficult to follow precisely because we have no way of knowing, in advance, whether a prospective sample recruit is a smoker or non-smoker. If, for example, one-third of all men in the population smoke, then we would expect to have to sample $6066 \times 3 = 18\,198$ men before arriving at a sample containing 6066 smokers. The excess number of nonsmokers could simply be rejected, although it may be more sensible to retain them in the sample, once questioned. A better approach is to allow for the expected imbalance through the parameter r, as the next example shows.

Example 8.14 If the proportion of men smoking is one-third, then in a random sample we would expect to find $n_1 = n/3$. Hence $n_2 = 2n/3$ and thus $r = n_1/n_2 = 0.5$. Using this new value for r in (8.14) and (8.15) for Example 8.13 gives

$$p_c = \frac{0.02065(0.5 \times 1.4 + 1)}{1.5} = 0.02340$$

$$n = \frac{1.5}{0.5 \times 0.4^2 \times 0.02065^2}\left[1.6449\sqrt{1.5 \times 0.02340 \times 0.97660}\right.$$
$$\left. + 1.2816\sqrt{0.02891 \times 0.97109 + 0.5 \times 0.02065 \times 0.97935}\right]^2$$

$$= 13543.30.$$

Rounding up gives a total sample size requirement of 13 544. We would expect that, after sampling, about a third of these would be nonsmokers. Notice that 13 544 is not exactly divisible by 3, but any further rounding up would not be justifiable because we cannot guarantee the exact proportion of smokers.

When we wish to make inferences about relative risks, and related quantities, the number of events that we will observe drives the accuracy of the results more than the number at risk, in the sense that adding one more person at risk will make less difference to the power than adding one more event. The number of events is implicitly included in the formulae here, as the numerator of the proportion of events, π, in the reference group; for example, in (8.14). In certain situations the number of events may be treated as the main parameter, rather than the sample size. It may even make sense to design the study to last until a certain number of events have been observed.

8.6.1   Using a table of sample sizes

Table B.9 gives values for the overall sample size when equal numbers are allocated to each group ($r = 1$). Although unequal allocation is not uncommon, equal allocation is by far the most usual, especially in intervention studies.

Example 8.15 At a smoking cessation clinic, the failure rate for the standard method of therapy used is 20%. Trials of a new method of helping smokers to quit are to be carried out, and the investigator concerned has specified that he wishes to detect when the new method has 40% of the chance of failure that the standard method has, with a probability of 0.90. If a two-sided 5% significance test is used with equal allocation to 'standard' and 'new' methods, what sample size is required?

Here $\pi = 0.20$ and $\lambda = 0.40$. This relative risk is to be detected with 90% power using a two-sided 5% test, so that Table B.9(c) is appropriate (treating as a one-sided $2\frac{1}{2}$% test). The sample size required is 342 (171 in each treatment group). Approximately the same result comes from (8.14).

Figure 8.6 shows how n varies when the relative risk that is to be detected with 90% power varies between 0.6 and 0.9 in the context of the preceding example. The shape of the curve is similar to that of Figure 8.5, but with two differences. First, the curve here looks like the mirror image of the previous one because now we are considering alternative hypotheses that specify reductions, rather than increases, compared against the null.

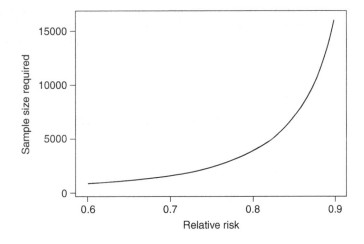

Figure 8.6. Sample size against relative risk to be detected for Example 8.15.

Second, the values for n are considerably bigger. As with single-sample tests for proportions, large numbers are required to detect small differences between proportions (that is, relative risks close to unity). This is also obvious from study of Table B.9.

In the literature there are several alternatives to (8.14), including simplifications and potential improvements. The latter group includes Casagrande et al. (1978), who use Fisher's exact test. See Fleiss et al. (2003) for a review.

8.6.2 Power and minimum detectable relative risk

A formula for z_β (and hence power) is easily derived from (8.14) to be

$$z_\beta = \frac{\pi(\lambda-1)\sqrt{nr} - z_\alpha(r+1)\sqrt{p_c(1-p_c)}}{\sqrt{(r+1)(\lambda\pi(1-\lambda\pi)+r\pi(1-\pi))}}$$

when $\lambda > 1$. If $\lambda < 1$, simply replace $\lambda - 1$ by $1 - \lambda$ in the leading term in the numerator. We cannot, however, invert (8.14) to provide a formula for the minimum detectable relative risk, λ. Instead, we can use an approximate method. This derives from the simplification to (8.14) used by Pocock (1983). The approximate value for λ turns out to be

$$\lambda \simeq \frac{1}{2a}\left[b \pm \sqrt{b^2 - 4ac}\right], \tag{8.16}$$

where

$$a = Y + \pi Z$$
$$b = 2Y + Z$$
$$c = Y - r(1 - \pi)Z,$$

in which

$$Y = rn\pi^2$$
$$Z = (r + 1)\pi(z_\alpha + z_\beta)^2.$$

This formula should be reasonably accurate when $r = 1$ but may be in considerable error when r is very large or very small (Woodward, 1992).

Example 8.16 Consider the cohort study of Example 8.13. Suppose that the investigators decide that they can afford a sample size of 12132, but no more. What is the minimum relative risk that they can expect to be able to detect with 90% power (all else as before)?

We know from Example 8.13 that the answer should be about 1.4. Using (8.16), we do indeed get $\lambda = 1.4$. This arises from

$$Y = 12132 \times 0.02065^2 = 5.1734,$$

$$Z = 2 \times 0.02065(1.6449 + 1.2816)^2 = 0.35371,$$

$$a = 5.1734 + 0.02065 \times 0.35371 = 5.1807,$$

$$b = 2 \times 5.1734 + 0.35371 = 10.7005,$$

$$c = 5.1734 - (1 - 0.02065)0.35371 = 4.8270$$

$$\lambda \simeq \frac{10.7005 \pm \sqrt{10.7005^2 - 4 \times 5.1807 \times 4.8270}}{2 \times 5.1734}$$

$$= 1.40 \text{ (taking the positive root)}.$$

Note that the negative root gives a value below unity. If we were dealing with a potentially protective factor, this would be the result of interest.

8.7   Case–control studies

A case–control study typically aims to compare the disease incidence or prevalence between two groups: those exposed to some risk factor of interest and those not exposed. Hence, the aim will be to test the hypotheses

$$H_0 : \pi_1 = \pi_2$$

$$H_1 : \pi_1/\pi_2 = \lambda$$

where the probabilities π_1 and π_2 are explicitly,

$$\pi_1 = p\left(\text{Disease}|\text{Exposed}\right)$$

$$\pi_2 = p\left(\text{Disease}|\text{Not exposed}\right),$$

and λ is, as usual, the relative risk; as in Section 8.2. As earlier, the vertical bar is read as 'given'; π_1 is thus 'the probability of disease given exposure to the risk factor'.

This is exactly the same formulation of hypotheses as in Section 8.6, with one crucial difference: here, we cannot test H_0 directly because we have no means of estimating either π_1 or π_2. This is due to the design of the case–control study, which does not allow for such estimation (Section 6.2.1). Instead, what we can do is to test the hypotheses

$$H_0^* : \pi_1^* = \pi_2^*$$

$$H_1^* : \pi_1^*/\pi_2^* = \lambda^*$$

where
$$\pi_1^* = p(\text{Exposed}|\text{Disease}) = p(\text{Exposed}|\text{Case}),$$
$$\pi_2^* = p(\text{Exposed}|\text{No disease}) = p(\text{Exposed}|\text{Control})$$

(assuming no bias), because the case–control study samples from the populations of those diseased and those not diseased. The outcome of the analysis is now exposure rather than disease.

We are not interested in the items involved in H_0^* and H_1^*, but luckily π_1^* and π_2^* turn out to have simple expressions in terms of λ (which is what we *are* interested in) and $P = p(\text{Exposure})$, the prevalence of the risk factor. Using a theorem of probability known as Bayes' theorem (Clarke and Cooke, 2004), we obtain

$$\pi_1^* = \frac{\lambda P}{1 + (\lambda - 1)P}$$

and

$$\pi_2^* \simeq P. \tag{8.17}$$

Thus we have

$$\lambda^* \simeq \frac{\lambda}{1 + (\lambda - 1)P}. \tag{8.18}$$

Approximation (8.17) will be good if the disease is rare amongst those exposed to the risk factor (and amongst the population in general). It is an exact result if the null hypothesis ($H_0 : \pi_1 = \pi_2$) is true. See Schlesselman (1974) or Woodward (1992) for details.

Using (8.17) and (8.18) in (8.14) and (8.15), for the test of H_0^* against H_1^*, gives

$$n = \frac{(r+1)(1 + (\lambda-1)P)^2}{rP^2(P-1)^2(\lambda-1)^2} \left[z_\alpha \sqrt{(r+1)p_c^*(1-p_c^*)} \right.$$
$$\left. + z_\beta \sqrt{\frac{\lambda P(1-P)}{[1 + (\lambda-1)P]^2} + rP(1-P)} \right]^2 \tag{8.19}$$

where

$$p_c^* = \frac{P}{r+1} \left(\frac{r\lambda}{1 + (\lambda-1)P} + 1 \right) \tag{8.20}$$

for a one-sided test. As usual, replace z_α by $z_{\alpha/2}$ for a two-sided test. Notice that the sample size depends upon P, the population exposure prevalence, λ, the relative risk that it is important to detect and r, the case : control ratio. As we have seen (in Section 6.2.1), a case–control study can only estimate the odds ratio. The approximation used in (8.17) ensures that the odds ratio is a good approximation to the relative risk. Hence, strictly we are considering the sample size needed to detect an *approximate* relative risk in a case–control study.

Example 8.17 A case–control study of the relationship between smoking and CHD is planned. A sample of men with newly diagnosed CHD will be compared for smoking status (smoker/non-smoker) with a sample of controls. Assuming an equal number of cases and controls, how many are needed to detect an approximate relative risk of 2.0 with 90% power using a two-sided 5% test? Government surveys have estimated that 30% of the male population are smokers.

Here $P = 0.3$, $r = 1$, $\lambda = 2$, $z_{\alpha/2} = 1.96$ and $z_\beta = 1.2816$ (see Table 8.1). Substituting into (8.20) gives

$$p_c^* = \frac{0.3}{2} \left(\frac{2}{1 + 0.3} + 1 \right) = 0.3808.$$

Then, by (8.19),

$$n = \frac{(2)(1.3)^2}{(0.3)^2(-0.7)^2}\left[1.96\sqrt{(2)(0.3808)(0.6192)} + 1.2816\sqrt{\frac{(2)(0.3)(0.7)}{(1.3)^2} + (0.3)(0.7)}\right]^2$$

$$= 375.6.$$

So we should take 188 cases and 188 controls — that is, 376 individuals in all.

8.7.1   Using a table of sample sizes

The result of the last example may be obtained more easily from Table B.10. Here, we need Table B.10(c), 5th column and 17th row to obtain the result. Schlesselman (1982) gives a comprehensive collection of tables for use in calculating sample size for case–control studies.

8.7.2   Power and minimum detectable relative risk

A formula for z_β is easily derived from (8.19). First calculate

$$M = \left|\frac{(\lambda-1)(P-1)}{1+(\lambda-1)P}\right|. \tag{8.21}$$

Then

$$z_\beta = \frac{\dfrac{MP\sqrt{nr}}{\sqrt{r+1}} - z_\alpha\sqrt{(r+1)p_c^*\left(1-p_c^*\right)}}{\sqrt{\dfrac{\lambda P(1-P)}{\left[1+(\lambda-1)P\right]^2} + rP(1-P)}}, \tag{8.22}$$

from which we may calculate the power. As in Section 8.6, we cannot invert (8.19) directly to get an expression for λ. Instead, we can use a similar argument to that which gave rise to (8.16) and thus obtain an approximate result,

$$\lambda \simeq 1 + \frac{-b \pm \sqrt{b^2 - 4a(r+1)}}{2a},$$

where

$$a = rP^2 - \frac{nrP(1-P)}{\left(z_\alpha + z_\beta\right)^2(r+1)}$$

$$b = 1 + 2rP.$$

Example 8.18 In the situation of Example 8.17, suppose that we wish to find the power to detect an approximate relative risk of 2 using a two-sided 5% test when 188 cases and 940 controls are available (a 1 : 5 case : control ratio). Assume a 30% prevalence of smoking once more.

Here, $P = 0.3$, $\lambda = 2$, $z_{\alpha/2} = 1.96$, $n = 188 + 940 = 1128$ and $r = 188/940 = 0.2$. Substituting into (8.21),

$$M = \left| \frac{(2-1)(0.3-1)}{1+(2-1)0.3} \right| = \left| -0.5385 \right| = 0.5385.$$

Also, from (8.20),

$$p_c^* = \frac{0.3}{(0.2+1)} \left(\frac{0.2 \times 2}{1 + (2-1)0.3} + 1 \right) = 0.3269.$$

With these results, (8.22) becomes

$$z_\beta = \frac{\dfrac{0.5385 \times 0.3\sqrt{1128 \times 0.2}}{\sqrt{0.2+1}} - 1.96\sqrt{(0.2+1)0.3269 \times 0.6731}}{\sqrt{\dfrac{2 \times 0.3 \times 0.7}{[1+(2-1)0.3]^2} + 0.2 \times 0.3 \times 0.7}} = 2.24.$$

From Table B.1, we see that the probability of a standard normal value below 2.24 is about 0.987. Hence, the power of the test, with the given sample size allocation, is approximately 99%.

The result of Example 8.18 is included in Figure 6.2. We saw there that the power increases, but with a diminishing rate of return, as the number of controls increases, given a fixed number of cases.

To complete the interpretation, consider varying the allocation ratio, r, keeping the *overall* sample size fixed. That is the situation in which we anticipate being able to interview only so many people, but we wish to consider how many of these should be taken from the available cases (assuming a large supply). Figure 8.7 shows the

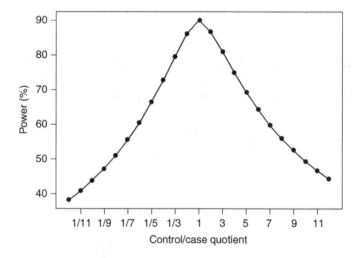

Figure 8.7. Power against control/case quotient. This shows the power to detect an approximate relative risk of 2 when the risk factor has a prevalence of 30%, a two-sided 5% significance test is to be used and the overall sample size (cases plus controls) is fixed at 376.

result within the context of Example 8.17, taking the overall sample size to be fixed at 376. Note that r is the reciprocal of the control/case quotient shown in Figure 8.7 (which is used for compatibility with Figure 6.2). Figure 8.7 illustrates situations in which the number of cases is an integer multiple of the number of controls (very unlikely in practice) or the number of controls is an integer multiple of the number of cases. The integers used are from 1 to 12.

As suggested in Section 8.4.3, Figure 8.7 shows that optimum allocation (maximum power) occurs where $r = 1$ (equal allocation). When the number of cases is fixed, we can always do better by recruiting more controls; however, when the overall number of cases plus controls is fixed, we cannot do better than to use equal allocation (compare Figure 6.2 with Figure 8.7).

8.7.3 Comparison with cohort studies

In most practical situations, a case–control study requires a much smaller sample size than does a cohort study for the same problem. Consider, for example, a cohort study for the smoking and CHD problem of Example 8.17, such as that described in Example 8.13. To be able to calculate an equivalent value for n in a cohort study, we need an estimate of π, the chance of a coronary event (morbid or mortal) amongst nonsmokers. Let us suppose that the cohort study is to last 10 years, and for this period π is estimated from a previous study to be 0.09. Notice that P, the prevalence of smoking, does not affect the value for n in a cohort study. Conversely, π does not affect the value for n in a case–control study.

Table 8.2 compares n for the two study designs over a range of values for the relative risk (or at least its approximate value from a case–control study). This illustrates the great advantage, in terms of sample size requirements, of a case-control study when the relative risk to be detected is small. In fact, coronary disease is not as rare as many diseases that are the subject of case–control studies. As Schlesselman (1974) shows, there are even greater savings with very rare diseases.

8.7.4 Matched studies

As discussed in Section 6.5, matching can improve the efficiency of a case–control study; in other words, we may be able to detect the same approximate relative risk

Table 8.2. Sample size requirements to detect a given relative risk with 90% power using two-sided 5% significance tests for cohort and case–control studies.

Relative risk	Cohort study[a]	Case–control study[b]
1.1	44 398	21 632
1.2	11 568	5 820
1.3	5 346	2 774
1.4	3 122	1 668
1.5	2 070	1 138
2.0	602	376
3.0	188	146

[a] Using (8.14), assuming an incidence of 0.09 for the nonfactor group.
[b] Using (8.19), assuming a prevalence of 0.3 for the risk factor.

with the same power using rather fewer subjects. In this case, the sample size for an unmatched study acts as an upper limit for the matched sample size. However, unfortunately this is not always true because the matched study must discard any concordant sets (Section 6.6). In a matched study in which the number of concordant sets is very large, we could even find a larger sample size requirement under matching. In addition, matching may require several potential controls to be rejected due to lack of matching properties. This is, in a sense, a component of sample size, although we shall not consider it further here.

For paired (1 : 1 matched) studies, we saw, in Section 6.6.1, that the test of the null hypothesis $\psi = 1$ is the same as the test of $\phi = 0.5$, where ϕ is the proportion of discordant pairs that have an exposed case. It will be simple to deal with ϕ because this is a single proportion, as already analysed in Section 8.5. The relationship between ψ and ϕ is given by (6.9), $\psi = \phi/(1 - \phi)$. Let the alternative hypothesis be that the approximate relative risk is λ. Taking the odds ratio as this approximate relative risk and using (6.9), under H_1, $\phi = \lambda/(1 + \lambda)$. Hence, to test for the usual null hypothesis of no effect against the alternative that the approximate relative risk is λ, we, instead, can test $H_0 : \phi = 0.5$ versus $H_1 : \phi = \lambda/(1 + \lambda)$. This is the form of hypotheses assumed in Section 8.5 where $\pi_0 = 0.5$ and $\pi_1 = \lambda/(1 + \lambda)$ and hence

$$d = \pi_1 - \pi_0 = \frac{\lambda}{1 + \lambda} - \frac{1}{2} = \frac{\lambda - 1}{2(\lambda + 1)}.$$

Substituting these results into (8.13) gives

$$d_p = \frac{\left[z_\alpha(\lambda + 1) + 2z_\beta\sqrt{\lambda} \right]^2}{(\lambda - 1)^2}. \tag{8.23}$$

This result is labelled d_p, rather than n, with the notation of Section 6.6.1 in mind, because it tells us the number of discordant pairs required. When sampling for the pair-matched case–control study, the total sample size shall include concordant pairs as well. Let the probability of a discordant pair be π_d and let n_p be the total number of pairs sampled. Then $\pi_d = d_p/n_p$ and thus $n_p = d_p/\pi_d$. The total sample size is thus

$$n = 2d_p \big/ \pi_d. \tag{8.24}$$

We can substitute (8.23) into (8.24) to arrive at the required sample size, provided we know π_d or can at least find a reasonable estimate of it. The problem is that the chance of a discordant pair is rarely known, to any reasonable degree of approximation, before the study begins. The exception is when the results of a similar, paired study are available. Contrast this with the situation in an unmatched study when we only need an estimate of the prevalence of the risk factor, which is often easily obtained, perhaps from publications of the national statistics office.

Some accounts of this topic avoid the problem by assuming approximate independence to exposure within matched pairs, but this is unlikely to be true in practice. More useful suggestions involve alternative formulations that require estimation of some unknown parameter concerned with matching (Fleiss and Levin, 1988). For instance, Donner and Li (1990) give a formulation that depends upon the value of Cohen's kappa (Section 2.9.2) for the members of matched pairs.

Example 8.19 Consider Example 8.17 again, but this time suppose that a matched 1 : 1 case–control study is envisaged. A previous study has suggested that the chance of a discordant pair is about 0.5. Assuming that, as before, an approximate relative risk of 2 is to be found with 90% power using a two-sided 5% test, (8.23) gives

$$d_p = \frac{\left[1.96(2 + 1) + 2 \times 1.2816\sqrt{2}\right]^2}{(2 - 1)^2} = 90.34.$$

Substituting this into (8.24) gives

$$n = 2 \times 90.34/0.5 = 361.4.$$

Hence, after rounding up, 362 individuals are required — that is, 181 matched pairs. This gives a saving of 14 compared with the unmatched version of Example 8.17.

For 1 : *c* matched studies, an approximate result for the total sample size is

$$n_c = \frac{(c + 1)^2}{4c} n \tag{8.25}$$

where n is as given by (8.24) for the paired situation. To see the relationship between the number of matched 1 : *c* sets, s_c, and the number of matched pairs, s_1, keeping type I error and power fixed, note that $s_1 = n/2$ and s_c = number of cases amongst the n_c people = $n_c/(c + 1)$. Hence,

$$s_c = \frac{c + 1}{2c} s_1. \tag{8.26}$$

Since the basic unit of observation in a matched study is the matched set (Section 6.6 and Section 10.12.2), it is not surprising to find that (8.26) is the result of Ury's measure of relative efficiency when comparing one to *c* matched controls (Section 6.5.3).

Example 8.20 In Example 8.19, we estimated that 361.4 subjects would be required to satisfy the requirements of the paired study. If, instead, a 1 : 3 matched study was envisaged, this would require, from (8.25), approximately

$$n_3 = \frac{(3 + 1)^2}{4 \times 3} \times 361.4 = 481.9,$$

rounded to 484 (the next highest multiple of $c + 1 = 4$), subjects. Since a quarter of these would be cases, we should need to recruit 121 cases and thus 363 controls. Note that the 181 pairs required in Example 8.19 has become 121 matched 1 : 3 sets here; this difference agrees with the result of (8.26):

$$\frac{4}{2 \times 3} \times 181 = 121$$

to the nearest whole number.

In Example 8.19, 181 cases and 181 controls were required, giving 362 in all. When the matching fraction is tripled, 60 fewer cases are required but 182 more controls, to achieve the same power. If cases are expensive to obtain, but controls are plentiful, this may well be worthwhile. However, the overall sample size has increased by $484 - 362 = 122$, so the paired study will be a better option if cases and controls are each in adequate supply and equally expensive to deal with.

For a discussion of sample size in case–control studies with variable matching fractions, see Walter (1980b). Note that (8.25) may also be applied to unmatched studies in which it generally provides an excellent approximation, for the relative sample sizes when there are c and 1 controls, to the 'exact' result obtainable from double use of (8.19).

8.8 Complex sampling designs

As discussed in Section 1.8.2, samples are sometimes drawn using stratification and/or clustering, in which case a **complex sampling design** has been used. This has a fundamental effect on sample size requirements, compared with the situation assumed throughout most of this chapter (and, indeed, the book), simple random sampling. Although a full discussion is beyond the scope of this book, note that we should expect sensible stratification to decrease the required sample size, but clustering to increase it, to maintain the same power.

Survey statisticians define the **design effect** (usually denoted 'deff') to be the ratio of the variance of an estimate derived from a complex sampling design to the variance of an estimate of the same thing derived from a simple random sample of the same size. This can be used as a factor for weighting up the sample size. That is, we calculate the sample size from the equations given earlier in this chapter (for simple random sampling) and multiply this by deff to obtain the sample size for the complex design. Formulae for deff for particular complex sampling designs are available from textbooks on sample survey methods, such as Cochran (1977).

As an example, we shall look at one such design here, the cluster design in which the number of individuals per cluster is constant. For instance, in Example 8.1 it could be that the 50 men were drawn using a cluster sample design with 10 men from each of five provinces (provinces are then the clusters). In this situation, an approximate result when there are many clusters is:

$$\text{deff} = 1 + (m - 1)\rho_{\text{icc}} \qquad (8.27)$$

where m is the number of individuals per cluster and ρ_{icc} is the **intracluster correlation coefficient**, which is the correlation between pairs of subjects in the same cluster. The general concept of correlation is discussed in Section 9.3.2. As long as we have an idea of the likely value for ρ_{icc}, perhaps from previous studies, we can derive the required sample size by multiplying the equivalent sample size for a simple random sample by the result of (8.27). An estimate of ρ_{icc}, using data from a previous study, may be obtained by a one-way analysis of variance (Section 9.2.2), where the groups are the clusters, as

$$\rho_{\text{icc}} = \frac{MSB - MSW}{MSB + (m-1)MSW}. \qquad (8.28)$$

Here MSB is the between-cluster mean square and MSW is the within-cluster mean square. Note that we would require this previous study to have clusters that may reasonably be assumed to be similar in terms of internal variability. This is unlikely if they were, for instance, much smaller (or larger) geographical units than in the study being designed (ρ_{icc} is likely to decrease with size, as the individuals get further apart). If the number per cluster varies a moderate amount, we might replace m by the mean number per cluster in (8.27). Unfortunately, other definitions of the sample intracluster correlation coefficient exist besides (8.28) (Muller and Buttner, 1994), and this sometimes leads to confusion.

The preceding paragraph is relevant when a cluster randomised trial (Section 7.4.2) is being designed. Several authors have explored the sample size problem for such trial designs in more detail than here, such as Reading et al. (2000), who modify (8.27) to allow for variations in cluster sizes. Campbell et al. (2001) includes a review. It is clear, from (8.27), that small values of ρ_{icc} have a huge impact on sample size even when m is small. For instance, the overall sample size is virtually doubled, compared with trials randomised at the individual level, when we choose 20 individuals from each cluster for an intracluster correlation coefficient of only 0.05, which is often the kind of level one sees in real life.

In an exploration of the effects of cluster randomisation in a general practice (primary care) setting, Campbell et al. (2000) show how total sample size (and thus number of practices) required varies with ρ_{icc} (varied between 0.01 and 0.15) and the number of individuals recruited per practice. For the most extreme realistic example they consider (cluster randomisation with 100 patients per practice and $\rho_{icc} = 0.15$), the total sample size was about 3200, compared with just below 200 for individual randomisation, taking the same power and other requirements, showing the potentially huge impact of clustering upon sample size.

8.9   Concluding remarks

This chapter provides a set of equations that give approximate sample size requirements in the most straightforward situations that arise in epidemiological research. The one common requirement in each section of this chapter is for the epidemiologist to specify the difference, or sometimes relative risk, that she or he wishes to be able to detect with some high probability (usually 0.90 or 0.95). This requires careful thought. Often the researcher will begin by being overoptimistic, specifying a difference so small that it requires an enormous sample to have a good chance of detecting it. Usually the value ultimately decided upon is some compromise between various objectives, including conserving resources. The ultimate decision may only be obtained after a few trial calculations. In this context, the 'inverse' formulae for power and minimum detectable difference (relative risk) included in this chapter may well be useful. It is quite possible that the value for n needed to be able to detect the difference that we would really like to find with high probability is beyond our resources. This problem has no easy solution: we must find more resources or accept reduced power.

Throughout, we have assumed that sample size may be determined by considering only one variable of interest. Frequently, the subsequent dataset will include several variables; for instance, we might be planning a lifestyle survey that will measure height, weight, blood pressure, cholesterol, daily cigarette consumption and several other things. We might well find that the optimal value of n for analysing height, say, is considerably different from that for analysing cholesterol. Similarly, there could be several end-points of interest in the subsequent dataset; for example, the cohort phase of the Scottish Heart Health Study recorded coronary events as well as deaths from all causes (Section 5.1.3).

If there are multiple criteria, the value for n might be calculated for each criterion. The maximum of all these gives the value for n that satisfies all requirements. This will often be far more than is needed for some of the criteria and hence may be considered too wasteful. An alternative approach is to pick the most important criterion and use this alone. Thus, if the effect of cholesterol on coronary death is considered to be the most crucial question in the lifestyle survey, we would determine n from considering this relationship alone.

A limitation with the equations provided in this chapter is that they make no allowance for confounding variables. That is, they consider only unadjusted comparisons. In general, the issue of allowing for confounding in sample size estimation is complex (Haneuse et al., 2012). However, a simple approximate method (Hsieh et al., 1998) is to take the sample size for the unadjusted formulae given in this chapter and multiply by $1/(1 - R^2)$, where R^2 is the coefficient of determination from a regression model (Section 9.7) which regresses the index variable on the confounders. The degree of error in this approximation is considered by Schoenfeld and Borenstein (2005).

We should remember that the equations for sample size are based upon probabilities (through the power). There can be no absolute guarantee that the important difference will be detected, when it does exist, even with a very high power specification. All we can say is that we will run very little risk of missing it when we specify a high value for the power. The higher the power is, the less the risk. Sample size evaluation is not an exact science, even when some so-called exact methods are used, because assumptions made (such as normal distributions) may be violated by the data ultimately collected. Often we can regard the sample size computed only as a reasonable guide. Furthermore, if there is a strong possibility that some individuals will drop out before the end of the study (a common occurrence in cohort and intervention studies), then it would be wise to increase the nominal study size accordingly.

Exercises

8.1   Vitamin A supplementation is known to confer resistance to infectious diseases in developing countries, although the precise mechanism is unclear. To seek to explain the mechanism, a group of healthy children will be given vitamin A supplements for a long period. At baseline, and at the end of the supplementation period, urine samples will be taken from all the children and neopterin excretion measured. The current level of neopterin is estimated as 600 mmol per millomole of creatinine, and the standard deviation of change due to supplementation has been estimated (from a small pilot sample) to be 200 mmol/mmol creatinine.

   (i)   Suppose that a drop of 10% in neopterin is considered a meaningful difference, which it is wished to find with 95% power using a two-sided 1% test. How many children should be recruited?

   (ii)   Suppose that resources allow only 150 children to be given the supplements. What is the chance of detecting a drop of 10% in neopterin with a 1% two-sided test?

   (iii) If 150 children are recruited, what is the smallest percentage reduction in neopterin that we can expect to detect with 95% power using a 1% two-sided test?

8.2   Suppose that you decided to instigate a study to compare the mean body mass index (BMI) of smokers and nonsmokers. You plan to use a one-sided 5% significance test of the null hypothesis of no difference against the alternative that smokers have a lower BMI. From past experience the standard deviation of BMI values is known to be about 4 kg/m^2.

(i)   What sample size would you use to be 95% sure of detecting when smokers have a BMI that is 1 kg/m^2 lower (assuming an equal number of smokers and nonsmokers is recruited)?

(ii)   If resources allow only 600 subjects to be recruited, what is the anticipated power for detecting a difference of 1 kg/m^2 (assuming an equal number of smokers and nonsmokers)?

(iii) If 200 smokers and 400 nonsmokers were recruited, what would be the anticipated power for detecting a difference of 1 kg/m^2?

(iv)   Suppose, now, that an alternative type of study is envisaged. Subjects who intend to give up smoking are to be recruited and their BMI will be recorded before, and several years after, giving up. If the conditions of the test to be applied to the subsequent data are as in (i) (that is, a difference of 1 kg/m^2 is to be detected with 95% power using a 5% one-sided test), under what condition does this design require fewer BMI recordings to be made than does the design used in (i)? You should assume that no subjects are 'lost' over time.

8.3   In Example 8.13 and Example 8.14, one-sided tests were used, rather than the more usual two-sided test. How do the sample size requirements change if a two-sided test is used in each case?

8.4   Basnayake et al. (1983) proposed an intervention study to test the hypothesis that Sri Lankan women are more suited to low-dose oral contraceptives (OCs). Women were to be randomly allocated to use either Norinyl (a standard-dose OC) or Brevicon (a low-dose OC). The aim is to determine the percentage of women continuing to use their allocated OC 12 months after entering the study.

(i)   Suggest suitable inclusion and exclusion criteria for entering the study.

(ii)   Suppose that the investigators wish to be 90% sure of detecting when the percentage of women continuing with the contraceptive after 12 months is 10% higher in the Brevicon group than in the Norinyl group. The 12-month continuation percentage amongst Norinyl users in previous studies was found to be 55%. In this study, a two-sided 5% significance test will be used, with an equal number in each treatment group. How many women should be entered into the study (assuming no loss during follow-up)? How many should be entered if 5% can be expected to be lost to follow-up within 12 months?

(iii) Do you have any criticisms of using only the 12-month continuation percentage to compare the properties of the two OCs? State any other measures that you would wish to consider.

8.5   Researchers at a health promotions unit plan a study of the relationship between taking diuretics and falling amongst old people. They believe that diuretics may be a risk factor for falling because they reduce blood pressure. In their study, the researchers plan to get pharmacists, in chemist shops, to ask old people whether they have fallen in the past year at the time that they issue them prescribed medication. Two variables will be recorded for each elderly customer: whether she or he has received diuretics and whether she or he has experienced a serious fall in the past year, both with yes/no responses. Altogether, 2000 subjects will be recruited.

(i)   The researchers estimate that one third of elderly people not taking diuretics will have experienced a serious fall within the previous year. Estimate the power of the test, assuming equal numbers in each group, to detect when the chance of a serious fall is 20% higher amongst those who have received diuretics, using a two-sided 5% significance test.

(ii)   Discuss any problems that you foresee for the proposed study.

8.6   To investigate the health effects of coffee drinking, a research team plans to carry out an epidemiological study. Because coronary heart disease (CHD) is the leading cause of death within the population to be studied, this is chosen as the basis for the sample size calculation. It is known that the CHD incidence amongst noncoffee drinkers is 2.3 per 100 and that 40% of the population drink coffee (here taken as regular consumption of four or more cups per day).

Find the sample size required (assuming equal-sized groups) to carry out a two-sided 5% significance test of the null hypothesis of no association between coffee drinking and CHD, given that the team wish to be 95% sure of detecting whenever coffee drinking (at least approximately) doubles the risk of CHD, using:

(i)   a cohort study.

(ii)   an unmatched case–control study.

It is also known that the risk of a specific type of cancer amongst noncoffee drinkers is eight per thousand.

(iii)   How does the sample size requirement change in (i) and (ii) if the cancer is chosen as the basis for the sample size calculation instead of CHD (all else kept unchanged)?

8.7   An unmatched case–control study is to be carried out to ascertain the effect of occupation on the chance of testicular cancer. Cases are to be new referrals to a hospital in a particular area; controls will be recruited amongst patients in the same hospitals with any one of a number of prespecified acceptable diagnoses. Each subject will be interviewed, or his records will be consulted, to discover his current or last employment. The various types of employment recorded will subsequently be combined into a number of mutually exclusive groups. Odds ratios will be calculated to compare each occupation group (in turn) with all the rest combined. An odds ratio (approximate relative risk) of 2 is considered so important that it should not be missed when a two-sided 1% significance test is used. In the time available, the investigators anticipate recruiting 400 cases. If necessary, they estimate that they could recruit up to 1600 controls.

What is the power for detecting an odds ratio of 2 for occupation groups that (i) 5%, (ii) 10% and (iii) 20% of the national male adult population belong to, when equal numbers of cases and controls (400 of each) are used?

What are the equivalent results for occupation groups that (iv) 5%, (v) 10% and (vi) 20% belong to when all 1600 controls are used (together with the 400 cases)?

(vii)   From your results, what recommendations would you make for the design of the study?

8.8   Schlesselman (1974) describes an unmatched case–control study of conotruncal malformations in the baby and use of oral contraceptives by the mother. He assumes that 30% of all women use oral contraceptives, and that a 5%

two-sided test is to be used with equal numbers in the two groups. Since the values of the parameters are all the same as here, Example 8.17 shows that 376 subjects (188 cases and 188 controls) are needed to detect an odds ratio (approximate relative risk) of 2 with 90% power.

(i)   What is the smallest odds ratio greater than unity that one can expect to detect with 90% power using four times as many subjects (that is, 1504 subjects)?

(ii)   Keeping the total number of subjects as 1504, produce a plot of the power against the smallest detectable odds ratio, varying the latter between 1.30 and 1.50. Interpret your graph.

CHAPTER 9

Modelling quantitative outcome variables

9.1   Statistical models

A statistical model has, at its root, a mathematical representation of the relationship between one variable, called the **outcome** or **y variable**, and one or more **explanatory** or **x variable**. For example, in the problem of finding a relationship between a smoker's daily cigarette consumption and the blood nicotine of her or his nonsmoking spouse, y is the blood nicotine and x is the cigarette consumption.

Many models have the simple form,

$$y = \frac{\text{systematic}}{\text{component}} + \frac{\text{random}}{\text{error}},$$

where the systematic component (but not the random error) is a mathematical function of the explanatory variables. The first aim of a modelling procedure will be to estimate the systematic component. This is achieved by analysing data from several subjects (smokers and their spouses in our example). We then obtain **fitted** or **predicted values**, expressed (as with other estimates) using the 'hat' notation:

$$\hat{y} = \frac{\text{systematic}}{\text{component}}.$$

Fitted values can be used to make epidemiological statements about the apparent relationship between y and the other variable(s) — for example, a prediction of how much blood nicotine is derived, on average, from any specific number of cigarettes smoked by the spouse. These predictions will clearly be incorrect by the amount of random error. For example, passive smoking may take place at a different rate for different people, even when each is exposed to the same basic conditions, if only due to physiological differences.

It is crucial that the model fitting ensures that the left-over random component really is random, and does not contain any further systematic component that could be removed and incorporated within $\hat{y}$. For accurate predictions, we also require the random error to be small; to reduce it, we may need to take account of further explanatory variables in the systematic (explained) part of the model. For example, blood nicotine may also depend upon the strength of the cigarette smoked. Consequently post-fitting model checking is advised (Section 9.8).

In this chapter, we shall consider models for a quantitative outcome variable (such as the blood nicotine example). We shall assume, virtually throughout the chapter, that the random error has a normal probability distribution with zero mean and constant variance and that each individual data item is independent of all others. Some alternatives are discussed briefly in Section 9.11 and Section 9.12.

The models are generally classified into two types: analysis of variance (ANOVA) models, for which the explanatory variables are categorical; and regression models, for which the explanatory variables are quantitative. A common approach will be used, leading to the general linear model, which allows explanatory variables of either type (Section 9.6).

9.2   One categorical explanatory variable

Models with a solitary categorical explanatory variable are called **one-way ANOVA** models. It will be convenient to introduce them here in terms of hypothesis testing, although the estimation procedures that follow are generally more useful in practice.

9.2.1   The hypotheses to be tested

In Section 2.7.3 we saw how to use the t test to compare two means, where the null hypothesis is that the two population means are equal. The one-way ANOVA extends this to provide a test of the null hypothesis that ℓ means are equal (for $\ell \geq 2$). As with the pooled t test, the one-way ANOVA will assume that there is equal variance in each of the ℓ groups. A simple hypothetical example will be used to introduce the underlying concepts of the methodology.

Example 9.1 Suppose that a study of the effects of a diet lacking in meat has recruited six vegans, six lacto-vegetarians and six people with an unrestricted diet (omnivores). The data are presented in Table 9.1, and may be downloaded from the web site for this book (see Appendix A). There are three groups; the null hypothesis is

$$\mu_1 = \mu_2 = \mu_3,$$

where the subscript 1 is for omnivores, 2 for vegetarians and 3 for vegans and each μ denotes a population mean for cholesterol. The alternative hypothesis is that at least one of the means is different from the others.

Table 9.1. Data from a hypothetical study of the effect of diet, showing total serum cholesterol (mmol/l) by type of diet for 18 different people.

Subject no. (within group)	Diet group			
	Omnivores	Vegetarians	Vegans	Total
1	6.35	5.92	6.01	
2	6.47	6.03	5.42	
3	6.09	5.81	5.44	
4	6.37	6.07	5.82	
5	6.11	5.73	5.73	
6	6.50	6.11	5.62	
Total	37.89	35.67	34.04	107.60
Mean	6.32	5.95	5.67	5.98

In general, with ℓ groups, we write the hypotheses as

$$H_0 : \mu_1 = \mu_2 = \ ... \ = \mu_\ell$$

$$H_1 : \mu_i \neq \mu_k \ \text{ for some } i \text{ and } k.$$

9.2.2 Construction of the ANOVA table

In order to provide formulae for the one-way ANOVA, we shall need to introduce some mathematical notation. Even when the arithmetic will be done by a computer package, interpretation of the methodology and the results requires some insight into the underlying mathematical formulation.

Let y_{ij} be the outcome for the jth subject in the ith group. For instance, in Example 9.1 the cholesterol reading for the fourth subject in the vegan group (group 3) is $y_{34} = 5.82$, from Table 9.1. If we let $\bar{y}$ be the overall sample mean and $\bar{y}_i$ be the sample mean in group i, then we can equate each y_{ij} to a combination of $\bar{y}$ and $\bar{y}_i$ through

$$y_{ij} = \bar{y} + (\bar{y}_i - \bar{y}) + (y_{ij} - \bar{y}_i). \tag{9.1}$$

In words, (9.1) says

$$\text{observation} = \begin{array}{l} \text{overall} \\ \text{mean} \end{array} + \begin{array}{l} \text{difference between} \\ \text{specific and overall mean} \end{array}$$

$$+ \begin{array}{l} \text{difference between} \\ \text{observation and specific mean.} \end{array}$$

Removing the brackets and cancelling terms that are both added and subtracted on the right-hand side makes the truth of (9.1) obvious. Applied to an example from Table 9.1: for the first subject in the omnivore group, we have

$$6.35 = 5.98 + (6.32 - 5.98) + (6.35 - 6.32)$$

$$= 5.98 + 0.34 + 0.03.$$

Subtracting $\bar{y}$ from both sides of (9.1) gives

$$(y_{ij} - \bar{y}) = (\bar{y}_i - \bar{y}) + (y_{ij} - \bar{y}_i).$$

When both sides of this expression are squared and then summed over the i and j subscripts, it turns out (after some algebraic manipulation) that

$$\sum_i \sum_j (y_{ij} - \bar{y})^2 = \sum_i \sum_j (\bar{y}_i - \bar{y})^2 + \sum_i \sum_j (y_{ij} - \bar{y}_i)^2,$$

which can also be written as

$$\sum_i \sum_j (y_{ij} - \bar{y})^2 = \sum_i n_i (\bar{y}_i - \bar{y})^2 + \sum_i \sum_j (y_{ij} - \bar{y}_i)^2, \tag{9.2}$$

where n_i is the number of observations in group i ($n_i = 6$ for each value of i in Example 9.1). Often n_i is called the number of **replicates** in group i. In words, (9.2) is represented as

$$\begin{array}{c} \text{total sum} \\ \text{of squares} \end{array} = \begin{array}{c} \text{group sum} \\ \text{of squares} \end{array} + \begin{array}{c} \text{error sum} \\ \text{of squares} \end{array}.$$

This is the fundamental breakdown provided in the one-way ANOVA. The **total sum of squares** is the sum of squares (SS) of all deviations from the overall mean, sometimes called the **corrected sum of squares**. This is a measure of the overall variation in cholesterol from person to person, in the context of Example 9.1. The **group sum of squares** (often called the **treatment sum of squares** in an experimental situation) measures variation between the group-specific sample means, because it is based upon the $\bar{y}_i - \bar{y}$ differences. If H_0 is true, we should expect this to be relatively small. The **error** (or **residual**) **sum of squares** simply measures the variation remaining after accounting for the variation between group means. This is sometimes called a **within-group sum of squares** because it is based upon the $y_{ij} - \bar{y}_i$ differences, which are differences between the observations and their mean within group i.

In speaking of the individual sums of squares as measures of variation based on squared differences, we are led into consideration of average measures as in the derivation of the variance (Section 2.6.3). Just as for the variance, (2.9), we should divide the SS by the appropriate degrees of freedom if we are to define an average measure. As in (2.9), the appropriate d.f. for the total SS is $n - 1$ (the number of observations less 1, equal to 17 in Example 9.1). Similarly, the group SS has $\ell - 1$ d.f. where ℓ is the number of groups ($\ell - 1 = 2$ in Example 9.1). This follows from the fact that when we know $\ell - 1$ of the group-specific means, assuming that the overall mean is known, we can calculate the final mean by subtraction (Section 2.6.3). For the error SS, each within-group measure of variation has $n_i - 1$ d.f., leading to $\sum(n_i - 1) = n - \ell$ d.f. overall. Example 9.1 has $18 - 3 = 15$ d.f. for error.

When the SS is divided by its d.f., the result is called a **mean square** (MS). We shall use the symbol s_e^2 to represent the error MS; this emphasises the fact that this is a measure of variation, just like the overall sample variance, s^2. The error MS is the residual variation in the y variable after accounting for the variation due to the group differences. Finally, the ratio of the group to the error mean squares is called the **F ratio** or **variance ratio**.

The general algebraic form of the ANOVA table is given by Table 9.2. By convention, the total MS (which is the variance for the y variable) is omitted from the ANOVA table. Table 9.2 is arithmetically demanding to prepare and a far easier construction

Table 9.2. One-way ANOVA table for ℓ groups when n_i observations are taken from the ith group: basic algebraic form.

Source of variation	Sum of squares (SS)	Degrees of freedom (d.f)	Mean square	F ratio
Groups	$\sum n_i(\bar{y}_i - \bar{y})^2$	$\ell - 1$	$s_g^2 = \text{SS}/\text{d.f.}$	s_g^2/s_e^2
Error	$\sum\sum(y_{ij} - \bar{y}_i)^2$	$n - \ell$	$s_e^2 = \text{SS}/\text{d.f.}$	
Total	$\sum\sum(y_{ij} - \bar{y})^2$	$n - 1$		

Table 9.3. One-way ANOVA table for ℓ groups when n_i observations are taken from the ith group: computational form.

Source of variation	Sum of squares (SS)	Degrees of freedom (d.f.)	Mean square	F ratio
Groups	$\sum \dfrac{T_i^2}{n_i} - \dfrac{T^2}{n}$	$\ell - 1$	$s_g^2 = \text{SS}/\text{d.f.}$	s_g^2/s_e^2
Error	by subtraction	by subtraction	$s_e^2 = \text{SS}/\text{d.f.}$	
Total	$\sum\sum y_{ij}^2 - \dfrac{T^2}{n}$	$n - 1$		

for hand calculation is given by Table 9.3. In this, equivalent expressions for the group and total SS are given, and the error SS and d.f. are found by subtracting the group component from the total. Table 9.3 requires the following additional definitions:

$$T_i = \sum_j y_{ij},$$

$$T = \sum_i T_i.$$

Hence, T_i is the total of the observations obtained from group i and T is the overall grand total of the sample values of the outcome variable, y. The term T^2/n, which is subtracted in both the group and the total SS in Table 9.3, is called the **correction factor**.

Example 9.2 We shall now apply the formulae given in Table 9.3 to the data of Table 9.1. Note that summary averages and totals already appear in Table 9.1. Here $\ell = 3$ and $n_i = 6$ for each of the three values for i. The correction factor is

$$T^2/n = 107.60^2/18 = 643.209.$$

The group SS is

$$\frac{37.89^2}{6} + \frac{35.67^2}{6} + \frac{34.04^2}{6} - 643.209 = 1.245.$$

The total SS requires calculation of $\sum\sum y_{ij}^2$. This is found by squaring each data item in Table 9.1 and summing the 18 squares. The total SS is thus

$$644.984 - 643.209 = 1.775.$$

Then, by subtraction, the error SS is

$$1.775 - 1.245 = 0.530.$$

The group d.f. is $3 - 1 = 2$; the total d.f. is $18 - 1 = 17$, and hence the error d.f. is $17 - 2 = 15$ (as noted earlier).

The group MS is thus $1.245/2 = 0.623$ and the error MS is $0.530/15 = 0.035$. The F ratio is $0.623/0.035 = 17.8$. The formal ANOVA table is given as Table 9.4.

Table 9.4. ANOVA table for cholesterol in Example 9.1 and Example 9.2.

Source of variation	Sum of squares	Degrees of freedom	Mean square	F ratio
Diets	1.245	2	0.623	17.8
Error	0.530	15	0.035	
Total	1.775	17		

9.2.3 How the ANOVA table is used

To construct a test of significance for the null hypothesis that all means are equal, we need to consider the average sums of squares, that is, the mean squares. The error MS is an average of the individual variances within groups and is essentially a generalisation of the pooled estimate of variance in a two-sample t test: see (2.16). It provides an estimate of the 'background variation' against which other components of variance can be compared. Here the only other component is that due to groups.

The F ratio compares the size of the group MS to the error MS. This should be small when H_0 is true (all population means are equal); large values are evidence against H_0. Precisely, we need to compare the F ratio against the F distribution with first d.f. given by the group d.f. and second d.f. given by the error d.f. This test requires one-sided critical values, such as those given in Table B.5. Hence, we can read off values directly from this table in ANOVA problems.

From Table 9.4, we test the hypothesis of no difference in mean cholesterol between diet groups by comparing 17.8 with $F_{2,15}$. Table B.5(e) shows that the 0.1% critical value of $F_{2,15}$ is 11.3. Hence, the test is significant for $p < 0.001$; there is a real difference in mean cholesterol by diet. Often the p value is added as an extra column to the ANOVA table, as we shall do subsequently.

9.2.4 Estimation of group means

As we have seen, the ANOVA provides an overall test of equality of several means. Usually, we shall also be interested in the size of the specific means.

The sample mean for group i, $\bar{y}_i$, is a straightforward estimate of the population mean for group i. To obtain a confidence interval for this mean, we could apply (2.11) to the subset of the entire data that originates from group i. However, provided that the ANOVA assumption of equal variance in each group is correct, a better estimate of this underlying variance is given by s_e^2 rather than the sample variance in group i. Hence, the confidence interval for μ_i, obtained by replacing s^2 with s_e^2 in (2.11), is

$$\bar{y}_i \pm t_{n-\ell} s_e / \sqrt{n_i} . \tag{9.3}$$

Notice that t is on $n - \ell$ d.f. in (9.3) because the error MS, s_e^2, has $n - \ell$ d.f. We evaluate $t_{n-\ell}$ at the required percentage level. In (9.3), $s_e/\sqrt{n_i}$ is the estimated standard error (s.e.) of $\bar{y}_i$ from the ANOVA model.

Example 9.3 For the hypothetical data in Table 9.1, the error MS is found from Table 9.4 to be 0.035. Each group has the same number of observations and hence each group sample mean has the same s.e. $= \sqrt{0.035}/\sqrt{6} = 0.076$. From Table B.4, the 5% critical value of t_{15} is 2.13. To

Table 9.5. Estimated mean
cholesterol (mmol/l) with 95%
confidence interval for each diet
group: data from Table 9.1.

Diet group	Mean (95% CI)
Omnivores	6.32 (6.16, 6.48)
Vegetarians	5.95 (5.79, 6.11)
Vegans	5.67 (5.51, 5.83)

complete the components of (9.3), sample means are taken from Table 9.1. The results are
shown in Table 9.5. Vegans are estimated to have the lowest blood cholesterol and omnivores
the highest.

9.2.5   Comparison of group means

The F test in the ANOVA tells us whether all the population means may be considered
equal. Whatever the result of this test, we often wish to compare specific pairs of group
means. For instance, from Example 9.2, we have seen that a significant difference exists
among the cholesterol means in the three diet groups, but we might still be interested
in knowing whether vegan and vegetarian means are significantly different. The F test
only tells us whether the whole set of means deviates significantly from the overall
mean. It is quite possible to have a significant F test but a nonsignificant particular
pairwise comparison. Conversely, we might have a nonsignificant F and yet a pair of
means that are significantly different. In the latter case, we could have one mean above,
but not significantly different from, the overall mean (for all the data from the ℓ groups)
and the second mean below, but again not significantly different from, the overall mean.

To estimate the difference between two specific population means, say, $\mu_i - \mu_k$, we
simply compute $\bar{y}_i - \bar{y}_k$. To construct a confidence interval, we adapt (2.15) and (2.18),
just as in Section 9.2.4, to obtain

$$\bar{y}_i - \bar{y}_k \pm t_{n-\ell}\, \hat{se}, \tag{9.4}$$

where the estimated standard error of $\bar{y}_i - \bar{y}_k$ is

$$\hat{se} = s_e \sqrt{1/n_i + 1/n_k}\,. \tag{9.5}$$

A t test (Section 2.7.3) follows from computation of $(\bar{y}_i - \bar{y}_k)/\hat{se}$, which is compared
against the t distribution on the error d.f. ($n - \ell$ d.f.).

Example 9.4 To compare vegetarian and vegan diets for the data of Table 9.1, from Table 9.4
and (9.5) we find

$$\hat{se} = \sqrt{0.035\left(1/6 + 1/6\right)} = 0.108.$$

As seen in Example 9.3, the 5% critical value of $t_{n-\ell} = t_{15}$ is 2.13. Thus, from (9.4), the 95%
confidence interval for the difference between these means is given by

$$5.95 - 5.67 \pm 2.13 \times 0.108,$$

that is, 0.28 ± 0.23 or $(0.05, 0.51)$. We test this difference by comparing $0.28/0.108 = 2.59$ with t_{15}. The p value is 0.02, so there is indeed evidence of a difference in vegetarian and vegan cholesterol means.

An incorrect procedure, sometimes applied when comparing mean values in epidemiology, is to construct the two individual confidence intervals and reject the null hypothesis only if they fail to overlap. Comparing the overlapping vegetarian and vegan confidence intervals in Table 9.5 with the result of Example 9.4 demonstrates the error. This underlines the fact that differences should be compared, as in this section, by taking account of their correct standard error, which, in turn, determines the length of the confidence interval.

When making pairwise comparisons, we need to beware of the possibility of bias. For instance, if we calculate the sample means and *then* decide to compare the two groups with the largest and smallest means, we know (all else being equal) that we are more likely to find a significant result than when other groups are compared. To prevent such bias, only preplanned comparisons should be made — that is, contrasts specified *before* data collection. Furthermore, we can expect, just by chance, to find at least one significant result if enough pairwise comparisons are made. This is easily proven from basic probability theory. A test carried out at the 5% level of significance has a probability of 5/100 of rejecting the null hypothesis (that the two means are equal) when it is true. For the three-group data of Table 9.1 we could carry out three pairwise tests. The chance of at least one of these rejecting a null hypothesis when all three null hypotheses are true is $1 - (95/100)^3 = 0.14$, which is far bigger than the nominal 0.05. In general, with m comparisons, this becomes $1 - (95/100)^m$. There is a better than even chance of at least one significant result when m exceeds 13.

Various solutions have been suggested for this problem of **multiple comparisons** (see Steel and Torrie, 1980). The simplest is the **Bonferroni rule**, which states that when m comparisons are made, the p value for each individual test should be multiplied by m. Thus, if Example 9.4 described just one of three comparison tests carried out with the dietary data, then the p value would be recomputed as $3 \times 0.02 = 0.06$. Using this method, we would now conclude that the difference between vegetarian and vegan cholesterol levels was not significant at the 5% level.

Two problems with the Bonferroni method are that it often gives values above unity and that it is conservative (tends to lead to nonsignificance). In general, it is best to restrict the number of comparisons to a small number, not to exceed the degrees of freedom $(\ell - 1)$, and then report the p values without the correction but possibly with a warning note. If many tests are necessary, a more extreme significance level than that usually taken (say, 0.1% rather than 5%) might be taken as the 'cut-point' for decision making. Using the Bonferroni rule, we would adopt an adjusted significance level of s/m where s is the nominal significance level (say, 5%) and m is the number of comparisons.

9.2.6   *Fitted values*

Often it is useful to consider the fitted (i.e., predicted) values determined by a statistical model. To do this, we need to consider the mathematical form of the model. In this section, we shall derive mathematical expressions for fitted values.

One-way ANOVA assumes that the only systematic component of the model is that due to groups. Note that group membership is a categorical variable (for example, diet has three alphabetic levels in Example 9.1). To be able to provide a mathematical expression for the model that is easily understandable and generalisable, we shall use a set of dummy variables to represent groups.

A **dummy** or **indicator variable** takes only two values: zero or unity. It takes the value unity when the 'parent' categorical variable attains some prespecified level, and the value zero in all other circumstances. The full set of dummy variables has one variable for each level of the categorical variable. Thus, in the dietary example, the full set of dummy variables is

$$x^{(1)} = \begin{cases} 1 \text{ for omnivores} \\ 0 \text{ otherwise,} \end{cases} \qquad x^{(2)} = \begin{cases} 1 \text{ for vegetarians} \\ 0 \text{ otherwise,} \end{cases}$$

$$x^{(3)} = \begin{cases} 1 \text{ for vegans} \\ 0 \text{ otherwise.} \end{cases}$$

Note the use of superscripts to identify specific dummy variables.

The ANOVA model for the diet example is

$$y = \alpha + \beta^{(1)}x^{(1)} + \beta^{(2)}x^{(2)} + \beta^{(3)}x^{(3)} + \varepsilon, \tag{9.6}$$

where α and the set $\{\beta^{(i)}\}$ — often called the **beta coefficients** — are unknown parameters. As usual, ε is the random component which (like y) varies from person to person; everything else in (9.6) is the systematic part of the model. For simplicity, unlike (9.1) and (9.2), the i and j subscripts are suppressed in (9.6).

The α and $\{\beta^{(i)}\}$ parameters are estimated by the principle of **least squares**. We call their estimates a and $\{b^{(i)}\}$, respectively. These are the values in the estimated systematic part of the model expressed by (9.6), that is,

$$\hat{y} = a + b^{(1)}x^{(1)} + b^{(2)}x^{(2)} + b^{(3)}x^{(3)} \tag{9.7}$$

that minimise the sum of squared differences between the true and fitted values, $\Sigma(y - \hat{y})^2$. Least squares ensures that the total, and thus the average, distance between the true and predicted value is as small as possible. Squares are required for the same reason that they are required when calculating the variance (Section 2.6.3) — that is, to avoid cancelling out of positive and negative differences. See Clarke and Cooke (2004) for mathematical details.

The fitted values — that is, the values of y predicted from the model — are given by (9.7). Since only one x value will be nonzero at any one time, (9.7) can be written in a more extensive, but more understandable, form by considering the three dietary groups separately:

for omnivores, $x^{(1)} = 1$, $x^{(2)} = 0$ and $x^{(3)} = 0$; hence, the fitted value is

$$\hat{y}_{\text{omnivore}} = a + b^{(1)};$$

for vegetarians, $x^{(1)} = 0$, $x^{(2)} = 1$ and $x^{(3)} = 0$, giving

$$\hat{y}_{\text{vegetarian}} = a + b^{(2)};$$

for vegans, $x^{(1)} = 0$, $x^{(2)} = 0$ and $x^{(3)} = 1$, giving

$$\hat{y}_{\text{vegan}} = a + b^{(3)}.$$

Notice that the one-way ANOVA model for this example can produce only three different predicted values because it assumes that, apart from random error, cholesterol is solely determined by diet.

One complication arises in the model specification, (9.7). We have four unknown parameters (a, $b^{(1)}$, $b^{(2)}$ and $b^{(3)}$), but we are estimating only three fitted values. This means that we cannot (mathematically) find values for the parameters unless we introduce a **linear constraint** upon their values. The constraint that we shall adopt concerns the 'b' parameters only and has the general form

$$\sum_{i=1}^{3} w^{(i)} b^{(i)} = w$$

for the dietary example. The $\{w^{(i)}\}$ are a set of weights and w is a scaling factor. A consequence of the necessity for such a constraint is that we need only two dummy variables to determine all the fitted values. This is another way of saying that diet, with three levels, has only 2 d.f. The full expression, (9.7) is said to be **overparametrised**.

The general form of the ℓ-group one-way ANOVA model is

$$y = \alpha + \beta^{(1)} x^{(1)} + \beta^{(2)} x^{(2)} + \; ... \; + \beta^{(\ell)} x^{(\ell)} + \varepsilon. \tag{9.8}$$

The general form of the fitted values from an ℓ-group one-way ANOVA is

$$\hat{y} = a + b^{(1)} x^{(1)} + b^{(2)} x^{(2)} + \; ... \; + b^{(\ell)} x^{(\ell)}, \tag{9.9}$$

where

$$x^{(i)} = \begin{cases} 1 & \text{if the group variable attains its } i\text{th level} \\ 0 & \text{otherwise} \end{cases}$$

and

$$\sum_{i=1}^{\ell} w^{(i)} b^{(i)} = w, \tag{9.10}$$

for some $\{w^{(i)}\}$ and w.

Various choices can be made for $\{w^{(i)}\}$ and w. In statistical textbooks it is usual to take $w^{(i)} = n_i$ for each i (that is, the weight is the sample size within group i) and $w = 0$. Then the linear constraint, (9.10), becomes

$$\sum_{i=1}^{\ell} n_i b^{(i)} = 0.$$

The great advantage of this choice is that it makes α become μ and $\beta^{(i)}$ become $\mu_i - \mu$ in (9.8) and thus a becomes $\bar{y}$ and $b^{(i)}$ becomes $\bar{y}_i - \bar{y}$ in (9.9). These parameters have a direct interpretation as the overall mean and the deviation of the ith group mean from this overall mean.

9.2.7 Using computer packages

Many commercial software packages will fit one-way ANOVA models. Statistical soft-ware packages usually allow one-way ANOVA models to be fitted in at least three ways. First, using a procedure specific to ANOVA problems (where the explanatory variables are categorical). PROC ANOVA in SAS and the ONEWAY and ANOVA routines in Stata fall into this category. Second, using a routine developed for a regression analysis (Section 9.3), such as PROC REG in SAS and REGRESS in Stata. Since regression procedures are designed for continuous explanatory variables, an extra step is required. Either the user must set up $\ell-1$ dummy variables (for a categorical variable with ℓ levels) and supply these to the computer routine (this works with regression procedures in any package); or the user has to tell the package that the explanatory variable is, instead, categorical (this works in Stata's REGRESS: the categorical variable must be declared using an 'i.' prefix — this notation is understood to mean 'treat this variable as categorical' in many Stata routines). Third, using a general linear models procedure (Section 9.6), that allows both categorical and con-tinuous explanatory variables, such as PROC GENMOD in SAS. Again, categorical variables need to be declared as such: in SAS this is achieved by use of a CLASS statement. In most of this chapter we shall see results only, for simplicity, from PROC GLM in SAS, although the first computer listing (Output 9.1) is split in two to show both SAS and Stata results for the same problem. The SAS programs used, as well as Stata alternatives, are available from the web site for this book — see Appendix A.

Unfortunately, different packages adopt different choices for $\{w^{(i)}\}$ and w in (9.10). For instance, Stata takes $w^{(1)} = 1$ and all other $w^{(i)}$ and w to be zero. Put simply, this constraint is

$$b^{(1)} = 0.$$

We shall mostly be viewing output from SAS which adopts the convention that $w^{(\ell)} = 1$ and all other $w^{(i)}$ and w are zero; that is,

$$b^{(\ell)} = 0.$$

So SAS fixes the parameter for the last level of a categorical variable to be zero, whereas Stata fixes the first to be zero.

Many users of SPSS will find that a more complex constraint has been used (although SPSS will allow user-defined constraints, as does Stata, with its 'ib.' prefix). This is the so-called 'deviation contrast': $w^{(i)} = 1$ for all i and $w = 0$. With this, (9.10) becomes

$$\sum_{i=1}^{\ell} b^{(i)} = 0.$$

SPSS then prints out results for the first $\ell - 1$ levels, leaving the user to compute the last b parameter (if required) as

$$b^{(\ell)} = -\sum_{i=1}^{\ell-1} b^{(i)}.$$

Table 9.6. Parameter estimates and fitted values (to two
decimal places) for three different model formulations;
data from Table 9.1.

Parameter/diet	Method		
	SAS[a]	Stata[a]	Textbook[b]
Parameter estimates			
a	5.67	6.32	5.98
$b^{(1)}$	0.64	0	0.34
$b^{(2)}$	0.27	−0.37	−0.03
$b^{(3)}$	0	−0.64	−0.31
Fitted values[c]			
Omnivores	6.31	6.32	6.32
Vegetarians	5.94	5.95	5.95
Vegans	5.67	5.67	5.67

[a] As described in Section 9.2.7.
[b] As defined at the end of Section 9.2.6.
[c] From (9.7), using the appropriate parameter estimates.

Whichever method is used, we shall arrive at the same fitted values, as Table 9.6 demonstrates (apart from rounding error) for the dietary data. However, it is crucial to discover which method the package selected has used. This is necessary for various tasks, not only the determination of fitted values (several examples appear later). If in doubt, we can run a simple example, such as Example 9.1, through the package. Note that SPSS values for the dietary example's $\{b^{(i)}\}$ will be the same as the 'textbook' because n_i is constant in this example.

Apart from rounding error, the fitted values shown in Table 9.6 are simply the sample means for the three dietary groups, as given in Table 9.1. Thus the most likely outcome for any future (for example) vegan is the mean of all vegans currently observed. The simplicity of this obvious result should not be viewed with cynicism! The methodology of this and the previous subsection is easily generalisable and demonstrably does give sensible results in the present context.

Output 9.1A shows SAS results for Example 9.1 from using the SAS general linear models procedure, PROC GLM. CHOLEST is the name chosen for the variable that holds cholesterol values. DIET was read in using the codes 1 = omnivore; 2 = vegetarian; 3 = vegan. Notice that (apart from rounding) the ANOVA table has the same numbers as in Table 9.4. SAS provides several decimal places, almost certainly too many for publication purposes. On the other hand, Table 9.4 is almost certainly too brief to provide accuracy in further calculations. Note how SAS alerts the user to the fact that the linear constraint used is not unique, although the message is somewhat cryptic. In future listings from SAS reproduced here, this message will be suppressed (although the 'B' warnings will be retained). Parameter estimates from Output 9.1A have been incorporated into Table 9.6. SAS denotes the parameter a as the 'intercept'; this has a more direct meaning in regression (Section 9.3.1). Along with each parameter estimate (except $b^{(3)}$, which is fixed to be zero) SAS gives its estimated standard error and a test that the parameter is zero. This is a t test (taking the error d.f. from

Output 9.1A. SAS PROC GLM results for Example 9.1 and Example 9.2.

Dependent variable: cholest

Source	DF	Sum of squares	Mean square	F value	Pr > F
Model	2	1.24487778	0.62243889	17.62	0.0001
Error	15	0.52983333	0.03532222		
Corrected total	17	1.77471111			

Parameter	Estimate		Standard error	t value	Pr > |t|
Intercept	5.673333333	B	0.07672703	73.94	<.0001
diet 1	0.641666667	B	0.10850841	5.91	<.0001
diet 2	0.271666667	B	0.10850841	2.50	0.0243
diet 3	0.000000000	B	.	.	.

Note: The X′X matrix has been found to be singular, and a generalised inverse was used to solve the normal equations. Terms whose estimates are followed by the letter 'B' are not uniquely estimable.

Output 9.1B. Stata ANOVA results for Example 9.1 and Example 9.2.

```
      Source |       SS          df       MS              Number of obs =        18
-------------+------------------------------              F(  2,    15) =     17.62
       Model |  1.24487738       2  .622438692            Prob > F       =   0.0001
    Residual |  .529833405      15  .035322227            R-squared      =   0.7015
-------------+------------------------------              Adj R-squared  =   0.6616
       Total |  1.77471079      17  .104394752            Root MSE       =   .18794

------------------------------------------------------------------------------
     cholest |      Coef.   Std. Err.      t    P>|t|     [95% Conf. Interval]
-------------+----------------------------------------------------------------
        diet |
          2  |  -.3699999   .1085084    -3.41   0.004    -.6012801   -.1387197
          3  |  -.6416666   .1085084    -5.91   0.000    -.8729468   -.4103864
             |
       _cons |      6.315    .076727    82.30   0.000      6.15146    6.47854
------------------------------------------------------------------------------
```

the ANOVA table) using the test statistic, $T = $ estimate/$\hat{se}$. Although these tests can be useful, they do require careful interpretation. From (9.7) we can show that

$$a = \hat{y}_{\text{vegan}},$$

$$b^{(1)} = \hat{y}_{\text{omnivore}} - \hat{y}_{\text{vegan}},$$

$$b^{(2)} = \hat{y}_{\text{vegetarian}} - \hat{y}_{\text{vegan}},$$

because of the SAS constraint $b^{(3)} = 0$. Hence, a is the predicted cholesterol value for vegans while $b^{(1)}$ and $b^{(2)}$ are estimates of the difference in cholesterol between each of the other two groups and vegans. Due to the SAS constraint, and to its being labelled as the last of the three groups, the vegan group is the **base** or **reference group**. Hence, the t tests show that the vegan mean is significantly different from zero ($p < 0.0001$); there is a significant difference between the omnivore and vegan means ($p < 0.0001$); and there is a significant difference between the vegetarian and vegan means ($p = 0.0243$). The last of these three tests agrees with Example 9.4.

If we wish to see all the group means (fitted values) with associated statistics and test all possible differences using SAS, we should issue a subcommand for PROC GLM to display the least squares means (Section 9.4.6).

Output 9.1B gives the results from using the ANOVA routine in Stata. Values in the ANOVA table are just as in Output 9.1A. As has been mentioned, unlike SAS, the lowest level of DIET (the value 1, for omnivores) is automatically taken as the base level. All the same, as shown by Table 9.6, the predicted values in each dietary group come out to be the same. Notice that Stata uses the label '_cons' for the intercept, or constant, term.

9.3 One quantitative explanatory variable

9.3.1 Simple linear regression

Like a one-way ANOVA, a **simple linear regression** (SLR) model relates the outcome variable, y, to a single explanatory variable, x. The only difference is that x is now a quantitative variable. For instance, whereas a one-way ANOVA model is suitable for relating serum cholesterol to type of diet (Example 9.1), an SLR model might relate serum cholesterol to dietary cholesterol intake (a continuous measure).

The SLR model is

$$y = \alpha + \beta x + \varepsilon, \tag{9.11}$$

where α and β are unknown parameters and, as usual, ε is the random error, which is assumed to have a standard normal distribution. The primary aim of an SLR analysis is to produce estimates a and b for α and β, respectively. That is, the fitted SLR line is

$$\hat{y} = a + bx. \tag{9.12}$$

This fitted model is best understood from a diagram (Figure 9.1). We call this a *linear* regression model because the x–y relationship is modelled to follow a straight line; *simple* linear regression is linear regression with only one x variable.

The parameter a is called the **intercept** because it is the value of y when $x = 0$, when the fitted line intercepts the y (vertical) axis. The parameter b is the **slope** of the fitted line; the line goes up b units for each unit increase in x. If b is negative, then the line slopes downward from left to right, and y will then decrease as x increases.

We can use the method of least squares to produce the estimates a and b from observed data on n pairs of (x, y) observations. Clarke and Cooke (2004) show these estimates to be

$$b = S_{xy}/S_{xx}, \tag{9.13}$$

$$a = \bar{y} - b\bar{x} = \left(\sum y/n\right) - b\left(\sum x/n\right), \tag{9.14}$$

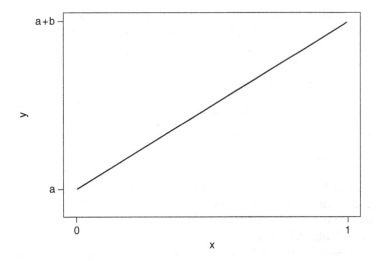

Figure 9.1. The simple linear regression model when x varies between 0 and 1.

where

$$S_{xx} = \sum_{i=1}^{n}(x - \bar{x})^2 \qquad (9.15)$$

and

$$S_{xy} = \sum_{i=1}^{n}(x - \bar{x})(y - \bar{y}). \qquad (9.16)$$

In fact, S_{xx} has already been defined as (2.10), in the definition of the sample variance of the x values. Here, we shall be interested in the sample variance of the y values, and an additional definition to be made is

$$S_{yy} = \sum_{i=1}^{n}(y - \bar{y})^2. \qquad (9.17)$$

From (2.9) we can see that the sample variance of the x values is $S_{xx}/(n-1)$ and that the sample variance of the y values is $S_{yy}/(n-1)$. We define $S_{xy}/(n-1)$ to be the sample **covariance** between the x and y variables. Whereas the variance measures how a single variable varies from observation to observation (ignoring any other variables), the covariance measures how two variables vary together (Section 9.3.2).

As is clear from (9.12), the SLR model predicts y from x. To be precise, we are assuming that when x is fixed at a specific value, the value of y is random, but with a systematic component which depends linearly upon x. Notice that if we decide subsequently that we should rather predict x from y, we *cannot* use the same fitted model. Instead we would need to fit a new SLR model in which the roles of y and x are interchanged. This will, in general, produce a different fitted line.

Just as when x is a categorical variable, it can be shown that (9.11) splits the overall variation in y into two components: that explained by regression on x and the error (residual, or unexplained, variation). We can summarise this split using the same

Table 9.7. Analysis of variance table for simple linear regression.

Source of variation	Sum of squares (SS)	Degrees of freedom (d.f.)	Mean square	F ratio
Regression on x	S_{xy}^2/S_{xx}	1	$s_r^2 = \text{SS}/\text{d.f.}$	s_r^2/s_e^2
Error	$S_{yy} - \left(S_{xy}^2/S_{xx}\right)$	$n-2$	$s_e^2 = \text{SS}/\text{d.f.}$	
Total	S_{yy}	$n-1$		

presentation as in Section 9.2.2, an ANOVA table: Table 9.7. Apart from the different formulae for all sums of squares and d.f., except those for the total, Table 9.7 is essentially identical to Table 9.2.

To compute Table 9.7 by hand, we should calculate S_{xx}, S_{xy} and S_{yy} — not from (9.15) to (9.17) — but rather from the following equivalent expressions, which are easier to deal with:

$$S_{xx} = \sum x^2 - \left(\sum x\right)^2 / n, \tag{9.18}$$

$$S_{xy} = \sum xy - \left(\sum x\right)\left(\sum y\right) / n, \tag{9.19}$$

$$S_{yy} = \sum y^2 - \left(\sum y\right)^2 / n. \tag{9.20}$$

Also note that the error SS is simply the total SS minus the regression SS.

By analogy with the one-way ANOVA model, the F ratio from Table 9.7 should be compared with one-sided F values on $(1, n-2)$ d.f. This produces a test of $\beta = 0$, the null hypothesis that the slope of the regression line is zero. If the result is significant (say, at the 5% level), the regression is said to be 'significant'. If $\beta = 0$, x has no role in predicting y because, in this case, (9.12) generates fitted values,

$$\hat{y} = a,$$

which are the same whatever the value of x. The fitted model then describes a horizontal straight line.

The **coefficient of determination**,

$$r^2 = \text{regression SS}/\text{total SS}, \tag{9.21}$$

measures how successful the regression has been. It is often multiplied by 100 so as to express the percentage of the variation in y that has been explained by regression on x. For SLR, the square root of r^2 is the correlation (Section 9.3.2).

Since a and b are sample-based estimates of α and β, we can specify their precision using confidence intervals. Respectively, these confidence intervals are

$$a \pm t_{n-2}\, \hat{\text{se}}(a) \tag{9.22}$$

$$b \pm t_{n-2}\, \hat{\text{se}}(b), \tag{9.23}$$

where the estimated standard errors are

$$\hat{se}(a) = \sqrt{s_e^2 \left\{ \frac{1}{n} + \frac{\bar{x}^2}{S_{xx}} \right\}} \tag{9.24}$$

$$\hat{se}(b) = \sqrt{s_e^2 / S_{xx}}, \tag{9.25}$$

and t_{n-2} is the appropriate critical value from the t distribution with the error d.f.

We can also test the null hypothesis that the intercept is zero, $H_0 : \alpha = 0$. This would be useful when we want to see whether the absence of x (that is, $x = 0$) is associated with the absence of y ($y = 0$). In practical applications, this is by no means always a sensible test to make. When it is sensible, we compute the test statistic

$$a/\hat{se}(a), \tag{9.26}$$

to be compared with t_{n-2}. Similarly, to test $H_0 : \beta = 0$, we compute

$$b/\hat{se}(b), \tag{9.27}$$

which is also to be compared with t_{n-2}. Notice that (9.27) tests the same thing as the F ratio in Table 9.7. The square of (9.27) is the F ratio and the square of (two-sided) t_{n-2} is (one-sided) $F_{1,n-2}$. In general, F and t tests are equivalent only when the F test has one for its first d.f. and has its second d.f. in common with the corresponding t test.

A regression model is often used for making predictions, which are easily obtained from (9.12). Suppose we wish to predict y for an individual whose x value is x_0. From (9.12), the predicted value is

$$\hat{y}_0 = a + bx_0. \tag{9.28}$$

We can attach confidence limits to our prediction. The confidence interval is

$$\hat{y}_0 \pm t_{n-2} \, \hat{se}(\hat{y}_0), \tag{9.29}$$

where the estimated standard error of the predicted value is

$$\hat{se}(\hat{y}_0) = \sqrt{s_e^2 \left\{ 1 + \frac{1}{n} + \frac{(x_0 - \bar{x})^2}{S_{xx}} \right\}}. \tag{9.30}$$

Another possibility is to predict the mean value of y over all individuals whose x value is x_0. That is, on average what value can y be expected to take when $x = x_0$? The predicted value is the same as before,

$$\hat{\bar{y}}_0 = \hat{y}_0,$$

where $\hat{y}_0$ is given by (9.28), but the confidence interval is

$$\hat{\bar{y}}_0 \pm t_{n-2} \, \hat{se}(\hat{\bar{y}}_0), \tag{9.31}$$

where

$$\hat{se}\left(\hat{\bar{y}}_0\right) = \sqrt{s_e^2 \left\{ \frac{1}{n} + \frac{\left(x_0 - \bar{x}\right)^2}{S_{xx}} \right\}}. \tag{9.32}$$

Notice that (9.30) and (9.32) will get smaller as the sample size, n, increases, just as we should expect. They will also be smaller for a chosen x_0 that is closer to $\bar{x}$ and will increase as x_0 moves away from $\bar{x}$ equally in either direction. This makes intuitive sense: the most accurate prediction is at the centre of the observed values and the least accurate are at the peripheries. A prediction at a value of x_0 beyond the range of observed data is sure to be of dubious quality because we can never be sure that the linear relationship holds in these uncharted regions. This is reflected in the large standard error, and thus wide confidence interval, for such a prediction.

Example 9.5 Table 9.8 shows data on the relationship between sugar consumption and dental caries in the 61 developing countries for which data were available to Woodward and Walker (1994). Sugar consumption was derived from government and industry sources and the average number of decayed, missing or filled teeth (DMFT) at age 12 was obtained from the WHO Oral Disease Data Bank, where the results of national surveys were compiled. Each of these surveys was carried out at some time between 1979 and 1990; sugar consumption has been averaged over the 5 (or sometimes fewer) years previous to the year of the DMFT survey.

The data in Table 9.8 are plotted in Figure 9.2. This type of diagram is called a **scatterplot**. From this scatterplot, we see that caries does seem to increase with sugar consumption, although the relationship is not strong due to the high variation in DMFT for small variations in sugar consumption.

The interesting epidemiological question is whether increased sugar consumption leads to caries, rather than the other way around, so we shall regress DMFT on sugar (as suggested by Figure 9.2). Thus DMFT is the y variable and sugar is the x variable.

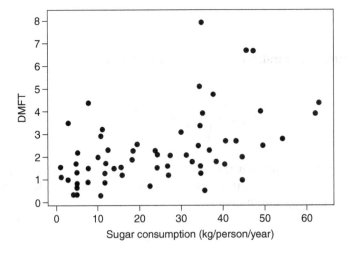

Figure 9.2. DMFT against sugar consumption in developing countries; data from Table 9.8.

Table 9.8. Estimates of mean DMFT at age 12 years and mean sugar consumption (kg/head of population/year) in 61 developing countries.

Country	Sugar	DMFT	Country	Sugar	DMFT
Algeria	36.60	2.3	Kuwait	44.63	2.0
Angola	12.00	1.7	Madagascar	7.76	4.4
Argentina	34.56	3.4	Malawi	7.56	0.9
Bahamas	34.40	1.6	Malaysia	35.10	3.9
Bahrain	34.86	1.3	Maldives	31.42	2.1
Bangladesh	2.88	3.5	Mali	5.00	2.2
Barbados	63.02	4.4	Morocco	32.68	1.8
Belize	49.02	4.0	Myanmar	1.44	1.1
Botswana	35.60	0.5	Niger	4.68	1.7
Brazil	46.98	6.7	Nigeria	10.15	2.0
Cameroon	7.56	1.5	Pakistan	16.02	1.2
China, PR	4.66	0.7	Philippines	23.93	2.2
Colombia	37.76	4.8	Saudi Arabia	38.66	1.8
Congo, DR	2.66	1.0	Senegal	14.26	1.5
Cuba	62.14	3.9	Sierra Leone	4.84	1.3
Cyprus	34.10	2.5	Singapore	49.56	2.5
El Salvador	34.44	5.1	Somalia	11.82	1.3
Ethiopia	3.92	0.4	Sri Lanka	18.10	1.9
Fiji	54.24	2.8	Sudan	24.16	2.1
Gambia	26.56	1.6	Syria	40.18	1.7
Ghana	4.36	0.4	Tanzania	4.72	0.6
Guatemala	35.30	8.1	Thailand	15.34	1.5
Guyana	40.65	2.7	Togo	10.70	0.3
Haiti	11.17	3.2	Tunisia	27.30	2.1
Hong Kong	24.18	1.5	Uganda	0.97	1.5
Indonesia	12.50	2.3	Western Samoa	19.10	2.5
Iraq	43.00	2.7	Yemen, AR	30.00	3.1
Ivory Coast	10.74	2.9	Yemen, PDR	22.32	0.7
Jamaica	45.98	6.7	Zambia	18.53	2.3
Jordan	44.44	1.0	Zimbabwe	27.00	1.2
Korea, Rep.	11.56	0.9			

Note: These data, together with the data in Table 9.18, may be downloaded from the book's web site; see Appendix A.

Source: Woodward, M. and Walker, A.R.P. (1994), *Br. Dent. J.*, 176, 297–302.

From Table 9.8, $n = 61$ and

$$\sum x = 1499.77, \qquad \sum y = 141.50,$$

$$\sum x^2 = 53463.2923, \qquad \sum y^2 = 479.51,$$

$$\sum xy = 4258.303.$$

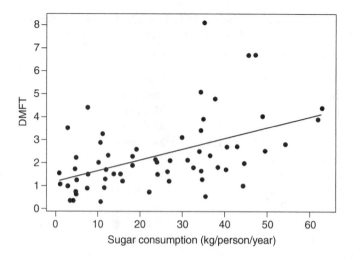

Figure 9.3. DMFT against sugar consumption in developing countries, showing the fitted simple linear regression line.

From (9.18) and (9.19),

$$S_{xx} = 53463.2923 - 1499.77^2/61 = 16589.357,$$

$$S_{xy} = 4258.303 - 1499.77 \times 141.50/61 = 779.32833.$$

Thus, from (9.13) and (9.14),

$$b = 779.32833/16589.357 = 0.0469776,$$

$$a = 141.50/61 - 0.0469776 \times 1499.77/61 = 1.16466.$$

Hence, after rounding, the fitted regression line is

$$y = 1.165 + 0.0470x.$$

As b is positive, the line predicts that y will increase with increasing x. This can be seen from Figure 9.3, in which the fitted line has been superimposed over the raw data.

To construct the ANOVA table, we use (9.20) to obtain

$$S_{yy} = 479.51 - 141.50^2/61 = 151.27639.$$

Then Table 9.9 is obtained using the formulae from Table 9.7.

From this, we see that $r^2 = 36.609/151.276 = 0.242$, using (9.21). Hence, just over 24% of the country-to-country variation in DMFT is due to differences in sugar consumption. The remaining

Table 9.9. Analysis of variance table for DMFT; developing countries.

Source of variation	Sum of squares	Degrees of freedom	Mean square	F ratio	p value
Regression on sugar	36.609	1	36.609	18.84	<0.0001
Error	114.667	59	1.9435		
Total	151.276	60			

76% may be attributed to other factors, presumably to include the fluoride content of the water drunk, dental hygiene practice and other aspects of diet. At this point, the major weakness of the data for exploring causality is worth noting: because the data are merely national averages, we cannot link specific individual outcomes for sugar consumption and caries (Section 1.7.1). An additional problem here is that sugar consumption relates to everyone, whereas DMFT is recorded only for 12-year-olds.

Using (9.25), we find the estimated standard error of the slope of the fitted regression line to be

$$\sqrt{1.9435/16589.357} = 0.0108237.$$

To obtain a 95% confidence interval for the slope from (9.23), we require the two-sided 5% critical value of t_{59}. From the T.INV.2T function in Excel this was found to be 2.001. Hence, the interval is

$$0.0469776 \pm 2.001 \times 0.0108237,$$

that is, 0.0470 ± 0.0217 or $(0.0253, 0.0687)$. If we wish, we can test the null hypothesis that the true slope, β, is zero using (9.27),

$$0.0469776/0.0108237 = 4.34.$$

Compared against $t_{59} = 2.001$, this is highly significant. From Table B.4, $p < 0.001$, using the nearest available d.f. of 60. In fact the p value, found from the T.DIST.2T function in Excel is even below 0.0001. Hence, there is real evidence to refute the assertion that DMFT does not increase with sugar consumption. The regression is significant at the 0.01% level.

Note that the alternative F test, based on the analysis of variance table (Table 9.9), gives the same result. The square of the t statistic is $4.34^2 = 18.84$, which is the F ratio given in Table 9.9. Comparing 18.84 with $F_{1,59}$ clearly will give a p value of somewhere below 0.001, by reference to the first column, last row of Table B.5(e).

Using (9.24), we find the estimated standard error of the intercept of the fitted regression line to be

$$\sqrt{1.9435\left\{\frac{1}{61} + \frac{\left(1499.77/61\right)^2}{16589.357}\right\}} = 0.3204,$$

leading to a 95% confidence interval for the intercept of

$$1.16466 \pm 2.001 \times 0.3204,$$

that is, 1.165 ± 0.641 or $(0.524, 1.806)$, using (9.22). To formally test the null hypothesis that the intercept is zero, we use (9.26) to obtain the test statistic

$$1.16466/0.3204 = 3.63.$$

Compared against t_{59}, this is highly significant ($p = 0.0006$). Hence, there is evidence to reject the null hypothesis; when sugar consumption is zero, we can, nevertheless, expect average DMFT to be nonzero in developing countries.

Output 9.2 shows the results obtained when SAS PROC GLM was used to analyse the sugar data. The results agree with the preceding calculations (apart from rounding error in certain cases). PROC GLM labels the regression SS as the 'model SS' and the slope is labelled SUGAR, showing that this is the parameter that multiplies this particular x variable.

Output 9.2. SAS PROC GLM results for Example 9.5.

Dependent variable: dmft

Source	DF	Sum of squares	Mean square	F value	Pr > F
Model	1	36.6090514	36.6090514	18.84	<.0001
Error	59	114.6673421	1.9435143		
Corrected total	60	151.2763934			

Parameter	Estimate	Standard error	t value	Pr > |t|
Intercept	1.164680383	0.32043887	3.63	0.0006
sugar	0.046976241	0.01082375	4.34	<.0001

To illustrate the use of regression for prediction, suppose we know that another developing country has an average annual sugar consumption of 35 kg per head of population. We then wish to predict its DMFT. In (9.28) and (9.30) this requires taking $x_0 = 35$. The predicted DMFT is, from (9.28),

$$1.16466 + 0.0469776 \times 35 = 2.8089,$$

which rounds off to 2.81. This agrees with a rough evaluation by eye, using the fitted line in Figure 9.3. From (9.30) the estimated standard error of this prediction is

$$\sqrt{1.9435\left\{1 + \frac{1}{61} + \frac{\left(35 - 1499.77/61\right)^2}{16589.357}\right\}} = 1.4100.$$

The 95% confidence interval for the prediction is, from (9.29),

$$2.8089 \pm 2.001 \times 1.4100,$$

that is, 2.81 ± 2.82 or $(-0.01, 5.63)$. This illustrates the large error in predicting individual values, especially when they are not close to the mean (which is around 25 in this case).

Suppose, instead, that we wish to predict the average DMFT over *all* countries with an average annual sugar consumption of 35 kg/head. This predicted mean value would still be 2.81, but the estimated standard error of this prediction is found, from (9.32), as

$$\sqrt{1.9435\left\{\frac{1}{61} + \frac{\left(35 - 1499.77/61\right)^2}{16589.357}\right\}} = 0.2111.$$

The 95% confidence interval for the predicted average is, from (9.31),

$$2.8089 \pm 2.001 \times 0.2111,$$

that is, 2.81 ± 0.42 or $(2.39, 3.23)$. Since we are now considering errors in predicting an average over several countries, this interval is considerably smaller than that found earlier for predicting the outcome for an individual country. Figure 9.4 shows the boundaries of the 95% confidence intervals for the average predictions at all values of sugar within the range of the observed data in Table 9.8. The predictions are simply the fitted SLR line. As anticipated, the minimum interval is for the prediction when sugar consumption takes its mean value in the observed dataset. As the sugar value, at which prediction is made, moves away from this mean, the interval increases in size.

9.3.2   Correlation

A topic closely related to simple linear regression is that of correlation. **Pearson's product-moment correlation coefficient** is a measure of linear association

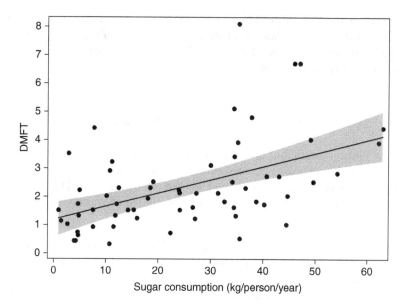

Figure 9.4. DMFT against sugar consumption in developing countries, showing predicted mean values and their 95% confidence limits.

between two quantitative variables, y and x. It is defined as the covariance divided by the square root of the product of the two variances. Its sample value is defined, using (9.15) through (9.17), as

$$r = \frac{S_{xy}}{\sqrt{S_{xx}S_{yy}}}. \tag{9.33}$$

The correlation coefficient takes the value -1 for perfectly negatively correlated data, where y goes down as x goes up in a perfect straight line: see Figure 9.5(a). For perfectly positively correlated data, as in Figure 9.5(b), it takes the value unity. The nearer to zero is the correlation coefficient, the less linear association there is between the two variables. Table B.11 gives values of r that provide just sufficient evidence of a nonzero correlation for various sample sizes. Statistical computer packages will produce exact p values.

As the choice of symbol suggests, the correlation coefficient, r, is the square root of the coefficient of determination, r^2, as defined by (9.21). Hence, for Example 9.5,

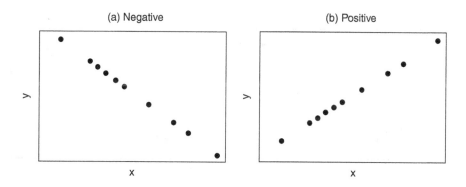

Figure 9.5. Perfect (a) negative and (b) positive correlation.

the correlation coefficient is $\sqrt{0.242} = 0.49$. Here $n = 61$; Table B.11 shows that $p < 0.001$, so there is strong evidence to refute the hypothesis of a lack of linear association between sugar consumption and DMFT in developing countries.

Examination of (9.13) and (9.33) shows that

$$r = b\sqrt{\frac{S_{xx}}{S_{yy}}} = b\left\{\frac{\text{standard deviation of } x \text{ values}}{\text{standard deviation of } y \text{ values}}\right\},$$

so that the correlation coefficient and slope of the regression line must vary together. Also, the test for the null hypothesis of a zero correlation must give the same result as the test for $\beta = 0$ (that is, no regression), as indeed we have found for the DMFT–sugar data.

Although correlation is a useful summary measure of a relationship, it has drawbacks:

- Even when the relationship is linear, it tells us nothing about the placement of the line; thus, unlike regression, it cannot be used for prediction.
- A significant correlation merely means that we cannot conclude complete absence of any linear relationship. With the size of the datasets common in epidemiology, correlations of below ± 0.1 may turn out to be significant at extreme levels of significance. This is sometimes erroneously referred to as 'strong correlation'.
- The significance test assumes that the two variables have a two-dimensional normal distribution. This is not easy to confirm, although it is usually assumed if the x and the y variables are reasonably symmetric (perhaps after a transformation).
- The correlation coefficient can give a misleading summary in certain special circumstances. This includes the cases shown by Figure 9.6.

Figure 9.6(a) illustrates the case when an outlier is present. There is clearly a negative relationship for the observations without the outlier, and yet application of (9.33) leads to a correlation of $r = 0.97$, quite close to perfect positive correlation. Figure 9.6(b) illustrates the case in which the observations cluster into two subsets. Although evidence does not indicate that y is related to x in either subgroup, the correlation is 0.99. Notice that the SLR model would also be inappropriate in these cases; transformations (Section 9.3.3) or subgroup analyses may be worth considering when straightforward correlation and SLR are inappropriate. These examples illustrate the need for a scatterplot before deciding upon an appropriate analysis strategy. When the

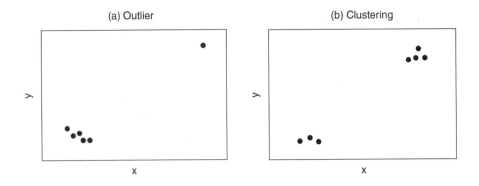

Figure 9.6. Two situations in which use of Pearson's correlation coefficient would be inappropriate.

dataset is huge, some summarization may be required, such as plotting average y values within certain ranges (such as the intervals between quantiles) of the x variable.

If we wish to quantify by how much y and x go up (or down) together, without specifying that the relationship follows a straight line, we can use (9.33) with the x and y values replaced by their ranks. The result is called **Spearman's correlation coefficient**. Thus, if the data followed a perfect exponential curve (see Figure 9.7(c)), Spearman's correlation would be exactly one, whereas Pearson's would be positive, but somewhat below unity. For the data of Table 9.8, we find Spearman's correlation coefficient by ranking the 61 y values (i.e., Togo = 1, ..., Guatemala = 61) and ranking the 61 x values (i.e., Uganda = 1, ..., Barbados = 61). We then apply (9.33) with the x ranks taking the place of x and the y ranks replacing y, to give a result of 0.53, slightly bigger than the Pearson correlation.

Spearman's correlation is used, rather than Pearson's, when the x or y data are highly non-normal (including when the data naturally occur in an ordinal form) and transformation cannot help. It is an example of a nonparametric correlation coefficient. If the sample size is even moderately large (say, above 30), Table B.11 may be used to assess the significance of Spearman's correlation. Conover (1998) gives exact values for use in hypothesis tests when $n \leq 30$.

Further details about correlation, including simple formulae for confidence intervals, are given by Clarke and Cook (2004).

9.3.3   Nonlinear regression

In Section 9.3.1 we assumed that the relationship between the two quantitative variables being related is linear. Although this is unlikely ever to be exactly true, except in artificial circumstances, it is often a working approximation in epidemiology. Some relationships are, however, certainly not linear and it would then be misleading to describe them by means of linear regression lines. For example, many epidemiological relationships are subject to 'diminishing returns': y increases with x at a continually decreasing rate (see Figure 9.7(d)).

Nonlinear regression models may be fitted, although their theory, computation and interpretation can be complex (see Bates and Watts, 1988 and Seber and Wild, 2003). In some cases, we can find a linear equivalent to the nonlinear model through transformation. Only this simple situation will be considered here.

All nonlinear modelling procedures begin with inspection of the scatterplot. From this, with some mathematical insight, we hope to deduce the appropriate form of the relationship. For example, if the points on the plot seem to follow the exponential curve (Figure 9.7(c)),

$$\hat{y} = A \exp(Bx), \tag{9.34}$$

for some parameters A and B, then this is the nonlinear model to fit.

The transformation method works by manipulating the nonlinear formula until it takes the linear form. For instance, taking logarithms (to the exponential base) of both sides in (9.34) gives

$$\log_e \hat{y} = a + bx, \tag{9.35}$$

which is of the linear form (9.12) if we consider $\log_e y$ as the outcome variable. Here, $a = \log_e A$ and $b = B$. We use the SLR model to fit the nonlinear model by regressing $\log_e y$ on x.

The only drawbacks with this simple procedure are that not all nonlinear formulae are linearisable and we must assume that, after transformation, the random error is

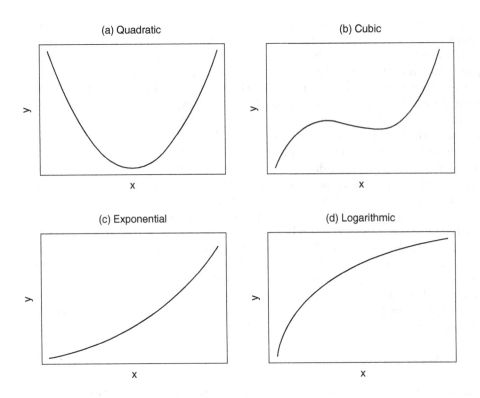

Figure 9.7. Some examples of nonlinear relationships: (a) $y = A + Bx + Cx^2$; (b) $y = A + Bx + Cx^2 + Dx^3$; (c) $y = A\exp(Bx)$; (d) $y = A + B\log(x)$.

both normally distributed and additive. For instance, the true values corresponding to (9.35) must satisfy

$$\log_e y = \alpha + \beta x + \varepsilon,$$

with α, β and the error term, ε, defined as usual. This assumption of additive normal error is often unreasonable (see Section 9.8 for methods of checking). Sometimes this causes us to switch to an alternative type of regression (Chapter 10 and Chapter 11) or to fit, from first principles, a nonlinear model with additive normal errors on the original scale. The latter might be attempted, for example, using the procedure PROC NLIN in the SAS package. Other possible approaches are discussed in Section 9.10.

As a guide to choosing an appropriate nonlinear equation, Figure 9.7 shows some examples that have been found useful in epidemiological research. Figure 9.7(a) and Figure 9.7(b) are examples of **polynomials**: equations involving integer powers of x. The **quadratic**, with terms up to x^2, is a second-degree polynomial; the **cubic** is a third-degree polynomial. The first-degree polynomial is the straight line. Polynomials give rise to curves in which the number of turning points is equal to the degree of the polynomial minus one. Thus, the quadratic has one turning point.

Each example in Figure 9.7 uses values of the parameters (A, B, etc.) which ensure that y increases as x increases for the biggest values of x. Each curve can be flipped over by changing the sign of one or more of the parameters. Each example in Figure 9.7 may be linearised, although the polynomials require a multiple linear regression model (Section 9.7), in which the explanatory variables are the powers of x.

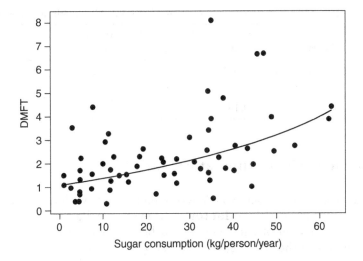

Figure 9.8. DMFT against sugar consumption in developing countries, showing the fitted regression curve from the log model.

Example 9.6 In Example 9.5, we saw how dental caries depend upon sugar consumption through a linear regression model. In fact, careful scrutiny of Figure 9.2 shows that the linear regression model is not entirely satisfactory for the data given in Table 9.8 (see also Section 9.8), and so a range of nonlinear models was considered. One of these was the 'log model', (9.35), which regresses $\log_e$(DMFT) on sugar. To fit this, we simply find logs (to base e, although any other base could be used) of all the DMFT values in Table 9.8 and then apply (9.13) to (9.16), taking y as $\log_e$(DMFT) and x as sugar consumption. This results in the fitted regression line

$$\hat{y} = 0.096 + 0.0214x.$$

To obtain the predicted DMFT score at a given value of x, say, $x = x_0$, we find the antilog (exponent) of the predicted y; thus our prediction is

$$\exp\left\{0.096 + 0.0214x_0\right\}.$$

Figure 9.8 shows the predicted DMFT values for each value of sugar consumption within the observed range. As expected, we now have a fitted curve. Comparing Figure 9.8 with Figure 9.3, the log model does seem to have captured the pattern of the data slightly better. This type of comparison is generally best made through residual plots (Section 9.8).

Table 9.10 gives the ANOVA for the log model. Using (9.21) we find $r^2 = 7.5933/29.1424 = 0.261$. Unfortunately, we cannot compare this directly with the r^2 from Table 9.9 (which is smaller), so as to conclude that the log model gives a better fit to the data, because the transformation alters the interpretation of r^2 on the original scale. Instead, see Example 9.13 for a comparison of the two models. See Kvålseth (1985) and Scott and Wild (1991) for a discussion of the r^2 problem and Flanders *et al.* (1992) for a general discussion of epidemiological linear regression models with transformations.

It is possible that some other nonlinear model might do better for the DMFT data, although it is clear from Figure 9.2 that no mathematical relationship will model the observed DMFT–sugar relationship closely. Considerably better prediction is likely only when other explanatory variables are introduced into the model.

Table 9.10. Analysis of variance table for $\log_e$(DMFT); developing countries.

Source of variation	Sum of squares	Degrees of freedom	Mean square	F ratio	p value
Regression on sugar	7.5933	1	7.5933	20.79	<0.0001
Error	21.5491	59	0.3652		
Total	29.1424	60			

9.4   Two categorical explanatory variables

In Section 9.2 we saw how a one-way ANOVA model deals with data that are classified by a single categorical variable or **factor** (as it is often called in this application). The next most complex model of this type would be one with two factors. For example, suppose that we know the sex of each of the subjects identified in Table 9.1. We could then analyse the data to see whether sex or type of diet, or both, influence blood cholesterol. This leads to a **two-way ANOVA**.

9.4.1   Model specification

By analogy with (9.6), the two-way ANOVA model for one factor (x_1) with ℓ levels and a second (x_2) with m levels may be written as

$$y = \alpha + \beta_1^{(1)}x_1^{(1)} + \beta_1^{(2)}x_1^{(2)} + \cdots + \beta_1^{(\ell)}x_1^{(\ell)}$$
$$+ \beta_2^{(1)}x_2^{(1)} + \beta_2^{(2)}x_2^{(2)} + \cdots + \beta_2^{(m)}x_2^{(m)} + \varepsilon.$$

As always, y and ε are the outcome variable and random error, respectively. The $\{\beta_1^{(i)}\}$ are a set of ℓ parameters representing the effects of each of the levels of x_1 and $\{\beta_2^{(i)}\}$ are m parameters representing x_2. The $\{x_1^{(i)}\}$ and $\{x_2^{(i)}\}$ are two sets of dummy variables. The intercept term, α, is often written as β_0 to emphasise that it is just another parameter that needs to be estimated. We shall adopt this convention from now on.

As usual, we shall denote the estimated βs as bs. For example, the fitted values from the two-way ANOVA model for the dietary data of Table 9.1 (when sex is known) are given by

$$\hat{y} = b_0 + b_1^{(1)}x_1^{(1)} + b_1^{(2)}x_1^{(2)} + b_1^{(3)}x_1^{(3)} + b_2^{(1)}x_2^{(1)} + b_2^{(2)}x_2^{(2)}, \qquad (9.36)$$

where

$$x_1^{(1)} = \begin{cases} 1 & \text{for omnivores} \\ 0 & \text{otherwise} \end{cases}$$

$$x_1^{(2)} = \begin{cases} 1 & \text{for vegetarians} \\ 0 & \text{otherwise} \end{cases}$$

$$x_1^{(3)} = \begin{cases} 1 & \text{for vegans} \\ 0 & \text{otherwise} \end{cases}$$

$$x_2^{(1)} = \begin{cases} 1 & \text{for men} \\ 0 & \text{for women} \end{cases}$$

$$x_2^{(2)} = \begin{cases} 1 & \text{for women} \\ 0 & \text{for men.} \end{cases}$$

To be able to fix the bs, we need to introduce constraints upon their values, just as in Section 9.2.6. Here we define one constraint for the b_1s and another for the b_2s. Both will have the general form of (9.10).

9.4.2 Model fitting

From now on, we shall assume that a computer package is available to do the model fitting. The output produced will depend upon the package, and sometimes the particular procedure chosen within the package, when a choice is possible. The user will need to supply the computer procedure with information about y, x_1 and x_2 for each observation. Additionally, she or he may need to use the data manipulation facilities within the package to set up two sets of dummy variables (Section 10.4.3), or may need to declare, to the routine that fits models, that x_1 and x_2 are factors. In the latter case, the package will automatically choose its own constraints upon the b_1s and b_2s, as explained in Section 9.2.7. For example, when PROC GLM in SAS is told that x_1 and x_2 are CLASS variables, it sets the parameters corresponding to the last levels of x_1 and x_2 to zero; that is, $b_1^{(\ell)} = 0$ and $b_2^{(m)} = 0$.

9.4.3 Balanced data

The data are **balanced** if each level of one factor occurs the same number of times within each level of the second factor. Equivalently, each factor combination must occur the same number of times. Thus, in Table 9.1, when we introduce sex as a further factor, the data would be balanced if half of the subjects in each diet group were male. We would then have three replicates of each of the $3 \times 2 = 6$ factor combinations; for instance there would be three male vegetarians.

The great advantage of balanced data is that we get independent estimates of the effect of each factor (see Example 9.8). This is a great help in the interpretation of results and leads to simple computation procedures (Clarke and Kempson, 1997). However, epidemiological research rarely produces balanced data by chance; this is normally achieved through design. The only situation in which such a design is common is an intervention study. Even then, drop-outs (leading to missing values) can destroy the designed balance.

Most nonstatistical commercial software that fits two-way ANOVA models will deal only with balanced data. Due to the simplicity of balance, several specialist statistical packages include a routine that deals only with balanced data. Such routines are straightforward to use and will not be considered further here. An example (mentioned previously) is PROC ANOVA in SAS.

9.4.4 Unbalanced data

As just indicated, unbalanced data are the norm in observational epidemiology (surveys, cohort and case–control studies). In this case, we shall not be able to assess the separate effects of the two factors simultaneously. Instead, we can assess their combined effect, through a one-way ANOVA in which the 'group SS' will now be called the **model SS**. For a two-way study, without consideration of interaction, the model d.f. will be $(\ell - 1) + (m - 1)$; this is the sum of the d.f. for the x_1 and x_2 factors.

The combined effect is, however, of limited epidemiological interest; really, we would like to split it into its components. We can do this only by considering the factors sequentially, allowing for what went before. The effect of the first factor entered into the model is then obtained unconditionally, but the second is evaluated after allowing for the first. 'Bar notation' is used to specify conditional effects, as in 'second|first' (see Table 9.12 for an example). Sequential fitting gives rise to a **sequential ANOVA** table in which the model SS is split into two components called the **sequential SS** (or, in SAS, the **Type I SS**). The sequential SS will sum to the model SS.

One problem with the sequential approach is that the factors are treated in a different way, which may compromise the interpretation. An alternative is to consider the effect of each factor after allowing for the other. This leads to **cross-adjusted SS** (called **Type III SS** by SAS and **partial SS** by Stata), which will not total to the model SS (unless the data are balanced). The cross-adjusted approach is used when t tests are provided for the β parameters within computer output: for instance, in the two-way ANOVA results at the end of Output 9.9.

Since the cross-adjusted SS and the second of the sequential SS measure the effect of one variable adjusted for the other, they give a means for adjustment to deal with confounding (Chapter 4). This topic will be considered further in Section 9.9.

The SAS package prints Type I and III SS by default. The Type II SS may also be useful. These are like the Type III SS except that the cross-adjustment now excludes any interaction terms. The ANOVA routine in Stata prints cross-adjusted SS by default.

Example 9.7 For the data in Table 9.1, suppose that subjects 1, 2, 4, 5 and 6 in the omnivore group, subject 6 in the vegetarian group and subject 1 in the vegan group are men; all others are women. This is illustrated by Table 9.11. The data were read into SAS and the two-way

Table 9.11. Serum total cholesterol (mmol/l) by sex and type of diet.

	Diet group		
	Omnivores	Vegetarians	Vegans
Male			
	6.35	6.11	6.01
	6.47		
	6.37		
	6.11		
	6.50		
Mean	6.360	6.110	6.010
Female			
	6.09	5.92	5.42
		6.03	5.44
		5.81	5.82
		6.07	5.73
		5.73	5.62
Mean	6.090	5.912	5.606
Overall mean	6.315	5.945	5.673

Output 9.3. SAS PROC GLM results for Example 9.7.

Dependent variable: cholest

Source	DF	Sum of squares	Mean square	F value	Pr > F
Model	3	1.45609556	0.48536519	21.33	<.0001
Error	14	0.31861556	0.02275825		
Corrected total	17	1.77471111			

Source	DF	Type I SS	Mean square	F value	Pr > F
diet	2	1.24487778	0.62243889	27.35	<.0001
sex	1	0.21121778	0.21121778	9.28	0.0087

Source	DF	Type III SS	Mean square	F value	Pr > F
diet	2	0.44904678	0.22452339	9.87	0.0021
sex	1	0.21121778	0.21121778	9.28	0.0087

Table 9.12. Sequential ANOVA table for Example 9.7.

Source of variation	Sum of squares	Degrees of freedom	Mean square	F ratio	p value
Diet	1.2449	2	0.6224	27.3	<0.0001
Sex|diet	0.2112	1	0.2112	9.3	0.009
Error	0.3186	14	0.0228		
Total	1.7747	17			

ANOVA model was fitted using PROC GLM. The results appear as Output 9.3 (here SAS results are given without the table of parameter estimates).

The Type I (sequential) and Type III (cross-adjusted) SS list the variables in the order fitted in the model; here DIET was fitted first. The Type I and III SS for the final (second) term fitted (SEX) must always be the same, and thus provide the same test, as indeed they do here: SEX has a significant effect ($p = 0.0087$) even after the effect of diet has been accounted for. The Type I and III SS, as well as associated tests, for DIET differ: DIET is highly significant ($p < 0.0001$) when considered alone, but not as significant ($p = 0.0021$) when considered in the presence of SEX. Here, some of the effect of diet on cholesterol is explained by the effect of sex: the nonmeat eaters tend to be female, whilst men tend to have higher values of cholesterol (see Table 9.11).

Notice that the Type I SS correctly sum to the model SS, which has three degrees of freedom (two for diet plus one for sex). Table 9.12 is the sequential ANOVA table constructed from Output 9.3 (with rounded values). This shows how the Type I SS split the entire 'model' source of variation into two components, with associated tests based on the usual F ratios using the error MS as the denominator. The error d.f. is most easily understood as the total d.f. less the d.f. of each of the two factors.

Of course, the order of fitting terms into the model could be altered so that SEX comes first. This would give rise to a different sequential ANOVA table including a test for the effect of sex uncorrected for diet. When using software that does not give cross-adjusted (Type III) SS, we must be careful to enter terms into the model in the appropriate order.

Example 9.8 Suppose, instead, that the first three subjects within each diet group in Table 9.1 were male and the rest were female. Output 9.4 gives the results from fitting a two-way

Output 9.4. SAS PROC GLM results for Example 9.8.

Dependent variable: cholest

Source	DF	Sum of squares	Mean square	F value	Pr > F
Model	3	1.25990000	0.41996667	11.42	0.0005
Error	14	0.51481111	0.03677222		
Corrected total	17	1.77471111			

Source	DF	Type I SS	Mean square	F value	Pr > F
diet	2	1.24487778	0.62243889	16.93	0.0002
sex	1	0.01502222	0.01502222	0.41	0.5330

Source	DF	Type III SS	Mean square	F value	Pr > F
diet	2	1.24487778	0.62243889	16.93	0.0002
sex	1	0.01502222	0.01502222	0.41	0.5330

ANOVA to this data structure. The data are now balanced, so the Type I and III SS are equal and both add to the model SS. The effects of sex and diet can be simultaneously evaluated: diet has a significant effect on cholesterol ($p = 0.0002$) but sex has no discernible effect ($p = 0.5330$).

9.4.5 Fitted values

As in Section 9.2.7, we can use the parameter estimates produced by the computer package to find the fitted values (model predictions). For instance, Table 9.13 shows the parameter estimates, as produced by SAS PROC GLM, for Example 9.7. Notice that the final parameter in each of the two sets is zero because this is the constraint imposed by SAS. Other packages may use different rules, although the method presented here would still be applicable. Results, such as those in Table 9.13, need to be substituted into (9.36). For example, consider the fitted value for male omnivores. Here $x_1^{(1)} = 1$, $x_2^{(1)} = 1$ and all other xs are zero. Hence, in (9.36),

$$\hat{y} = 5.62489 + 0.44789 + 0.29067 = 6.3635.$$

For female omnivores, the corresponding sum is

$$\hat{y} = 5.62489 + 0.44789 + 0 = 6.0728.$$

These and the remaining predictions are shown in Table 9.14. Notice that these results differ from the sex-specific dietary group sample means shown in Table 9.11.

Table 9.13. Parameter estimates produced by SAS for Example 9.7.

Intercept b_0	Diet			Sex	
	$b_1^{(1)}$	$b_1^{(2)}$	$b_1^{(3)}$	$b_2^{(1)}$	$b_2^{(2)}$
5.62489	0.44789	0.27167	0	0.29067	0

Table 9.14. Fitted values for Example 9.7.

Sex	Diet group		
	Omnivore	Vegetarians	Vegans
Male	6.3634	6.1872	5.9156
Female	6.0728	5.8966	5.6249

9.4.6 Least squares means

Fitted values give predictions for the average values in the cross-classes (see Table 9.14), but we often wish to have predictions for one (or both) of the factors alone. We do this by averaging out the effect of the other factor, using the fitted values. Since the fitted values are based on least squares estimation, we call these averaged-out values **least squares means**. They are also known as **adjusted means**.

Consider finding the average effect of each diet from the data in Table 9.14; that is, averaging diet over the sexes. A logical way to do this is by weighting the cross-classified fitted values in Table 9.14 according to the observed frequencies overall, called the **observed margins**. Since there are 7 men and 11 women in the dataset of Example 9.7, the weights are 7 and 11, respectively. This gives us least squares means: for omnivores, $(6.3634 \times 7 + 6.0728 \times 11)/18 = 6.19$; for vegetarians, $(6.1872 \times 7 + 5.8966 \times 11)/18 = 6.01$; for vegans, $(5.9156 \times 7 + 5.6249 \times 11)/18 = 5.74$. These are interpreted as the predicted values of cholesterol for each diet group after taking account of the effect of sex. Hence, if sex were considered a confounder, these could be called confounder-adjusted estimates (Section 9.9). Notice that these adjusted estimates differ from the overall means given in Table 9.11, indicating that sex has had some effect. Although they are of less practical sense here, similarly we could work out least squares means for sex, adjusted for diet.

Sometimes it is sensible to test whether a least squares mean is zero. More often, in epidemiology, we wish to compare least squares means. Computer procedures, such as SAS PROC GLM, and the LINCOM command in Stata, are available to do this. Output 9.5 shows SAS results for diet in Example 9.7 (here the DIET codes are 1 = omnivore; 2 = vegetarian; 3 = vegan, as before). Notice that the cholesterol means agree with the rounded values derived above. All means are significantly different from zero ($p < 0.0001$), but this is only to be expected: no one has zero cholesterol. Of more interest are the comparative tests; after allowing for sex effects, we see that vegans have significantly lower cholesterol than omnivores ($p = 0.0010$) and vegetarians ($p = 0.0075$). As mentioned in Section 9.2.5, caution is generally advisable with such multiple testing.

An alternative way of computing least squares means is to weight the cross-classified fitted values equally, called the **balanced margins** method. Applying this method to the data of Example 9.7, using the fitted values of Table 9.14, gives us least squares means: for omnivores, $(6.3634 + 6.0728)/2 = 6.22$; for vegetarians, $(6.1872 + 5.8966)/2 = 6.04$; for vegans, $(5.9156 + 5.6249)/2 = 5.77$. These are similar, but not identical, to those given earlier. Other weightings would be possible; for example, weights that reflect the sex structure of the US. This is similar to the issue of choosing a standard population when deriving adjusted rates (Section 4.5); this idea is developed further in Section 10.16.1. In practice, the method using observed margins is probably used most often. This may be because it generalises straightforwardly to the method of least squares estimation when we have at least one continuous variable, in addition to the index categorical variable — we evaluate the fitted values at the mean values of the continuous variables (see Example 9.16).

Output 9.5. Further SAS PROC GLM results for
Example 9.7.

Diet	cholest LSMEAN	Standard error	Pr > |t|	LSMEAN number
1	6.18581481	0.07477450	<.0001	1
2	6.00959259	0.06513515	<.0001	2
3	5.73792593	0.06513515	<.0001	3

Least squares means for effect diet Pr > |t| for H0: LSMean(i)=LSMean(j) Dependent variable: cholest			
i/j	1	2	3
1		0.1246	0.0010
2	0.1246		0.0075
3	0.0010	0.0075	

9.4.7   Interaction

In Section 4.7, the basic concepts of interaction were introduced. In the current context, an interaction would occur if the mean effect of one factor differed depending upon the value of the second factor. In Example 9.7, there would be a different average effect of diet on blood cholesterol for men and women.

The two-way ANOVA discussed so far can be extended to include an interaction. Interaction terms are simply the cross-multiplied terms of the constituent main effects. Thus, if the two main effects have ℓ and m levels, respectively, we define the interaction by the ℓm new x variables derived as the cross-products of the dummy variables representing the main effects.

For example, we can extend (9.36) to include a sex-by-diet interaction by creating variables,

$$x_3^{(11)} = x_1^{(1)}x_2^{(1)} \qquad x_3^{(21)} = x_1^{(2)}x_2^{(1)} \qquad x_3^{(31)} = x_1^{(3)}x_2^{(1)}$$

$$x_3^{(12)} = x_1^{(1)}x_2^{(2)} \qquad x_3^{(22)} = x_1^{(2)}x_2^{(2)} \qquad x_3^{(32)} = x_1^{(3)}x_2^{(2)},$$

each of which is to be multiplied by a corresponding b_3 parameter in the fitted model. For instance, using the definition of $x_1^{(1)}$ and $x_2^{(1)}$ given in Section 9.4.1,

$$x_3^{(11)} = \begin{cases} 1 \text{ if } x_1 = 1 \text{ and } x_2 = 1 \\ \text{otherwise}; \end{cases}$$

so $x_3^{(11)}$ is unity only for male omnivores; otherwise it is zero. The fitted two-way ANOVA model with interaction for this example is

$$\hat{y} = b_0 + b_1^{(1)}x_1^{(1)} + b_1^{(2)}x_1^{(2)} + b_1^{(3)}x_1^{(3)} + b_2^{(1)}x_2^{(1)} + b_2^{(2)}x_2^{(2)}$$
$$+ b_3^{(11)}x_3^{(11)} + b_3^{(21)}x_3^{(21)} + b_3^{(31)}x_3^{(31)} + b_3^{(12)}x_3^{(12)} + b_3^{(22)}x_3^{(22)} + b_3^{(32)}x_3^{(32)}. \tag{9.37}$$

The interaction can be fitted using dummy variables exactly as suggested here (Section 10.9) or by including an interaction term in a model declaration made to a procedure

Output 9.6. SAS PROC GLM results for Example 9.9.

Source	DF	Type I SS	Mean square	F value	Pr > F
diet	2	1.24487778	0.62243889	24.86	<.0001
sex	1	0.21121778	0.21121778	8.44	0.0132
diet*sex	2	0.01821556	0.00910778	0.36	0.7024

Parameter	Estimate		Standard error	t value	Pr > |t|
Intercept	5.606000000	B	0.07075780	79.23	<.0001
diet 1	0.484000000	B	0.17332051	2.79	0.0163
diet 2	0.306000000	B	0.10006664	3.06	0.0099
diet 3	0.000000000	B	.	.	.
sex 1	0.404000000	B	0.17332051	2.33	0.0380
sex 2	0.000000000	B	.	.	.
diet*sex 1 1	−0.134000000	B	0.24511222	−0.55	0.5946
diet*sex 1 2	0.000000000	B	.	.	.
diet*sex 2 1	−0.206000000	B	0.24511222	−0.84	0.4171
diet*sex 2 2	0.000000000	B	.	.	.
diet*sex 3 1	0.000000000	B	.	.	.
diet*sex 3 2	0.000000000	B	.	.	.

that recognises factors and interactions, such as PROC GLM in SAS and both ANOVA and REGRESS in Stata. As before, constraints will need to be made to enable estimation, and we must know which method the computer package uses. In general, because the first factor has $\ell - 1$ d.f. and the second has $m - 1$, the interaction, defined through their product, has $(\ell - 1)(m - 1)$ d.f. Since ℓm terms are used to define the interaction, we therefore need to introduce $\ell m - (\ell - 1)(m - 1) = \ell + m - 1$ independent linear constraints.

SAS sets the parameter for the last level of a factor (CLASS variable) to zero; thus, it also sets the corresponding interaction parameters to zero. That is, $b_3^{(ij)}$ is fixed at zero when i takes the last level of x_1 or j takes the last level of x_2. By contrast, in Stata the first levels are set to zero by default and hence $b_3^{(ij)}$ is zero when i takes the first level of x_1 or j takes the first level of x_2. Other packages will have similar rules. Fitted values, and thus least squares means, from a two-way ANOVA model with interaction simply reproduce the observed sample means (given in Table 9.11 in our running example).

Example 9.9 Output 9.6 shows the Type I SS and parameter estimates from fitting the two-way ANOVA model with interaction to the data of Table 9.11. There is no significant interaction ($p = 0.7024$) in this case. Notice that, for example, the fitted value for male omnivores (DIET = 1; SEX = 1) is found from picking out all the appropriate terms in (9.37); that is, with rounding,

$$5.606 + 0.484 + 0.404 - 0.134 = 6.360.$$

As anticipated, this is the sample mean for male omnivores given in Table 9.11.

9.5 Model building

When we have two factors, the two-way ANOVA model is not necessarily the appropriate one for the data. An interesting epidemiological question is whether a simpler one-way ANOVA will suffice. If it will, then we can say that one of the two factors is sufficient for predicting the quantitative outcome variable.

Five possible models could be adopted when two factors have been observed: the **empty** (or **null**) model (that with no factors); the two one-way ANOVA models; the two-way ANOVA; and the two-way with interaction. In epidemiological research, we may often find it useful to fit all possible models because this provides insight into the relationships between the factors and the outcome variable, and gives precise information for model selection. The empty model, which assumes that no factors have any effect (that is, $\hat{y} = \bar{y}$), is so simple that it is generally unnecessary to fit it. Having fitted all the models, we sometimes wish to decide upon one model that is, in some sense, 'best'. We can use F tests from ANOVA tables to help make our decision.

Thus, for the balanced data of Example 9.8, we would reject the two-factor model, and conclude that the simpler one-way model with diet alone will suffice (that is, sex can be ignored in determining cholesterol). However, notice that we have not tested for an interaction in Example 9.8; it would be dangerous to delete a variable before considering its role within interactions.

Whenever we fit an ANOVA model that includes all possible interactions between all the factors included in the model, the fitted values must equal the sample means, because no source of variation is left unaccounted for, between groups. This has already been seen in the one-way ANOVA of Section 9.2.7 (where there can be no interactions) and the two-way ANOVA with interaction of Section 9.4.7.

Example 9.10 Table 9.15 gives data from a random sample of 150 subjects from the Scottish Heart Health Study (SHHS). We wish to see how body mass index (BMI) depends upon cigarette smoking history and a person's sex. Table 9.16 gives some summary statistics calculated from Table 9.15.

Taking BMI as the y variable, sex as x_1 and smoking as x_2, we have four possible (nonempty) models:

1. y versus x_1 (BMI depends upon sex alone).
2. y versus x_2 (BMI depends upon smoking alone).
3. y versus x_1 and x_2 (BMI depends upon sex and smoking).
4. y versus x_1, x_2 and their interaction (BMI depends upon smoking status in a different way for men and women).

Models 1 and 2 are one-way ANOVA models; model 3 is a two-way (unbalanced) ANOVA and model 4 is a two-way ANOVA with interaction.

We could fit models 1 and 2 using formulae given in Section 9.2, where ℓ (the number of groups) is 2 and 3, respectively. Instead of this, we shall view SAS output. The data from Table 9.15 were read into SAS; Outputs 9.7 and 9.8 show excerpts from the SAS results from fitting models 1 and 2, respectively. As both are one-term models (they have a single x variable), Type I and III sums of squares and mean squares are irrelevant; they simply repeat the model SS and MS, and so are omitted here. Parameter estimates are easily interpreted by reference to the marginal (row and column) totals of Table 9.16 (see Section 9.2.7 for explanation).

The F test in Output 9.7 shows that sex is important as a predictor of BMI (it is only just nonsignificant at the customary 5% significance level; $p = 0.0512$). Output 9.8 shows that smoking is very significant ($p = 0.0019$). Hence, both sex and smoking are needed in the absence of the other.

Output 9.9 gives the results of fitting model 3. The model SS has three degrees of freedom, made up of one from SEX (because it has two levels) and two from SMOKING (because it has three levels). The model terms are significant ($p = 0.0004$) when taken together, but this fact does not lead to a simple epidemiological interpretation. We need to break up the SS (and d.f.) in order to provide useful results.

The first break-up gives the Type I (sequential) SS. The x terms SEX and SMOKING were introduced in this order and so the Type I SS shows the effect of SEX alone and then the effect of SMOKING after accounting for SEX. Both are significant at the 5% level. Thus, SEX is a

Table 9.15. BMI (kg/m²), sex and cigarette smoking status for a random sample of 150 subjects in the SHHS. Codes for sex are 1 = male, 2 = female. Codes for smoking are 1 = current, 2 = ex, 3 = never.

BMI	Sex	Smoking status	BMI	Sex	Smoking status	BMI	Sex	Smoking status
30.25	1	3	24.34	1	2	29.01	1	3
24.16	1	3	26.85	1	2	24.74	1	1
23.29	1	1	26.75	1	1	28.73	1	1
24.11	1	1	26.58	1	2	25.95	1	3
21.20	1	1	28.65	1	2	27.10	1	1
26.67	1	2	24.46	1	3	28.03	1	2
25.93	1	2	24.57	1	2	24.45	1	1
26.59	1	3	19.72	1	1	20.55	1	1
21.72	1	2	30.85	1	3	23.80	1	2
25.10	1	1	25.26	1	3	32.18	1	3
27.78	1	1	27.18	1	2	25.39	2	3
25.07	2	2	25.16	2	2	28.38	1	3
21.45	2	1	32.87	2	3	25.22	2	3
23.53	2	1	23.50	2	3	26.03	2	2
22.94	2	1	34.85	2	2	25.56	2	2
22.03	2	3	23.88	2	2	26.90	2	2
27.12	2	2	26.72	2	3	26.90	2	3
24.39	2	2	26.85	1	1	25.96	2	3
24.24	2	2	26.02	2	1	24.75	2	1
28.35	2	2	20.80	1	3	21.45	2	1
27.03	2	3	28.34	1	1	22.55	1	3
30.12	2	3	24.00	2	1	25.96	1	3
27.97	1	3	28.84	2	3	23.80	2	3
24.77	2	1	26.35	1	1	21.91	2	2
23.89	1	3	22.77	2	3	20.55	2	3
19.29	2	1	18.72	2	3	21.61	2	2
24.24	2	3	26.13	2	1	24.52	2	2
22.46	2	2	20.32	2	1	22.38	2	2
26.44	2	3	25.56	2	3	24.46	2	2
23.44	2	1	23.05	2	1	23.83	2	1
28.09	1	3	25.01	1	1	29.00	1	2
28.67	1	2	15.55	1	1	25.31	1	2
26.99	1	2	24.34	1	1	23.30	1	1
31.31	1	2	22.57	1	2	24.91	1	1
25.83	1	1	29.03	1	2	29.48	1	2
29.37	1	1	23.99	1	1	29.04	1	1
28.96	1	2	27.16	1	1	24.82	1	1
21.91	1	2	25.88	1	2	24.05	1	3
32.42	1	1	28.74	1	2	33.08	1	3
25.22	1	3	24.76	1	2	31.96	1	1
35.74	1	2	31.21	1	1	26.51	1	3
29.71	1	3	24.90	1	2	19.96	1	1
29.94	2	3	25.39	2	1	30.12	2	3
33.95	2	3	25.15	2	1	32.02	2	3
21.17	2	1	33.75	2	3	22.77	2	3
20.57	2	1	21.91	2	1	22.52	2	1
20.81	2	1	27.14	2	2	28.16	2	1
29.27	2	3	21.36	2	3	28.80	2	3
32.05	2	3	24.01	2	1	27.46	1	1
26.61	2	3	22.94	2	1	24.91	2	3

Note: These data may be downloaded; see Appendix A.

Table 9.16. Mean BMI (kg/m^2) by cigarette smoking status and sex (sample size given in brackets); data from Table 9.15.

Smoking status	Sex		
	1 (Male)	2 (Female)	Total
1 (Current)	25.53 (31)	23.23 (24)	24.53 (55)
2 (Ex)	26.83 (26)	25.34 (18)	26.22 (44)
3 (Never)	26.90 (21)	26.74 (30)	26.81 (51)
Total	26.33 (78)	25.22 (72)	25.80 (150)

Output 9.7. SAS PROC GLM results for Example 9.10, model 1.

Dependent variable: bmi

Source	DF	Sum of squares	Mean square	F value	Pr > F
Model	1	46.279129	46.279129	3.86	0.0512
Error	148	1772.354349	11.975367		
Corrected total	149	1818.633477			

Parameter	Estimate		Standard error	t value	Pr > |t|
Intercept	25.22000000	B	0.40782906	61.84	<.0001
sex 1	1.11179487	B	0.56555715	1.97	0.0512
sex 2	0.00000000	B	.	.	.

Output 9.8. SAS PROC GLM results for Example 9.10, model 2.

Dependent variable: bmi

Source	DF	Sum of squares	Mean square	F value	Pr > F
Model	2	148.472524	74.236262	6.53	0.0019
Error	147	1670.160954	11.361639		
Corrected total	149	1818.633477			

Parameter	Estimate		Standard error	t value	Pr > |t|
Intercept	26.80647059	B	0.47199284	56.79	<.0001
smoking 1	−2.27937968	B	0.65524995	−3.48	0.0007
smoking 2	−0.58828877	B	0.69353897	−0.85	0.3977
smoking 3	0.00000000	B	.	.	.

useful predictor by itself and SMOKING is useful even when we have accounted for SEX. The sequential ANOVA table, constructed from the SAS results, is given as Table 9.17.

The Type III (cross-adjusted) SS show the effect of SEX accounting for SMOKING, and SMOKING accounting for SEX. The latter, of course, repeats the corresponding Type I result. The new result here is that SEX is important even when we know SMOKING (indeed it is even more important since $p = 0.0158$ now, rather than 0.0420).

Notice that the model SS in Output 9.9 is greater than the sum of those in Output 9.7 and Output 9.8 (214.04 > 46.28 + 148.47), showing that sex and smoking do not act independently. Indeed, they seem to act antagonistically (Section 4.7), explaining the increasing significance of

Output 9.9. SAS PROC GLM results for Example 9.10, model 3.

Dependent variable: bmi

Source	DF	Sum of squares	Mean square	F value	Pr > F
Model	3	214.039970	71.346657	6.49	0.0004
Error	146	1604.593507	10.990366		
Corrected total	149	1818.633477			

Source	DF	Type I SS	Mean square	F value	Pr > F
sex	1	46.2791286	46.2791286	4.21	0.0420
smoking	2	167.7608418	83.8804209	7.63	0.0007

Source	DF	Type III SS	Mean square	F value	Pr > F
sex	1	65.5674469	65.5674469	5.97	0.0158
smoking	2	167.7608418	83.8804209	7.63	0.0007

Parameter	Estimate		Standard error	t value	Pr > |t|
Intercept	26.25471312	B	0.51626231	50.86	<.0001
sex 1	1.33998243	B	0.54860663	2.44	0.0158
sex 2	0.00000000	B	.	.	.
smoking 1	−2.48288503	B	0.64981850	−3.82	0.0002
smoking 2	−0.82833910	B	0.68915699	−1.20	0.2313
smoking 3	0.00000000	B	.	.	.

Table 9.17. Sequential ANOVA table for BMI (kg/m^2); data from Table 9.15, results taken from Output 9.9.

Source of variation	Sum of squares	Degrees of freedom	Mean square	F ratio	p value
Sex	46.28	1	46.28	4.21	0.04
Smoking | sex	167.76	2	83.88	7.63	0.0007
Error	1604.59	146	10.99		
Total	1818.63	149			

sex after accounting for smoking. The model SS in Output 9.7 is, as it should be, the Type I SS for SEX in Output 9.9 and the two Type I SS correctly add to the model SS in Output 9.9.

Output 9.10 is for model 4. The crucial test in this listing is that for the SMOKING by SEX interaction (written with an asterisk in SAS notation) after accounting for the two constituent main effects. As this was introduced last into the model, the result can be read either from the Type I or Type III SS. Otherwise the Type III SS have no useful interpretation here. The interaction is clearly not significant ($p = 0.2595$); therefore, we conclude that smoking status does not act differently on BMI for men and women. Although we will thus reject model 4, for completeness the parameter estimates have been shown. Notice the effect of the SAS rule, that the parameter for the last level of any group is set to zero, on these estimates. We can find fitted values for any combination of SEX and SMOKING by picking out and adding the appropriate terms. For example, for female never-smokers (SMOKING = 3; SEX = 2), the predicted BMI (in rounded figures) is

$$26.74 + 0 + 0 + 0 = 26.74 \text{ kg/m}^2.$$

Output 9.10. SAS PROC GLM results for Example 9.10, model 4.

Dependent variable: bmi

Source	DF	Sum of squares	Mean square	F value	Pr > F
Model	5	243.823372	48.764674	4.46	0.0008
Error	144	1574.810105	10.936181		
Corrected total	149	1818.633477			

Source	DF	Type I SS	Mean square	F value	Pr > F
sex	1	46.2791286	46.2791286	4.23	0.0415
smoking	2	167.7608418	83.8804209	7.67	0.0007
sex*smoking	2	29.7834014	14.8917007	1.36	0.2595

Source	DF	Type III SS	Mean square	F value	Pr > F
sex	1	62.7066646	62.7066646	5.73	0.0179
smoking	2	162.4050180	81.2025090	7.43	0.0009
sex*smoking	2	29.7834014	14.8917007	1.36	0.2595

Parameter	Estimate		Standard error	t value	Pr > |t|
Intercept	26.74033333	B	0.60377096	44.29	<.0001
sex 1	0.16061905	B	0.94090909	0.17	0.8647
sex 2	0.00000000	B	.	.	.
smoking 1	−3.50700000	B	0.90565645	−3.87	0.0002
smoking 2	−1.40533333	B	0.98595385	−1.43	0.1562
smoking 3	0.00000000	B	.	.	.
sex*smoking 1 1	2.13475730	B	1.30144695	1.64	0.1031
sex*smoking 1 2	1.33399634	B	1.38329241	0.96	0.3365
sex*smoking 1 3	0.00000000	B	.	.	.
sex*smoking 2 1	0.00000000	B	.	.	.
sex*smoking 2 2	0.00000000	B	.	.	.
sex*smoking 2 3	0.00000000	B	.	.	.

This requires the least complex arithmetic. One of the most complex examples is for male ex-smokers (SMOKING = 2; SEX = 1) giving

$$26.74 + 0.16 - 1.41 + 1.33 = 26.82 \text{ kg/m}^2.$$

Apart from rounding error, all six fitted values generated this way must agree with the cross-classified group sample means shown in Table 9.16, as they do.

Although we have built up the model from simplest to most complex, a sounder strategy would be to start with model 4 and only work 'backwards' if the interaction is not significant. This can save unnecessary work.

Given our results, we conclude that person-to-person variation in BMI depends upon both the person's sex and smoking status, each of which is still important after the other has been accounted for (that is, model 3 is 'best'). Supposing that it is the effect of smoking (and giving up smoking) that is of key interest, it would be useful to see least squares means for smoking after correcting for the sex effect. These are sensible summaries of the effect of smoking, given that there is no evidence of a sex interaction in this case.

To obtain these, model 3 was refitted, this time requesting SAS to show least squares means for smoking. Results are shown in Output 9.11. In fact, these are broadly similar to the uncorrected,

Output 9.11. SAS PROC GLM results from refitting Example 9.10, model 3, with terms in reverse order.

Source	DF	Type I SS	Mean square	F value	Pr > F
smoking	2	148.4725235	74.2362618	6.75	0.0016
sex	1	65.5674469	65.5674469	5.97	0.0158

Smoking	bmi LSMEAN	Standard error	Pr > |t|	LSMEAN number
1	24.4686189	0.4476583	<.0001	1
2	26.1231649	0.5012927	<.0001	2
3	26.9515040	0.4679991	<.0001	3

Least squares means for effect smoking Pr > |t| for H0: LSMean(i)=LSMean(j) Dependent variable: bmi			
i/j	1	2	3
1		0.0148	0.0002
2	0.0148		0.2313
3	0.0002	0.2313	

raw means in Table 9.16, although the difference between current and never smokers is increased. Smoking appears to provide a benefit in reducing BMI, much of which goes after quitting. See Bolton–Smith and Woodward (1997) for an analysis of the complete SHHS dataset.

So as to provide further insight, Output 9.11 has been generated by introducing the terms into the model in the opposite order to that used for Output 9.9. Both fit the same model, model 3, and hence almost all the SAS results are identical and are not presented here. The exception is the sequential SS display, which is shown. As they must, the two Type I SS sum to the model SS in Output 9.9; the SMOKING Type I SS is the same as the model SS in Output 9.8; the SEX given SMOKING Type I SS is the same as the equivalent Type III SS in Output 9.9.

9.6 General linear models

In Section 9.2 we introduced a model using a single categorical variable, which was generalised to deal with two categorical variables in Section 9.4. We could now go on to generalise the model for a single quantitative variable given in Section 9.3.1. However, the similarity of the models and the ANOVA tables in Section 9.2 and Section 9.3 show this to be unnecessary. Both models take the form

$$y = \alpha + \beta x + \varepsilon,$$

except that a categorical x variable needs to be represented by a set of dummy variables and associated β parameters. That is, βx needs to be expanded out.

A bivariable linear regression model takes the form

$$y = \beta_0 + \beta_1 x_1 + \beta_2 x_2 + \varepsilon, \tag{9.38}$$

which is exactly as for the two-way ANOVA model, except that the latter expands $\beta_1 x_1$ and $\beta_2 x_2$ into their component sets (Section 9.4.1). The bivariable regression ANOVA table, sequential and cross-adjusted SS have exactly the same interpretation as in Section 9.4, and model building proceeds as in Section 9.5. Interaction is represented as the product of the x_1 and x_2 variables. Fitted values are generated in a similar way (see Example 9.14) but now go up gradually, rather than in steps.

From now on, we shall deliberately blur the distinction between categorical and quantitative variables in the right-hand side of the model equation. We shall consider models in which the variables can be of either type. Provided the model is linear in structure and the error is additive and normally distributed, as in (9.38), then we call such models **general linear models**. Notice that these should not be confused with generalised linear models which, for one thing, allow the error to be non-normal (Chapter 10). A general linear model is a special case of a generalised linear model.

Much of the terminology from general linear models arises from regression analysis. For example, the parameters (multipliers of the x variables) in (9.36) and (9.38) are called **partial regression coefficients**, meaning that they represent the effect of the corresponding x variable, when all other x variables are kept fixed. In a sense, all ANOVA models *are* regression models, once the dummy variables are defined. Thus, (9.36) is a linear regression model with five x variables and (9.37) is a linear regression model with eleven x variables. The only difference is that the x variables must be bound in sets within an ANOVA model: it makes no sense to fit a subset of the dummy variables for one particular categorical variable.

When the explanatory variable of major interest is quantitative, but in the analysis we assess the confounding or interaction effects of a subsidiary categorical explanatory variable, the procedure is called a **comparison of regressions** (Example 9.11). When the explanatory variable of major interest is categorical and the subsidiary is quantitative, we call this an **analysis of covariance**. However, these terms are largely redundant and reflect the separate historical development of ANOVA and regression models. Stata acknowledges the common root of regression and ANOVA models by both allowing categorical variables to be analysed within its flagship regression command, REGRESS, when these variables are given an 'i.' prefix (as has already been noted) and by allowing continuous variables to be analysed within its flagship analysis of variance command, ANOVA, when these variables are given a 'c.' prefix.

Example 9.11 The publication used in Example 9.5 gave separate results for developing and industrialised countries. Table 9.18 shows the data for the 29 industrialised countries considered in the paper. Taking this together with Table 9.8, we have 90 observations on national sugar consumption and dental caries.

Since we found a better regression fit when the logarithm of DMFT was regressed on sugar for developing countries (Example 9.6), we shall take the y variable to be $\log_e(\text{DMFT})$ in this example. There are two x variables: let x_1 = sugar consumption and x_2 = type of country. Four regression models will be considered:

1. y versus x_1 (DMFT depends upon sugar alone).
2. y versus x_2 (DMFT depends upon type of country alone).
3. y versus x_1 and x_2 (DMFT depends upon sugar and type of country).
4. y versus x_1, x_2 and their interaction (DMFT depends upon sugar in a different way in developing and industrialised nations).

Model 1 is a simple linear regression model fitted to the 90 (developing and industrialised) observations. Model 2 is a one-way analysis of variance model for a factor with two levels. Model 3 is a general linear model with two variables, one of which is quantitative and the other categorical. Model 4 is another general linear model, but with an interaction term added.

The four models were fitted in SAS PROC GLM, having declared TYPE (of country) as a CLASS variable. LOGDMFT was defined as $\log_e(\text{DMFT})$ and fitted as the y variable. Results are given as Output 9.12 to Output 9.15. Although we shall ultimately choose only one of the

Table 9.18. Estimates of mean DMFT at age 12 years and mean sugar consumption (kg/head of population/year) in 29 industrialised countries.

Country	Sugar	DMFT	Country	Sugar	DMFT
Albania	22.16	3.4	Japan	23.32	4.9
Australia	49.96	2.0	Malta	47.62	1.6
Austria	47.32	4.4	Netherlands	53.54	2.5
Belgium	40.86	3.1	New Zealand	50.16	2.4
Canada	42.12	4.3	Norway	41.28	2.7
Czechoslovakia	49.92	3.6	Poland	49.28	4.4
Denmark	48.28	1.6	Portugal	33.48	3.2
Finland	41.96	2.0	Sweden	45.60	2.2
France	37.40	3.0	Switzerland	44.98	2.4
Germany, West	39.42	5.2	Turkey	28.32	2.7
Greece	33.30	4.4	UK	43.95	3.1
Hungary	48.98	5.0	USA	32.14	1.8
Iceland	51.62	6.6	USSR	48.92	3.0
Ireland	48.56	2.9	Yugoslavia	37.86	6.1
Italy	30.74	3.0			

Source: Woodward, M. and Walker, A.R.P. (1994), *Br. Dent. J.*, 176, 297–302.

Output 9.12. SAS PROC GLM results for Example 9.11, model 1.

Dependent variable: logdmft

Source	DF	Sum of squares	Mean square	F value	Pr > F
Model	1	10.97728939	10.97728939	34.99	<.0001
Error	88	27.60682128	0.31371388		
Corrected total	89	38.58411068			

Parameter	Estimate	Standard error	t value	Pr > |t|
Intercept	0.1511479867	0.12292940	1.23	0.2221
sugar	0.0211598620	0.00357711	5.92	<.0001

models to represent our data, each model will be described in turn, so as to provide interpretation of SAS output and to illustrate differences between the models.

Output 9.12 gives the fitted linear regression model (after rounding) as

$$\hat{y} = 0.1511 + 0.0212\, x_1,$$

which is illustrated by Figure 9.9(a). Since this is a one-term model, the Type I and Type III (sequential and cross-adjusted) SS and MS are both equal to the model SS and MS, and so are not shown. The slope is significantly different from zero ($p < 0.0001$). However, the intercept is not significantly different from zero at the 5% level ($p = 0.2221$).

Output 9.13 gives the results of fitting the one-way ANOVA model. We can interpret the parameter estimates given in Output 9.13 only if we know how the categorical variable x_2 (TYPE) was read into SAS. In fact, TYPE took the value 1 for industrialised and 2 for developing countries in the dataset read into SAS. Hence the fitted model (after rounding) defined by the estimates at the bottom of Output 9.13 is

$$\hat{y} = 0.6215 + 0.5196x_2^{(1)} + 0x_2^{(2)}$$

Output 9.13. SAS PROC GLM results for Example 9.11, model 2.

Dependent variable: logdmft

Source	DF	Sum of squares	Mean square	F value	Pr > F
Model	1	5.30737923	5.30737923	14.04	0.0003
Error	88	33.27673144	0.37814468		
Corrected total	89	38.58411068			

Parameter	Estimate		Standard error	t value	Pr > |t|
Intercept	0.6215250932	B	0.07873432	7.89	<.0001
type 1	0.5196338074	B	0.13870315	3.75	0.0003
type 2	0.0000000000	B	.	.	.

where

$$x_2^{(1)} = \begin{cases} 1 \text{ for industrialised countries} \\ 0 \text{ for developing countries,} \end{cases}$$

$$x_2^{(2)} = \begin{cases} 1 \text{ for developing countries} \\ 0 \text{ for industrialised countries.} \end{cases}$$

The predicted y for industrialised countries is thus

$$\hat{y} = 0.6215 + 0.5196 + 0 = 1.1411,$$

and for developing countries is

$$\hat{y} = 0.6215 + 0 + 0 = 0.6215.$$

Thus $\log_e$(DMFT) and, consequently, DMFT itself are higher in industrialised countries. This difference is significant ($p = 0.0003$) according to the two equivalent tests shown in Output 9.13. These two tests are an F test on (1, 88) d.f. and a t test on 88 d.f. As explained in Section 9.3.1, these two tests are equivalent because the first d.f. for F is 1 and the second is equal to the d.f. for the t test. The intercept, which is now the predicted $\log_e$(DMFT) value for developing countries, is significantly different from zero ($p < 0.0001$). Figure 9.9(b) illustrates the fitted model.

Output 9.14 shows results for model 3. The fitted two-variable model (after rounding from Output 9.14) is

$$\hat{y} = 0.1703 + 0.0184 \, x_1 + 0.2032 x_2^{(1)} + 0 x_2^{(2)},$$

where $x_2^{(1)}$ and $x_2^{(2)}$ are as before. Hence, for industrialised countries (where $x_2^{(1)} = 1$ and $x_2^{(2)} = 0$) we have

$$\hat{y} = 0.1703 + 0.0184 x_1 + 0.2032 + 0 = 0.3735 + 0.0184 x_1.$$

For developing countries (where $x_2^{(1)} = 0$ and $x_2^{(2)} = 1$),

$$\hat{y} = 0.1703 + 0.0184 x_1 + 0 + 0 = 0.1703 + 0.0184 x_1.$$

Figure 9.9(c) illustrates this fitted model (a 'parallel lines' model).

In Output 9.14, the model SS of 11.60 (rounded) splits sequentially into 10.98 (for SUGAR) and 0.62 (for TYPE given SUGAR). SUGAR, the first term entered into the model, is highly

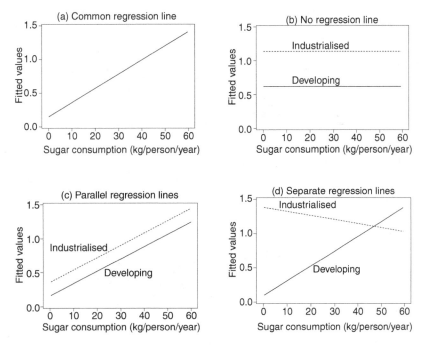

Figure 9.9. Fitted values against sugar consumption (a) to (d) for models 1 to 4, respectively, as specified in the text.

Output 9.14. SAS PROC GLM results for Example 9.11, model 3.

Dependent variable: logdmft

Source	DF	Sum of squares	Mean square	F value	Pr > F
Model	2	11.59555941	5.79777971	18.69	<.0001
Error	87	26.98855126	0.31021323		
Corrected total	89	38.58411068			

Source	DF	Type I SS	Mean square	F value	Pr > F
sugar	1	10.97728939	10.97728939	35.39	<.0001
type	1	0.61827002	0.61827002	1.99	0.1616

Source	DF	Type III SS	Mean square	F value	Pr > F
sugar	1	6.28818018	6.28818018	20.27	<.0001
type	1	0.61827002	0.61827002	1.99	0.1616

Parameter	Estimate		Standard error	t value	Pr > |t|
Intercept	0.1703433216	B	0.12299546	1.38	0.1696
sugar	0.0183506278		0.00407585	4.50	<.0001
type 1	0.2032214738	B	0.14394967	1.41	0.1616
type 2	0.0000000000	B	.	.	.

Output 9.15. SAS PROC GLM results for Example 9.11, model 4.

Dependent variable: logdmft

Source	DF	Sum of squares	Mean square	F value	Pr > F
Model	3	12.97276317	4.32425439	14.52	<.0001
Error	86	25.61134750	0.29780637		
Corrected total	89	38.58411068			

Source	DF	Type I SS	Mean square	F value	Pr > F
sugar	1	10.97728939	10.97728939	36.86	<.0001
type	1	0.61827002	0.61827002	2.08	0.1533
sugar*type	1	1.37720376	1.37720376	4.62	0.0343

Parameter	Estimate		Standard error	t value	Pr > |t|
Intercept	0.095506602	B	0.12543488	0.76	0.4485
sugar	0.021394414	B	0.00423693	5.05	<.0001
type 1	1.291599971	B	0.52539846	2.46	0.0160
type 2	0.000000000	B	.	.	.
sugar*type 1	−0.027274207	B	0.01268294	−2.15	0.0343
sugar*type 2	0.000000000	B	.	.	.

significant ($p < 0.0001$) by itself, but TYPE is not significant ($p = 0.1616$) after accounting for SUGAR. The Type III SS show that SUGAR is still highly significant after accounting for TYPE. Hence, we do not seem to require TYPE, once we know SUGAR, to predict LOGDMFT. This is despite the fact that TYPE is a significant predictor when taken in isolation (as seen in Output 9.13).

Output 9.15 shows results for model 4. The fitted model when the interaction between the x terms is included is obtained from Output 9.15 (after rounding) as

$$\hat{y} = 0.0955 + 0.0214x_1 + 1.2916x_2^{(1)} + 0x_2^{(2)} - 0.0273x_1 x_2^{(1)} + 0x_1 x_2^{(2)},$$

with $x_2^{(1)}$ and $x_2^{(2)}$ as before. Hence, for industrialised countries (where $x_2^{(1)} = 1$ and $x_2^{(2)} = 0$), we have

$$\hat{y} = 0.0955 + 0.0214x_1 + 1.2916 - 0.0273x_1 = 1.3871 - 0.0059x_1.$$

For developing countries (where $x_2^{(1)} = 0$ and $x_2^{(2)} = 1$),

$$\hat{y} = 0.0955 + 0.0214x_1.$$

The fitted model (a 'separate lines' model) is illustrated by Figure 9.9(d).

The Type III SS are not useful here (and so are not shown) because we would not wish to consider either main effect after accounting for their interaction. The Type I SS show, crucially, that the interaction *is* significant at the 5% level ($p = 0.03$), after accounting for the two main effects. That is, the interaction truly adds to the predictive power of the model. Hence, model 4 is the one to adopt: $\log_e(\text{DMFT})$ and thus DMFT itself depend upon sugar in a different way in the two types of countries. Since the slope for industrialised countries is virtually zero, it seems that DMFT has a relationship with sugar only in developing countries. This is an example of a unilateral interaction (Section 4.7). The epidemiological explanation for this may be the greater use of fluoride toothpastes, and other dental hygiene products, in more developed nations.

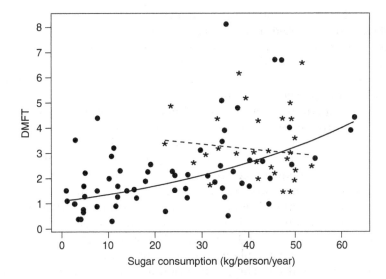

Figure 9.10. DMFT against sugar consumption, showing the fitted curves from model 4 in the text. Asterisks and dashed line denote industrialised countries; dots and solid line denote developing countries.

Due to the significant interaction, prediction depends upon type of country even though its main effect is not significant, after accounting for the effect of sugar, in Output 9.14 and Output 9.15. It would *not* be correct to drop this nonsignificant main effect from the model because it still contributes to the interaction.

To emphasise the effect of using $\log_e$(DMFT) as the dependent variable, Figure 9.10 shows the predicted values from the best model, model 4, on the original scale. The observed values are also given for comparison. Fitted values are shown only for the observed ranges of sugar consumptions.

9.7 Several explanatory variables

So far we have been restricted to one or two explanatory variables in our models. The principles thus established for model interpretation and evaluation carry over to the multiple-variable (or multivariable) situation, which is common in epidemiology. For instance, we can evaluate the importance of a specific explanatory variable, adjusting for the effect of several others which are confounding variables, by fitting it together with the confounders in the multivariable model. We shall return to this issue in Section 9.9.

A more complex situation is one in which we have several candidate risk factors and we wish to know which of them is required to predict the outcome variable. For instance, we could have five risk factors (say x_1 to x_5) but we wish to know whether some subset of the five will suffice for predicting y. Those variables not in the selected subset may be omitted because they have no real relationship with y, or because they are highly correlated with one or more of the selected variables.

Most statistical computer packages include automatic routines to select an appropriate subset of explanatory variables. These operate on the principle of parsimony; precise details are given by Draper and Smith (1998). One *modus operandi* would be to begin by fitting all the separate single-variable models that relate y to an x variable and select that x variable which gives the most highly significant result (from its one-way ANOVA table). Provided this most significant result is more extreme than some predetermined level (say 5%), we enter the variable into our selected subset and continue.

At the second stage, we could test each other variable for an effect conditional on the variable already selected (using F tests from the sequential ANOVAs) and select that which is most significant, provided that one is significant at 5%. At the next stage, we evaluate each remaining variable conditional on these first two selected, etc. We stop when we fail to find a significant addition. This is a simple kind of **forward selection** procedure. **Backward selection** works in the reverse order, starting with all explanatory variables and deleting (if possible) the least important at each stage. **Stepwise selection** is a mixture of these two approaches; as such it may also be used as a generic name for these automatic selection methods.

Automatic selection procedures have the advantage of simplicity of operation. However, they are not guaranteed to find the 'best' model in any statistical sense. More importantly, they may prevent the researcher from understanding her or his data completely. For example, it will not be clear how interrelationships between the variables affect the epidemiological interpretation. Often researchers treat the selected subset as the only variables that have any effect on the outcome variable, failing to recognise that an excluded variable may still be important when some of the selected variables are not adjusted for. The justification for adjustments should be epidemiological rather than statistical. Other problems are discussed by Greenland (1989).

Unfortunately, the alternative, to fit all possible models, can be a daunting task. For instance, even if we ignore interactions, with five explanatory variables there are 31 models to fit (5 with one x variable, 10 with two, 10 with three, 5 with four and 1 with all five). When we consider that we could have anything up to five-way interactions as well, the number of models appears to be prohibitively large. However, we can often reduce the scale of the problem by using our experience (to delete uninteresting or unlikely combinations), common sense (perhaps to delete multiway interactions because they are extremely difficult to interpret) or by thinking carefully about what we wish to achieve (for instance, we may always want certain variables, such as age and sex, in the model because they are fundamental confounders). Furthermore, modern computing facilities make it particularly easy to fit several models to the same set of data with little effort.

Supposing that we can fit all the models that interest us, how should we compare them (perhaps to find the best overall model)? A common mistake is to do this through the coefficient of determination (the ratio of the model to the total SS, often multiplied by 100). When many variables are involved, this is usually called the R^2 **statistic**, to distinguish it from the corresponding r^2 statistic, which involves only one explanatory variable: (9.21). Unfortunately, R^2 will *always* grow as extra explanatory variables are added to the model. This is a mathematical certainty, whatever the importance of the added variable. Thus, for quantitative explanatory variables, R^2 can be used only to compare models with the same number of terms.

Various statistics have been proposed to replace R^2 when comparing models with different degrees of freedom (Montgomery and Peck, 2012). Many computer packages produce an **adjusted R^2** to serve this purpose; effectively, it corrects R^2 for the d.f. A simple and effective method of comparison is to find the model with the smallest error MS. As this is the unexplained variation standardised by its d.f., it will serve as an overall measure of lack of explanatory power. Often models with slightly higher error MS but fewer x terms are compared with the minimum error MS model through sequential ANOVA table F tests, so as to enable nonsignificant terms to be deleted. Hence, a more parsimonious model may result.

As described in Section 9.6, when the multiple variable model includes categorical variables we should consider the set of dummy variables for any one categorical variable to be bound together. We either keep or delete the entire set from a model; the sets should not be broken up. If all the variables are quantitative, we have a

multiple regression model. This title is sometimes used for any many-variable general linear model. Epidemiological investigators often use 'multivariate analysis' as a synonym for multiple regression (of any kind). This practice should be avoided because the term has a different meaning in statistics.

Example 9.12 Bolton–Smith *et al.* (1991) use data from the SHHS to ascertain dietary and nondietary predictors of high-density lipoprotein (HDL) cholesterol. Here some of their analyses are reproduced using further survey data unavailable at the time of their report, but using fewer variables and restricting the analysis to men. The data to be used are records of serum HDL cholesterol, age, alcohol, dietary cholesterol and fibre consumption for 4897 men. These data may be downloaded; see Appendix A.

As a first step to exploring the relationship between the variables (which are all quantitative), consider Table 9.19. We see that the outcome variable, HDL cholesterol, is highly correlated only with alcohol. Although there are significant correlations with cholesterol and (negatively) with fibre, the actual correlations are low. There are reasonably high negative correlations between alcohol and both age and fibre, and positive correlations between cholesterol and both alcohol and fibre.

We might consider that age is really a confounding variable; we would then like to assess the effect of dietary risk factors after having allowed for age. We might then wish to look at **partial correlation coefficients:** correlations between the other variables adjusted for age. These may be found as the correlations between the residuals (Section 9.8) from the separate SLRs of each of the other four variables on age. Statistical computer packages will produce the partial correlations by more direct methods. Continuing, we may then fit all possible regressions with the proviso that age is present in all models.

Rather than do this, we shall treat age just as for the other three explanatory variables. Table 9.20 gives the results of all the regression fits. Using the R^2 criterion within subsets of models that have the same number of variables, the best one-variable model regresses HDL cholesterol on alcohol (as we already know from Table 9.19); the best two-variable model has the x variables alcohol and age; and the best three-variable model has alcohol, age and cholesterol. As they must, these models also have the lowest error MS within their set. Overall, the best model seems to be that with alcohol and age because it has the lowest error MS of all.

We should consider whether the age plus alcohol model might be replaced by something simpler (that is, with fewer variables). In this case, a simpler model could be one with only a single x variable, and the sensible choice, from such models, is that with alcohol alone because this is the SLR model with highest R^2 (by far). To make the comparison, we fit the bivariable regression model with age and alcohol (with some software, it may be necessary to fit alcohol first so that we can ascertain whether age has a significant *extra* effect). The sequential ANOVA table is given as Table 9.21. From this, we see that age is necessary after allowing for alcohol (although alcohol is clearly much more important). Thus, the alcohol plus age model is considered to be the best for predicting HDL cholesterol in men. From Table 9.20, we see that age and alcohol together explain about 11% of the person-to-person variation in HDL cholesterol.

Table 9.19. Pearson correlation matrix for serum HDL cholesterol, age and alcohol, cholesterol and fibre consumption; SHHS men.

	HDL	Age	Alcohol	Cholesterol	Fibre
HDL	1	*−0.006*	0.328	0.058	−0.041
Age		1	−0.124	−0.033	*−0.017*
Alcohol			1	0.146	−0.133
Cholesterol				1	0.102
Fibre					1

Note: Values given in italics are not significantly different from zero ($p > 0.05$).

Table 9.20. Results of fitting all possible (nonempty) regression models, using age (years), consumption of alcohol (units/week), cholesterol (mg/day) and fibre (g/day) to predict HDL cholesterol (mmol/l); SHHS men.

Number of x variables	R^2 (%)	Error mean square	Intercept	Age	Alcohol	Cholesterol	Fibre
					Estimates		
1	0.0037	0.13478	1.3839	-0.00039			
1	**10.7632**	0.12027	1.2607		0.00622		
1	0.3309	0.13434	1.3106			0.00014	
1	0.1714	0.13455	1.4086				-0.00206
2	**10.8859**	**0.12013**	1.1477	0.00225	0.00630		
2	0.3327	0.13436	1.3239	-0.00027		0.00014	
2	0.1759	0.13457	1.4301	-0.00043			-0.00206
2	10.7729	0.12029	1.2518		0.00619	0.00002	
2	10.7637	0.12030	1.2583		0.00622		0.00011
2	0.5569	0.13406	1.3566			0.00015	-0.00238
3	**10.8966**	0.12014	1.1379	0.00226	0.00628	0.00002	
3	10.8870	0.12016	1.1435	0.00226	0.00631		0.00017
3	0.5592	0.13408	1.3721	-0.00031		0.00015	-0.00238
3	10.7730	0.12031	1.2508		0.00620	0.00002	0.00005
4	**10.8970**	0.12017	1.1355	0.00226	0.00628	0.00002	0.00011

Note: Values given in bold are the best (see text for criteria).

Table 9.21. Sequential ANOVA table for Example 9.12.

Source of variation	Sum of squares	Degrees of freedom	Mean square	F ratio	p value
Alcohol	71.01	1	71.01	591.10	<0.0001
Age | alcohol	0.81	1	0.81	6.74	0.0095
Error	587.94	4894	0.12		
Total	659.76	4896			

Notice that, just because alcohol plus age gives the best model, our analyses show that this does *not* mean that cholesterol and fibre have no effect on HDL cholesterol. Indeed, they have a stronger statistical effect than age when taken alone, according to Table 9.19. From Table 9.20, we can see that their statistical effect is removed by alcohol. The epidemiological conclusions that we can reach depend upon our understanding of the causal pathways (Section 4.3). If we can assume that heavier drinking just happens to go with a diet relatively high in cholesterol and low in fibre, then we might conclude that the (small) effects of cholesterol and fibre are explained by confounding with alcohol.

Having fitted all the models, we can see precisely how the variables interrelate. Of particular interest here is the variable age. From Table 9.20, we see that it is significant (and then has a positive effect) only when considered with alcohol; indeed, it has a small negative effect unless alcohol is allowed for. From Table 9.19, we would not even consider it further if we based our analysis on simple correlations, and yet it has appeared in the 'best' model.

Another point of interest is the effect of alcohol; this is all but unchanged regardless of which other variables are allowed for in the analysis. Hence, no variables act as confounders for alcohol. Alcohol is not only the strongest predictor of HDL cholesterol, but its effect is not influenced by any of the other explanatory variables considered.

9.7.1 Information criteria

One drawback with the use of the minimum mean square error to choose between models is that the method is not applicable with other common classes of models, such as the logistic, binomial, Poisson and Cox models of later chapters. A more general approach is to use **information criteria**, the two most commonly used of which are the Akaike Information Criterion (AIC) (Akaike, 1974) and the Bayesian Information Criterion (BIC) (Schwarz, 1978). Which is the best is a subject of debate, and depends upon the context. With general linear models, the AIC has superior theoretical qualities. However, the difference between what the AIC and the BIC identifies as the best model is unlikely to be very different, in that the explanatory variables included in each 'best' model are usually similar.

The two criteria are generally defined as $AIC = 2p - 2\log_e \hat{L}$ and $BIC = p\log_e n - 2\log_e \hat{L}$. As always, n is the sample size. $\hat{L}$ is the fitted likelihood for the model under consideration, a measure of goodness-of-fit (Section 10.7) and p is the number of explanatory parameters fitted (including the intercept). This is equal to one plus the number of explanatory variables fitted if all are continuous variables, such as in Example 9.12. A categorical variable with ℓ levels contributes $\ell - 1$ to the value of p (since $\ell - 1$ dummy variables are required to fit the categorical variable: see Section 9.2.6). Although this statistic is seldom reported in general linear modelling, we can obtain the likelihood for a general linear model using any computer procedure designed for the generalised linear model — an extension of the general linear model which is not restricted to assuming a normal distribution for the data (Section 10.6). Such procedures may well also provide the AIC and BIC automatically.

We can define a general information criterion as $cp - 2\log\hat{L}$, which will be the AIC when $c = 2$ and the BIC when $c = \log_e n$. The cp portion of the general information criterion measures the complexity of the model since it increases as more variables are entered; this is referred to as a **penalty**. The other portion measures the goodness-of-fit of the particular model under consideration. Taking one portion from the other gives a result which balances complexity against accuracy, which is the basic idea behind information criteria. Since the penalty is given a positive weight, and goodness-of-fit is given a negative weight, the best model is that with the smallest information criterion. As AIC $-$ BIC $= p(2 - \log_e n)$, and since $\log_e n$ will be larger than 2 when n exceeds 7, the BIC will increase more than the AIC as extra predictors are entered into the model. That is, the AIC and BIC statistics measure accuracy in the same way, but the BIC approach gives a greater penalty to the addition of extra terms in the model. Consequently, the best model identified by the BIC often contains fewer explanatory variables than the best model identified by the AIC.

As when using the mean square error, the best model identified by an information criterion may not be the final model that is adopted for clinical use. As we saw in Example 9.12, it is sensible to also consider other models, especially those that are less complex (i.e., with smaller p). In practice, the final model may be chosen with regard to non-statistical properties of potential explanatory variables, such as ease of acquisition.

Example 9.13 Consider variable selection in Example 9.12 anew. Each of the 16 possible models was fitted and the likelihoods obtained from a computer package. From the results, the AIC and BIC were obtained: see Table 9.22. Both criteria gave the same best model amongst the subsets containing the same number of explanatory variables, as would be expected. However, the overall best model according to the BIC contains only alcohol, whereas the best according to the AIC also contains age. These are the same two models that were singled out for consideration in Example 9.12.

Table 9.22. Akaike and Bayesian Information Criteria for Example 9.13 ($n = 4897$). The 'best' model (lowest AIC/BIC) within each set (where the sets are defined by the number of explanatory variables fitted) has its AIC/BIC shown in bold, and the overall best models have their AIC/BIC boxed.

age	alcohol	cholest	fibre	Number of x terms	p	$\log_e \hat{L}$	AIC	BIC
				0	1	−2040.50478	**4083.0094**	**4089.5060**
X				1	2	−2040.41509	4084.8301	4097.8230
	X			1	2	−1761.67645	**3527.3527**	**3540.3460** (boxed)
		X		1	2	−2032.38866	4068.7772	4081.7700
			X	1	2	−2036.30493	4076.6100	4089.6030
X	X			2	3	−1758.30905	**3522.6183** (boxed)	3542.1070
X		X		2	3	−2032.34606	4070.6920	4090.1810
X			X	2	3	−2036.19286	4078.3856	4097.8750
	X	X		2	3	−1761.41239	3528.8247	3548.3140
	X		X	2	3	−1761.66311	3529.3262	3548.8450
		X	X	2	3	−2026.83206	4059.6639	4079.1530
X	X	X		3	4	−1758.01545	**3524.0310**	**3550.0160**
X	X		X	3	4	−1758.27723	3524.5545	3550.5400
X		X	X	3	4	−2026.77488	4061.5498	4087.5350
	X	X	X	3	4	−1761.40967	3530.8193	3556.8050
X	X	X	X	4	5	−1758.00285	**3526.0055**	**3558.4880**

Since information criteria are only used in a relative sense, the absolute results for any one model have no meaning. For example, multiplying each AIC statistic in Table 9.22 by a constant, or adding a constant to each statistic, will have no effect on which model is best, either within a set or overall. As a consequence, when obtaining the AIC and BIC statistics directly from computer packages, the numerical results obtained for any one model may not agree with those obtained from using the formulae given here, although the way these numbers are used will be the same. For example, PROC GENMOD is the standard procedure in SAS for handling generalised linear models (Chapter 10); as mentioned already, this includes the general linear model. The AIC and BIC results it produces take a value of p that is one more than the number of explanatory terms fitted: thus the SAS code for Example 9.13, available from the web site for this book, gives AIC results that are two more, and BIC results that are $\log_e(4897)$ bigger, than appear in Table 9.22. The likelihoods PROC GENMOD produces are shown in Table 9.22. The corresponding GLM routine in Stata, again, gives the likelihoods shown in Table 9.22, but different (transformed) results for the AIC and BIC. However, the definitions of AIC and BIC given above are used by the post-estimation (ESTAT IC) command which can be used after the GLM command (again, see the code given on the web site for this book).

As indicated from the outset, the AIC and BIC may be used in many regression contexts, some of which require generalisations of the definitions above. In every case, practical use of the criteria is as described here. For an example of their use in a different context see Example 10.16.

9.7.2   Boosted regression

With the emergence of large datasets with many variables, for example in genomic research, a number of innovative methods for determining associations have been developed, and are still being developed. Many of these involve the use of a training set, to develop models of association, and a validation set, to test the models, which are obtained by splitting the observed dataset. In the regression context, these are often called **boosting** methods. In its generality, boosting is an extremely flexible method of model selection. Although this methodology is rarely used in epidemiology at the time of writing, it is an efficient method for model selection and is certainly worthy of consideration for use with large datasets. Schonlau (2005) describes a Stata plug-in which applies the boosting method of Hastie *et al.* (2001).

9.8   Model checking

As indicated in Section 9.1, the model adopted should have isolated the systematic and random components of the outcome variable. After fitting the model, we can see how successful we have been by examining the differences between the observed and fitted values, $y - \hat{y}$. These errors generated by the model are called the **residuals**. If the model has been successful, the residuals will be both relatively small and truly random. Furthermore, because we have assumed (when developing significance tests, etc.) that the random error has a normal distribution with zero mean and constant variance, the residuals should be a random sample from this distribution.

A very useful way of examining the residuals is to plot them against the fitted values; the resultant diagram is called a **residual plot**. If the residual plot shows an obvious pattern, such as the points appearing to make a 'U' shape, then the residuals have a systematic component. This violates the assumption of the model, and suggests that a different model should be fitted (perhaps a quadratic regression in the example of the 'U' shape cited). If the residual plot shows one or more very large, or very small, values, we should be concerned about the effect of the corresponding x–y values as **outliers**. These are points a long way from the fitted line (should it have been drawn on the original scatterplot). They may have seriously affected the fit of the regression line and will certainly have inflated the error MS. It is always worth checking outliers in case they have been wrongly recorded, or in case they come from a source so special that it might sensibly be considered separately.

Since size may be hard to judge objectively, the residuals are often divided by their standard error before their examination begins. The standard error is estimated by the square root of the error MS from the ANOVA table for the model. Hence, the **standardised residuals** are

$$(y - \hat{y})/s_e \tag{9.39}$$

for each observation. The standardised residuals should follow the standard normal distribution if the model is 'good'. Hence, we expect only 5% of their values to exceed ±1.96, from Table B.2. Any standardised residual that is less than −1.96 or greater than 1.96 may be considered an outlier. We can check the normality assumption by constructing a normal plot (Section 2.7.1) of the residuals or the standardised residuals.

Example 9.14 For the sugar and caries data from developing countries, as analysed in Example 9.5, we have the observed, y, values in Table 9.8. The fitted values (estimated systematic component) come from the regression line

$$\hat{y} = 1.165 + 0.0470x.$$

To calculate the residuals (estimated random component), one for each country, we find $\hat{y}$ and subtract the result from the corresponding y. For instance, the fitted value for Algeria ($x = 36.60$) is

$$\hat{y} = 1.165 + 0.0470 \times 36.60 = 2.89.$$

The residual is thus

$$y - \hat{y} = 2.3 - 2.89 = -0.59.$$

On Figure 9.3, we could measure this residual by sending up a vertical line at a sugar consumption of 36.60. The vertical distance between the dot (observed value) and the line (fitted value) is 0.59. This residual is negative because the dot lies below the fitted regression line.

From Table 9.9, the error MS is $s_e^2 = 1.9435$. From (9.39), the standardised residual for Algeria is

$$-0.59/\sqrt{1.9435} = -0.42.$$

Figure 9.11 shows the residual plot, using standardised residuals, including a useful reference line at zero. The point for Algeria has coordinates (2.89, −0.42). There is evidence of a slight increase in residual variability with increasing $\hat{y}$. There is one very large standardised residual (that for Guatemala). We have no reason to suppose that this is based on erroneous data, nor

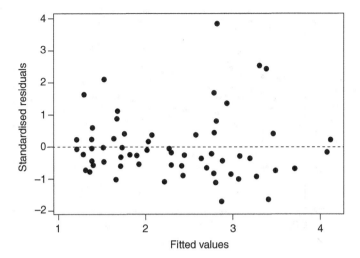

Figure 9.11. Residual plot for the simple linear regression model of Example 9.5 (DMFT on original scale).

any other good reason to treat this country separately. Three other countries also provide outliers. Since all four are positive outliers (beyond +1.96), the residual plot is unbalanced with roughly two-thirds of standardised residuals taking negative values.

Figure 9.12 is the normal plot for this problem. Here there is obvious curvature, akin to an elongated 'S' shape. We conclude that the standardised residuals do not arise from the required standard normal distribution.

Figure 9.13 and Figure 9.14 show equivalents to the last two plots, for log transformed DMFT regressed on sugar, as in Example 9.6. In Figure 9.13, we see a random pattern in the residuals with no one gross outlier nor any indication of growth of residual variation, unlike before; also 30 residuals are negative and 31 are positive, so there is no imbalance, unlike before. However, there are still a number of outliers. The pattern of Figure 9.14 is fairly close to a straight line, although a problem exists in the tails.

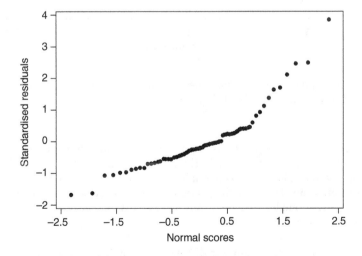

Figure 9.12. Normal plot for the standardised residuals from the simple linear regression model of Example 9.5 (DMFT on original scale).

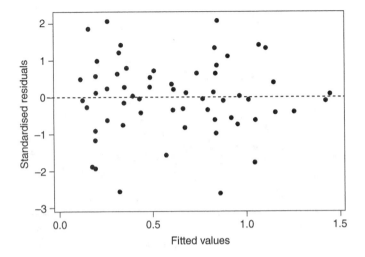

Figure 9.13. Residual plot for the transformed simple linear regression model of Example 9.6 (DMFT on log scale).

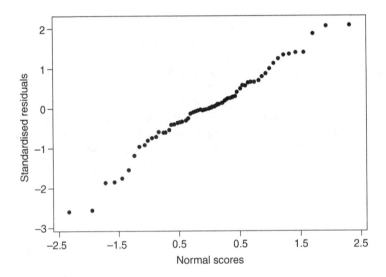

Figure 9.14. Normal plot for the standardised residuals from the transformed simple linear regression model of Example 9.6 (DMFT on log scale).

We can conclude that the log model is slightly better than the model on the original scale. The log regression model seems to satisfy the model requirements reasonably well. As noted in Example 9.6, a better model may be available; we can find out only by trial-and-error fitting and residual examination. However, inspection of the scatterplot, Figure 9.2, shows that no very precise regression model can be fitted to these data because of what appears to be substantial random error.

Residual plots will look somewhat different when ANOVA models have been fitted. Since fitted values go up in steps (at the levels of the group variable(s)) there will be several residuals for each fitted value. Hence, the residual plot will be a series of columns of points. Problems with the model would be diagnosed if the columns had very different averages or dispersions.

Another issue when considering the fit of quantitative explanatory variables is that of **influence**. An influential value is one that has a serious impact on the regression parameter estimates; that is, where the line sits (for simple linear regression). If we draw an analogy with a see-saw (teeter-totter), where a child exerts greater turning moment the further she or he sits from the centre, we see that it is extreme values of x (far from their mean) that exert greatest influence on the regression fit — for example, the x values of over 60 kg of sugar per head per annum in Figure 9.2 (from Cuba and Barbados). An objective measure of influence is **Cook's distance**, computed by many statistical software packages. See Cook and Weisberg (1982) for details.

For further details of the theory of model checking, see Belsley *et al.* (1980) and Draper and Smith (1998). More applied accounts are given by Chatterjee and Price (2000) and Montgomery and Peck (2012).

9.9   Confounding

In most of the preceding, we have assumed that all the explanatory variables are of equal status. If, instead, one of them is the variable of interest and the rest are confounders, it is unlikely to be sensible to think about the 'best' model, as in Section 9.5 and Section 9.7. Instead, we may well wish to fit the variable of interest alone, then with certain important confounders and finally with all confounders and compare the results, just as was done in a different context in Table 4.8.

Example 9.15 Table 9.23 shows hypothetical data on systolic blood pressure (SBP) collected from 36 individuals, 26 of whom are regular users of a certain chilli sauce. The researchers hypothesised that the chilli sauce, being of high sodium content, would promote raised blood pressure amongst its users. However, the mean difference in SBP between users and non-users, 4.35 mmHg, was not sufficiently high, in this small sample, to be formally significant after fitting a general linear model to these data (or a simple t test, which is an equivalent procedure in this case): the standard error of the mean difference is 2.53 and the p value is 0.095.

Several, but by no means all, of the sample of people taken were known to be African Americans (AAs), who have a well-known tendency for relatively high blood pressure. Furthermore, different ethnicities may well tend towards different affinities for chilli sauce. Hence ethnicity may be a confounding factor in the association between chilli sauce use and SBP. Table 9.24 shows the data split by the three ethnic groups represented in the study, together with some useful summary statistics. The prevalence of use of the chilli sauce is greatest in Mexican Americans (MAs) and least in AAs. The mean SBP goes the other way — least in MAs and greatest in AAs. Within each ethnic group, the effect of chilli sauce on SBP is reasonably consistent, between 5.00 and 6.19 mmHg. Notice that each stratified level of effect is greater than the effect when ethnicity is ignored, seen in Table 9.23, of 4.35 mmHg. A general linear model (a two-way ANOVA model gives an equivalent

Table 9.23. Systolic blood pressure (mmHg) for regular users and non-users of a chilli sauce.

		Mean
Chilli sauce	126, 131, 128, 130, 123, 137, 135, 136, 148, 123	131.70
No chilli sauce	118, 128, 113, 131, 123, 122, 125, 127, 117, 138, 130, 125, 131, 124, 133, 123, 135, 119, 140, 128, 132, 126, 128, 130, 130, 135	127.35
Difference in means		4.35

Table 9.24. Systolic blood pressure (mmHg) for regular users and non-users of a chilli sauce, by ethnicity.

	Mexican Americans	Whites	African Americans
Chilli sauce	126, 131	128, 130, 123, 137	135, 136, 148, 123
No chilli sauce	118, 128	113, 131, 123, 122, 125, 127, 117, 138	130, 125, 131, 124, 133, 123, 135, 119, 140, 128, 132, 126, 128, 130, 130, 135
Percentage chilli	50%	33%	20%
Mean	125.75	126.17	130.55
Mean: chilli	128.50	129.50	135.50
Mean: no chilli	123.00	124.50	129.31
Difference in means	5.50	5.00	6.19

procedure in this case) was fitted using PROC GLM in SAS, with SBP as the outcome variable and chilli sauce use and ethnicity as the explanatory variables. The effect of chilli sauce adjusted for race was estimated by the difference between the least squares means (Section 9.4.6), with and without chilli sauce use, as 5.63 mmHg. Notice that this, as might be expected, is within the range covered by 5.00 to 6.19. The standard error of this effect (i.e., the adjusted mean difference) is 2.45 mmHg and the corresponding test has a p value of 0.03.

In this example, ethnicity clearly confounds the chilli sauce — SBP relationship since taking account of the confounding increases the estimated effect substantially, whilst the form of conceivable causal associations seems to satisfy the conditions of Figure 4.5. For a pictorial view of the effects estimated, before and after adjustment, see Figure 9.15. This figure also serves to

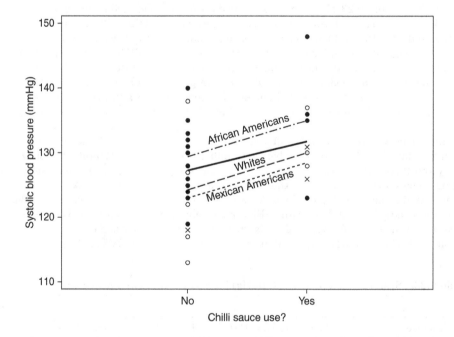

Figure 9.15. Fitted values from (a) the model predicting systolic blood pressure from chilli sauce use alone (solid line); and (b) the model predicting systolic blood pressure from both chilli sauce use and ethnicity: Example 9.15. Mexican Americans are represented by crosses; Whites are represented by open circles; and African Americans are represented by closed circles (some symbols are hidden due to overlaps).

emphasize the underlying concordance between classical regression and ANOVA models, and hence the application of both within the general linear model. Although neither explanatory variable considered here is continuous, the effect of chilli sauce can be envisaged as the slope of the line joining the means of chilli sauce users and non-users. This type of display is usually reserved for regression models, but can also be used for categorical explanatory variables — the key difference is that the scatterplot now consists of columns of points, rather than having a wide horizontal spread. Figure 9.15 has a single (solid) line for the overall effect of chilli sauce (ignoring race) and three intermittent lines for the stratified effects, by race. Since the latter are the fitted values (Section 9.4.5) from the model with just the main effects of chilli sauce and race, the lines are necessarily parallel (i.e., we have only allowed for confounding). If, instead, we fitted a model to examine interaction (by including the cross-product terms of chilli sauce and ethnicity, with two d.f.), the fitted lines would be divergent. When such a model was fitted (Section 9.4.7) there was no evidence of interaction ($p = 0.98$), as we should expect from the similar differences in SBP by ethnicity seen in Table 9.24 and the small sample size.

As far as the practitioner is concerned, the process of adjusting for a confounder using statistical modelling within a computer package is very easy. Whereas the basic model (without the confounder) requires fitting just the index variable of interest (chilli sauce in Example 9.15), the confounding model requires simply adding the supposed confounder (ethnicity in the example). The outcome variable stays the same. Example 9.16, following, gives a second example using real data. When there are many confounders, the process is easily generalised. One note of caution is that this simple approach only works if the relationships are modelled appropriately. In most cases in practice, linear relationships are assumed but rarely tested thoroughly for continuous confounding variables, in contrast to the index variable.

Example 9.16 We shall now consider an example that is part of an investigation reported by McDonagh *et al.* (1997). This followed an intriguing suggestion by Patel *et al.* (1995) that *Helicobacter pylori* infection may be related to the level of plasma fibrinogen. McDonagh *et al.* (1997) used data from the third Glasgow MONICA survey, first, to see if this relationship held in their data and, second, to see whether it could be explained by confounding. Here we shall consider only the MONICA data for men, of whom 510 had their fibrinogen and *H. pylori* status recorded. These data may be downloaded; see Appendix A.

Initially, fibrinogen was compared amongst men who had and did not have *H. pylori*. Results are given in Table 9.25. In this table, the *Q*s are the quartiles (defined in Section 2.6.1). Since there is clear right skew in these data, all further analyses were carried out on log-transformed fibrinogen. The 95% confidence interval for the difference between the two $\log_e$(fibrinogen) means (positive − negative) is (0.01, 0.10). The test to compare log means has a *p* value of 0.012. Hence, *H. pylori* status does, indeed, appear to be related to fibrinogen: men with positive *H. pylori* have higher values.

Age is a potential confounding factor in the relationship between *H. pylori* and fibrinogen, because both variables are known to increase with age. For the MONICA data, this is confirmed because the Pearson correlation between age and $\log_e$(fibrinogen) is 0.34, whilst summary statistics for age by *H. pylori* status, given in Table 9.26, show that those with the infection are, on average, a few years older.

Table 9.25. Fibrinogen (g/l) by *H. pylori* status; MONICA men.

H. pylori status	n	Mean (s.e.)	Q_1	Q_2	Q_3
Positive	361	2.93 (0.038)	2.43	2.84	3.35
Negative	149	2.76 (0.059)	2.33	2.55	3.07

Note: s.e. = standard error.

Table 9.26. Age (in years) by *H. pylori* status; MONICA men.

H. pylori status	n	Mean (s.e.)	Q_1	Q_2	Q_3
Positive	361	53.4 (0.71)	42	55	65
Negative	149	47.0 (1.10)	37	46	57

Note: s.e. = standard error.

Table 9.27. $\log_e$(fibrinogen) mean (with standard error in parentheses) by age group and *H. pylori* status; MONICA men.

Age group (years)	n	*H. pylori* status Positive	*H. pylori* status Negative	p value
25–34	65	0.86 (0.041)	0.87 (0.033)	0.86
35–44	100	0.99 (0.032)	0.97 (0.030)	0.60
45–54	107	1.00 (0.024)	1.00 (0.039)	0.99
55–64	122	1.10 (0.022)	1.10 (0.052)	0.89
65–74	116	1.13 (0.025)	1.03 (0.059)	0.09

To explore the effect of age further, $\log_e$(fibrinogen) and *H. pylori* were compared within each separate 10-year age group. The MONICA study sampled people aged from 25 to 74 years, so there are five age groups. Results for $\log_e$(fibrinogen) are given in Table 9.27. This suggests that *H. pylori* status has no age-specific effect on fibrinogen. Hence, we can expect to find no effect of *H. pylori* on fibrinogen levels, after adjustment for age.

To adjust the relationship between $\log_e$(fibrinogen) and *H. pylori* for age, the model

$$y = \beta_0 + \beta_1 x_1 + \beta_2^{(1)} x_2^{(1)} + \beta_2^{(2)} x_2^{(2)} + \varepsilon$$

was fitted, where x_1 is age; x_2 represents *H. pylori* status; y is $\log_e$(fibrinogen) and ε is the random error. The dummy variables for *H. pylori* are

$$x_2^{(1)} = \begin{cases} 1 & \text{for negatives} \\ 0 & \text{for positives,} \end{cases} \qquad x_2^{(2)} = \begin{cases} 1 & \text{for positives} \\ 0 & \text{for negatives.} \end{cases}$$

PROC GLM in SAS produced the following fitted model:

$$\hat{y} = 0.7319 + 0.0059x_1 - 0.0206x_2^{(1)} + 0x_2^{(2)}$$

with sequential ANOVA table as given by Table 9.28. The key line here is that for *H. pylori* given age. Since the F test has a p value of 0.36, we can conclude that there is no difference

Table 9.28. Sequential ANOVA table for $\log_e$(fibrinogen: Example 9.16.

Source of variation	Sum of squares	Degrees of freedom	Mean square	F ratio	p value
Age	3.459	1	3.459	66.86	<0.0001
H. pylori|age	0.043	1	0.043	0.83	0.36
Error	26.229	507	0.052		
Total	29.730	509			

between the average $\log_e$(fibrinogen) levels by *H. pylori* status, after allowing for age. Hence, the relationship seen earlier can be explained by both variables changing with increasing age.

Age-adjusted $\log_e$(fibrinogen) means by *H. pylori* status come from calculating the fitted values, $\hat{y}$, for each level of *H. pylori*, x_2. For *H. pylori* negatives, we have

$$\hat{y} = 0.7319 + 0.0059x_1 - 0.0206 = 0.7113 + 0.0059\,x_1;$$

and for *H. pylori* positives,

$$\hat{y} = 0.7319 + 0.0059x_1.$$

To obtain age-adjusted (least squares) means by *H. pylori* status, we then evaluate $\hat{y}$ at the mean age in the sample; that is, we find fitted values keeping age fixed at its mean. Since the mean age of the 510 MONICA men was 51.56, the age-adjusted $\log_e$(fibrinogen) means are, for *H. pylori* negatives,

$$0.7113 + 0.0059 \times 51.56 = 1.01;$$

and for *H. pylori* positives,

$$0.7319 + 0.0059 \times 51.56 = 1.03,$$

which are very similar. This emphasizes the lack of association between fibrinogen and *H. pylori* after allowing for the effect of age. Notice the different ways in which least squares means are calculated when adjusting for a quantitative variable, such as age, compared with a categorical variable, such as sex (Section 9.4.6).

We can, of course, obtain these least squares means directly from PROC GLM in SAS. As we have seen previously, this also gives the standard error of the least squares means. We can use these to find a 95% confidence interval for the age-adjusted mean $\log_e$(fibrinogen) as

$$\text{least squares mean} \pm 1.96 \times \text{standard error} \tag{9.40}$$

for each *H. pylori* group. We can find the corresponding interval for fibrinogen (on the original scale) by back-transformation; in this case, we raise the lower and upper limits in (9.40) to the exponential power.

One final point to make is that we have taken fibrinogen to be the outcome variable. It *may* be that the epidemiological hypothesis is that fibrinogen (and age) determines the risk of *H. pylori*. Although the basic principles of dealing with the confounder (age) will remain the same, it would not be sensible to fit a general linear model with *H. pylori* as the outcome variable, because this variable is binary and certainly not normally distributed. The correct approach is described in Chapter 10.

9.9.1 Adjustment using residuals

Given a suitable computer package, the easiest way to adjust for a single confounder is through sequential ANOVA and least squares means from a bivariable model. An alternative procedure that uses only single-variable models is worth reporting, as an aid to interpretation.

To explain this method, suppose that we wish to find the effect of x on the outcome variable, y, adjusting for the confounder, c. We proceed by fitting the model that relates y to c; call this model's residuals e_y. Then we fit the model that relates x to c; call these residuals e_x. Confounder-adjusted results then come from fitting the model that relates e_y to e_x. Thus, whereas the unadjusted analysis stems from the model that fits

x to y, the adjusted analysis stems from the model that fits the x residuals to the y residuals. Both residuals measure the remaining effect *after* taking account of the confounding variable, and so we have a logical method for removing the effect of confounding from the x–y relationship.

The residuals method leads to the same result as the bivariable (or, in general, many-variable) modelling approach using sequential sums of squares and fitted values, in the context of general linear models. This method was applied to Example 9.15, using PROC GLM in SAS repeatedly. Race was the c variable, chilli sauce the x variable and SBP the y variable. The estimated beta coefficient for chilli was, indeed, the same by both methods (using the SAS code available on the web site for this book).

The residuals method does not generalise to other statistical modelling situations, such as those met in Chapters 10 and 11, whereas the method of adjustment by adding confounders so as to make the single-variable, unadjusted, model into a multivariable model does. Hence the residual method has little practical utility.

9.10   Splines

In Section 9.3.3 the issue of non-linear associations was raised and addressed through transformations. An alternative approach is to abandon the idea of a single model that fits across the entire range of the explanatory variable and, instead, fit a specific model within intervals. An attractive way of doing this is to use a **spline**. In general a spline is a set of polynomial functions that are 'tied' together so that they meet at key points within the range of the explanatory variable, known as the **knots**. If k knots are chosen, there will be $k + 1$ components to the spline. The simplest type of spline is a **linear spline**: a collection of linear functions which differ within the intervals between the chosen knots. Another name for a linear spline is a **piecewise-linear function**.

Example 9.17 Consider the sugar-DMFT data of Table 9.8. Suppose that knots are chosen at 12 and 34 kg/person/year, these being the approximate tertiles of sugar consumption. In this case $k = 2$ and thus we require three spline components, one in each of the ranges: minimum to 12, 12 to 34 and 34 to maximum, where the minimum and maximum are the lowest and highest values for sugar. To allow for extrapolation, these extremes might be taken as zero and infinity, but clearly the fitting process will be restricted to the observed range of data. We can define the spline as $s = s_1 + s_2 + s_3$ where

$$s_1 = \begin{cases} x \text{ if } x \le 12 \\ 12 \text{ if } x > 12 \end{cases}$$

$$s_2 = \begin{cases} 0 \text{ if } x \le 12 \\ x - 12 \text{ if } 12 < x \le 34 \\ 22 \text{ if } x > 34 \end{cases}$$

$$s_3 = \begin{cases} 0 \text{ if } x \le 34 \\ x - 34 \text{ if } x > 34, \end{cases}$$

and x is sugar. With this representation, $s = x$; that is, x has simply been re-expressed. To demonstrate that this is so, Table 9.29 has been constructed with a few representative values for x (including values outside the observed range). Hence we can regress DMFT on sugar by regressing DMFT on s_1, s_2 and s_3 taken together. The results of fitting this three-variable linear

Table 9.29. Demonstration that the linear spline function, s, is equal to the observed values, x for Example 9.17.

Sugar, x	s_1	s_2	s_3	$s = \sum s_i$
0	0	0	0	0
6	6	0	0	6
12	12	0	0	12
23	12	11	0	23
34	12	22	0	34
50	12	22	16	50
100	12	22	66	100

regression in Stata are shown as Output 9.16 and Figure 9.16 shows the spline fit, with a shaded 95% confidence interval for the mean predicted DMFT from this model.

The fitted model here, by the method of least squares, is

$$DMFT = 1.381432 + 0.0200691s_1 + 0.0505495s_2 + 0.052371s_3.$$

Notice that this can be rewritten as an equation in x (sugar) using the definition of the 's' terms above.

The output and figure both show the break in the fitted line when sugar takes the value 12 kg/person/year (the first knot). The key feature in any linear spline model is the change in the slopes, as fitted through regression, below and above the knots. Here the fitted slope changes from about 0.02 to 0.05, so the rate of change of DMFT with sugar has increased between the lowest and middle thirds of sugar consumption. From the output we can see that the fitted slope has barely altered at the second, and final, knot. Indeed, the change is not perceivable on the plot. So the best-fitting straight-line relationship is essentially the same within the two highest thirds of sugar consumption. Looking at the overall fit in Figure 9.16 we see only slight deviation from a single straight line, which is much the same finding as from Figure 9.8 where a log model was fitted to these data.

Output 9.16. Results from Stata when fitting the linear spline model for DMFT: Example 9.17.

Source	SS	df	MS			
				Number of obs =		61
				F(3, 57) =		6.15
Model	36.9723451	3	12.324115	Prob > F	=	0.0011
Residual	114.304052	57	2.00533424	R-squared	=	0.2444
				Adj R-squared	=	0.2046
Total	151.276397	60	2.52127328	Root MSE	=	1.4161

dmft	Coef.	Std. Err.	t	P>|t|	[95% Conf. Interval]	
s1	.0200691	.0720272	0.28	0.782	-.1241629	.164301
s2	.0505495	.0270027	1.87	0.066	-.0035224	.1046214
s3	.0523711	.0324927	1.61	0.113	-.0126944	.1174365
_cons	1.381432	.6253947	2.21	0.031	.1291004	2.633763

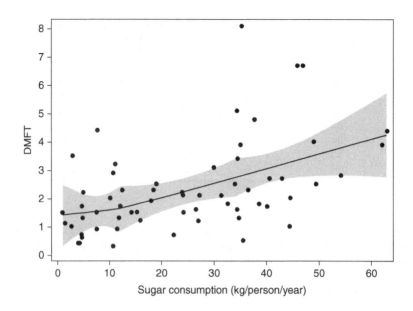

Figure 9.16. Fitted values (and 95% confidence intervals) for DMFT from a linear spline model for sugar data (with knots at 12 and 34 kg/person/year), plus the observed data: Example 9.17.

The general method for constructing a linear spline with k knots, m_1 to m_k, is a generalisation of that used in Example 9.17:

$$s_1 = \begin{cases} x \text{ if } x \leq m_1 \\ m_1 \text{ if } x > m_1 \end{cases}$$

$$s_i = \begin{cases} 0 \text{ if } x \leq m_{i-1} \\ x - m_{i-1} \text{ if } m_{i-1} < x \leq m_i \\ m_i - m_{i-1} \text{ if } x > m_i \end{cases}$$

$$s_{k+1} = \begin{cases} 0 \text{ if } x \leq m_k \\ x - m_k \text{ if } x > m_k, \end{cases}$$

where i runs from 2 to k in the middle term. These definitions make $\sum s = x$ within each interval between the knots (and thus overall), joining successive spline components at the intervening knot in the resultant plot.

Stata has a convenient routine for spline construction, MKSPLINE. The file to produce Output 9.16, available from the web site for this book, computes linear splines both using the formula given in Example 9.17 and using MKSPLINE: both are the same. Since comparison of slopes is such a common feature of a linear spline analysis, Stata has a subcommand, MARGIN, which can be used with MKSPLINE to transform the spline parameters so as to provide output which shows, for all but the first spline component, changes in slopes compared to the previous component. When this subcommand was used, Output 9.17 was produced: the components are now called sug1, sug2 and sug3 to differentiate them from s1, s2 and s3 (in Output 9.16). As already explained, sug1 = s1; sug2 = s2 − s1; sug3 = s3 − s2. From Output 9.17 we can see that there is no significant difference ($p = 0.74$) between the slopes below and above

Output 9.17. Results from Stata when fitting the linear spline model for DMFT with parameters that estimate differences in slopes.

dmft	Coef.	Std. Err.	t	P>|t|	[95% Conf. Interval]	
sug1	.0200691	.0720272	0.28	0.782	-.1241629	.164301
sug2	.0304804	.0908535	0.34	0.738	-.1514505	.2124114
sug3	.0018216	.0511946	0.04	0.972	-.1006939	.104337
_cons	1.381432	.6253947	2.21	0.031	.1291004	2.633763

the first knot, 12, as well as below and above the second knot, 34 ($p = 0.97$). So, it seems here that our two-knot linear spline is not fundamentally better than the single line model of Example 9.5.

Notice that the confidence limits in Figure 9.16 make up a string of three "bow-tie" patterns (with a degree of overlap). This reflects the fitting of three linear components of the spline, and is a generalisation of the shape of confidence intervals seen for a single straight line fit, as exemplified by Figure 9.4.

9.10.1 Choice of knots

A drawback with the spline approach is that the pattern that emerges when plotting will change as the number of knots change, as well as according to the choice of where the knots are placed. In interpreting plots using splines we should always be cognisant of the effect of these decisions, which should be effectively communicated. Most importantly, we should not over-emphasise the role of any chosen knot when considering thresholds, particularly risk thresholds in situations where the outcome variable relates to the chance of a disease (Section 10.10.3). Since our modelling process has only allowed the fitted line to change direction at the knots, it is not appropriate to report any knot as a proven threshold on the basis of the current analysis. We cannot know whether the change in direction would be sharper either before or after any chosen knot. Since the findings are so much affected by the choice of knots, it is crucial that these are chosen, *a priori,* in an objective way.

Sometimes the knots will be chosen because they represent meaningful thresholds; for example, values that are considered to be clinically relevant, generally because these are thresholds used in the past to make decisions about when to give treatments. An example of this is the analyses of risks associated with levels of estimated glomerular filtration rate by Matsushita *et al.* (2010), who chose the knots as the risk thresholds already used by nephrologists. Otherwise the number of knots should be chosen with regard to the sample size since, as the number of knots increases, the fitted line will get more and more jumpy until it reflects sampling variation as much as the systematic pattern underlying the data. In practice, it is rare to find more than nine knots used. When the knots are not fixed according to some specific criteria relating to the data, placement of the knots is generally made so as either to make the intervals between them constant or to evenly distribute the observed data values between them, as was done — at least, roughly — in Example 9.17. The MKSPLINE command has both options. Strategic advice regarding the positioning of knots is provided by Harrell (2001). In principle, the issues concerned with placing the knots are the same as those for choosing cut-points when cutting a quantitative variable into categories.

9.10.2   Other types of splines

Whilst linear splines are generally used to fit regression models, other (more complex) types of splines are generally used to provide smooth representations of data from a scatterplot. With a sensible choice of the number of knots, this enables the researcher to understand the underlying systematic pattern in the data and thus, for example, to see whether a linear regression model appears to be a reasonable choice for deriving predictions or making other inferences.

The simplest type of spline that can achieve such smoothing is the **cubic spline**, which is made of components which are third-degree (or lower) polynomials. In general the linear spline will show sharp changes in direction, akin to a twig when snapped, but still intact, whereas a cubic spline will show curvature, more akin to the look of a pliant material, such as plasticine, when bent. The most popular type of cubic spline is the **restricted cubic spline**, sometimes called the **natural spline**. This is the same as the general cubic spline, except that the two extreme splines are linear. Such a restriction is sensible because of the absence of any information regarding curvature beyond the range of the data. Besides providing useful visual interpretations of associations, restricted cubic splines can be useful for making extrapolations, in which case the extreme knots are placed at the extremities of the sample data.

Example 9.18 Figure 9.17 and Figure 9.18 show linear and restricted cubic splines, respectively, fitted to the data from Example 9.12 using MKSPLINE in Stata. Here the final model of that example has been used, i.e., HDL-cholesterol is regressed on alcohol and age. However, here alcohol has been fitted as a spline; in both the case of the linear and restricted cubic spline, the knots were placed at the quartiles of alcohol (2, 10 and 24 units/week). The fits of the two models are very similar, but the curvature in the cubic spline model (except beyond the extreme knots) is in contrast to the sharp bend in the linear spline. Notice how the extreme skew in

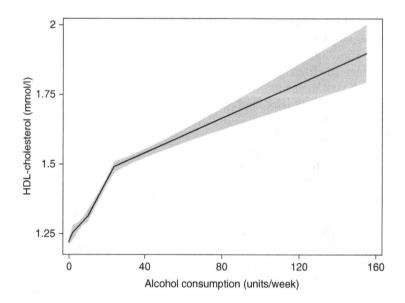

Figure 9.17. Predicted values (and 95% confidence intervals) for HDL-cholesterol from a linear spline model for alcohol (with knots at 2, 10 and 24 units/week), adjusted for age: Example 9.18.

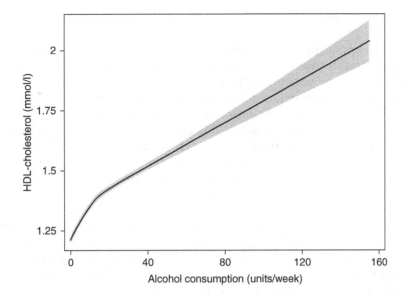

Figure 9.18. Predicted values (and 95% confidence intervals) for HDL-cholesterol from a restricted cubic spline model for alcohol (with knots at 2, 10 and 24 units/week), adjusted for age: Example 9.18.

alcohol levels has pushed all the 'action' to a small part of its range; it might be considered worthwhile to use at least one more knot above the third quartile.

In order to produce each of these two plots of fitted values, the second predictor, age, needed to be set at a constant value. The natural choice is to take this value to be the mean in the observed data, which is 49.64 years. This is just as when computing least squares means — see Example 9.16. Thus, Figure 9.17 and Figure 9.18 show predictions for men of average age; for shorthand these are called 'age-adjusted' values.

Figure 9.17 and Figure 9.18 strongly suggest that the association between alcohol consumption and HDL-cholesterol is non-linear, and thus we can improve on the 'final' model of Example 9.12. Indeed, a quadratic term in alcohol is a significant ($p < 0.001$) predictor of HDL-cholesterol for these data, adjusting for age and the linear term for alcohol. Hence either a spline or a quadratic model in alcohol would be a better choice than the linear model. Another option worth considering would be to fit **fractional polynomials** of alcohol. Fractional polynomials are polynomials in whole and fractional powers of the explanatory variable (Royston and Altman, 1994), which are able to take on a wide range of shapes. Stata has a FRACPOLY routine to create the best fractional polynomial fit between an explanatory and an outcome variable.

Beyond the cubic spline, there are other types of spline which are better for smoothing, or more flexible. A general type of spline with great flexibility is the **basis spline**, generally known as the **B-spline.** This can be obtained from Stata using a user-defined procedure, BSPLINE, which may be downloaded (Newson, 2000). The details of B-splines are beyond the scope of this book: see de Boor (1978) for a thorough exposition of this and other aspects of splines. Another approach to smoothing patterns arising from scatterplots is to use locally weighted scatterplot smoothing (LOWESS) (Cleveland, 1979), which is also easy to apply in Stata.

9.11   Panel data

Sometimes epidemiological investigations involve the collection of several results for the outcome variable from the same individuals. In general, such data are called **panel data**, where the panels are the individual subjects. In this case, the individual data values are no longer independent, since measures from the same individual will be correlated. Two types of panel data are common. First, where the outcome variable is recorded on the same individual at different points in time (**longitudinal data**) and, second, where a set of repeated results — for example, multiple measures of blood pressure — are taken from the same individual at a given point in time. A combination of the two is also possible. Panels can also be clusters of subjects, such as families, or of other types of observational units.

Panel data can be analysed using several statistical techniques, but we have only room to cover one briefly in this book — **generalised estimating equations (GEEs)**. See Brown and Prescott (2006) for a practical account of alternative methods. The theory behind GEEs is beyond our scope, but they are essentially an extension of the generalised linear model (which is used throughout most of Chapter 10), and which has already been mentioned earlier in this chapter. Indeed, SAS embeds GEEs into its flagship generalised linear model routine, GENMOD. Here we shall only view results from the XTGEE routine in Stata, which was written specifically for GEEs. In every case in this section, both the data and the Stata program which produced the output can be downloaded (see Appendix A). Hardin and Hilbe (2013) give a brief historical perspective and both theoretical and practical details of GEEs. On a more general level, a comprehensive mathematical account of how to deal with panel data is given by Diggle *et al.* (2002).

The key limitation of GEEs, compared to some other methods for dealing with panel data, is that they produce only population-averaged results. That is, inferences can only be made for the 'average' individual, rather than specific individuals. Similarly, they are not suited to investigations of sources of variability, which is sometimes of interest when data have a hierarchical structure. In most cases in epidemiology, the GEE approach is sufficient. It also has the benefit of being usable for modelling proportions and rates (Chapter 10), as well as quantitative outcome variables. An additional feature of a GEE, compared to a general, or a generalised, linear model is that we need to assume a form for the within-subject (within-panels, in general) correlations — we shall still assume that results from different subjects are uncorrelated. Results of GEEs can change when a different correlation structure is assumed. Packages, such as SAS and Stata, allow the user to choose her or his own correlation structure (often called the **working correlation structure**), but experience suggests that it is much more important to choose *some* structure than to ignore it altogether and proceed with a general linear model, which assumes an **independent correlation** structure with zero correlations between different data items within a panel. In the examples following, we shall always assume **exchangeable correlation**, which is when each pair of different results, within each panel, has the same non-zero correlation. This is the default in XTGEE. However, to protect against making the wrong choice, it is useful to take **robust estimates** (White, 1982) of standard errors, which give correct standard errors (but have no control over bias) even when the model assumed is incorrect. We can also use a generalisation of the AIC (Section 9.7.1), called the quasilikelihood under the independence model criterion (QIC), suggested by Pan (2001), to choose between correlation structures. PROC GENMOD returns this automatically when a GEE model is invoked. A variation on this, which imposes a penalty for additional variables, is the QICu which allows us to choose between models.

As with the AIC and BIC (Section 9.7.1), smaller values are best. QICu is also given by PROC GENMOD. In Stata, a user-supplied routine, QIC, may be used to obtain QIC and QICu.

An additional feature of panel data is that they may be structured in two ways. First, the 'long-and-thin' method, wherein each data item defines a separate row in the database; each panel will have multiple rows. The database must then have an identification variable which defines the panel — often called a 'subject ID'. This enables different data items to be linked within the same panel. Second, the 'short-and-fat' method, wherein each panel has a single row which contains all the data relating to that panel. The variable names will then need to distinguish, for example, the first from the second measure of each particular variable. We shall assume the long-and-thin method here, which is ideal for GEE analyses.

Here we shall look at three examples of the application of GEEs, which introduce the essential concepts. All of these involve longitudinal data. The simplest type of longitudinal data arises from a before-and-after study, which is typically, and most effectively, analysed by a paired t test.

Example 9.19 The data from the Alloa Study, shown in Table 2.15, were entered into Stata as three columns: subject ID, time (1 or 2; before or after cholesterol screening) and total cholesterol value. Output 9.18 shows the results from fitting a GEE which regresses cholesterol on time, declaring ID as the panel. The estimate, 95% confidence interval and p value are the same, or very nearly so, as found using a paired t test in Example 2.11.

As explained, the correlation structure assumed here (and in Example 9.20 and Example 9.21) is the exchangeable structure which only requires a single parameter. Here the value of this, estimated by XTGEE, was 0.90, which is (unsurprisingly) what is found from computing the correlation between the cholesterol results at the first and second visit, taking the data in short-and-fat form. If we had assumed an independent correlation structure in the GEE model this would be (virtually) equivalent to using a two-sample t test.

Output 9.18. Stata XTGEE results for the Alloa Study data: Example 9.19.

GEE population-averaged model		Number of obs	=	88
Group variable:	id	Number of groups	=	44
Link:	identity	Obs per group: min =		2
Family:	Gaussian	avg =		2.0
Correlation:	exchangeable	max =		2
		Wald chi2(1)	=	4.07
Scale parameter:	1.521545	Prob > chi2	=	0.0436

(Std. Err. adjusted for clustering on id)

tc	Coef.	Robust Std. Err.	z	P>|z|	[95% Conf. Interval]	
time	-.1699999	.0842268	-2.02	0.044	-.3350815	-.0049184
_cons	6.011364	.2115851	28.41	0.000	5.596664	6.426063

Another study design from a previous chapter that produces longitudinal data is the cross-over trial. In this case, the GEE approach has the advantage of being generalisable to more complex cross-overs, for instance with three or more study periods and types/levels of intervention, or even to trials where one intervention is managed using a parallel group design and the other by a cross-over.

Example 9.20 The Aspergesic trial data of Table 7.5 were read into Stata as five columns: subject ID, period (1 or 2), group (1 or 2), treatment (ibuprofen or Aspergesic) and pain score. Regressing pain score on treatment, period and their interaction, in XTGEE, gave a test statistic of -0.59 ($p = 0.55$, when compared to the standard normal), for the treatment by period interaction, which is essentially the same as the test statistic of -0.60 derived for the same test, by a different method, in Example 7.9. Regressing pain on treatment gave a test statistic of 1.46 ($p = 0.145$), comparable to the value of 1.44 derived in Example 7.9. Similarly, the estimate and confidence interval for the treatment and period effects are virtually the same as in Example 7.9.

Finally, we shall consider a parallel group trial where the outcome is measured several times during follow-up. In this situation, it may well be sensible to choose a working correlation structure where the correlations diminish as the observations move further apart. One way of doing this is to use a simple autoregressive correlation structure in which the correlations between different data items, within a panel, are of the form ρ^d for some value of ρ which is less than unity and d is the distance in time (e.g., the number of days) between the two data items under consideration. Then, the greater the distance, the smaller is the correlation. In the next example, several correlation structures were tried: the conclusions stayed the same as when the exchangeable structure was used, for which results are shown.

Example 9.21 Salt is thought to be a major determinant of high blood pressure. In many countries, much of the daily intake of salt comes from bread. Girgis *et al.* (2003) describe an intervention study of consumer acceptability of gradual reduction in the salt content of bread. Subjects ($n = 110$) were randomly assigned to the reduced salt or normal salt (control) bread groups; treatment allocation was blinded. Those in the reduced salt group received specially baked bread: each week, for 5 weeks, the salt content of this bread was 5% less than in the previous week. The process started with bread of normal salt content in week one. Thus, by the end of the study they were eating bread with 25% less salt than at the beginning. Those in the control group received bread of a constant, normal salt level for 6 weeks.

Subjects completed a questionnaire each week. Amongst other things, each week the subjects were asked to rate (on a scale of 0 to 100) the acceptability of the bread they had been eating in the previous week. This generated six responses from each subject, collected at evenly spaced intervals in time. The research question these data are to answer is, 'Does acceptability of bread change, over time, in a different way when salt content is manipulated?' Assuming that straight lines are reasonable models for the data, this is a problem of comparison of regression lines; if there was only one observation per week in each group we could directly apply the material of Section 9.6. However, in reality there are 110 regression lines, one for each subject, which split into two groups. The research question is interpreted to ask whether the average slopes differ between the two groups.

To address this problem, first note that descriptive analyses suggest that acceptability scores are reasonably well approximated by a normal distribution. We might fit, just as we would without the repeated observations, the model relating acceptability score to time (in weeks), experimental group and their interaction — the 'separate lines regression model' (Section 9.6). Output 9.19 shows the results.

If the slopes of the regression lines (acceptability versus time) are different (at the 5% level), then the interaction p value should be below 0.05, which it clearly is not ($p = 0.952$). We thus conclude that gradual reduction of salt has no effect on changes in acceptability of bread over a 6-week period.

It is instructive to see what would happen if we ignored the unit of replication (subjects) in these data. Output 9.20 shows the results of fitting the same model as before, but now taking mean acceptability (the variable ACCEPT_MEAN) at each time as the outcome variable

— that is, after the data have been collapsed down to 12 observations, one for each group at each of the 6 weeks, by averaging over subjects. Comparing Output 9.19 and Output 9.20 shows, as expected, that when we ignore the replications we get similar estimates, but the standard errors are much too large, reflecting the loss of information. Output 9.20 gives a perfectly valid analysis, but it is far from ideal. An incorrect analysis would be to apply a general linear model to the original bread salt data, which would assume independence between all 613 observations (110 × 6, less missing values), which clearly cannot be true because each individual contributes several scores.

Output 9.19. Stata XTGEE results for the bread salt data of Example 9.21.

```
GEE population-averaged model            Number of obs      =      613

Group variable:                subject   Number of groups   =      109

Link:                         identity   Obs per group: min =        1

Family:                       Gaussian                 avg =      5.6

Correlation:              exchangeable                 max =        6

                                         Wald chi2(3)       =     1.78

Scale parameter:              474.4962   Prob > chi2        =   0.6195

                    (Std. Err. adjusted for clustering on subject)
```

accept	Coef.	Robust Std. Err.	z	P>|z|	[95% Conf. Interval]	
1.treat	2.810524	3.668219	0.77	0.444	-4.379053	10.0001
week	.3083311	.6400002	0.48	0.630	-.9460463	1.562709
treat#c.week						
1	.0520065	.8554733	0.06	0.952	-1.62469	1.728703
_cons	51.72696	2.726814	18.97	0.000	46.38251	57.07142

Output 9.20 Stata REGRESS results for the bread salt data of Example 9.21, using mean values.

accept_mean	Coef.	Std. Err.	t	P>|t|	[95% Conf. Interval]	
1.treat	2.478869	6.028226	0.41	0.692	-11.42224	16.37998
week	.2666585	1.094534	0.24	0.814	-2.257343	2.790659
treat#c.week						
1	.0009036	1.547905	0.00	1.000	-3.568573	3.57038
_cons	51.96881	4.262599	12.19	0.000	42.13924	61.79838

As with all data analyses, GEE analyses should begin with exploratory plots to understand the data structure. With longitudinal data, since it can be difficult to see the patterns in plots with overlapping time series (for instance, the 110 sets of joined data points, or the regression lines fitted to them, in Example 9.21), it can be useful to plot results for a random set of individuals. Assuming individual regression lines are plotted when there are more than two time points, the result will look like one of the panels of Figure 7.5. Such a plot is called a **spaghetti plot**, although this term can have different meanings. Usually data from between six and ten individuals are shown on a spaghetti plot, together with the overall mean.

9.12   Non-normal alternatives

With the exception of Spearman's correlation coefficient, all the foregoing procedures in this chapter assume that data, or at least the residuals from the model fitted to the data, arise from a normal distribution. Alternative methods exist for cases in which normality may not be reasonably assumed, or induced by transformation. As with Spearman's correlation, several of these utilize the ranks of the data. One example is the **Kruskal–Wallis test**, which is a direct generalization of the two-sample Wilcoxon test (Section 2.8.2) to cover several samples. Just as the Wilcoxon test is a nonparametric (distribution-free) alternative to the t test, so the Kruskal–Wallis test is a nonparametric alternative to the one-way ANOVA.

Several nonparametric alternatives to the methods of this chapter are described by Conover (1999); Härdle (1990) is concerned solely with nonparametric regression. As described in Section 2.8.2, these methods will be less powerful than the methods given earlier in this chapter when normality is (at least roughly) true. Other approaches to dealing with lack of normality and other problems with model assumptions are described by Tiku *et al.* (1986) and Birkes and Dodge (1993).

Due to space limitations, we shall consider only the Kruskal–Wallis test here. This requires data to be classified into ℓ groups, as in the one-way ANOVA. The null hypothesis can be taken as 'the distributions are the same in all the groups', and the alternative is 'at least one distribution is different'. When $\ell = 2$, the Kruskal–Wallis test reduces to the Wilcoxon test of Section 2.8.2. As with the Wilcoxon test, we begin by ranking the entire set of data. Let R_{ij} be the rank of the jth subject in group i; n_i be the size of group i; $n = \Sigma_i n_i$ be the total sample size and $T_i = \Sigma R_{ij}$ be the sum of ranks for group i. If there are no tied ranks, the Kruskal–Wallis test statistic is

$$\frac{12}{n(n+1)} \sum_{i=1}^{\ell} \frac{T_i^2}{n_i} - 3(n+1). \tag{9.41}$$

When there are ties, we take the average rank for each tied rank in a set (as in Section 2.8.2) and compute

$$d = \frac{1}{n-1} \left\{ \sum_{i=1}^{\ell} \sum_{j=1}^{n_i} R_{ij}^2 - \frac{(n+1)^2 n}{4} \right\}. \tag{9.42}$$

The test statistic is then

$$\frac{1}{d}\left\{\sum_{i=1}^{\ell}\frac{T_i^2}{n_i}-\frac{(n+1)^2 n}{4}\right\}. \tag{9.43}$$

If there are few ties, then (9.41) is a reasonable approximation to (9.43). Whether (9.41) or (9.43) is used, the Kruskal–Wallis test statistic is compared against chi-square on $\ell - 1$ d.f. However, this is an approximate procedure; for small sample sizes an exact procedure is preferable (see Iman $et\ al.$, 1975).

Example 9.22 Consider the dietary data of Table 9.1. This time we shall test whether serum total cholesterol differs between dietary groups without assuming any specific probability distribution. The entire data were ranked in ascending order; Table 9.30 shows the results, arranged as in Table 9.1.

Here, $n = 18$ and $n_i = 6$ for $i = 1, 2, 3$; thus

$$\sum\frac{T_i^2}{n_i}=\frac{91.5^2}{6}+\frac{53^2}{6}+\frac{26.5^2}{6}=1980.5833.$$

Ignoring the presence of ties, the relatively simple formula, (9.41), gives the test statistic

$$\frac{12}{18\times19}\times 1980.5833 - 3\times 19 = 12.49.$$

Alternatively, we can use the more complex procedure, which does take account of the ties. We require

$$\sum\sum R_{ij}^2 = 15^2 + 17^2 + \cdots + 3^2 = 2108;$$

$$(n+1)^2 n/4 = 19^2 \times 18/4 = 1624.5.$$

Then, using (9.42),

$$d = \frac{1}{17}(2108-1624.5) = 28.4412.$$

Table 9.30. Ranks for the dietary data of Table 9.1.

Subject no. (within group)	Diet group		
	Omnivores	Vegetarians	Vegans
1	15	8	9
2	17	10	1
3	12	6	2
4	16	11	7
5	13.5	4.5	4.5
6	18	13.5	3
Total	91.5	53	26.5

The test statistic, (9.43), is thus

$$\frac{1}{28.4412}(1980.5833 - 1624.5) = 12.52.$$

In this case, with 4/18 tied ranks, the two approaches give virtually the same result. In both cases, comparing the test statistic with χ_2^2 leads to a p value of 0.02. Hence, there is a real difference in cholesterol distributions between dietary groups. Compare this to the p value of less than 0.001, reported in Section 9.2.3, for the corresponding one-way ANOVA.

Exercises

(Some of these exercises require the use of a computer package with appropriate procedures.)

9.1   Use one-way ANOVA to test whether the mean cholesterol is the same for those with and without coronary heart disease in the Scottish Heart Health Study (SHHS) data of Table 2.10. Compare your result with that of Example 2.10.

9.2   For the Glasgow MONICA data introduced in Exercise 2.4, construct the one-way ANOVA table for protein S by alcohol group.
  (i)   Use this to test whether mean protein S differs between the five alcohol groups.
  (ii)   Find a 99% confidence interval for the mean protein S for nondrinkers.
  (iii) Find a 99% confidence interval for the difference between mean protein S in heavy and nondrinkers.
  (iv)   Test whether the distribution of protein S differs among the five alcohol groups using a Kruskal–Wallis test. Compare the result with that of (i).

9.3   In a case–control study of coronary heart disease (CHD) and consumption of hydrogenated marine oils, Thomas (1992) obtained fat specimens at necropsy from 136 men who died from CHD and another 95 men who died from other, unrelated, causes. Data were collected from nine areas of England and Wales. He published a sequential ANOVA table for the percentage hydrogenated menhaden in adipose tissue, part of which is given here.

Source of variation	Sum of squares
Areas	2.3203
Case–control status | areas	0.4089
Interaction | main effects	0.1675
Error	
Total	10.3117

  (i)   Complete the ANOVA table, including the test results.
  (ii)   Interpret your results.
  (iii) Is there any prior analysis that you would have wished to perform before constructing the ANOVA table?

9.4 Data have been collected from 12 people in a study of how smoking affects the desire for healthy eating. Each person's smoking status was recorded: two were never smokers; four were ex-smokers; three were classified as light smokers and three as heavy smokers. Consumption of antioxidant vitamins was also recorded, measured on a combined and standardised scale. The one-way ANOVA model relating antioxidant score to smoking status was fitted using three computer packages and by hand calculation using the method given in a statistics textbook (you do not need to know how any of these methods work to be able to answer the questions). The fitted model (in each case) was:

$$\hat{y} = a + b^{(1)}x^{(1)} + b^{(2)}x^{(2)} + b^{(3)}x^{(3)} + b^{(4)}x^{(4)},$$

where all terms are as in (9.9) and superscripts 1 through 4 denote never, ex-, light and heavy smokers, respectively. The four sets of parameter estimate results follow.

Parameter estimates	GENSTAT	SAS	SPSS	Textbook
a	1.8	0.3	1.025	1.0
$b^{(1)}$	0	1.5	0.775	0.8
$b^{(2)}$	−0.3	1.2	0.475	0.5
$b^{(3)}$	−1.3	0.2	−0.525	−0.5
$b^{(4)}$	−1.5	0	−0.725	−0.7

(i) Confirm that all four methods give the same fitted values (estimated means) for the antioxidant score in each smoking group. Write down these fitted values.

(ii) What must the observed mean antioxidant scores have been in each smoking group?

(iii) Use your results in (ii) to compute the total observed antioxidant score for each smoking group. Add these together and divide by 12 to find the overall mean score. Check that this agrees with the appropriate value in the 'Textbook' column in the table.

(iv) Suppose that a new computer package becomes available, which chooses the constraint upon the b parameters that $b^{(2)} = 0$. Write down the set of parameter estimates that this package would produce for the problem described here.

9.5 Refer to the epilepsy data of Table C.8 in Appendix C.

(i) Fit a two-way ANOVA model without interaction to the BO test results. Give the sequential ANOVA table with diagnosis introduced first. Interpret your results.

(ii) Find the standardised residuals from the model fitted in (i). Plot these against the fitted values. Also produce a normal plot of the standardised residuals. Identify any unusual values.

(iii) Find the fitted values from the model of (i). Use these to calculate the least-squares BO test means by duration of treatment, adjusted for diagnosis.

(iv) Fit the two-way ANOVA model with interaction. Is there any evidence of interaction?

(v) Define a new variable, 'combination', which specifies the combination of diagnosis and duration for each child (for example, children 1, 4 and 11 make up the group with the combination of PS and one year's duration). Fit the one-way ANOVA model that relates BO test to combination. Show that the combination sum of squares is equal to the sum of the three sequential sums of squares for the model of (iv).

9.6 Kiechl *et al.* (1996) give observed and adjusted mean values for γ-glutamyl-transferase (U/l) by alcohol status (average daily consumption in grams) for 820 subjects in a cross-sectional survey carried out in Bruneck, Italy. Results are shown in the following table.

Alcohol group (g)	Observed	Adjusted[a]
Abstainers	14.9	17.9
1–50	17.4	18.6
51–99	31.8	30.0
≥100	40.2	38.4

[a] For sex, age, smoking, body mass index, physical activity and social status.

Discuss the consequences of these results with regard to the use of γ-glutamyl-transferase as a biochemical marker of alcohol consumption.

9.7 For the Glasgow MONICA data introduced in Exercise 2.4:
(i) Plot protein S against protein C.
(ii) Find the Pearson correlation between protein C and protein S.
(iii) Repeat (i), but after transforming protein C by using the inverse reciprocal transformation defined in Section 2.8.1. How much difference has this made? Test the null hypothesis that the correlation is zero. Why is it more likely that the test is valid when this transformed variable is used?
(iv) Find the Spearman correlation between protein C and protein S. How would this result alter if protein C were first transformed?
(v) Fit the simple linear regression of protein S (the y variable) on protein C. Test for a significant regression using an F test and specify the coefficient of determination.
(vi) Calculate the standardised residuals and fitted values for each observation from (v). Hence construct a residual plot. Does this suggest any problems with the model?
(vii) Find the normal scores of the standardised residuals. Use these to construct a normal plot. What does this tell you, and why is this result important in the current context?
(viii) Test the null hypothesis that the true intercept (for the regression model) is zero.
(ix) Find a 95% confidence interval for the true intercept.
(x) Test the null hypothesis that the true slope is zero using a t test. Compare your results with the F test in (v).
(xi) Find a 95% confidence interval for the true slope.
(xii) Predict protein S when protein C is 100 iu/dl. Give a 95% confidence interval for this prediction.
(xiii) Predict the mean value of protein S for all men with a protein C value of 100 iu/dl. Give a 95% confidence interval for this prediction.

9.8 For the SHHS data of Table 2.10, regress systolic on diastolic blood pressure. Identify any regression outlier using standardised residuals. Refit the model with the outlier removed.

9.9 Cotinine is an objective biochemical marker of tobacco smoke inhalation. For the SHHS data of Table 2.10, plot cotinine against self-reported daily cigarette consumption. Discuss the problems of using standard simple linear regression analysis with these data to predict the average amount of cotinine per cigarette smoked.

9.10 Consider the ozone exposure data of Table C.9 (see Appendix C). It would be of interest to establish whether age, height and weight are important predictors of ozone exposure effects. This will assist in the efficient design of future studies of ozone exposure. Fit the three possible simple linear regression models to the data of Table C.9 in order to address this issue. What do you conclude?

9.11 Refer to the anorexia data of Table C.10.
   (i)   Estimate the mean BPI for cases and for controls.
   (ii)   Compare the two distributions (cases and controls) using boxplots.
   (iii)   Do your results in (i) and (ii) support the researchers' prior hypothesis that cases have a lower BPI? Consider the danger involved in carrying out a one-sided test, as this prior hypothesis might suggest. Test the null hypothesis that cases and controls have the same BPI, using a two-sided test.
   (iv)   One possible confounding variable in this example is the true width, because the relative error in perception (that is, the BPI) might differ with increasing body size. Plot BPI against true width, marking cases and controls with different symbols or colours. Does BPI seem to change with true width? If so, how? Does it appear that a different regression line will be required for cases and controls?
   (v)   From a general linear model, test the effect of case–control status adjusted for true width.
   (vi)   Write down the equation of the fitted bivariable model from (v). Find the mean true width. Hence compute the least squares means (adjusted for true width) for cases and controls.
   (vii)   Fit the simple linear regressions of (a) BPI on true width; (b) case–control status on true width. Find the (raw) residuals from (a) and (b) and fit the simple linear regression of the (a) residuals on the (b) residuals. Compare the slope parameter from this model with that for case–control status in (vi). You should find a close relationship: why?
   (viii) Compare the results in (v) and (vii) with those in (ii) and (iii). What effect has adjustment for true width had? Are there any other potential confounding variables that may be worth considering, if data were available?

9.12 Returning to the MONICA data of Exercise 9.2, fit all the remaining general linear models (without interaction) to predict protein S from any of age, alcohol group and protein C. Summarise your overall findings. Does any of these three variables have an important effect in the presence of the other two?

9.13 Using the SHHS data in Table 2.10, fit all possible multiple regression models (without interactions) that predict serum total cholesterol (the y variable) from diastolic blood pressure, systolic blood pressure, alcohol, carbon monoxide and cotinine. Scrutinise your results to understand how the x variables act in conjunction. For these data, which is the 'best' multiple regression model for cholesterol? What percentage of variation does it explain?

9.14 For the U.K. population data of Table C.11, fit the simple linear regression of population on year. Calculate the r^2 statistic. Is this model a good fit to the data? Note that it will be easier to fit 'year' as 1, 2, 3, ..., allowing for the missing year at 1941.

9.15 The bread salt data of Example 9.21 (available from this book's web site) include a score for flavour (on a 0 to 100 scale), similar to that for acceptability. Fit GEE models to the flavour data to test whether there is (a) an effect of treatment group, adjusted for time and (b) an interaction between group and time. Try different assumptions about the pattern of correlations within patients, and see how these affect the conclusions of these hypothesis tests.

CHAPTER 10

Modelling binary outcome data

10.1 Introduction

In epidemiology we are most often concerned with deciding how a risk factor is related to disease (or death). If we decide to develop statistical models to represent the relationship between risk factor and disease, it is natural to take the risk factor as the x variable and the disease outcome as the y variable in the model (Section 9.1). Implicitly, it is the x variable that is a potential cause of the y variable and not vice versa.

Consider, now, the nature of this y variable. In the most straightforward situation, it measures whether or not the individual concerned has contracted the disease; hence, it is a binary variable. Raw data, collected from n individuals, will be of the form of Table 10.1 in which the risk factor values may be quantitative or qualitative. If we consolidate the data, by counting how often disease occurs at each distinct value of x, we obtain the alternative view of the data given in Table 10.2, in which each risk factor value (assumed to be ℓ in all) appears only once. This format will be assumed, for now.

Table 10.1. Raw data on risk factor values and disease outcome.

Risk factor value	Disease?
x_1	yes
x_2	no
.	.
.	.
.	.
x_n	no

Table 10.2. Grouped data on risk factor values and disease outcome.

Risk factor value	Number with disease	Total number	Proportion with disease
x_1	e_1	n_1	r_1
x_2	e_2	n_2	r_2
.	.	.	.
.	.	.	.
.	.	.	.
x_ℓ	e_ℓ	n_ℓ	r_ℓ

Table 10.3. Prevalent *H. pylori* and occupational social class amongst men in north Glasgow; third MONICA survey.

		Number		Proportion with
Occupational social class (rank)		With *H. pylori*	Total	*H. pylori*
I	Nonmanual, professional (1)	10	38	0.26
II	Nonmanual, intermediate (2)	40	86	0.46
IIIn	Nonmanual, skilled (3)	36	57	0.63
IIIm	Manual, skilled (4)	226	300	0.75
IV	Manual, partially skilled (5)	83	108	0.77
V	Manual, unskilled (6)	60	73	0.82

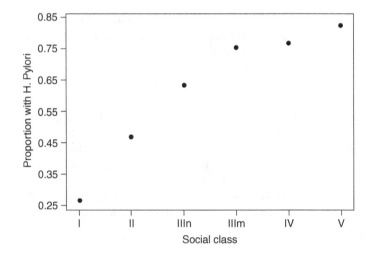

Figure 10.1. Prevalent *Helicobacter pylori* against occupational social class amongst men in north Glasgow; third MONICA survey.

Of the n_i people with the ith risk factor value x_i, e_i have the disease, giving a proportion with disease of $r_i = e_i/n_i$. This notation is chosen with epidemiological practice in mind, and is consistent with earlier chapters of this book. The proportion of people who experience an event (e_i/n_i) will give the risk (r_i) of disease for people with the ith value of the risk factor. With a continuous risk factor, the risk factor variable may be grouped so as to produce large numbers for the n_i. The problem of modelling disease outcome may now be seen to be one of modelling the relationship between r and x.

Example 10.1 Table 10.3 shows data from the *Helicobacter pylori* study of McDonagh *et al.* (1997) described in Example 9.16. Figure 10.1 shows a scatterplot of the proportion with prevalent disease against social class. In the main, the chance of *H. pylori* seems to increase as we go across the social classifications (that is, with increasing deprivation). We might seek to quantify this relationship through a regression model.

Example 10.2 The Scottish Heart Health Study (SHHS) recruited 5754 men aged 40 to 59. Table 10.4 shows the number and percentage of deaths within an average of 7.7 years of follow-up, by age of man at baseline (time of recruitment). Although we have seen in Section 5.2 that some subjects were observed for longer durations than others in the SHHS, we shall ignore these differences throughout this chapter: that is, we will treat the SHHS as a fixed cohort (this restriction is lifted in Chapter 11).

The data are illustrated by Figure 10.2. There is clearly a tendency for risk of death to increase with age, as would be expected, but some individual age groups have more (or fewer) deaths than would be expected according to the general pattern. Presumably this is due to random variation. Regression modelling should be useful to summarise the relationship shown in Table 10.4 and to smooth out the random variation.

Table 10.4. Deaths by age at baseline; SHHS men.

Age (years)	Number Dying	Total	Percentage dying
40	1	251	0.4
41	12	317	3.8
42	13	309	4.2
43	6	285	2.1
44	10	236	4.2
45	8	254	3.1
46	10	277	3.6
47	12	278	4.3
48	10	285	3.5
49	14	276	5.1
50	15	274	5.5
51	14	296	4.7
52	19	305	6.2
53	36	341	10.6
54	26	305	8.5
55	21	276	7.6
56	28	325	8.6
57	41	302	13.6
58	38	260	14.6
59	49	302	16.2

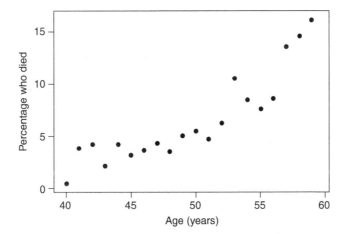

Figure 10.2. Percentage of deaths against age at baseline; SHHS men.

10.2   Problems with standard regression models

The relationship between r and x could be modelled using simple linear regression (or, because x could be qualitative, more generally by the general linear model), as described in Chapter 9. Computationally, this is quite possible, but three problems cause this approach to be inappropriate.

10.2.1   The r–x relationship may well not be linear

Proportions (including risks) must lie between 0 and 1 inclusive. When the observed proportions scan most of this allowable range, as in Table 10.3, the pattern in the scatterplot is generally nonlinear, as in Figure 10.1. This is because of a tendency toward 'squashing up' as proportions approach the asymptotes (barriers) at 0 or 1. The problem is not so acute in Figure 10.2 because the percentages (restricted to be between 0 and 100) cover only a small part of the allowable range. Nevertheless, some levelling out at the left-hand side may be seen.

10.2.2   Predicted values of the risk may be outside the valid range

The fitted linear regression model for r regressed on x is given by (9.12) as

$$\hat{r} = a + bx.$$

This can lead to predictions of risks that are negative or are greater than unity, and thus impossible.

Example 10.3 Fitting a linear regression line to the data in Table 10.4 and Figure 10.2, using (9.13) and (9.14), gives the equation,

$$\hat{r} = -25.394 + 0.645 \times \text{age}.$$

Here both the constant and slope are highly significant ($p < 0.001$) and the model explains 97% of the variation in risk. Hence, the regression model appears to be very successful. However, suppose the model were to be used to predict the risk of death for someone aged 39. This prediction would be

$$\hat{r} = -25.394 + 0.645 \times 39 = -0.239,$$

a negative risk! To be fair, extrapolation from regression lines is never a good idea. However, here we are extrapolating only by 1 year and we would hope that the regression model would behave well this close to the observed range of ages. Furthermore, similar problems are found with confidence limits for predicted risks *within* the range of the observed data for this example. With other datasets, the predicted risks can take impossible values even within the range of observations.

10.2.3   The error distribution is not normal

In simple linear regression, we fit the model

$$r = \alpha + \beta x + \varepsilon,$$

where ε arises from a standard normal distribution. This is (9.11) but where the y variable is the proportion with the disease (the risk). Proportions are not likely to have a normal distribution; they are likely to arise from a binomial distribution. We would expect to detect this lack of normality if we carried out model checking (Section 9.8), for instance, in the situation of Example 10.3.

If we ignore this problem, we can still fit the simple linear regression model, but any inferences drawn from it would be inaccurate. For example, the confidence interval for the slope of the regression line is calculated using t statistics, which make an assumption of normality. Furthermore, simple linear regression assumes that each observation is equally precise and thus should be given equal weight. The proportion $r_i = e_i/n_i$ will have estimated variance $r_i(1 - r_i)/n_i$ (the binomial variance), which is certainly not constant for all i, even if the sample sizes within each level, n_i, are fixed.

One way around the distributional problem may be to transform the data; if the n_i are all reasonably similar the arcsine square root transformation (Section 2.8.1) should be useful because this makes the variance reasonably constant. However, this method is, at best, approximate.

10.3   Logistic regression

Figure 10.3 shows the shape of the logistic function,

$$y = \left\{1 + \exp(-b_0 - b_1 x)\right\}^{-1}, \tag{10.1}$$

relating some variable, y, to another variable, x, through the constants b_0 and b_1. The elongated S shape of the logistic function is a good match to the types of relationship we wish to measure: solving the problem of Section 10.2.1. There is an asymptote at $y = 0$ and at $y = 1$, solving the problem of Section 10.2.2. Hence, the fitted regression equation,

$$\hat{r} = \left\{1 + \exp(-b_0 - b_1 x)\right\}^{-1}, \tag{10.2}$$

where, as usual, $\hat{r}$ is the fitted (or predicted) value, b_0 is the sample estimate of the true 'intercept', β_0, and b_1 is the sample estimate of the true 'slope', β_1, should provide a useful model in the current context, provided we can treat the random variation appropriately. As far as the practitioner is concerned, this simply means telling the computer that the data have binomial, rather than normal, error, when using standard commercial software, thus solving the problem of Section 10.2.3. Such software will

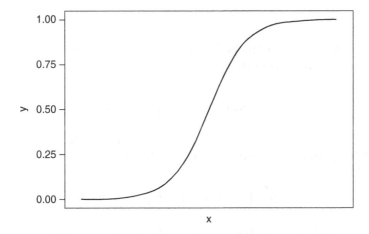

Figure 10.3. The logistic function, defined by (10.1).

produce maximum likelihood estimates (Clayton and Hills, 1993) of the β coefficients using iterative calculations.

We can manipulate (10.2) into:

$$\log_e\left(\frac{\hat{r}}{1-\hat{r}}\right) = b_0 + b_1 x, \tag{10.3}$$

which is the most often quoted form of the logistic regression equation. The left-hand side of (10.3) is called the **logit**. By reference to Section 3.2, we see that the logit is the log of the odds of disease. Hence, the logistic regression model postulates a relationship between the log odds of disease and the risk factor. This makes this model of key importance in epidemiology. The right-hand side of (10.3) is exactly as for a simple linear regression model and is called the **linear predictor**. Note that (10.3) should strictly be called the 'simple linear logistic regression' equation because there is only one x variable, and it is assumed to have a linear effect on the logit.

The odds of disease, for any specified value of x, come from raising the result of (10.3), with b_0 and b_1 supplied by a computer package, to the power e. Suppose that we wished to estimate the odds ratio, ψ, for $x = x_1$ compared with $x = x_0$. Thus, in the context of Example 10.2, we might wish to find the odds of death for a man aged 59 compared with a man aged 40. Here, $x_1 = 59$ and $x_0 = 40$. Obviously, we could do this by calculating the two separate odds, from (10.3), and dividing. A better method is to use the fact that the log of a ratio is the difference between the logs of the two components of that ratio, and hence

$$\log(\hat{\psi}) = \log\left(\hat{odds}_1/\hat{odds}_0\right) = \log(\hat{odds})_1 - \log(\hat{odds})_0$$

$$= \hat{logit}_1 - \hat{logit}_0$$

$$= b_0 + b_1 x_1 - \left(b_0 + b_1 x_0\right)$$

$$= b_1\left(x_1 - x_0\right),$$

so that

$$\hat{\psi} = \exp\left\{b_1\left(x_1 - x_0\right)\right\}. \tag{10.4}$$

That is, the odds ratio (x_1 compared with x_0) is the exponent of the slope parameter (b_1) times the difference between x_1 and x_0. Its estimated standard error is

$$\hat{se}\left(\log \hat{\psi}\right) = \left(x_1 - x_0\right)\hat{se}\left(b_1\right), \tag{10.5}$$

where $\hat{se}(b_1)$ is the estimated standard error of b_1, to be supplied by computer software. Hence, the 95% confidence interval for ψ has limits

$$\exp\left\{b_1\left(x_1 - x_0\right) \pm 1.96\left(x_1 - x_0\right)\hat{se}\left(b_1\right)\right\}. \tag{10.6}$$

Standard errors, and thus confidence intervals, are more difficult to obtain for odds, risk and relative risk: see Section 10.4.1.

10.4   Interpretation of logistic regression coefficients

In this section we shall consider how to use the estimates of the logistic regression coefficients to make useful inferences in epidemiological research. We shall consider four different types of x variable: binary, quantitative, categorical and ordinal.

10.4.1 Binary risk factors

Example 10.4 Consider the data from the EGAT study given in Table 3.2. These data were entered into SAS and analysed through PROC GENMOD, one of the SAS procedures that may be used to fit logistic regression models. The equivalent procedure in Stata is GLM. Part of the output is given in Table 10.5. Similar output would be expected from other statistical packages. This tells us that the model

$$\hat{\text{logit}} = -4.8326 + 1.0324x \tag{10.7}$$

has been fitted. To interpret this, we need to know that the codes used for smoking status, the x variable, were

$$x = \begin{cases} 1 & \text{for smokers} \\ 0 & \text{for nonsmokers.} \end{cases}$$

From (10.4), the odds ratio for a cardiovascular death, comparing smokers with nonsmokers, is

$$\exp\{1.0324(1-0)\} = \exp(1.0324) = 2.808.$$

Thus, the odds ratio for exposure compared with nonexposure is particularly easy to derive when exposure is coded as 1 and nonexposure as 0 in the logistic regression model. All we have to do is to raise the slope parameter estimate, b_1, to the power e.

Also, from Table 10.5, the estimated standard error of this log odds ratio is 0.3165. From (10.6), an approximate 95% confidence limit for the odds ratio may be calculated as

$$\exp\{1.0324 \pm 1.96 \times 0.3165\};$$

that is, (1.510, 5.221).

We can also use (10.7) to find the odds, if so desired. The odds of a cardiovascular death come directly from (10.7), because the logit is the log odds. For smokers ($x = 1$), the log odds are

$$-4.8326 + 1.0324 \times 1 = -3.8002,$$

giving odds of 0.0224. For nonsmokers ($x = 0$), the odds are

$$\exp(-4.8326 + 0) = 0.0080.$$

Table 10.5. Excerpt derived from SAS output for Example 10.4.

Parameter	Estimate	Standard error
INTERCEPT	−4.8326	0.2592
SMOKING	1.0324	0.3165

In the last example, we can also estimate the risk, r, of a cardiovascular death for smokers, from (10.2) and (10.7). That is,

$$\hat{r} = \left\{1 + \exp(4.8326 - 1.0324 \times 1)\right\}^{-1} = 0.0219.$$

In fact, it is slightly easier to note that

$$\hat{r} = \left\{1 + \exp(-\hat{\text{logit}})\right\}^{-1}. \tag{10.8}$$

So, for nonsmokers,

$$\hat{r} = \left\{1 + \exp(4.8326)\right\}^{-1} = 0.0079.$$

The estimated relative risk for smokers compared with nonsmokers is then most easily found as the ratio: $0.0219/0.0079 = 2.77$. Note that all the answers given here agree with those found by simple methods in Example 3.1 and Example 3.2.

Standard errors, and thus confidence limits, for odds are generally not straightforward to obtain. This is because they may involve more than one regression parameter, and, because the parameters are not independent, **covariances** between parameters need to be accounted for. For example, the variance of the logit when $x = 1$ (smokers in Example 10.4) is

$$V(b_0) + V(b_1) + 2C(b_0, b_1),$$

where the Vs denote variances and C denotes covariance. SAS PROC GENMOD, GLM in Stata and other computer software can be asked to produce the estimated **variance–covariance matrix** (sometimes simply called the **covariance matrix**) of parameter estimates. This is a square matrix with both rows and columns labelled by the parameters. Diagonal elements are the covariances of each parameter with itself; that is, the variances. Off-diagonals are the covariances; as these are equal above and below the diagonal, only one of them needs to be reported. In Example 10.4, the estimated variance–covariance matrix is given by Table 10.6. From this,

$$\hat{V}\left(\hat{\text{logit}}_{\text{smokers}}\right) = 0.06720 + 0.10018 + 2 \times -0.06720 = 0.03298$$

and so

$$\hat{\text{se}}\left(\hat{\text{logit}}_{\text{smokers}}\right) = \sqrt{0.03298} = 0.1816,$$

Table 10.6. Variance–covariance matrix for Example 10.4.

	b_0	b_1
b_0	0.06720	−0.06720
b_1		0.10018

and the 95% confidence interval for the odds of a coronary event amongst smokers is thus

$$\exp\left\{-3.8002 \pm 1.96 \times 0.1816\right\},$$

which is (0.016, 0.032).

Standard errors of risks and relative risks are difficult to obtain because they are nonlinear functions of the regression parameters, b_0 and b_1. In general, the variance of a nonlinear function is *not* the same function of the variances. Thus, in Example 10.4, even if we know var(risk$_{\text{smokers}}$) and var(risk$_{\text{nonsmokers}}$), we cannot easily find the variance of λ, the relative risk for smokers compared with nonsmokers, because

$$\text{var}(\lambda) \neq \text{var}\left(\text{risk}_{\text{smokers}}\right)\Big/\text{var}\left(\text{risk}_{\text{nonsmokers}}\right).$$

As a consequence, only *approximate* standard errors of risk and relative risk may be derived. Even these are messy to derive and consequently are omitted here. Hence, it is best to use odds ratios (and odds, if required) as the outcome measures whenever logistic regression is used, whatever the form of the explanatory variable. To model risk and relative risk directly, see Section 10.16.

10.4.2 Quantitative risk factors

Example 10.5 Consider the data in Table 10.4. The parameter estimates from using SAS PROC GENMOD with these data are presented in Table 10.7.

Hence the fitted model is:

$$\hat{\text{logit}} = -8.4056 + 0.1126x, \tag{10.9}$$

where the logit is the log odds of death and x is the age of the man. The interpretation of $b_1 = 0.1126$ is very easy in this case; it is simply the slope of the regression line, directly analogous to the situation in simple linear regression. Reference to (10.4) shows that for each increase in age of 1 year, the logit is estimated to increase by 0.1126. Figure 10.4 illustrates observed and fitted logit values and percentages. The logistic regression has smoothed out the irregularities (particularly at age 40) in the observed data. This may be easier to see from the logits, where the fitted values necessarily follow a straight line. However, interpretation is more immediate for the percentages. Observed logits are calculated from the definition of odds, (3.8); fitted percentages (risks multiplied by 100) come from (10.2).

To best understand the practical implications of the fitted model, we should transform the fitted logits. For example, we have already posed the question, 'What is the odds ratio for men aged 59 relative to age 40?' From (10.4) and (10.9), this is

$$\hat{\psi} = \exp\{0.1126(59 - 40)\} = 8.49.$$

Table 10.7. Results produced by SAS for Example 10.5.

Parameter	Estimate	Standard error
INTERCEPT	−8.4056	0.5507
AGE	0.1126	0.0104

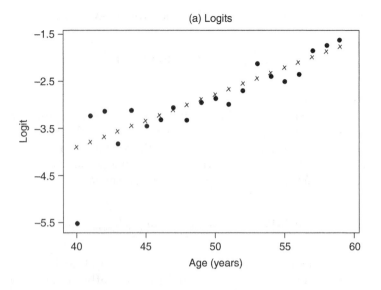

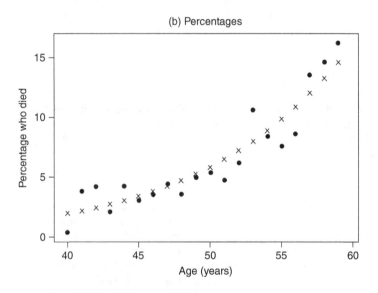

Figure 10.4. Observed and fitted (a) logits and (b) percentages, from a logistic regression model for the data in Table 10.4. Observed values are indicated by dots, fitted values by crosses.

Men aged 59 are approximately eight and a half times as likely to die in the next 7.7 years as those aged 40. To calculate the 95% confidence interval for ψ, we use (10.6), substituting the estimated value of $se(b_1) = 0.0104$ from Table 10.7,

$$\exp\{0.1126(59-40) \pm 1.96(59 - 40)0.0104\},$$

or (5.77, 12.51). Thus, we are 95% confident that the interval from 5.77 to 12.51 contains the true odds ratio.

10.4.3 Categorical risk factors

When the x variable is categorical with ℓ levels, the fitted logistic regression model becomes

$$\text{lo\hat{g}it} = b_0 + b_1^{(1)}x^{(1)} + b_1^{(2)}x^{(2)} + \cdots + b_1^{(\ell)}x^{(\ell)}, \tag{10.10}$$

where each $x^{(i)}$ variable is defined as

$$x^{(i)} = \begin{cases} 1 & \text{if } x \text{ takes its } i\text{th level} \\ 0 & \text{otherwise.} \end{cases}$$

That is, the $\{x^{(i)}\}$ are dummy variables (Section 9.2.6), which together represent the variable x. In fact, because x will have $\ell - 1$ degrees of freedom, these $x^{(i)}$ variables cannot be independent because there are ℓ of them. Hence, they must be fitted subject to one, arbitrary, linear constraint, just as in Section 9.2.6. We will see the effect of the choice of constraint in Example 10.6. From (10.10), the estimated logit for level i is

$$\text{lo\hat{g}it}^{(i)} = b_0 + b_1^{(i)},$$

subject to the linear constraint chosen.

Then the odds ratio for level i compared with level j, which we shall call $\psi^{(ij)}$, may be found in much the same way as (10.4) was derived from (10.3). That is,

$$\text{lo\hat{g}it}^{(i)} - \text{lo\hat{g}it}^{(j)} = b_1^{(i)} - b_1^{(j)},$$

whence

$$\hat{\psi}^{(ij)} = \exp\left(b_1^{(i)} - b_1^{(j)}\right). \tag{10.11}$$

Furthermore,

$$\text{se}\left(\text{lo\hat{g}it}^{(i)} - \text{lo\hat{g}it}^{(j)}\right) = \sqrt{V\left(b_1^{(i)}\right) + V\left(b_1^{(j)}\right) - 2C\left(b_1^{(i)}, b_1^{(j)}\right)}. \tag{10.12}$$

Unfortunately, this requires knowledge of $C\left(b_1^{(i)}, b_1^{(j)}\right)$. In the special case when $b_1^{(j)} = 0$, (10.11) and (10.12) reduce to the much simpler forms:

$$\hat{\psi}^{(ij)} = \exp\left(b_1^{(i)}\right) \tag{10.13}$$

$$\text{se}\left(\text{lo\hat{g}it}^{(i)} - \text{lo\hat{g}it}^{(j)}\right) = \text{se}\left(b_1^{(i)}\right). \tag{10.14}$$

Whether (10.12) or (10.14) is used, the 95% confidence interval for $\psi^{(ij)}$ is

$$\exp\left\{\left(b_1^{(i)} - b_1^{(j)}\right) \pm 1.96 \; \hat{se}\left(\hat{logit}^{(i)} - \hat{logit}^{(j)}\right)\right\}. \qquad (10.15)$$

Example 10.6 The data in Table 10.3 are for an explanatory variable (social class) with six categorical levels. In such cases odds ratios, to summarize the relationship between risk factor and disease status, may be defined in several ways. For example, any one of the six social class levels could be defined as the base level and all other classes would be compared with this reference. This gives rise to five prevalence odds ratios. Any other choice of base would give five different odds ratios, although appropriate multiplication of these would reproduce the original set (Section 3.6).

When categorical variables are fitted in computer packages, the natural choice of base level will vary with the package chosen (Section 9.2.7). The data in Table 10.3 were fitted in SAS PROC GENMOD by entering the social class rank from Table 10.3 as the variable RANK, declared as a categorical variable (CLASS variable in SAS notation). The parameter estimates produced are presented in Table 10.8. That is, the fitted model is, by reference to (10.10),

$$\hat{logit} = 1.5294 - 2.5590x^{(1)} - 1.6692x^{(2)} - 0.9904x^{(3)}$$

$$-0.4129x^{(4)} - 0.3294x^{(5)} + 0x^{(6)},$$

where

$$x^{(i)} = \begin{cases} 1 & \text{if the social class rank is } i \\ 0 & \text{otherwise} \end{cases}$$

are the relevant dummy variables and the computer package has supplied values for the $\left\{b_1^{(i)}\right\}$.

From this, we can see, as previously explained in Section 9.2.7, that SAS fixes the parameter for the *last* level of any categorical variable to be zero. This implies that the linear constraint imposed by SAS on (10.10) is $b_1^{(\ell)} = 0$. Consequently SAS expects odds ratios to be calculated relative to the *highest* level; that is, the social class with rank = 6 is the base. Hence, for example, the odds ratio contrasting social class IIIn (rank 3) to social class V (rank 6) is, from (10.13),

$$\hat{\psi}^{(36)} = \exp(-0.9904) = 0.371,$$

with 95% confidence interval, from (10.14) and (10.15),

$$\exp(-0.9904 \pm 1.96 \times 0.4111)$$

or (0.166, 0.831). Other odds ratios, relative to social class V are similarly easy to derive.

Table 10.8. Results produced by SAS for Example 10.6.

Parameter	Estimate	Standard error
INTERCEPT	1.5294	0.3059
RANK 1	−2.5590	0.4789
RANK 2	−1.6692	0.3746
RANK 3	−0.9904	0.4111
RANK 4	−0.4129	0.3340
RANK 5	−0.3294	0.3816
RANK 6	0.0000	0.0000

Suppose that we prefer our odds ratios to use the first social class as the base. This might be because we expect this class to have the lowest prevalence odds and we find comparisons against the 'lowest' group easier to interpret. For example, consider comparing social class II (rank 2) to social class I (rank 1). From (10.11),

$$\hat{\psi}^{(21)} = \exp\left(b_1^{(2)} - b_1^{(1)}\right) = \exp(-1.6692 - (-2.5590))$$

$$= e^{0.8898} = 2.43.$$

An alternative way of deriving this from the table of parameter estimates is to notice that

$$\hat{\psi}^{(21)} = \hat{\psi}^{(26)}\hat{\psi}^{(61)} = \hat{\psi}^{(26)}\big/\hat{\psi}^{(16)}$$

$$= \exp(-1.6692)\big/\exp(-2.5590)$$

$$= \exp\left(-1.6692 - (-2.5590)\right),$$

as before.

To obtain the 95% confidence interval for $\hat{\psi}^{(21)}$, we need first to obtain the estimated variance–covariance matrix. The matrix produced by SAS PROC GENMOD is presented as Table 10.9. Note that $b_1^{(6)}$ is fixed by SAS, so has no variance.

Then, by (10.12),

$$\hat{se}\left(\text{lo}\hat{g}\text{it}^{(2)} - \text{lo}\hat{g}\text{it}^{(1)}\right) = \sqrt{0.14033 + 0.22930 - 2(0.09359)} = 0.4271.$$

Thus the 95% confidence interval for $\hat{\psi}^{(21)}$ is, from (10.15),

$$\exp(-1.6692 - (-2.5590) \pm 1.96 \times 0.4271),$$

that is, $\exp(0.8898 \pm 0.8371)$ or (1.05, 5.62).

As may be seen from Example 10.6, having a 'slope' parameter of zero for the chosen base level offers a great advantage. As a consequence, it is sensible to force the computer package to do this, and so avoid the more extensive calculations made at the end of Example 10.6. To be able to force the most convenient mode of fitting, we must know the linear constraint used by whatever computer package we choose to adopt. For instance, we have seen that SAS PROC GENMOD fixes the last level to have a 'slope' parameter of zero, $b^{(\ell)} = 0$. As we saw in Section 9.2.7, some packages

Table 10.9. Variance–covariance matrix produced by SAS for Example 10.6.

	b_0	$b_1^{(1)}$	$b_1^{(2)}$	$b_1^{(3)}$	$b_1^{(4)}$	$b_1^{(5)}$
b_0	0.09359	−0.09359	−0.09359	−0.09359	−0.09359	−0.09359
$b_1^{(1)}$		0.22930	0.09359	0.09359	0.09359	0.09359
$b_1^{(2)}$			0.14033	0.09359	0.09359	0.09359
$b_1^{(3)}$				0.16899	0.09359	0.09359
$b_1^{(4)}$					0.11153	0.09359
$b_1^{(5)}$						0.14564

Table 10.10. Social class coding (SOCLASS) suitable for treating lowest rank (RANK) as the base group when considered as a CLASS variable in SAS.

Social class	RANK	SOCLASS
I	1	7
II	2	2
IIIn	3	3
IIIm	4	4
IV	5	5
V	6	6

(including Stata), by contrast, will fix the *first* level to have a slope parameter of zero, $b^{(1)} = 0$. Hence, the estimate and estimated standard error of $\psi^{(21)}$ for Example 10.6 would come directly from these packages, only requiring RANK to be declared as a categorical variable. Some computer routines allow the user a degree of choice in setting the base level. In Stata this works through the 'ib#.' operator, where # is the base level of choice. Without such a facility, there are two ways to force the chosen package to use a base that is not the one that the package automatically chooses when the levels are entered in their natural order. The easiest way is to present the package with levels of the x variable that are appropriately reordered.

Example 10.7 Consider the problem at the end of Example 10.6 again, and suppose that SAS PROC GENMOD is to be used. So as to use social class I as the base for all the odds ratios, we can use the coding in Table 10.10 for the new variable SOCLASS derived from the old variable RANK.

The lowest RANK is now the highest SOCLASS; everything else is left unaltered. The parameter estimates from SAS for the logistic regression using SOCLASS are shown in Table 10.11. Now, from (10.13), (10.14) and (10.15), we see immediately that

$$\hat{\psi}^{(21)} = \exp(0.8899) = 2.43,$$

with a 95% confidence interval of

$$\exp(0.8899 \pm 1.96 \times 0.4271)$$

Table 10.11. Results produced by SAS for Example 10.7.

Parameter	Estimate	Standard error
INTERCEPT	−1.0296	0.3684
SOCLASS 2	0.8899	0.4271
SOCLASS 3	1.5686	0.4595
SOCLASS 4	2.1461	0.3920
SOCLASS 5	2.2296	0.4333
SOCLASS 6	2.5590	0.4789
SOCLASS 7	0.0000	0.0000

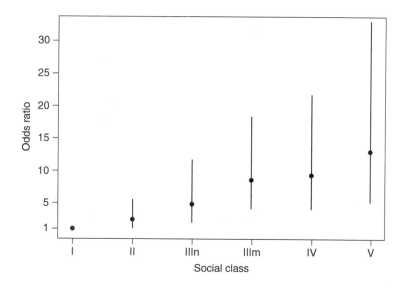

Figure 10.5. Prevalence odds ratios (with 95% confidence intervals) for *H. pylori* by social class group.

or (1.05, 5.62) as before. Indeed, all $\hat{\psi}^{(i1)}$ are easy to deal with; the complete set of odds ratios and their 95% confidence intervals are shown in Figure 10.5. Keeping the odds for social class I fixed as 1, we can see how the prevalence odds ratio of *H. pylori* increases with 'increasing' social class (increasing deprivation).

The other way to change the default choice of base is to employ dummy variables. SAS PROC GENMOD, GLM in Stata (with an "i." prefix) and other computer routines allow the explanatory variable to be declared as categorical. Several other computer packages, or individual procedures, do not have this facility. When using such software, categorical variables must be defined as a set of dummy variables. Even when a categorical declaration *is* available, we can choose not to make this declaration, because the linear constraint used is inconvenient, and define convenient dummy variables instead. Given a categorical variable with ℓ levels, we shall need to define and fit $\ell - 1$ dummy variables (Section 9.2.6).

Example 10.8 Consider, again, the problem of calculating odds ratios relative to the base of social class I for Example 10.6. This time SAS PROC GENMOD was used without the CLASS declaration to denote RANK (Example 10.6) or SOCLASS (Example 10.7) as categorical. Instead five dummy variables, X2 to X6, were defined out of the original RANK variable; Xi will have value 1 if RANK = i and 0 otherwise. The consequent dataset, arising from Table 10.3, for input to SAS is given as Table 10.12, where E is the number with disease and N is the total number

Table 10.12. Data for Example 10.8 including dummy variables for social class (X2 to X6).

RANK	X2	X3	X4	X5	X6	E	N
1	0	0	0	0	0	10	38
2	1	0	0	0	0	40	86
3	0	1	0	0	0	36	57
4	0	0	1	0	0	226	300
5	0	0	0	1	0	83	108
6	0	0	0	0	1	60	73

Table 10.13. Results produced by SAS for
Example 10.8.

Parameter	Estimate	Standard error
INTERCEPT	−1.0296	0.3684
X2	0.8899	0.4271
X3	1.5686	0.4595
X4	2.1461	0.3920
X5	2.2296	0.4333
X6	2.5590	0.4789

at each level. Note that, for example, X4 is zero unless RANK = 4. The five explanatory variables, X2 to X6, were fitted using PROC GENMOD. Table 10.13 gives the results, which are exactly as in Table 10.11, as they should be.

10.4.4 Ordinal risk factors

Our logistic regression models for Table 10.3 have, so far, ignored the ordering of the categories (levels). It might be sensible to consider a logistic regression model for the ranks, rather than the categories they represent. This requires treating 'rank' as a quantitative measure; we may then proceed exactly as in Section 10.4.2.

Example 10.9 The *H. pylori* data in Table 10.3 were, once more, analysed with SAS PROC GENMOD, but now treating RANK as continuous (that is to say, no CLASS declaration was made and dummy variables were not defined). The estimated intercept is −1.0893 and slope is 0.5037. Hence, the model fitted is

$$\hat{\text{logit}} = -1.0893 + 0.5037x,$$

where x is the rank. Notice that this implies a linear trend in the log odds by increasing rank score (Figure 10.6(a)); hence, this is a linear trend model of a certain kind.

If we consider the odds ratio for a unit increase in the rank score, (10.4) gives

$$\hat{\psi} = e^{0.5037} = 1.65.$$

Hence, we estimate that the odds go up by a factor of 1.65 (i.e., by 65%) for each step along the social scale. That is, we have fitted a model for a constant multiplicative increase in odds by social class. This is emphasized by Figure 10.6(b). The odds ratio for a step of s units is 1.65^s. Recall that, due to the way occupational social class groups are defined, a higher numbered group represents increased deprivation.

If the ordinal (linear trend) model is adequate, we would expect the estimates of the odds from this model to be close to those from the categorical model (where they are not assumed to have a fixed relationship with each other) fitted in Example 10.7. For example, from Table 10.13, the odds in social class IIIn (rank 3) are exp (−1.0296 + 1.5686) = 1.71 for the categorical model (from Table 10.13) and exp (−1.0893 + 0.5037 × 3) = 1.52 for the ordinal model, which are fairly close. Since the odds ratio is scaled so that its value in the base group (social class I) is unity, separately for each model, we cannot expect close agreement when comparing sizes of odds ratios in Figure 10.5 and Figure 10.6(b) even when the linear trend model is appropriate. Thus, the odds ratio for social class IIIn compared with I is 4.80 for the categorical model but only 2.74 for the ordinal model;

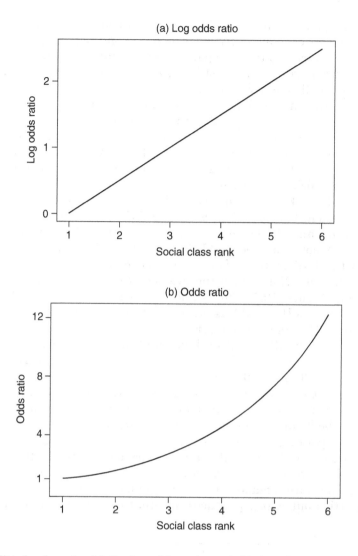

Figure 10.6. Fitted values for (a) the log odds ratio; and (b) the odds ratio, when social class I (rank = 1) is fixed to have an odds of unity.

this difference does not prove lack of appropriateness of the linear trend assumption. We consider the goodness of fit of the ordinal model in Example 10.28.

10.4.5 Floating absolute risks

Whenever the explanatory variable is ordinal, such as social class in the preceding examples or when a continuous variable has been split into a set of ordinal groups (see Section 3.6.1), interpretation of the trend through plots of odds ratios and confidence intervals for each level, such as Figure 10.5, is somewhat complex. This is because, as is illustrated by Example 10.6, each confidence interval depends upon variation arising from the base level as well as the level against which it is plotted. Often the result is wide confidence intervals that are likely to overlap even when there is real trend in the data. For display purposes, this may not be satisfactory.

To avoid this problem, it is possible to apply a transformation to the set of $\ell - 1$ parameter estimates comparing other levels to the base, and the corresponding variance–covariance matrix, so that the parameter estimates remain unchanged and the covariances reduce to zero (or at least become very small) but, as a make-weight, the base level, which really has zero variance, now has a nonzero 'quasi-variance' attached to it. Effectively, this means that the entire variation, illustrated by the set of confidence intervals, is redistributed so that the base level now gets a confidence interval and the other confidence intervals shrink in size. The resulting estimates are called **floating absolute risks** (FARs) (Easton *et al.,* 1991). Assuming normal distributions, when the covariances are zero the FARs are independent of each other, unlike the odds ratios from which they derive.

Figure 10.7 shows FARs for the social class example. Here the vertical label has been left as it was in Figure 10.5 because the FAR estimates are just reproductions of the odds ratios, and the latter have a more exact, and more widely understood, interpretation. A note has been added to say that the confidence intervals were derived from the FAR method. This is the recommended way of labelling graphs produced in this way. Notice how the eye sees the trend more easily from Figure 10.7 than from Figure 10.5. Furthermore, the significant ($p < 0.05$) difference between social classes IIIn and V is much more easily spotted from Figure 10.7 than from Figure 10.5. The confidence interval for $\hat{\psi}^{(36)}$ in Example 10.6 shows that this odds ratio really is significant (it excludes unity). The transformation made to the variance–covariance matrix makes the off-diagonal elements, corresponding to all but the first row of Table 10.9, zero.

FAR methodology is not specific to logistic regression; indeed, in practice it has been more often applied to survival models, such as those met in Chapter 11. Estimates may be 'floated' around any base group or around any numerical value. Another of its advantages is that changes of base do not require recalculation of standard errors as would normally be necessary (see Example 10.6). However, the FAR approach has two major disadvantages (Greenland *et al.,* 1999; Arbogast, 2005). First, the transformation made is not unique and could be replaced by another with similar properties but which produces different confidence limits. Second, due to

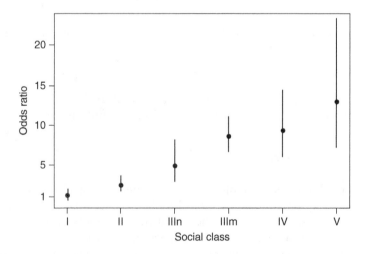

Figure 10.7. Prevalence odds ratios (with 95% confidence limits calculated using the floating absolute risk method) for *H. pylori* by social class group.

the way they are computed, the FAR confidence limits only have a definition in terms of the complete set of levels of the risk factor taken together. Looking at any level in isolation, the confidence limits have no interpretation. Thus, for example, we cannot say that the confidence interval for social class IV in Figure 10.7 represents anything about that specific social class, whereas we know that 95% of the time the corresponding interval in Figure 10.5 will include the true odds ratio for social class IV compared with social class I.

A further drawback is that the covariances will not always come out to be exactly zero, as they did in the preceding social class example; typically, this occurs when confounding variables are accounted for. Although they should still be negligible in size, the FARs will then be not strictly independent. These problems have limited widespread application of the method. However, it does warrant consideration as a descriptive tool, particularly when the reference group is small or has few events. For an example of the use of FARs, see Asia Pacific Cohort Studies Collaboration (2003a). A SAS routine to calculate FARs and their confidence intervals is available to download from the web site for this book (Appendix A).

10.5   Generic data

Up to now we have assumed that the data are supplied to the computer package in a grouped form (as in Table 10.2). However, as mentioned at the outset in Section 10.1, raw data are usually ungrouped, simply recording the risk factor level and disease status for each individual separately. This is called the **generic**, **case-by-case** or **binary data** format, as represented by Table 10.1.

In practice, generic data are easier to deal with than grouped data; it is simply easier to describe the methodology using the grouped format. With generic data, we code our disease status variable to be 1 if disease is present and 0 if disease is absent. We can fit logistic regression models just as before, except that, in the notation of Section 10.1, $n_i = 1$ for each i (each individual),

$$e_i = \begin{cases} 1 & \text{if individual } i \text{ has the disease} \\ 0 & \text{else} \end{cases}$$

and hence $r_i = e_i/n_i = e_i$.

Example 10.10 Table 10.4 presents a summarised version of the SHHS data on age and death. The original database for the study is, conceptually, a rectangular matrix of individuals against variables. When we select out the age and death status variables only, we obtain a matrix with 5754 rows and two columns (AGE and DEATH, coded as 0 for no, 1 for yes). These data are available to be downloaded; see Appendix A. A third column made up of 5754 entries of the number 1 was defined as the risk denominator (although with both SAS and Stata this is unnecessary since the outcome variable (DEATH in this example) is already coded 1 for an event and 0 for a non-event). These three columns then take the place of the first three columns in Table 10.4, although age will now have many duplicate values and will not be sorted in order. These three columns of generic data can be input to a computer package and a logistic regression model fitted.

SAS PROC GENMOD was used in this way. Output 10.1A gives part of the full output. The estimates and their standard errors will be seen to agree with those found using the grouped data of Table 10.4, as presented in Table 10.7. The degrees of freedom column in Output 10.1A is redundant here and in all future examples, except that it will show a result of zero when

Output 10.1A. SAS PROC GENMOD results for Example 10.10.

Analysis of parameter estimates							
Parameter	DF	Estimate	Standard error	Wald 95% confidence limits		Chi-square	Pr > ChiSq
Intercept	1	−8.4056	0.5507	−9.4849	−7.3263	233.00	<.0001
age	1	0.1126	0.0104	0.0922	0.1330	116.92	<.0001

Output 10.1B. Stata GLM results for Example 10.10.

death	Coef.	OIM Std. Err.	z	P>|z|	[95% Conf. Interval]	
age	.1125569	.0104094	10.81	0.000	.0921549	.1329589
_cons	-8.405635	.550676	-15.26	0.000	-9.48494	-7.32633

the corresponding parameter is fixed to be zero. The chi-square test given in Output 10.1A is explained in Section 10.7.6.

Output 10.1B shows the results corresponding to Output 10.A from GLM in Stata. The two outputs are equivalent, although there are four differences in the numerical display from Stata, compared with SAS. First, Stata has a general policy of showing the intercept term last in its displays of regression coefficients, labelled '_cons' (as in Output 9.1B). Second, Stata has used more decimal places for all but the p value. Third, Stata has used a standard normal test rather than the chi-square test, on one degree of freedom, used by SAS. The two tests will give the same p value. Fourth, Stata labels a p value of <0.001 as "0.000".

As Example 10.10 demonstrates, we get the same estimates from generic and grouped data. There will be differences when we consider tests of goodness of fit of logistic regression models in Section 10.7.

10.6   Multiple logistic regression models

Just as with standard regression models, logistic models may be specified with several explanatory variables, rather than only one. Given k explanatory variables, the multiple logistic regression model is, by analogy with (10.3),

$$\log_e\left(\frac{\hat{r}}{1-\hat{r}}\right) = b_0 + b_1 x_1 + b_2 x_2 + \cdots + b_k x_k,$$

where $\hat{r}$ is the estimated risk of disease. The right-hand side of the model equation is now a multiple linear predictor.

If, say, x_i is a categorical variable with ℓ levels, then we replace $b_i x_i$ with

$$b_i^{(1)} x_i^{(1)} + b_i^{(2)} x_i^{(2)} + \cdots + b_i^{(\ell)} x_i^{(\ell)},$$

where

$$x_i^{(j)} = \begin{cases} 1 \text{ if } x_i = x_i^{(j)} \text{ (i.e., } x_i \text{ takes its } j\text{th level)} \\ 0 \text{ otherwise} \end{cases}$$

subject to an arbitrary linear constraint (such as $b_i^{(1)} = 0$). All this, apart from the differences identified in Section 10.3, is exactly as for general linear models (Chapter 9). Logistic regression is an example of a **generalised linear model** (McCullagh and Nelder, 1989), a class of models that includes the general linear model (standard regression and analysis of variance).

Multiple-variable logistic models are dealt with in much the same way as single-variable models, but (as with multiple-variable general linear models) allow for a wider range of inferences. Basic analyses are now explained by example.

Example 10.11 Table 10.14 presents data on coronary heart disease (CHD), blood pressure and cholesterol from the cohort phase of the SHHS. As in Example 10.2, we are considering this as a fixed cohort study with a follow-up period of 7.7 years. This time, data are shown only for the 4095 men with no evidence of CHD at baseline, for whom systolic blood pressure and serum total cholesterol were measured. The blood pressure and cholesterol groups chosen in Table 10.14 are the fifths for the entire set of male data — that is, before those with CHD at baseline were deleted.

These data were read into SAS, denoting the systolic blood pressure (SBP) variable as SBP5TH and the total cholesterol variable as CHOL5TH. They were then analysed in PROC GENMOD, fixing the lowest level of each of SBP5TH and CHOL5TH to have a log odds ratio of zero (odds ratio of unity). The parameter estimates produced by SAS (after relabelling, as explained in Section 10.4.3) are given in Table 10.15.

Table 10.14. Ratio of CHD events to total number by systolic blood pressure (SBP) and cholesterol fifths for men in SHHS who were free of CHD at baseline.

SBP (mmHg)	Serum total cholesterol (mmol/l)				
	≤5.41	5.42–6.01	6.02–6.56	6.57–7.31	>7.31
≤118	1/190	0/183	4/178	8/157	4/132
119–127	2/203	2/175	6/167	10/166	11/137
128–136	5/173	9/176	9/181	8/167	11/164
137–148	5/139	3/156	10/154	13/174	16/174
>148	5/123	8/123	12/144	13/179	23/180

Table 10.15. Estimates for Example 10.11, as produced by SAS.

Parameter		Estimate
INTERCEPT		−4.5995
SBP5TH	1	0.0000
SBP5TH	2	0.6092
SBP5TH	3	0.8697
SBP5TH	4	1.0297
SBP5TH	5	1.3425
CHOL5TH	1	0.0000
CHOL5TH	2	0.2089
CHOL5TH	3	0.8229
CHOL5TH	4	1.0066
CHOL5TH	5	1.2957

From Table 10.15, the fitted model is

$$\hat{\text{logit}} = -4.5995 + 0x_1^{(1)} + 0.6092x_1^{(2)} + 0.8697x_1^{(3)} + 1.0297x_1^{(4)}$$

$$+ 1.3425x_1^{(5)} + 0x_2^{(1)} + 0.2089x_2^{(2)} + 0.8229x_2^{(3)} \qquad (10.16)$$

$$+ 1.0066x_2^{(4)} + 1.2957x_2^{(5)},$$

where $x_1^{(i)}$ represents the ith level of SBP and $x_2^{(i)}$ represents the ith level of cholesterol, for i running from 1 to 5 in rank order in each case. Since the highest estimate is for the highest fifth in each case, we can immediately see that it is most risky to be in the top fifth of both SBP and cholesterol.

We can estimate the log odds of CHD for a man in the highest level of SBP (>148 mmHg) and highest level of cholesterol (>7.31 mmol/l) to be, from (10.16),

$$\hat{\text{logit}} = -4.5995 + 1.3425 + 1.2957 = -1.9613.$$

The odds are thus $e^{-1.9613} = 0.1407$.

We can estimate the risk for a man in this extreme group, using (10.8), to be

$$\hat{r} = \{1 + \exp(1.9613)\}^{-1} = 0.1233.$$

So the chance of a coronary event in a follow-up period of 7.7 years is estimated to be 0.1233 (i.e., about 12%) for middle-aged Scotsmen who are in the highest 20% of both SBP and cholesterol.

We can estimate the log odds ratio for a man in the combination of highest levels (5, 5) relative to the combination of lowest levels (1, 1) (SBP $\leq$ 118 mmHg; cholesterol $\leq$ 5.41 mmol/l) from (10.16) as

$$\log(\hat{\psi}) = \hat{\text{logit}}^{(5,5)} - \hat{\text{logit}}^{(1,1)}$$

$$= (-4.5995 + 1.3425 + 1.2957) - (-4.5995)$$

$$= 1.3425 + 1.2957 = 2.6382,$$

whence the odds ratio is $e^{2.6382} = 14.0$. Notice that the constant term (-4.5995) simply cancels out, as it must do whenever any odds ratio is calculated.

The relative risk for the same contrast is

$$\hat{r}^{(5,5)} / \hat{r}^{(1,1)}$$

which turns out to be $0.1233/0.009957 = 12.4$. Notice that this is similar to the odds ratio, as would be expected because CHD is reasonably unusual, even in the high-risk group.

It is interesting to see how the two risk factors behave when varied alone, to compare with the combined effect seen already. From Table 10.15, the odds ratio comparing level 5 of SBP to level 1, keeping cholesterol fixed, is $e^{1.3425} = 3.8$. It is quite correct to ignore all the estimates for cholesterol in deriving this. To see this, consider the odds ratio for the last fifth compared with the first fifth for SBP, keeping cholesterol fixed at its third fifth. This is the same as finding the odds ratio for the combination of (SBP, cholesterol) as (5, 3) relative to (1, 3). From (10.16),

$$\hat{\text{logit}}^{(5,3)} = -4.5995 + 1.3425 + 0.8229$$

$$\hat{\text{logit}}^{(1,3)} = -4.5995 + 0 + 0.8229.$$

Hence, log odds ratio $= \hat{\text{logit}}^{(5,3)} - \hat{\text{logit}}^{(1,3)} = 1.3425$ and $\psi = e^{1.3425}$, as stated. The constant term and the slope parameter for level 3 of cholesterol have cancelled out.

Similarly, for comparing between extreme levels of cholesterol, keeping SBP fixed, the odds ratio is $e^{1.2957} = 3.7$. Notice that $3.8 \times 3.7 = 14.1$, which is very similar to the combined odds ratio of 14.0 found earlier. In fact, the difference is merely due to rounding error, since here no interaction has been fitted (see Section 4.8.2 and Section 10.9).

Confidence intervals for comparisons in which only one variable's levels are varied follow exactly as in Section 10.4.3. When the levels of two (or more) variables are varied, we shall need the variance–covariance matrix. For instance, the standard error of the log odds ratio comparing (5, 5) to (1, 1) in Example 10.11 is

$$se\left\{\hat{logit}^{(5,5)} - \hat{logit}^{(1,1)}\right\} = se\left\{b_0 + b_1^{(5)} + b_2^{(5)} - \left(b_0 + b_1^{(1)} + b_2^{(1)}\right)\right\}$$

$$= se\left\{b_1^{(5)} + b_2^{(5)}\right\}$$

$$= \sqrt{V\left(b_1^{(5)}\right) + V\left(b_2^{(5)}\right) + 2C\left(b_1^{(5)}, b_2^{(5)}\right)}.$$

Using this, the 95% confidence interval is, as usual,

$$\text{estimate} \pm 1.96 \, \hat{se}.$$

Example 10.12 A rather more substantial example than the last is provided by fitting six risk factors for the SHHS data on men with no prior history of CHD. This time SBP and cholesterol were fitted as quantitative variables because Table 10.15 suggests that both of their effects are linear (see also Section 10.7.5). The other variables fitted were age, body mass index (BMI: weight/square of height), smoking status and self-reported activity in leisure. Age and BMI are quantitative; smoking is coded as 1 = never smoked; 2 = ex-smoker; 3 = current smoker. Activity in leisure is also categorical, coded as 1 = active; 2 = average; 3 = inactive. As in Example 10.11, any man for whom at least one variable has a missing value is not included (see Chapter 14 for methods to impute missing values). The data used are available for downloading; see Appendix A.

With so many variables, it is very time consuming to create the multiway table (which needs to be six dimensional here) corresponding to Table 10.14. Furthermore, the quantitative variables would give rise to huge tables because we are not grouping them here. Hence, the data were input to SAS in generic form: 4049 lines, each containing data for the seven variables, AGE, TOTCHOL, BMI, SYSTOL, SMOKING, ACTIVITY and CHD, where

$$CHD = \begin{cases} 1 & \text{if the individual has a CHD event} \\ 0 & \text{if not} \end{cases}$$

and the variables have obvious names. PROC GENMOD was used to fit the logistic regression model with base levels 1 (active) for activity in leisure and 1 (never smoked) for smoking status. As explained in Section 10.5, a further column consisting of 4049 copies of the number 1 was created to hold the n_i. The parameter estimates produced are given in Table 10.16. The fitted model is thus

$$\hat{logit} = -10.1076 + 0.0171x_1 + 0.3071x_2 + 0.0417x_3$$

$$+ 0.0204x_4 + 0x_5^{(1)} + 0.3225x_5^{(2)} + 0.7296x_5^{(3)} \tag{10.17}$$

$$+ 0x_6^{(1)} - 0.1904x_6^{(2)} - 0.1011x_6^{(3)},$$

where the x variables and units of measurement are as defined in Table 10.16.

Table 10.16. Parameter estimates for Example 10.12, as produced by SAS.

Variable name/symbol		Units of measurement/code	Parameter estimate
—	INTERCEPT	—	−10.1076
x_1	AGE	years	0.0171
x_2	TOTCHOL	mmol/l	0.3071
x_3	BMI	kg/m^2	0.0417
x_4	SYSTOL	mmHg	0.0204
$x_5^{(1)}$	SMOKING 1	never-smoker	0.0000
$x_5^{(2)}$	SMOKING 2	ex-smoker	0.3225
$x_5^{(3)}$	SMOKING 3	current smoker	0.7296
$x_6^{(1)}$	ACTIVITY 1	active	0.0000
$x_6^{(2)}$	ACTIVITY 2	average	−0.1904
$x_6^{(3)}$	ACTIVITY 3	inactive	−0.1011

As in the single-variable situation, the parameter for a quantitative variable represents the increase in log odds for a unit increase in the variable, but now keeping all other variables fixed. Hence, the increase in log odds for an increase of 1 mmol/l in cholesterol, keeping the other five variables fixed, is 0.3071; the log odds for an increase of 2 mmol/l in cholesterol, keeping all else fixed, is $2 \times 0.3071 = 0.6142$; the odds ratio for a cholesterol of $x + s$ relative to x, keeping all else fixed, is $\exp(0.3071s)$, regardless of the value of x.

Similar interpretations follow for categorical variables. Thus, 0.3225 is the log odds ratio for ex-smokers compared with never-smokers, keeping all the other five variables fixed at some arbitrary values. Notice that the negative signs for estimates of ACTIVITY give unexpected inferences in our example: those who are average and inactive have lower odds of CHD than those who are active in their leisure time. This may be a result of bias caused by self-assessment of activity level.

As in Example 10.11, we can use the multiple logistic regression model to make inferences about combinations of variable outcomes. For example, the log odds for a 50-year-old active male ex-smoker who is currently free of CHD and has a serum total cholesterol value of 6.0 mmol/l, BMI of 25 kg/m^2 and SBP of 125 mmHg is

$$\hat{\text{logit}} = -10.1076 + 0.0171 \times 50 + 0.3071 \times 6.0$$

$$+ 0.0417 \times 25 + 0.0204 \times 125 + 0.3225 + 0 = -3.4950,$$

from which the odds are $e^{-3.495} = 0.030$ and, using (10.8), the risk is $\{1 + e^{3.495}\}^{-1} = 0.029$. Hence, we expect around 3% of such men to experience a coronary event during a period of 7.7 years.

Consider a similar man with all as before, except that he is a current smoker and has an SBP of 150. The log odds for such a man compared with the previous type is easily found by finding the difference in logits, ignoring any terms that must cancel out:

$$0.0204(150 - 125) + 0.7296 - 0.3225 = 0.9171.$$

Thus $\hat{\psi} = e^{0.9171} = 2.50$. The second type of man has two and a half times the odds of a CHD event, compared with the first type.

10.7 Tests of hypotheses

So far we have considered only the issue of estimating the effect of a risk factor upon disease outcome in our discussion of logistic regression. As in other branches of statistical analysis, we will often be interested in whether the effect observed is attributable to chance. Three particular types of hypothesis will be described here: tests of goodness of fit of the overall model; tests of effect of any one risk factor contained within the model; and tests of the linear effect of ordered categorical risk factors.

Most of these tests use a quantity called the **deviance**, which is calculated whenever a generalised linear model is fitted by a statistical computer package. The deviance, in turn, is calculated from the **likelihood**, which is a measure of how likely a particular model is, given the observed data. Complete details and many examples are given in Clayton and Hills (1993). The deviance is, essentially, a measure of the difference between the postulated model and the model that, by definition, is a perfect fit to the data (called the **full**, or **saturated**, model). To be precise, it is given by

$$D = -2\{\log \hat{L} - \log \hat{L}_F\},$$

where L is the likelihood for the postulated model and L_F is the likelihood for the full model. The larger the value of the deviance, the greater the difference between the likelihood of the current model and that of the model that has perfect fit. When the data have a normal distribution (the general linear model), the deviance is the residual sum of squares.

As far as the practical epidemiologist is concerned, the deviance may be regarded simply as a test statistic, akin to Student's t statistic, the chi-square statistic and many others. The interested reader is referred to McCullagh and Nelder (1989) for a full explanation and to Collett (2002) for an explanation in the context of logistic regression.

10.7.1 Goodness of fit for grouped data

If the data are grouped — that is, not in generic form — the deviance of the model can be used to test for goodness of fit of the model to the data: the model deviance is compared with chi-square on the model deviance degrees of freedom (d.f.). Table 10.17 shows the model deviance and d.f. for all the examples used so far. The d.f. for a model deviance is calculated just as for the error term in the general linear model; that is,

d.f. = number of data items

– number of independent parameters in the fitted model,

Table 10.17. Model deviance and brief descriptions for all prior examples.

Example number	Brief description	Type of Variable	Type of Data	Model Deviance	Model d.f.	Model p value[a]
10.1/6/7/8	MONICA *H. pylori*	categorical	grouped	0	0	—
10.9	MONICA *H. pylori*	quantitative	grouped	6.55	4	0.17
10.2/3/5	SHHS deaths	quantitative	grouped	23.46	18	0.17
10.10	SHHS deaths	quantitative	generic	2683.67	5752	—
10.4	EGAT	categorical	grouped	0	0	—
10.11	SHHS CHD	categorical	grouped	18.86	16	0.28
10.12	SHHS CHD	both	generic	1481.34	4040	—

[a] p values are found from a computer package, comparing the deviance to chi-square with d.f. as for the deviance.

where the number of independent parameters is 1 for the intercept (constant) term, 1 for a quantitative variable and $\ell - 1$ for a categorical variable with ℓ levels. Each of the 'data items' corresponds to a distinct definition of n (denominator for the calculation of risk). For example, there are 20 data items in Example 10.2. Table 10.18 shows how the d.f. for the deviance is calculated for each of the seven examples listed in Table 10.17. With generic data format (Example 10.10 and Example 10.12), the number of data items is simply the sample size.

We cannot use the model deviance to test goodness of fit when the data are analysed in generic form (Section 10.7.2); hence, no p value is given in Table 10.17 for Example 10.10 and Example 10.12. However, notice that the deviance and d.f. are quite different for Example 10.5 and Example 10.10, which (as we have already seen) produce the same fitted models. The model deviance is similarly of no use when it turns out to be zero. In fact, this signifies that the full model must have been fitted. This is always the case when a single categorical variable is recorded and fitted to grouped data, as in Example 10.4 and Example 10.6. As Table 10.18 shows, we have 'used up' all the degrees of freedom in the models fitted in these examples; no other sources of variability remain. By definition, such models have perfect fit and goodness of fit is not an issue.

For Example 10.5, Example 10.9 and Example 10.11, we can test for goodness of fit. In Example 10.5 and Example 10.9 a quantitative variable is used to summarize the effect of the x variable; this does *not* give rise to a full model because there is remaining variation about the fitted line (Figure 10.4). Neither of these models has a significant deviance ($p > 0.10$) and hence we may conclude that there is no evidence of lack of fit.

In Example 10.11 the remaining variation, not modelled, is the interaction between SBP and cholesterol. This interaction will have $(5-1)(5-1) = 16$ d.f. because both SBP and cholesterol have five levels. However, again $p > 0.10$, so we conclude that there is no evidence that the model with only the two main effects is an unsatisfactory fit to the data.

Table 10.18. Derivation of d.f. for model deviances.

Example number	Number of data items	Variables (no. of independent parameters)	Difference = d.f.
10.1/6/7/8	6	constant (1) social class (5)	$6 - 1 - 5 = 0$
10.9	6	constant (1) social class (1)	$6 - 1 - 1 = 4$
10.2/3/5	20	constant (1) age (1)	$20 - 1 - 1 = 18$
10.10	5754	constant (1) age (1)	$5754 - 1 - 1 = 5752$
10.4	2	constant (1) smoking (1)	$2 - 1 - 1 = 0$
10.11	25	constant (1) SBP (4) cholesterol (4)	$25 - 1 - 4 - 4 = 16$
10.12	4049	constant (1) age (1) cholesterol (1) BMI (1) SBP (1) smoking (2) activity (2)	$4049 - 1 - 1 - 1 - 1 - 1 - 2 - 2 = 4040$

If lack of fit is found, we might suspect that further explanatory variables are needed to predict disease, or that we have, in some way, inadequately modelled the effect of the current variables; for example, transformations might be needed or important interactions might be missing. Important outliers may also be in the data. Section 10.11.1 discusses how we might identify certain specific problems with the model. If we have ruled out all such issues, another possibility is that the assumption of binomial variation (Section 10.2.3) is incorrect. Then, when the model deviance is much greater than its degrees of freedom, we have **overdispersion**. This general term is applicable to various statistical models. In the logistic regression context, overdispersion is also called **extra-binomial variation**. The simplest way to deal with this is by using a dispersion parameter, which multiplies the standard binomial variance (Williams, 1982). Many commercial computer routines, including PROC GENMOD in SAS, will allow such a parameter to be included in the specification of the logistic model.

Although it is comforting to find absence of evidence for lack of fit through the summary test on the model deviance, this does not necessarily mean that the fit cannot be improved, for example, through transformations of the explanatory variables. Model checking is still essential (Section 10.11). Indeed, tests of goodness of fit are really of limited use; generally, it is much more meaningful to test for specific effects (Section 10.7.3).

10.7.2 Goodness of fit for generic data

When the data are in generic form, the deviance no longer has an approximate chi-square distribution and thus the test of goodness of fit described in Section 10.7.1 cannot be applied. Since the problem arises due to the sparse nature of the data, an obvious way to seek to address this problem is to group the generic data in some way. Hosmer and Lemeshow (2000) suggest the use of ordinal groups based on the estimated risks (Section 10.4.1) from the logistic regression model. Typically 10 such groups are defined, using the deciles of the probabilities to define the class intervals. The Hosmer–Lemeshow test compares the observed number of people with disease amongst subjects in each group with that expected according to the average risk within the group, across all the groups. This test, which involves use of the chi-square distribution once again, is available from leading statistical packages; PROC LOGISTIC in SAS has an option for the test and the LOGISTIC routine in Stata has a post-estimation command ESTAT, GOF with a similar utility. A significant result, say at the 5% level, implies lack of fit of the model. As with generic data, a nonsignificant result certainly does not mean that no further model checking is required.

10.7.3 Effect of a risk factor

Now we consider a test of the effect of a risk factor, rather than the adequacy of the overall model that contains this risk factor and other terms (including the constant). As a preliminary, the concept of model **nesting** will be defined: model A is said to be nested within model B if model B contains all the variables of model A plus at least one other. In this context, the constant is thought of as a variable. Examples of nesting are given in Table 10.19.

When model A is nested within model B, we can test the hypothesis that the extra terms in B have no additional effect by calculating the difference between the deviances of models A and B, denoted ΔD, and comparing this with chi-square on

Table 10.19. Some examples of nesting (model A is nested within model B).

Example number	Model A	Model B
10.6	constant	constant + social class
10.11	constant + SBP	constant + SBP + cholesterol
10.12	constant + age + cholesterol + BMI + smoking	constant + age + cholesterol + BMI + SBP + smoking + activity in leisure

d.f. given by the difference in d.f., denoted Δd.f., between the two models. This procedure (relying upon an approximate theoretical derivation) works for generic, as well as grouped, data.

Example 10.13 We return to the *H. pylori* and social class data of Table 10.3, as analysed in Examples 10.6 to Example 10.8. We will be interested in knowing whether a man's social class has any effect on his chance of having *H. pylori*. So far, we have fitted the model that assumes that it does:

$$\hat{\text{logit}} = b_0 + b_1^{(1)}x^{(1)} + b_1^{(2)}x^{(2)} + b_1^{(3)}x^{(3)} + b_1^{(4)}x^{(4)} + b_1^{(5)}x^{(5)} + b_1^{(6)}x^{(6)}. \tag{10.18}$$

Let us consider the null hypothesis, $H_0 : b_1^{(j)} = 0$ for all j, against the alternative, $H_1 :$ some $b_1^{(j)} \neq 0$. The null hypothesis states that no social class has any effect on the log odds of *H. pylori* different to the overall average effect (encapsulated by the constant term). Under H_0,

$$\hat{\text{logit}} = b_0, \tag{10.19}$$

which is equivalent to saying that each social class has the same effect. Model (10.19) is clearly nested within model (10.18); the difference between them is the set of variables for the risk factor 'social class'. In Example 10.6, we found that (10.18) is

$$\hat{\text{logit}} = 1.5294 - 2.5590x^{(1)} - 1.6692x^{(2)}$$
$$- 0.9904x^{(3)} - 0.4129x^{(4)} - 0.3294x^{(5)},$$

and the deviance for this model is 0 on 0 d.f. (see Table 10.17 and Table 10.18, or simply note that this is the full model). Fitting (10.19) gives

$$\hat{\text{logit}} = 0.7876,$$

with deviance 64.44 on 5 d.f. Notice that the b_0 in model (10.19) is different from that in model (10.18); just because the models are nested certainly does not suggest that the estimates of any common effects are, in any way, close. Here

$$\Delta D = 64.44 \text{ on } \Delta\text{d.f.} = 5 \text{ d.f.}$$

Comparing to χ_5^2, the *p* value for this is below 0.0001. Hence, the test is extremely significant; we reject H_0 and conclude that there is, indeed, some effect of social class.

Table 10.20. Analysis of deviance table for Example 10.14.

Model	D	d.f.
1 Constant	94.58	24
2 Constant + SBP	56.73	20
3 Constant + cholesterol	49.48	20
4 Constant + SBP + cholesterol	18.86	16

Note: D = deviance.

Example 10.14 Consider Example 10.11 once more. Four models (not involving interactions) may be fitted:

1. $\hat{\text{logit}} = b_0$

2. $\hat{\text{logit}} = b_0 + b_1^{(1)}x_1^{(1)} + b_1^{(2)}x_1^{(2)} + b_1^{(3)}x_1^{(3)} + b_1^{(4)}x_1^{(4)} + b_1^{(5)}x_1^{(5)}$

3. $\hat{\text{logit}} = b_0 + b_2^{(1)}x_2^{(1)} + b_2^{(2)}x_2^{(2)} + b_2^{(3)}x_2^{(3)} + b_2^{(4)}x_2^{(4)} + b_2^{(5)}x_2^{(5)}$

4. $\hat{\text{logit}} = b_0 + b_1^{(1)}x_1^{(1)} + b_1^{(2)}x_1^{(2)} + b_1^{(3)}x_1^{(3)} + b_1^{(4)}x_1^{(4)} + b_1^{(5)}x_1^{(5)}$

   $+ b_2^{(1)}x_2^{(1)} + b_2^{(2)}x_2^{(2)} + b_2^{(3)}x_2^{(3)} + b_2^{(4)}x_2^{(4)} + b_2^{(5)}x_2^{(5)},$

where x_1 = SBP and x_2 = cholesterol, each fitted as a categorical variable with five levels. Similar to the last example, $b_j^{(i)}$ will vary from model to model for each value of i and j because it represents the effect of $x_j^{(i)}$ adjusted for all other variables included in the specific model. Results of fitting these models may be presented in an **analysis of deviance table** (Table 10.20).

We can assess the significance of SBP by comparing models 1 and 2; cholesterol by comparing models 1 and 3; SBP and cholesterol together by comparing models 1 and 4; SBP *over and above* cholesterol by comparing models 3 and 4; cholesterol *over and above* SBP by comparing models 2 and 4. As in Section 9.5, this gives us scope for answering several types of questions that are common in epidemiology.

Results are given in Table 10.21. In this table, the vertical line means 'given', as is standard notation (used elsewhere in this book). The p values come from comparing ΔD with χ^2 on Δd.f. Notice that the Δd.f. are as would be expected in each case: four when one of the five-level effects is assessed and eight when both are assessed. In general, the assessment of one variable at a time will be more illuminating than multiple assessments (such as that on 8 d.f. given here). Hence, future analysis of deviance tables will show only ΔD for single effects.

All of the tests are highly significant, implying that both variables have an effect on CHD, whether or not the effect of the other is already accounted for. However, notice that whenever we analyse two variables together, we might also consider their interaction (Section 10.9).

Example 10.15 Turning now to Example 10.12, there are six risk factors, and hence 64 possible models that could be fitted (without interactions). We could use an automatic variable selection algorithm to choose a 'best' model, but (as in Section 9.7) more insight will be gained by building the final model rather more carefully.

Consider, first, the raw effects of each of the six variables. To assess these, we fit the constant alone and then the constant plus each variable in turn. Subtracting each other

Table 10.21. Further analysis of deviance table for Example 10.14.

Effect	ΔD	Δd.f.	p value
SBP	94.58 − 56.73 = 37.85	24 − 20 = 4	<0.0001
Cholesterol	94.58 − 49.48 = 45.10	24 − 20 = 4	<0.0001
SBP + cholesterol	94.58 − 18.86 = 75.72	24 − 16 = 8	<0.0001
SBP | cholesterol	49.48 − 18.86 = 30.62	20 − 16 = 4	<0.0001
Cholesterol | SBP	56.73 − 18.86 = 37.87	20 − 16 = 4	<0.0001

Table 10.22. First analysis of deviance table for Example 10.15.

Model	Fit details		Test details			
	D	d.f.	ΔD^a	Δd.f.^{a}	p value	Effect
Constant	1569.37	4048	—	—	—	
Constant + AGE	1563.46	4047	5.91	1	0.015	AGE
Constant + TOTCHOL	1534.56	4047	34.81	1	<0.0001	TOTCHOL
Constant + BMI	1560.43	4047	8.94	1	0.003	BMI
Constant + SYSTOL	1528.01	4047	41.36	1	<0.0001	SYSTOL
Constant + SMOKING	1556.22	4046	13.15	2	0.0014	SMOKING
Constant + ACTIVITY	1569.06	4046	0.31	2	0.86	ACTIVITY

^{a} Relative to the first model.

deviance obtained from the first and comparing to χ^2 with Δd.f. degrees of freedom gives the required tests (Table 10.22).

From this we can conclude that activity in leisure is not an important risk factor: its effect is nowhere near significant because $p \gg 0.05$. In fact, this is comforting, because (as already noted) the estimates found in Example 10.12 are not what would be expected: those who are average in activity were found to have the least, and those who are active the most, risk of CHD. Now we know that the differences are explainable by chance variation. It could well be that self-reported level of activity is simply not a very accurate measure of the true level of activity.

All the remaining variables are significant ($p < 0.05$). Of these, age seems to be the least important, perhaps because of the restricted age range and because prevalent cases of CHD were excluded. Total cholesterol and systolic blood pressure are the most important.

Next, we consider fitting the model with the five variables that have significance when taken alone and deleting one variable at a time to see whether that variable is needed in the presence of the remainder (Table 10.23). We see that age is not significant ($p = 0.22$) in the presence of the other four variables. If we take strict 5% significance, BMI may also be dropped, but because it is almost significant ($p = 0.057$) in the presence of the remaining four, and is very significant by itself, we shall keep it in our predictive model. Total cholesterol, systolic blood pressure and smoking status are all highly significant in the presence of each other, age and BMI.

Continuing by fitting the four variables that seem important, and then dropping terms one by one, gives Table 10.24 (here the first row repeats results from the previous analysis of deviance table). The results are almost exactly as before, as far as p values are concerned. If we use the 6.2% significance level, all four remaining variables are significant in the presence of the other three, so none can be dropped.

As a final step, we should try bringing 'activity' back into the model; adding that to the four previously chosen gives a nonsignificant ΔD ($p = 0.58$). Hence, we conclude that the model that best represents the log odds of CHD is that found from fitting total cholesterol, BMI, systolic blood pressure and smoking. The fitted model turns out to be

$$\hat{\text{logit}} = -9.4572 + 0.3035(\text{TOTCHOL}) + 0.0401(\text{BMI})$$

$$+ 0.0214(\text{SYSTOL}) + 0.3291(\text{ex}) + 0.7094(\text{current}),$$

where 'ex' = 1 only for ex-smokers and 'current' = 1 only for current smokers.

10.7.4   Information criteria

The last example involved a variable selection process. As discussed in Section 9.7.1, one approach to such problems is to use the Akaike Information Criterion (AIC) or the Bayesian Information Criterion (BIC). As in other regression problems, the model with the minimum AIC or BIC is, by these criteria, the best. Computer routines, including PROC LOGISTIC and PROC GENMOD in SAS and GLM in Stata, produce

Table 10.23. Second analysis of deviance table for Example 10.15.

Model (each including the constant)	Fit details		Test details			
	D	d.f.	ΔD^a	Δd.f.^{a}	p value	Effect
AGE + TOTCHOL + BMI + SYSTOL + SMOKING	1482.47	4042	—	—	—	
TOTCHOL + BMI + SYSTOL + SMOKING	1484.00	4043	1.53	1	0.22	AGE|others
AGE + BMI + SYSTOL + SMOKING	1507.72	4043	25.25	1	<0.0001	TOTCHOL|others
AGE + TOTCHOL + SYSTOL + SMOKING	1486.09	4043	3.62	1	0.057	BMI|others
AGE + TOTCHOL + BMI + SMOKING	1509.03	4043	26.56	1	<0.0001	SYSTOL|others
AGE + TOTCHOL + BMI + SYSTOL	1496.34	4044	13.87	2	0.001	SMOKING|others

a Relative to the first model.

Table 10.24. Third analysis of deviance table for Example 10.15.

Model (each including the constant)	Fit details		Test details			
	D	d.f.	ΔD^a	Δd.f.^{a}	p value	Effect
TOTCHOL + BMI + SYSTOL + SMOKING	1484.00	4043	—	—	—	
BMI + SYSTOL + SMOKING	1509.00	4044	25.00	1	<0.0001	TOTCHOL|others
TOTCHOL + SYSTOL + SMOKING	1487.48	4044	3.48	1	0.062	BMI|others
TOTCHOL + BMI + SMOKING	1515.37	4044	31.37	1	<0.0001	SYSTOL|others
TOTCHOL + BMI + SYSTOL	1497.40	4045	13.40	2	0.001	SMOKING|others

a Relative to the first model.

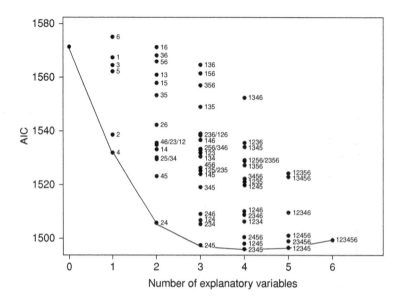

Figure 10.8. Akaike information criteria (AIC) for Example 10.15, produced using PROC GEN-MOD in SAS. The labels are: 1 = age; 2 = serum total cholesterol; 3 = body mass index; 4 = systolic blood pressure; 5 = smoking; 6 = physical activity. The lines join the "best" models (lowest AIC) within each set (where the sets are defined by the number of explanatory variables fitted).

AIC and BIC automatically. Information criteria statistics can be compared between models that are not nested, unlike deviances. However, they have the disadvantage of not leading to a simple hypothesis test, unlike deviances.

Example 10.16. Using PROC GENMOD in SAS, the AIC and BIC were quantified for all 64 models in Example 10.15. Figure 10.8 plots the AIC for each model. From this, we can see that the minimum AIC within each set with the same number of explanatory variables fitted (by definition, excepting the null model) always includes systolic blood pressure (labelled as 4). The next most commonly occurring variable is cholesterol, which pairs with systolic blood pressure in the best two-variable model and stays within each successively more complex model. Age (surprisingly, given the literature on CHD risk factors) and physical activity clearly have relatively little explanatory power, whether or not the other variables are allowed for. The overall best model, by the AIC, has cholesterol, BMI, systolic blood pressure and smoking. In general, we may wish to continue by testing whether any of these variables could be dropped due to lacking significance in the presence of the others — the figure suggests that BMI would be the most likely candidate to be dropped. Here this has already been done in Example 10.15; clearly the results from this and that example are consistent. BIC results are not shown here, but this criterion identified the same global and within-set minima as did AIC.

10.7.5 Tests for linearity and nonlinearity

In Section 10.4.4 we saw how to fit a linear trend in the log odds for an ordered categorical explanatory variable. We can test for the significance of the linear trend, just as for other logistic regression models. We can go further. Since the linear trend model specifies a summary (1 d.f.) relationship (straight line) between the ℓ levels of the ordered categorical variable (on $\ell - 1$ d.f.), the linear trend model is nested within the overall model. The ΔD between the two models can be used to test for nonlinearity, when compared with chi-square on $\ell - 2$ d.f.

Table 10.25. Analysis of deviance table for Example 10.17.

Model	Fit details		Test details			
	D	d.f.	ΔD	Δd.f.	p value	Effect
1 Constant	64.44	5	—	—	—	
2 Constant + social class	0	0	64.44	5	<0.0001	social class
3 Constant + linear trend	6.46	4	57.98[a]	1	<0.0001	linear trend
			6.46[b]	4	0.17	nonlinearity

[a] Relative to model 1.
[b] Relative to model 2.

Example 10.17 For the *H. pylori* data of Table 10.3, social class was fitted as a categorical variable in Example 10.6 and as an ordinal variable in Example 10.9 (the model that assumes a linear trend on the log scale). The analysis of deviance table for the combined analysis (which repeats some results from Example 10.13) is given as Table 10.25. Here, two ΔDs are calculated using the linear trend model. These are the test statistic for linear trend: deviance of the linear model subtracted from the deviance of the constant model; and the test statistic for nonlinearity: deviance of linear trend model less the deviance of the categorical model. In fact, because the categorical model happens to be the full model in this example, the latter is also the test for goodness of fit of the linear trend model, which is intuitively reasonable. Clearly, social class has a significant effect (upon prevalence of *H. pylori*), and the effect seems to be well summarized by a linear trend, because there is no evidence of nonlinearity ($p = 0.17$).

However, we have to be careful when we use such a general test for nonlinearity. Consider a single explanatory variable, x. The nonlinearity is a combination of several effects and can be broken down into distinct polynomial components (Section 9.3.3). These components, each with 1 d.f., are the effects of different powers of x — that is x^2, x^3, etc. It may be that one (or more) of these is significant, but when its effect is combined into the total, this is swamped by the nonsignificant (usually higher order) terms.

In Example 10.6, there does seem to be some curvature in the response; although *H. pylori* undoubtedly goes up with social class, the prevalence has a local peak in the middle classes (Figure 10.1). This may be explained by a second-degree polynomial (quadratic) term, x^2. A quadratic curve has one turning point, either a U shape or its reverse (Figure 9.7(a)). If the quadratic term is significant but the linear is not, then the outcome variable goes up and then down, or vice versa. Such responses are relatively unusual in epidemiology, but Section 3.6.3 gives one example. In Figure 10.1, it appears that an inverted U shape is superimposed on a straight line so that the upward trend has a 'wobble'. Some other types of nonlinearity might be modelled by using a transformation, exactly as for normal regression models (Section 9.3.3).

Example 10.18 To test for all polynomial effects in Example 10.17, the quintic polynomial (highest order possible because social class has five degrees of freedom) was fitted, along with all polynomials of lower orders. Let x denote the social class rank, as defined in Example 10.9, and c = constant. Results are given in Table 10.26. Note that the sum of the ΔDs for all the nonlinear effects (x^2, x^3, x^4 and x^5) in Table 10.26 is 5.76 + 0.05 + 0.43 + 0.22 = 6.46, the ΔD for nonlinearity found in Table 10.25. All we have done here is to partition this ΔD, and its Δd.f., into four components, each representing a different type of effect.

The significant effects here are x and x^2. Hence the quadratic model

$$\hat{\text{logit}} = b_0 + b_1 x + b_2 x^2$$

Table 10.26. Analysis of deviance table for Example 10.18.

Model	Fit details		Test details			
	D	d.f.	ΔD[a]	Δd.f.[a]	p value	Effect
c	64.44	5	—	—	—	
$c + x$	6.46	4	57.98	1	<0.0001	linear
$c + x + x^2$	0.70	3	5.76	1	0.02	quadratic
$c + x + x^2 + x^3$	0.65	2	0.05	1	0.82	cubic
$c + x + x^2 + x^3 + x^4$	0.22	1	0.43	1	0.51	quartic
$c + x + x^2 + x^3 + x^4 + x^5$	0	0	0.22	1	0.64	quintic

[a] Relative to the polynomial model of one less degree.

is suggested. The global test for nonlinearity in Example 10.17 has been misleading. After fitting the model to determine the b coefficients, Figure 10.9 was produced. Observed and expected values are reasonably close, as we would hope (see also Example 10.28).

Epidemiologists often split quantitative variables into categories before analysis, typically using quintiles (as in Example 10.11) or some other percentiles. This is because the consequent set of odds ratios is easy to understand and gives a greater insight into the risk profile than if the variables were left in their raw form (Section 10.10.2). Tests for linear trend then explore, as in Example 10.17, whether there is a linear effect on the log scale, from (say) fifth to fifth. If the variable is very skewed, this does not imply that there is a linear trend across the true range of the data, because the quintiles are then not even approximately equally spaced over this range. If the idea is to explore possible linearity in the variable, probably to ascertain whether it would be appropriate to fit it in its raw, quantitative form, then the coded values used for the ordinal variable should be an appropriate summary of the categorical groups, such as the medians of each fifth (as suggested in Section 3.6.2) in the context of Example 10.11. Notice that it would not be correct to compare the deviances for the models with the variable in grouped and ungrouped (quantitative) form because these are not nested models. The general issue explored here is also considered in Section 10.10.

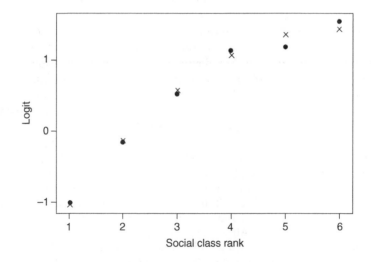

Figure 10.9. Observed (from a categorical model) and expected (from a quadratic model) logits for *H. pylori* by social class group. Observed values are indicated by dots, expected values by crosses.

10.7.6 Tests based upon estimates and their standard errors

In Section 10.4 to Section 10.6, we saw several examples in which an estimate was quoted with its estimated standard error. Provided that the estimator is approximately normally distributed, we can use this information (as in other statistical procedures) to provide a simple approximate test of the null hypothesis that the true value of the parameter estimated is zero, adjusting for all other effects in the model. We compare

$$\left(\frac{\text{estimate}}{\hat{se}} \right)^2$$

with chi-square with 1 d.f. This is sometimes called a **Wald test**, corresponding to the Wald label given to confidence limits in most of the SAS outputs of this chapter. The process is often equivalent to calculating the confidence interval and checking whether zero is inside it. The result is generally slightly different from the recommended method using deviances. In practice, the difference is unlikely to be important unless more fundamental problems are present, such as a very small sample size.

Example 10.19 In Example 10.6, we found the 95% confidence interval for the logit that compares social class II to social class I to be $0.8898 \pm 0.8371 = (0.053, 1.727)$. As zero is outside this interval, we can conclude that there is a significant difference ($p < 0.05$) in the prevalence of *H. pylori* between these two social class groups. We can be more precise by looking at the square of the ratio between the estimate and its estimated standard error, $(0.8898/0.4271)^2 = 4.34$, giving a p value of 0.037 when compared with χ_1^2.

Notice that we could also use the confidence interval for the odds ratio, rather than the logit, but in this case a significant result is a consequence of *unity* lying outside the confidence interval.

Example 10.20 The Analysis of Parameter Estimates produced by SAS for Example 10.12 is given as Output 10.2. SMOKING 4 and ACTIVITY 4 are the relabelled *lowest* levels (never-smoker and active, respectively), as explained in Example 10.7. Here, SAS has done the necessary division and squaring to obtain the chi-square test statistics (using more decimal places than shown for the individual components). For the quantitative variables (age, total cholesterol, BMI and SBP), and indeed any variable (with the exception of the constant) that has 1 d.f., the tests shown are directly comparable to the ΔD in dropping that term from the model fitted.

Output 10.2. SAS PROC GENMOD results for Example 10.20.

Analysis of parameter estimates							
Parameter	DF	Estimate	Standard error	Wald 95% confidence limits		Chi-square	Pr > ChiSq
Intercept	1	−10.1076	0.9972	−12.0620	−8.1532	102.75	<.0001
age	1	0.0171	0.0136	−0.0096	0.0438	1.57	0.2096
totchol	1	0.3071	0.0597	0.1901	0.4241	26.47	<.0001
bmi	1	0.0417	0.0214	−0.0002	0.0835	3.80	0.0513
systol	1	0.0204	0.0038	0.0129	0.0279	28.41	<.0001
smoking	2	1	0.3225	0.2506	−0.1686	0.8137	1.66	0.1980
smoking	3	1	0.7296	0.2192	0.3000	1.1592	11.08	0.0009
smoking	4	0	0.0000	0.0000	0.0000	0.0000	.	.
activity	2	1	−0.1904	0.1801	−0.5433	0.1625	1.12	0.2903
activity	3	1	−0.1011	0.2335	−0.5586	0.3565	0.19	0.6651
activity	4	0	0.0000	0.0000	0.0000	0.0000	.	.

For instance, in Table 10.17 we saw that the deviance for the model of Example 10.12 is 1481.34 on 4040 d.f. When BMI was dropped from the model — that is, the remaining four variables were fitted — the deviance grew to 1485.04 on 4041 d.f. Thus, $\Delta D = 3.70$, slightly smaller than the value 3.80 given for the Wald test in Output 10.2. Similarly, the p value from the ΔD test is slightly bigger at 0.0544, compared with 0.0513, although differences in the third decimal place are not at all important.

For variables with more than 1 d.f. (smoking and activity in the example), the chi-square test statistics give a set of 1 d.f. tests that partition the entire d.f., rather like the polynomial partition in Example 10.18. Here, because of the SAS rules and the labelling of levels adopted, other levels of the categorical variables are contrasted with the lowest level. We can see that the only significant ($p < 0.05$) difference in CHD risk is between SMOKING 3 (current smokers) and SMOKING 4 (never-smokers). It would also be possible to construct a Wald test on $\ell - 1$ d.f. to test the significance of all ℓ levels of a categorical variable together, or indeed to test multiple explanatory variables together, if that was meaningful.

We can use the 'Estimate' and 'Wald 95% confidence limits' columns to see that the odds ratio for current smokers compared with never-smokers is $\exp(0.7296) = 2.07$ with 95% confidence interval $(\exp(0.3000), \exp(1.1592)) = (1.35, 3.19)$. Note that this 'Estimate' column was previously used to create Table 10.16.

10.7.7 Problems with missing values

In all the examples used here, the issue of missing values has not arisen because anyone with any missing value has been deleted in all examples. In most large-scale epidemiological investigations, some values are missing, and we must be careful how we deal with them. It is assumed that a method for imputing missing values is not to be used and, instead, the standard method of deleting observations with missing values is to be used. See Chapter 14 for a discourse on missing values.

Often we build up multiple regression models by getting so far and then wondering if a newly introduced variable will alter the inference. If this new variable has missing values that lead us to delete additional observations, then we *cannot* compare the deviance of the extended model with any model that has gone before. This is because the models with differing sets of observations (subjects) are not nested. Instead, we shall need to refit previous models, possibly including that with the constant alone, using only individuals with complete data. These will provide suitable reference models for calculation of ΔD.

10.8 Confounding

As with general linear models, adjustment for confounding variables is achieved through logistic modelling by fitting the confounder with the risk factor (Section 9.9). Comparison of deviances, for the model with the confounder against the model with the confounder plus the risk factor, gives an indication of whether the risk factor is still important after allowing for the confounder. Comparison of odds ratios from the models with the risk factor alone, and with the confounder added, indicates the effect of the confounder. No formal significance test to see whether a potential confounder is truly a confounder exists; this is not entirely a statistical issue. However, we could reasonably conclude no confounding in the study at hand if the odds ratios, unadjusted and adjusted, were very similar.

Example 10.21 Consider the problem of Example 10.11 and Example 10.14 again. Suppose we wished to consider SBP as a potential confounding factor for the cholesterol–CHD relationship. We obtain a test of the null hypothesis that cholesterol has no effect on CHD after adjustment

Table 10.27. CHD odds ratios for cholesterol, unadjusted and adjusted for systolic blood pressure, for men in SHHS who were free of CHD at baseline.

Serum total cholesterol fifth	Odds ratio	
	Unadjusted	Adjusted
1	1	1
2	1.25	1.23
3	2.36	2.28
4	2.96	2.74
5	4.05	3.65

for SBP by comparing models 2 and 4 in Example 10.14. As we have already seen, this involves a test on the difference in deviances, which turns out to be extremely significant ($p < 0.0001$). Thus, SBP does not remove the effect of cholesterol (as already seen in Example 10.14), and we can judge that cholesterol has an effect over and above that of SBP.

This is not sufficient for us to conclude that SBP does not confound the cholesterol–CHD relationship: it could still be that the magnitude of the relationship is altered appreciably (or even the direction changed) by the presence or absence of SBP. To consider this, we could look at the odds ratios for fifths of cholesterol with and without adjustment for SBP. Parameter estimates from fitting statistical models produced by computer packages (unless specifically stated otherwise) always adjust each term for all other terms fitted, and in Example 10.11 the only terms fitted (besides the constant) are cholesterol and SBP fifths. Note that this is model 4 in Example 10.14. Thus, the cholesterol estimates given in Table 10.15 are adjusted for SBP, and vice versa. To get unadjusted estimates, we fit model 3 of Example 10.14 again. Results are given in Table 10.27. For ease of interpretation, odds ratios are shown (slope parameter estimates raised to the power e).

The two sets of odds ratios are very similar (in both cases the base odds ratio is, of course, fixed at unity). There is little evidence of any important confounding effect. Nevertheless, the adjusted odds ratios are smaller; accounting for another major coronary risk factor has attenuated the effect of cholesterol. We would expect this because of a tendency for unhealthy lifestyle factors to cluster together.

10.9 Interaction

As with general linear models, we deal with interaction by introducing one or more terms into the logistic regression model that are the cross-multiplications of the constituent variables. Here, we shall consider interactions involving two variables. Higher order interactions would be defined, and dealt with, in a similar way. In turn, we shall consider interactions between two categorical variables, a quantitative and a categorical variable and (briefly) two quantitative variables. Interaction in logistic regression models means heterogeneity in the odds ratios, in the sense explained in Section 4.8.2. As discussed in Section 4.9, whenever an interaction turns out to be significant, the main effects of the constituent terms (for example, simple one-factor odds ratios) are likely to be misleading, and thus should not be reported.

10.9.1 Between two categorical variables

We can define a categorical variable, A, with ℓ levels by $\ell - 1$ dummy variables (Section 10.4.3). Given a second categorical variable, B, with m levels and therefore $m - 1$ dummy variables, the interaction is represented by the set of $(\ell - 1)(m - 1)$ variables

Table 10.28. CHD status, after follow-up of 7.7 years, by Bortner score
quarter at baseline for those in SHHS with Bortner score measured
who were free of CHD at baseline.

| Quarter of | Male | | Female | | |
Bortner score	No CHD	CHD	No CHD	CHD	Total
1 (≤144)	1022	57 (5.3%)	915	30 (3.2%)	2024
2 (145–169)	918	56 (5.8%)	1081	20 (1.8%)	2075
3 (170–194)	927	39 (4.0%)	1066	10 (0.9%)	2042
4 (>194)	1022	46 (4.3%)	938	10 (1.0%)	2016
Total	3889	198 (4.8%)	4000	70 (1.7%)	8157

formed by cross-multiplication of the two individual sets of dummy variables. The
interaction has $(\ell - 1)(m - 1)$ d.f. We test by calculating ΔD for the model that includes
the two main effects (A and B) compared with the model that includes these and the
interaction (written $A*B$).

Example 10.22 Table 10.28 shows some more data from the SHHS, this time for both sexes.
Bortner score (Bortner, 1969) is a measure of personality (Type A behaviour). Although a high
Bortner score has been thought to be a bad thing, Table 10.28 shows that the opposite is true
in the SHHS. CHD incidence seems to come down with increasing Bortner score, but much
more rapidly for women. Hence, we might suspect an interaction between Bortner score and
sex. We will test this using dummy variables, taking Bortner score in grouped form, grouping
being by quarters (as in the table).
    Dummy variables, X1 to X3 for Bortner quarter and X4 for sex, are defined in Table 10.29. The
interaction variables, X5 to X7, defined by cross-multiplying the relevant components of Table 10.29,
are given in Table 10.30. Table 10.31 shows the consequent full dataset; the number with CHD
positive is the number of events (denoted e in Section 10.1) out of n trials (sample size for the

Table 10.29. Dummy variables for
Bortner score and for sex.

Bortner quarter	X1	X2	X3	Sex	X4
1	0	0	0	female	0
2	1	0	0	male	1
3	0	1	0		
4	0	0	1		

Table 10.30. Interaction variables for Bortner score by sex
(derived from Table 10.29).

| Bortner quarter | X5 Sex | | X6 Sex | | X7 Sex | |
	Female	Male	Female	Male	Female	Male
1	0	0	0	0	0	0
2	0	1	0	0	0	0
3	0	0	0	1	0	0
4	0	0	0	0	0	1

Table 10.31. Specification of data (M = male; F = female).

		Dummy variables representing								
		Bortner quarter			Sex	Interaction				
Bortner quarter	Sex	X1	X2	X3	X4	X5	X6	X7	CHD Positive	n
1	M	0	0	0	1	0	0	0	57	1079
1	F	0	0	0	0	0	0	0	30	945
2	M	1	0	0	1	1	0	0	56	974
2	F	1	0	0	0	0	0	0	20	1101
3	M	0	1	0	1	0	1	0	39	966
3	F	0	1	0	0	0	0	0	10	1076
4	M	0	0	1	1	0	0	1	46	1068
4	F	0	0	1	0	0	0	0	10	948

Bortner quarter/sex group). Table 10.32 is the analysis of deviance table for these data. All effects are significant ($p < 0.05$), including the interaction. Hence model 5 should be adopted:

$$\hat{\text{logit}} = b_0 + b_1\text{X1} + b_2\text{X2} + b_2\text{X3} + b_4\text{X4} + b_5\text{X5} + b_6\text{X6} + b_7\text{X7}$$

and the odds ratios will thus be examined separately for the two sexes. The $\{b_i\}$ produced by SAS PROC GENMOD are presented in Table 10.33.

Consider the fitted logit for Bortner quarter 1, male sex. By Table 10.31, X4 = 1 and all other X variables are zero. Hence, the logit is

$$-3.4177 + 0.5313 \times 1.$$

Continuing in this fashion, we can produce all the logits. A sensible set of odds ratios to summarize the findings would be comparisons of the other three Bortner quarters against the first, separately for each sex. As usual, log odds ratios are the differences between the logit for the numerator and denominator of the odds ratio. For example, the log odds ratio for Bortner 4 versus 1, male sex, is

$$\left\{-3.4177 + (-1.1234 \times 1) + 0.5313 \times 1 + 0.9090 \times 1\right\} - \left\{-3.4177 + 0.5313 \times 1\right\}$$

$$= -1.1234 + 0.9090 = -0.2144.$$

Table 10.32. Analysis of deviance table for Example 10.22.

	Fit details		Test details			
Model	D	d.f.	ΔD	Δd.f.	p value	Effect
1 Constant	86.63	7	—	—	—	
2 Constant + X1 to X3	72.49	4	14.14[a]	3	0.003	Bortner
3 Constant + X4	21.40	6	65.23[a]	1	<0.0001	sex
4 Constant + X1 to X4	8.15	3	64.34[b]	1	<0.0001	sex|Bortner
			13.25[c]	3	0.004	Bortner|sex
5 Constant + X1 to X7	0	0	8.15[d]	3	0.043	interaction|Bortner, sex

[a] Relative to model 1.
[b] Relative to model 2.
[c] Relative to model 3.
[d] Relative to model 4.

Table 10.33. Parameter estimates for model 5 in Table 10.32, as produced by SAS.

Parameter	Estimate	Standard error
INTERCEPT	−3.4177	0.1855
X1	−0.5722	0.2921
X2	−1.2514	0.3679
X3	−1.1234	0.3681
X4	0.5313	0.2301
X5	0.6618	0.3505
X6	0.9694	0.4250
X7	0.9090	0.4204

Table 10.34. Odds ratios (95% confidence intervals) by sex and Bortner quarter for SHHS subjects who were free of CHD at baseline.

Bortner quarter	Sex	
	Male	Female
1	1	1
2	1.09 (0.75, 1.60)	0.56 (0.32, 1.00)
3	0.75 (0.50, 1.12)	0.29 (0.14, 0.59)
4	0.81 (0.54, 1.20)	0.33 (0.16, 0.67)

Notice that the constant and sex terms cancel out. Continuing in this way, we find the complete set of log odds ratios and hence odds ratios. Table 10.34 shows the latter, together with associated confidence intervals.

Confidence intervals for female odds ratios (relative to Bortner quarter 1) are easy to construct because each is calculated from only one b parameter. For instance, from Table 10.33, the log odds ratio for Bortner 4 versus 1, female sex, is −1.1234 with estimated standard error 0.3681, giving a 95% confidence interval for the odds ratio of

$$\exp(-1.1234 \pm 1.96 \times 0.3681).$$

Calculation of confidence intervals for the male odds ratios is more complex because each involves two b parameters. For instance, we have already seen this when finding the estimated odds ratio for Bortner 4 versus 1, where all but two terms cancelled out. In this situation, we need to have the variance–covariance matrix, as in Example 10.6. Alternatively, we could refit model 5 using a new definition of X4 that makes X4 = 1 for females and 0 for males (X5 to X7 will also change as a consequence). Then it is the male standard errors, rather than the female, that can be calculated directly from the standard errors of the b. This method will be described in detail in Example 10.23.

Our conclusion from Table 10.34 is that Bortner score has little effect on the incidence of CHD for men, but increasing score implies decreasing risk (with the highest two quarters virtually the same) for women: a unilateral interaction.

If the computer package used allows interactions to be specified as part of the model directly *and* allows categorical variables to be declared, then much work can be saved because the dummy variables do not need to be constructed. SAS PROC GENMOD was used in this way, defining BORT to be the Bortner quarter, except that the first quarter has BORT = 5 so as to make it the reference group (Example 10.7). Sex was read in as SEX = 1 for men and 2 for women; the CLASS declaration was used for BORT and for SEX; and BORT*SEX was included in the model statement. Output 10.3 shows the parameter estimates produced when model 5 of Table 10.32 was fitted. The nonzero parameter estimates and their standard errors are exactly as in Table 10.33, as they should be.

Output 10.3. SAS PROC GENMOD results for Example 10.22, model 5.

Analysis of parameter estimates								
Parameter			DF	Estimate	Standard error	Wald 95% confidence limits		Chi-square	Pr > ChiSq
Intercept			1	−3.4177	0.1855	−3.7814	−3.0541	339.30	<.0001
bort	2		1	−0.5722	0.2921	−1.1448	0.0004	3.84	0.0502
bort	3		1	−1.2514	0.3679	−1.9725	−0.5302	11.57	0.0007
bort	4		1	−1.1234	0.3681	−1.8449	−0.4020	9.32	0.0023
bort	5		0	0.0000	0.0000	0.0000	0.0000	.	.
sex	1		1	0.5313	0.2301	0.0803	0.9823	5.33	0.0210
sex	2		0	0.0000	0.0000	0.0000	0.0000	.	.
bort*sex	2	1	1	0.6618	0.3505	−0.0251	1.3487	3.57	0.0590
bort*sex	2	2	0	0.0000	0.0000	0.0000	0.0000	.	.
bort*sex	3	1	1	0.9694	0.4250	0.1365	1.8024	5.20	0.0225
bort*sex	3	2	0	0.0000	0.0000	0.0000	0.0000	.	.
bort*sex	4	1	1	0.9090	0.4204	0.0851	1.7330	4.68	0.0306
bort*sex	4	2	0	0.0000	0.0000	0.0000	0.0000	.	.
bort*sex	5	1	0	0.0000	0.0000	0.0000	0.0000	.	.
bort*sex	5	2	0	0.0000	0.0000	0.0000	0.0000	.	.

10.9.2 *Between a quantitative and a categorical variable*

When one variable is quantitative and the other is categorical (with ℓ levels), the interaction is represented by the set of variables defined by the product of the quantitative variable and each of the dummy variables for the categorical variable. We shall need to define $\ell - 1$ interaction dummy variables because the interaction has $\ell - 1$ d.f.

Example 10.23 The problem of Example 10.22 could have been addressed by retaining Bortner score in its original quantitative form. Using the generic form of the data, the set of models from before was refitted with quantitative Bortner score using SAS PROC GENMOD. Sex was declared as a CLASS (categorical) variable with values 1 for men and 2 for women. Results are shown in Table 10.35. The data may be downloaded; see Appendix A.

As in the previous example, all effects are significant (note that the unadjusted effect of sex is just as in Table 10.32, apart from rounding error). Hence, the interaction needs to be accounted for; model 5 is the 'best'. SAS results for model 5 are given as Output 10.4. The fitted model is

$$\hat{\text{logit}} = b_0 + b_1^{(1)}\text{SEX}^{(1)} + b_1^{(2)}\text{SEX}^{(2)} + b_2 x + b_3^{(1)}\text{SEX}^{(1)} x + b_3^{(2)}\text{SEX}^{(2)} x, \tag{10.20}$$

where x = Bortner score and

$$\text{SEX}^{(1)} = \begin{cases} 1 \text{ for men} \\ 0 \text{ for women} \end{cases} \qquad \text{SEX}^{(2)} = \begin{cases} 1 \text{ for women} \\ 0 \text{ for men.} \end{cases}$$

In the special parameterisation used by SAS, the last levels of everything arising from a CLASS statement, including terms that contribute to interactions, are set to zero. Hence, SEX 2 (the code for women) and BORTNER*SEX 2 are set to zero in Output 10.4. The general logit for men is, from (10.20),

$$\hat{\text{logit}}_{\text{M}} = b_0 + b_1^{(1)} + b_2 x + b_3^{(1)} x$$

$$= \left(b_0 + b_1^{(1)}\right) + \left(b_2 + b_3^{(1)}\right) x$$

Table 10.35. Analysis of deviance table for Example 10.23.

Model	Fit details				Test details	
	D	d.f.	ΔD	Δd.f.	p value	Effect
1 Constant	2357.88	8156	—	—	—	
2 Constant + Bortner	2347.61	8155	10.27^a	1	0.001	Bortner
3 Constant + sex	2292.66	8155	65.22^a	1	<0.0001	sex
4 Constant + sex + Bortner	2283.07	8154	64.54^b	1	<0.0001	sex|Bortner
			9.59^c	1	0.002	Bortner|sex
5 Constant + sex + Bortner + Bortner*sex	2274.58	8153	8.49^d	1	0.004	interaction|Bortner, sex

[a] Relative to model 1.
[b] Relative to model 2.
[c] Relative to model 3.
[d] Relative to model 4.

Output 10.4. SAS PROC GENMOD results for Example 10.23, model 5.

Analysis of parameter estimates								
Parameter		DF	Estimate	Standard error	Wald 95% confidence limits		Chi-square	Pr > ChiSq
Intercept		1	−1.9644	0.4982	−2.9409	−0.9879	15.55	<.0001
sex	1	1	−0.6266	0.5821	−1.7675	0.5144	1.16	0.2818
sex	2	0	0.0000	0.0000	0.0000	0.0000	.	.
bortner		1	−0.0129	0.0032	−0.0192	−0.0067	16.57	<.0001
bortner*sex	1	1	0.0106	0.0036	0.0035	0.0178	8.54	0.0035
bortner*sex	2	0	0.0000	0.0000	0.0000	0.0000	.	.

and the general logit for women is:

$$\hat{\text{logit}}_F = \left(b_0 + b_1^{(2)}\right) + \left(b_2 + b_3^{(2)}\right)x.$$

In this example, these become:

$$\hat{\text{logit}}_M = (-1.9644 - 0.6266) + (-0.0129 + 0.0106)x$$

$$= -2.5910 - 0.0023x$$

$$\hat{\text{logit}}_F = (-1.9644 + 0) + (-0.0129 + 0)x$$

$$= -1.9644 - 0.0129x.$$

We have two straight lines of different intercept and slope. The odds ratios for a unit increase in x are then

$$\hat{\psi}_M = \exp(-0.0023) = 0.998$$

for men and

$$\hat{\psi}_F = \exp(-0.0129) = 0.987$$

for women, because the constant term will cancel out when the appropriate logits are subtracted.

Just as in Example 10.22, the confidence interval is easy to obtain for any odds ratio that uses one only of the b parameters in its estimation. Here, female odds ratios only use b_2 (all other terms are fixed to be zero or cancel out). Thus, from Output 10.4, the 95% confidence interval for a unit increase in Bortner score for women is obtained from the 'Estimate' and 'Standard error' columns as

$$\exp(-0.0129 \pm 1.96 \times 0.0032)$$

or from the 'Wald 95% Confidence Limits' columns as $(\exp(-0.0192), \exp(-0.0067))$, both of which give $(0.981, 0.993)$.

Since any odds ratio for men uses b_2 and $b_3^{(1)}$, we either need the variance–covariance matrix or to refit the model but this time forcing the male sex to be the last, in numerical order, entered to SAS. We will use the latter method. Similar 'tricks' will work with other packages.

If we define a new variable,

$$\text{SEX2} = 3 - \text{SEX},$$

Output 10.5. Further SAS PROC GENMOD results for Example 10.23, model 5, using a different variable to represent sex compared with that in Output 10.4.

Analysis of parameter estimates							
Parameter		DF	Estimate	Standard error	Wald 95% confidence limits		Chi-square	Pr > ChiSq
Intercept		1	−2.5910	0.3011	−3.1810	−2.0009	74.06	<.0001
sex2	1	1	0.6266	0.5821	−0.5144	1.7675	1.16	0.2818
sex2	2	0	0.0000	0.0000	0.0000	0.0000	.	.
bortner		1	−0.0023	0.0018	−0.0058	0.0011	1.72	0.1903
bortner*sex2	1	1	−0.0106	0.0036	−0.0178	−0.0035	8.54	0.0035
bortner*sex2	2	0	0.0000	0.0000	0.0000	0.0000	.	.
Scale		0	1.0000	0.0000	1.0000	1.0000		

then

$$SEX2 = 3 - 1 = 2 \text{ when } SEX = 1 \text{ (men)}$$

$$SEX2 = 3 - 2 = 1 \text{ when } SEX = 2 \text{ (women)}$$

so that SEX2 takes its highest level for men. SAS will, consequently, fix the parameter estimates for men to be zero.

Results from SAS are given as Output 10.5. Notice how the parameters involving sex in Output 10.4 and Output 10.5 have a different sign, but the same magnitude. Other parameter estimates are completely different, although the fitted model will turn out to be exactly the same as before. Straightaway we see that

$$\hat{\psi}_M = \exp(-0.0023) = 0.998$$

(just as before), with 95% confidence interval,

$$\exp(-0.0023 \pm 1.96 \times 0.0018)$$

or $(\exp(-0.0058), \exp(0.0011))$, both of which give $(0.994, 1.001)$. Both the male and the female odds ratios indicate a drop of odds with increasing Bortner score, but the rate of decrease is greater for women. The trend is significant ($p < 0.05$) only for women (from checking whether the 95% confidence interval contains unity). This agrees with the findings in Example 10.22.

10.9.3 Between two quantitative variables

Interactions between two quantitative variables are easy to fit: the $A*B$ interaction is literally the product of A and B, on a case-by-case basis. Using a computer package, if variable A is in one column and B in another, we simply ask the package to multiply the two columns to form the interaction variable's column. However, such interactions may be difficult to interpret: a significant result means that there is a linear effect of $A \times B$ after allowing for linear effects of both A and B. Generally, it is more helpful to categorise either variable, or both the variables, and proceed as in Section 10.9.1 or 10.9.2.

10.10 Dealing with a quantitative explanatory variable

We have already seen how we can fit quantitative 'x' variables in logistic regression models, including how to do tests for non-linearity, but further consideration of descriptive approaches to this common issue in epidemiology, including the use of splines, will be useful.

10.10.1 Linear form

In medical research, most often two approaches to modelling quantitative variables are used: either treat the variable in its basic quantitative (often continuous) form, or divide it into a small number of mutually exclusive and exhaustive groups and analyse as if the original variable was categorical. For instance, systolic blood pressure (SBP) was taken as a quantitative variable in Example 10.12, but as a categorical variable in Example 10.11. Often both approaches are used in a single research publication.

We have already seen how to fit a variable in linear form (Examples 10.3 and 10.5). Fitting a logistic regression model for the log odds of CHD on SBP taken as a continuous variable (i.e., just as it comes from the database) in Example 10.12 gives the model:

$$\hat{\text{logit}} = -6.236367 + 0.0237823\,(\text{SYSTOL}),$$

where SYSTOL is the quantitative variable which holds SBP. In a similar way to Example 10.5, this means that for every one extra unit (mmHg) of SBP, the odds of CHD increases by a factor of 1.024 or 2.4% (because $1.024 = \exp(0.0237823)$). If we prefer, we could (say) state our conclusion in terms of units of 5 mmHg, in which case we find $\exp(5 \times 0.0237823) = 1.126$, and conclude that the odds increases by 12.6% for every extra 5 mmHg. The 95% confidence limits of the odds ratio for a 5 mmHg increase are computed as $\exp(5 \times \text{estimate} \pm 1.96 \times 5 \times \text{SE})$, where 'estimate' and 'SE' are the estimate and standard error for the logit, as produced by computer packages. Notice that multiplication by 5 needs to be done before taking exponents, as was done similarly for the difference of 10 years of age in Example 10.5. The effect that has been estimated is called the **linear effect** of SBP. However, since the effect of SBP on the odds of CHD has been modelled on the logarithmic scale, the effect is linear for the logit (i.e., log odds), and so it is log-linear for the odds. When we utilise a linear effect, we implicitly assume that the effect is homogeneous across the range of the 'x' variable (as explained in Example 10.12).

As in the above example, we often prefer to state the linear effect for an s unit difference (see also Example 10.9), rather than a single-unit difference. This might be to avoid small numbers in the log odds ratios (equivalent to odds ratios with many zeros following unity) or because we wish to compare several odds ratios, for a diverse set of risk factors, on a standardised scale. To do the latter, a common convention is to take s to be the standard deviation (SD) of the risk factor in the observed dataset. Then all odds ratios will be for a one SD increase.

10.10.2 Categorical form

If the quantitative variable is to be analysed in categories, the first decision to be made is how to define these categories. To avoid bias, these should be chosen *a priori*. Three main ways of choosing the groupings to be used are: to divide the observed range of the variable into equal intervals; to use existing clinical guidelines; and to divide into equal-sized groups. The latter is best in a statistical sense, since it spreads the data across the groups evenly and thus gives tighter confidence intervals and better power for comparisons between groups. We can divide into equal-sized groups either according to the sample size or to the number of events. The former method is most popular, and makes most sense when there are several outcomes to be analysed. The latter method is usually better, in terms of achieving tighter confidence intervals.

A final decision, when the categories are to be defined by the data, is how many groups to use? Three groups is the minimum required to be able to show a trend, but if the sample size and number of events are large enough, more information on the true shape of the association can be gleaned from using more groups. In most cases, three, four or five groups are used, making the categories the thirds, fourths (or quarters) and fifths, respectively. As emphasised elsewhere in this book, it is technically incorrect to call these the tertiles, quartiles and quintiles, respectively, since these are the end-points of their respective groups. Nevertheless, this unfortunate mix of terminology is rife in medical journals. The scope for confusion in such usage is obvious when we consider that, for example, there are three thirds but only two tertiles. In rare cases there are enough data to use up to ten equal-sized groups, the tenths. Random error comes into play more strongly as the number of groups goes up, and thus chance perturbations in general patterns become more likely. Consequently, we have to play off the advantage of greater capacity to determine underlying patterns against the disadvantage of greater chance of false leads when more groups are employed.

Example 10.24 Table 10.36 shows estimates from the logistic regression on SBP, when grouped into quarters. The variable SBP4 takes the values 1, 2, 3 and 4 according to whether the corresponding SBP value lies within the first, second, third or fourth quarter. In fact, because of clustering of SBP values in these data, the quarters are not exactly equal; for example, there are 85 values of 121 mmHg, which is the first quartile (the other two quartiles are 131 and 143). This technicality is unimportant. As in earlier examples, the confidence interval for the logit is found as the estimate $\pm 1.96 \times$ SE and the estimates and confidence interval for the odds ratio are found by raising the corresponding logit results to the exponential power. There is no odds ratio computed for the first value of SBP, as this is the base group. Such results, for the odds ratio, are typically presented in graphical form with equal spaces between the four results (including the base value of 1, with no confidence limits). However, this ignores the fact that the SBP values are, in general, not equally distributed within the quarters; typically the middle two quarters span a relatively small interval compared to the highest quarter because the latter is unbounded. Hence a more informative, but not such an attractive, display of the results would be produced by plotting the odds ratios against the medians of the quarters.

The same analysis was done with the quarters defined by the events; that is, the quarters were defined using the quartiles of SBP amongst only those with a CHD event during follow-up. These quartiles are 128, 138 and 151 mmHg; as would be expected for a risk factor which has a positive association with the outcome variable, these are all greater than the corresponding quartiles for the entire data. Also as expected, the percentage of people in each 'event quarter' decreases with increasing quarter (from 41% in the first quarter to 16% in the fourth), but each group experienced (at least, approximately) the same number of events (about 50). Table 10.37 shows the results from fitting a logistic model with this definition of groups. The pattern of the odds ratios is much the same as in Table 10.36, although the odds ratio comparing the fourth

Table 10.36. Logistic regression of CHD on systolic blood pressure by quarters of subjects.

	CHD	n	logit			Odds ratio (95% CI)
			Estimate	SE	95% CI	
Intercept			−3.74526	0.202349	(−4.142, −3.349)	
1st quarter	25	1083	0			1
2nd quarter	39	960	0.58336	0.260138	(0.074, 1.093)	1.79 (1.08, 2.98)
3rd quarter	56	995	0.92580	0.244678	(0.446, 1.405)	2.52 (1.56, 4.08)
4th quarter	76	1011	1.23545	0.234889	(0.775, 1.696)	3.44 (2.17, 5.45)

CI = confidence interval; SE = standard error.

Table 10.37. Logistic regression of CHD on systolic blood pressure by quarters of events.

| | CHD | n | logit | | | Odds ratio (95% CI) |
			Estimate	SE	95% CI	
Intercept			−3.51713	0.146464	(−3.804, −3.230)	
1st quarter	48	1665	0			1
2nd quarter	47	946	0.56599	0.209382	(0.156, 0.976)	1.76 (1.17, 2.65)
3rd quarter	50	805	0.80243	0.206824	(0.397, 1.208)	2.23 (1.49, 3.35)
4th quarter	51	633	1.08248	0.206828	(0.677, 1.488)	2.95 (1.97, 4.43)

CI = confidence interval; SE = standard error.

and first quarter has come out less extreme. The confidence intervals are of a more consistent size and are all narrower in Table 10.37 than in Table 10.36; the easiest way to see this is to compare the standard errors for the logit. Hence this method of dividing SBP is statistically superior because the inferences are more precise. Whether this is more relevant to practice is another matter.

10.10.3 Linear spline form

Although categorical models produce results that have a simple interpretation, and are familiar to regular readers of medical journals, they are relatively crude. As already indicated, many authors combine a categorical description of the association between the quantitative variable of interest and the disease outcome with results from fitting a linear model, as illustrated earlier in this section, or sometimes a trend model across the categories (see Section 10.7.5). This is fine if the association really is linear (on the log scale), but the categorical analysis is not the best way of assessing this. As explained in Section 9.10, a linear spline model is a good tool for exploring associations with quantitative variables.

Example 10.25 Using Stata, a linear spline model with knots at the three quartiles for SBP was fitted to the same dataset used repeatedly in this section. The results appear in Table 10.38. Each slope (the log odds for a 1 mmHg higher SBP) in the spline is positive; although only one is

Table 10.38. Logistic regression of CHD on a systolic blood pressure linear spline with knots at the three quartiles.

| | Slope | | | Differences between slopes | | |
	Estimate	SE	p value	Estimate	SE	p value
Intercept	−10.26870	3.892244	0.008			
SBP ≤ 121	0.05686	0.033307	0.09			
121 < SBP ≤ 131	0.04757	0.032482	0.14	−0.00929	0.057449	0.87
131 < SBP ≤ 143	0.00821	0.021839	0.71	−0.03935	0.049035	0.42
SBP > 143	0.02031	0.007044	0.004	0.01210	0.026099	0.64

SBP = systolic blood pressure (mmHg); SE = standard error.

significantly different from zero, note that the power for detecting significance at the 5% level within any component of the spline is limited. There is no significant difference between one slope and the next (the smallest of all the p values is 0.42), so there is no reason to doubt that the association is linear; any differences are attributable to chance.

At this point, it is instructive to consider the predicted (fitted) values from the three models for SBP taken together: see Figure 10.10, panels (a), (b) and (d). For added insight, the 95% confidence intervals for these predictions were also computed (easily obtainable from computer packages, such as Stata, which was used here) and plotted. Panels (b) and (d) give the most interesting comparison, and hence these have been placed one under the other: the breaks in each thus correspond vertically. Whilst predictions from the categorical model go up in steps, the spline model has graduated increases; effectively, the categorical model averages the spline model between each pair of consecutive knots. Looking at the confidence limits, the accuracy of prediction from the categorical model is equal at, for example, 150 and 230 mmHg; in the spline model the former is far more precisely estimated than the latter. Given that 150 is well within the range of the data, but the data are sparse beyond 200 mmHg (the 99.75th percentile), intuitively we would expect some difference in precision. However, the very nature of the categorical model is to assume equal status of each value within any specific category. The linear fit shows the 'bow-tie' shape typical of fitted values (similar to Figure 9.4), and the spline model shows a juxtaposition of several bow-ties.

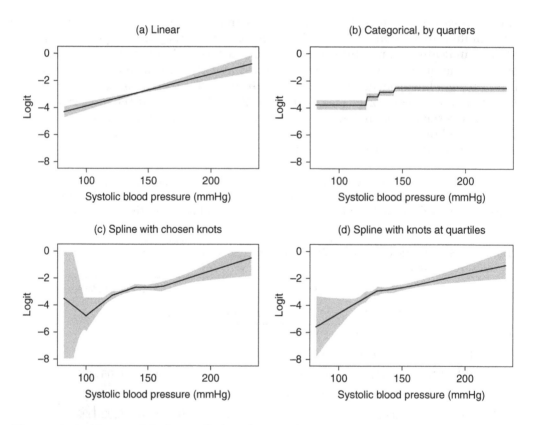

Figure 10.10. Four models for predicting the log odds (logit) of coronary heart disease from the level of systolic blood pressure. Shaded regions are 95% confidence intervals for the predicted log odds (panel (c) has a truncated vertical scale).

In this example, most likely we would choose to adopt the linear model as the "best" due to its simplicity. However, a word of warning is necessary: the spline model depends upon its knots. To show this, Figure 10.10(c) was drawn from a spline model with knots placed at 100, 120, 140 and 160 mmHg. Here clinical guidelines (current in the US at the time of writing) were used to fix the last three knots, whilst 100 was chosen to fit the sequence. Also, 100 is a round, low value, but not low enough for there to be too few at or below it to allow reasonable estimation (here there are 53 observations). With these splines there is a clear "kick up" in log odds (and thus in the risk of CHD) as SBP decreases below 100 mmHg. This is consistent with several published articles that have suggested a 'J-shaped' association between blood pressure and cardiovascular risk. However, there are not really enough data at low levels of SBP to draw a conclusion of a J-shape here (for instance, the p value comparing the slope below and just above 100 is 0.54 in these data). This illustrates a drawback with splines: even when the overall pattern is linear in one direction, there may be piecewise-linear sections of the spline which go in the opposite direction, purely by chance. The visual impact of this (without more intensive investigation) is far more likely to lead to rejection of a simple, consistent overall association than when ordered categorical groupings are used. As far as our data are concerned, we can still conclude an overall log-linear association between SBP and the odds of CHD because of the p value of 0.54 quoted above. Even if the p value had been significant, less than 2% of men had SBP values as low as 100 mmHg and so the consequence of not accounting for the proposed non-linearity in practice is likely to be small.

In many examples in this chapter, quantitative variables are fitted just as they come, which, as we have seen, means that a linear association has been assumed. This is often quite a reasonable assumption, as in the last example, or it may be acceptable as a working model. Sometimes it is patently not a reasonable assumption, even in approximate terms.

Example 10.26 Consider data from the PROGRESS randomised controlled trial of blood pressure reduction (McMahon *et al.*, 2001), which is available on the web site for this book. These data come from 3005 patients who have previously suffered a stroke or transient ischaemic attack. We shall only look at the subjects from this trial who received the placebo treatment. Over a follow-period of 4.1 years, 413 of the patients had a (recurrent) stroke. In this case we are interested in seeing how the estimated glomerular filtration rate (eGFR) is associated with the odds of stroke during the trial.

Output 10.6 is an extract from Stata output when fitting linear and spline (with knots at the two tertiles) to these data. The spline model was fitted twice: parameterised by the components of the spline, and parameterised by the difference in slopes (see Section 9.10) subsequent to the first slope. Figure 10.11 shows the two fitted models together. The naïve straight-line model, with a slope for the logit of −0.015, is suggesting that the odds of stroke decrease by 1.5% (i.e., $100 \times (1 - \exp(-0.015))$) for every extra unit (ml/min/1.73 m^2) of eGFR. However, this clearly misses the kink in the association in the lower range of eGFR. The results from the spline model suggest that the logit increases at a non-significant rate of 0.004 per unit until eGFR reaches 66 ml/min/1.73 m^2 (the first knot), after which it declines at a significant rate of 0.033 per unit, making a slight (non-significant) change at 82 ml/min/1.73 m^2 (the second knot). Of course, these 'change points' — one that appears to be active and one that is inactive — are simply the ones we have chosen to explore. We cannot pinpoint the one important change in response to have occurred at 66 ml/min/1.73 m^2, but we can certainly conclude that there is evidence of a non-linear association and that the linear model is not suitable for these data. The linear model overestimates the relative odds of stroke, comparing a higher to a lower eGFR, in the majority of its observed range.

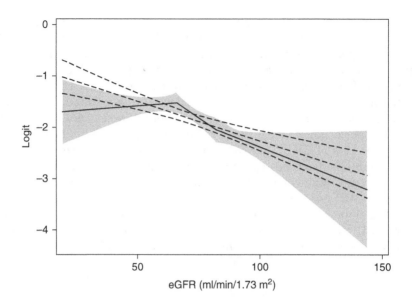

Figure 10.11. Linear model with 95% confidence interval (dashed lines), and linear spline model with two knots at the thirds (solid line) together with a shaded 95% confidence interval, for Example 10.26.

Output 10.6. Stata results for Example 10.26. The explanatory variable is EGFR, which is expressed as a linear spline (on the log scale) with two knots (SP1, SP2 and SP3 being the three components of the spline) and STROKE is the outcome variable.

(i) Linear model

stroke	Coef.	OIM Std. Err.	z	P>|z|	[95% Conf. Interval]	
egfr	-.0153916	.0030171	-5.10	0.000	-.0213049	-.0094782
_cons	-.7194951	.2202935	-3.27	0.001	-1.151262	-.2877278

(ii) Spline model; (a) parameterised directly

stroke	Coef.	OIM Std. Err.	z	P>|z|	[95% Conf. Interval]	
sp1	.0037335	.0082569	0.45	0.651	-.0124498	.0199168
sp2	-.0328144	.0113979	-2.88	0.004	-.0551539	-.0104748
sp3	-.0187772	.0107677	-1.74	0.081	-.0398816	.0023271
_cons	-1.765907	.4782059	-3.69	0.000	-2.703174	-.828641

(iii) Spline model; (b) parameterized as differences in slopes

stroke	Coef.	OIM Std. Err.	z	P>|z|	[95% Conf. Interval]	
sp1	.0037335	.0082569	0.45	0.651	-.0124498	.0199168
sp2	-.0365479	.0172084	-2.12	0.034	-.0702757	-.0028202
sp3	.0140371	.0196438	0.71	0.475	-.0244641	.0525383
_cons	-1.765907	.4782059	-3.69	0.000	-2.703174	-.828641

10.10.4 *Generalisations*

The issues raised about modelling quantitative explanatory variables here are much the same in any regression application, whilst the splines are defined without regard to the outcome variable, and are thus independent of the modelling process. Hence there is not a great difference between the way splines are used here and in Section 9.10. For instance, if confounding variables are to be taken account of, an adjusted spline model can be fitted by simply adding the confounding variables to the list of parameters in the model and then the spline can be plotted for people at average levels of all the confounders (or for some other suitable standard) as in Figure 9.18. Similarly, cubic and other types of splines can be used in logistic regression modelling just as in regression models for quantitative outcomes. Looking ahead, splines can also be used in exactly the same way for the survival models that are the subject of Chapter 11.

10.11 Model checking

10.11.1 *Residuals*

In Section 10.7.1 and Section 10.7.2, we saw how to test for goodness of fit. As noted there, such tests are insufficient to determine whether the model is appropriate. Just as in general linear models (Section 9.8), we need also to examine model residuals. In this section we shall illustrate only residual analysis for grouped data. When the data are generic, the residuals will, by definition, be of a special binary form, requiring a more complex interpretation (Collett, 2002).

There are several different types of residual that have been suggested for use with logistic regression models. The simplest is the **raw residual**. Using the definition of e_i in Section 10.1, the ith raw residual, resid_i, is

$$\text{resid}_i = \text{observed}_i - \text{expected}_i = e_i - \hat{e}_i \tag{10.21}$$

as in general linear models. In logistic regression,

$$\hat{e}_i = n_i \hat{r}_i, \tag{10.22}$$

where $\hat{r}_i$ is the predicted risk from the model.

Unfortunately, the raw residual is difficult to interpret because its size depends on the variability of both e_i and $\hat{e}_i$. Various ways of standardising the raw residual have been suggested; see Collett (2002) for an extensive description. One of these leads to the **deviance residual**, which is derived from components of the deviance. The ith deviance residual is

$$\text{devres}_i = \left\{\text{sign}\left[\text{resid}_i\right]\right\}\left\{\sqrt{2e_i \log_e\left(\frac{e_i}{\hat{e}_i}\right) + 2(n_i - e_i)\log_e\left(\frac{n_i - e_i}{n_i - \hat{e}_i}\right)}\right\}, \tag{10.23}$$

where the first term on the right-hand side denotes that we take the sign of the deviance residual to be the sign of the ith residual. Then

$$\text{model deviance} = \sum(\text{devres}_i)^2.$$

Much more useful is the **standardised deviance residual** defined by

$$\text{stdevres}_i = d_i \Big/ \sqrt{\left(1 - h_i\right)}, \tag{10.24}$$

where

$$h_i = n_i \hat{r}_i \left(1 - \hat{r}_i\right) \text{V}\left(\widehat{\text{logit}}_i\right). \tag{10.25}$$

Here we introduce h_i, called the **leverage**. The standardised deviance residuals have variance unity and so are easy to interpret for size. Furthermore, provided the n_i are not small, these residuals will, approximately, have a standard normal distribution when the model is correct. Thus, we might investigate stdevres values larger than 1.96 or less than -1.96, the upper and lower 2½% percentage points from the standard normal distribution. Some computer packages will produce residuals automatically; with others they will need to be derived from any of (10.21) to (10.25).

Whichever residuals are chosen, we expect to find values close to zero and without any systematic pattern for the model to be acceptable. As in general linear models, we can check for systematic patterns by plotting the residuals. In logistic modelling, residuals are often plotted against the observation number (giving an **index plot**), the linear predictor and/or each explanatory variable. The latter two will be equivalent if there is only one explanatory variable. The plots will identify any observations with large residuals (outliers). The great advantage of standardised deviance residuals (as with standardised residuals in general linear models) is that we have limits to guide our subjective concept of size.

Example 10.27 We shall carry out model checking of Example 10.5.

First we evaluate, as a specific example, residuals for the first observation (men aged 40). Here $i = 1$ and, by observation (Table 10.4), $e_1 = 1$ and $n_1 = 251$. By (10.2) and using the estimates from Table 10.7, the predicted risk of death,

$$\hat{r}_1 = \left\{1 + \exp(8.4056 - (0.1126)(40)\right\}^{-1} = 0.019809.$$

By (10.22) and Table 10.4, the predicted number of deaths, $\hat{e}_1 = 251 \times 0.019809 = 4.972$. Then, by (10.21) and Table 10.4, the raw residual, $\text{resid}_1 = 1 - 4.972 = -3.972$. Then, by (10.23), the deviance residual,

$$\text{devres}_1 = -\sqrt{2 \times 1 \times \log_e\left(\frac{1}{4.972}\right) + (2)(251 - 1)\log_e\left(\frac{251 - 1}{251 - 4.972}\right)}$$

$$= -2.191.$$

To obtain the leverage, h_1, we need the variance of $\widehat{\text{logit}}_1$. We can get this from the estimated variance–covariance matrix of model parameters as

$$\text{V}(b_0 + b_1 x) = \text{V}(b_0) + x^2 \text{V}(b_1) + 2x \text{C}(b_0, b_1),$$

where $x = 40$. For brevity, we simply quote the answer here to be 0.020207. Then, by (10.25), $h_1 = 251 \times 0.019809(1 - 0.019809)0.020207 = 0.098480$. Finally, by (10.24), the first standardised deviance residual,

$$\text{stdevres}_1 = -2.191 \Big/ \left(\sqrt{1 - 0.098480} \right) = -2.31.$$

Table 10.39 shows the full set of residuals of the three types mentioned, plus observed and expected deaths. This analysis has been done using a computer retaining a considerable number of decimal places. Consequently the results for age 40 are slightly more accurate than those just derived.

The three residuals always have the same sign, but the rank ordering for raw residuals is quite different from the other two. Consideration of Figure 10.4(a) would lead us to expect the first residual to be the largest. Whilst it is for the other two, it is nowhere near the largest (in absolute terms) amongst the raw residuals. This illustrates the problem with raw residuals. The first standardised deviance residual is less than -1.96, indicating a real problem with the model. The result for age 40 is an outlier.

As a consequence, men of age 40 were deleted and the model refitted. To predict deaths for men aged 41 to 59 the fitted model turned out to be

$$\hat{\text{logit}} = -8.0827 + 0.1067x,$$

where x = age. Compare this with (10.9).

Table 10.39. Residuals and death statistics for the model fitted in Example 10.5.

| Age | Number of deaths | | Residuals | | |
	Observed	Expected	Raw	Deviance	Standardised deviance
40	1	4.96	−3.96	−2.19	−2.30
41	12	7.00	5.00	1.74	1.85
42	13	7.62	5.38	1.80	1.91
43	6	7.84	−1.84	−0.69	−0.73
44	10	7.24	2.76	0.99	1.03
45	8	8.69	−0.69	−0.24	−0.25
46	10	10.56	−0.56	−0.18	−0.18
47	12	11.81	0.19	0.06	0.06
48	10	13.48	−3.48	−1.02	−1.05
49	14	14.53	−0.53	−0.14	−0.15
50	15	16.04	−1.04	−0.27	−0.28
51	14	19.26	−5.26	−1.30	−1.34
52	19	22.04	−3.04	−0.69	−0.71
53	36	27.34	8.66	1.65	1.72
54	26	27.10	−1.10	−0.22	−0.23
55	21	27.16	−6.16	−1.29	−1.35
56	28	35.38	−7.38	−1.36	−1.46
57	41	36.32	4.68	0.81	0.89
58	38	34.50	3.50	0.63	0.70
59	49	44.15	4.85	0.78	0.91

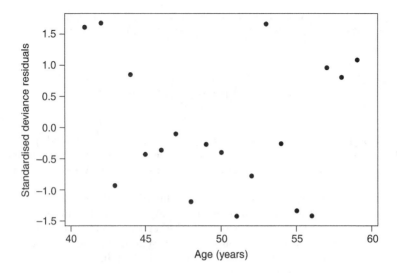

Figure 10.12. Standardised deviance residuals against age for a logistic regression model fitted to the data of Table 10.4, after first omitting age 40 years.

Figure 10.12 shows the standardised deviance residuals plotted against age for this revised model. There are no unusually extreme residuals, nor any obvious patterns. The logistic regression model seems to produce adequate predictions of chances of death for men aged 41 to 59 years.

Example 10.28 In Example 10.18, we saw the inadequacy of the linear model for predicting *H. pylori* prevalence by social class. Figure 10.13(a) shows the plot of standardised deviance residuals against social class for this model. The upside-down U pattern is obvious, suggesting that the systematic effect of social class has not yet been captured fully. Figure 10.13(b) shows the same plot for the quadratic model; this model is acceptable because there is no pattern (and no unacceptably large residuals).

10.11.2 *Influential observations*

As in general linear models, outliers are not the only kind of problematic observations. Additional diagnostic tests are required to identify those observations with a substantial impact on the fit of the logistic model. Refer to Collett (2002) for details and examples.

10.12 Measurement error

Although the classical regression methods of theoretical epidemiology assume that the explanatory and outcome variables are perfectly recorded, in practice measurement error is common. Sometimes this error can be systematic, for instance where a weighing scale has been poorly calibrated so that it gives values that are too low. By and large, this type of error, once detected, is easy to correct, without subsequent loss of fidelity of the analyses, and should be avoidable. Random measurement error — that is, unpredictable variation, lower or higher than the true value — is more troublesome, typically being more difficult or costly to detect and correct. If the random

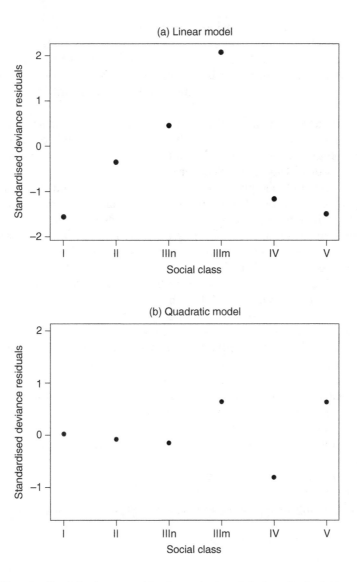

Figure 10.13. Standardised deviance residuals against social class for logistic regression models with (a) only a linear term; and (b) linear and quadratic terms, using the data of Table 10.3.

error is in the outcome variable we can expect greater variability in the association between the explanatory and outcome variables than there would be with no error. The result will be loss of power and a greater chance of not detecting a true association by failing to find a result significant. If the random error is in the explanatory variable the result will be a bias towards a null estimate of association (so-called **regression dilution bias**); that is, we are likely to conclude that the association is weaker than it truly is. An example of this, which can be addressed quantitatively, follows.

10.12.1 Regression to the mean

In many cohort and intervention studies, some of the continuous measurements taken at baseline are taken again from at least a subset of the original study population some time into the follow-up period. When this happens, we would expect to find that, on average, the second (repeat) readings are closer to the overall mean than were the first (baseline) readings. This is a manifestation of the phenomenon known as **regression to the mean**, an issue common to several types of medical study; several examples are given by Bland and Altman (1994) and Morton and Torgerson (2003).

In this setting, regression to the mean works through reducing the range of the distribution of the risk factor as time goes by. Taking the example of blood pressure, those with extremely high values at baseline will tend to be found, on remeasurement, to have lower values, closer to the mean blood pressure. This occurs because some people will usually have moderate blood pressure but, due to natural variation within subjects, just happened to have a high blood pressure at the time of observation. On the other hand, it is unlikely (although not impossible) that these people with extremely high blood pressure values at baseline really have even higher usual blood pressures than were recorded, simply because they are already towards the top of the distribution. The same is true, but in the opposite direction, for those towards the bottom of the distribution; they can be expected to return somewhat higher values at the second survey. In general, the result is that analyses of the relationship between disease and the baseline values of the risk factor (the basic measure of any cohort study) underestimate the relationship between disease and the usual values of this risk factor.

This is easy to see from a contrived example. Suppose everyone in a population is recorded, at baseline, as having systolic blood pressure values of 110, 120 or 130 mmHg, and that an equal number of people has each of these three values. Suppose that the log odds of disease is perfectly linearly related to these recorded blood pressures, as in Figure 10.14. Now suppose that, on remeasurement, those with 110 mmHg recorded at baseline now take their usual values of 115 and those with 130 now take their usual values of 125, due to regression to the mean; those with 120, already in the middle of the distribution, stay as they were.

The result is illustrated by Figure 10.14. The line that relates disease to usual blood pressure has a steeper slope than that relating disease to baseline blood pressure. Hence, by using baseline blood pressure, we underestimate the strength of the association, compared with the association we would find between disease and usual blood pressure; i.e., we have regression dilution error.

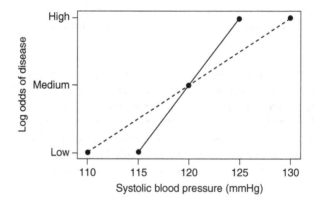

Figure 10.14. Relationship between disease and both baseline (solid line) and usual (dashed line) systolic blood pressure in a hypothetical cohort study.

Table 10.40. Mean systolic blood pressure at
baseline and 3 years later in the Fletcher
Challenge reliability study, by tenth of the
baseline values.

Tenth at baseline	Systolic blood pressure (mmHg)		
	Baseline	Repeat	Difference
1	101.4	109.6	−8.2
2	108.2	116.0	−7.8
3	111.2	116.1	−4.9
4	116.3	118.8	−2.5
5	119.0	122.1	−3.1
6	121.1	123.3	−2.2
7	126.3	127.6	−1.3
8	130.5	130.0	0.5
9	136.1	134.9	1.2
10	148.4	142.6	5.8

Example 10.29 The Fletcher Challenge Study (MacMahon *et al.*, 1995) is a cohort study of similar size (over 10 000 people), and with similar aims, to the SHHS cohort used as a source of examples throughout this book. One major difference is that the Fletcher Challenge investigators incorporated a repeat survey of a random sample of around 2000 subjects into the design of their study, specifically so as to be able to correct for regression dilution bias. This repeat survey on a subsample, sometimes called a **reliability study**, was carried out 3 years after baseline.

Table 10.40 shows first (baseline) and second (repeat) systolic blood pressure means by tenth of the distribution at baseline for the 1503 people from whom blood pressure measurements were obtained in both surveys. This shows a classic instance of regression to the mean; second values tend to be higher than first for those who started very low, and smaller than first for those who started very high. Furthermore, the magnitude of the difference gets progressively smaller as we move up the tenth, apart from the anomaly in the fifth tenth (explained by sampling variation — because of clustering of blood pressure values, only 42 people were assigned to this tenth). As the distribution of differences is clearly skewed towards the lower tenths, at least one other factor, besides regression to the mean, is likely to have contributed to the change in the blood pressure distribution. Systolic blood pressure is known to rise with age, so the most obvious factor would be ageing.

10.12.2 Correcting for regression dilution

One way of correcting for regression dilution bias is to use a reliability study to calculate an **attenuation coefficient**, which estimates the degree of attenuation caused by the bias (Frost and Thompson, 2000). We then proceed by carrying out a standard analysis (such as through regression), relating disease to baseline values of the risk factor for all subjects. The overall measure of association (e.g., the slope of the line relating the logit to the continuous risk factor) is then multiplied by this attenuation coefficient to produce an estimate of the association between disease and usual values of the risk factor. Normally, this attenuation factor will be greater than one, due to regression to the mean. However, for a factor such as height amongst middle-aged people, which has little temporal variation and often has little measurement error, it would be expected to be approximately one (that is, there is no regression dilution bias). The attenuation coefficient could also be below one, but this would be unusual.

Since the reliability study is analysed independently of the data in the main study (that used to estimate the logit), it is possible for the reliability study to be a fraction of the size of the main study, provided it is a representative sample, as in the case of the Fletcher Challenge Study (Example 10.29). Furthermore, the same attenuation coefficient can be applied when different disease outcomes are considered and when different risk models are used (e.g., when the survival models of Chapter 11 are used), as well as logistic regression.

A simple way of deriving the attenuation coefficient is described by MacMahon et al. (1990), referred to here as the **MacMahon–Peto** method. The baseline values are divided into a number of mutually exclusive and exhaustive groups. The means of the baseline values in the lowest and highest groups are evaluated, and their difference computed. Then the means of the repeat sample values for individuals who fall in these two groups are evaluated, and their difference is also computed. The MacMahon–Peto attenuation coefficient is the ratio of the first to the second difference. We can do these computations for the Fletcher Challenge Study from the summary data shown in Table 10.40. Here the attenuation coefficient is

$$\frac{148.4 - 101.4}{142.6 - 109.6} = \frac{47.0}{33.0} = 1.42.$$

Suppose the Fletcher Challenge Study data were used to estimate the association between stroke and systolic blood pressure. We thus correct for regression dilution bias by multiplying the log odds ratio for stroke, associated with an increase of one unit (mmHg) in baseline systolic blood pressure, by 1.42. The result is interpreted as the log odds ratio for stroke for a 1 mmHg increase in usual systolic blood pressure. Providing the reliability study is large (say, involving more than 100 people) we can correct the standard error of the log odds ratio, and thus construct regression dilution-adjusted confidence intervals, by multiplying the baseline standard error by the same amount.

An alternative to the nonparametric MacMahon–Peto method is to fit a simple linear regression model (Section 9.3.1) with repeat measures as the y variable and baseline measures as the x variable. The attenuation coefficient is then the reciprocal of the regression slope. This has the disadvantage of requiring the usual assumptions of standard regression models, such as normally distributed data, but has the advantage that it does not require arbitrary grouping structures, such as the tenths used in the MacMahon–Peto calculation here. Practical experience suggests that the two approaches give similar results. For instance, fitting this regression model to the raw data from the Fletcher Challenge Study (those data used to create Table 10.40) gave an attenuation coefficient of 1.43, virtually identical to the MacMahon–Peto value. Both these methods can give misleading results when important confounding factors are included in the logistic (or alternative) regression model for the main study. Unlike the MacMahon–Peto method, the regression approach may be extended to cope with this situation (Rosner et al., 1990; Carroll et al., 2006). Measurement error in confounding variables can also be expected to have an effect on inferences for the index explanatory variable (Philips and Davey Smith, 1992).

When using attenuation coefficients, we should take account of the time elapsed from baseline to the end of data collection in the main study. Clarke et al. (1999) show that the attenuation coefficient tends to get bigger as time goes by. Using data from the Framingham Study, their analysis gives attenuation coefficients for systolic blood pressure of 1.5 after 6 years, 1.9 after 16 years and 2.9 after 26 years, to be compared with 1.4 after 3 years for the Fletcher Challenge Study. For the most meaningful correction, it is best to time the reliability study about half-way through the follow-up interval.

An attenuation coefficient calculated from one study may be used in another study that has no internal capacity for correcting for regression dilution bias (that is, no repeat measures). This is reasonable if the study populations, settings and follow-up periods are similar. When, for example, laboratory methods used to derive the risk factor are liable to differ, we should be cautious of such extrapolation.

Sometimes the risks associated with the continuous risk factor are described by dividing the values derived at baseline into a number of mutually exclusive and exhaustive groups (as in Example 10.11, Example 10.22 and Example 10.25) and plotting odds ratios (or log odds ratios) against the averages of these groups. In the plot, we can adjust for regression dilution using the MacMahon–Peto approach by plotting (say) odds ratios for the baseline groups against the means of these same groups in the repeat sample. Thus, if our groups are fifths (as in Example 10.11), we plot the odds ratios associated with each of the baseline fifths against the sample means for these baseline fifths in the repeat sample. Using the regression method of correction, we fit separate regression lines for each baseline group, thus generating an attenuation coefficient for each group. We then adjust the position of the average for any group on the x axis of the plot by multiplying this average by the group's attenuation coefficient. In the plots, whatever method of correction is used, we label the x axis as 'usual' values of the risk factor. See Asia Pacific Cohort Studies Collaboration (2003a) for an example.

The discussion so far has assumed that only one resurvey of the study population will take place, but sometimes several are undertaken. We might then simply calculate attenuation coefficients for different periods of follow-up (as in Clarke et al., 1999), which requires no new methodology. Alternatively, we might pool all the repeat surveys and calculate a single attenuation coefficient through a generalised estimating equation model (Section 9.11) used to regress the several repeat measures on the baseline value. This is another generalisation of the regression approach to correction for regression dilution. Again, Asia Pacific Cohort Studies Collaboration (2003a) provides an example.

10.13   Case–control studies

Logistic regression may be used to analyse case–control studies; however, just as when only descriptive statistics are used, the range of analyses possible is restricted. Matched studies, whatever the design framework, require special analyses (matched cohort studies are considered in Section 10.17.8).

10.13.1   Unmatched studies

Suppose that we define case–control status to be the outcome variable, with a case outcome taken to be the positive event, and exposure status to be the explanatory variable. Then we can analyse the case–control study by logistic regression in much the same way as for data arising by cross-sectional survey, cohort study or intervention. The only proviso is that we *cannot* construct estimates of the risk, relative risk or odds of disease. In the context of logistic regression, this is proved mathematically by Collett (2002). Hence, (10.8) does not hold and, whilst (10.3) still defines the logit, the logit is no longer the log odds (more precisely, it is no longer a valid estimate of the population log odds).

Table 10.41. Sun protection during childhood against case–control status for cutaneous melanoma.

Sun protection?	Cases	Controls	Total
Yes	99	132	231
No	303	290	593

What we *can* do is estimate the odds ratio, exactly as for any other type of study design; for instance, (10.4) is still usable. Similarly, procedures for testing with deviances and model checking described earlier still hold good. Thus, as long as we make all inferences in terms of odds ratios, which is the natural thing to do using a logistic model in any case, unmatched case–control studies give no new problem. Notice that all these comments are consistent with the material of Section 6.2.1.

Example 10.30 The data of Table 6.2 (showing case–control status for melanoma and sun protection status) are presented in Table 10.41, this being of the typical format of this chapter. In the notation of Table 10.2, Cases = e and Total = n. SAS PROC GENMOD returned the following estimate (and estimated standard error) for protection: −0.3315 ($\hat{se} = 0.1563$). This gives the estimated odds ratio as exp(−0.3315) = 0.72, with 95% confidence interval

$$\exp(-0.3315 \pm 1.96 \times 0.1563)$$

or (0.53, 0.98), which agrees with the result found without using the logistic regression model in Example 6.3.

The Δdeviance for comparing the model with sun protection status to the empty model (with a constant term only) is 4.53 on 1 d.f. ($p = 0.03$). This result is very similar to the chi-square test statistic of 4.19 ($p = 0.04$) reported in Example 6.3.

When several exposure variables are present, possibly in addition to confounding and interaction variables, we simply take each to be an explanatory variable in a multiple logistic regression model (as usual). If any of the explanatory variables is continuous, we would normally wish to analyse the data in generic form. The outcome variable would then take the value 1 for cases and 0 for controls.

10.13.2 Matched studies

Matched studies are analysed using **conditional logistic regression models**. These are obtained from maximum likelihood analysis, conditioning on the observed set of explanatory variables in any one matched set being allocated to that set, although not necessarily to the same individuals within the set (Breslow and Day, 1993). In general, this leads to relatively complex analyses (Breslow *et al.*, 1978), including special methods for checking model fit (Hosmer and Lemeshow, 2000), and special computer routines are needed. In the special case of 1 : 1 matching, the conditional likelihood can be reduced to the standard likelihood, and thus standard logistic regression procedures can be used (Collett, 2002). In SAS, matched analyses may be carried out using PROC PHREG, a procedure designed primarily for use with Cox regression (Section 11.6), provided that the DISCRETE option is selected. In Stata, the CLOGIT routine is applicable. Whatever package is used, it will be necessary to declare the matching information, usually by defining a unique number for each matched set.

Example 10.31 The paired data of Table 6.11 were read into SAS in generic form: for each individual the set (pair) number (1 to 109), case–control status (1 = case; 0 = control) and family history status (1 = yes; 0 = no) were read. The conditional logistic regression analysis performed by PROC PHREG gave the following estimate (and estimated standard error) for family history: 0.733969 (s̃e = 0.35119). This gives the estimated odds ratio as exp(0.733969) = 2.08, with 95% confidence interval

$$\exp(0.733969 \pm 1.96 \times 0.35119)$$

or (1.05, 4.15). The odds ratio is exactly as given in Example 6.8, although the confidence interval is slightly narrower than the exact interval found previously. The test results also turn out to be very similar to those found in Example 6.8. Note that there is really no need to include any of the concordant pairs in the data input and analysis.

Example 10.32 In Example 6.11, we analysed data from a many : many matched case–control study of myocardial infarction (MI). As well as the risk factor, D-dimer (recorded as low/high), a number of potential confounding variables were available for each study participant. One of these was systolic blood pressure (SBP). In Section 6.6.4, we saw how to determine the effect of D-dimer on MI (case–control status). Now we shall also see how to assess the adjusted effect of D-dimer, accounting for the effect of SBP. Table 10.42 shows the data required as input to the computer; as in Table 6.19, the sets have been sorted by increasing size.

Three conditional logistic regression models were fitted using PROC PHREG: D-dimer alone; SBP alone; and both together. The minus-twice log likelihoods (Section 10.7) for these models were reported as 96.966, 92.899 and 92.713, respectively; furthermore, the empty model (reported automatically by PROC PHREG) has the value 97.239.

D-dimer, with two levels, has 1 d.f. Hence, we may test for D-dimer, unadjusted and adjusted, by comparing 97.239 − 96.966 = 0.273 and 92.899 − 92.713 = 0.186, respectively, with χ_1^2. Clearly neither is significant at any reasonable level. Hence, we may conclude that D-dimer appears to have no effect on MI, whether or not we adjust for SBP. The estimated odds ratio (with 95% confidence interval) is 1.26 (0.53, 2.96) unadjusted and 1.22 (0.50, 2.94) adjusted, showing that adjustment has no real effect. Notice that the continuous variable SBP is a significant risk factor for MI in its own right because its effect is evaluated from comparing 97.239 − 92.899 = 4.34 with χ_1^2 ($p = 0.04$).

The unadjusted results from maximum likelihood methodology recorded here are similar to the Mantel–Haenszel results given in Example 6.11. The test statistic is slightly bigger than the continuity-corrected test statistic in Example 6.11, although without the continuity correction the two results are only 0.001 apart. The estimate and lower confidence limit for ψ are identical; the upper limit is 2.96, compared with 3.02 in Example 6.11.

10.14   Outcomes with several levels

Up to now, we have assumed that disease outcome is measured as 'yes' or 'no'. In some instances, it may be possible to define the severity of disease — for example, 'no', 'little', 'moderate', or 'severe' disease and 'death'. Then the outcome is ordinal; the y variable is an ordered categorical variable. Although this is outside the intended scope of this chapter, it is so closely related to the preceding material that it is appropriate to consider this situation here.

Armstrong and Sloan (1989) give an example of an ordered categorical outcome variable arising from a study of miners exposed to tremolite fibres, in which the outcome is the profusion of small opacities on a chest x-ray recorded on a 12-point ordered scale. Hastie *et al.* (1989) give a similar example in which a combined osteoporosis score is constructed for each subject from individual grades of osteoporosis

Table 10.42. Results from a matched case–control study of MI. Case–control status is 0 for a control and 1 for a case; D-dimer status is 0 for low and 1 for high (exposed); SBP = systolic blood pressure.

Set no.	Case/ control	D-dimer status	SBP (mmHg)	Set no.	Case/ control	D-dimer status	SBP (mmHg)
1	0	0	142	15	0	1	147
1	0	1	105	15	0	1	163
1	1	0	142	15	0	1	206
2	0	0	131	15	0	0	152
2	0	0	117	15	0	1	143
2	0	0	120	15	0	0	120
2	1	0	130	15	0	1	180
3	0	0	126	15	1	1	200
3	0	1	109	15	1	0	147
3	0	0	103	16	0	0	163
3	1	1	179	16	0	0	147
4	0	1	138	16	0	0	143
4	0	1	124	16	0	0	123
4	0	1	136	16	0	1	153
4	1	1	147	16	1	0	148
5	0	1	127	16	1	1	127
5	0	1	143	16	0	1	155
5	0	1	136	16	0	0	149
5	0	0	160	17	1	1	156
5	1	0	127	17	0	0	159
6	0	1	155	17	0	1	190
6	0	1	125	17	0	1	131
6	0	0	184	17	0	1	152
6	0	0	165	17	0	1	164
6	1	1	177	17	0	1	160
7	0	1	123	17	0	1	135
7	0	1	139	17	0	1	169
7	1	0	133	17	1	0	137
7	0	0	153	18	0	1	174
7	0	0	131	18	1	1	141
8	0	0	154	18	0	0	137
8	0	0	138	18	0	0	144
8	0	1	164	18	0	0	152
8	1	0	150	18	0	0	150
8	0	0	161	18	0	0	185
9	0	0	113	18	0	1	134
9	0	1	125	18	1	1	134
9	1	1	112	18	0	1	134
9	0	1	150	19	0	0	122
9	0	1	139	19	0	0	141
10	0	0	125	19	0	0	130
10	0	1	130	19	0	0	142
10	0	0	151	19	0	1	131
10	0	0	129	19	0	0	140
10	1	1	152	19	1	0	146
11	0	0	129	19	0	0	122

(continued)

Table 10.42. Results from a matched case–control study of MI. Case–control status is 0 for a control and 1 for a case; D-dimer status is 0 for low and 1 for high (exposed); SBP = systolic blood pressure. (Continued)

Set no.	Case/ control	D-dimer status	SBP (mmHg)	Set no.	Case/ control	D-dimer status	SBP (mmHg)
11	0	0	92	19	0	1	136
11	1	0	131	19	0	0	129
11	0	1	137	19	0	1	153
11	0	0	105	19	0	1	140
12	0	0	109	19	1	1	181
12	0	0	108	19	1	0	207
12	0	0	139	20	0	1	148
12	0	1	110	20	0	0	125
12	1	1	129	20	0	0	147
13	0	1	113	20	0	1	142
13	0	0	161	20	0	0	134
13	0	0	121	20	0	1	128
13	0	0	104	20	1	1	132
13	1	0	131	20	0	0	143
14	0	1	151	20	0	1	144
14	0	0	117	20	1	0	189
14	0	0	120	20	0	1	134
14	0	0	135	20	0	1	149
14	0	1	181	20	0	1	111
14	0	1	171	20	0	1	113
14	0	0	148	20	1	1	115
14	1	1	145				

Note: These data may be downloaded; see Appendix A.

of the sacrium, ilium, pelvis and ischium. In such cases, standard regression modelling is inappropriate because the y variable is not normally distributed. Nonparametric procedures such as the two-sample Wilcoxon test (Section 2.8.2) are applicable, but cannot make allowance for several explanatory variables, as would a statistical model. It would be possible to collapse the outcomes into a binary variable — for example, below 6 and above 6 for the problem of Armstrong and Sloan (1989) — and then use logistic regression modelling. However, this would throw away information on the precise severity of disease.

What is required is a modelling procedure that falls somewhere between standard and logistic regression. Several such models for ordered categorical outcomes have been suggested (Agresti, 1996). One of these is the **proportional odds model** (McCullagh, 1980), which is easy to fit using commercial software, such as SAS and Stata.

10.14.1 The proportional odds assumption

Consider a simple problem in which each individual is recorded as exposed or unexposed to a solitary risk factor. This is just as in Section 10.4.1, but now disease severity is recorded, say, on a ℓ-point ordinal scale. Table 10.43 shows the form of the data: this is a direct extension of Table 3.1.

Table 10.43. Disease severity (D_ℓ most; D_1 least) against risk factor status.

Risk factor status	Disease severity					Total
	D_ℓ	$D_{\ell-1}$	...	D_2	D_1	
Exposed	e_ℓ	$e_{\ell-1}$		e_2	e_1	
Not exposed	u_ℓ	$u_{\ell-1}$		u_2	u_1	
Total						n

Consider combining the severity classes (D) into two groups. For example, we could take D_ℓ by itself as one group and the rest ($D_{\ell-1}$ to D_1) as the other. Then Table 10.43 would reduce to Table 3.1 such that

$$a = e_\ell \quad b = e_1 + e_2 + \cdots + e_{\ell-1}$$

$$c = u_\ell \quad d = u_1 + u_2 + \cdots + u_{\ell-1}.$$

We could then apply (3.9) to find the odds ratio for most severe disease status (perhaps death) against any less severe disease status (perhaps survival) as

$$\psi_\ell = \frac{e_\ell \left(u_1 + u_2 + \cdots + u_{\ell-1} \right)}{\left(e_1 + e_2 + \cdots + e_{\ell-1} \right) u_\ell}. \tag{10.26}$$

We can group columns of Table 10.43 in $\ell - 1$ other ways so as to produce 2×2 tables (each akin to Table 3.1) with 'more severe' in the left-hand and 'less severe' in the right-hand column. We simply keep moving the point of separation one step to the right each time within the D columns of Table 10.43. Each time an odds ratio may be calculated just as for (10.26): the odds ratio for the j most severe classes of disease versus the $\ell - j$ least severe is, from (3.9),

$$\psi_{\ell-j+1} = \frac{\left(e_{\ell-j+1} + e_{\ell-j+2} + \cdots + e_\ell \right)\left(u_1 + u_2 + \cdots + u_{\ell-j} \right)}{\left(e_1 + e_2 + \cdots + e_{\ell-j} \right)\left(u_{\ell-j+1} + u_{\ell-j+2} + \cdots + u_\ell \right)}. \tag{10.27}$$

The proportional odds assumption is that (10.27) is the same whatever the value of j (here, j varies from 1 to $\ell - 1$). That is, the relative odds of more severe disease are the same, whatever the definition of 'more severe'.

Example 10.33 Woodward *et al.* (1995) describe an application of the proportional odds method to CHD prevalence for the baseline SHHS. Prevalent CHD was defined on a four-point graded scale: MI; angina grade II; angina grade I; and no CHD (in decreasing order of severity). In several previous analyses, the three grades of CHD had been combined and logistic regression analysis used. The new analysis made use of the more detailed information about the extent of disease.

Here we will develop a proportional odds analysis of parental history (before age 60) of CHD as a risk factor for CHD in men, one of several factors looked at by Woodward *et al.* (1995). Table 10.44 shows baseline CHD severity against parental history status for every man in the

Table 10.44. Prevalent CHD against parental history of CHD; SHHS men.

Parental history of CHD?	MI	Angina II	Angina I	No CHD	Total
Yes	104	17	45	830	996
No	192	30	122	3376	3720
Total	296	47	167	4206	4716

SHHS from whom the relevant information was obtained. Note that this includes data from three Scottish districts that were unavailable to Woodward *et al.* (1995).

To check the proportional odds assumption, we (conceptually) divide the disease columns of Table 10.44 into (i) MI versus the rest; (ii) MI plus angina II versus angina I plus no CHD; and (iii) any CHD versus no CHD. This produces the following tables:

(i)	104	892	(ii)	121	875	(iii)	166	830
	192	3528		222	3498		344	3376

Then we can calculate the three odds ratios from (3.9) or (10.27) as: (i) 2.14; (ii) 2.18; and (iii) 1.96. These are reasonably similar and we can conclude that the proportional odds assumption seems to be acceptable. We might report some kind of average of these three as *the* odds ratio for CHD severity (Example 10.34). Certainly men whose parents had CHD are more likely to have a relatively severe form of CHD themselves.

10.14.2 The proportional odds model

The proportional odds regression model is a direct generalisation of the logistic regression model, using the proportional odds assumption. Suppose, as before, there are ℓ disease severity categories. Logistic regression could then be used to model $\ell - 1$ logits (just as (10.27) defines $\ell - 1$ odds ratios). These are combined in the proportional odds model: the ith logit is estimated as

$$\hat{\text{logit}}_i = b_{0i} + b_1 x, \quad i = 1, 2, ..., \ell - 1. \tag{10.28}$$

Notice that the constant term, b_{0i}, varies with i (the choice of threshold amongst the disease categories), but the slope parameter, b_1, is independent of i. The latter is the mathematical encapsulation of the proportional odds assumption.

If several risk factors or confounders are present, possibly plus interaction terms, the proportional odds model is a multiple regression version of (10.28):

$$\hat{\text{logit}}_i = b_{0i} + b_1 x_1 + b_2 x_2 + \cdots + b_k x_k \quad i = 1, 2, ..., \ell - 1, \tag{10.29}$$

for some $k > 1$.

Computer packages will give estimates of the b coefficients and model deviances, which are used exactly as in Section 10.7. The SAS procedure PROC LOGISTIC, and the Stata procedure OLOGIT, will fit proportional odds models. PROC LOGISTIC also prints out the result of a formal test (described by Peterson, 1990) of the proportional odds assumption. Since this test appears to be very sensitive to small departures from the assumption, only very extreme significance levels (such as $p < 0.01$) should be used as evidence to reject the proportional odds assumption with large samples.

Example 10.34 SAS PROC LOGISTIC was used to analyse the data of Example 10.33. The data were entered into SAS with CHD severity coded in rank order (MI coded as 4,..., no CHD as 1). Results appear in Output 10.7. Note that the binary explanatory variable, parental CHD (PARNTS = 1 if yes, 0 if no), was not declared as a categorical variable. If it had been, because of the SAS rule for categorical variables (Section 9.2.7), the estimate would have been the negative of what appears in Output 10.7.

First, we can see that the test of the proportional odds assumption is not significant ($p = 0.2964$), so we have an objective justification for our analysis. The maximum likelihood estimates include INTERCEPT terms, which are the three separate b_{oi} in (10.28). Of more interest is the PARNTS line, which tells us that the estimate of b_1 in (10.28) is 0.6843, which gives an odds ratio of $e^{0.6843} = 1.982$. This is the estimated odds ratio for more severe CHD, comparing those with, to those without, parental history of CHD. This is an average (although not a simple arithmetic mean) of the three individual odds ratios calculated in Example 10.33.

We can use the INTERCEPT terms to estimate odds or risks if these are meaningful. For example, the logit for all CHD versus no CHD, for those with parental history of CHD is, by (10.28),

$$-2.2858 + 0.6843 \times 1 = -1.6015,$$

where INTERCEPT 3 is chosen because all CHD : no CHD is the third split (Example 10.33). Then, by (10.8), the estimated prevalence risk is

$$\hat{r} = \left\{1 + \exp(1.6015)\right\}^{-1} = 0.17.$$

Since we have fitted the full model, we can check this from Table 10.44 (or its third split). Observed data give the prevalence of CHD for those with parental history of CHD:

$$\left(104 + 17 + 45\right)\big/996 = 166\big/996 = 0.17,$$

as anticipated.

Output 10.7. SAS PROC LOGISTIC results for Example 10.34.

Score test for the proportional odds assumption		
Chi-square	DF	Pr > ChiSq
2.4323	2	0.2964

Analysis of maximum likelihood estimates						
Parameter		DF	Estimate	Standard error	Wald chi-square	Pr > ChiSq
Intercept	1	1	−2.8844	0.0683	1783.7104	<.0001
Intercept	2	1	−2.7251	0.0647	1771.6565	<.0001
Intercept	3	1	−2.2858	0.0566	1629.7621	<.0001
parnts		1	0.6843	0.1017	45.3103	<.0001

10.14.3 Multinomial regression

If the outcome variable is categorical with several levels, and these levels have no natural order, a **multinomial regression** (sometimes called a **polytomous regression**) model is appropriate (Biesheuvel *et al.*, 2008). These can also be fitted using PROC LOGISTIC in SAS; in Stata, the MLOGIT routine is used. With this model there are contrasts between the levels of both the outcome and the explanatory variable(s). However, for any one contrast between levels of the outcome variable, interpretation follows that for logistic regression.

10.15 Longitudinal data

Just as we saw in Section 9.11 for a continuous outcome variable, when the binary outcome variable is recorded repeatedly for the same individual (that is, the data are longitudinal), we should allow for this by using a modelling procedure that includes within-subject correlations, such as generalised estimating equations (GEEs). As in Section 9.11, this is a special case of panel data. Details are beyond the scope of this book and concepts will be demonstrated only through a concise example. As ever, plots are required to guide the analysis in practice.

Example 10.35 The questionnaire used in the bread salt study of Example 9.21 asked whether the individual concerned felt that the bread she or he had been eating in the last week had a different degree of saltiness to the bread eaten in the previous week (the data may be downloaded; see Appendix A). This question was asked each week from weeks 2 to 6, giving five responses from each individual (except where missing values occurred). The primary research question in this study (Girgis *et al.*, 2003) was whether the responses to the 'change in saltiness' question were the same in each study group: intervention (weekly 5% salt reduction) and control. As in the published analyses, an exchangeable correlation structure will be assumed in the GEE model. For these data, reasonable alternative assumptions made no substantive difference to the conclusions, although this is not always true.

Output 10.8 shows the results from SAS, having fitted the model relating the log odds of a positive response to the question, 'Has there been a change in saltiness?' to treatment group. We see that there is no evidence of a difference between groups ($p = 0.8412$). Note that SAS has taken 'R' (the code for the reduced salt, intervention, group) to be the reference group because this is the last of the two in alphabetical order, but this is not the natural choice. As usual, we reverse the sign of the regression coefficient for group, as well as raising to the exponential power, to obtain the odds ratio of a positive response to the saltiness question, comparing those taking reduced salt to those not, of $\exp(0.0480) = 1.05$ with 95% confidence interval ($\exp(-0.4213)$, $\exp(0.5172)$). Thus, the odds of someone thinking that the bread she or he was eating had a different salt content is only marginally greater when the bread had 5% less salt content than when it had no change. That is, gradual reduction in salt content seems to be virtually undetectable over the period of the study. Notice that this simple analysis takes no account of the time at which the question was asked; as in Example 9.21, it would be easy to add time to the model in some appropriate way.

Output 10.8. SAS PROC GENMOD results for Example 10.35.

Analysis of GEE parameter estimates							
Empirical standard error estimates							
Parameter		Estimate	Standard error	95% confidence limits		Z	Pr > |Z|
Intercept		0.1381	0.1662	−0.1878	0.4639	0.83	0.4063
group	C	−0.0480	0.2394	−0.5172	0.4213	−0.20	0.8412
group	R	0.0000	0.0000	0.0000	0.0000	.	.

10.16 Binomial regression

At the start of this chapter the problem of regression modeling for binary data was introduced and the solution to this problem was presented through the use of logistic regression, which gives results for odds ratios. This approach works very well, both theoretically and, from experience, across a wide range of applications. However, it does not satisfy needs if the goal is to obtain relative risks adjusting for confounding variables. Whilst (10.8) can be used to obtain a risk from an odds exactly in the unadjusted case, from which a relative risk easily follows from an odds ratio, the result is not exact when confounding is allowed for. Furthermore, as discussed in Section 10.4.1, only an approximate 95% confidence interval for the risk and relative risk can be obtained from a logistic regression model.

A more direct method for obtaining risks and relative risks is available through **binomial models**. Whereas the logistic model has the form

$$\log_e\left(\frac{\hat{r}}{1-\hat{r}}\right) = b_0 + b_1 x_1 + b_2 x_2 + \cdots + b_k x_k, \tag{10.30}$$

for k explanatory variables, where r is the risk of an outcome (as earlier in this chapter), the binomial model is

$$\log_e(\hat{r}) = b_0 + b_1 x_1 + b_2 x_2 + \cdots + b_k x_k. \tag{10.31}$$

Hence, whereas the logistic model produces results directly for the logit (i.e., the log odds) the binomial model produces results for the log risk. Unsurprisingly, the latter makes it easier to produce inferences for the risk and relative risk. Note that, because the binomial model, as defined above, uses a log transformation (or **link**), it is sometimes called the **log-binomial model**. In Section 10.16.2 we shall use a binomial model without the log transformation (i.e., with what is called the **identity link**).

Fitting binomial models to data using proprietary software that handles generalised linear models, such as PROC GENMOD in SAS or the GLM command in Stata, requires telling the software that the random variability is binomial (just as for the logistic model) and that the linear predictor relates to the log of the outcome (unlike logistic regression where a logit link is involved between the outcome and the linear predictor). Otherwise, all follows just as for logistic regression, barring the interpretation of the result.

Example 10.36 Consider the data of Table 10.14, relating systolic blood pressure and cholesterol, by fifths, to CHD. Table 10.45 shows the results from fitting both logistic and binomial models to these data (in each case, fitting the model with both predictors but no interaction) in SAS (and Stata). As will be seen, the mutually adjusted odd ratios and relative risks are much the same, which is just as would be expected for a rare disease (Section 3.3). Furthermore, the test statistics for comparing nested models are virtually identical between the two approaches.

In Example 10.36, changing to a binomial model serves little purpose, because the index disease is rare and only relative measures of chance are considered (as has been the case almost exclusively throughout this chapter). When the disease is not rare, the odds ratio will not generally be a good estimate of the relative risk, whilst (as already indicated) when confounding is allowed for, the simple way of moving from an odds to a risk does not work. Both of these issues are illustrated by the next example. This example derives from a cross-sectional study, so that prevalences and prevalence ratios will be computed,

Table 10.45. Odds ratios (from logistic regression) and relative risks (from binomial regression) for CHD for the data of Table 10.14.

	Fifth	Odds ratio (95% CI)	Relative risk (95% CI)
Systolic blood pressure	1	1	1
	2	1.84 (1.01, 3.35)	1.81 (1.01, 3.23)
	3	2.39 (1.34, 4.23)	2.29 (1.32, 3.99)
	4	2.80 (1.59, 4.93)	2.68 (1.55, 4.62)
	5	3.83 (2.21, 6.63)	3.56 (2.10, 6.04)
Serum total cholesterol	1	1	1
	2	1.23 (0.66, 2.32)	1.23 (0.66, 2.27)
	3	2.28 (1.29, 4.00)	2.20 (1.28, 3.80)
	4	2.74 (1.58, 4.73)	2.60 (1.54, 4.41)
	5	3.65 (2.14, 6.23)	3.41 (2.04, 5.70)

CI = confidence interval.

rather than risk and relative risk – the same distinction holds for odds and odds ratios, but will be suppressed for simplicity of exposition. In fact, the material of this section has greater importance in cross-sectional studies than in cohort studies. This is because prevalence is frequently found to be common, whereas incidence is more often rare.

Example 10.37 Consider the data of Example 9.16, and suppose the aim of the study is to investigate whether high values of fibrinogen are associated with a high prevalence of *H. pylori*. Using the data for Example 9.16 provided on the web site for this book, Table 10.46 was constructed. Age is included as a potential confounding variable, as in Example 9.16. For simplicity, as with fibrinogen, this has been dichotomised here. Prevalence and odds were calculated using the standard formulae of Chapter 3; note that the unadjusted prevalence ratio is $0.7770/0.6307 = 1.232$ and the odds ratio is $3.4833/1.7079 = 2.039$, which are very different.

These data were entered into SAS and analysed using PROC GENMOD both through logistic and binomial regression. Results for fibrinogen were obtained with and without adjustment for age, in each case, by fitting the four models itemised in Table 10.47.

Table 10.46. Fibrinogen, age and *H. pylori* prevalence for men in Example 10.37. High fibrinogen is defined as ≥ 2.7 g/l; older age is ≥ 50 years.

		H. pylori	No *H. pylori*	Prevalence	Odds
High fibrinogen	Older age	161	33	0.8299	4.8788
High fibrinogen	Younger age	48	27	0.6400	1.7778
Low fibrinogen	Older age	73	26	0.7374	2.8077
Low fibrinogen	Younger age	79	63	0.5563	1.2540
High fibrinogen		209	60	0.7770	3.4833
Low fibrinogen		152	89	0.6307	1.7079

Table 10.47. Models fitted using SAS PROC GENMOD in Example 10.37. Notation as in the general expressions, (10.30) and (10.31): r is the prevalence, b_0 is the intercept, b_1 is a dummy variable for fibrinogen, x_1 (high = 1; low = 0) and b_2 is a dummy variable for age, x_2 (1 = older; 0 = younger).

Type of model	Logistic regression	Binomial regression
Unadjusted	(1) $\log_e(\hat{r}/(1 - \hat{r})) = b_0 + b_1 x_1$	(2) $\log_e(\hat{r}) = b_0 + b_1 x_1$
Adjusted for age	(3) $\log_e(\hat{r}/(1 - \hat{r})) = b_0 + b_1 x_1 + b_2 x_2$	(4) $\log_e(\hat{r}) = b_0 + b_1 x_1 + b_2 x_2$

Table 10.48. Results from fitting PROC GENMOD in SAS for Example 10.37. Model numbers and algebraic terms correspond to Table 10.47.

| Model fitted | Parameters | | | Prevalence[a] | | Prevalence ratio |
	Intercept b_0	Fibrinogen b_1	Age b_2	High fibrinogen	Low fibrinogen	
(1) Unadjusted logistic	0.5352	0.7127	—	0.7769	0.6307	1.232
(2) Unadjusted binomial	−0.4609	0.2085	—	0.7769	0.6307	1.232
(3) Adjusted logistic	0.1934	0.4496	0.9002	0.8239	0.7491	1.100
(4) Adjusted binomial	−0.5796	0.1240	0.2705	0.8310	0.7341	1.132

[a] For logistic models, calculated using (10.8); for binomial models, found directly from parameters; the prevalence shown in the adjusted model is for older people.

We will use both logistic and binomial models to estimate the prevalence of *H. pylori* for an older person who has high fibrinogen and for an older person who has low fibrinogen (to conserve space, the corresponding prevalences for younger people are omitted). Also we shall find the prevalence ratio for high versus low fibrinogen from both models.

Table 10.48, left side, gives all the relevant parameters taken from fitting models to the data in Table 10.46. The right side of the table has been computed differently for logistic and binomial models. For binomial models, the parameter values have been inserted into the fitted values, taking $x_1 = 1$ for high fibrinogen, $x_1 = 0$ for low fibrinogen and (in the adjusted model only) $x_2 = 1$ for older age. Taking the exponent of the result gives the (estimated) prevalence. Apart from negligible rounding error, these are the true results, by comparison with Table 10.46. For logistic models, exactly the same substitutions were made, but the result is now the logit. For the unadjusted model, putting the logit into (10.8) correctly gives the prevalence just as for the binomial, both for those with high and low fibrinogen. However, using (10.8) for the adjusted model gives different results to the true results from the binomial model. Results from the logistic model can be viewed as approximate.

In a logistic regression model (without an interaction term), the odds ratio (comparing levels of the index risk factor) is the same whatever the values of the confounding variables (as illustrated by Example 10.11). In a binomial model, the same is true for the relative risk. However, if we use (10.8) on a multivariable logistic model we will obtain different results for the relative risk depending upon the values of the confounding variables. Thus, in Example 10.37, when the adjusted relative risk is estimated at younger ages (i.e., $x_2 = 0$) the result from the binomial model is 1.132, just as in Table 10.48, but from the logistic model, via (10.8), the result is 1.196, somewhat higher than the 1.100 found when conditioning on the subjects being older men. This further illustrates the inappropriateness of using (10.8), except in the case of a single explanatory variable, and thus the value of the binomial model.

So far the issue of estimating variability has not been considered. The next example shows how to estimate the variability of the estimated relative risk from binomial regression, a problem which does not have an exact solution in the context of logistic regression (Section 10.4.1).

Example 10.38 In Example 3.1 we estimated the risk of a cardiovascular death for smokers in EGAT to be 0.021877 with a 95% confidence interval of (0.01426, 0.02949) and the relative risk for smokers versus nonsmokers to be 2.7682 (1.500, 5.108). Consider how to derive these using computer output from a binomial model fitted to the EGAT data, as presented in Table 3.2.

Table 10.49 shows results from SAS PROC GENMOD used with a log link and binomial distribution. Here SMOKING was coded as 1 for smokers and 0 for nonsmokers, as in Example 10.4.

Table 10.49. Excerpt derived from SAS
output for Example 10.38.

Parameter	Estimate	Standard error
INTERCEPT	−4.8405	0.2572
SMOKING	1.0182	0.3126

Table 10.50. Variance-covariance matrix for Example 10.38.

	INTERCEPT (b_0)	SMOKING (b_1)
INTERCEPT (b_0)	0.06614	−0.06614
SMOKING (b_1)		0.09769

This implies that the fitted model is

$$\log_e(\hat{r}_{\text{smokers}}) = -4.8405 + 1.0182\,(\text{SMOKING}).$$

Hence the estimated risk for smokers (SMOKING = 1) is exp(−4.8405 + 1.0182 × 1) = exp(−3.8223) = 0.021877, as expected. To obtain the confidence interval, we first need to find the standard error of the log risk. To obtain this we need the variance-covariance matrix, just as we saw for logistic regression in Section 10.4.1. In this case, SAS gave the matrix presented as Table 10.50.

From the methodology of Section 10.4.1, the variance of the log risk is $V(b_0) + V(b_1) + 2C(b_0, b_1)$, where V represents variance and C represents covariance. This is estimated here as 0.06614 + 0.09769 + 2 × −0.06614 = 0.03155. The estimated standard error of the log risk is thus the square root of this, 0.177623. Hence the usual ('Wald') normal-based 95% confidence interval for the log risk is 0.021877 ± 1.96 × 0.03155 = (−4.17044, −3.47416). Finally, raising each limit to the exponential power gives a 95% confidence interval for the risk for smokers as (0.0154, 0.0310), very close to the answers given above from Chapter 3.

For completeness, the risk for nonsmokers (i.e., SMOKING = 0) is derived from Table 10.49 simply as exp(b_0) = exp(−4.8405) = 0.007903. The corresponding 95% confidence interval, also directly from Table 10.49, is

$$(\exp(-4.8405 - 1.96 \times 0.2572),\ \exp(-4.8405 + 1.96 \times 0.2572)) = (0.00477, 0.01308).$$

Finally, we can derive the estimated relative risk as the ratio of the risks for smokers and nonsmokers, as just derived, giving 0.021877/0.007903 = 2.77, just as found in Example 3.1. As with the risk for nonsmokers, but not the risk for smokers, we can obtain a confidence interval for the relative risk without requiring the variance-covariance matrix, since

$$\log(\text{relative risk}) = \log(\text{risk}_{\text{smokers}}) - \log(\text{risk}_{\text{nonsmokers}}) = b_0 + (1)(b_1) - (b_0 + (0)(b_1)) = b_1.$$

This corresponds to the methodology for obtaining the odds ratio from logistic regression models outlined in Section 10.3. Thus the 95% confidence interval for the relative risk is

$$(\exp(1.0182 - 1.96 \times 0.3126,\ \exp(1.0182 + 1.96 \times 0.3126) = (1.50, 5.11),$$

as reported in Example 3.1.

10.16.1   Adjusted risks

When we wish to adjust a relative risk for a confounding variable, or variables, binomial regression may be used in just the same way as has been described earlier in this chapter for the odds ratio. All that is required is to include the confounders in the regression model. We can take the idea one step further and also adjust a risk for confounders. It is unusual to want to do this for the odds, although it could be achieved using logistic regression. The extra complexity when adjusting for risk, as opposed to a relative risk, is that we have to specify what set of values of the confounding variable will be utilised when computing the adjusted risk. That is, in the language of Section 4.5, we need to state the standard population to be used. In fact, the problem of adjusting a risk is analogous to that of adjusting a mean, which was discussed in Section 9.4.6 and Section 9.9.

Example 10.39 The data from Table 4.6 were read into SAS and analysed using a binomial model. The fitted model from PROC GENMOD was

$$\log_e(\hat{r}) = -3.6171 + 0.4388(\text{SMOKING}) + 0.2645(\text{HOUSING}). \quad (10.32)$$

Here SMOKING is 1 for a smoker and 0 for a nonsmoker; and HOUSING is 1 for renters and 0 for owner–occupiers. Table 10.51 reproduces the raw data with the estimates from (10.32) included, before and after exponentiation.

We can get the relative risk for renting versus owning, adjusted for smoking, by exponentiating the estimated beta coefficient for HOUSING in (10.32), which is $\exp(0.2645) = 1.30$. This follows, by analogy, from the way we estimated the odds ratio from fitted logistic models, for instance in Example 10.11. Otherwise, we could get these results by computing the risk ratio from the bivariable binomial model for smokers (0.05427/0.04166), or for nonsmokers (0.03499/0.02686), taking results shown in Table 10.51. The equality of these two results emphasises that the values taken by the confounding variable (here, smoking) do not need to be accounted for when adjusting a relative risk, unlike the situation for risks. The standard error produced by PROC GENMOD for the adjusted log relative risk (i.e., that corresponding to the estimate, 0.2645) is 0.1583, and thus the estimated 95% confidence interval for the smoking-adjusted relative risk is $\exp(0.2645 \pm 1.96 \times 0.1583) = (0.96, 1.78)$.

As a footnote, the Mantel–Haenszel adjusted relative risk for this example was also found, in Example 4.10, to be the same, 1.30. However, in general Mantel–Haenszel and maximum-likelihood estimates will differ. A further similarity in this case is that the standard error of 0.1612 found for the Mantel–Haenszel equivalent in Example 4.10 is similar to the 0.1583 found from fitting a binomial model. Thus confidence limits will thus also be similar.

Now consider estimating the risk for renters in Example 10.39. We have two risks for renters in the final column of Table 10.51: one for each outcome of the confounding

Table 10.51. Data from Table 4.6 and fitted values from the binomial model.

Housing tenure	Confounder	Raw data			Binomial results	
		CHD events	n	Risk[a]	Log risk	Risk[b]
Owner–occupier	Nonsmoker	48	1770	0.02712	−3.6171	0.02686
Renter	Nonsmoker	33	956	0.03452	−3.3526	0.03499
Owner–occupier	Smoker	29	707	0.04102	−3.1783	0.04166
Renter	Smoker	52	950	0.05474	−2.9138	0.05427

[a] From basic formula, (3.1);
[b] From (10.32).

variable. To combine these to get a single value we need to weight these two values in some way. To see how to do this, a general formula for a weighted mean estimate, and its corresponding standard error (SE), will first be described.

In general, the weighted mean of k estimates, $\hat{\theta}_1, \hat{\theta}_1, \ldots \hat{\theta}_k$, when the weights are $w_1, w_2, \ldots w_k$, respectively, is

$$\hat{\theta} = \frac{\sum w_i \hat{\theta}_i}{\sum w_i}. \tag{10.33}$$

The form of the estimate, $\hat{\theta}_i$, from stratum i will vary by application. To obtain the estimated SE of this weighted estimate we need to first obtain the variances for each $\hat{\theta}_i$, call this $\hat{var}(\theta_i)$, then use the general formula for the SE of a weighted average of k estimates:

$$SE = \frac{\sqrt{\sum w_i^2 \hat{var}(\theta_i)}}{\sum w_i}, \tag{10.34}$$

where the sums run from 1 to k. Weighted averages are used in many applications, and have been implicitly used previously in this book (where the general formulae were by-passed for simplicity).

For our current problem, $k = 2$, and the simple approach would be to replace the general estimate, $\hat{\theta}_i$, by the risk. In practice, it is easier, and more accurate when considering confidence intervals (as discussed later), to standardise on the log scale, using the estimates produced by the binomial model directly. That is, use $\log_e(r_i)$ in (10.33) and (10.34) and then exponentiate results for the estimate and its confidence limits at the final stage.

Three reasonable possibilities for weighting are: (i) take all the weights to be the same (**balanced**, or **equal weighting**); (ii) weight according to the distribution of the confounder (the so-called **observed margins**) in the study population; (iii) weight according to the distribution of the confounder in some external population (which could be some hypothetical ideal), as was done in Example 4.6.

Returning to Example 10.39: using (i), the log standardised risk for renters is, from the log risks in Table 10.51, $(-3.3526 + (-2.9138))/2 = -3.1332$, giving a standardised risk of $\exp(-3.1332) = 0.04358$. Using (ii), the log standardised risk is $(-3.3526 \times 2726 + (-2.9138) \times 1657/(2726 + 1657) = -3.3526 \times 0.3781 + (-2.9138) \times 0.6219 = -3.1867$, noting that (from Table 10.51) the study population contains 1657 smokers out of a total population of 4383 men (i.e., the prevalence of smoking is 0.3781). So the standardised risk using method (ii) is $\exp(-3.1867) = 0.04131$. A similar calculation follows when an external population is used as the standard. As the answers from using methods (i) and (ii) are different, it is clear that we must specify which standard population has been used when expressing standardised risks. For completeness, notice that standardised risks for owner–occupiers follow in exactly the same way: as 0.03345 and 0.03171, respectively. As they should, the ratios of standardised risks using both methods gives the adjusted relative risk of 1.30, found earlier.

A more direct method for obtaining the standardised risk is to use (10.32) directly. For method (i) we evaluate $\log_e(\hat{r})$ using (10.32) when SMOKING is given the value 0.5, for each of renters and owner–occupiers. For method (ii) we use (10.32) when SMOKING takes the value of its prevalence, 0.3781, again for each level of HOUSING. To show this works in the latter case: for renters (HOUSING = 1), (10.32) gives $-3.6171 + 0.4388 \times 0.3781 + 0.2645 \times 1 = -3.1867$; for owner–occupiers (HOUSING = 0), (10.32) gives $-3.6171 + 0.4388 \times 0.6219 = -3.4512$. Exponentiating these outcomes gives results of 0.04131 and 0.03171, just as before. In the usual parlance of regression models, this kind of process is generally called adjustment, so a reasonable alternative name for these results is **adjusted risks**.

It is now useful to consider the general situation of several confounding variables, some of which are continuous. We can easily generalise method (ii) to take the parameters from the model and use them to find $\log_e(\hat{r})$ for an average member of the study population with regard to the confounding variables. That is, the linear predictor, (10.31), is evaluated when the x variables (for all but the index risk factor) are taken to have the mean value for any continuous variable, and to take the value of the proportion for any binary variable, including dummy variables which would be defined, as a set, for any multi-level categorical variable. Since the proportion is a special type of mean (for a variable that takes the values 0 and 1), the overall result is for an average profile in the study population. Method (iii) would simply require the same procedure, but using means from an external population. Method (i) does not lend itself so readily to such a generalisation, but may be modified to require evaluating $\log_e(\hat{r})$ in (10.31) when each categorical variable takes the value $1/c$, where c is the number of groups for that variable, and each continuous variable takes its mean value. This is the approach used by SAS PROC GENMOD, applied through the LSMEANS statement, just as is described in a different context in Section 9.4.6. It may be useful to think of methods (i) – (iii) together as adjustment to a standard population, where the standard population is: (i) a population with the same means as the study population except that categorical variables are taken to have equal prevalence at all levels; (ii) the study population; and (iii) some external population.

Very often the computer package being used will give the confidence interval for an adjusted risk, at least using methods (i) or (ii), automatically; for example, see the SAS PROC GENMOD program for Example 10.39 on the web site for this book. Otherwise some tedious algebra and computation may be necessary. To show how this works, some results for Example 10.39 will be derived from first principles. Suppose that we wish to find a 95% confidence interval for the smoking-adjusted risks in Example 10.39 using the overall study population as the standard. We have already seen that, since the prevalence of smoking overall is 0.3781, from (10.31), the estimated adjusted log risk for renters (HOUSING = 1) is

$$\text{adj}(r_{\text{renters}}) = \log_e(\hat{r}) = b_0 + b_1 \overline{(\text{SMOKING})} + b_2(1) = b_0 + 0.3781b_1 + b_2.$$

To obtain the variance of this we need to know a general result from statistical theory. Suppose we have three random variables, X, Y and Z, and three constants, a, b and c, and we want to know the variance of $aX + bY + cZ$. Extending the notation of Section 10.4.1,

$$V(aX + bY = cZ) = a^2V(X) + b^2V(Y) + c^2V(Z) + 2abC(X, Y) + 2acC(X, Z) + 2bcC(Y, Z).$$

From this general result,

$$V(\text{adj}(r_{\text{renters}})) = \hat{V}(b_0) + (0.3781)^2\,\hat{V}(b_1) + \hat{V}(b_2) + 2 \times 0.3781 \times \hat{C}(b_0, b_1) + \\ 2\hat{C}(b_0, b_2) + 2 \times 0.3781 \times \hat{C}(b_1, b_2). \tag{10.35}$$

Table 10.52 shows the variance–covariance matrix given by PROC GENMOD for Example 10.39. Substituting values from Table 10.52 into (10.35) gives an estimated

Table 10.52. Variance–covariance matrix for Example 10.39.

	b_0	b_1	b_2
Intercept, b_0	0.01629	−0.009644	−0.01040
Smoking, b_1		0.02496	−0.005608
Housing tenure, b_2			0.02504

variance of 0.0125793. Assuming a normal approximation gives a 95% confidence interval for the adjusted risk of

$$\exp(-3.1867 \pm 1.96 \times \sqrt{0.0125793}) = (0.0332, 0.0515).$$

The equivalent result for owner–occupiers is easier to obtain, as (0.0254, 0.0395), since it only involves two regression parameters.

To use any other standard population, in this simple case of a single binary confounder, we simply replace 0.3781 by the required alternative parameter in (10.35). For example, a balanced standard population would require a value of 0.5, which results in 95% confidence intervals of (0.0353, 0.0538) for renters and (0.0268, 0.0418) for owner–occupiers. As should be expected, given the results found for the estimated risks, the confidence intervals vary with the chosen standard.

The contrast between the classical demographic idea of standardisation described in Section 4.5, which is based on tabulated data, and statistical adjustment, based on generic data, is worth consideration. The former uses an interaction model applied to the risks (because the demographic method, as applied in Example 4.8, uses the observed risks in each cross-classification of the data), whereas the latter uses a main effects model applied to the log risks. When we fit a regression model with all interactions to tabular (i.e., categorical) data, this is the full model, and hence the estimated risks from the model must equal the observed risks. When there is no interaction between the confounder(s) and the index risk factor, it is acceptable to use a main effects model; as discussed in Section 4.9, when there is interaction, we should not be considering adjustment for confounding. In Example 10.39 there is no evidence of an interaction ($p = 0.88$).

Finally, note that it is possible to use similar methods to derive standardised risks from logistic, rather than binomial models (see Flanders and Rhodes, 1987). As already expressed in Section 10.4.1, the problem with using this approach is that the variance estimates will then only be approximations.

10.16.2 Risk differences

Binomial models also allow easy calculation of a risk difference and its confidence interval. To obtain these from standard software we fit a binomial model with the identity link (rather than the log link used up to now in this chapter). The result will be the fitted model,

$$\hat{r} = b_0 + b_1 x_1 + b_2 x_2 + \cdots + b_k x_k.$$

By analogy to what we have already seen for logistic regression and binary regression with a log link, when a binary model is fitted with an identity link, the risk difference for variable x_1, adjusted for all other x variables, will be b_1 and the 95%

Table 10.53. Fitted coefficients from two binomial models with identity link, as fitted to the data of Table 4.6

	Single-variable model		Dual-variable model	
	Estimate	Standard error	Estimate	Standard error
Intercept	0.0311	0.0035	0.0265	0.0036
Smoking	–	–	0.0168	0.0064
Housing	0.0135	0.0059	0.0094	0.0060

confidence interval for this estimate will be $b_1 \pm 1.96 \times \mathrm{SE}(b_1)$, where SE is the standard error. When x is a categorical variable with more than two levels, a set of risk differences, again adjusted for all other x variables, will be found from the b coefficients corresponding to the partition of x into dummy variables.

Example 10.40 Table 10.53 includes the parameter estimates returned by applying PROC GENMOD with binomial variation and identity link to the raw data in Table 10.51. Two different models were fitted: the simple model with housing tenure alone and the model with both smoking status and housing tenure.

From the single-variable (i.e., unadjusted) model, the estimated risk for housing tenure = 0 (owner–occupiers) is 0.0311 and for housing tenure = 1 (renters) is 0.0311 + 0.0135 = 0.0446; these are as reported in Table 4.5. The risk difference, renters minus owner–occupiers, is 0.0135. A 95% confidence interval for this difference is 0.0135 ± 1.96 × 0.0059 = (0.0019, 0.0251). The same result can be found, to three decimal places, by applying (2.5).

From the bivariable (i.e., adjusted) model, the estimated smoking-adjusted risk difference is 0.0094 and the corresponding 95% confidence interval is 0.0094 ± 1.96 × 0.0060 = (–0.0024, 0.0212).

Notice that the estimated risks from the bivariable model in Example 10.40 are: for renters who do not smoke, 0.0265 + 0.0094 = 0.0359; for renters who smoke, 0.0265 + 0.0168 + 0.0094 = 0.0527; for owner–occupiers who do not smoke, 0.0265; and for owner–occupiers who smoke, 0.0265 + 0.0168 = 0.0433. These are all different (although not greatly so) from the estimated risks given in the right-hand side of Table 10.51, even though these were also produced by a bivariable model. This emphasises that the fitted values from a statistical model depend upon the assumptions made when using that model; here we are assuming that effects are additive, whereas previously we assumed that they are multiplicative. Not surprisingly, hypothesis tests for the effect of an index variable over and above that of a confounder, may, likewise, give different answers under the different assumptions. Furthermore, as already discussed in Section 4.8.4, the same issues arise when dealing with interactions. Notice that when full models expressing all sources of variability are fitted for both additive (identity link) and multiplicative (log link) models (for example, the model with smoking status, housing tenure and their interaction in Example 10.39 and Example 10.40), the fitted values must inevitably be the same: both will equal the observed values. In this situation the modeling process would only be useful to determine the effect of interaction, which will inevitably differ between additive and multiplicative models.

Risk differences may be expressed per unit time, such as per year, or (to avoid small numbers) as differences, for example, in percentages per year.

10.16.3 Problems with binomial models

We have now seen that the binomial regression model can be an extremely useful one for modeling binary data. Why, then, does this chapter concentrate on another model, the logistic, which cannot provide such direct measures of risk, relative risk and risk difference?

One reason is that, unlike the logistic model, the binomial model is not applicable to case–control data, because risk is not estimable from such data (Section 6.2). However, Greenland (2004) shows how external information may sometimes be used to circumvent this problem.

To understand a second problem with binomial models, refer to Section 10.2 where three major problems were discussed regarding the use of a standard (normal-based) regression model to model risks or percentages. The logistic regression model solves all three problems; the binomial model solves two but fails on the third: predicted values of the risk may be outside the valid range — see Section 10.2.2. To see this, consider a single-variable binomial model with log link. In this situation, (10.31) gives estimated risks as

$$\hat{r} = \exp(b_0 + b_1 x_1).$$

The linear predictor will give rise to a nonsensical prediction whenever $b_0 + b_1 x_1 > 0$, i.e.,

$$x_1 > -(b_0/b_1). \tag{10.36}$$

Example 10.41 The binomial model (with log link) was fitted to the data in Table 10.4 (available on the web site for this book) on the risk of death within 7.7 years according to current age. The fitted model was

$$\log_e(\hat{r}) = -8.1053 + 0.1051(\text{AGE}).$$

From (10.36), estimates of the risk, r, will be outside of the acceptable range whenever age is greater than $8.1053/0.1051 = 77.12$. For instance, suppose we wish to estimate the risk of death within 7.7 years for someone aged 80 years. From the fitted model, the predicted risk would be $\exp(-8.1053 + 0.1051 \times 80) = 1.35$, or 135%. Clearly, this is nonsense.

As in Example 10.3 (where Table 10.4 is presented), it should be emphasised that the particular estimate derived here involves extrapolation and there is no suggestion of a problem within the range of the data. For the corresponding binomial model with identity link the problem is exactly as illustrated by Example 10.3.

A third problem is that the iterative procedure needed to fit binomial models does not always converge to a proper solution. Software that fits these models should produce a warning whenever this occurs. Such problems are most likely to occur when data are analysed in generic form and when there are many confounding variables within the fitted model — each tends to produce **sparse data**, meaning data where some combinations of values for the explanatory variables are taken by small numbers of subjects. It may be possible to get around this problem by forcing the software to make additional iterations or to use a more sensible starting position for the iterative process than the default one chosen by the software: this is done by a SAS macro available from http://www.hsph.harvard.edu/faculty/donna-spiegelman/files/relrisk9.pdf. Another class of solutions to the problem is to make the data less sparse by converting continuous confounders into ordinal variables (e.g., grouping by fifths), by removing confounders (for example, those that are highly correlated with others) from the model or by combining categories of the categorical variables. Of course, these latter solutions may not be acceptable on the grounds that they differ from the researcher's conceptual model.

Yet another approach to solving convergence issues is to use the COPY algorithm described by Petersen and Deddens (2008).

Otherwise, we can abandon the binomial approach completely and, instead, fit the required model using **generalised estimating equation (GEE) Poisson regression**, available in all leading statistical packages. Zou (2004) describes the ideas behind the use of the GEE Poisson model and concludes that this model is generally acceptable for modelling risks. However, in most (but not all) situations, the binomial model is likely to be slightly better than the GEE Poisson in terms of bias, power and/or correct coverage of 95% confidence intervals: see Petersen and Deddens (2008), Skov *et al.* (1998) and Zhou (2004). Also the GEE Poisson, unlike the binomial, can give rise to fitted values of the outcome variable, corresponding to observed values of the explanatory variables, that exceed unity.

In SAS, a GEE Poisson model can be fitted using PROC GENMOD, as for binomial and logistic models, with a log link, but now specifying a Poisson distribution as well as declaring each individual subject in the database to act as a panel variable (Section 9.11). In this application GEE Poisson regression should be applied with robust standard errors (Section 9.11), which are derived using the observed variability in the data rather than the variability predicted by the underlying Poisson model. When applying SAS as described, robust estimates are given by default. Stata's GEE routine, XTGEE, requires similar Poisson, log link and panel declarations, but now a request for robust standard errors is required.

Example 10.42 A set of data with six risk factors for CHD was introduced in Example 10.12, and is available on the web site for this book. In this earlier example, and subsequent developments, logistic regression models were fitted to these data and odds ratios presented. We now consider binary regression models and relative risks for these data. In particular, we shall develop the model with all six predictors.

In this case, when a binomial model was fitted to these data using PROC GENMOD in SAS, the algorithm did not converge. Hence a GEE Poisson model was fitted instead. Table 10.54 shows the GEE Poisson results from SAS, tabulated to the right of results derived from logistic regression (the odds ratios shown are the exponents of the corresponding estimates in Table 10.16). It may be seen that the two sets of results are very similar; indeed, several statistics are the same, to two decimal places. This is because CHD is a rare occurrence in these data (196 of 4049 men, or 5%, had a CHD event during follow-up).

Table 10.54. Odds ratios (from logistic regression) and relative risks (from GEE Poisson regression), and associated statistics (CI = confidence interval), for the data of Example 10.12.

	Odds ratio		Relative risk	
Variable	Estimate (95% CI)	p value	Estimate (95% CI)	p value
Age (years)	1.02 (0.99, 1.04)	0.21	1.02 (0.99, 1.04)	0.19
Total cholesterol (mmol/l)	1.36 (1.21, 1.53)	<0.0001	1.32 (1.20, 1.45)	<0.0001
Body mass index (kg/m^2)	1.04 (1.00, 1.09)	0.05	1.04 (1.00, 1.08)	0.04
Systolic blood pressure (mmHg)	1.02 (1.01, 1.03)	<0.0001	1.02 (1.01, 1.03)	<0.0001
Never smoking (base)	1		1	
Ex-smoking	1.38 (0.84, 2.26)	0.20	1.36 (0.85, 2.15)	0.20
Current smoking	2.07 (1.35, 3.19)	0.0009	1.98 (1.33, 2.97)	0.0008
Inactive (base)	1		1	
Active	0.83 (0.58, 1.18)	0.29	0.84 (0.61, 1.17)	0.30
Average activity	0.90 (0.57, 1.43)	0.67	0.91 (0.59, 1.40)	0.67

Suppose, now, that we wish to derive adjusted risks by smoking status; that is, risks that adjust for all the other variables in Table 10.54. As explained in Section 10.16.1, a simple, and logical, way to do this is to take the fitted model and evaluate it when all these other variables take their mean values in the study population; i.e., marginal weighting. Using the parameters from the Poisson GEE model supplied by SAS, the fitted model is

$$\log_e(\hat{r}) = -9.6080 + 0.0162(\text{AGE}) + 0.2793(\text{TOTCHOL}) + 0.0386(\text{BMI})$$
$$+ 0.0187(\text{SYSTOL}) + 0.3042(\text{ex}) + 0.6854(\text{current}) + (-0.1734)(\text{active})$$
$$+ (-0.0925)(\text{average}),$$

using the same notation as in Example 10.12 and Example 10.15, with obvious extensions. As discussed earlier, the coefficients in this model are the logs of the relative risks tabulated in the right-hand side of Table 10.54. In these data, the mean age, cholesterol, body mass index and systolic blood pressure are, respectively, 49.17 years, 6.36 mmol/l, 25.97 kg/m² and 133.22 mmHg. The prevalence of being active is 0.2440 and of having average activity is 0.5913. Hence the adjusted log risks for never smokers, ex-smokers and current smokers are, respectively,

$$\log_e(\hat{r}_{\text{never smokers}}) = -9.6080 + 0.0162 \times 49.17 + 0.2793 \times 6.36 + 0.0386 \times 25.97$$
$$+ 0.0187 \times 133.22 + (-0.1734) \times 0.2440 + (-0.0925) \times 0.5913 = -3.6611;$$

$$\log_e(\hat{r}_{\text{ex-smokers}}) = -9.6080 + 0.0162 \times 49.17 + 0.2793 \times 6.36 + 0.0386 \times 25.97$$
$$+ 0.0187 \times 133.22 + 0.3042 \times 1 + (-0.1734) \times 0.2440 + (-0.0925) \times 0.5913 = -3.3570;$$

$$\log_e(\hat{r}_{\text{current smokers}}) = -9.6080 + 0.0162 \times 49.17 + 0.2793 \times 6.36 + 0.0386 \times 25.97$$
$$+ 0.0187 \times 133.22 + 0.6854 \times 1 + (-0.1734) \times 0.2440 + (-0.0925) \times 0.5913 = -2.9757.$$

Notice that each of these was calculated from the raw data on the web site for this book, using more decimals than are given in intermediate results. To get adjusted risks we raise each to the exponential power, giving answers of 0.02570, 0.03484 and 0.05101, respectively. Since the average follow-up of the cohort was 7.7 years, we might reinterpret these as the adjusted annual risks of CHD for never, ex- and current smokers of 3.34, 4.52 and 6.62 per thousand, respectively.

Computation of standard errors for these three estimates is rather more work, since several variance and covariance terms need to be dealt with. Using the LSMEANS statement, with an OM option to request marginal weighting, in PROC GENMOD, the 95% confidence intervals corresponding to the annual risks per thousand were found as (2.32, 4.80), (3.37, 6.07) and (5.50, 7.97) for never, ex-and current smokers, respectively.

Interestingly, unlike PROC GENMOD in SAS (version 9.3), the GLM routine in Stata, fitting a binomial model to these data, did converge using the default convergence criteria. The results obtained were very similar to those shown in the right side of Table 10.54. Using Stata's XTGEE routine to fit a GEE Poisson model to the same data gave exactly the same results as shown in the right side of Table 10.54.

As a final word on this example, recall that it may not make sense to adjust smoking for some of the variables included here, depending upon the causal pathways envisaged.

In Section 11.10 Poisson regression will be introduced as a way to deal with censoring in follow-up data. It is important to recognise that this is different from GEE Poisson regression. The use of 'simple' Poisson regression models will produce standard errors and p values that are too large when modeling risks.

10.17   Propensity scoring

As was emphasised in Chapter 1, intervention studies are better than cohort studies at investigating causality. In Chapter 7 we saw that the randomised controlled trial (RCT) is the gold standard intervention study design. This is because, when appropriately designed and conducted, the RCT most effectively controls the thorny issues of confounding and bias by randomly allocating the treatment (be it a drug or otherwise) to subjects. In Section 1.8.1, Doll and Hill's historical cohort study of smoking was said to be a necessary alternative to the more desirable intervention study because it was unethical to assign smoking as a randomised treatment. However, suppose we could draw two samples, of smokers and nonsmokers, who were equally likely to have taken up smoking — some chose to do so and some did not, but otherwise they are identical. We follow them up, recording incident events, as in a classical cohort study. In this situation we would have a 'natural experiment', akin to the essential conditions of a RCT. Construction of such a natural experiment is the underlying aim of propensity scoring, a methodology introduced by Rosenbaum and Rubin (1983).

The **propensity score** (PS) is defined to be the probability of exposure (e.g., to smoking) given the observed data on other variables, which we shall refer to as the covariates. Provided we have a valid estimate of the PS, which requires observation of all the appropriate covariates, then anyone with the same PS has an equal chance of being exposed. Four methods for using PSs in epidemiology will first be introduced in broad detail, motivated by a simple example using hypothetical data. Details of how methods should be applied in practice follow later, applied to a more realistic example using real data.

10.17.1   Pair-matched propensity scores

The most intuitive method of using PSs to make inferences is to treat the PS as a matching variable. For instance, suppose we take a set of pairs of smokers and nonsmokers, wherein each member of the pair has the same PS. We then have a natural experiment, similar to a RCT with an equal number in each arm. Analogous to a RCT, this matching is done independently of the outcome provided the 'controls' (the non-exposed) are selected as matches at random. We want matching to be independent of the outcome of interest, because otherwise our estimates of exposure–outcome associations would be biased. This could be achieved with more reliance by carrying out the matching at baseline, before outcome events occur. An added bonus would be that only the matched pairs need then be followed up (or have their records searched in a retrospective cohort study). Provided we use an analytic method that appropriately allows for the matching, we have a study design that, theoretically, is as protected from confounding and bias as the RCT. We shall thus refer to the result from a PS analysis as an estimate of the **causal effect** of the exposure.

Example 10.43 Consider the data of Table 9.24 (reproduced here as Table 10.55, for ease of reference) where the exposure is chilli sauce use and the outcome is systolic blood pressure (SBP). The aim of the study is to determine whether chilli sauce is a potential cause of raised SBP (see Example 9.15). There is only one covariate here: ethnicity. As the table shows, 50% of Mexican Americans (MAs) are chilli sauce users, and hence the PS for MAs is 0.5. Similarly, the PS for Whites is 0.33, and for African Americans (AAs) is 0.2. To define the PS pairs we need to match each exposed person with an unexposed person with the

Table 10.55. Systolic blood pressure (mmHg) for regular users and non-users of a chilli sauce, by ethnicity: data reproduced from Table 9.24.

	Mexican Americans	Whites	African Americans
Chilli sauce	126, 131	128, 130, 123, 137	135, 136, 148, 123
No chilli sauce	118, 128	113, 131, 123, 122, 125, 127, 117, 138	130, 125, 131, 124, 133, 123, 135, 119, 140, 128, 132, 120, 128, 130, 130, 135

Table 10.56. Paired data constructed from Table 10.55. SBP = systolic blood pressure (mmHg).

Pair	1	2	3	4	5	6	7	8	9	10
Propensity score	0.5	0.5	0.33	0.33	0.33	0.33	0.2	0.2	0.2	0.2
Chilli sauce: SBP	126	131	128	130	123	137	135	136	148	123
No chilli sauce: SBP	128	118	125	127	117	138	123	135	119	133
Difference in SBP	−2	13	3	3	6	−1	12	1	29	−10

same PS. Here this simply means finding a match within each ethnic group. Take the first person, a MA with SBP of 126 mmHg. She or he must be matched with a MA who is unexposed: the choices are the persons with SBPs of 118 or 128 mmHg. At random, the person with a SBP of 128 was chosen. Continuing this way, matching by PS within ethnic group, Table 10.56 shows the random matches chosen for each of the ten exposed subjects. To estimate the effect of chilli sauce consumption we find the differences within each pair and average, as in a paired t test. Using the methods of Section 2.7.4, the estimated effect of chilli sauce is to raise SBP by 5.40 mmHg with a standard error of 3.37 mmHg ($p = 0.14$). This estimate is comparable with that obtained from adjustment using modelling in Example 9.15, but the standard error is larger, and the p value consequently less extreme, because of the smaller sample used here.

It is clear that a lot of data have been wasted in Example 10.43 — as is manifested by the comparison of standard errors made at the end of the example. Three further methods of propensity scoring each use all the data, or at least all of the data barring outliers (Section 10.17.6).

10.17.2 Stratified propensity scores

The second PS method we shall consider is to **stratify on the PS**. In Example 10.43 there are three strata defined by the PS — because there is only one covariate in this example, these strata are uniquely defined by ethnicity. Within each strata we take all the available SBP measures and find the difference in means between those exposed and unexposed. Under the basic assumption of propensity scoring, these individuals are all equally likely to have used the chilli sauce and hence the difference in means is an unbiased estimate of the effect of chilli sauce in the particular ethnic group. Averaging over the three estimates gives an overall estimate of the causal effect of the chilli sauce on SBP. Weighted averaging is routinely used, as specified by (10.33) and (10.34); the most intuitive type of weighting is according to the size of the stratum. In our chilli sauce example the outcome of interest is a mean and so the general estimate, $\hat{\theta}_i$, in (10.33) and (10.34) is the ith sample mean. When the outcome is a relative risk it is usual to use (10.33) and (10.34) after a natural log transformation, so that the derivation of an associated confidence interval and significance test can more reasonably invoke a normal approximation (a similar transformation was used in Section 3.1 and Section 10.16.1). The same transformation is usual for several other summary statistics, such as odds ratios and hazard ratios (Chapter 11). In propensity scoring, often the weights in (10.33) and (10.34) are taken to be the stratum sample sizes.

From Table 9.24 we see that the three differences in means are 5.5, 5 and 6.19 mmHg for AM, White and AA groups, respectively. Weighting these by their sample sizes, 4, 12 and 20, respectively, using (10.33) where $k = 3$, gives a result of 5.7153: the estimated causal effect of chilli sauce is to raise SBP by about 5.72 mmHg. The three sample SEs are 5.590, 4.454 and 3.546 mmHg. Using (10.34), the required SE is thus

$$\sqrt{((4 \times 5.590)^2 + (12 \times 4.545)^2 + (20 \times 3.546)^2)/36} = 2.5440 \,\text{mmHg}$$

(using extra decimal places than shown here, for greater accuracy). If desired, a Wald test for a null causal effect of the chilli sauce can be constructed from this: compare $(5.7153/2.5440)^2 = 5.047$ to chi-square with 1 d.f., giving a p value of 0.025.

10.17.3 Weighting by the inverse propensity score

Another method of using the PS to control for confounding is to consider hypothetical, or pseudo, samples that would be expected when all people are exposed to the effect of interest (e.g., chilli sauce) and when all are not. If we construct such pseudo samples in a fair (i.e., unbiased) way then the causal effect of chilli sauce may be estimated as the difference between the mean outcomes in the two pseudo samples. Such a fair construction can be achieved by considering each value of the propensity score separately.

Example 10.44 Consider Whites (PS = 0.33) in Table 10.55. First, think about the pseudo population who are all exposed to chilli sauce. For every White exposed there are two Whites unexposed, according to the PS. In reality there are four exposed Whites, so our pseudo Exposed Whites sample should have the actual four unexposed Whites plus another $2 \times 4 = 8$ Whites who were unexposed in reality, but will be exposed in the pseudo sample. We do not know their real values, because they were never really exposed to chilli sauce. Our best estimate of the outcomes for all these eight is the mean outcome amongst the four Whites who were observed to be exposed. Hence the pseudo Exposed Whites sample consists of the four original values plus eight pseudo copies of the mean of these original four (see the Exposed Whites cell of Table 10.57). Now consider the pseudo Unexposed Whites sample. According to the PS, there is one exposed White for every two unexposed. In reality there are eight unexposed Whites, so our pseudo Unexposed Whites sample should have the actual eight unexposed Whites plus another $(1/2) \times 8 = 4$ Whites who are exposed in reality, but will be unexposed in the pseudo sample. Again, we can never know their true results, but can estimate each of them as the mean of the eight truly unexposed outcomes. Hence the pseudo Unexposed Whites sample consists of the eight original values plus four pseudo values, each of which is the mean of the eight original unexposed values (see the Unexposed Whites cell of Table 10.57).

Similar operations fill in the remainder of Table 10.57. Each of the two pseudo samples (made up of observed and added values) has four MAs, twelve Whites and twenty AAs, as in the real sample. We can then do all the sums in this table and add across the rows to get a sum of outcomes in the Exposed pseudo sample of 4778, and thus a mean effect of 4778/36 = 132.722. In the Unexposed pseudo sample the corresponding mean effect is 4572.25/36 = 127.007. The causal effect of the chilli sauce is thus estimated to be 132.722 − 127.007 = 5.72 mmHg.

Table 10.57 also includes the number of times each true observation appears in each pseudo sample: the weights for the individual observations (not to be confused

Table 10.57. Pseudo samples, and resultant weights, from Table 10.55.

	Mexican Americans (PS = 0.5)	Whites (PS = 0.33)	African Americans (PS = 0.2)
Exposed (to chilli)			
Observed	126, 131	128, 130, 123, 137	135, 136, 148, 123
Added	$2 \times (126 + 131)/2$	$8 \times (128 + 130 + 123 + 137)/4$	$16 \times (135 + 136 + 148 + 123)/4$
Total weight[a]	2	3	5
Unexposed (no chilli)			
Observed	118, 128	113, 131, 123, 122, 125, 127, 117, 138	130, 125, 131, 124, 133, 123, 135, 119, 140, 128, 132, 126, 128, 130, 130, 135
Added	$2 \times (118 + 131)/2$	$4 \times (113 + \cdots + 138)/8$	$4 \times (130 + \cdots + 135)/16$
Total weight[a]	2	1.5	1.25

[a] Number of times each true observation in the exposure/ethnicity cross-class contributes to the pseudo sample.

PS = propensity score

with the weights for the means in stratified propensity scores). These weights must be the same for each person with the same PS and using these weights simplifies the arithmetic used in estimation. Furthermore, a little thought, and some mental arithmetic, shows that the weight given to each exposed person in the real data is 1/PS and the weight given to each unexposed person is 1/(1 − PS). In general this will be the case, and thus the method of estimation described here is called **inverse propensity score weighting**. This may be conveniently applied using weighted regression, which is routinely available in all statistical software packages (e.g., by adding a WEIGHT option to PROC REG in SAS). Fitting the weighted regression of SBP on chilli sauce use (coded 0 for no and 1 for yes) in PROC REG gave the estimate 5.72 (as above) with a SE of 2.47 ($p = 0.03$). Since estimates are derived from what would be expected if the opposite exposure to that observed had pertained, the method used here is termed **counterfactual**.

10.17.4 Adjusting for the propensity score

The easiest method of using the PS to obtain an estimate of the causal effect of exposure is to fit a regression model that predicts the outcome from the PS and the exposure. This PS method mimics the classical method of adjustment by regression; the only difference is that the effect of many confounders is considered to be subsumed within the solitary variable that is the PS. In our running example, using PROC REG with chilli sauce use (CHILLI) coded, again, as 0 for no and 1 for yes, the fitted model was

$$\text{SBP} = 134.172 + (-25.845)(\text{PS}) + 5.626(\text{CHILLI}).$$

The estimated causal effect of chilli sauce is thus 5.63. The corresponding SE reported by SAS was 2.44, for a p value of 0.03.

10.17.5   Deriving the propensity score

Except in simple situations, such as Example 10.43, the usual method for estimating the PS is via logistic regression (which explains why the subject is included in this chapter), although other approaches are possible. The basic idea is to regress the logit of exposure on covariates and then use (10.8) to estimate the probability of exposure. The set of covariates should include all confounding variables, including (if necessary) their interactions; otherwise, estimates of causal effects will be biased. Additionally, inclusion of covariates only related to outcome, not exposure, is expected to be beneficial because this should reduce the variance of the final estimate of the causal effect of exposure. Inclusion of variables only related to exposure, not outcome, is expected to have the opposite effect.

Of course, in practice we can only adjust for what has actually been measured or, more precisely, what we can measure before we need to find the PS. Also, we are clearly limited in our knowledge of what is a confounder in any given situation. Expert advice can ameliorate the latter problem, but experts are not infallible. This is the inherent weakness in a PS analysis (as it is in classical adjustment for confounders by regression), compared to a RCT which is virtually guaranteed, with large numbers, to not only balance known confounding variables but also unknown confounders.

Example 10.45 Suppose we wish to determine whether heavy drinking (of alcohol) appears to be a causal factor for cancer. Although different relationships with alcohol would be anticipated for different cancer sites (breast, stomach, etc.), in this example we shall take all sites together. The web site for this book contains data for all men (excluding those with missing values) in the Scottish Heart Health Study (SHHS), using a longer follow-up (median of almost 24 years) than in previous examples. Table 10.58 shows the basic data. Heavy drinking was defined as an intake above 20g per day, as estimated from a food frequency questionnaire (see Bolton–Smith *et al.*, 1991). Three other variables are included in this dataset: age, cigarette smoking status (yes/no) and social status (measured using a continuous variable, specific to Scotland, called the Scottish Index of Multiple Deprivation (SIMD), which decreases with increasing social deprivation). These can be assumed, for the sake of this example, to be the three sole confounding variables in the alcohol–cancer relationship.

Propensity scores were estimated using PROC LOGISTIC in SAS, regressing the logit for being a heavy drinker on age, smoking and SIMD score. The fitted model was

$$\hat{\text{logit}} = 1.1012 + (-0.0391)(\text{AGE}) + 0.0137(\text{SIMD}) + 0.3329(\text{SMOKER}),$$

where SMOKER = 1 for current smokers and 0 otherwise. The estimated probability of being a heavy drinker (the PS) may be derived from this estimated logit, for each person, using (10.8) — which SAS can be asked to apply automatically. The mean PS was 0.399; the minimum, median and maximum values were 0.226, 0.389 and 0.731, respectively.

Table 10.58. Heavy drinking related to cancer in the SHHS

Heavy drinker at entry?	Cancer death during follow-up?			Risk
	Yes	No	Total	
Yes	280	1730	2010	0.139
No	382	2652	3034	0.126
Total	662	4382	5044	0.131

10.17.6 Propensity score outliers

For the PS method to be a valid approach to assessing causality, each subject must have some chance of exposure and some chance of non-exposure. However, it is not inconceivable that, in any particular population, some people may never have the chance of being exposed to some particular factor (for example, practicing Catholics and birth control) and some may never have the chance to avoid exposure. The obvious thing to do in these situations is to remove these people from the analysis. More generally, in PS analyses it is usual to exclude anyone who lies outside the overlapping ranges of the two PS distributions: the **PS outliers**. The remaining sample is said to be in **common support**. If the matching design of Section 10.16.1 is adopted it will not even be possible to find a match for PS outliers in the exposure group — similarly, PS outliers in the unexposed group will never be chosen as a match — and hence exclusions are inevitable. Naturally, such exclusions have implications for the generality of the inferences that can be made from the study.

10.17.7 Conduct of the matched design

Should the matched design be adopted, in practice it will often not be appropriate to match on exact PS values because the PS distribution will be too sparse. In this situation, subjects should be matched as closely as possible. Often 'close' matching is done sequentially: the first exposed subject to be matched is chosen at random, as are subsequent exposed subjects until all have been considered. At each stage, matches are chosen from amongst all remaining (unmatched) unexposed subjects — although matching with replacement is sometimes used. This one-by-one approach to matching ignores the fact that a match found at any particular stage might be more closely matched by an exposed subject considered at a later stage. Hence this approach is called **greedy matching**.

Two greedy matching algorithms are popular. The **caliper method** requires pre-specification of the maximum distance (the 'caliper width'), between the PS of the exposed person and her or his match, that will be allowed. Austin (2011) suggests using a caliper width of 0.2 standard deviations of the logit of the PS. For each exposed person in turn, we can either take the first match we find (within the specified caliper width) or take the best possible: that with the smallest difference in PS from the index exposed subject (called the **nearest neighbour**). The other most popular scheme is the $k \to 1$ **digit matching method** (see Austin, 2007), which is most easily described by example. Suppose we choose k to be five. For each exposed person in turn, we then first try to match this exposed subject to an unexposed subject on the first five decimals (remember that the PS is a probability and thus lies between 0 and 1): e.g., 0.1543498761 and 0.154340986 match on the first five decimals. If no match is found then we try to match on the first four decimals, etc. as far as $k = 1$. With both of these matching schemes we can end up with no match, in which case the exposed person is dropped from the analysis.

Several other methods have been suggested, including some that find the nearest neighbour match for all exposed subjects (with no maximum threshold imposed on the level of agreement) and some that seek to obtain an overall best match, such as by minimising the overall average difference between the PS of exposed subjects and their matches. Also, instead of picking one unexposed subject per exposed subject, we could expand the overall sample size of our study by taking multiple 'controls' for each exposure, thus producing PS-matched sets rather than pairs (one set for each exposed person). However, Austin (2010) recommends using either 1 : 1 or 1 : 2 matching, because when more matches are sought the increased bias caused by increased lack of agreement in PS between the exposed and unexposed subjects tends to outweigh the decreased variance of estimates arising from using more subjects. Several authors have written routines to carry out matching in SAS, Stata and other packages. For example, the PSMATCH2 routine in Stata, available for download by itself and incorporated in the TEFFECTS command in base Stata, allows use of several matching schemes.

Once the matches have been established, we should compare the exposed and unexposed groups in the matched dataset (which will typically be much smaller than the original dataset) for balance in each of the covariates. This is an essential step before analyses begin, to ensure that any important systematic differences between the two groups has been removed, at least as far as we can ascertain from the available data. Although imbalance in any covariate within specific matched pairs, or sets, is to be expected, exposed and unexposed people should be similar in distribution for all covariates, as in a large RCT.

Checking for balance in covariates can be done in several ways. The simplest is a comparison of average values (or percentages for binary variables, or relative frequencies for categorical variables) between the exposed and unexposed subjects. Austin (2009) suggests computing the effect size (see Section 13.4.4) to provide a summary comparison, further suggesting that an effect size of over 10% should be viewed as problematic. More comprehensive comparisons are better; for instance we might compare the five-number and/or two-number summaries (see Chapter 2). Graphical displays, such as boxplots or quantile–quantile plots, are especially useful. Since we would also expect the relationships between covariates to be similar in both the groups, we might also compare pairwise correlations between those exposed and unexposed. See Austin (2009) for further suggestions.

Just as with a RCT, exact balance in all covariates is not guaranteed even with the best matching scheme; chance imbalances can occur, and are more likely to be important in small samples. Our discussion of balance so far has assumed that a matched design has been adopted, but similar issues ensue when a stratified PS design is used. We then seek balance in covariate distributions within each stratum. In this case we can only expect to find reasonable balance when the strata are large. This requires a reasonably large sample size overall, as well as no one stratum being extremely small. In order to spread the sample size evenly, strata are often defined using percentiles, typically the quintiles, of the PS distribution. When acceptable balance has not been achieved, we might try an alternative matching, or stratification, scheme or a *post-hoc* adjustment in a regression model used to estimate the causal effect of exposure.

10.17.8   Analysis of the matched design

Propensity scores naturally arise in cohort studies, so that when the matched PS study design is used we need to consider how to analyse matched cohort studies. If the outcome variable in the study is quantitative, the paired t test, as used in Example 10.43, is the obvious method of choice. If the outcome variable is non-normal, the one-sample Wilcoxon test, applied to within-pair differences, might be used instead.

Binary outcomes (the subject of this chapter) require further consideration. In Section 6.6.1 we considered pair-matched case–control studies. If we envisage making inferences about an odds ratio, the methods of Section 6.6.1 can be used directly, taking 'case' status as a positive outcome and 'control' as negative (e.g., d_1 in Table 6.10 is the number of pairs in which the exposed person has experienced an event but her or his unexposed partner has not). To clarify this, Table 10.59 reproduces Table 6.10 with

Table 10.59. Display of results from a paired cohort study.

Exposed subject has an event?	Unexposed subject has an event?	
	Yes	No
Yes	c_1	d_1
No	d_2	c_2

labels appropriate to cohort studies. However, there are theoretical problems with the use of an odds ratio in the current context, concerning the different results that are found when using the so-called **marginal** method of analysis used in Section 6.6.1 and a so-called **conditional**, or **population-averaged** analysis which deals directly with individual pairs, rather than the summary table across all pairs, Table 10.59. This problem, called a lack of **collapsibility**, is well illustrated by Agresti and Min (2004). So, some authors consider that it is better to use relative risks, or risk differences, which (like the paired difference in means) exhibit the property of collapsibility. Using the notation of Table 10.59, from first principles (see Section 3.1), the estimated risk of an event amongst the exposed is the number of exposed people who have an event divided by the number of exposed people, $(c_1 + d_1)/n$, where n is the total number of exposed people, which must also be the number of unexposed people and the number of pairs, since $1:1$ matching is applied. Hence $n = c_1 + c_2 + d_1 + d_2$. Similarly, the estimated risk of an event amongst the unexposed is $(c_1 + d_2)/n$. Thus the estimated relative risk in a paired cohort study, exposed versus unexposed, is

$$\hat{\lambda} = (c_1 + d_1)/(c_1 + d_2) \tag{10.37}$$

and the corresponding estimated risk difference is $(d_1 - d_2)/n$. Agresti and Min (2004) give the variance of $\log_e \hat{\lambda}$ as

$$\frac{d}{(c_1 + d_2)(c_1 + d_1)}, \tag{10.38}$$

and the variance of the risk difference as

$$\frac{d - ((d_1 - d_2)^2/n)}{n^2},$$

where $d = d_1 + d_2$, the total number of discordant pairs, as in Section 6.6.1.

If the matching is done on a $1:$ many basis, a straightforward analytic approach would be to use a generalised estimating equation model, taking the matched set as the panel variable. If the outcome is survival time, Austin (2008) recommends using stratified (on match pairs or sets) Cox models (Chapter 11). These modelling approaches also allow us to carry out adjustments, just as with standard regression modelling, should this be desired — perhaps to allow for a variable that was omitted from the PS.

10.17.9 Case studies

Case studies which address the issues covered in the last few pages are provided by Austin and Mamdani (2006) and Willamson et al. (2012). A case study based on Example 10.45 follows.

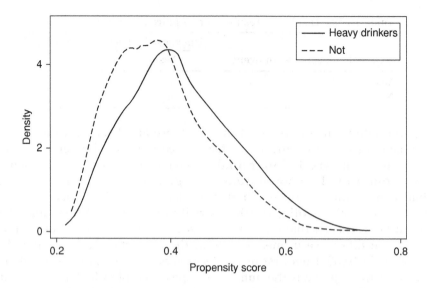

Figure 10.15. Kernel density plots of propensity scores by heavy drinking status.

Example 10.46 Consider estimating the association between heavy drinking and cancer using the data introduced in Example 10.45, wherein the PSs were estimated. From Table 10.58 we see that, partially because of the long follow-up, cancer deaths are not rare and hence the odds ratio cannot necessarily be expected to provide a good estimate of the relative risk here (although, because the two risks are similar, in this example the overall unadjusted odds ratio, 1.12, turns out to be virtually the same as the relative risk, 1.11). For this reason, as well as the theoretical issue concerned with odds ratios mentioned in Section 10.17.8, analyses will be based on binomial regression. First, classical regression analyses were run, to provide a benchmark comparison. Using PROC GENMOD is SAS, the relative risks (95% confidence intervals) for cancer, heavy drinkers versus not, were 1.11 (0.96, 1.28); $p = 0.17$ (unadjusted) and 1.16 (1.00, 1.33); $p = 0.04$ (adjusted for age, smoking and SIMD).

Next, a simple $5 \rightarrow 1$ greedy digit matching algorithm (using SAS code from Parsons, 2001) was employed to try to find a match for each of the 2010 heavy drinkers. Suitable matches were found for 1944. Figure 10.15 shows the PS distributions for heavy drinkers and their PS-matched non-heavy drinkers. There is a small non-overlapping range and hence the issue of PS outliers is unlikely to be important here. Table 10.60 shows the agreement between the three covariates in the whole sample and in the matched sample; Figure 10.16 illustrates the SIMD score, as an example of how such comparisons may be presented. Although not perfect, the agreement between those who are, and are not, heavy drinkers is, as would be anticipated, much better in the matched sample.

Table 10.60. Summary statistics for all men in the SHHS and in the PS-matched sample, by heavy drinking status (values for n are: heavy drinkers/not).

Covariate	Drinking	All ($n = 2010/3034$)	Matched ($n = 1944/1944$)
Age (years): mean (SD)	Heavy	49.00 (5.72)	49.17 (5.70)
	Not	50.29 (5.79)	49.14 (5.75)
SIMD score: mean (SD)	Heavy	24.65 (19.1)	23.43 (18.0)
	Not	20.08 (15.9)	23.03 (17.5)
Smoker: %	Heavy	44.43	42.95
	Not	33.85	43.11

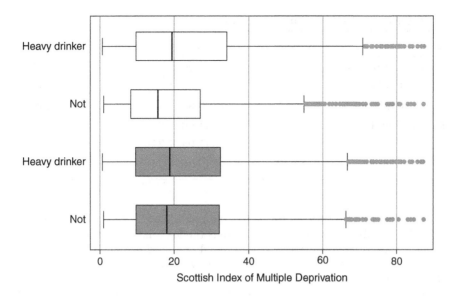

Figure 10.16. Boxplots for the Scottish Index of Multiple Deprivation by heavy drinking status. The transparent boxes are for the original, full, dataset ($n = 5044$) and the filled boxes are for the PS-matched sample ($n = 3888$).

Table 10.61 shows the results for the pair-matched PS design. Applying (10.37) to this table gives an estimated relative risk of 1.1695; applying (10.38) gives an estimated variance of the log relative risk of 0.00697. The 95% confidence limit for the relative risk is thus $\exp(\log_e(1.1695) \pm 1.96 \times \sqrt{0.00697}) = (0.99, 1.38)$, similar to the results from adjusted regression analysis. For a Wald test of no causal effect of heavy drinking, the test statistic is $\{\log_e(1.1695)\}^2/0.00697 = 3.52$, giving a p value of 0.06.

Next, the PSs were divided into their equal fifths. Table 10.62 shows the results from applying PROC GENMOD to fit the binomial model with heavy drinking (yes/no) as the sole explanatory

Table 10.61. Results for a pair-matched analysis: Example 10.46.

Heavy drinker dies from cancer?	Non-heavy drinker dies from cancer?	
	Yes	No
Yes	29	247
No	207	1461

Table 10.62. Results by strata and interim totals for stratified PS analysis. RR = relative risk; SE = standard error.

Stratum (fifth)	log RR	SE	Events	n	$n \times$ log RR	$(n \times$ SE$)^2$
1	−0.0244	0.1589	165	1008	−24.5952	25654.81
2	0.2714	0.1626	135	1009	273.8426	26916.80
3	0.2016	0.1763	115	1009	203.4144	31643.68
4	0.2103	0.1755	115	1009	212.1927	31357.15
5	0.0506	0.1628	132	1009	51.0554	26983.06
Total			662	5044	715.9099	142555.50

Table 10.63. Full set of results for Example 10.46.

Method	Relative risk (95% confidence interval)	p value
Unadjusted regression	1.11 (0.96, 1.28)	0.17
Adjusted regression	1.16 (1.00, 1.33)	0.04
Pair-matched by PS	1.17 (0.99, 1.38)	0.06
Stratified by PS	1.15 (1.00, 1.33)	0.06
Weighted by inverse PS	1.15 (1.04, 1.27)	0.007
Adjusted for PS	1.15 (0.99, 1.33)	0.06

variable, separately in each fifth. Substituting the results into (10.33) and (10.34), where the weight, w, is the sample size, n, and the estimate is the log relative risk, per stratum, gives an estimated log relative risk of 0.1419 with estimated standard error of 0.0749. The estimated relative risk (95% confidence interval) and p value for a test of no effect then follow as 1.15 (1.00, 1.33) and 0.06, respectively.

To complete the full set of results, presented in Table 10.63, an inverse-PS weighted binomial model and a PS-adjusted binomial model for heavy drinking were each fitted. Clearly, all methods that deal with controlling for the covariates give similar answers, even if they do not always stay on the same side of the conventional 5% threshold for significance.

A clear drawback of the matching approach is that different matching algorithms are likely to give different results. For example, the algorithm used in Example 10.46 only identified matches for 1944 heavy drinkers. An alternative algorithm that finds the closest match (in the PS) for all 2010 heavy drinkers might be preferred.

To explore this, the PSMATCH2 routine was run in Stata (the program used is available from the web site for this book) to select nearest neighbour matches for all heavy drinkers in Example 10.46. Using (10.37) and (10.38), the estimated causal effect of heavy drinking (with 95% confidence interval) was 1.14 (0.97, 1.34). Compared to the pair-matched result in Table 10.63, this confidence interval is, as anticipated (because n is bigger), slightly narrower. On the other hand, the mean absolute (i.e., ignoring the sign) difference in PSs in the 2010 pairs is 0.0093; the maximum absolute difference is 0.304, which indicates a particularly poor match. Amongst the 1944 pairs used in Example 10.46, the mean absolute difference was only 0.0012, with a maximum of 0.082. Hence the smaller relative risk, 1.14, from the nearest neighbour matches, compared to the 1.17 from the $5 \rightarrow 1$ digit match, 1.17, shown in Table 10.63 may reflect greater bias in the former.

10.17.10 Interpretation of effects

So far we have taken it for granted that each of the four PS methods, as introduced, estimate the same causal effect (of exposure). In fact, they do not. In most cases, one of two causal effects is likely to be of interest: the effect of the exposure overall or the effect of the exposure amongst those exposed. Taking the paradigm of a hypothetical alternative population with different exposures — the counterfactual idea — underlying the idea of propensity scoring, the former is the difference between the expected outcome if everyone was exposed and the expected outcome if everyone was unexposed, called the **average treatment effect (ATE)** by many authors (although 'exposure' is a more general term than 'treated'). The latter is the difference between the observed mean outcome and the expected outcome if all were unexposed within the sub-population that is really exposed, called the **average treatment effect amongst the treated (ATT)**. A third causal effect, that of exposure amongst those unexposed is defined similarly, and called the **average treatment effect amongst the untreated (ATU)**, but is rarely of interest. The three causal effects may differ and whichever should be estimated depends on the aim of the study. The PSMATCH2 routine in Stata finds the ATT (for mean or risk differences) by default, but can alternatively be programmed to produce each of the other two causal effects.

Of the four PS methods, as they were introduced and used in the examples here, the matching method estimates the ATT, the stratification and inverse weighing methods estimate the ATE and the adjustment method estimates neither. The inverse-weighting method is the easiest to explain, since this was derived here using a counterfactual argument wherein both exposed and unexposed people had a counter-factual and thus it must be that the ATE was estimated: recall that the weights derived were 1/PS and 1/(1 − PS) for the exposed and unexposed, respectively. If we gave a weight of unity to those exposed (to treat those people as observed) and gave a weight to unexposed people of PS/(1 − PS), we would estimate the ATT; if we gave a weight to the unexposed of unity and gave a weight of (1 − PS)/PS to the exposed, we would estimate the ATU. The stratification method, as introduced here, estimates the ATE because the strata are weighted by the number of subjects within them; if we weighted by the number of exposed subjects in the strata we would estimate the ATT; if we weighted by the number of unexposed subjects we would estimate the ATU. The matching method, again as introduced here, estimates the ATT because a match is found for each exposed person from amongst the unexposed; if a match were found for each unexposed person from those exposed then the ATU would be estimated; if a match were found for everyone, the ATE would be estimated. To use the adjustment method to estimate the three specific causal effects we need to add a PS by exposure interaction term to the regression model. ATE, ATT and ATU then follow from finding the effect of exposure at the mean value of the PS, the mean value of the PS amongst those exposed and the mean value of the PS amongst those not exposed, respectively. See Williamson *et al.* (2012) for more details.

10.17.11 Problems with estimating uncertainty

In the computations for Example 10.45 it was assumed that the PS is a fixed quantity. Of course, this is not true: the PS values were obtained from a logistic model in Example 10.45, and thus are subject to random error. To obtain a precise estimate of the standard error of a causal effect we need to take this into account. One way of doing this is to use bootstrapping (see Chapter 14), which may be used in conjuction with many commands in Stata.

10.17.12 Propensity scores in practice

Here, four methods for estimating causal effects have been presented. At the time of writing, there is no clear best method of the four, whilst research into better methods proceeds. In the two examples we have considered, all four PS methods give similar results to classical adjustment methods using regression. This is in line with most reports in the literature; for example, Stürmer *et al.* (2006) found that only 9 of 69 comparisons of PS methods with classical regression adjustment, when estimating the same exposure effect, were importantly different. So why should PS methods be useful?

First, consider a comparison with RCTs. Repeating what has already been said, PS methods are a direct alternative to the RCT whenever the latter is unethical or infeasible.

Most applications of PS methods involve retrospective use of large databases already in existence, such as medical insurance databases or other routinely collected data. Then the PS approach will save time and money, compared to a RCT. An example is the comparison of the risk of cardiovascular disease when taking two different medications for glycaemic control, amongst subjects with diabetes, by Roumie *et al.* (2012). The authors conducted a 1 : 1 matched PS design by utilizing existing US Veterans Health Administration databases, which hold data on exposure and covariates, linked to Medicare files, which hold data on events, including cardiovascular disease. To run a comparable RCT would cost hundreds of millions of dollars and likely require at least five years of prospective follow-up. Another advantage of the PS method over the RCT is its avoidance of the issue of generalisability which is often in question with an RCT because of its inclusion and exclusion criteria (Section 7.1.2). On the other hand, RCTs and PS-based observational studies may produce different results, for the same question, and it may not be clear why. For instance, Dahabreh *et al.* (2012) compared results from studies that used PS and RCT designs for the same 17 therapeutic interventions for acute coronary syndromes and found that, for the majority of the interventions, the PS designs estimated a more extreme benefit. Perhaps differences are due to the greater generalisability of the PS design (e.g., the RCTs tended to underestimate benefit because they omitted very sick patients), or perhaps the PS designs were poorly conducted (e.g., they tended to omit important covariates and this led to an overall overestimate of benefit). If the PS design is well conducted and analysed, with all confounders accounted for, the PS design may even be more reliable than the RCT for general application; but a key limitation is that we can virtually never be sure that all confounders *have* been considered.

Second, consider a comparison of the PS method with adjustment by regression. The PS approach has a clear advantage when there are many variables that we wish to control for, but the sample size, or number of events observed, is not large. Although there are no hard and fast rules, it has been suggested that the number of variables that are included in a multiple regression model for continuous outcomes should not be more than a tenth of the sample size, and for binary event outcomes, not more than a tenth of the number of events. If not, then some regressors (i.e., covariates in the current context) need to be dropped. Propensity scoring effectively reduces a set of covariates to a single variable, the PS, and thus circumvents any problem in this regard. Another advantage of the propensity scoring approach is that the 'adjustment model' (i.e., the covariate selection) is determined without reference to the outcomes, and hence is not as susceptible to bias as would be a classical regression study where certain covariates might be thrown out of the final adjusted model because the results are not in line with expectation. Indeed, the PSs can be computed at baseline, before any outcomes are available. The propensity scoring approach may also reasonably be claimed to be less susceptible to model misspecification than a classical regression approach; although the PS itself is the result of a modelling process we have easy ways of checking whether balance in covariates has been achieved, and it essentially doesn't matter how we arrived at this balance. Finally, the propensity scoring approach is designed to focus specifically on a particular exposure from the point of view of an experiment, which focuses attention on such issues as the relative make-up of those unexposed and exposed, including issues of overall balance and whether ranges coincide. Such issues are generally forsaken in regression modelling. Nevertheless, applied results from PS analyses are often presented alongside traditional analyses using regression adjustment for confirmatory purposes; for example in the study previously mentioned by Roumie *et al.* (2012), which found similar results using both methods.

Further reading on propensity scoring might usefully focus on the overview given by Williamson *et al.* (2012), which has been a model for some of the preceding text, and the textbook by Guo and Fraser (2010), which covers applications in Stata. The web site http://www.biostat.jhsph.edu/~estuart/propensityscoresoftware.html has an inventory of software that can be used in propensity scoring.

Exercises

(Most of these exercises require a computer package with appropriate procedures.)

10.1   For the data of Exercise 3.1, find the odds of cardiovascular death for binge beer drinkers and for nonbingers, and the odds ratio comparing the former to the latter, using a logistic regression model. Also, find 95% confidence limits for the odds ratio and test the null hypothesis that the odds ratio is unity. Compare your results with those in Exercise 3.1.

10.2   A 12-year study of coronary heart disease (CHD) collected data from men aged 35 to 54 years. Five variables are available for analysis: CHD outcome (yes/no); age group (35–39/40–44/45–49/50–54 years); diastolic blood pressure (mmHg); serum total cholesterol (mmol/l); cigarette smoking status (never/current/ex). When a logistic regression model was fitted to these data, with CHD as the outcome variable, the following parameter estimates were found:

Effect	Estimate
Constant (intercept)	−5.777
Age 35–39	0
Age 40–44	1.102
Age 45–49	1.275
Age 50–54	2.070
Diastolic blood pressure	−0.0006598
Serum total cholesterol	0.2414
Never smoked	0
Current smoker	1.190
Ex-smoker	0.7942
Age 40–44*current smoker	−0.4746
Age 40–44*ex-smoker	−0.7009
Age 45–49*current smoker	−0.2109
Age 45–49*ex-smoker	0.4739
Age 50–54*current smoker	−0.6831
Age 50–54*ex-smoker	0.06005

Note: * denotes an interaction.

(i)   Which levels of the two categorical explanatory variables have been fixed as the base, or reference, levels?

(ii)   From the fitted model, estimate the odds ratio of CHD for a man aged 47 who currently smokes cigarettes compared with a man of the same age who has never smoked cigarettes.

(iii) From the fitted model, estimate the probability that a man aged 47 who currently smokes cigarettes, has a diastolic blood pressure of 90 mmHg and a serum total cholesterol level of 6.20 mmol/l will develop CHD within 12 years.

10.3   In a survey of the prevalence of asthma in schoolchildren, Strachan (1988) calculated a bronchial liability index as the forced expiratory volume in 1 second after exercise divided by that before exercise. Results for the liability index, classified by whether mould was in the child's room, were presented as ratios of number with wheeze in the past year divided by total number of children, as follows.

Liability index	No mould	Mould
<0.8	17/35	3/5
0.8–0.89	7/63	4/9
0.9–0.99	34/383	10/30
≥1.0	20/303	5/34

Using logistic regression models,

(i) Ignoring liability index altogether, find an odds ratio for mould compared with no mould, together with a 95% confidence interval.

(ii) Confirm that mould and liability index do not interact in their effect upon asthma.

(iii) Find the odds ratio for mould compared with no mould, together with a 95% confidence interval, adjusting for liability index. Compare your answer with that in (i). Interpret the result.

(iv) Find odds ratios for the liability index groups, taking the '<0.8' group as base, adjusting for mould status. Give 95% confidence limits in each case.

(v) Test whether there appears to be a linear effect across the four liability groups, adjusting for mould status. Estimate and interpret the linear effect. Give a 95% confidence interval for the estimate.

10.4 Refer to the data in Table C.1 (see Appendix C). In the following, use logistic regression models.

(i) Find prevalence risks, odds, relative risk and odds ratio (high versus low) by factor IX status for each sex group. Give 95% confidence intervals for the odds ratios. Test for an association between factor IX and cardiovascular disease (CVD) for each sex separately using model deviances. Compare your answers with those for Exercise 3.4.

(ii) Find an age-adjusted, a sex-adjusted and an age/sex-adjusted odds ratio for high versus low factor IX status. Compare your results with those for Exercise 4.7.

(iii) Test for a sex by factor IX, and an age group by factor IX, interaction. Compare your answers with those for Exercise 4.7.

(iv) Check whether there is a three-way interaction between sex, age group and factor IX status in predicting CVD.

10.5 Swan (1986) gives the following data from a study of infant respiratory disease. Each cell of the table shows the number out of so many observed children who developed bronchitis or pneumonia in their first year of life, classified by sex and type of feeding (with the risk in parentheses).

Sex	Bottle only	Breast + supplement	Breast only
Boys	77/458 (0.17)	19/147 (0.13)	47/494 (0.10)
Girls	48/384 (0.13)	16/127 (0.13)	31/464 (0.07)

The major question of interest is whether the risk of illness is affected by the type of feeding. Also, is the risk the same for both sexes and, if there are differences between the feeding groups, are they the same for boys and girls?

(i)   Fit all possible linear logistic regression models to the data. Use your
        results to answer all the preceding questions through significance testing.
        Summarize your findings using odds ratios with 95% confidence intervals.
(ii)   Fit the model with explanatory variables sex and type of feeding (but
        no interaction). Calculate the residuals, deviance residuals and stan-
        dardised deviance residuals and comment on the results.

10.6   Saetta *et al.* (1991) carried out a prospective, single-blind experiment to
        determine whether gastric content is forced into the small bowel when gas-
        tric-emptying procedures are employed with people who have poisoned them-
        selves. Each of 60 subjects was asked to swallow 20 barium-impregnated
        polythene pellets. Of the 60, 20 received a gastric lavage, 20 received induced
        emesis and 20 (controls) received no gastric decontamination. The number
        of residual pellets, counted by x-ray, in the intestine after ingestion for each
        subject was, for the induced emesis group:

$$0, 15, 2, 0, 0, 15, 1, 16, 0, 1, 1, 0, 6, 0, 0, 1, 0, 16, 7, 11;$$

for the gastric lavage group:

$$9, 3, 4, 15, 3, 5, 0, 0, 2, 11, 0, 0, 0, 0, 7, 5, 9, 0, 0, 0;$$

and for the control group:

$$0, 9, 0, 0, 4, 5, 0, 0, 13, 0, 0, 12, 0, 0, 1, 0, 4, 4, 6, 7.$$

(i)   Is there a significant difference between treatment groups?
(ii)   Is the control group significantly different from the other two?

10.7   A cohort study has been carried out to investigate the supposed health benefits
        of consuming antioxidant vitamins. A large number of men were studied: at
        baseline their daily antioxidant vitamin consumption (denoted AOX in the
        following tables) was categorised as 1 = low; 2 = medium; 3 = high. Also, at
        baseline, their daily alcohol consumption (ALC: 1 = none; 2 = occasional
        drinker; 3 = moderate drinker; 4 = heavy drinker) and smoking status (SMO:
        1 = nonsmoker; 2 = current smoker) were recorded. Over a 10-year follow-up
        period, each death amongst the cohort was recorded. Logistic regression anal-
        ysis was used to analyse the data.

(i)   When the following sets of explanatory variables were fitted using a
        computer package, the following deviances were found:

Terms fitted	Deviance
Constant only	309.62
AOX	211.38
SMO	227.43
ALC	270.01
AOX + SMO	173.28
AOX + ALC	195.53
AOX + SMO + ALC	171.84
AOX + SMO + AOX*SMO	144.09

Notes: * denotes an interaction. All models
include a constant term (intercept).

Write a report to describe the findings, including a table to show the results of appropriate significance tests. Would you suggest any other models be fitted? If so, state which models and what you would hope to discover by fitting them.

(ii)   When the last model in the preceding table was fitted, the package also produced the estimates and estimated variance–covariance matrix shown next. Here the package has been forced to take AOX = 1 and SMO = 1 as the reference groups for antioxidants and smoking, respectively. The number in parentheses denotes the level of the variable. The parameters corresponding to the first level must be zero.

Estimates

Parameter	Estimate	Standard error
Constant	−2.38	0.16
AOX(2)	−0.37	0.22
AOX(3)	−0.91	0.34
SMO(2)	1.19	0.18
AOX(2)*SMO(2)	−0.31	0.37
AOX(3)*SMO(2)	−0.94	0.38

Variance–covariance matrix

	Constant	AOX(2)	AOX(3)	SMO(2)	AOX(2)*SMO(2)	AOX(3)*SMO(2)
Constant	0.026					
AOX(2)	−0.041	0.048				
AOX(3)	−0.052	0.017	0.116			
SMO(2)	−0.080	0.038	0.041	0.032		
AOX(2)*SMO(2)	−0.011	0.057	0.059	0.064	0.137	
AOX(3)*SMO(2)	−0.003	0.043	0.071	0.019	−0.008	0.144

Estimate the odds ratios, and find the corresponding 95% confidence limits, for antioxidant vitamin consumption, using low consumption as the base, for smokers and nonsmokers separately.

10.8   A researcher has carried out a case–control study of risk factors for leukaemia amongst children. He has been told, by a colleague, that he should be using logistic regression to analyse his data. He remembers, from his days at medical school, how to calculate chi-square significance tests and relative risks from contingency tables, and he has done this for all the variables (potential risk factors) in his dataset (both continuous and categorical). He comes to you for help, and asks two questions:

(i)   'What is the advantage of using logistic regression rather than simple chi-square tests and relative risks?'

(ii)   'How can I interpret the results of a logistic regression analysis obtained from the SAS package?'

How would you answer these questions?

10.9   Heinrich et al. (1994) describe a study of the effects of fibrinogen on CHD in which healthy men aged 40 to 65 were followed up for 6 years. In the paper, the ratio of CHD events to total numbers is given for subgroups defined by equal thirds of fibrinogen and LDL cholesterol, one of several other variables measured in the study that may affect the fibrinogen–CHD relationship. These ratios are presented here (taking account of a revision subsequent to initial publication).

Fibrinogen third	LDL cholesterol third		
	Lowest	Middle	Highest
Lowest	5/263	3/215	9/186
Middle	5/230	6/219	14/213
Highest	3/178	8/217	27/262

Analyse the data and write a short report of your findings so as to address the study aim.

10.10 Repeat the analysis of Exercise 6.1, the unmatched case–control study of oral contraceptive use and breast cancer, using logistic regression modelling. Compare results.

10.11 Repeat the analysis of Example 6.4, the unmatched case–control study of ethnicity and *E. coli*, using logistic regression modelling. Compare results.

10.12 Repeat the analysis of Example 6.9, the 1 : 5 matched case–control study of BCG vaccination and tuberculosis, using logistic regression modelling. Compare results.

10.13 Refer to the venous thromboembolism matched case–control study of Exercise 6.12.

(i) Use logistic regression to repeat the analysis of Exercise 6.12. Compare results.

(ii) The associated dataset also includes data on body mass index (BMI), a potential confounding factor in the relationship between HRT and venous thromboembolism. Test for a significant effect of HRT on venous thromboembolism, adjusting for BMI. Estimate the odds ratio for HRT users versus nonusers, adjusting for BMI. Does BMI appear to have a strong confounding effect?

10.14 A colleague plans to undertake a study to investigate the risk factors for Creutzfeldt–Jakob disease, which is a very rare disease. He comes to you to seek advice before he begins data collection. What follows is a series of questions that he asks you. In each case, you should answer the question and provide a brief justification of your answer.

(i) 'I plan to do a case–control study. Is this a suitable choice of design? If not, what should I do instead?'

(ii) 'I am considering calculating a series of relative risks for each risk factor I measure. Is this sensible? If not, what should I do instead?'

(iii) 'I am pretty sure that an individual's age affects his chance of having Creutzfeldt–Jakob disease, and age is related to several of the risk factors in which I am interested. Thus, I was thinking of doing separate analyses for each age group. The only problem is that the numbers are likely to get rather small. What can I do to avoid this problem?'

(iv) 'I suspect that a couple of my risk factors act differently for men and women. Is it OK to give a simple average value over the sexes in these cases, or should I do some sort of weighting?'

(v) 'Once I have done all the analyses you have suggested to me, how should I present my results?'

10.15 Rework Example 10.22 to estimate relative risks using binomial regression.
- (i) Show that the analysis of the deviance table is very similar to Table 10.32.
- (ii) Show that the relative risks are very similar to the odds ratios in Table 10.34.

10.16 Rework Example 10.22 to estimate risk differences using binomial regression.
- (i) Find the 'best' model.
- (ii) Draw a conclusion from the differences between the 'best' model here and in Exercise 10.15.
- (iii) Find the sex-adjusted risk differences by Bortner score quarter, and corresponding 95% confidence intervals, taking the lowest quarter as the reference group.

10.17 Taking the data of Example 10.23, fitting models that include sex, Bortner score and their interaction, estimate
- (i) The odds ratios (with 95% confidence intervals) for a 100-unit increase in Bortner score for men and women separately.
- (ii) The relative risks (with 95% confidence intervals) for a 100-unit increase in Bortner score for men and women separately, using a binomial model.
- (iii) The relative risks (with 95% confidence intervals) for a 100-unit increase in Bortner score for men and women separately, using a Poisson GEE model.
- (iv) Compare your answers to (i) – (iii) and explain how they relate to the estimates derived in Example 10.23.

10.18 Suppose that a goal of the Scottish Heart Health Study was to estimate the difference in the risks of coronary heart disease between current smokers and those who have never smoked, during the first 7.7 years of follow-up, after allowing for confounding. Using the data on the web site for this book, that first appeared in Example 10.12, use propensity scoring to address this goal. To do this, assume that age, systolic blood pressure, total cholesterol and body mass index are the only variables required in the propensity score (that is, use the data available, taking no account of activity as well as having deleted ex-smokers). As in Example 10.12, treat this study as a fixed cohort. In each case below, use the same computational methods as in Example 10.46 and give the estimate, 95% confidence interval and p value.
- (i) Use stratification of the propensity score according to its fifths.
- (ii) Use inverse propensity score-weighted binomial regression
- (iii) Use propensity score-adjusted binomial regression.

10.19 The web site for this book has a link to a pair-matched dataset created from the data used in Exercise 10.18.
- (i) Using this dataset, find the estimate, 95% confidence interval and p value for the current smoker versus never-smoker risk difference using propensity score matching.
- (ii) Compare your answers with those in Exercise 10.18, and draw conclusions.
- (iii) Comment on the utility of propensity scoring in this context.
- (iv) Carry out any descriptive evaluations of the matching process that you feel are appropriate.
- (v) If possible, produce better matched samples and compare your new results with earlier results.

CHAPTER 11

Modelling follow-up data

11.1 Introduction

In this chapter we consider statistical models for data collected from follow-up (cohort or intervention) studies that involve censoring or when, even in the absence of censoring, the time to an event is regarded as the outcome variable of interest. Following from the basic ideas introduced in Chapter 5, models for survival data occupy Section 11.2 to Section 11.9 and models for person-years data are found in Section 11.10. The final section, Section 11.11, describes a variant on the logistic regression model introduced in Chapter 10.

11.1.1 Models for survival data

Two types of regression models for survival data are in general use in epidemiology: *parametric* and *semiparametric*. Parametric models require a theoretical probability model to be specified for the data. Two useful probability models are introduced in Section 11.4; these are used to create parametric regression models in Section 11.7. The Cox proportional hazards regression model is defined in Section 11.5 and Section 11.6. This makes no probability distribution assumption. The reader who wishes only to use the Cox model can omit Section 11.4, Section 11.7 and parts of Section 11.8.

11.2 Basic functions of survival time

11.2.1 The survival function

In Section 5.3 we defined the estimated survival function, which may be calculated from observed survival data, as the estimated cumulative probability of survival. If we let T be the random variable denoting the survival time, then the survival function, S, evaluated at some specific time, t, is

$$S(t) = P(T > t). \tag{11.1}$$

That is, $S(t)$ gives the probability that survival time (follow-up duration without an event) exceeds t time units.

11.2.2 The hazard function

The **hazard** is the instantaneous probability of failure (the opposite to survival) within the next small interval of time, having already survived to the start of the interval. As an illustration, consider the entire human life span and take the event of interest to be

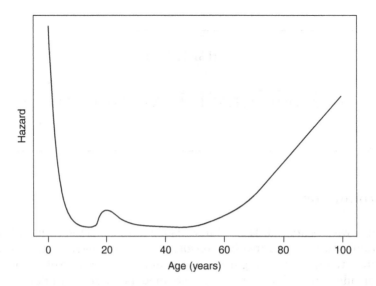

Figure 11.1. Idealised hazard function for human death across the entire human life span (assumed to peak at age 100).

death from any cause. The chance of death within the next small interval of time will be relatively high for a newborn baby but will progressively decrease for children who have already survived past the early days of high risk. For older children and young to middle-aged adults, the chance of death in the next small interval of time should be fairly constant, although slight variations may occur, for example, due to death from misadventure amongst older teenagers. For older adults, the chance of death will be expected to increase with age, due to increasing frailty. Hence, we might expect to see, at least approximately, the hazard function shown in Figure 11.1, in which survival time is age (time since birth). This is a graph of the **hazard function**, or a **hazard plot**.

The precise mathematical definition of the hazard evaluated at time t, $h(t)$, is given by Collett (2003). In words, it is the probability of failure during an interval of time, conditional upon survival to the start of the interval (time t), divided by the size of the interval, in the limit as the size of the interval tends to zero.

11.3   Estimating the hazard function

We shall now consider how to estimate the hazard function from observed data. This will complement the methods for estimation of the survival function given in Chapter 5. As its definition suggests, the hazard is a special type of rate (Section 3.8), and the three methods of calculation described here use this fact in their derivation.

11.3.1   Kaplan–Meier estimation

In Section 5.4 we saw how to estimate the survival function by the Kaplan–Meier (KM) method. The same approach can be used to estimate the hazard function under the assumption that the hazard is constant between successive failure times in the observed data set. These failure times are the distinct times at which events (for example, deaths) occur; when two or more events occur at the same time, they all define the same failure time.

As in Chapter 5, let e_t be the number of events at time t, where t is one of the failure times, and let n_t be the number at risk (that is, survivors) at time t. Now suppose that the next failure time (in rank order) is u_t time units away. We will then estimate the hazard during the time interval from t to $t + u_t$ to be the risk per unit time during the interval,

$$h_t = \frac{e_t}{n_t u_t}. \tag{11.2}$$

This defines a step function that can change (up or down) at successive failure times. Strictly speaking, t is the time *just before* the e_t events occur (just as in Section 5.4). If there were no repeated failure times, e_t would always be 1.

Example 11.1 Karkavelas *et al.* (1995) give the following survival times (in rank order) for 27 subjects with glioblastoma multiforme:

$$10, 12, 13, 15, 16, 20, 20, 24, 24, 26, 26, 27, 39, 42,$$

$$45, 45, 48, 52, 58, 60, 61, 62, 73, 75, 77, 104, 120.$$

Survival time is recorded as the number of weeks between initiation of cisplatin treatment and death. No subjects were recorded as being censored. Table 11.1 shows the failure times together with the estimated survival and hazard functions and the elements used in their calculation through using (5.3) and (11.2). The two functions are plotted in Figure 11.2 and Figure 11.3.

Table 11.1. Data and survival and hazard function estimation for subjects with glioblastoma multiforme.

Time (t)	Survivors (n_t)	Deaths (e_t)	Interval (u_t)	Survival (s_t)	Hazard (h_t)
0	27	0	10	1	0
10	27	1	2	0.9630	0.0185
12	26	1	1	0.9259	0.0385
13	25	1	2	0.8889	0.0200
15	24	1	1	0.8519	0.0417
16	23	1	4	0.8148	0.0109
20	22	2	4	0.7407	0.0227
24	20	2	2	0.6667	0.0500
26	18	2	1	0.5926	0.1111
27	16	1	12	0.5556	0.0052
39	15	1	3	0.5185	0.0222
42	14	1	3	0.4815	0.0238
45	13	2	3	0.4074	0.0513
48	11	1	4	0.3704	0.0227
52	10	1	6	0.3333	0.0167
58	9	1	2	0.2963	0.0556
60	8	1	1	0.2593	0.1250
61	7	1	1	0.2222	0.1429
62	6	1	11	0.1852	0.0152
73	5	1	2	0.1481	0.1000
75	4	1	2	0.1111	0.1250
77	3	1	27	0.0741	0.0123
104	2	1	16	0.0370	0.0313
120	1	1		0	

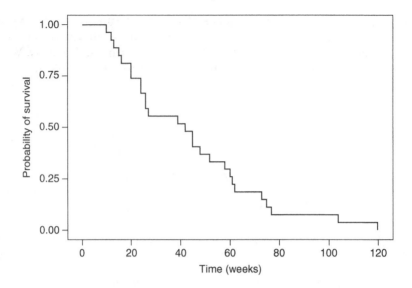

Figure 11.2. Estimated survival function for subjects with glioblastoma multiforme.

The survival plot (Figure 11.2) shows a rapid drop in estimated survival probability up to week 27, with 46% loss between weeks 10 and 27. Thereafter, there is little attrition for 18 weeks until the former pattern is re-established, but with somewhat less consistency. A long 'tail' appears in the survival plot because of the relatively long survival of the last couple of subjects. The hazard plot (Figure 11.3) necessarily mirrors these changes. The hazards appear to be very different over time; the hazard (for death) is greatest in the periods around 25, 60 and 75 weeks and broadly seems to increase with increasing survival time.

11.3.2   Person-time estimation

One disadvantage with the KM approach is that the hazard function tends to be spiked, as in Figure 11.3. An alternative approach is first to divide the time continuum into a

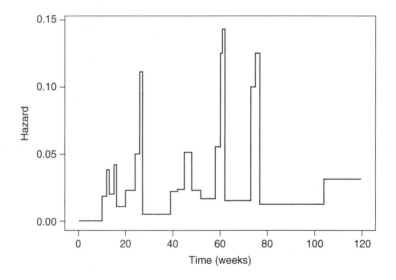

Figure 11.3. Estimated hazard function for subjects with glioblastoma multiforme.

number of intervals (as in a life table) and then take the person-years event rate, (5.18), as the estimate of the hazard within any particular interval. Since time may be recorded in some unit other than years, we shall take (5.18) to be the person-time event rate in this context. Provided that the intervals are larger, on average, than the durations between failure times, this method will tend to produce a smoother hazard plot, which is easier to interpret.

Example 11.2 Suppose that the survival times in Example 11.1 were grouped into 10-week intervals: 0 to 9, 10 to 19, 20 to 29 weeks,... The estimated hazard (for instance) during the second of these intervals is, by (5.18), the number of deaths, e, divided by the number of person-weeks, y. From Table 11.1, $e = 5$. Person-time is easier to calculate separately for those who survive the interval and those who die within the interval (and, when they exist, those who are censored within the interval). The components are then summed. From Table 11.1, we see that deaths occur in weeks 10, 12, 13, 15 and 16. Thus the person-weeks for deaths within the second interval is $0 + 2 + 3 + 5 + 6 = 16$. The number of person-weeks for survivors is calculated as the number of survivors (to week 20) times the length of the interval: $22 \times 10 = 220$. Hence, the estimated hazard (per week) in the second interval is

$$h_t = \frac{5}{16 + 220} = 0.0212.$$

This is roughly in line with the individual hazards given for times between 10 and 19 weeks in Table 11.1, as it must be. When the complete set of such hazards is plotted, they show a similar overall pattern to that seen in Figure 11.3, although with fewer 'bumps'.

11.3.3   Actuarial estimation

When survival analysis is performed using the life table approach with the actuarial approximation, (5.8), we can find an estimate of the hazard that is analogous to (11.2). Suppose now that u_t is the length of the interval in the life table that begins at time t. Taking e_t as in (11.2) and n_t^* as in (5.8), we find the average number of person-time units at risk in the interval beginning at t to be $(n_t^* - \frac{1}{2} e_t)u_t$. This leads to an estimated hazard of

$$h_t = \frac{e_t}{\left(n_t^* - \frac{1}{2} e_t\right)u_t}. \tag{11.3}$$

Example 11.3 The hazard in the first year of follow-up for men in the Scottish Heart Health Study (SHHS) whose type of housing accommodation is known may be estimated from Table 5.3. Here $t = 0$ and $n_0^* = 4398.5$, $e_0 = 17$ and $u_0 = 365$ (in days). Hence, by (11.3), the estimated hazard in the first year is

$$h_0 = \frac{17}{\left(4398.5 - 17/2\right)\left(365\right)} = 0.00001061.$$

We then assume that this estimate applies to each of the first 365 days after baseline. Notice that we could have taken $u_0 = 1$, which would give a hazard per year; daily rates are more in keeping with the hazard as an instantaneous failure rate.

Given that we have the individual event and censoring times (from Example 5.6), a more accurate picture of daily hazard (allowing it to vary) may be obtained for the problem of Example 11.3 from applying (11.2). Calculations then mirror those used in Table 11.1 except that n_t now decreases due to censoring as well as events. Alternatively, we could apply (5.18) on a person-day basis. We shall not consider actuarial methods in the remainder of this chapter because these are inferior when we have complete survival information.

11.3.4   The cumulative hazard

Another useful concept in survival analysis is the **cumulative hazard**. This can be estimated by the **Nelson–Aalen** (NA) estimate: the sum of the failure probabilities at all times up to and including the current time, t. That is,

$$\sum_{i \leq t} \frac{e_i}{n_i},$$

where n and e are, respectively, the number at risk at the start and the number of events in each interval of the life table, as defined in Section 5.3, or at each event time, as in the KM construction where each row of the life table is for a distinct event time. For example, for the data in Table 11.1, the NA estimate at $t = 10$ is $1/27 = 0.0370$; at $t = 12$ is $0.0370 + (1/26) = 0.0755$; at $t = 13$ is $0.0755 + (1/25) = 0.1155$, etc. Unlike the KM estimate, the NA estimate is not estimating a probability and can take values in excess of unity.

11.4   Probability models

One approach to modelling survival data is to construct a realistic probability model that seems to fit the data reasonably well. Inferences, such as predictions of average survival time (for example, average time to death), may then be made from the probability model. As in other applications, the advantages are that the probability model has a mathematical form, which may be manipulated as required, and has a smoother form than the observed data. In this context, predictions of intermediate survival probabilities (at times between the observed values) would be made from a smooth curve rather than a step function (such as Figure 5.8). This seems a sensible approach to interpolation.

11.4.1   The probability density and cumulative distribution functions

Suppose, now, that we seek to define a probability distribution for survival time — that is, a complete prediction of the survival probabilities at all possible times. Any probability distribution may be specified by its **probability density function** (p.d.f.), denoted f, or its **cumulative distribution function** (c.d.f.), F. In survival analysis $f(t)$, the p.d.f. evaluated at time t, is the probability that an event occurs within a very small interval of time following time t. This differs from the hazard function in that the latter is evaluated only for those people who have already survived to time t; that is, the hazard is a conditional probability.

A graphical plot of $f(t)$ against t gives an **event density** curve. Mathematically, F is the integral of f, that is, the area (to the left of a fixed point) under the event density curve. For example, the p.d.f. of the normal distribution is illustrated by Figure 2.13.

Table B.1 gives the values from the c.d.f. of the standard normal distribution. Data-based analogues of these two theoretical concepts are, respectively, the histogram and the area under the histogram to the left of any fixed point divided by the total area enclosed by the histogram.

Consider a probability distribution, which represents survival data. By definition, the c.d.f. evaluated at time t is

$$F(t) = P(T \le t) \tag{11.4}$$

so that the area under the p.d.f. to the left of t is the probability of a survival time of t or less. Now (11.1) and (11.4) show that $S(t)$ and $F(t)$ are complementary probabilities; that is,

$$S(t) = 1 - F(t). \tag{11.5}$$

Since the total area under a p.d.f. curve is always unity, (11.5) requires $S(t)$ to be the area to the right of the point t under the p.d.f. curve. Figure 11.4 shows the relationships between S, f and F for an arbitrary probability model for survival time. Different models will produce different curves and hence different enclosed areas to the left or right. A number of useful relationships between $h(t)$ and $S(t)$, $f(t)$ and $F(t)$ may be derived, such as

$$h(t) = f(t) / S(t). \tag{11.6}$$

The **cumulative hazard function**, $H(t)$, in probabilistic terms, is the integral of the hazard function and is related to the survival function through

$$H(t) = -\log_e\{S(t)\}.$$

We have seen that $H(t)$ can be estimated by the NA estimate and $S(t)$ by the KM estimate. The same equation holds approximately when these estimators are substituted in the above formula for the data in Table 11.1.

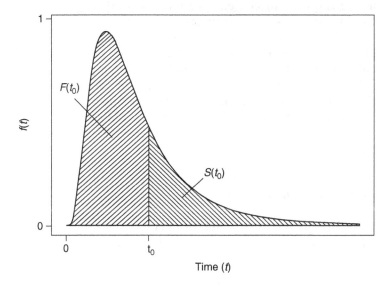

Figure 11.4. Relationship between the survival function, $S(t)$; the probability density function, $f(t)$; and the cumulative distribution function, $F(t)$, for survival times, t. $S(t)$ and $F(t)$ are evaluated at a specific time $t = t_0$.

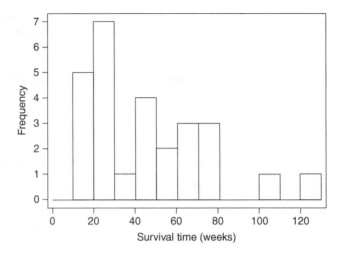

Figure 11.5. Histogram of the survival times for 27 subjects with glioblastoma multiforme.

11.4.2 Choosing a model

Due to its pre-eminence in statistics, the obvious probability model to consider first is the normal distribution. This would be a particularly easy model to deal with because of the values of $F(t)$ given, at least after standardisation, by Table B.1. However, the normal distribution is unsuitable because survival times tend to have a skewed distribution. For example, Figure 11.5 shows the histogram of the survival times from Example 11.1. The symmetrical normal curve of Figure 2.13 would not be a good fit to these data.

We seek a probability distribution whose shape mirrors that of typical survival data — a situation directly analogous to that met in Section 10.2 for data in the form of proportions. In the current context, we have several ways in which a candidate probability distribution could be investigated for goodness of fit. As we have just seen, one method is to look at the shape of the curve, defined by the p.d.f., and compare with the outline of a histogram of the data. Another is to calculate the survival function, S, defined by the probability distribution and compare this with the observed survival function. A third is to compare the shape of the theoretical and observed hazard functions. Due to the mathematical relationships between the different functions of survival time, such as (11.6), we should be able to take any of these three approaches and still be able to specify the fitted survival and hazard functions, the p.d.f. and c.d.f. (as required).

11.4.3 The exponential distribution

The simplest realistic probability model for survival times assumes that they follow an **exponential** distribution. The exponential has p.d.f.

$$f(t) = \lambda e^{-\lambda t}, \tag{11.7}$$

for $t \geq 0$, where λ is a constant that could be estimated from observed data. Throughout this chapter, λ is used to represent an unknown parameter for a probability distribution (as is common in the current context); this should not be confused with its use as the relative risk elsewhere in the book. By calculus, we may use (11.7) to show that

$$F(t) = 1 - e^{-\lambda t}$$

and hence, by (11.5),

$$S(t) = e^{-\lambda t}. \tag{11.8}$$

Also, by substituting (11.7) and (11.8) into (11.6), we obtain

$$h(t) = \lambda. \tag{11.9}$$

Figure 11.6 shows the shape of the three functions defined by (11.7) to (11.9) for an arbitrary choice of λ. The exponential p.d.f., $f(t)$, captures the right skewness, which is typical of survival data. In fact, this $f(t)$ has extreme right skew. The exponential survival function, $S(t)$, has the essential elements of the observed survival plots that we have seen in Chapter 5: it takes the value 1 at $t = 0$; it is nonincreasing as t increases; and it is never negative. However, the latter two properties would hold whatever the probability model chosen. The exponential hazard function, $h(t)$, defines a straight line with zero slope. Both $f(t)$ and $h(t)$ take the value λ when $t = 0$.

Notice that $h(t)$ does not depend upon time, t. This means that whenever we adopt the exponential distribution, we are assuming that the hazard is constant at all follow-up times. According to Figure 11.1, this might be a reasonable assumption if we wish to model time to death amongst young to middle-aged adults. In many practical applications of survival analysis in epidemiology, this is an unreasonable restriction and consequently the exponential distribution is rarely used, despite its attractive simplicity.

Since the mean of the exponential distribution is $1/\lambda$ (Clarke and Cooke, 2004), the mean survival time is assumed to be $1/\lambda$ whenever we adopt the exponential model

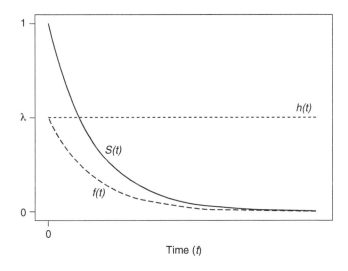

Figure 11.6. Probability density function, $f(t)$; survival function, $S(t)$; and hazard function, $h(t)$, for the exponential distribution.

for survival time. This gives a simple way of estimating λ from sample data when there is no censoring; we estimate λ by

$$\hat{\lambda} = 1/\bar{t}, \qquad (11.10)$$

where $\bar{t}$ is the mean of the observed survival times. When there is censoring, we estimate λ by

$$\hat{\lambda} = e \Big/ \sum t_i$$

where e is the total number of events and $\sum t_i$ is the sum of all the follow-up times, survival times for those who experience an event and censoring times for those who are censored. As with (11.10), this gives a maximum likelihood estimate for λ.

If we wish to summarise exponentially distributed survival data, we should use the median rather than the mean, due to the skewness. The median survival time from the exponential model is easily found. Let t_m be the median survival time. Then

$$S(t_m) = 0.5,$$

because half of the subjects will have survival times above the median. Then, by (11.8),

$$0.5 = e^{-\lambda t_m},$$

leading to the result

$$t_m = \frac{1}{\lambda} \log_e(2) = \frac{0.69315}{\lambda}. \qquad (11.11)$$

Other percentiles may be derived in a similar way.

Example 11.4 To fit an exponential distribution to the data given in Example 11.1 (where there is no censoring) we first find the sample mean of the survival times,

$$\bar{t} = (10 + 12 + 13 + \cdots + 120)/27 = 44.22.$$

Then, by (11.10),

$$\hat{\lambda} = 1/44.22 = 0.0226.$$

The model p.d.f. is thus, from (11.7),

$$f(t) = (0.0226)e^{-0.0226t};$$

the survival function is, from (11.8),

$$S(t) = e^{-0.0226t};$$

and the (constant) hazard function is, from (11.9),

$$h(t) = 0.0226.$$

From (11.11), the median survival time from the exponential model is

$$t_m = 0.69315/0.0226 = 30.7 \text{ weeks.}$$

We could evaluate the goodness of fit of the exponential model in Example 11.4 by comparing the plot of $S(t)$ with Figure 11.2. We delay such a comparison to Example 11.5. A further graphical test is described in Section 11.8.1. The theoretical hazard and probability density functions cannot be compared with their observed analogues (Figure 11.3 and Figure 11.5) in terms of size because the scales used are different. However, they can be compared for shape. The exponential assumption of constant hazard does not seem to agree with Figure 11.3, where there appears to be some tendency for the hazard to grow with time. Furthermore, the histogram of Figure 11.5 suggests a peak that is offset from the left edge, unlike the exponential p.d.f. shown in Figure 11.6. Notice also that the median survival time from the exponential model is well below the sample median of 42 weeks, which may be calculated from the raw data given in Example 11.1. There is, then, evidence that the exponential model is inappropriate for the glioblastoma multiforme data.

11.4.4   The Weibull distribution

A common probability model for survival data employs the **Weibull** distribution. This distribution has p.d.f.

$$f(t) = \lambda\gamma\left(t^{\gamma-1}\right)\exp\left\{-\lambda\left(t^\gamma\right)\right\}, \tag{11.12}$$

for $t \geq 0$, where λ and γ are constants that may be estimated from sample data. λ is called the **scale parameter** and γ is the **shape parameter**. Figure 11.7 illustrates the different shapes that the Weibull p.d.f. can take as γ changes. It is the great

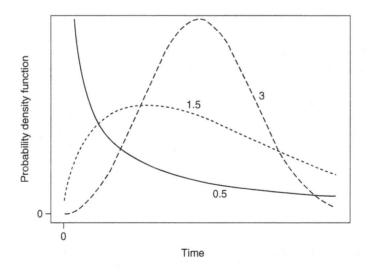

Figure 11.7. The probability density function for the Weibull distribution with $\gamma = 0.5$, 1.5 and 3.

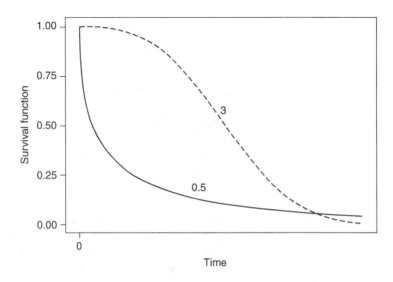

Figure 11.8. The survival function for the Weibull distribution with $\gamma = 0.5$ and 3.

flexibility of the Weibull that makes it such a useful probability model. Notice that some values of γ reproduce the typical right skew of survival data.

The survival function corresponding to (11.12) is

$$S(t) = \exp\left\{-\lambda\left(t^{\gamma}\right)\right\}. \tag{11.13}$$

Figure 11.8 shows the Weibull survival functions for two values of γ chosen so as to illustrate the two major types of curvature possible with the model.

The hazard function corresponding to (11.12) and (11.13) is

$$h(t) = \lambda\gamma\left(t^{\gamma-1}\right), \tag{11.14}$$

which encompasses a wide range of shapes as γ changes (see Figure 11.9), including decreasing ($\gamma < 1$), increasing ($\gamma > 1$) and static ($\gamma = 1$) hazards.

When $\gamma = 1$, (11.12) to (11.14) reduce to (11.7) to (11.9), respectively. This shows that the exponential is simply a special case of the Weibull: one in which the shape parameter is unity. This can also be seen from comparing the straight line for $\gamma = 1$, which crosses the vertical axis at λ, in Figure 11.9 with the exponential hazard function shown in Figure 11.6.

The median survival time, according to the Weibull model, is found from (11.13) to be

$$t_m = \left\{\frac{0.69315}{\lambda}\right\}^{1/\gamma}. \tag{11.15}$$

The estimation of λ and γ for the Weibull model is, unfortunately, not as straightforward as the estimation procedure for the exponential (described in Section 11.4.3). An iterative approach is necessary to find the maximum likelihood estimates. Normally,

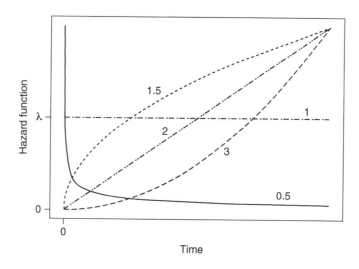

Figure 11.9. The hazard function for the Weibull distribution with $\gamma = 0.5$, 1, 1.5, 2 and 3.

this is done by computer, although Parmar and Machin (2006) give a numerical example. Some commercial statistical packages adopt a generalised approach to fitting various probability distributions which uses a **log-linear representation** (Collett, 2003). Essentially, this means that a different, but equivalent, formulation of the Weibull is used rather than (11.12) to (11.14). This new formulation is, for the hazard function,

$$h(t) = \frac{1}{\xi}\left(t^{\frac{1}{\xi}-1}\right)\exp(-\alpha/\xi). \qquad (11.16)$$

Comparing (11.16) to (11.14), we see that

$$\lambda = \exp\left(-\alpha/\xi\right),$$
$$\gamma = 1/\xi, \qquad (11.17)$$

so that it is reasonably simple to convert from one formulation to the other. PROC LIFEREG in the SAS package uses the representation in (11.16) and refers to α as the 'intercept' and ξ as (confusingly) the 'scale' parameter. In recent versions of SAS, the shape parameter, γ, is also given in the default output, together with a different scale parameter (the exponent of the intercept, α). The STREG routine in Stata, which fits a range of parametric models for survival data with Weibull as the default, uses the symbol p to represent γ and has an intercept ("_cons") term which is $\log_e\lambda$.

Example 11.5 A Weibull model was fitted to the data in Example 11.1 using SAS PROC LIFEREG. The output included estimates of the intercept (3.9075) and the scale (0.5973). Taking these as α and ξ in (11.17) gives

$$\lambda = \exp(-3.9075/0.5973) = 0.00144,$$

$$\gamma = 1/0.5973 = 1.674.$$

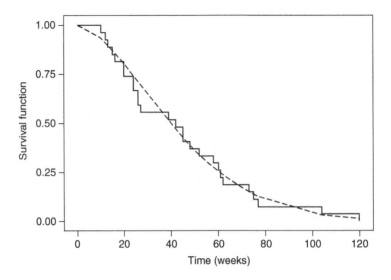

Figure 11.10. Observed (solid line) and Weibull (dashed line) survival functions for the glio-blastoma multiforme data.

Thus, the fitted Weibull model for the glioblastoma multiforme data has, by (11.12) to (11.15),

$$f(t) = 0.00241t^{0.674}\exp(-0.00144t^{1.674}),$$

$$S(t) = \exp(-0.00144t^{1.674}),$$

$$h(t) = 0.00241t^{0.674},$$

$$t_m = 40.0 \text{ weeks.}$$

Figure 11.10 shows the observed (as in Figure 11.2) and fitted (Weibull) survival functions. These seem to be in close agreement. Further support for the Weibull model in this example comes from comparing Figure 11.7, which suggests a right-skewed p.d.f curve when γ is around 1.5 (as here), with Figure 11.5. The fitted hazard function increases with increasing t, which broadly agrees with Figure 11.3. Finally, the Weibull median survival time is quite close to the observed value, calculated from Example 11.1, of 42 weeks.

Another graphical test of the suitability of the Weibull is given in Section 11.8.1, where we shall also compare the exponential and Weibull fits. It appears (by informal comparison with Example 11.4) that the Weibull is a better fit to the glioblastoma multiforme data than is the exponential.

11.4.5 Other probability models

The Weibull and its special case, the exponential, are the most common probability distributions used to model survival data. However, despite its flexibility, the Weibull cannot reproduce all possible shapes. For example, it cannot produce a hazard that rises to a peak and then falls. Other probability distributions may capture such shapes; the **log–logistic** distribution is a possible model for the example just raised. See Collett (2003) for details of the log–logistic model and other possible probability models for survival data.

11.5   Proportional hazards regression models

11.5.1   Comparing two groups

When two groups are to be compared (say, those exposed and those unexposed to some risk factor), an assumption often made in survival analysis is that the ratio of the group-specific hazards (say, exposed divided by unexposed) is the same at all possible survival times. This is called the **proportional hazards** (PH) assumption. We have already encountered this in the context of the log-rank test in Section 5.5.3; here we use the PH assumption in the definition of regression models. An example of PH would occur in the study of survival across the entire human life span (as in Figure 11.1) if two racial groups were studied and the hazard for death at any particular time for those in one racial group was always the same multiple of the hazard at the equivalent age in the other group.

Let the hazards in the two groups at time t be $h_0(t)$ and $h_1(t)$. Then PH implies that

$$\frac{h_1(t)}{h_0(t)} = \phi \tag{11.18}$$

at all survival times, t. Here, ϕ is a constant that is invariant over time. This constant is called the **hazard ratio** or **relative hazard**. The hazard that appears in the denominator, $h_0(t)$, is called the **baseline hazard**. A plot of the logarithm of the hazard against time, showing the two groups separately, would produce parallel curves separated by a distance of $\log(\phi)$.

Since hazards are always positive, a more convenient expression for the hazard ratio is

$$\phi = e^\beta,$$

where β is some parameter that has no restrictions (that is, it could be negative or positive) and so is easier to deal with. Equivalently,

$$\log_e \phi = \beta. \tag{11.19}$$

11.5.2   Comparing several groups

When several (say, ℓ) groups are to be compared (for example, the ℓ distinct levels of a risk factor), we choose one of the groups to be the base group and compare all other groups against this one. The PH assumption then becomes

$$\frac{h_i(t)}{h_0(t)} = \phi^{(i)}, \tag{11.20}$$

where $i = 1, 2, ..., \ell - 1$. That is, the hazard ratio comparing group i to group 0 is a constant, independent of time, but that constant may vary with the choice of the comparison group (that used in the numerator of the ratio). Figure 11.11 illustrates the PH assumption for four groups. The curve shown is an arbitrary choice, but the log hazards must stay parallel (that is, the vertical separation between the curves must stay constant).

As in the two-group situation, we prefer to let

$$\phi^{(i)} = \exp\left(\beta^{(i)}\right)$$

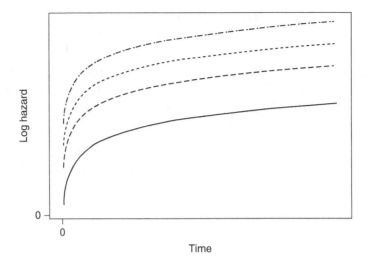

Figure 11.11. The proportional hazards assumption for a categorical risk factor with four levels.

for some unrestricted parameter $\beta^{(i)}$. Hence,

$$\log_e \phi^{(i)} = \beta^{(i)}, \tag{11.21}$$

for $i = 1, 2, \ldots, \ell - 1$. Rather than having $\ell - 1$ equations, the set of equations making up (11.21) may be rewritten as

$$\log_e \phi = \beta^{(1)} x^{(1)} + \beta^{(2)} x^{(2)} + \cdots + \beta^{(\ell-1)} x^{(\ell-1)}, \tag{11.22}$$

where

$$x^{(i)} = \begin{cases} 1 & \text{if the comparison group} = i \\ 0 & \text{otherwise.} \end{cases} \tag{11.23}$$

This defines a linear regression model for the logarithm of the hazard ratio, where the dummy variables $\{x^{(i)}\}$ are the explanatory variables and $\{\beta^{(i)}\}$ are the 'slope' parameters. Notice that this linear model has no intercept term, unlike the general linear model for normally distributed data (see, for example, (9.8)). No intercept is necessary here provided that we are concerned only with estimating ϕ, because it is subsumed within the baseline hazard. That is, (11.20) and (11.22) give

$$\log_e\{h_i(t)\} = \log_e\{h_0(t)\} + \beta^{(1)} x^{(1)} + \beta^{(2)} x^{(2)} + \cdots + \beta^{(\ell-1)} x^{(\ell-1)},$$

so that a constant added to (11.22) could be eliminated by a redefinition of $h_0(t)$.

When sample data are available, we may use them to find an estimate, $b^{(i)}$, of $\beta^{(i)}$ for all i. The logarithm of the hazard ratio is then estimated to be, by comparison with (11.22),

$$\log_e \hat{\phi} = b^{(1)} x^{(1)} + b^{(2)} x^{(2)} + \cdots + b^{(\ell-1)} x^{(\ell-1)}. \tag{11.24}$$

To fit the model, we would first have to set up the dummy variables defined by (11.23). That is, for anyone in group i (for $i > 0$) each x variable takes the value zero except for $x^{(i)}$, which takes the value unity. Some computer packages will do this automatically after being given key commands, just as we saw for logistic regression in Section 10.4.3. For those in the base group, $x^{(i)} = 0$ for all i, because then (11.20) and (11.22) give, for the comparison of the base group with itself,

$$\log_e \phi = \log_e \phi^{(0)} = \log_e \left\{ \frac{h_0(t)}{h_0(t)} \right\} = \log_e \{1\} = 0 + 0 + \cdots + 0 = 0,$$

which is consistent because $\log(1) = 0$.

Different PH models make different assumptions about $h_0(t)$, the baseline hazard. This leads to different estimates of the $\{\beta^{(i)}\}$. One approach is to assume a particular probability distribution model for $h_0(t)$; in Section 11.7, we shall assume the Weibull model. An alternative approach is to leave $h_0(t)$ totally unspecified; this leads to the Cox model of Section 11.6. Whichever approach is used, there is much in common as far as data analysis is concerned. The remainder of this section will be concerned with useful common methodology; specific examples are dealt with in Section 11.6 and Section 11.7. The PH assumption is tested in Section 11.8.

Using (11.23) and (11.24), the hazard ratio for group i compared with group 0 is estimated by

$$\hat{\phi} = \hat{\phi}^{(i)} = \exp\{b^{(i)} \times 1\} = \exp\{b^{(i)}\}. \tag{11.25}$$

An approximate 95% confidence interval for $\beta^{(i)}$ is given by

$$b^{(i)} \pm 1.96 \hat{se}\left(b^{(i)} \right),$$

and hence an approximate 95% confidence interval for $\phi^{(i)}$ is given by

$$\exp\left\{ b^{(i)} \pm 1.96 \hat{se}\left(b^{(i)} \right) \right\}, \tag{11.26}$$

where, as usual, $\hat{se}$ denotes the estimated standard error.

Notice that (11.18) and (11.19) are special cases of (11.20) and (11.21) where i can only take one value. If we let $b^{(1)} = b$ and $x^{(1)} = x$, then, when $\ell = 2$, (11.24) becomes

$$\log_e \hat{\phi} = bx, \tag{11.27}$$

where the dummy variable x takes the value unity for group 1 and zero for group 0.

11.5.3   Modelling with a quantitative variable

When the single explanatory variable is quantitative, the PH model is (11.27) where x represents the continuous variable. The baseline hazard is the hazard when $x = 0$ since then (11.27) gives

$$\log_e \hat{\phi} = \log_e \left\{ \frac{\hat{h}_0(t)}{\hat{h}_0(t)} \right\} = \log_e \{1\} = b \times 0 = 0,$$

where $\hat{h}$ is the estimated hazard.

The slope parameter, b, estimates the amount by which $\log_e \phi$ goes up as x increases from 0 to 1. That is, b estimates the amount by which the log hazard at $x = 1$ exceeds the log hazard at $x = 0$. The PH assumption requires that this amount be the same at all survival times.

Since the hazard at $x = 0$ may be difficult to interpret, we may wish to redefine the baseline hazard by setting $z = x - \bar{x}$ and taking z as the explanatory variable. The baseline hazard will then be for $x = \bar{x}$ and ϕ will measure hazards relative to the hazard at the average value of x.

Note that, by applying (11.27) at two specific values of x, s units apart, and raising the difference to the exponential power, the estimated hazard ratio for an increase in x of s units is

$$\exp(bs). \tag{11.28}$$

An approximate 95% confidence interval for this hazard ratio is given by

$$\exp\left\{ bs \pm 1.96s\left(\hat{se}(b) \right) \right\}. \tag{11.29}$$

All the material in Section 10.10 can be easily adapted to survival analysis.

11.5.4   Modelling with several variables

When there is more than one explanatory variable, we can define a multiple PH regression model. With k variables this is

$$\log_e \hat{\phi} = b_1 x_1 + b_2 x_2 + \cdots + b_k x_k. \tag{11.30}$$

Some of these x variables may be categorical, in which case a set of dummy variables may be defined, as in (11.23), and used to represent them (a different set is needed for each different categorical variable). This is exactly as we have seen already for general linear models (Chapter 9) and logistic regression (Chapter 10). The baseline hazard in (11.30) is the hazard for someone whose quantitative variables all take the value zero and who is in the base group for each of the categorical variables.

Example 11.6 Suppose $k = 3$; x_1 represents the categorical variable 'alcohol status' (nondrinkers/light drinkers/heavy drinkers); x_2 represents age and x_3 represents body mass index (BMI, defined as weight divided by the square of height). By reference to (11.23), two dummy variables are needed to represent x_1. For instance,

$$x_1^{(1)} = \begin{cases} 1 \text{ for moderate drinkers} \\ 0 \text{ otherwise,} \end{cases}$$

$$x_1^{(2)} = \begin{cases} 1 \text{ for heavy drinkers} \\ 0 \text{ otherwise.} \end{cases}$$

The PH regression model, (11.30), is

$$\log_e \hat{\phi} = b_1^{(1)} x_1^{(1)} + b_1^{(2)} x_1^{(2)} + b_2 x_2 + b_3 x_3,$$

and the baseline hazard is for those nondrinkers who have age zero and body mass index zero. Since there zero values are meaningless, we may choose to transform x_2 and x_3 as suggested in Section 11.5.3.

Once we have the values for $\{b_i\}$ (and their estimated standard errors), from a computer package, we can calculate an estimated hazard ratio (and 95% confidence interval) corresponding to any x variable, just as in Section 11.5.2 or Section 11.5.3, depending upon the form of x. The only difference here is that this would be the hazard ratio when all other x variables are fixed (at any values or levels). That is, we obtain *adjusted* hazard ratios.

Interactions are modelled by including appropriate terms in (11.30), just as in Section 9.4.7 and Section 10.9. For instance, the interaction between alcohol status and age in Example 11.6 is modelled by two new x variables: $x_4^{(1)} = x_1^{(1)} x_2$ and $x_4^{(2)} = x_1^{(2)} x_2$. The interaction between BMI and age requires only one new term, $x_5 = x_2 x_3$. The estimated hazard ratios for combinations of outcomes of risk factors relative to base combinations follow by picking out from the linear model for $\log_e \hat{\phi}$ those terms that are both nonzero and do not appear in both the numerator and denominator hazard (and thus cancel out). See Section 10.9 for more details.

We can compare nested models (defined in Section 10.7.3) through the **likelihood ratio test**. For each model to be considered, this requires calculation of the statistic $-2\log L$, where L is the likelihood function evaluated at the values of the maximum likelihood estimates of all parameters in the model. If L_v is the likelihood for a model with v terms and L_{v+u} is the likelihood for a model with the same v terms plus a further u terms, then, under the null hypothesis that the β coefficients for all these extra u terms are zero,

$$\Delta = -2\log L_v - (-2\log L_{v+u}) \tag{11.31}$$

follows a chi-square distribution with u d.f. Hence, we can test whether these u terms are needed in the model, adjusting for the effect of the other v terms, by comparing (11.31) against χ_u^2.

In Example 11.6, we might wish to test for the effect of BMI (x_3), adjusting for alcohol status and age (x_1 and x_2). This involves comparing the model with all four terms against that with three terms (the two dummy variables for x_1 plus the quantitative variable x_2). Here, $v = 3$, $u + v = 4$ and hence we compare Δ with χ_1^2.

Notice that this procedure mimics that of Section 10.7.3 in which (11.31) defines ΔD. Collett (2003) explains why $-2\log L$ should not be called a deviance in the current context. Nevertheless, the distinction is unnecessary in practical applications. Alternatives to the likelihood ratio test in survival analysis are reviewed by Parmar and Machin (2006).

11.5.5 Left-censoring

As we saw in Chapter 1, a key issue in epidemiology is whether the risk factor is a potential cause of the outcome, and we can have much more confidence in concluding that a relationship is causal if we can be sure that the potential cause precedes the outcome. In a cohort study we can ensure that the value of the risk factor recorded at baseline precedes the overt form of the outcome disease by excluding all subjects with the disease at baseline; that is, by studying disease incidence. We did this in many previous examples with real-life data, such as Example 4.3. Sometimes, however, a latent form of the disease, or even some other disease, may have altered the risk factor prior to study baseline. For instance, when we study the relationship between body mass index (BMI) and cancer in a cohort study, it may be that pre-existing latent cancer (yet to manifest itself) led to loss of body weight before the study started. The consequence might be that a misleading 'J'-shaped relationship is found between BMI and cancer, leading to an erroneous conclusion that a low BMI leads to a higher risk of cancer than does a moderate level.

As there is often no information on pre-existing latent disease, epidemiologists sometimes compute hazard ratios, at least in a sensitivity analysis, with follow-up counted from some way (typically 2–5 years) into the observation period: an example of **left-censoring** (the usual form of censoring, illustrated by Figure 5.2, is **right-censoring**). In other words, any event within the first period, when the latent disease would be expected to develop into overt disease, is ignored. Since the period left-censored is arbitrary, and power will be lower than when using all the data, such analyses require cautious interpretation.

11.6   The Cox proportional hazards model

The PH model introduced by Cox (1972) is the most widely used regression model in survival analysis. Its great advantage is that it requires no particular form for the survival times; in particular, the baseline hazard is unspecified. The theory behind the Cox approach is explained by Collett (2003) and set within a general epidemiological modelling context by Clayton and Hills (1993). Here we are purely concerned with its use in practice. As the Cox approach requires iterative calculations to fit the model, practical applications require use of a computer. All leading commercial statistical software packages have Cox regression procedures; we shall view only results from SAS. Within SAS, Cox regression is carried out by the procedure PROC PHREG. In Stata, STCOX is used.

Example 11.7 The patients with glioblastoma multiforme who were the subject of Example 11.1 were classified according to cellularity in Karkavelas *et al.* (1995). The survival times (in weeks) for those with low cellularity (below 300 nuclei) were

$$12, 15, 16, 20, 24, 26, 27, 39, 42, 45, 45, 58, 60, 61, 62, 73, 77, 104, 120;$$

for those with high cellularity (300 nuclei or more) survival times were

$$10, 13, 20, 24, 26, 48, 52, 75.$$

A variable defining group membership (CELLULAR = 1 for low and 2 for high) and another for survival time were read into SAS PROC PHREG. Output 11.1 shows part of the default SAS output.

Notice that the binary explanatory variable CELLULAR has been read in as if it were a quantitative variable (we can always do this with a binary variable). The slope parameter, b, will thus estimate the effect of a unit increase in CELLULAR: 2 versus 1, or high versus low.

Here $b = 0.55791$ and $\hat{s}e(b) = 0.43710$. From (11.28), when $s = 1$, the estimated hazard ratio is

$$\exp(0.55791) = 1.747,$$

as shown in the right-hand column of Analysis of maximum likelihood estimates in Output 11.1.

From (11.29), the 95% confidence interval for the hazard ratio is

$$\exp(0.557912 \pm 1.96 \times 0.43710),$$

that is, $\exp(0.557912 \pm 0.856716)$ or $(0.74, 4.11)$. Hence, we estimate that the hazard, at any time, is 1.75 times greater for those with high, compared with low, cellularity. However, the wide confidence interval contains unity, so we cannot claim that there is sufficient evidence to conclude any difference in risk by type of cellularity with this small data set. SAS PROC PHREG

Output 11.1. SAS PROC PHREG results for Example 11.7.

Model fit statistics		
Criterion	Without covariates	With covariates
–2 LOG L	129.585	128.064

Testing global null hypothesis: BETA = 0			
Test	Chi-square	DF	Pr > ChiSq
Likelihood ratio	1.5213	1	0.2174

Analysis of maximum likelihood estimates						
Variable	DF	Parameter estimate	Standard error	Chi-square	Pr > ChiSq	Hazard ratio
cellular	1	0.55791	0.43710	1.6292	0.2018	1.747

can be made to calculate and show the confidence interval directly; such results will be included in all future PHREG outputs.

The remainder of Output 11.1 provides two tests of the null hypothesis that the hazard ratio is unity. The likelihood ratio test is the difference in $-2\log L$ (where L is the likelihood) on adding the variable (or 'covariate') CELLULAR to the null model (that with no explanatory variables); that is, $129.585 - 128.064 = 1.5213$ (note that SAS rounds the difference to an extra decimal place). The p value for the likelihood ratio test is shown to be 0.2174. An alternative is the Wald test (Section 10.7.6); the square of the estimate of β divided by its standard error compared against chi-square with 1 d.f. SAS shows the p value for this test to be 0.2018, very similar to the likelihood ratio test result.

The glioblastoma multiforme dataset has the advantages, to an introductory account, of being small and not involving censoring; however, epidemiological studies rarely have either of these qualities. The remaining examples concerning the Cox model will use the extensive SHHS data set, in which the majority of subjects are censored. In Chapter 10 we ignored the fact that baseline times varied between subjects and treated the SHHS as a simple fixed cohort. Here we use the information on true survival times — elapsed time from recruitment to an event or censoring — just as we did in Chapter 5.

We shall now carry out Cox regression analyses of the problems already described by Example 10.11 and Example 10.14 (in Example 11.8); Example 10.12 and Example 10.15 (in Example 11.10); Example 10.22 (in Example 11.11) and Example 10.23 (in Example 11.12). In each case, the data used are available for downloading; see Appendix A. What we shall find, throughout, is that the estimates and confidence intervals for the hazard ratio are very similar to those found earlier for the odds ratio. Similarly, the likelihood ratio test results are mostly very similar to the results from analysis of deviance tables found in the corresponding examples of Chapter 10. The agreements are due to the nature of the SHHS (see the discussion in Section 5.2), and cannot be expected in general. See Section 14.5 for a general method for comparing odds ratios and hazard ratios. These are formally compared using SHHS data in Example 14.9.

Example 11.8 Consider the analysis of serum total cholesterol and systolic blood pressure (SBP) as risk factors for coronary heart disease (CHD) for men who were free of CHD at baseline in the SHHS. Cholesterol and SBP have been divided into their fifths (as in Table 10.14). Here, we have a multiple regression problem with two explanatory variables, both of which are categorical with five groups. The baseline hazard will be chosen as that for someone in the lowest fifth of both cholesterol and SBP. Dummy variables (as in Section 10.4.3) CHOL2,

CHOL3, CHOL4 and CHOL5 were defined for cholesterol, and similarly SBP2, SBP3, SBP4 and SBP5 for SBP. For instance,

$$\text{CHOL3} = \begin{cases} 1 \text{ for someone in the 3rd cholesterol fifth} \\ 0 \text{ otherwise} \end{cases}$$

and

$$\text{SBP4} = \begin{cases} 1 \text{ for someone in the 4th SBP fifth} \\ 0 \text{ otherwise.} \end{cases}$$

There are three possible Cox models for the logarithm of the hazard ratio, as specified by (11.30): first, the model with cholesterol alone; then the model with SBP alone; and finally the model with both. Note that we are not considering interactions here.

As we saw in Example 11.7, SAS PROC PHREG returns the value of Δ in (11.31) for comparing the current model against the null model. By differencing the Δs for two models that we wish to compare, we can produce a new Δ that is appropriate for the required comparison. For instance, Table 11.2 shows the 'Δ versus null' likelihood ratio test values returned by SAS PROC PHREG. These are differenced to produce the contrasts required: SBP alone; cholesterol alone (both requiring no further differencing), and the adjusted effects (cholesterol adjusted for SBP and vice versa). Similar differencing is required for the d.f.

All effects in Table 11.2 are highly significant. Thus, we conclude that both cholesterol and SBP have an important effect on the hazard for CHD; neither removes the effect of the other. That is, we require the following model:

$$\log_e \hat{\phi} = b_1^{(2)}\text{CHOL2} + b_1^{(3)}\text{CHOL3} + b_1^{(4)}\text{CHOL4} + b_1^{(5)}\text{CHOL5} +$$

$$b_2^{(2)}\text{SBP2} + b_2^{(3)}\text{SBP3} + b_2^{(4)}\text{SBP4} + b_2^{(5)}\text{SBP5}.$$

This is model 3 in Table 11.2. The parameter estimates supplied by SAS are shown in Output 11.2. Notice that the four levels of each risk factor, other than the base level, are numbered 2 to 5 here rather than 1 to 4, as used in (11.22) and elsewhere. These numbers are arbitrary; the base group is defined by the dummy variables (all dummy variables in a set take the value zero when the base level of that set is attained).

To clarify what SAS has produced, Table 11.3 gives the complete set of estimated hazard ratios and 95% confidence intervals obtained from the final two columns of Output 11.2. To get these columns from the columns showing the parameter estimates and their estimated standard errors, SAS has used (11.25) and (11.26).

The estimates of the 'slope' parameters in Output 11.2 and Table 10.15 are fairly close. The chi-square test statistics in Table 11.2 (Δ) and Table 10.21 (ΔD) are also similar, despite the use of grouped data in Example 10.14.

Table 11.2. Likelihood ratio test results for Example 11.8.

Model	Δ versus null (d.f.)	Test details			
		Δ	d.f.	p value	Effect
1 SBP	39.017 (4)	39.017	4	<0.0001	SBP
2 Cholesterol	45.026 (4)	45.026	4	<0.0001	cholesterol
3 SBP + cholesterol	76.508 (8)	37.491[a]	4	<0.0001	cholesterol|SBP
		31.482[b]	4	<0.0001	SBP|cholesterol

[a] Relative to model 1.
[b] Relative to model 2.

Output 11.2. SAS PROC PHREG results for Example 11.8, model 3.

							95% Hazard ratio	
Variable	DF	Parameter estimate	Standard error	Chi-square	Pr > ChiSq	Hazard ratio	confidence limits	
sbp2	1	0.60228	0.30181	3.9823	0.0460	1.826	1.011	3.300
sbp3	1	0.85006	0.28755	8.7394	0.0031	2.340	1.332	4.111
sbp4	1	1.00789	0.28337	12.6507	0.0004	2.740	1.572	4.774
sbp5	1	1.32801	0.27493	23.3323	<.0001	3.774	2.202	6.468
chol2	1	0.20250	0.31789	0.4058	0.5241	1.224	0.657	2.283
chol3	1	0.80416	0.28292	8.0791	0.0045	2.235	1.284	3.891
chol4	1	0.97593	0.27402	12.6842	0.0004	2.654	1.551	4.540
chol5	1	1.25631	0.26722	22.1031	<.0001	3.512	2.080	5.930

Analysis of maximum likelihood estimates

Table 11.3. Estimated CHD hazard ratios (95% confidence intervals) for serum total cholesterol (base = 1st fifth) and systolic blood pressure (base = 1st fifth) for SHHS men who were free of CHD at baseline.

Fifth	Serum total cholesterol	Systolic blood pressure
1	1	1
2	1.22 (0.66, 2.28)	1.83 (1.01, 3.30)
3	2.24 (1.28, 3.89)	2.34 (1.33, 4.11)
4	2.65 (1.55, 4.54)	2.74 (1.57, 4.77)
5	3.51 (2.08, 5.93)	3.77 (2.20, 6.47)

An attractive way of presenting results from a Cox (or other) survival model, when a categorical risk factor is of prime interest, is to show the estimated survival function separately for each level of the categorical predictor. This is similar to a KM plot, such as Figure 5.5, but where survival probabilities arise from a model. To do this the baseline hazard needs to be specified. Although this is not part of the Cox model framework, an estimated baseline hazard can be found, and may be obtained from commercial software, such as PROC PHREG in SAS and STCOX in Stata: see Section 13.3.3. When a multiple regression model has been fitted, the survival probabilities can be presented at fixed values of the other covariates (i.e., excepting the index categorical variable). For example, Figure 11.12 shows the estimated survival probabilities derived from Example 11.8 for the five equal fifths of cholesterol, shown for men within the middle fifth of SBP. Thus, after controlling for SBP, we can see that the highest three fifths of cholesterol separate from each other, and the lowest two fifths, within 2 years. The lowest two fifths intertwine before separating after around 6 years of observation. Since (from Table 11.3) the risk is higher when SBP is higher, choosing a lower level of SBP as the reference will cause all the curves to move up (better survival) and choosing a higher level will cause them to move down (lower survival). The shapes, and relative positions, of the five plots will stay the same. Such plots are easily produced, as was this plot, from the STS GRAPH command in Stata, following fitting the Cox model using STCOX.

Table 11.3 suggests that there is a dose–response effect for both cholesterol and SBP. The evidence for causality would be strengthened by considering a linear trend effect for each variable. To demonstrate this idea we shall, for simplicity, consider only the linear trend for SBP here.

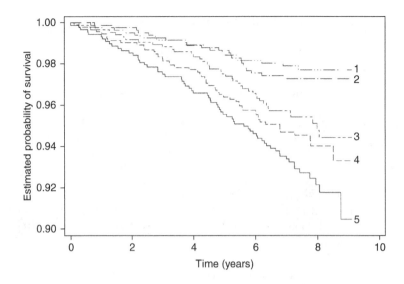

Figure 11.12. Estimated survival probabilities for coronary heart disease by fifth of serum total cholesterol, adjusted for systolic blood pressure and evaluated for men in the middle 20% of the systolic blood pressure distribution: Example 11.8. The numbers labelling the lines denote the equal fifths of cholesterol (e.g., 1 refers to the lowest 20%).

Example 11.9 By analogy with Section 10.7.5, we can represent the linear trend in the log hazard ratio of SBP by introducing a quantitative variable to represent the SBP fifths. For simplicity, we take this variable (SBP5TH in Output 11.3) to be 1 in the first fifth of SBP, 2 in the second fifth, etc.

Output 11.3 gives an extract from the results when SBP5TH was fitted as the only explanatory variable in a Cox model using SAS. From this we see that the likelihood ratio test, comparing the linear trend to the null model, is significant ($p < 0.0001$). Hence, there is evidence of a linear trend in the log hazard ratio by increasing fifth of SBP. The Δ value comparing the categorical SBP (model 1 in Table 11.2) with the linear is $39.017 - 37.7899 = 1.227$. Comparing this to chi-square on $4 - 1 = 3$ d.f., we get a test for a nonlinear response of SBP on CHD. Here this is not significant and, furthermore, Δ is so small that no specific polynomial effect can be

Output 11.3. SAS PROC PHREG results for Example 11.9.

Model fit statistics		
Criterion	Without covariates	With covariates
−2 LOG L	3247.392	3209.603

Testing global null hypothesis: BETA = 0			
Test	Chi-square	DF	Pr > ChiSq
Likelihood ratio	37.7899	1	<.0001

Analysis of maximum likelihood estimates							
Variable	DF	Parameter estimate	Standard error	Chi-square	Pr > ChiSq	Hazard ratio	95% Hazard ratio confidence limits	
sbp5th	1	0.32026	0.05345	35.9064	<.0001	1.377	1.240	1.530

important (unlike in Example 10.17). Thus, we conclude that the effect of SBP upon CHD acts through a linear trend on the log scale; from Output 11.3 the hazard for CHD is estimated to be multiplied by 1.38 (to two decimal places) when one SBP fifth is compared with the next lowest. A 95% confidence interval for this multiplicative constant is (1.24, 1.53). As anticipated from the likelihood ratio test, this interval excludes unity.

Example 11.10 A more substantial example to the last one, again taking men in the SHHS with no CHD at baseline and with no missing values (n = 4049), comes from fitting the model

$$
\begin{aligned}
\log_e \hat{\phi} = {} & b_1 x_1 + b_2 x_2 + b_3 x_3 + b_4 x_4 + b_5^{(2)} x_5^{(2)} + b_5^{(3)} x_5^{(3)} \\
& + b_6^{(2)} x_6^{(2)} + b_6^{(3)} x_6^{(3)},
\end{aligned}
\tag{11.32}
$$

where x_1 = age (in years); x_2 = serum total cholesterol (mmol/l); x_3 = BMI (kg/m^2); x_4 = SBP (mmHg), $x_5^{(2)}$ and $x_5^{(3)}$ are two dummy variables representing smoking status (never/ex/current) and $x_6^{(2)}$ and $x_6^{(3)}$ are two dummy variables representing activity in leisure (active/average/inactive):

$$
x_5^{(2)} = \begin{cases} 1 & \text{for ex-smokers} \\ 0 & \text{otherwise,} \end{cases} \qquad
x_5^{(3)} = \begin{cases} 1 & \text{for current smokers} \\ 0 & \text{otherwise,} \end{cases}
$$

$$
x_6^{(2)} = \begin{cases} 1 & \text{for average activity} \\ 0 & \text{otherwise,} \end{cases} \qquad
x_6^{(3)} = \begin{cases} 1 & \text{for the inactive} \\ 0 & \text{otherwise.} \end{cases}
$$

The baseline hazard is the hazard for subjects with $x_1 = x_2 = x_3 = x_4 = 0$ who have never smoked and are active in their leisure time. Output 11.4 gives the results from fitting (11.32) using SAS PROC PHREG. As declared to SAS: x_1 = AGE; x_2 = TOTCHOL; x_3 = BMI; x_4 = SYSTOL; $x_5^{(2)}$ = SMOKE2; $x_5^{(3)}$ = SMOKE3; $x_6^{(2)}$ = ACT2 and $x_6^{(3)}$ = ACT3 in (11.32).

As an example of the interpretation of parameters for quantitative variables, consider the variable 'total cholesterol'. Output 11.4 shows that the estimated hazard ratio for comparing two people of the same age, with the same BMI, same systolic blood pressure, same smoking habit and same self-reported leisure activity level, when one person has a cholesterol value one unit (1 mmol/l) higher than the other, is 1.331 (higher cholesterol compared with lower). We are 95% sure that the interval (1.195, 1.483) covers the true multiple-adjusted hazard ratio for a unit increase in cholesterol. Such one-unit hazard ratios (and confidence intervals) may (alternatively) be obtained from the parameter estimates and standard errors using (11.28) and (11.29) with $s = 1$.

Output 11.4. SAS PROC PHREG results for Example 11.10.

							95% Hazard ratio confidence limits	
Variable	DF	Parameter estimate	Standard error	Chi-square	Pr > ChiSq	Hazard ratio		
age	1	0.01802	0.01318	1.8711	0.1713	1.018	0.992	1.045
totchol	1	0.28606	0.05499	27.0584	<.0001	1.331	1.195	1.483
bmi	1	0.03810	0.02052	3.4486	0.0633	1.039	0.998	1.081
systol	1	0.02005	0.00364	30.3474	<.0001	1.020	1.013	1.028
smoke2	1	0.31211	0.24409	1.6350	0.2010	1.366	0.847	2.205
smoke3	1	0.69989	0.21344	10.7523	0.0010	2.014	1.325	3.059
act2	1	−0.18858	0.17315	1.1861	0.2761	0.828	0.590	1.163
act3	1	−0.10975	0.22417	0.2397	0.6244	0.896	0.577	1.390

Analysis of maximum likelihood estimates

The Wald tests in Output 11.4 suggest that some of the explanatory variables are unnecessary, at least in the presence of others, for predicting CHD. Certainly age and leisure activity seem likely to be redundant. We do not attempt a model building analysis here; see Example 10.15 and Example 10.16 for examples of methodical approaches, which could equally well be applied here.

Example 11.11 We now use the SHHS data to investigate whether there is an interaction between sex and Bortner personality score in the determination of the coronary hazard for those free of CHD at baseline. Here we consider Bortner score represented by its quarters (as in Table 10.28), so we shall be fitting an interaction between two categorical variables.

The four levels of Bortner score were fitted using the three dummy variables BORT2, BORT3 and BORT4, which represent contrasts with the first quarter (that is, they are the variables X1, X2 and X3 in Table 10.29). Sex was fitted as the variable SEX1, which is unity for men and zero for women (X4 in Table 10.29). The interaction between them requires three more dummy variables, which are most easily found by multiplying BORT2 by SEX1; BORT3 by SEX1 and BORT4 by SEX1 (to create X5 to X7 in Table 10.30). The derived variables were called BOR2SEX1, BOR3SEX1 and BOR4SEX1 within the computer program.

Here, four Cox models may be fitted: Bortner score alone; sex alone; both variables; and the full model including both variables and their interaction. Results of model fitting appear in Table 11.4. From this we conclude that all effects are important. Since there is a significant Bortner score by sex interaction, we cannot assess the two risk factors separately (Section 4.9). Output 11.5 gives the results from fitting the full model, (4).

From Output 11.5, we can easily determine hazard ratios for Bortner score, comparing each other quarter with the first, for each sex group separately. All we need do is to pick out the BORT and interaction terms that are nonzero for the particular Bortner–sex combination that we wish to compare with the first Bortner quarter of the same sex group, just as in Example 10.22. For instance, the male hazard ratio for Bortner quarter 4 versus Bortner quarter 1 is

$$\exp(-1.11231 + 0.88817) = 0.80.$$

The corresponding female hazard ratio is

$$\exp(-1.11231) = 0.33,$$

as shown directly by SAS. The female hazard ratio does not require the BOR4SEX1 interaction term because the corresponding x variable is defined to be zero when SEX1 = 0 (that is, for females).

Table 11.4. Likelihood ratio test results for Example 11.11.

Model	Δ versus null (d.f.)	Test details			
		Δ	d.f.	p value	Effect
1 Bortner (BORT2+BORT3+BORT4)	14.61 (3)	14.61	3	0.002	Bortner
2 Sex (SEX1)	65.46 (1)	65.46	1	<0.0001	sex
3 Bortner + sex (BORT2+BORT3+BORT4+ SEX1)	79.29 (4)	64.68[a]	1	<0.0001	sex|Bortner
		13.83[b]	3	0.003	Bortner|sex
4 Bortner*sex (all variables)	87.44 (7)	8.15[c]	3	0.043	interaction| Bortner, sex

Note: Model 4 includes the two constituent main effects.
[a] Relative to model 1.
[b] Relative to model 2.
[c] Relative to model 3.

Output 11.5. SAS PROC PHREG results for Example 11.11, model 4.

Variable	DF	Parameter estimate	Standard error	Chi-square	Pr > ChiSq	Hazard ratio	95% Hazard ratio confidence limits	
bort2	1	−0.57632	0.28868	3.9857	0.0459	0.562	0.319	0.990
bort3	1	−1.24407	0.36515	11.6076	0.0007	0.288	0.141	0.590
bort4	1	−1.11231	0.36515	9.2791	0.0023	0.329	0.161	0.673
sex1	1	0.52449	0.22556	5.4069	0.0201	1.690	1.086	2.629
bor2sex1	1	0.66799	0.34458	3.7579	0.0526	1.950	0.993	3.832
bor3sex1	1	0.95283	0.42014	5.1433	0.0233	2.593	1.138	5.908
bor4sex1	1	0.88817	0.41547	4.5699	0.0325	2.431	1.077	5.488

Analysis of maximum likelihood estimates

As they involve only one term, confidence intervals for female hazard ratios are easy to compute from Output 11.5. Thus, the female hazard ratio comparing Bortner quarter 4 with quarter 1 has 95% confidence interval

$$\exp(-1.11231 \pm 1.96 \times 0.36515)$$

or (0.16, 0.67), as shown directly by SAS. Similarly, we can obtain the other two female hazard ratios with Bortner quarter 1 as base.

For men, because the log hazard ratio estimates are the sum of two terms, each corresponding variance is the sum of two variances plus twice the covariance (as in the example given in Section 10.6). Output 11.5 does not include the covariances, which are not produced by default within SAS (but see Example 11.12). Rather than asking for them and carrying out computations with covariances, a short-cut procedure was adopted just as in Example 10.23. Sex was fitted as SEX2, which is unity for women and zero for men, rather than as the previously defined SEX1. The interaction terms were then recalculated as BOR2SEX2 = BORT2 × SEX2, etc., and model 4 in Table 11.4 was refitted. Results appear as Output 11.6. In this, the terms involving sex (main effect and interaction) must have the same magnitude but opposite sign compared with Output 11.5. The estimates of hazard ratios from this output will turn out to be exactly as before; for instance, the Bortner 4 versus 1 hazard ratio for men is

$$\exp(-0.22413) = 0.80,$$

Output 11.6. Further SAS PROC PHREG results for Example 11.11, model 4, using a different variable to represent sex compared with that used in Output 11.5.

Variable	DF	Parameter estimate	Standard error	Chi-square	Pr > ChiSq	Hazard ratio	95% Hazard ratio confidence limits	
bort2	1	0.09167	0.18815	0.2374	0.6261	1.096	0.758	1.585
bort3	1	−0.29124	0.20782	1.9640	0.1611	0.747	0.497	1.123
bort4	1	−0.22413	0.19820	1.2788	0.2581	0.799	0.542	1.179
sex2	1	−0.52449	0.22556	5.4069	0.0201	0.592	0.380	0.921
bor2sex2	1	−0.66799	0.34458	3.7579	0.0526	0.513	0.261	1.007
bor3sex2	1	−0.95283	0.42014	5.1433	0.0233	0.386	0.169	0.879
bor4sex2	1	−0.88817	0.41547	4.5699	0.0325	0.411	0.182	0.929

Analysis of maximum likelihood estimates

Table 11.5. Hazard ratios (95% confidence intervals) by sex and Bortner quarter for SHHS subjects who were free of CHD at baseline.

Quarter of Bortner score	Sex	
	Male	Female
1	1	1
2	1.10 (0.76, 1.59)	0.56 (0.32, 0.99)
3	0.75 (0.50, 1.12)	0.29 (0.14, 0.59)
4	0.80 (0.54, 1.18)	0.33 (0.16, 0.67)

which SAS gives directly; for women, it is

$$\exp(-0.22413 - 0.88817) = 0.33,$$

as before. For men (but not women), 95% confidence intervals are read directly from Output 11.6. For instance, the male Bortner 4 versus 1 confidence interval is (0.54, 1.18).

The full set of hazard ratios and confidence intervals is given in Table 11.5. The numerical results are very similar to those in Table 10.34 and the conclusions are thus identical: Bortner score has little effect on the risk of CHD for men but has a negative relationship for women.

Example 11.12 Bortner score is measured as a quantitative variable in the SHHS, so it is possible to repeat Example 11.11 using the raw, ungrouped form of Bortner score. Taking BORTNER as the variable that measures Bortner score and SEX1, as in Example 11.11, to be the dummy variable for sex, the interaction between the quantitative and categorical variables is modelled as BORTSEX1 = BORTNER × SEX1. That is, the interaction is represented by a single explanatory variable that takes the value of the Bortner score for men and zero for women. As in Example 11.11, four models for the hazard ratio are possible, one of which is the 'sex only' model, which is exactly as in Example 11.11. Table 11.6 gives results of model fitting; model 4 is required to predict the hazard ratio for a coronary event, and parameter estimates from fitting it with PROC PHREG are shown in Output 11.7. This time the estimated variance–covariance matrix is included.

The estimated hazard ratio and 95% confidence interval for an increase of one unit in the Bortner score for women is read directly as 0.987 (0.981, 0.993). For men, the corresponding

Table 11.6. Likelihood ratio test results for Example 11.12.

Model	Δ versus null (d.f.)	Test details			
		Δ	d.f.	p value	Effect
1 Bortner (BORTNER)	10.81 (1)	10.81	1	0.001	Bortner
2 Sex (SEX1)	65.46 (1)	65.46	1	<0.0001	sex
3 Bortner + sex (BORTNER + SEX1)	75.58 (2)	64.77[a]	1	<0.0001	sex|Bortner
		10.12[b]	1	0.002	Bortner|sex
4 Bortner*sex (BORTNER + SEX1 + BORTSEX1)	84.02 (3)	8.44[c]	1	0.004	interaction| Bortner, sex

Note: Model 4 includes the two constituent main effects.

[a] Relative to model 1.
[b] Relative to model 2.
[c] Relative to model 3.

Output 11.7. SAS PROC PHREG results for Example 11.12, model 4.

							95% Hazard ratio	
Variable	DF	Parameter estimate	Standard error	Chi-square	Pr > ChiSq	Hazard ratio	confidence limits	
bortner	1	−0.01292	0.00314	16.9106	<.0001	0.987	0.981	0.993
sex1	1	−0.61260	0.57226	1.1459	0.2844	0.542	0.177	1.664
bortsex1	1	0.01047	0.00358	8.5248	0.0035	1.011	1.003	1.018

Analysis of maximum likelihood estimates

Estimated covariance matrix			
Variable	bortner	sex1	bortsex1
bortner	0.0000098748	0.0014968052	−.0000098747
sex1	0.0014968052	0.3274803765	−.0019885262
bortsex1	−.0000098747	−.0019885262	0.0000128502

estimate is easy to produce as exp(−0.01292 + 0.01047) = 0.998. The estimated standard error is obtained by picking out the relevant terms from the Estimated covariance matrix in Output 11.7, as in Section 10.4.3. That is,

$$\sqrt{0.0000098748 + 0.0000128502 + 2(-0.0000098747)} = 0.00173,$$

giving a 95% confidence interval for the hazard ratio of

$$\exp\{(-0.01292 + 0.01047) \pm 1.96 \times 0.00173)\}$$

or (0.994, 1.001). Hence, the hazard for CHD comes down slightly as Bortner score goes up for each sex, but the effect for men is explainable by chance variation (because unity is in the 95% confidence interval).

11.6.1 Time-dependent covariates

In all the examples so far we have assumed that the explanatory variables, or **covariates**, are fixed at baseline. In some situations, we may have updates on the values of these variables, or perhaps just a subset of them, as the study progresses. This situation is quite common in intervention studies, when subjects are invited to attend at clinics every few months. At each clinic, a number of health checks may be carried out — for example, the current size of a tumour may be measured. In cohort studies, the initial study questionnaire may be readministered every few years to discover the latest smoking habit, diet, activity level, etc. of each study participant. In occupational cohort studies, the current exposure to suspected toxic substances, as well as other information, could be recorded regularly. In survival analysis, explanatory variables with such updated information are called **time-dependent covariates**.

Cox (1972) showed that such variables may be included in his regression model. The most recent value of a time-dependent covariate is used at each specific time in the model. This is not necessarily a directly observed value; it could, for example, be the maximum value of a variable observed so far or the difference between the current maximum and minimum values.

Consider a time-dependent covariate $x(t)$ that takes the value 1 if the risk factor is present, and 0 if absent, at time t. For example, $x(t)$ might record whether a subject is a smoker at time t. The Cox regression model for the log hazard ratio then assumes

$$\log_e \hat{\phi} = b_1 x_1 + b_2 x_2 + \cdots + b_k x_k + bx(t), \tag{11.33}$$

where $x_1, x_2, \ldots, x_k$ are a set of fixed covariates, as in (11.30). The hazard ratio for someone who smokes at time t compared with someone who does not, with all other variables fixed, is then estimated to be

$$\hat{\phi} = \exp(b),$$

just as in the case where x represents a fixed covariate. Similarly, when x is a quantitative variable, such as blood pressure,

$$\hat{\phi} = \exp(bs)$$

will estimate the hazard ratio for an increase in s units of blood pressure, as in (11.28). We can test for the significance of $x(t)$ by comparing minus twice log likelihoods for the models with and without this term, just as when all the covariates are fixed at baseline.

Because (11.33) depends upon t, the hazard ratio is allowed to vary over time whenever time-dependent covariates are included in a model. For this and other reasons, time-dependent proportional hazards models can be difficult to interpret (Altman and De Stavola, 1994). A simple example of their use is provided by Collett (2003).

11.6.2   Recurrent events

In Section 9.11 and Section 10.15, we have seen situations in which observations on the outcome variable are repeated over time. The equivalent situation in the current context occurs when survival times are recorded, for the same individual, between successive events of the same type that this individual experiences. Examples would be times between recurrent ischaemic strokes and between bouts of infection.

Although several approaches to this problem based on the Cox model have been suggested, the simplest and most popular is that due to Andersen and Gill (1982). The basic **Andersen–Gill model** essentially treats each time period between successive events as a separate observation within the Cox model. Thus, someone with two events would contribute three observations: time to the first event (not censored); time to second event (not censored); and time following the second event (censored). Different people will contribute different numbers of observations to the model. This model is easy to deal with because it requires only the same software as for the standard Cox model. The disadvantage is that the implicit assumption that preceding events have no effect on the hazard of a future event may be false; hence variations on this simple approach have been suggested. See Therneau and Grambsch (2000) for more information.

11.7   The Weibull proportional hazards model

The Weibull proportional hazards model assumes that the survival times in the base group follow a Weibull distribution. That is, from (11.14), the baseline hazard is

$$h_0(t) = \lambda \gamma \left(t^{\gamma - 1} \right), \tag{11.34}$$

for some values of λ and γ. The Weibull parameters λ and γ may be estimated from observed data; thus, we estimate the baseline hazard directly. Under the PH assumption, (11.18), when two groups are compared, the hazard in the numerator (comparison) group is

$$h_1(t) = \phi h_0(t),$$

where ϕ is the hazard ratio. Hence,

$$h_1(t) = \phi \lambda \gamma \left(t^{\gamma - 1} \right). \tag{11.35}$$

By reference to (11.14), we can see that (11.35) is in the form of a Weibull hazard with scale parameter $\phi\lambda$ and shape parameter γ. Hence, if $h_0(t)$ has a Weibull form and the hazards are proportional (that is, time-homogeneous), then $h_1(t)$ also has a Weibull form with the same shape parameter.

Generalisations from this two-group comparison to the other situations covered by Section 11.5 show that all hazards will turn out to have the Weibull form with the same shape parameter throughout. Figure 11.11 actually shows log hazards from four Weibull distributions, each of which has $\gamma = 3$ but a different λ. In Example 11.6, when a Weibull PH model is used, the hazard for a 50-year-old heavy drinker with a BMI of 28.2 is estimated as

$$\exp\left(b_1^{(2)} + 50 b_2 + 28.2 b_3 \right) \lambda \gamma \left(t^{\gamma - 1} \right).$$

When a Weibull PH model is used, we estimate λ and γ, as well as all the β regression ('slope') parameters. Maximum likelihood estimation requires iterative calculation, so a statistical computer package is required.

We shall view results from the SAS routine PROC LIFEREG. This fits a range of probability models (including the exponential), although the Weibull PH model is the default. Exponential models are dealt with similarly to Weibull models, so only Weibull models (with greater applicability) are described here. One snag with PROC LIFEREG is the log-linear representation used, as mentioned in Section 11.4.4. Due to this, the regression parameters produced by SAS, which we shall call $\{B_i\}$, must be transformed to produce the regression parameters $\{b_i\}$ introduced in Section 11.5. This is achieved through the general result,

$$b_i = -B_i / \xi, \tag{11.36}$$

where ξ is the SAS PROC LIFEREG scale parameter. The estimated standard error of b_i is

$$\hat{se}\left(b_i \right) = \frac{1}{\xi^2} \sqrt{ \xi^2 V\left(B_i \right) + B_i^2 \, V\left(\xi \right) - 2\xi B_i C\left(\xi, B_i \right) }, \tag{11.37}$$

as shown by Collett (2003). As usual, V denotes the variance and C the covariance, as found in the estimated variance–covariance matrix. Using STREG in Stata, the estimates and confidence limits are output directly.

We shall now illustrate the use of Weibull PH models through some of the same examples used for Cox regression in Section 11.6. Since model selection and hazard ratio interpretation follow in an identical way to the Cox model, only the first two examples from Section 11.6 (Example 11.7 and Example 11.8) will be reanalysed. All results will be found to be very similar to those from the analogous Cox analysis; however, this is not the case in general because the imposition of the Weibull form may produce different inferences. In Section 11.8, we shall consider how to check whether the Weibull PH form is appropriate; if it is, we would anticipate hazard ratio estimates similar to those when the Cox model is used.

Example 11.13 A Weibull PH regression model was fitted to the cellularity group data of Example 11.7 using SAS PROC LIFEREG. In the source file (available to be downloaded; see Appendix A) the variable CELLULARITY was coded as 1 for low, and 2 for high, cellularity. In order to force SAS to take the hazard for low cellularity as the baseline hazard, the transformation

$$\text{CELLULAR} = 5 - \text{CELLULARITY}$$

was used. Thus, low cellularity gets the new code $5 - 1 = 4$ and high cellularity gets the new code $5 - 2 = 3$. By the standard SAS rules, when CELLULAR was fitted as a categorical (CLASS) variable, the highest level (CELLULAR = 4; low cellularity) is the base group (as required). Output 11.8 gives the results from fitting CELLULAR.

The model fitted is

$$\log_e \hat{\phi} = bx,$$

where

$$x = \begin{cases} 1 & \text{for high cellularity} \\ 0 & \text{for low cellularity.} \end{cases}$$

We pick out the SAS regression parameter, B, as the coefficient for high cellularity (CELLULAR = 3) in Output 11.8. From this output:

$$\hat{\alpha} = 4.0040 \qquad V(\hat{\alpha}) = 0.018755$$

$$\hat{\xi} = 0.5745 \qquad V(\hat{\xi}) = 0.007316$$

$$B = -0.3635 \qquad V(B) = 0.058634$$

$$C(\hat{\xi}, B) = -0.000272.$$

Output 11.8. SAS PROC LIFEREG results for Example 11.13.

Analysis of Parameter Estimates							
Parameter	DF		Estimate	Standard error	95% Confidence limits		Chi-square	Pr > ChiSq
Intercept		1	4.0040	0.1369	3.7355	4.2724	854.80	<.0001
cellular	3	1	−0.3635	0.2421	−0.8381	0.1111	2.25	0.1333
cellular	4	0	0.0000	.	.	.	.	.
Scale		1	0.5745	0.0855	0.4291	0.7692		
Weibull shape		1	1.7407	0.2592	1.3001	2.3305		

Estimated covariance matrix			
	Intercept	cellular3	Scale
Intercept	0.018755	−0.017252	−0.003183
cellular3	−0.017252	0.058634	−0.000272
Scale	−0.003183	−0.000272	0.007316

By (11.17),

$$\hat{\lambda} = \exp\left(-4.0040/0.5745\right) = 0.00094$$

$$\hat{\gamma} = 1/0.5745 = 1.7407.$$

The fourth decimal place in the preceding has been corrected using the result given in Output 11.8 as the 'Weibull shape' estimate.

By (11.36),

$$b = -\left(-0.3635\right)/0.5745 = 0.6327.$$

By (11.37),

$$\hat{se}(b) = \left(\sqrt{0.019352 + 0.0009667 - 0.0001136}\right)/0.330050 = 0.4307.$$

Then, by (11.25) and (11.26), the estimated hazard ratio (high versus low cellularity) is $\hat{\phi} = \exp(0.6327) = 1.88$ with 95% confidence interval

$$\exp(0.6327 \pm 1.96 \times 0.4307)$$

or (0.81, 4.38). The estimated hazard function for those with low cellularity is the estimated baseline hazard, (11.34),

$$(0.00094)(1.7407)t^{0.7407} = 0.001636t^{0.7407},$$

and the estimated hazard function for high cellularity is, from (11.35),

$$\hat{\phi} \times 0.001636t^{0.7407} = 0.00308t^{0.7407}.$$

If we wish, we can also specify the fitted survival functions for each group from (11.13). For low and high cellularity, respectively, these are

$$\exp\left\{-\hat{\lambda}\left(t^{\hat{\gamma}}\right)\right\} = \exp\left(-0.00094t^{1.7407}\right)$$

and

$$\exp\left\{-\hat{\phi}\hat{\lambda}\left(t^{\hat{\gamma}}\right)\right\} = \exp\left(-0.00177t^{1.7407}\right).$$

So that these can be compared with the observed survival functions, KM estimates of the two survival functions were calculated and plotted together with these fitted functions. The results are shown in Figure 11.13. Agreement is quite good, suggesting that the Weibull model is reasonable. However, a curve and a step function are hard to compare by eye; an easier graphical test may be found in Section 11.8.1.

As with Cox models, nested Weibull PH regression models are best compared through Δ as defined by (11.31). We can test the effect of cellularity in Example 11.13 by finding the difference in minus twice log likelihoods of the Weibull model with cellularity as the explanatory variable and the Weibull model with no explanatory variables (the null model). The latter has already been described in Example 11.5, because this is the model of a single Weibull form for the entire glioblastoma multiforme

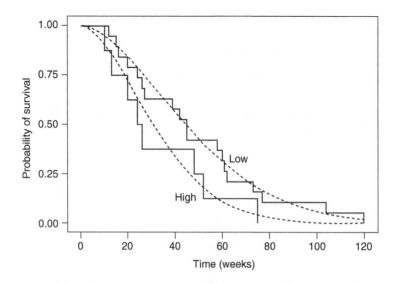

Figure 11.13. Observed (solid line) and Weibull (dashed line) survival functions by cellularity; glioblastoma multiforme data.

data set. In this example, $\Delta = 1.977$ (from computer output not shown); comparing this to χ_1^2 leads to the conclusion that cellularity has no significant effect ($p > 0.1$). This is consistent with the chi-square test for CELLULAR given in Output 11.8 ($p = 0.1333$) and with the finding in Example 11.7.

As the foregoing shows, provided that we do not wish to use the model to estimate the baseline hazard and are content with comparative measures of chance, there is little difference in the way Cox and Weibull PH regression models are interpreted. An example of a multiple regression survival model with quantitative variables will illustrate this further.

Example 11.14 Output 11.9 shows the results of fitting a Weibull PH model to the problem of Example 11.10 using PROC LIFEREG. Table 11.7 copies the B coefficients from Output 11.9 and

Output 11.9.   SAS PROC LIFEREG results for Example 11.14.

Analysis of Parameter Estimates								
Parameter		DF	Estimate	Standard error	95% Confidence limits		Chi-square	Pr > ChiSq
Intercept		1	15.7827	0.9241	13.9715	17.5939	291.69	<.0001
age		1	−0.0142	0.0105	−0.0347	0.0064	1.82	0.1778
totchol		1	−0.2273	0.0464	−0.3182	−0.1364	24.02	<.0001
bmi		1	−0.0304	0.0164	−0.0626	0.0018	3.43	0.0639
systol		1	−0.0160	0.0031	−0.0220	−0.0100	26.96	<.0001
smoking	2	1	−0.2490	0.1944	−0.6300	0.1321	1.64	0.2004
smoking	3	1	−0.5546	0.1737	−0.8951	−0.2141	10.19	0.0014
smoking	4	0	0.0000	.	.	.	.	.
activity	2	1	0.1519	0.1377	−0.1180	0.4219	1.22	0.2700
activity	3	1	0.0916	0.1779	−0.2571	0.4404	0.27	0.6065
activity	4	0	0.0000	.	.	.	.	.
Scale		1	0.7935	0.0556	0.6917	0.9103		
Weibull shape		1	1.2602	0.0883	1.0985	1.4457		

Table 11.7. Interpretation of parameter estimates in Output 11.9.

| Explanatory | Regression coefficients | | Estimated hazard ratio | |
variable	B	b	$\hat{\phi}$	Effect[a]
Age	−0.0142	0.0178	1.02	increase of 1 year
Total cholesterol	−0.2273	0.2864	1.33	increase of 1 mmol/l
Body mass index	−0.0304	0.0384	1.04	increase of 1 kg/m^2
Systolic blood pressure	−0.0160	0.0202	1.02	increase of 1 mmHg
Smoking	−0.2490	0.3137	1.37	ex- versus never-smoker
	−0.5546	0.6989	2.01	current versus never-smoker
Leisure activity	0.1519	−0.1915	0.83	average versus active
	0.0916	−0.1155	0.89	inactive versus active

[a] Adjusted for all other explanatory variables.

uses (11.36) and then either (11.25) or (11.28) to produce the remaining numerical columns. A complete analysis accounts for sample-to-sample variation, through (11.37) and (11.26) or (11.29); nested models are compared using (11.31). However, the inferences obtained turn out to be very similar to those in Example 11.10 and, in general terms, Example 10.12 and Example 10.15.

11.8 Model checking

In the last few sections, we have assumed proportional hazards and/or a Weibull (or exponential) form for the survival data. We now consider some procedures that enable these assumptions to be checked. Such procedures should always be carried out before a particular model is accepted.

11.8.1 Log cumulative hazard plots

The **log cumulative hazard** (LCH) function (sometimes called the **integrated hazard function**) is

$$H(t) = \log_e\left\{-\log_e S(t)\right\}. \tag{11.38}$$

A plot of the estimated LCH function against the logarithm of survival time (the **LCH plot**) may be used to check both the proportional hazards assumption and the assumption of a Weibull (or exponential) distribution for survival data, as required.

Consider, first, the following one-sample problem: a set of survival data is available and we wish to check whether the Weibull distribution provides an appropriate probability model. Substituting the Weibull survival function, (11.13), into (11.38) gives

$$H(t) = \log_e \lambda + \gamma \log_e t, \tag{11.39}$$

which is the equation of a straight line. Hence, if we obtain observed values of the LCH and plot these against the logarithm of survival time, we expect to find a straight line if the Weibull assumption is correct. Moreover, (11.39) shows that the slope of this line will provide an estimate of γ and the intercept will provide an estimate of $\log_e(\lambda)$. In general, these will be only rough estimates, so the maximum likelihood estimates are much preferred. Nevertheless, if the slope of the line is around unity, we can conclude that an exponential model will suffice (because a Weibull with $\gamma = 1$ is an exponential).

Example 11.15 In Example 11.5 we fitted a Weibull distribution to the glioblastoma multiforme data. Now we shall use the LCH plot to check the assumption that the Weibull is appropriate. First, we need to calculate the observed LCH values using (11.38) with the observed survival probabilities in the right-hand side. In Table 11.1, we have the KM estimates of $S(t)$; these are reproduced in Table 11.8, together with the estimated LCH function from substituting these into (11.38). Since there are 23 distinct survival times, Table 11.8 has 23 rows. However, because log (0) is undefined, the LCH function cannot be evaluated at the final survival time (120 weeks). The remaining 22 pairs of LCH versus log time values are plotted in Figure 11.14.

Figure 11.14 shows a reasonable approximation to a straight line, so the Weibull model seems acceptable. To consider whether the simpler exponential model is sufficient, we need to judge whether the slope of the approximating line is around unity. This may be done by eye or by fitting a least-squares linear regression line to the data (as enumerated in Table 11.8). The latter, using (9.13), produced a slope of 1.69, well above 1.0. Hence, there is evidence to reject the exponential model. Notice that the slope estimate of γ is not dissimilar to the maximum likelihood estimate of 1.674 found in Example 11.5. The intercept of −6.52 from the simple linear regression fit (using (9.14)) leads to an estimate of $\log_e(-6.52) = 0.00147$ for λ. This is also in good agreement with the corresponding estimate in Example 11.5.

Table 11.8. LCH plot calculations for Example 11.15.

Time (weeks)	log (time)	Estimated P (survival)	LCH
10	2.30	0.9630	−3.277
12	2.48	0.9259	−2.565
13	2.56	0.8889	−2.139
15	2.71	0.8519	−1.830
16	2.77	0.8148	−1.586
20	3.00	0.7407	−1.204
24	3.18	0.6667	−0.903
26	3.26	0.5926	−0.648
27	3.30	0.5556	−0.531
39	3.66	0.5185	−0.420
42	3.74	0.4815	−0.313
45	3.81	0.4074	−0.108
48	3.87	0.3704	−0.007
52	3.95	0.3333	0.094
58	4.06	0.2963	0.196
60	4.09	0.2593	0.300
61	4.11	0.2222	0.408
62	4.13	0.1852	0.523
73	4.29	0.1481	0.467
75	4.32	0.1111	0.787
77	4.34	0.0741	0.957
104	4.64	0.0370	1.193
120	4.79	0.0000	—

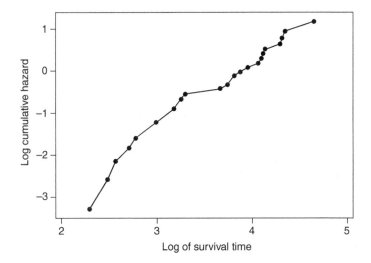

Figure 11.14. LCH plot for the glioblastoma multiforme data (note that time was measured in weeks).

Consider, now, the two-sample problem in which we wish to assume that the hazards are proportional. If we let $H_1(t)$ be the LCH function for the comparison group and $H_0(t)$ be the LCH function for the base group (that is, the baseline LCH), then under the PH assumption, (11.18),

$$H_1(t) = \phi H_0(t),$$

from which it may be shown that

$$H_1(t) = \log_e \phi + H_0(t), \tag{11.40}$$

for any survival time t. Hence, a joint plot of the two estimated LCH functions against log time should produce parallel curves if the PH assumption is valid. By (11.40), the vertical separation of the two curves in the LCH plot will provide an estimate of $\log_e \phi$, although the maximum likelihood estimate from fitting the PH model is more reliable.

If the baseline hazard has the Weibull form, then (11.39) shows that the two-group LCH plot will produce parallel *lines*. Hence, parallel relationships suggest that a Cox PH regression model may be used; if the relationships are straight lines, then a Weibull PH regression model may be used instead. Furthermore, if the parallel straight lines have slope unity, then the exponential PH model will suffice.

Example 11.16 In Example 11.7 and Example 11.13, we used PH regression models to compare low and high cellularity groups. To check the PH assumption for this problem, KM estimates (Section 5.4) are first obtained for each cellularity group. These are then used to calculate the corresponding estimated LCHs as in Table 11.8, but now separately by cellularity group. Logarithms need to be calculated for each observed survival time, again as in Table 11.8, again for each group separately.

These steps were carried out; Figure 11.15 shows the results. This LCH plot gives a good approximation to two parallel lines and hence a Weibull PH regression model is acceptable. Since the condition for a Cox model is less strenuous, this model is a possible alternative.

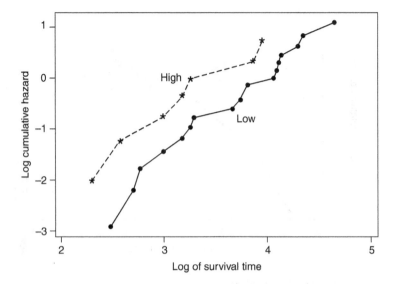

Figure 11.15. LCH plot for the glioblastoma multiforme data showing low and high cellularity groups separately (note that time was measured in weeks).

When there are several groups, the PH assumption requires a set of parallel relationships; again the Weibull and PH assumptions together require parallel lines. Calculations are straightforward as a generalisation of the two-sample problem. Quantitative variables would need to be grouped at the outset.

Example 11.17 Figure 11.16 gives the LCH plot for cholesterol fifths in the SHHS, as used in Example 11.8 (that is, for men with no CHD symptoms at baseline). A particular feature of this plot is the long line from the left for the third fifth. However, this is caused by the sole individual who had a CHD event on the first day of follow-up (so that log(time) = log(1) = 0). The remaining values produce reasonably parallel lines, except that the bottom two fifths seem to intertwine. Hence, there is no strong reason to reject a Cox or Weibull PH model for comparing cholesterol

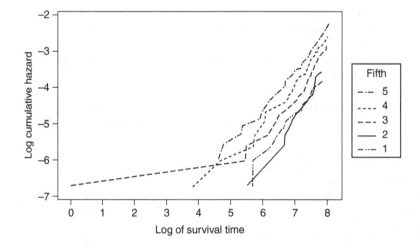

Figure 11.16. LCH plot for cholesterol fifths for SHHS men free of CHD at baseline (note that time was measured in years).

fifths, although we would expect similar hazards in the two lowest fifths, as indeed we found in Example 11.8 (there, after adjustment for blood pressure). The rank order of the LCH values in Figure 11.16 will correspond with the rank order of the hazards.

In general, we should be concerned about the PH assumption whenever the lines (or curves) run at different angles — particularly when they cross. However, as Example 11.17 shows, lines can cross due to unusual values, particularly early event outliers, or due to similar hazards, where the hazard ratio stays near unity but moves slightly above or below unity as time increases. Sampling variation can produce more subtle perturbations from parallel relationships. Hence, the LCH plot has its limitations as a diagnostic tool; it would be better to combine it with at least one of the objective methods that follow.

11.8.2   An objective test of proportional hazards for the Cox model

An objective test of the PH assumption for the Cox model may be obtained by introducing a time-dependent covariate. This follows from our observation, in Section 11.6.1, that the hazard may vary over time (thus violating the PH assumption) when a time-dependent covariate is included in the Cox model.

Consider an explanatory variable x_1 that we wish to test for PH within the Cox model. Define a new variable, x_2, as the product of x_1 and time: $x_2 = x_1 t$. Then fit the time-dependent Cox regression model

$$\log_e \phi = \beta_1 x_1 + \beta_2 x_2(t), \tag{11.41}$$

where x_2 is written as $x_2(t)$ to show that it varies with time. We then compare the fits of (11.41) and the model with the fixed covariate x_1 alone. A significant difference implies that the hazards associated with x_1 are not proportional. Values of β_2 larger than zero imply that the hazard ratio increases with time: $\beta_2 < 0$ suggests that the hazard ratio decreases with time and $\beta_2 = 0$ is consistent with PH.

Example 11.18 In Example 11.7 we assumed that the hazards for cellularity were proportional when a Cox model was used. To test this, the variable representing cellularity (coded 1 for low and 2 for high) was multiplied by time. Calling this product x_2 and calling the cellularity variable x_1, the Cox model (11.41) was fitted in SAS. The value of minus twice the log likelihood was returned as 128.019. This is to be compared with the equivalent value when x_1 is fitted alone, 128.064 from Output 11.1. The difference, $\Delta = 0.045$, is not significant ($p > 0.10$) upon comparison with χ_1^2. The estimated value of β_2 is -0.0047, so the hazard ratio (high versus low) appears to decrease slightly with time, but not in any important way.

One drawback with the test introduced here is that it is, as with all models involving time-dependent covariates, computationally demanding. Matters can be improved by taking $x_2 = x_1(t - t_m)$ where t_m is the median survival time, or $x_2 = x_1 \log(t)$. Even then, data sets with a large number of observations, such as the SHHS, require a powerful computer to fit (11.41) within a reasonable amount of time.

11.8.3   An objective test of proportional hazards for the Weibull model

As we saw in Section 11.7, the Weibull PH model requires the Weibull hazards for each group to have the same shape parameter. Hence, a test for a common shape parameter will provide a test of the PH assumption.

Consider an explanatory variable with ℓ groups. We fit separate Weibull models to the data for each separate group. The sum of the minus twice log likelihoods for these individual fits gives the measure of fit for the overall model with distinct shape parameters for each group. This is to be subtracted from the value of minus twice log likelihood for the Weibull PH regression model for the entire data (that is, using a common shape parameter for each group). The difference is compared against chi-square with $\ell - 1$ d.f.

Example 11.19 In Example 11.13 we assumed that the hazards for cellularity were proportional when a Weibull model was used. To test this, Weibull models were fitted to the low and high cellularity data separately. The values of minus twice log likelihood derived from SAS PROC LIFEREG output were 37.50 and 16.46, respectively. The value of minus twice log likelihood from fitting the PH model for cellularity to the entire data set (as in Example 11.13) was 53.98. Hence, we compare $53.98 - (37.50 + 16.46) = 0.02$ with χ^2_1. As the result is clearly nonsignificant, we can conclude that there is no evidence that a different shape parameter is required for each group. Hence, there is no evidence against PH.

11.8.4   Residuals and influence

As with other modelling procedures, model checking should include consideration of residuals and influential values. Various types of residual have been suggested for the Cox and Weibull models, and most computer packages that fit such models will produce residuals. However, interpretation is not easy, particularly because certain residuals may still have a pattern even when the fitted model is 'correct' and because censored and uncensored observations often cluster separately. An added problem with residuals from the Cox model is that they may depend upon the method used to approximate the baseline hazard (Section 11.3).

The interested reader is referred to the specialist textbooks by Kalbfleisch and Prentice (2002), Fleming and Harrington (1991) and Collett (2003). The latter gives a particularly good account of influential observations. Reviews of lack of fit methods for the Cox model are given by Kay (1984) and Le and Zelterman (1992).

11.8.5   Nonproportional hazards

When the PH assumption fails, more complex models, beyond our current scope, may be necessary. See the textbooks just referenced and Clayton and Cuzick (1985) for details.

One situation in which hazards are nonproportional is very easy to deal with, using the Cox approach, and deserves mention. This is when proportionality is lacking for one explanatory variable and yet all other explanatory variables act proportionately, and in the same way, within each of the strata formed by the 'problem' variable. The solution, which is easily applied using standard software for the Cox model, is to fit a **stratified Cox model**. A separate (unspecified) baseline hazard function is assumed here for each stratum of the 'problem' variable. Interpretation of the regression coefficients (the b parameters) follows just as for the standard Cox model. See Section 12.6 for an example of the use of the stratified Cox model.

11.9   Competing risk

As explained in Section 5.6, we may not want to treat people who are lost to follow-up due to having experienced certain types of events (not of the type of current interest) as censored, but instead treat these events as competing with the index event. Although the method for competing risk (CR) outlined in Section 5.6 works well for descriptive purposes, it is not suitable for regression modeling because of lack of specificity in relationships between the key parameters of survival models (Putter *et al.*, 2007; Bakoyannis and Touloumi, 2012). Fine and Gray (1999) suggested a simple regression model, similar to the Cox model, to address this situation. Their approach requires treating those with a competing event as not censored; that is, they are not removed from the life table as would be the case when CR is ignored. In the context of Example 5.6, suppose that the person lost to follow-up at 91 days had the competing event (say, death due to a non-CHD cause). The life table for this example, Table 5.5, would now, allowing for CR, have 4400 men at risk (of CHD) at 101 days, rather than 4399. Using this approach, a cumulative incidence function can be defined that does allow unique relationships between hazard and survival functions for any type of event. One technical issue is that Fine and Gray's distribution function does not have a proper probability distribution, because it does not integrate to unity. Consequently, this is called a **subdistribution function.** Like the Cox model, with its unspecified baseline hazard, the Fine and Gray model is semiparametric in nature, with unspecified baseline subdistribution hazards. Both models assume proportionality of effects of covariates, which should be tested for the Fine and Gray model, for example using the method suggested in Section 11.8.2. The interpretation of regression coefficients from the Fine and Gray model is similar to when the Cox model is used. However, unlike the typical situation with Cox models, interpretation of absolute effects is made though the cumulative risk of failure (as in Section 5.6), rather than survival.

In many practical situations the hazard and subdistribution hazard ratios turn out to be similar, generally because the competing event is relatively rare. As the next example shows, this is certainly not always true. Even when it is true, the cumulative risk of failure may still be quite different when evaluated from a Cox, and an equivalent Fine and Gray, model: we should expect estimated risks from the latter model to be smaller. In multiple regression models, differences between Cox hazard ratios and Fine and Gray subdistribution hazard ratios may be due to changes in the way confounding variables act on the index and competing events, rather than any direct differences on the exposure of key interest. For a succinct, but reasonably comprehensive account of modelling in CR analysis see Putter *et al.* (2007).

Implementation of Fine and Gray's model in SAS is as an option in PROC PHREG; in Stata, the STCRREG procedure may be used. Robust standard errors (Section 9.11) are preferred with this model, due to technicalities in the model's construction (Fine and Gray, 1999).

Example 11.20 The web site for this book has a link to the data from 160 men aged 65 years or older who took part in the World Health Organisation's MONICA surveys in Glasgow. Subjects were selected to be free of CVD at baseline. The variables included in this dataset are current (i.e., baseline) cigarette smoking (coded 1 for smokers and 0 for nonsmokers) and age, plus the time to an event or censoring and the nature of the event (classified as cardiovascular disease (CVD)), death from a non-CVD cause or censoring (event-free loss to follow-up) during a median follow-up period of about 11 years and a maximum of over 23 years. Amongst men who had both a CVD event and died from a non-CVD cause, the CVD event (and time to event) is that recorded. Of the 160 men, 83 had a CVD event and a further 48 had no CVD event but died from a cause other than CVD during follow-up (to the end of 2009). We wish to consider the (presumed) causal effects of smoking on CVD.

Output 11.10 Stata STCOX results for Example 11.20.

_t	Haz. Ratio	Std. Err.	z	P>|z|	[95% Conf. Interval]	
age	1.059852	.038593	1.60	0.110	.986847	1.138257
smoker	2.330337	.5413126	3.64	0.000	1.478066	3.67404

Output 11.11 Stata STCRREG results for Example 11.20 (SHR is the subdistribution hazard ratio).

_t	SHR	Robust Std. Err.	z	P>|z|	[95% Conf. Interval]	
age	1.035611	.0394801	0.92	0.359	.9610516	1.115955
smoker	1.698266	.3940784	2.28	0.022	1.077672	2.676239

The 'classic' approach to this issue, as used elsewhere in this chapter, is to treat death due to any cause except the index disease (CVD, here) as censoring. That is, anyone lost to follow-up due to emigration, being event-free at the close of the study or having a non-CVD death is censored. Output 11.10 shows the results of fitting the Cox model: from this we conclude that smoking multiplies the risk of CVD by 2.33 (i.e. the risk is about 133% higher for smokers than nonsmokers), having controlled for age. However, this is really a hypothetical result in the situation where another disease does not first lead to death. We might tell someone that smoking more than doubles your risk of CVD if you don't die from something else first. In practice, other diseases will intervene to prevent CVD from having the chance to occur in future. Furthermore, the subjects in this study are elderly, and thus at high risk of death. Finally, smoking is known to promote many diseases, in addition to CVD. Thus it makes good sense to consider non-CVD death as a competing event here.

Output 11.11 shows the results from fitting the Fine and Gray model to the same data. Notice that the hazard ratio column from Output 11.10 has been replaced by a subdistribution hazard ratio (SHR) column in Output 11.11. Now that we account for the fact that non-CVD deaths occur, and given that such (premature) deaths are more likely amongst smokers, the estimated relative risk of CVD, smokers compared to nonsmokers, is reduced to 1.70, after controlling for age. This reduction makes sense: some of the adverse effects of smoking are 'eaten up' by the competing event.

Figure 11.17 shows the estimated cumulative incidence under each of the models fitted, when evaluated at the average age of men in the study (about 69 years). Under both modeling assumptions the risk of CVD for smokers increases soon after observation starts, and there is a clear separation in risk between the two groups throughout observation. As expected, risks are considerably lower when intervening non-CVD mortality is allowed for: once a man has died from another cause he clearly has no chance of having a future CVD event.

11.9.1 Joint modeling of longitudinal and survival data

Another type of competing risk is where a quantitative or binary risk factor is being monitored over time, but death (or some other 'hard' outcome) may intervene

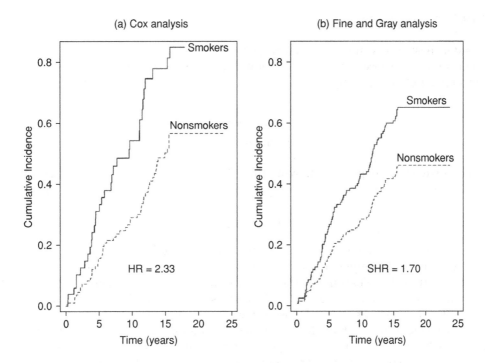

Figure 11.17. Cumulative incidence evaluated at the mean value of age from (a) Cox and (b) Fine and Gray competing risk analyses, showing results for smokers and nonsmokers separately. HR = hazard ratio; SHR = subdistribution hazard ratio.

to prevent future measurements. For instance, we might want to compare cognitive decline in old age, comparing a group who are regular drinkers with another group who are teetotallers. Anyone who dies during follow-up obviously cannot provide complete data, whilst their death may say something about the adverse effects of their drinking (or abstinence) on their cognition. In such situations it will often be possible to construct a meaningful composite outcome to study, such as 'death or a decrease of more than three points in the Mini-Mental State Examination' in the example. If this is not satisfactory, an alternative is to model the longitudinal and survival outcomes jointly: see Williamson *et al.* (2008) and Crowther *et al.* (2012).

11.10 Poisson regression

Suppose, now, that follow-up data are recorded in the form of the number of events and the number of person-years, as in Section 5.7, possibly disaggregated in some way (for example, by age group). A reasonable assumption is that the number of events follows a **Poisson** distribution because this is the appropriate probability model for counts of rare, independent events of any sort (Clarke and Cooke, 2004). With this assumption, we shall define regression models for person-years data. Subsequently, in Section 11.10.4, we will see how the same models may be used with a different type of data.

11.10.1 Simple regression

Consider, first, the situation in which person-years analysis is to be used to compare two groups: say, those 'unexposed' (group 1) and 'exposed' (group 2) to the risk factor of interest. Let the dummy explanatory variable x denote group membership:

$$x = \begin{cases} 1 \text{ for members of group 2} \\ 0 \text{ for members of group 1.} \end{cases} \tag{11.42}$$

Then we shall adopt the following linear model for the logarithm of the estimated person-years rate, $\hat{\rho}$:

$$\log_e \hat{\rho} = b_0 + b_1 x, \tag{11.43}$$

where b_0 and b_1 are some constants estimated from the observed data.

This is entirely analogous to the procedure in logistic regression in which some transformation of the estimated risk, $\hat{r}$, is assumed to have a linear relationship with the explanatory variable: see (10.3). We can use a statistical computer package to fit (11.43), taking account of the Poisson variation in the observed data, just as we fit the linear model for the transformed $\hat{r}$, accounting for the appropriate binomial variation, in Chapter 10. That is, like logistic regression (and 'normal' regression), Poisson regression is a special case of the generalised linear model. Thus we can fit Poisson models using PROC GENMOD in SAS or GLM in Stata. In addition, Stata has a POISSON routine that is specific to Poisson regression.

A further step is required to get (11.43) into the form of a generalised linear model. Since, by (5.18), $\hat{\rho} = e/y$, where e is the number of events and y is the number of person-years, then

$$\log_e \hat{\rho} = \log_e e - \log_e y,$$

so that (11.43) gives

$$\log_e e = \log_e y + b_0 + b_1 x. \tag{11.44}$$

Note that the e subscript in (11.44) refers to the base of the logarithm (as usual) and should not be confused with e standing for the number of events.

In (11.44) the term $\log_e y$ is called the **offset**. In general, an offset is an explanatory variable with a known regression parameter (here unity, because the variable $\log_e y$ is multiplied by 1), which consequently does not need to be estimated. In (11.44), the offset is the amount that must be added to the regression equation, $b_0 + b_1 x$, in order to estimate e for any given x. Thus, the regression prediction must be 'offset' by this amount. The offset will need to be declared to the computer package chosen to fit the Poisson regression model.

Usually, b_0 and b_1 in (11.44) are taken to be the maximum likelihood estimates for their population equivalents, as calculated by commercial software. Once we know b_0 and b_1, we would normally be most interested in estimating rates and relative rates. For the exposed group, (11.42) and (11.43) give

$$\log_e \hat{\rho}_2 = b_0 + b_1 \times 1 = b_0 + b_1, \tag{11.45}$$

and for the unexposed,

$$\log_e \hat{\rho}_1 = b_0 + b_1 \times 0 = b_0, \tag{11.46}$$

where $\hat{\rho}_2$ and $\hat{\rho}_1$ are the estimated event rates in the two groups. Hence,

$$\log_e \hat{\rho}_2 - \log_e \hat{\rho}_1 = b_1,$$

so that

$$\hat{\omega} = \hat{\rho}_2 / \hat{\rho}_1 = \exp(b_1) \tag{11.47}$$

is the estimated relative rate. Hence, we can find the rates and relative rate from the fitted regression parameters. Notice the similarity with the way the odds and odds ratio were found from logistic regression models in Section 10.4.1.

From (11.46), a 95% confidence interval for the unexposed rate is given by

$$\exp\left\{b_0 \pm 1.96 \hat{se}(b_0)\right\} \tag{11.48}$$

and, from (11.47), a 95% confidence interval for the relative rate is given by

$$\exp\left\{b_1 \pm 1.96 \hat{se}(b_1)\right\}, \tag{11.49}$$

both of which are easily found from standard computer output. Slightly more work is needed to find a confidence interval for the rate in the exposed group. From (11.45),

$$se(\log_e \hat{\rho}_2) = \sqrt{V(b_0) + V(b_1) + 2C(b_0, b_1)}, \tag{11.50}$$

leading to the 95% confidence interval for ρ_2 of

$$\exp\left\{(b_0 + b_1) \pm 1.96 \hat{se}(\log_e \hat{\rho}_2)\right\}. \tag{11.51}$$

We can then use the estimated variance–covariance matrix of the regression parameters use to evaluate (11.51).

Example 11.21 Consider the problem of comparing coronary event rates by housing tenure status in the SHHS. Tenure status (owner–occupiers = 2; renters = 1), the number of events and the number of person-years, as specified in the 'Total' segment of Table 5.14, were read into PROC GENMOD in SAS. Logarithms of the person-years, by tenure status, were calculated and declared as an offset. Poisson variation was also specified and the variance–covariance matrix was requested.

Output 11.12 is an extract from SAS. Here the SAS terms INTERCEPT and PRM1 refer to b_0 and TENURE 1 and PRM2 refer to b_1. By its standard rules (Section 9.2.7), SAS automatically fixes TENURE 2 (which is also referred to as the parameter PRM3) to be zero. We now substitute values from this output into the equations specified earlier.

Output 11.12. SAS PROC GENMOD results for Example 11.21.

Analysis of parameter estimates							
Parameter	DF	Estimate	Standard error	Wald 95% confidence limits		Chi-square	Pr > ChiSq
Intercept	1	−5.1866	0.0981	−5.3788	−4.9944	2797.69	<.0001
tenure	1 1	0.3705	0.1353	0.1053	0.6357	7.50	0.0062
tenure	2 0	0.0000	0.0000	0.0000	0.0000	.	.

Estimated covariance matrix		
Parameter	Prm1	Prm2
Prm1	0.009615	−0.009615
Prm2	−0.009615	0.01831

Parameter information		
Parameter	Effect	tenure
Prm1	Intercept	
Prm2	tenure	1
Prm3	tenure	2

From (11.47), $\hat{\omega} = \exp(b_1) = \exp(0.3705) = 1.45$. From (11.46), $\hat{\rho}_1 = \exp(−5.1866) = 0.00559 = 5.59$ per thousand per year, and from (11.45), $\hat{\rho}_2 = \exp(−5.1866 + 0.3705) = 8.10$ per thousand per year. Of course, $8.10/5.59 = 1.45$ as already found. Notice that the three estimates agree with the values obtained by simple arithmetic, using (5.18) as the standard definition, as given in the 'Total' segment of Table 5.13.

We can go further and calculate confidence intervals corresponding to the three estimates. From (11.49), the 95% confidence interval for ω, the relative coronary event rate (renters versus owner–occupiers), is

$$\exp(0.3705 \pm 1.96 \times 0.1353),$$

which we can also get from the SAS output as $(\exp(0.1053), \exp(0.6357))$. Either way, the result is (1.11, 1.89). Since unity is outside this interval, we reject the null hypothesis that housing tenure status has no effect on CHD at the 5% level of significance. Indeed, the p value for this test is $p = 0.0062$ from the right-hand column of Output 11.12 (but see Section 10.7.6).

From (11.48) the 95% confidence interval for ρ_1, the coronary event rate for owner–occupiers, is

$$\exp(−5.1866 \pm 1.96 \times 0.0981)$$

or (4.61, 6.78) per thousand per year. Again, we can also get this from raising the Wald 95% confidence limits columns to the exponential power. From (11.50) and the estimated variance–covariance matrix,

$$\hat{se}\left(\log_e \hat{\rho}_2\right) = \sqrt{0.009615 + 0.01831 + 2 \times (−0.009615)} = 0.09325.$$

Thus, (11.51) gives the 95% confidence interval for ρ_2, the coronary event rate for renters, as

$$\exp\{(−5.1866 + 0.3705) \pm 1.96 \times 0.09325\}$$

or (6.75, 9.72) per thousand per year.

When several (more than two) groups are to be compared, we replace x in (11.43) and (11.44) by a set of dummy variables. Results are then usually summarised by the set of relative rates (with confidence intervals), taking one group to be the base against which all others are compared. This requires repeated use of (11.47) and (11.49). The procedure is an exact analogue of that used to create a set of odds ratios in Section 10.4.3. Where appropriate, trends across the relative rates may be fitted by analogy with Section 10.4.4. In Example 11.24, we shall see a worked example of how to deal with a categorical variable, with four levels, in a Poisson regression analysis.

11.10.2 Multiple regression

The Poisson regression model may easily be extended to the situation of several explanatory variables. The basic form of the multiple Poisson regression model, by extending (11.43), is

$$\log_e \hat{\rho} = b_0 + b_1 x_1 + b_2 x_2 + \cdots + b_k x_k ,$$

where $x_1, x_2, \ldots, x_k$ are the k explanatory variables. Just as in other multiple regression models, each 'slope' parameter (b_i, for $i > 0$) represents the effect of its corresponding x variable upon the dependent variable ($\log_e \hat{\rho}$) keeping all other x variables fixed.

In particular, suppose x_k represents the exposure variable, a binary variable denoting group membership, just as in (11.42). That is,

$$x_k = \begin{cases} 1 & \text{for members of group 2 (exposed)} \\ 0 & \text{for members of group 1 (unexposed).} \end{cases}$$

All other x variables are confounding variables. Then, by reference to (11.47), the estimated relative rate for those exposed compared with those unexposed, adjusting for the confounders, is

$$\hat{\omega} = \exp\left(b_k\right) \tag{11.52}$$

with 95% confidence interval

$$\exp\left\{b_k \pm 1.96\,\hat{\text{se}}\left(b_k\right)\right\}, \tag{11.53}$$

as in (11.49). To allow for interactions, we simply let some of the xs be interaction terms, as in Section 10.9 and Section 11.6. This inevitably complicates the estimation procedure.

Comparison of two nested Poisson regression models is achieved by comparing the difference in deviance between models to chi-square with d.f. given by the difference in d.f. of the two models, in the same way as for logistic regression (Section 10.7.3).

Example 11.22 We have seen how to compare renters and owner–occupiers in the SHHS in Example 11.21. Now we consider the possible confounding effect of age, just as in the analysis of Example 5.14 where a MH analysis was used.

Table 11.9. Analysis of deviance table for Example 11.22. Each term adds to those in the previous row.

Terms in model	D	d.f.	ΔD	Δd.f.	p value
Constant	35.08	11	—	—	—
+ age	10.10	6	24.98	5	0.0001
+ tenure	3.66	5	6.44	1	0.011
+ age*tenure	0	0	3.66	5	0.60

Note: * denotes interaction; Δ denotes 'difference in'; D denotes deviance.

Data on age group (six in all), tenure status (renters/owner–occupiers), coronary events and person-years were input to SAS PROC GENMOD from Table 5.14 (this time omitting the 'Total' segment). The log of the person-years (in each age/tenure group) was used as an offset. An analysis of deviance was performed, each time adding one new term to those in the existing model; results are given in Table 11.9.

We conclude that age has an effect on the coronary rate; tenure status has an effect over and above that of age; and there is no difference in the effect of tenure across the age groups. This leads to adoption of the model

$$\log_e \hat{\rho} = b_0 + b_1(\text{age}) + b_2(\text{tenure}).$$

When this was fitted, SAS PROC GENMOD gave the results in Output 11.13. In the data input, TENURE = 1 denoted renters, TENURE = 2 denoted owner–occupiers and AGE took values from 1 to 6 according to the rank of the age group.

By (11.52), the estimated age-adjusted relative rate (renters compared with owner–occupiers) is exp(0.3439) = 1.41. This is, to two decimal places, the same as the MH estimate found in Example 5.14. By (11.53), the 95% confidence interval for the age-adjusted relative rate is

$$\exp(0.3439 \pm 1.96 \times 0.1356),$$

which can also be computed from Output 11.13 as exp((0.0783), exp(0.6096)), giving (1.08, 1.84). These, again, happen to agree precisely with the confidence limits found in Example 5.14. Note also that the p value of 0.0112 for TENURE 1 given for the Wald test in the right-hand column of Output 11.13 agrees with that ($p = 0.011$) found from the likelihood (analysis of deviance) test in Table 11.9.

Output 11.13. SAS PROC GENMOD results for Example 11.22.

Analysis of parameter estimates							
Parameter	DF		Estimate	Standard error	Wald 95% confidence limits		Chi-square	Pr > ChiSq
Intercept		1	−4.9564	0.4158	−5.7713	−4.1414	142.09	<.0001
age	1	1	−1.4992	0.6057	−2.6863	−0.3122	6.13	0.0133
age	2	1	−0.3723	0.4360	−1.2268	0.4823	0.73	0.3932
age	3	1	−0.2088	0.4297	−1.0510	0.6334	0.24	0.6270
age	4	1	−0.2300	0.4300	−1.0728	0.6127	0.29	0.5927
age	5	1	0.2304	0.4303	−0.6131	1.0738	0.29	0.5924
age	6	0	0.0000	0.0000	0.0000	0.0000	.	.
tenure	1	1	0.3439	0.1356	0.0783	0.6096	6.44	0.0112
tenure	2	0	0.0000	0.0000	0.0000	0.0000	.	.

As with simple regression models (Chapter 9), the preceding methodology is easily extended to cope with a risk factor that has several levels or a quantitative risk factor: see Example 11.24.

11.10.3 Comparison of standardised event ratios

Poisson regression may also be used to compare standardised event ratios (SERs), providing an alternative to the approach adopted in Section 5.7.3. Taking the variable x as in (11.42), consider the model

$$\log_e(\text{SER}) = b_0 + b_1 x, \tag{11.54}$$

where, as introduced in Section 4.5.2, SER $= e/E$ where e is the observed and E is the expected number of events (E having been calculated using some suitable standard population). Hence,

$$\log_e(\text{SER}) = \log_e e - \log_e E,$$

and thus (11.54) gives

$$\log_e e = \log_e E + b_0 + b_1 x. \tag{11.55}$$

Note that (11.54) and (11.55) are the same as (11.43) and (11.44) except that $\hat{\rho}$ has been replaced by SER in (11.54) and y has been replaced by E in (11.55). Provided that these changes are made, all other formulae in Section 11.10.1 and Section 11.10.2 transfer over. In particular, (11.47) and (11.49) suggest that an estimate for the relative SER is given by

$$\hat{\omega}_S = \exp\!\left(b_1\right), \tag{11.56}$$

with corresponding 95% confidence interval

$$\exp\!\left(b_1 \pm 1.96\,\hat{\text{se}}\!\left(b_1\right)\right). \tag{11.57}$$

Note that the Poisson multiple regression model now provides a means of adjusting standardised event ratios. Since standardisation is a form of adjustment, this produces a hybrid adjustment. For instance, age-standardised mortality ratios might be further adjusted, through modelling, for smoking status, if suitable data were available.

Example 11.23 SAS PROC GENMOD was used to analyse the hypothetical chemical company data of Example 5.13. Observed and expected numbers of deaths were entered for each company, and log of the expected number was declared as an offset. Codes for company were chosen so as to make the original company (of Example 5.10) the base group. Output 11.14 gives the results.

From (11.56), the estimated relative standardised mortality ratio is $\exp(-0.8849) = 0.413$, which agrees, as it should, with the value calculated from first principles in Example 5.13. From (11.57), the 95% confidence interval for the standardised event ratio is

$$\exp(-0.8849 \pm 1.96 \times 0.5227)$$

Output 11.14. SAS PROC GENMOD results for Example 11.23.

Analysis of parameter estimates							
Parameter		DF	Estimate	Standard error	Wald 95% confidence limits		Chi-square	Pr > ChiSq
Intercept		1	0.9889	0.5000	0.0089	1.9688	3.91	0.0480
company	0	1	−0.8849	0.5227	−1.9095	0.1396	2.87	0.0905
company	1	0	0.0000	0.0000	0.0000	0.0000	.	.

or (0.148, 1.150). Once again, this may also be derived from the Wald 95% confidence limits given by SAS. This confidence interval is narrower than the exact interval given in Example 5.13; the upper limit here is considerably smaller. This is explained by the small number of observed deaths (four) in the original chemical company, which compromises the approximation used here.

11.10.4 Routine or registration data

Although not concerned with follow-up data, this is the appropriate place to consider models for event rates arising from routine or registration data. This is where the estimated event rate is

$$\hat{\rho} = e/p,$$

where p is (typically) a mid-year population estimate, as in Section 3.8. Such rates may be modelled using Poisson regression. The rates are treated just as for follow-up (person-years) event rates except that p replaces y in (11.44) and all that follows in Section 11.10.1 and Section 11.10.2. To show this, an example will suffice.

Example 11.24 We shall now use the Poisson regression model to compare coronary event rates between the deprivation groups in north Glasgow using the MONICA data given in Table 4.9. For each of the 32 age/deprivation groups defined by Table 4.9, codes for age (1 to 8 in rank order) and deprivation group, mid-year population size and number of events were read into SAS. Deprivation group (the variable DEPGP) was coded so as to ensure that all slope parameters in the Poisson regression model represent comparisons with deprivation group I. As explained in Section 10.4.3, this may be achieved in SAS by coding group II as 2, III as 3, IV as 4 and I as 5 (or any other number larger than 4).

As in Example 11.22, various models were fitted using PROC GENMOD. Each fit used the log of the mid-year population as an offset. This time the unadjusted effect of deprivation group was tested as well as the age-adjusted effect. Table 11.10 gives the results.

From Table 11.10, we conclude that age has a big effect on the coronary rate; deprivation group has an effect both with and without taking account of age; and age does not modify the effect of deprivation on the coronary rate. This leads to adopting model 4,

$$\log_e \hat{\rho} = b_0 + b_1(\text{age}) + b_2(\text{depgp}).$$

When fitted, this produced Output 11.15 from PROC GENMOD. Note the huge estimated standard error for age group 1. This is because there are no events in age group 1 (25 to 29 years): see Table 4.9. Not surprisingly, SAS PROC GENMOD has not been able to estimate the effect for this group with reasonable precision. When large standard errors are found, there is usually some problem with model fitting. Such problems may be avoided by combining groups — for instance, age groups 1 and 2 in this example. For the effects that we are interested in, those for the deprivation groups, this modification makes very little difference here, so we shall proceed with the model as fitted in Output 11.15.

Table 11.10. Analysis of deviance table for Example 11.24.

Terms in model	D	d.f.	ΔD	Δd.f.	p value
1 Constant	697.79	31	—	—	—
2 Age	33.07	24	664.72[a]	7	<0.0001
3 depgp	662.87	28	34.92[a]	3	<0.0001
4 Age + depgp	13.46	21	19.61[b]	3	0.0002
5 Age*depgp	0	0	13.46[c]	21	0.89

Note: Model 5 includes the two constituent main effects.
[a] Relative to model 1.
[b] Relative to model 2.
[c] Relative to model 4.

Output 11.15. SAS PROC GENMOD results for Example 11.24, model 4.

Analysis of parameter estimates							
Parameter		DF	Estimate	Standard error	Wald 95% confidence limits		Chi-square	Pr > ChiSq
Intercept		1	−4.3850	0.1331	−4.6460	−4.1241	1084.67	<0.0001
age	1	1	−26.0795	25491.02	−49987.6	49935.41	0.00	0.9992
age	2	1	−5.5785	1.0028	−7.5440	−3.6130	30.94	<0.0001
age	3	1	−2.9358	0.3108	−3.5450	−2.3265	89.20	<0.0001
age	4	1	−1.7787	0.1923	−2.1557	−1.4018	85.55	<0.0001
age	5	1	−1.1739	0.1577	−1.4830	−0.8647	55.39	<0.0001
age	6	1	−0.9280	0.1411	−1.2046	−0.6514	43.25	<0.0001
age	7	1	−0.4503	0.1193	−0.6842	−0.2164	14.24	0.0002
age	8	0	0.0000	0.0000	0.0000	0.0000	.	.
depgp	2	1	0.2599	0.1526	−0.0392	0.5589	2.90	0.0886
depgp	3	1	0.4852	0.1450	0.2010	0.7694	11.19	0.0008
depgp	4	1	0.5724	0.1453	0.2877	0.8572	15.52	<0.0001
depgp	5	0	0.0000	0.0000	0.0000	0.0000	.	.

By reference to (11.52), the age-adjusted relative rate for deprivation group II versus group I is $\exp(0.2599) = 1.30$. The corresponding 95% confidence interval can be derived from (11.53) or the 'Wald' columns of Output 11.15 as (0.96, 1.75). The full set of estimated relative rates and confidence intervals is given in Table 11.11. Also shown are the relative SERs and corresponding 95% confidence intervals, each calculated from (5.22) and (5.23). Results by the two methods are in excellent agreement, despite the use of two different approaches to adjustment for age. Notice that, because a relative SER is a relative indirect standardised rate, the estimates of the relative SER in Table 11.11 are exactly as plotted for indirect standardisation in Figure 4.6.

Table 11.11. Relative rates (95% confidence intervals) for coronary events; north Glasgow men.

Deprivation group*	Poisson regression method	Relative SERs method
I	1	1
II	1.30 (0.96, 1.75)	1.29 (0.95, 1.77)
III	1.62 (1.22, 2.16)	1.62 (1.21, 2.18)
IV	1.77 (1.33, 2.36)	1.77 (1.32, 2.39)

* I is least disadvantaged; IV is most disadvantaged.

Table 11.12. Analysis of deviance table for dose–response
analysis (age-adjusted) in Example 11.24. The terms in the
model, besides age, refer to the assumed form of the deprivation
group effect.

Model	D	d.f.	ΔD	Δd.f.	p value
1 Age	33.07	24	—	—	—
2 Age + categorical	13.46	21	19.61[a]	3	0.0002
3 Age + linear	14.42	23	18.65[a]	1	<0.0001
4 Age + quadratic	13.52	22	0.90[b]	1	0.34
5 Age + cubic	13.46	21	0.06[c]	1	0.81

Note: The deviance and d.f. for the second and final models must be
the same.
[a] Relative to model 1.
[b] Relative to model 3.
[c] Relative to model 4.

Finally, rather than treating deprivation group as a categorical variable, we can take it as
ordinal and consider dose–response effects. This is appropriate here because the deprivation
group numbers indicate increasing relative deprivation. Through the Poisson regression model,
it is straightforward to fit a trend in the log relative rate.

As explained in Section 10.4.4 and Section 10.7.5, we fit the linear trend by defining a
quantitative variable that takes the values 1, 2, 3, 4 for successive deprivation groups I, II, III,
IV. Retaining the confounding variable (age) throughout, Table 11.12 gives the appropriate
analysis of deviance table. From this, we conclude that the log relative rate has a linear trend,
having allowed for age effects, and there is no evidence of any nonlinearity. Thus, increasing
deprivation has a constant additive effect on the log relative rate, and a constant multiplicative
effect on the relative rate, for coronary events.

When the linear trend model (model 3 in Table 11.12) was fitted in PROC GENMOD, the
parameter estimate (with estimated standard error) for the age-adjusted trend was found to
be 0.1868 (0.0436). The age-adjusted relative rate for any deprivation group compared with the
next most advantaged is thus $e^{0.1868} = 1.21$, with 95% confidence interval

$$\exp(0.1868 \pm 1.96 \times 0.0436),$$

or (1.11, 1.31).

11.10.5 Generic data

The examples using Poisson regression described here involve grouped data. As with
logistic regression (Section 10.5), generic data may also be used as input and will give
the same parameter estimates but different measures of fit (deviances). See McNeil
(1996) for a worked example.

Generic data input will be necessary when we wish to model a continuous
variable without first grouping it. When the model includes variables that alter
during follow-up, multiple records would be necessary for each subject. For example,
if we require relative rates by age group from generic data, we must define separate
observations (for entry to the computer package) for each age group for each person
(see also Section 11.11).

11.10.6   Model checking

Since Poisson regression is another member of the family of generalised linear models, not surprisingly the methods of model checking for logistic regression described in Section 10.7.1 and Section 10.11 may be adapted to the present context. In particular, with grouped data, the model deviance compared with chi-square on the model deviance d.f. gives a summary test for goodness of fit. Overdispersion is termed **extra-Poisson variation** in this context. Procedures for residuals and identifying influential observations follow similarly to logistic regression. Although formulae may vary, the results are used in precisely the same way. For example, SAS PROC GENMOD produces raw and deviance residuals for Poisson regression that are analogous to those described in Section 10.11.1.

11.11   Pooled logistic regression

An alternative to using survival models and, in some cases, to Poisson regression modelling, is to use a **pooled logistic regression** model. This is a logistic regression model, just as was described in Chapter 10, but where the observations ('lines' of data) are for every survival interval observed for every individual in the study. Here the survival intervals are predefined and would often be of equal length, such as single years of follow-up. For instance, in a mortality study that lasted 3 years, each participant could contribute up to three observations to the pooled logistic model: those who died in the first year donate one observation, those who died in the second year donate two observations and the rest contribute three observations. See Allison (1995) for a justification of the pooled logistic methodology and a detailed description of its application.

Pooled logistic regression is useful when the risk factor changes over time in a known way because it provides a direct means of incorporating such changes into the model. In this case, it is an alternative to the time-dependent Cox model (Section 11.6.1) and the Poisson regression model (Section 11.10.5). There are two situations in which risk factor values will be updated. The first is when repeat measurements of the risk factor are taken. For example, Barzi *et al.* (2003) describe a study of people who had recently suffered a nonfatal heart attack in which dietary intakes of fish, fruit, olive oil and vegetables were measured at baseline and then again at 6, 18 and 42 months after baseline. Pooled logistic regression models were used to analyse the relationship between consumption of each food and the risk of death. Here, there were four unequal survival periods, three between the four measurements and the final one lasting for an average of 3 years (to the closing date for analysis) after the 42-month dietary assessment. Consumption in each period was characterised as a time-weighted cumulative average of the frequency of consumption recorded at the start and end of the current and all preceding periods.

The second way in which risk factor values will be updated is when the risk factor naturally changes with time. For example, Gillespie *et al.* (1994) analysed a cohort study in which the goals included estimation of lung cancer risks for current smokers by number of years smoked, and for former smokers by number of years smoked and years since quitting. Details on smoking habits, such as years smoked and years since quitting, were only collected at baseline. Although no risk factor data were collected during follow-up, the number of years smoked, for smokers, and number of years since quitting, for ex-smokers, automatically increased by one for each extra year of follow-up, during which time deaths were recorded. This was easily allowed for in a pooled logistic regression model. Note, however, the assumption that smokers did not quit and former smokers did not revert to smoking during the follow-up.

Pooled logistic regression may also be useful when we wish to adjust for age in a study with a wide variation in follow-up times. In this case, adjustment for baseline age in a logistic or standard survival model may be unreliable because it is out of date in widely differently ways for different people. A pooled logistic model, like a time-dependent Cox model and a Poisson regression model used with person-years data, will allow adjustment for attained age, sometimes called 'age at risk', which is easy to compute for any follow-up survival period. This should provide better control for the confounding effects of age.

Example 11.25 As an example of how to apply the principles of pooled logistic regression, consider the SHHS housing tenure data once again. Table 5.4 indicates how many observations there will be when the basic data are expanded by year of follow-up. Looking at the owner–occupier group only, for simplicity, we see from this table that $2482 - 2472 = 10$ men experienced only (part of) the first year; $2472 - 2455 = 17$ experienced only the first two years; $2455 - 2434 = 21$ experienced only the first three years, etc. In total, then, the number of observations in the owner–occupier group in the expanded data will be:

$$\left(2482 - 2472\right) + 2 \times \left(2472 - 2455\right) + 3 \times \left(2455 - 2434\right) + \cdots$$
$$+ 9 \times \left(806 - 48\right) + 10 \times 48 = 19\ 966.$$

A similar computation for the renter group gives a result of 15 161 (actually, use of Table 5.4 gives one less; the difference is due to leap years, which were not allowed for here, for simplicity). Hence, there will be $19\ 966 + 15\ 161 = 35\ 127$ observations in the expanded data set.

To apply pooled logistic regression, the original data set (one observation per person; $n = 4402$) needs to be expanded, as explained previously, such that every one of the 35 127 observations consists of all the explanatory variables, set at the value they took at the start of the specific interval concerned for the specific individual concerned, plus a binary variable that records the CHD outcome (1 = CHD occurred; 0 = censored) at the end of the specific interval for the specific person.

For instance, suppose we wish to analyse housing tenure adjusted for age using pooled logistic regression. We then need to record tenure, age and CHD outcome for each observation in the expanded data set. Thus an individual in rented accommodation who begins the study at age 46 and dies of CHD in the fifth year of observation would donate the following five observations on tenure, age and CHD, respectively, to the expanded data set for pooled analysis:

Rented, 46, 0
Rented, 47, 0
Rented, 48, 0
Rented, 49, 0
Rented, 50, 1

This assumes that housing tenure status was not updated during the follow-up, for instance, by resurveying. Age, of course, increases by one in each successive year.

Before considering the result from a pooled logistic regression model, notice that, because housing tenure is not updated during follow-up and follow-up times are generally similar and not particularly long in the SHHS, pooled and ordinary logistic regression models should produce virtually the same result, even if the data structure and interpretation of the age adjustment are different. The odds ratio (95% confidence interval) from pooled logistic regression is 1.43 (1.09, 1.86); these results are, indeed, virtually identical to those obtained from logistic regression, 1.43 (1.09, 1.88). Notice that these results are also very similar to the earlier results (themselves the same) in Example 5.14 and Example 11.22 when MH methods and Poisson regression were applied to the grouped form of these data: 1.41 (1.08, 1.84).

Pooled logistic regression has the advantage of just being logistic regression applied to an expanded data set, thus not requiring any new methodology to produce estimates (the same PROC GENMOD statements in SAS were used for pooled and ordinary logistic regression analyses in Example 11.25). With time-dependent risk factors, it has the advantages of simplicity of application and interpretation compared with time-dependent Cox models, although when unequal intervals are used (as in Barzi *et al.*, 2003), some allowance for this must be made in the specification of the model. Furthermore, it provides a direct estimate of risk as well as the usual relative risk (or alternatives). For instance, in the application of Gillespie *et al.* (1994) mentioned earlier, age-specific estimates of the risk of lung cancer by number of years smoking, and by number of years since quitting for ex-smokers, were produced according to the number of cigarettes smoked per day. This led to estimations of the lung cancer risk a smoker of a certain age who smokes a certain number of cigarettes could have avoided by quitting at various earlier ages in her or his life. Such results are of great practical use in promoting smoking cessation.

Two disadvantages of the pooled logistic approach are the computer programming needed to expand the data set by survival period and the (often) huge size of the resultant data. Although Example 11.25 demonstrates that pooled logistic regression gives sensible results, it would not be the preferred method of analysis for the data of this example because of the simple structure of the observed data. Another disadvantage is that the exact times at which events occur are not used, yet such information will almost always be available whenever the model is used. One way around this is to use a **pooled Cox model**, which is a Cox model applied to the same expanded data set as required for the pooled logistic model, but for the addition of event or censoring times. In general, we can expect similar estimates of relative chance of disease from pooled logistic, pooled Cox, time-dependent Cox and Poisson regression models, when numbers are large but the event rates are low.

Exercises

(Most of these exercises require the use of a computer package with appropriate procedures.)

11.1 Find the two sets of actuarial estimates (using monthly intervals) of the hazard function for the Norwegian Multicentre Study data of Table C.5 (see Appendix C). Plot them on the same graph and comment on the results.

11.2 For the brain metastases data of Table C.2, treating anyone who did not die due to a tumour as censored,
   (i) Using the life table computed in Exercise 5.2 (i), estimate and plot the hazard function using the person-time and actuarial methods.
   (ii) Find the Kaplan–Meier estimates of the hazard function and plot them. Compare your result with that of (i).
   (iii) Fit an exponential distribution to the survival times. Record and plot the fitted hazard function.
   (iv) Fit a Weibull distribution to the survival times. Record and plot the fitted hazard function.
   (v) Use a LCH plot to test the exponential and Weibull assumptions.
   (vi) Compare survival experiences for those who have, and have not, received prior treatment using the Weibull and Cox proportional hazards regression models. For both approaches, find the hazard ratio for prior versus

no prior treatment and test for an effect of prior treatment, unadjusted and adjusted for age. Compare results with those of Exercise 5.2.

(vii) Use a LCH plot to check the proportional hazards assumption. Use the same plot to assess the assumption of separate Weibull distributions for the two treatment groups.

11.3 An investigation considered the effect of abnormal platelets on survival for 100 patients with multiple myeloma. Since age and sex were thought to be potential confounding variables, these were recorded. The following variables from the study were entered into a statistical software package: survival time (in months) from time of diagnosis: survival status (0 = alive; 1 = dead) at end of study; platelets (0 = abnormal; 1 = normal) at diagnosis; age (in years) at diagnosis; sex (1 = male; 2 = female). All explanatory variables were fitted as quantitative variables. Cox regression was used to analyse the data.

(i) When the explanatory variables platelets, sex and age were fitted, the parameter estimates and estimated standard errors were:

Variable	Estimate	Standard error
Platelets	−0.720	0.197
Age	−0.003	0.015
Sex	−0.307	0.083

Estimate the hazard ratio for platelets adjusted for age and sex, together with the corresponding 99% confidence interval. Interpret your result. From the model fitted, would the estimated hazard ratios for platelets be different for 40-year-old men and 50-year-old women? If so, by how much?

(ii) A further seven models were fitted to the data. The value of −2 log likelihood for each model fitted was:

Terms fitted	−2 log likelihood
Platelets	320.073
Age	311.747
Sex	321.814
Platelets + age	307.825
Platelets + sex	315.537
Platelets + age + sex	306.005
Platelets + age + sex + age*platelets	304.611
Platelets + age + sex + sex*platelets	306.000

Note: * denotes an interaction.

Stating the effect controlled for in each case, determine the role of age and sex as effect modifiers of the platelet–myeloma relationship and determine the effect of platelets on myeloma. Would you consider the model used in (i) the 'best'?

11.4 Refer to the lung cancer data of Exercise 2.2 (see the web site for this book) and use Cox regression models in the following:

(i) Fit the model that relates survival to education only, testing for the effect of education. Compare your result to that of Exercise 5.3 (iv). Add a time-dependent covariate, education multiplied by time, so as to test the basic assumption of this Cox model.

(ii)   Find estimated hazard ratios (with 95% confidence limits) to assess the effect of each of the six explanatory variables (including education) when considered individually. Take the group labelled '1' as the base group for each categorical variable.

(iii)   Continue so as to find the most appropriate Cox multiple regression model. Justify your choice.

11.5   Reanalyse the data given in Exercise 5.5 using Poisson regression: find relative rates with 95% confidence intervals, taking the lowest exposure group as base. Test for linear trend and for nonlinear polynomial relationships across the exposure groups, taking the mid-points of each exposure group as the 'scores' for the groups. You should assume a maximum dust exposure of 1200, so as to produce verifiable results.

11.6   For the smelter workers data in Table C.3, fit the appropriate Poisson regression model so as to determine the p value for the effect of exposure to arsenic, adjusting for age group and calendar period. Also find the adjusted relative rate for high versus low exposure, together with a 95% confidence interval. Compare your results with those of Exercise 5.8 (ii) and (iii).

11.7   Reanalyse the data given in Exercise 5.7: find a set of estimated relative rates with 95% confidence intervals using Poisson regression models for each vitamin (low intake = base) and compare with the results found in Exercise 5.7. Carry out tests for linear trend in the rates.

11.8   Berry (1983) gives the following observed and expected numbers of deaths due to lung cancer in men suffering from asbestosis. The data are disaggregated by the Pneumoconiosis Medical Panel at which the men were certified and the disability benefit awarded when first certified (the relative amount of compensation).

| | Number | |
Compensation	Observed	Expected
London panel		
Low	51	5.03
Medium	17	1.29
High	10	0.38
Cardiff panel		
Low	12	4.05
Medium	14	0.98
High	5	0.29

Fit all possible Poisson regression models, fitting (where appropriate) 'compensation' and 'panel' as categorical variables. Thus, test for all possible effects. Use your results to decide which (if any) of compensation, panel and their interaction are related to lung cancer death. Give a suitable set of standardised mortality ratios, together with 95% confidence intervals, to summarize your findings. Express these graphically.

11.9   Refer to the nasal cancer data of Table C.12, taking each explanatory variable as categorical.

(i)   Use Poisson regression to test the effect of age, year of first employment and duration of exposure.

    (ii)   Decide whether each of the three explanatory variables is important in the presence of the other two.

    (iii)   Give estimates and 95% confidence intervals for the adjusted relative rates.

11.10 For the lung cancer data of Exercise 2.2, fit all possible Cox models and produce a table showing the -2 log likelihood, Akaike Information Criterion (AIC) and Bayesian Information Criterion (BIC) for each model.

    (i)   Which model has the lowest value of each of these three measures of fit amongst models with 1, 2, 3, 4 and 5 predictor variables, respectively?

    (ii)   Display the AIC and BIC results for all models in a graph.

    (iii)   Which model is the best? Why?

    (iv)   Assuming that a parsimonious model is sought, which model is second best? Carry out an appropriate significance test to compare the best and second best models. What do you conclude?

CHAPTER 12

Meta-analysis

12.1 Reviewing evidence

In Chapter 2 to Chapter 11 we have seen how to design and analyse specific epidemiological studies. In this chapter, we discuss how to review the evidence of several studies, the totality ideally being all the available evidence on the association between the risk factor exposure and disease outcome of interest. Such reviews typically have two major aims:

1. To ascertain how much consistency the exposure–outcome relationship has across different studies. This addresses one of the key conditions for establishing causality in epidemiology (Section 1.6.3) — that of consistency, at least in a qualitative sense, in different study settings.
2. If appropriate, to combine the quantitative measures from the individual studies into a summary estimate (and corresponding measure of variation). Taking all relevant and appropriate studies together produces the maximum possible sample size (without new data collection), and hence must give the maximum possible precision, i.e., smallest possible confidence limits around the estimate.

The process of addressing these two aims is known as **meta-analysis**. Sometimes the term is used solely to refer to the pooling operation involved in (2) above, but this ignores the crucial question of whether pooling is really appropriate and how representative the overall pooled estimate is of the individual study estimates. In many situations, the finding that, say, a relative risk calculated in one study setting is very different from all others is just as useful as the knowledge of the overall 'best' estimate of relative risk. Consideration of what makes that one study special might suggest particular circumstances under which the exposure has a somewhat different effect or might identify a particular study design that tends to give biased answers.

Example 12.1 Lee (2001) compiled all available data, subject to some specified qualification criteria, from epidemiological studies that quantify the relationship between the type of cigarette smoked and lung cancer. Here we shall look at his collection of data from studies that compared those who had ever smoked hand-rolled cigarettes to those who had only ever smoked manufactured cigarettes. Lee identified 11 publications describing such studies: eight were case–control studies and three were cohort studies. Lee decided to separate the results, when both were available, from the same study, for men and women. Figure 12.1 displays Lee's data, showing the estimate of relative risk for each study and its 95% confidence interval; see Section 12.4.1 for a discussion of this type of diagram (called a **forest plot**). Since case–control studies cannot provide direct estimates of relative risk (Section 6.2.1), Lee has clearly assumed that the odds ratios from the case–control studies he found are good estimates of relative risk.

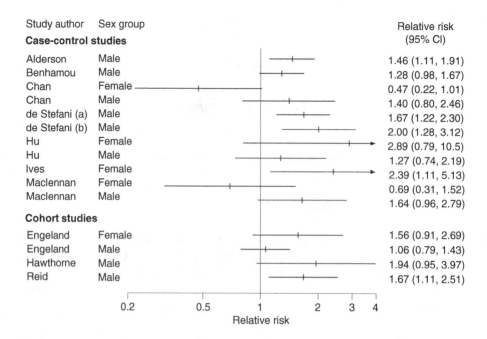

Figure 12.1. Forest plot showing the estimated lung cancer relative risks and 95% confidence intervals (CIs) for those who have ever smoked hand-rolled cigarettes compared to those who have only ever smoked manufactured cigarettes. Arrows denote limits of CIs beyond the extremes of the scale used.

Figure 12.1 is a simple, but informative, way of addressing aim (1) above. The first thing we notice from the figure is that all but two of the 15 sex-specific analyses found smoking hand-rolled cigarettes to be more hazardous than manufactured cigarettes. No studies found manufactured cigarettes to be significantly more risky than hand-rolled cigarettes at the usual 5% level, because the 95% confidence intervals straddle the line for a relative risk of one for both the studies with estimated relative risks less than one (although one of them is only marginally nonsignificant). Of the 13 studies with an estimated relative risk above one, only five had significant results at the 5% level.

This is a not untypical situation when meta-analysis is applied; in the published literature there is some uncertainty about the direction of effect and several studies where no conclusive evidence is presented. In extreme situations, it could be that every study of a particular exposure–disease relationship has been so small as to have insufficient power to detect a relative risk that would be medically important (see Chapter 8). In such situations, it is especially advantageous to continue the meta-analysis by pooling all the data together to derive an overall estimate, that is, addressing aim (2). As we shall see later, this is by no means always a sensible thing to do, but in the particular case of Example 12.1, a pooled relative risk was, indeed, quoted in the source paper.

Consideration of Example 12.1 brings to mind several issues: how did Lee compile his studies (how did he decide which studies were sensible to include and which were not); what are the differences in setting, design and methods of analysis between the studies he did select; and are some of the studies likely to be more reliable than others? Such issues are dealt with in Section 12.2. Most of the rest of the chapter is concerned with the quantitative side of meta-analysis. Specialist software packages are available for meta-analysis; most of the methods that appear in this chapter may be applied using the suite of routines that are readily downloadable to the Stata package (Sterne, 2009): see stata-press.com/data/mais.html.

12.1.1   The Cochrane Collaboration

Anyone considering meta-analysis, or even a simple descriptive review of an epidemiological association, would be well advised to consult the website of the Cochrane Collaboration: http://www.cochrane.org. This Collaboration was founded in the early 1990s to promote the development of critical review of evidence and to ensure that health care professionals have ready access to such reviews in order to be able to make well-informed decisions about health care and policy. The Collaboration has revolutionised the approach to medical research, particularly at the interface between research and practice. Collaborative review groups cover many of the major topics in medicine, whilst Cochrane Centres are in several countries. Just as with the statistical tools of meta-analysis, the Cochrane Collaboration was originally developed for application to randomised controlled clinical trials, but has since been extended to encompass epidemiological studies, diagnostic tests (Section 2.10) and other applications. The web site includes links to reviews, details of methodology and software.

12.2   Systematic review

Before we can carry out a meta-analysis, we need to compile the evidence. At the very least, this requires searching electronic databases of published literature to identify papers on the topic of interest. As we would like to identify all the relevant evidence, we may need to consider other sources of information, such as conference proceedings, government and corporate reports (so called 'grey literature'), web sites and personal communication with leading experts.

By far the best way to approach such information gathering is through a **systematic review**, by which is meant a formal, planned, objective review. Each step taken is documented in a protocol, to such an extent that another reviewer should be able to reproduce the findings, and the results are presented in a structured way, typically in tables. Systematic reviews include a **critical appraisal** wherein each study is considered for such things as potential sources of bias, generalisability and power to detect important effects. Only those studies considered relevant and valid would be taken forward into the meta-analysis. Taken together, systematic review and meta-analysis provide the basic elements of an **evidence-based approach** to medicine (Jenicek, 2003), epitomised in the Cochrane Collaboration. The idea here is that synthesis of all existing reliable and appropriate evidence provides the best possible background against which informed decisions can be made.

12.2.1   Designing a systematic review

The first step in a systematic review must be to define the aims precisely. For example, consider a review of obesity. Do we want to review all studies of obesity prevalence; all studies of the association between obesity and, say, coronary heart disease (CHD); all studies of interventions to reduce obesity, etc? Even if we can easily filter out non-epidemiological studies, such as case studies and laboratory experiments, we may still have an impossible task or, at least, stretch our resources too thinly, unless the precise demands of the review are established. Often this is best achieved through specification of the hypothesis to be addressed, for example, the null hypothesis that obesity is unrelated to CHD. This is the kind of hypothesis that we shall assume throughout this chapter.

Assuming the systematic review we have decided upon has not already been done, the next step is to consider whether there should be inclusion and exclusion criteria for our systematic review. For instance, we may be interested only in studies of the prevalence of obesity in developing countries, or in the last 10 years, or might decide, for practical reasons, to restrict to publications in English. We might well decide to exclude studies that fail to fulfill some quality criteria, such as those that do not use some essential measurement tool or those clearly so poorly designed as to be worthless because they are likely to have biased results (Section 12.2.2).

Next we must decide how we will identify the relevant studies. Generally, this will be through searches of electronic databases, typically including Medline (e.g., via PubMed: http://www.ncbi.nlm.nih. gov/PubMed). Some skill is required in the use of search terms so as to be exhaustive but not include totally irrelevant 'hits'. For an example, consider an analysis of the effect of different levels of cigarette tar on lung cancer (an issue also considered by Lee, 2001, in the paper giving rise to Example 12.1; see also National Cancer Institute, 2001). Searching an electronic medical database using the term 'tar' will identify, even in a single year, a range of publications that have no bearing upon the epidemiological issue at hand. For instance, TAR is used as an abbreviation for 'target achievement ratio' and 'traumatic aortic rupture', amongst other things. Even simultaneous searching with the terms 'tar' and 'lung cancer' may still identify studies relating products of industrial processes (e.g., coal tar) with lung cancer and may include animal experiments.

Searching can be improved by use of the National Library of Medicine medical subject heading (MeSH) terms, available on major medical databases. See Gault *et al.* (2002) for comments on the use of MeSH terms in practice. In some cases, we may find it useful to use truncated search terms, which allow for words with different endings that have the same importance in our search. For example, in PubMed Medline, an asterisk is used as a wildcard, so the search term 'epidemiol*' would identify uses of 'epidemiology', 'epidemiological' and 'epidemiologic' as well as certain foreign-language variations.

The point of the search will be to identify all material relevant to our hypothesis (or hypotheses) and to omit anything that is clearly irrelevant or does not satisfy the qualification criteria. In most cases, this is begun on-line using titles and, where available, abstracts and completed by review of the complete publication or report. Reasons for excluding studies should be recorded, especially when they are rejected for reasons of quality. This is often achieved through simple checklists (data sheets) completed for all studies, which are subsequently summarised in a table in the final report of the systematic review. Multiple publications from the same study must be consolidated and duplications avoided. If possible, decisions to include or exclude should be ratified by a second person.

The studies accepted for the review will require summarisation. A convenient way of doing this is through a **data extraction table**, showing such things as authors, setting, design, sample size, major results relevant to the hypothesis, conclusions drawn and comments on quality (Section 12.2.2). Some reviews include a score of study quality (Section 12.7). Studies that are themselves reviews would normally be included, but only 'new' information would be extracted. Data extraction tables form the core of the descriptive outcome from systematic reviews; text will normally be added to draw overall conclusions in final reports.

If sufficient quantitative information is available and this is a goal of our review, we may continue by summarising the numerical results. As mentioned already, this is the subject of following sections of this chapter. Some studies may have adequate design but be inappropriately analysed, in which case we might keep them in the systematic review but not be able to extract suitable data for subsequent quantitative summaries of evidence. This quantitative stage is not necessary, nor should it be seen as necessarily desirable. If there are few studies, or sufficient lack of uniformity in approach to bring into question the utility of any form of numerical summarisation (Section 12.4), we may reasonably decide to stop at the descriptive stage.

Details of all stages of systematic reviews, as well as example checklists, are available from the University of York, NHS Centre for Reviews and Dissemination (http://www.york.ac.uk/inst/crd/ report4.htm). Other sources of advice on how to undertake systematic reviews in epidemiology include Dickersin (2002) and Stroup *et al.* (2000). Guidelines for reporting systematic reviews (and meta-analyses) are given by Moher *et al.* (2009). The Cochrane handbook is available at http://handbook.cochrane.org/.

Example 12.2 Woodward *et al.* (2000) describe a systematic review of studies of mental disorder amongst those who committed homicide, this being one component of a comprehensive review of the epidemiology of mentally disordered offending (Badger *et al.*, 1999). The aim was to summarise all the international research since 1990 that gave quantitative information, based on more than 10 people, on mentally disordered homicide offenders (such as their demographic profile or trends in their numbers over time) and the link between psychiatric conditions and the act of committing homicide (such as odds ratios for homicide comparing the mentally disordered with all others).

A wide range of electronic databases was searched, including medical (such as Medline), social science and criminology databases, restricted to articles with at least an abstract written in English. These were searched using a wide range of search terms, including truncated terms. The search was extended to unpublished work through use of book catalogues, compilations of dissertation abstracts and searches of conference proceeding and 'grey literature' databases. Hand searches of leading journals and citation tracing were also part of the search strategy. A letter seeking information and advice was sent to authors of key articles identified in these searches and to known international experts, and was also distributed at an important conference. Personal contact, principally by e-mail, was found crucial to the success of the review, especially for identifying government publications and material in press.

Selection of material to review followed a three-step process (simplified here to cover only published academic papers). First, titles of all identified articles were read. When the titles clearly indicated that the corresponding paper would not be relevant (about 75% of the total), this paper was discarded. Second, abstracts were obtained for the remainder, where possible through electronic means. All were read and for those not relevant (about 60%) the papers were rejected. Third, for the remainder, complete papers were obtained for full review. A member of the review team read every article; translators were employed where necessary.

For each study, basic details were entered into a standard checklist, which served to ascertain that the study satisfied the conditions of the review protocol. If so, another standard form was completed which included questions on design, sample size, generalisability, dropout rate and diagnostic criteria. Any study deemed inadequate, for prespecified reasons of unreliable diagnosis, lack of specificity to the issue or poor design (suggesting biased results), as well as any duplicates (including preliminary versions of later reports), was excluded at this stage (10% of the exclusions were read by another team member as a check). These studies were listed with the reasons for exclusion. The remaining articles were summarised in a data extraction table; Table 12.1 shows a sample of two consecutive rows of this.

Altogether, 28 studies, from 10 countries, were included in the data extraction table and the final report; seven studies were read in full but excluded, most often because they reported results only for homicide followed by suicide, rather than just homicide. The final report included descriptive summaries of the 28 studies, grouped by general characteristics such as 'studies of trends' and 'studies of homicide recidivists'. It also included overall summaries of the epidemiological findings and discussed the shortfalls in the available data and how these might be addressed in future research.

Table 12.1. Portion of a summary table from a systematic review of mentally disordered homicide offenders.

Author	Aims of study	Characteristics of subjects	Instruments/ sources used	Main findings	Comments on quality	Conclusions drawn
Boscredon– Noé et al. (1997)	Analysis of trends in the number of mentally disordered homicide offenders over the period 1838–1995.	$n = 108$ men who committed homicide or tentative homicide and then were confined in the Albi psychiatric hospital in the mid-Pyrénées (southern France).	Hospital records	Annual rate of mentally disordered homicide offenders hospitalised remained constant at 0.23–0.30 per 100 000 per year. Family members are victims of the attack in 55% of cases; most often a woman who lives with the offender is the victim.	Changes in definitions and catchment areas over time may cause problems. Not every mentally disordered homicide offender is necessarily included.	No trends in mentally disordered homicide offenders over time. Family members often targeted.
Bourget and Bradford (1990)	Comparison of parental and other homicide offenders.	$n = 13$ (parental) $n = 48$ (other) cases referred to a forensic psychiatry service in Ottawa.	DSM-III-R	Mean age was 27 years (parental group) and 29 years (comparison group). 69% of parental group were female compared with 19% of others; 62% of parental group were married compared with 17% of others. Psychiatric diagnoses were similar in the two groups although only the parental group had any subjects with major depression (31%).	Only considers cases sent for psychiatric evaluation. Small numbers; power of 35%.	Murder of one's own children appears to be a multifaceted phenomenon. A preventative approach needs to consider the parents' potential to abuse, the vulnerability of the child and the presence of a crisis that might precipitate the abuse.

Note: The power shown is that for detecting a relative risk of 3 for a factor with 50% prevalence using a two-sided 5% test.

DSM-II-R = Diagnostic and Statistical Manual of Mental Disorders (revised third edition).

Source: Woodward *et al.* (2000).

12.2.2   Study quality

Inevitably, the studies compiled through a systematic, or a more informal, review will vary in quality. Part of the process of review is to identify such quality differentials and to report on them within the narrative of the data extraction summary. Quality assessment is clearly inescapable for systematic reviews which adopt a quality threshold below which studies will be rejected.

The earlier chapters of this book give a guide to assessing study quality. As far as study design goes, Section 1.8 determines the broad hierarchy: intervention studies generally give the most reliable information, cohort studies are second best and case–control studies third. This should not be read as saying that, for example, all cohort studies give more reliable inferences about the risk factor–disease relationship than all case–control studies, but just that this is to be expected in general. The specific circumstances of the problem at hand must also be a consideration. For example, the case–control methodology is better suited to studying the use of a mobile phone as a source of distraction leading to increased risk of a car crash than the cohort study approach, because only the former can study acute use as opposed to general use, not specific to the time of the accident. The preceding specialist chapters on particular study designs give general comments on subtypes of the major study designs in epidemiology.

Another quality issue is whether the study has been appropriately analysed. Again, reference to earlier chapters will provide the reader with the basic tools to answer this question. Aspects of this are whether appropriate control for confounding and tests for interaction have been carried out. Study conduct is also a crucial aspect of study quality: poor choice of controls, high rates of nonresponse and inadequate follow-up are examples of poor conduct because they are likely to have led to biased results. In reports of systematic reviews, we should also quantify the sampling error for each study, generally summarised by sample size, width of confidence interval or (as in Example 12.2) power to detect a specific effect. The latter two are more useful than sample size when comparing studies of varying designs. Sampling error is generally not, however, considered when determining quality scores (Section 12.7).

All the preceding issues are sometimes categorised as being about **internal validity**: how well has the specific study addressed the hypothesis of the review in its own setting? This may be contrasted with another broad dimension of quality, **external validity**. This includes considering how generalisable the results are to other settings. Typical examples would be where a study is restricted to men, or to hospital patients. It also includes consideration of the measurement tools used and the outcome measure. For instance, an international convention for recording diagnoses would generally be preferable to a local convention, and a true outcome measure would generally be preferable to a proxy.

A final quality issue concerns the publication (or alternative medium) that describes the study. If this is inadequate, perhaps because description of issues that help determine levels of bias is lacking, confidence limits (or standard errors) are not given for estimates, or details of how measurements (such as biochemical assays) were carried out are missing, then we would conclude that the information extracted is of poor quality by virtue of omission of such details.

Although a general epidemiologist will be able to describe all these aspects of quality, subject specialists are often required to turn such descriptions of specific aspects into assessments of quality. For example, only a subject expert would be able to judge whether adjustment for confounders has been appropriately performed.

12.3   A general approach to pooling

The basic idea of meta-analysis is to take a set of like quantities (such as relative risks) from a number of studies and to summarise them using some overall average of these quantities. This average could be a simple mean; however, this would give equal weight to all studies, so generally this would be unacceptable. For instance, we might prefer to give greater weight to a study with a larger sample size. Alternatively, we might have some idea of the quality of the individual studies and wish to give greater weight to a study with a higher quality score. Such considerations lead to the use of a weighted average in meta-analysis.

Suppose that there are k studies in the meta-analysis. The pooled summary of the estimates $\hat{\theta}_1, \hat{\theta}_2, ..., \hat{\theta}_k$ taken from the k studies is the weighted average

$$\hat{\theta}_{\text{pooled}} = \frac{\sum w_i \hat{\theta}_i}{\sum w_i}, \qquad (12.1)$$

where w_i is the weight given to the ith study (or, more strictly, the weight given to $\hat{\theta}_i$), and the summation runs over all k studies. (12.1) is a special case of the general formula for a weighted mean, (10.33).

To ascertain the reliability of the meta-analysis summary estimate, we should (as in all other applications in this book) calculate a corresponding measure of variation. The estimated standard error of the pooled estimate is

$$\hat{\text{se}}\left(\hat{\theta}_{\text{pooled}}\right) = \frac{\sqrt{\sum w_i^2 \hat{\text{var}}(\hat{\theta}_i)}}{\sum w_i}, \qquad (12.2)$$

where $\hat{\text{var}}(\hat{\theta}_i)$ is the estimated variance of $\hat{\theta}_i$. Again, (12.2) is a special case of the general formula, (10.34). To obtain confidence intervals for θ_{pooled} we shall assume that this arises from a normal distribution. The 95% confidence interval is then

$$\hat{\theta}_{\text{pooled}} \pm 1.96\,\hat{\text{se}}\left(\hat{\theta}_{\text{pooled}}\right). \qquad (12.3)$$

As usual, we replace 1.96 by other critical values from Table B.2 in order to obtain confidence intervals for different percentage levels.

As we have seen in Section 3.1 and Section 10.16, the distribution of the log relative risk is better approximated by a normal distribution than is the relative risk. Therefore, if we wished to pool relative risks (such as those in Example 12.1), we would do better to work with the log relative risks; that is, taking the quantity $\hat{\theta}_i$ to be the estimated log relative risk for study i, for all values of i. Having obtained the estimate and its confidence limits, from (12.1) and (12.3), we would usually back-transform to the raw scale — that is, raise the results to the exponential power (assuming logs to the base e have been used) before presentation. Besides relative risks, both odds ratios and hazard ratios should be dealt with on the log scale so as to improve the approximation to normality. See Section 12.3.7 for examples.

To test whether a pooled summary statistic is significantly different from zero, we compute the test statistic,

$$\hat{\theta}_{\text{pooled}} \Big/ \hat{\text{se}}\left(\hat{\theta}_{\text{pooled}}\right), \qquad (12.4)$$

and compare with the standard normal distribution (Table B.2). In the case of relative risks, odds ratios and hazard ratios, this is applied on the log scale where it tests, for instance, whether the log relative risk is zero (equivalent to testing whether the relative risk is one).

12.3.1 Inverse variance weighting

To use (12.2), (12.3) and (12.4), we need to decide upon the weights for each study. As the name suggests, the weights used in the **inverse variance** (IV) weighting scheme are

$$w_i = 1/\text{v}\hat{\text{a}}\text{r}(\hat{\theta}_i) \tag{12.5}$$

for $i = 1, 2, \ldots k$. The great advantage of this weighting scheme is that the variance of the pooled estimate is then as small as it could possibly be; that is, we get maximum precision for the main result of our meta-analysis. Not surprisingly, this is the most popular weighting scheme, but note that it takes no account of any differences in study quality, such as differential levels of bias error. Under IV weighting, (12.2) reduces to the simpler form

$$\hat{\text{se}}(\hat{\theta}_{\text{pooled}}) = 1/\sqrt{\sum w_i}, \tag{12.6}$$

which would then be plugged into (12.3). We shall assume IV weighting throughout Section 12.3, but consider some alternatives in Section 12.5 and Section 12.7.

12.3.2 Fixed effect and random effects

There are two basic approaches to meta-analysis: we assume a fixed effect or random effects. Whilst (12.1) to (12.6) apply in both cases, they differ in how the values of the estimated variances of the individual quantities to be pooled, $\text{v}\hat{\text{a}}\text{r}(\hat{\theta}_i)$, are computed (which determines the IV weights) and in how the principal result of the meta-analysis, the pooled estimate, (12.1), is interpreted.

A **fixed effect** meta-analysis is the most straightforward. It assumes that there is an overall true quantity that every study is estimating. Although most, if not all, studies miss this true result, the amount by which they miss is assumed to be purely due to sampling error. For instance, in Example 12.1, each study contributes a relative risk that is assumed to be an estimate of the true relative risk relating all who have ever smoked hand-rolled cigarettes to all who have smoked manufactured cigarettes only. It is just chance that some of the individual estimates are rather closer or further away from the (unknown) true relative risk. All else being equal, we do anticipate, of course, that larger studies will be rather closer to this true relative risk (see Section 12.8.1 for a development of this idea).

Random effects meta-analysis (DerSimonian and Laird, 1986) assumes that the true quantities from the individual studies have a probability distribution (usually assumed to be normal, for convenience). The pooled estimate, (12.1), then estimates the mean of the individual study-specific quantities. In the context of Example 12.1, each study is assumed to have a true relative risk, which is allowed to be different from the true relative risk in any other study. Meta-analysis techniques may be used to estimate the mean of all these true relative risks, and this is an estimate of the average relative risk comparing people who ever smoked hand-rolled cigarettes to people who have smoked nothing other than manufactured cigarettes. The pooled estimate now has two sources of sampling error: one due to within-study variation and one due to the variation between studies.

The meta-analysis literature of recent years is replete with discussion of the pros and cons associated with these two methods. One extreme argument is that unless the fixed effect assumption is correct, meta-analysis is meaningless; that is, the overall summary has no useful interpretation. This philosophy is consistent with thinking of the study as a variable that might interact with the exposure variable of interest (type of cigarette in Example 12.1). As stated in Section 4.9, when an interaction occurs, the main effects are meaningless — in this context, this means that if the true effect of exposure differs by study — it is fruitless to talk about some universal summary measure of the effect of exposure.

At the other extreme, it might be argued that it is unreasonable to assume that every epidemiological study of a given risk factor exposure and disease would estimate exactly the same quantity because of variations in study design and conduct. For instance, the inclusion criteria might differ and there could well be different relationships for different types of people. Relative risks relating those who have ever smoked hand-rolled cigarettes to those who have smoked only manufactured cigarettes might, for example, be different for studies using relatively younger people.

In some ways, the random effects assumption is the safe option. It produces confidence intervals that are never smaller than the corresponding fixed effect intervals, and thus allows more scope for uncertainty. If there is no between-study variation, the more complicated random effects estimate and corresponding confidence interval will simply collapse down to the fixed effect results. Unfortunately, the fixed and random effects estimates (as well as their confidence intervals) are usually not the same and may differ even when the between-study variation is fairly small.

Some authors avoid the problem of choice by including both fixed and random effects results in their meta-analysis, usually avoiding any explicit interpretation of the meaning of the separate values. Certainly this gives people of both philosophies the quantitative information they require. Others fix their chosen assumption *a priori* or base acceptance or rejection of the fixed effect assumption upon the evidence for heterogeneity in the observed data (Section 12.3.3). Whatever method of working is adopted, it is important that it is made clear to all potential users of the meta-analysis.

12.3.3   Quantifying heterogeneity

The decision about which method of meta-analysis to use depends upon whether we believe that the studies are homogeneous or heterogeneous with respect to the effect of exposure to the study variable on the disease of interest. If we believe that they are homogeneous, then the fixed effect approach is acceptable; if not, then we either conclude that pooling is undesirable or we accept the random effects approach. Either way, it would naturally be advantageous to quantify the degree of heterogeneity across the studies in the meta-analysis.

One way to do this is through a test of the null hypothesis of homogeneity, which may also be viewed as a test of lack of interaction between the study and the exposure. Suppose that the weighted average, (12.1), is calculated using some study-specific weights that ignore between-study variation, i.e., using fixed effect weights. Let the result of (12.1) with such weights be $\hat{\theta}_{FX}$. The homogeneity test statistic is then,

$$Q = \sum w_i \left(\hat{\theta}_i - \hat{\theta}_{FX} \right)^2, \tag{12.7}$$

where the summation runs from 1 to k (recall that k is the number of studies). This is to be compared with chi-square on $k - 1$ d.f. The test is derived under the assumption that IV weighting is used. Even when the pooled estimate, $\hat{\theta}_{FX}$, is derived using some other weighting scheme, it is still common to use (12.7) to test homogeneity (an example is given in Section 12.5.2).

The individual components of (12.7) represent the contributions of the corresponding studies to the test statistic, Q, which increases with increasing heterogeneity. That is, study i contributes

$$q_i^2 = w_i\left(\hat{\theta}_i - \hat{\theta}_{FX}\right)^2 \tag{12.8}$$

to the overall result. Examination of these components of heterogeneity gives useful information. Studies that suggest most strongly that they are really estimating something other than the overall (fixed effect) weighted mean will stand out as having the largest components.

The test of homogeneity should be used with caution because it will be subject to the limitations of all tests (Section 3.5.5). Since there are rarely a large number of studies to pool, a common issue in meta-analysis is whether the homogeneity test has sufficient power (Section 8.2) to be able to reach a reliable conclusion. For this reason, some people use a less extreme significance level than usual to reach a decision for this test. Typically, if 5% tests are taken as the norm, a 10% level is used as the cut-off for rejecting the null hypothesis of no heterogeneity. However, the justification for this 'correction' is dubious; the degree of correction is quite arbitrary and will lead to unacceptable levels of type I error when many studies are in the meta-analysis. Hence, it is not recommended as a standard rule. If, as is suggested, the statistical test is seen as a *guide* to aid decision making, the choice of a cut-off is hardly crucial.

Given the problems with the test, a better approach would be to estimate the degree of heterogeneity. Higgins and Thompson (2002) suggest two summary measures of heterogeneity, called H and I^2:

$$H = \sqrt{Q/(k-1)} \tag{12.9}$$

$$I^2 = 100\left(Q - (k-1)\right)/Q \tag{12.10}$$

$$= 100\left(1 - (1/H^2)\right), \tag{12.11}$$

both of which are defined only for $Q > k - 1$. If $Q \leq k - 1$, H is defined to be unity and I^2 to be zero. H corrects Q for its degrees of freedom, avoiding the difficulty of the p value for Q depending upon the number of studies in the meta-analysis. As Higgins *et al.* (2003) discuss, I^2 has a very useful interpretation as the percentage of variability across studies that is attributable to heterogeneity rather than chance.

Higgins and Thompson (2002) provide various methods for quantifying the uncertainty in H and I^2, the simplest of which uses test-based methods to compute the estimated standard error of the logarithm of H when $Q > k$ as

$$\hat{se}\left(\log_e H\right) = \frac{\log_e Q - \log_e(k-1)}{2\left(\sqrt{2Q} - \sqrt{2k-3}\right)} \tag{12.12}$$

and when $Q \leq k$ as

$$\hat{se}\left(\log_e H\right) = \sqrt{\frac{3(k-2)^2 - 1}{6(k-2)^3}} \; .$$

In both cases, 95% confidence limits for H are then (L, U) where

$$L = \exp\left\{\log_e H - 1.96 \; \hat{se}\left(\log_e H\right)\right\}$$
$$U = \exp\left\{\log_e H + 1.96 \; \hat{se}\left(\log_e H\right)\right\}.$$

$$(12.13)$$

When (12.13) gives values less than one, they are rounded up to one. A 95% confidence interval for I^2 is then easily derived from (12.11) as

$$\left(100\left(1 - \left(1/L^2\right)\right), \; 100\left(1 - \left(1/U^2\right)\right)\right).$$

$$(12.14)$$

When L or U is one, the corresponding limit for I^2 will automatically become zero. Of these two statistics, I^2 is preferable in practice because of its easy interpretation. I^2 may be compared across meta-analyses with different numbers of studies and using different metrics (relative risk, risk difference, etc.).

If we prefer to use a statistical method to choose between fixed and random effects based on the observed data, we could use I^2 to decide whether there is more than a critical level of heterogeneity by predefining an acceptable level. For instance, we might decide to accept a fixed effect approach when less than 25% of the variation is due to heterogeneity. Otherwise, we simply take I^2 as a useful companion to our pooled summary estimate.

In practice, the majority of authors of epidemiological meta-analyses conclude that important heterogeneity is likely to be present. This is not surprising given likely variations in study design, settings, measurements and ways with which confounding is dealt. Hence, random effects results are more common in published analyses.

12.3.4   *Estimating the between-study variance*

As we have seen, the essential difference between the fixed effect and random effects methods is that only the latter allows for between-study variation. The between-study variance, generally denoted τ^2, may be estimated (Sutton *et al.*, 2000) from the mean, $\overline{w}$, and variance, s_w^2, of the fixed effect weights. Consider the quantity,

$$D = \frac{k-1}{k\overline{w}}\left(k\overline{w}^2 - s_w^2\right).$$

$$(12.15)$$

If $Q > k - 1$, the estimated value of τ^2 is taken to be

$$\hat{\tau}^2 = (Q - k + 1)/D.$$

$$(12.16)$$

On the other hand, if $Q < k - 1$, we take $\hat{\tau}^2$ to be zero. In this latter case, no between-study variation is present and the random effects measures reduce to the fixed effect measures.

12.3.5 Calculating inverse variance weights

In Section 12.3.1 we have seen the formulae for the IV weight, (12.5), and its standard error, (12.6), for the ith study. As both depend upon the variance of the estimate from study i, the way we compute them differs for fixed and random effects meta-analysis.

Under the fixed effect assumption, everything is straightforward. The weight for study i is simply the inverse of the usual variance estimate calculated using the data collected in study i. For example, when dealing with log relative risks, we take the reciprocal of the square of the result of (3.5).

Under the random effects assumption, the estimated variance associated with study i should include a component for the between-study variation. That is, the weights now become

$$w_i^{(R)} = 1 \Big/ \Big(\big(1/w_i \big) + \hat{\tau}^2 \Big), \tag{12.17}$$

and (12.6) applies with $w_i^{(R)}$ replacing w_i. Due to the inclusion of a constant term, $\hat{\tau}^2$, in each calculation, the random effects weights will be more alike than their fixed effect counterparts. Random effects meta-analysis thus tends to give less extreme weights to larger studies, compared to fixed effect.

12.3.6 Calculating standard errors from confidence intervals

The methodology described so far assumes that the quantities to be pooled and their standard errors are directly available from all studies. If our only source of information about a particular study is its published account, we will, of course, be limited by what the authors decided to include. When a confidence interval is given, rather than a standard error, formulae given earlier in this book may often be used to estimate the missing standard error.

Example 12.3 The summary statistics given in Example 12.1 are estimates of relative risk and their 95% confidence intervals. These have been derived from various different values presented in the original study publications, but for our purposes we shall treat these as the only data available. To use the approach to pooling given in this section, we need to derive the corresponding set of log relative risks (straightforward to compute) and their standard errors. The latter come from taking logs of the lower confidence limit and noting that this is the log relative risk minus 1.96 times the required standard error. To see this, inspect (3.11) and (3.12). Thus, if we subtract the log lower limit from the log relative risk and divide by 1.96, we get the standard error. We should then do a similar operation using the upper confidence limit; now the estimated standard error is the log upper limit minus the log relative risk, all divided by 1.96. The two answers should be the same, but will generally differ due to rounding error. Our final best estimate is then the average of the two results.

As an example, consider the first study in Figure 12.1, Alderson. The estimated log relative risk is $\log_e(1.46) = 0.37844$. The log of the lower 95% confidence limit is $\log_e(1.11) = 0.10436$. The standard error is then estimated as

$$(0.37844 - 0.10436)/1.96 = 0.13984.$$

The log upper 95% limit is $\log_e(1.91) = 0.64710$. From this, the standard error is estimated as

$$(0.64710 - 0.37844)/1.96 = 0.13707.$$

Table 12.2. Estimates and standard errors to be pooled and consequent weights for the meta-analysis of data from Figure 12.1.

		Log relative risk		Weights	
Study author	Sex	Estimate	Standard error	Fixed effect	Random effects
Alderson	male	0.37844	0.13845	52.169	18.461
Benhamou	male	0.24686	0.13598	54.082	18.696
Chan	female	−0.75502	0.38880	6.615	5.372
Chan	male	0.33647	0.28656	12.178	8.539
de Stefani (a)	male	0.51282	0.16175	38.222	16.350
de Stefani (b)	male	0.69315	0.22729	19.357	11.540
Engeland	female	0.44469	0.27649	13.081	8.973
Engeland	male	0.05827	0.15138	43.638	17.267
Hawthorne	male	0.66269	0.36481	7.514	5.949
Hu	female	1.06126	0.65997	2.296	2.125
Hu	male	0.23902	0.27679	13.053	8.960
Ives	female	0.87129	0.39050	6.558	5.334
Maclennan	female	−0.37106	0.40559	6.079	5.013
Maclennan	male	0.49470	0.27216	13.501	9.169
Reid	male	0.51282	0.20814	23.083	12.768
Total				311.424	154.515

The two estimates of the same thing differ because the confidence intervals given in Lee (2001), reproduced in Example 12.1, are only given to two decimal places. The best estimate of the s.e. of the log relative risk is (0.13984 + 0.13707)/2 = 0.13845. Repeating these calculations for all studies produces the first and second data columns of Table 12.2, which give all the necessary information to begin pooling using the formulae given above (see Example 12.4).

The basic meta-analysis routine in Stata, METAN, allows for the use of either standard errors or confidence limits in the pooling process for the meta-analytic mean. However, whichever is used has to be the same for all studies.

12.3.7 Case studies

In principle, the IV weighting approach may be used to pool any kinds of like quantities. As already indicated, the methods given here assume a normal distribution, so we should apply a normalising transformation (see Section 2.8.1) when required, such as with relative risks, odds ratios and hazard ratios where log transforms should be used. In this section, we shall see two examples of how to handle meta-analyses with this common transformation.

Example 12.4 A fixed effect meta-analysis of the data in Example 12.1 uses the results from Example 12.3. To obtain the weights, we apply (12.5), which requires taking the reciprocal of the square of the second data column of Table 12.2. The results — the fixed effect weight for each study — are shown in the third data column of this table. Applying (12.1) gives the estimated pooled log relative risk as

$$\left\{ \left(52.169\right)\left(0.37844\right) + \left(54.082\right)\left(0.24686\right) + \cdots + \left(23.082\right)\left(0.51282\right) \right\} / 311.424$$

$$= 0.34064.$$

Applying (12.6) gives the estimated standard error of this as

$$1/\sqrt{311.424} = 0.05667.$$

From (12.3) we then get the 95% confidence limits as

$$0.34064 \pm 1.96 \times 0.05667 = (0.22957, 0.45171).$$

Going back to the raw scale, the estimated pooled relative risk is computed as exp(0.34064) with confidence limits (exp(0.22957), exp(0.45171)). The fixed effect IV weighted estimate (with 95% confidence interval) of the lung cancer relative risk for ever smoking hand-rolled cigarettes compared to smoking only manufactured cigarettes is thus 1.41 (1.26, 1.57).

A test of the null hypothesis that the pooled log relative risk is zero (i.e., the pooled relative risk is unity) comes from (12.4):

$$0.34064/0.05667 = 6.01.$$

From Table B.1, we can see that this is highly significant, $p < 0.0001$, so we reject the null hypothesis.

We can test the null hypothesis that the log relative risks (and hence the relative risks) are homogeneous across the studies from (12.7), computed here as

$$Q = \left(52.169\right)\left(0.37844 - 0.34064\right)^2 + \cdots + \left(23.082\right)\left(0.51282 - 0.34064\right)^2$$

$$= 23.689.$$

This is compared to chi-square on $(15 - 1) = 14$ d.f.; from a computer package, $p = 0.05$. To summarize the heterogeneity, we use (12.10): $I^2 = 100 \times (23.689 - 14)/23.689 = 40.9$. To compute 95% confidence limits for this percentage, we first use (12.12) (noting that $Q > k$) to get

$$\hat{se}\left(\log_e H\right) = \frac{\log_e(23.689) - \log_e(14)}{2\left(\sqrt{2 \times 23.689} - \sqrt{27}\right)} = 0.15588.$$

Then, from (12.9), $H = \sqrt{23.689/14} = 1.3008$. Substituting these values into (12.13) gives

$$L = \exp\left\{\log_e(1.3008) - 1.96 \times 0.15588\right\} = 0.9583,$$

which would be rounded up to one, and

$$U = \exp\left\{\log_e(1.3008) + 1.96 \times 0.15588\right\} = 1.7656.$$

Finally, from (12.14), 95% confidence limits for I^2 are

$$\left(0, \; 100 \times \left(1 - \left(1/(1.7656)^2\right)\right)\right) = (0, \; 67.9).$$

Hence, the percentage of variation across studies due to heterogeneity is estimated to be 41% with a 95% confidence interval of (0, 68%).

Before carrying out a random effects analysis, first note that the results will be just the same as for a fixed effect analysis if $Q < k - 1$ (Section 12.3.4). This is not the case here (Q is 23.689 and $k - 1$ is 14), so the two methods will differ. We proceed by first computing the mean and variance of the fixed effect weights, using (2.8) and (2.9) applied to the third data column of Table 12.2. The results are 20.762 and 307.929, respectively. Substituting into (12.15), we then compute

$$D = \frac{15-1}{15 \times 20.762}\left(15 \times (20.762)^2 - 307.929\right) = 276.82.$$

Then (12.16) gives the between-studies variance estimate of

$$\hat{\tau}^2 = (23.689 - 15 + 1)/276.82 = 0.03500.$$

The random effects weights come from (12.17) and are given in the final column of Table 12.2. For instance, the weight for the first study is

$$w_1^{(R)} = 1/\left(\left(1/52.169\right) + 0.03500\right) = 18.461.$$

Notice that, as expected, the random effects weights are less variable than the fixed effect (another illustration is provided by Example 12.5).

From here, the process follows exactly that already used for the fixed effect analysis; all that is different is the weights used. We apply (12.1), (12.6) and (12.3) in turn and raise the results of (12.1) and (12.3) to the exponential power. The random effects IV weighted estimate (with 95% confidence interval) of the lung cancer relative risk for ever smoking hand-rolled cigarettes compared to smoking only manufactured cigarettes thus turns out to be 1.42 (1.21, 1.66). Again, just as before, we can use (12.4) to obtain the test statistic for no association. Here the value is 4.34 ($p < 0.0001$), so there is evidence of a relationship between whether or not hand-rolled cigarettes have ever been smoked and the risk of lung cancer amongst those who have ever smoked.

Notice that, in this example, the fixed and random effects estimates are virtually identical, despite the homogeneity test being significant and the percentage of variance due to heterogeneity being non-negligible. Due to inclusion of between-studies variation, the random effects approach has produced wider confidence limits, although not dramatically so.

Example 12.5 In an overview of cohort studies in the Asia–Pacific region, data were compiled from nine studies with information on diabetes status (yes/no) at baseline and both fatal and nonfatal cerebrovascular disease during follow-up (Asia Pacific Cohort Studies Collaboration, 2003b). Table 12.3 shows some basic information from each study, including estimates of beta coefficients (logs of hazard ratios: those with diabetes compared to those without) and their estimated standard errors computed from Cox models (Section 11.6)

Although we ultimately wish to produce a pooled estimate of the hazard ratio, as already mentioned we shall achieve this through calculations on the log hazard ratios (i.e., the estimated beta coefficients) because they are better approximated by a normal distribution. It is thus convenient that most computer packages that fit Cox regression models automatically produce estimates of betas and their standard errors. For a graphical view of the individual studies and a peek ahead at the results of pooling, see Figure 12.2.

A fixed effect meta-analysis proceeds by first calculating the weights as the inverse variances of the beta estimates, using (12.5). This requires squaring the last column of Table 12.3 (to obtain the variances) and then taking reciprocals. Results are included in Table 12.4 in which the percentage contribution of each fixed effect weight is shown to aid interpretation. The Busselton and Singapore Heart studies (those with the smallest standard errors in Table 12.3) make the greatest contribution to the pooled estimate. In contrast, the CISCH and Civil Service

Table 12.3. Individual studies of diabetes and cerebrovascular disease (CBV) in the Asia–Pacific region.

Study name (location)	Diabetes CBV	Diabetes No CBV	No diabetes CBV	No diabetes No CBV	Estimates b	Estimates $se(b)$
Busselton Health Study (Australia)	17	85	454	4718	1.351	0.248
Capital Iron and Steel Company Hospital Cohort (CISCH) (PR China)	1	24	37	1736	0.770	1.013
Civil Service Workers Study (Japan)	1	52	8	2102	1.611	1.061
Fletcher Challenge Study (NZ)	7	251	77	9976	1.334	0.395
Ohasama Study (Japan)	8	216	46	1970	0.679	0.390
Seven Cities Cohort Study (PR China)	9	116	284	10264	1.468	0.340
Singapore National Health Survey (NHS)	20	300	24	2987	2.079	0.310
Singapore Thyroid and Heart Study	22	195	53	2072	1.852	0.255
Tanno/Soubetsu Study (Japan)	3	104	30	1677	0.509	0.606

studies have relatively little impact because they have relatively large standard errors, and thus less precise estimates.

The pooled estimate of beta is then, from (12.1), 1.48485. The standard error of this estimate comes from (12.6) as 0.121033. The fixed effect pooled estimate of the hazard ratio is $\exp(1.48485) = 4.41$; a 95% confidence interval comes from (12.3), taking exponents, i.e., $\exp(1.48485 \pm 1.96 \times 0.121033) = (3.48, 5.60)$.

The homogeneity test Q statistic is calculated, using (12.7), to be 13.56. Table 12.4 includes the individual components of Q, from (12.8), e.g., $q_1^2 = 16.2591 \times (1.351 - 1.48485)^2 = 0.2913$ for the Busselton study. The Ohasama and Singapore NHS studies make the largest contribution to heterogeneity. Two factors make each stand out in this respect: (1) distance between their beta estimate and the overall estimate and (2) the precision of their estimate (measured by the standard error). Table 12.3 shows that Singapore NHS has the highest log hazard ratio, so it makes sense that this should contribute highly to the measure of heterogeneity. At the other extreme, Ohasama does not have quite the smallest estimate, but its estimate has higher weight than does the study with the smallest estimate, Tanno/Soubetsu, due to its smaller standard error (greater precision). In contrast, the contribution to Q of the Seven Cities study is virtually zero because its estimate is very close to the overall pooled estimate.

When compared to chi-square on $9 - 1 = 8$ d.f., the Q statistic has a corresponding p value of 0.094 (derived from a computer package) and the percentage of variation across studies due to heterogeneity, I^2, (with 95% confidence interval) turns out to be 41% (0, 73%) using (12.9) to (12.14). Notice that this percentage is, quite by chance, exactly the same as in Example 12.4,

Table 12.4. Weights and components of the heterogeneity statistic for studies of diabetes and CBV.

Study name	Weights Fixed effect		Weights Random effects		Components of heterogeneity	
Busselton	16.2591	(23.8%)	6.2784	(18.4%)	0.2913	(2.1%)
CISCH	0.9745	(1.4%)	0.8897	(2.6%)	0.4980	(3.7%)
Civil Service	0.8883	(1.3%)	0.8173	(2.4%)	0.0141	(0.1%)
Fletcher Challenge	6.4092	(9.4%)	3.9402	(11.6%)	0.1459	(1.1%)
Ohasama	6.5746	(9.6%)	4.0020	(11.8%)	4.2695	(31.5%)
Seven Cities	8.6505	(12.7%)	4.6867	(13.8%)	0.0025	(0.0%)
Singapore NHS	10.4058	(15.2%)	5.1581	(15.1%)	3.6734	(27.1%)
Singapore Heart	15.3787	(22.5%)	6.1426	(18.0%)	2.0730	(15.3%)
Tanno/Soubetsu	2.7230	(4.0%)	2.1505	(6.3%)	2.5931	(19.1%)
Total	68.2637	(100.0%)	34.0655	(100.0%)	13.5608	(100.0%)

although the p value for the Q statistic is bigger here — suggesting an artificial difference in the Q p values due to fewer studies contributing here. The non-negligible Q p value and I^2 statistic give statistical justification to the choice of a random effects model.

For a random effects meta-analysis, we compute the estimate of between-studies variation, using (12.15) and (12.16) as $\hat{\tau}^2 = 0.09777$. The random effects weights then follow from (12.17) and are included in Table 12.4. These weights are then used in (12.1) to produce the random effects pooled estimate of beta, 1.42466, which in turn gives a hazard ratio of $\exp(1.42466) = 4.16$. The estimated standard error of this pooled estimate is 0.171334, from (12.6). Putting the results into (12.3) and taking exponents produces a 95% confidence interval for the random effects pooled estimate of the hazard ratio (those with diabetes compared to those without) of (2.97, 5.82).

A test of the null hypothesis of no association is equivalent to testing whether beta is zero. We could test this for fixed effect or for random effects estimates, using (12.4). For random effects, $1.42466/0.171334 = 8.315$. From Table B.1, this is statistically significant, even at extreme significance levels. As a hazard ratio of over 4 is certainly clinically important, we conclude that we have real evidence of an important association.

12.3.8   Pooling risk differences

Sometimes meta-analysis is used to pool risk differences, which do not require transformation before pooling. Given the individual exposed and unexposed group risks from each study, IV weighting is easily applied using the methods of Section 2.5.3 and Section 10.16.2. However, risk differences tend to be much more variable from study to study than are proportionate measures such as relative risk, odds ratio and hazard ratio. For one thing, length of follow-up will have an effect on risk in cohort and intervention studies. This may be overcome by changing to rates per year or per person-year, but other sources of variability are less easily dealt with.

For instance, whilst it may seem reasonable to assume that smokers of hand-rolled cigarettes will be so many more times likely to die from lung cancer as smokers of manufactured cigarettes in all situations, it is probably not reasonable to assume that smokers of hand-rolled cigarettes always have so much more risk than smokers of manufactured cigarettes. In a country in which smoking is not well established, so that there is not a long history of the habit, all smokers are likely to have low rates of lung cancer. Then the hand-rolled minus manufactured cigarette difference is sure to be small — much smaller than in a country where lung cancer rates are high due to established smoking habits. Even within a country, background rates of disease are likely to change over time.

Another example would be when some of the studies to be pooled are from occupational groups in which risks of disease are relatively low in both those exposed and unexposed to the factor of interest, due to the 'healthy worker effect' (Section 5.1.3); the remaining studies are based in general populations. Since risks are lower in the studies based on occupational groups, risk differences will also tend to be lower than in the other studies. Essentially, the problem is due to variations in disease incidence across studies, which is not such an important issue where relative risks, and other proportionate measures of chance of disease, are concerned.

In most instances in epidemiology, then, it is inappropriate to approach the problem of computing a pooled risk difference by direct means. However, we might consider an indirect approach, computing a summary risk difference for a standard population. To achieve this, we first pool relative risks (or some approximating measures) from the k studies in the meta-analysis and then calculate the pooled risk difference, exposed minus unexposed, Δ_{pooled}, as

$$\Delta_{\text{pooled}} = P\left(\lambda_{\text{pooled}} - 1\right),$$

where λ_{pooled} is the pooled relative risk and P is the risk of disease amongst those unexposed to the risk factor of interest in the standard population. Provided that we may assume P to be fixed, because it is an idealised parameter, confidence intervals follow by multiplying (12.3) by P. If the exposure is rare, P might be taken as a national annual morbidity or mortality rate. It may, alternatively, be useful to take a set of different values of P to represent the range of typical observations across different populations.

12.3.9 Pooling differences in mean values

When the outcome measure is continuous (as for a measurement such as blood pressure), rather than binary (as for a disease outcome), we would usually summarise the comparison between the two groups through the difference in their means (Section 2.7.3). In a cohort or intervention study, it is generally most appropriate to compare changes between the two groups during the study — that is, to compute final minus baseline differences (the deltas; see Example 7.1) and then compare the groups through the difference in the means of these deltas.

Suppose we have differences in means from a number of studies, which we desire to pool. Such pooling using IV weighting is straightforward: for each study, we take the estimate of the standard error of the difference in means, (2.15), and the weight for that study is simply the reciprocal of its square. This is satisfactory provided the scales are consistent across studies. When they are not consistent, the standardised mean effect size (Section 13.4.4) should be used, instead.

12.3.10 Other quantities

Although the most common parameters for pooling in epidemiology are covered in this chapter, epidemiologists may sometimes wish to pool other quantities. Remembering the possible need for transformation to approximate normality (Section 12.3.7), this can be achieved using IV weighting if the standard error can be computed using formulae given in earlier chapters of this book or elsewhere. Many of the specific topics described earlier in this book are the subject of specialist publications on meta-analysis. For example, Irwig et al. (1995) describe how to pool the results of diagnostic tests, and Elbourne et al. (2002) cover meta-analysis of cross-over trials. Specialist meta-analysis textbooks, such as Sutton et al. (2000) and Borenstein et al. (2009), consider a range of different quantities and methods, far beyond the scope of this single chapter.

12.3.11 Pooling mixed quantities

As stated in the introduction, meta-analysis seeks to pool like quantities. Sometimes the preceding review has compiled, from published works, mixtures of relative risks, odds ratios, relative rates and hazard ratios, each representing the relative chance of the same disease, comparing the same exposure to no exposure. Most researchers would call the common 'relative chance' the relative risk. Indeed, this was the case with the meta-analysis of Lee (2001), described in Example 12.1.

Provided that we are confident that the measures (and their standard errors) would not alter importantly if one of the alternative metrics were used, we can go ahead and pool, as in Example 12.4. Odds ratios should be close to relative risks when the disease is rare (Section 3.3.1), whilst relative rates and hazard ratios should each be close to relative risks when censoring is rare or evenly distributed between the exposure and no exposure groups. After his review, Lee (2001) decided that pooling was appropriate for the studies he selected.

A similar issue arises when some publications provide confounder-adjusted estimates and some provide unadjusted estimates (or several different adjustment sets are used: for an example, see Example 12.12). Again, pooling is straightforward, but requires prior consideration of whether such pooling is meaningful. Sometimes several types of adjusted estimates (and associated standard errors) may be available from some studies, and we must decide which adjusted estimate to use (if any) in our meta-analysis. Lee (2001) decided to pool estimates from the publications he collected that were adjusted for the maximum number of confounding variables. Consequently, the number of variables adjusted for ranged from none to six in Figure 12.1.

Although mixed quantities give no extra computational problems, clearly they incur a greater chance of heterogeneity. When we have decided that we are prepared to pool mixed quantities, a *post hoc* description of differences from study to study is absolutely crucial. This is the subject of the next section. If differences are great, we should abandon the single meta-analysis and revert to pooling subsets of quantities that are truly alike.

12.3.12 Dose-response meta-analysis

Published studies often present a set of odds ratios, or other metrics, for a quantitative risk factor across ordered categories, all relative to the chosen reference group. Unfortunately, these categories are often inconsistent; for instance, one author may have divided the risk factor into fifths, and another into quarters. Still other authors may have left the variable in its continuous form. A method of estimating dose–response from such disparate data, due to Greenland and Longnecker (1992), may be useful in this situation, to derive a pooled estimate of the dose–response effect. This may be implemented by the GLST routine, which can be downloaded to Stata.

12.4 Investigating heterogeneity

In the last section we have seen how individual studies may give estimates that differ from each other and from the overall pooled 'best' estimate, and how this variation may be summarised in a test of homogeneity and an estimate of the percentage of overall variation due to heterogeneity. In many respects, this aspect of meta-analysis is just as important as establishing the pooled estimate. In understanding the effect of a risk factor (or treatment in an intervention study), it is fundamental to be able to see how much, and in what way, the effect varies in different situations. This is true whether fixed or random effects are assumed. Thus a complete meta-analysis should include a description of study-to-study differences, as indeed was stated at the outset of this chapter.

When epidemiological studies are pooled, heterogeneity may well occur due to differences in study design, and this possibility should be investigated. A good example comes from a review of benzodiazepine use and the risk of hip fracture amongst the elderly (Cumming and Le Couteur, 2003). This found significantly ($p < 0.05$) elevated relative risk in all five cohort or population-based case–control studies identified in the review, but no significant effect in all four hospital-based case–control studies identified. Furthermore, the former group reported very consistent relative risks (around 1.5), whereas the three studies in the latter group that reported relative risks all gave values at or below one (one of the four studies did not specify the estimate).

As has been seen in earlier chapters, cohort studies would generally be more reliable than case–control studies. Also, use of population controls would generally give more reliable results than hospital controls in case–control studies (Section 6.4).

Thus we might expect that hospital-based case–control studies would give the least reliable results. In the hip fracture example, the probable explanation for the lack of effect in hospital studies is that elderly people in hospitals frequently use benzodiazepines, thus diluting the differential between cases of hip fracture and controls.

12.4.1   Forest plots

The simplest, and often most effective, way to look at study-to-study differences is through a **forest plot**, such as that in Figure 12.1. Most contemporary published meta-analyses include such a plot.

Example 12.6 A forest plot for the data of Example 12.5 is given as Figure 12.2. Unlike Figure 12.1, this uses the size of the plotting symbols to show the precision of the estimates by making the area of the square boxes proportional to the reciprocal of the variance of the estimate; i.e., the weight given to the study. Meta-analysis routines in computer packages will usually have such an automatic feature. The other additional feature is the diamond used to show the overall pooled estimates (both fixed and random effects are shown, for completeness). Here, the centre of the diamond is plotted at the estimate and the sides go out to the 95% confidence limits. Studies have been ordered according to the size of their confidence intervals so that studies providing the most precise estimates come closest to the summary diamonds. It is clear that the Busselton and Singapore Heart studies have the most precise estimates, although the Busselton estimate is much closer to the overall average.

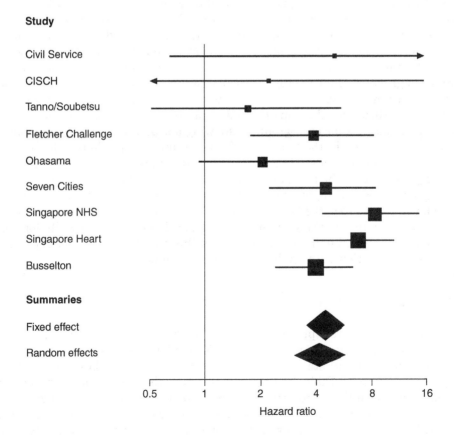

Figure 12.2. Forest plot for the data of Example 12.5. Boxes are drawn proportional to the inverse variance of the estimates. Arrows are as in Figure 12.1.

Another example of a forest plot, with design variations, follows later, as Figure 12.6. There are no fixed rules for what precise information forest plots should show. Essentially, they simply show a 'forest' of lines for confidence intervals with some indication of the estimate within each line. They have applications outside meta-analysis, such as for showing the odds ratios for disease of a range of different binary risk factors measured in the same study. Figure 14.8 provides another example. Although the style of boxes used in Figure 12.2 is the most conventional, the information conveyed by the size of each box is really just the reverse of what the corresponding confidence interval already shows, because the confidence interval increases with the standard error (the reciprocal of the square root of the weight). Hence, some authors prefer to draw boxes in proportion to another measure of relative study importance; when survival data are used, a sensible choice is the total number of events observed in the particular study. This was indeed used in the source paper for the diabetes data (Asia Pacific Cohort Studies Collaboration, 2003b).

Another point worthy of consideration is whether the boxes obscure the actual position of the estimate. This can be a real problem when the boxes are big, relative to the plotting space. Then, even though it can convey only one item of information, the use of standard symbols with a clear central point, such as those in Figure 12.1, may be better. Alternatively, light shading might be considered: see Figure 12.6. It is generally better to use log scales on the horizontal axis when showing results obtained from pooling on the log scale, as done in Figure 12.1 and Figure 12.2. This is because the log scale produces symmetric confidence intervals, which are easier to interpret, and because equal relative effects either side of 'no effect' appear as equal distances (for example, a halving of risk is as far from zero as is a doubling of risk, although on the opposite side).

Often, heterogeneity in meta-analyses is due to some kind of grouping effect. For instance, in Example 12.4 there might be important differences between case–control and cohort studies or between men and women; in Example 12.5, there might be a geographical grouping of effect sizes. If such an effect is suspected, it would be useful to subset the lines in the forest plot according to the groups, as was done for study design in Figure 12.1. Should a subgroup effect be apparent, it would make sense to present a separate meta-analysis for each group by showing a separate summary diamond under each subgroup's results in the forest plot. If the grouping variable is ordinal, such as a ranking score for quality of study (Section 12.7), the lines in the plot might be ordered accordingly. Notice that the grouping variable might be intrinsic to the studies, as is the case for study design, or might be one of the variables recorded within each study, as is the case for sex. Of course, the latter situation is applicable only when we can obtain the necessary data relating to the grouping variable, such as separate results for men and women. When published data are inadequate in this regard, further enquiry, usually by personal communication with study investigators, will be necessary.

12.4.2   Influence plots

One limitation of the forest plot is that it gives no direct representation of the amount of overall heterogeneity due to each study. To explore this aspect of the data, it is useful to examine the q^2 statistics, (12.8); for Example 12.5, these are given in the penultimate column of Table 12.4. However, when there are many studies, such a table may become difficult to interpret and a plot may be useful. Since the other important aspect of each study is the weight it provides, it can be helpful to produce a scatterplot of q^2 against w, the weight. For example, we might plot the % heterogeneity against the % weights from Table 12.4.

A better way of displaying the same information is to plot $\pm q$ against $\sqrt{w}$, where $\pm q$ is the square root of q^2, given a positive sign when the estimate from the study in question is greater than the fixed effect estimate, and a negative sign otherwise. Such a plot will be called an **influence plot**. An advantage of taking square roots before plotting is that the display is less skewed, and thus somewhat easier to interpret, than it would otherwise tend to be.

Under IV weighting and the null hypothesis of homogeneity, $\pm q$ is the standardised form (estimate minus its average divided by its standard error) of the estimate for the particular study in question. Thus, if there is homogeneity and the normal probability model is appropriate, we would expect 95% of all values of $\pm q$ to be between -1.96 and 1.96 (Section 2.7). Adding horizontal lines at the vertices ± 1.96 (which might just as well be plotted at ± 2, for simplicity) to the influence plot gives indicative boundaries outside which we might consider a study very influential in terms of the overall heterogeneity. A horizontal line at zero may also be useful, simply to separate studies that give estimates bigger or smaller than the overall fixed effect pooled estimate. On the horizontal scale, studies to the left are those with relatively small weights (imprecise estimates; large confidence intervals). Studies further to the right contribute more weight to the pooled meta-analysis estimate.

Use of different plotting styles for subgroups may help to show sources of heterogeneity. For instance, an influence plot for Example 12.1 could use different symbols for case–control and cohort studies or for men and women. We then inspect the influence plot for clusters of like symbols.

Example 12.7 Figure 12.3 is an influence plot for the diabetes data of Example 12.5. The Ohasama study is identified as unusual, as already commented upon in Example 12.5. Of course, this does not imply that anything is wrong with this study's data; it simply flags it as exceptionally influential in terms of rejecting the null hypothesis of no effect difference between

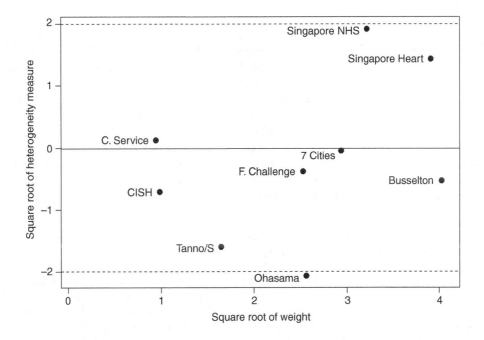

Figure 12.3. Influence plot for the diabetes data.

studies. Similarly, Figure 12.3 confirms other comments already made in Example 12.5. A noticeable feature in this plot, which may not be noticed in earlier views of the meta-data, is how the two Singapore studies cluster together, having a large influence on the pooled estimate (far to the right), tending to make it bigger (above the zero line), and making a large contribution to heterogeneity (far from the zero line). It is evident that, if these two studies should be excluded, we would obtain a lower estimate of the effect of diabetes and there would be more consistency between the remaining studies.

The influence plot is closely related to the **radial plot** (Galbraith, 1988), which some meta-analysis computer programs will produce. In essence, the radial plot is a plot of another type of standardised estimate from each study, $\sqrt{w}\,\hat{\theta}$, against the square root of the weight, $\sqrt{w}$. The horizontal axis is the same as on an influence plot, but the vertical scale differs by the addition of $\sqrt{w}\,\hat{\theta}_{pooled}$. Radial plots have some useful properties, but tend to be somewhat more difficult to understand, and certainly harder to draw with nonspecialist software, than are influence plots.

12.4.3 Sensitivity analyses

Whenever a study has been shown to be highly influential or to have a large weight, it would be sensible to rerun the meta-analysis with this study excluded. We would then need to decide whether to report both the overall and the restricted results. Similar sensitivity analyses are carried out for many other reasons in meta-analyses. They should be carried out, for example, whenever there is uncertainty in the methods used or when there are important known variations in study quality (Section 12.7).

12.4.4 Meta-regression

As we have seen, there are often situations wherein we speculate that an ancillary variable might account for the heterogeneity in the meta-data. So far, we have looked at descriptive techniques, which are useful when this variable is categorical or ordinal. When the ancillary variable is continuous, it will be useful to draw a scatterplot of the estimate from each study against this ancillary variable. If the extra variable is important in determining the effect of the response variable, we should see a pattern in the plot. Instead of drawing a standard scatterplot (such as Figure 9.2), it is better to draw the points in relative size to the weights of the different studies so as to emphasise the weighting principle behind meta-analysis. Scatter plots with points drawn in relative size according to some feature of each data point are collectively known as **bubble plots**. Many statistical computer packages produce such plots.

Example 12.8 The studies contributing to the meta-analysis of Example 12.5 varied in the age profiles of their subjects. The mean age, at study baseline, of subjects included in the published meta-analysis (Asia Pacific Cohort Studies Collaboration, 2003b) for each study was: Busselton 46.3; CISCH 53.9; Civil Service 44.2; Fletcher Challenge 44.4; Ohasama 59.5; Seven Cities 53.8; Singapore NHS 38.8; Singapore Heart 40.1; Tanno/Soubetsu 50.8 years. Figure 12.4 is a bubble plot (areas of circles drawn in proportion to fixed effect study weights) of estimated beta coefficient (log of hazard ratio) against mean age. There is an approximate linear relationship: it appears that the log hazard ratio declines with increasing age. Age differences in study populations seem to be a likely explanation of at least some of the heterogeneity in the studies of Example 12.5.

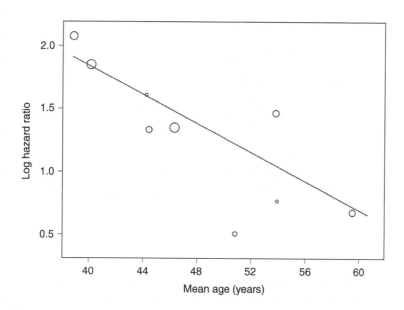

Figure 12.4. Bubble plot for the diabetes meta-analysis of Example 12.5, including the fixed effect regression line of Example 12.9.

When models involving ancillary variables are applied to meta-data, the process is called **meta-regression** (Thompson and Sharp, 1999). The fixed effect simple linear meta-regression model is

$$\hat{\theta} = a + \beta x + \varepsilon, \tag{12.18}$$

where x is the value of the ancillary variable (age in Example 12.8), θ is the quantity being pooled (the log hazard ratio in Example 12.8), α and β are the regression parameters and ε is the normally distributed random error, similar to (9.11). Although this model allows the value of $\hat{\theta}$ to vary between studies, it is still a fixed effect model because it assumes that the variation due to study is systematically predictable through x.

We can fit (12.18) exactly as for simple linear regression, but this would ignore the important aspect of the weight given to each study. Taking the general approach of meta-analysis (of Section 12.3), we fit (12.18) to the meta-data using a **weighted regression** approach. This is a straightforward extension of the least squares method of Section 9.3.1, incorporated in all leading statistical software packages. The weights should be taken as in the initial meta-analysis; here we shall assume IV weighting once more.

Besides using weighted least squares, one other change must be made when extending the simple linear regression methodology of Section 9.3.1 to meta-regression (see Higgins and Thompson, 2004). The standard error of the estimates of regression parameters should be divided by the square root of the mean square error from the (weighted) regression analysis of variance table, s_e (see Table 9.7). That is, to estimate the meta-regression standard errors of α and β, we extract the standard errors given by standard statistical software and divide each by s_e. With these revised values, we can use (9.22) and (9.23) to give confidence intervals about the regression parameters and use (9.26) and (9.27) to test the null hypotheses that each, in turn, is zero. In most cases, the intercept, α, is of little interest and inferences are restricted to the slope parameter, β.

Table 12.5. Analysis of variance table for weighted regression in
Example 12.9.

Source of variation	Sum of squares	Degrees of freedom	Mean square
Regression on age	9.5956	1	9.5956
Error	3.9652	7	0.5665
Total	13.5608	8	

Example 12.9 Applying a weighted least squares regression analysis to Example 12.8, where the weights were the reciprocal of the variance, using a computer package, produced an estimate of slope, −0.05710, with standard error, 0.01387. The intercept was estimated as 4.1150. Thus the fitted line

$$\hat{\theta} = 4.1150 - 0.0570x$$

was that added to Figure 12.4; the log hazard ratio is estimated to decrease by 0.057 for every extra year of life. The analysis of variance table is given as Table 12.5. From these results, we find the standard error of the estimated meta-regression slope to be $0.01387/\sqrt{0.5665} = 0.01843$. Substituting this result into (9.22), a 95% confidence interval for the slope is

$$-0.05710 \pm 2.36 \times 0.01843 = -0.057 \pm 0.043,$$

where 2.36 is the value from the t distribution on 7 d.f. (see Table B.4). We can test the null hypothesis of no change in the log hazard ratio as age increases from (9.27), the estimate divided by its standard error: here $-0.0570/0.01843 = -3.098$. By inspection of Table B.4, we see that this is significant on 7 d.f., $p < 0.02$. Thus, we conclude that differences in age have, indeed, systematically affected the beta coefficients and thus the cerebrovascular disease hazard ratios for those with, compared to those without, diabetes. We would expect less heterogeneity in a meta-analysis of age-adjusted hazard ratios. Sensibly, the published meta-analysis (Asia Pacific Cohort Studies Collaboration, 2003b) adjusted for age.

We can easily extend the one-variable fixed effect meta-regression approach to deal with many ancillary variables, any of which may be categorical; we simply fit the general linear model of Section 9.6, using weighted least squares and adjusting the standard errors of model coefficients, as above. This gives a general method for identifying factors that contribute to the heterogeneity between studies. If we can obtain estimates from each study which adjust for these factors, we might consider a revised meta-analysis using adjusted estimates (and standard errors). Otherwise, we report the factors as part of our discussion of why the pooled meta-analysis estimate might be inadequate to cover all situations.

In this description, we have restricted ourselves to fixed effect meta-regression. As shown, this is a simple extension of the material of Chapter 9. Random effects meta-regression adds a further random component to (12.18), allowing for further sources of heterogeneity beyond that explained by the predictors in the regression model. The methods are beyond the scope of this book but are applied by the METAREG command in Stata, which is straightforward to use; see the program for Example 12.9 on the web site for this book. See Berkey *et al.* (1995) and Thompson and Sharp (1999) for technical details.

Higgins and Thompson (2004) show that a fixed effect meta-regression gives, unsurprisingly, unreliable p values in the presence of heterogeneity. Less intuitive is their finding that random effects meta-regression gives inflated false positive rates (i.e., the

p values returned are artificially low; tests evaluated at the nominal 5% level of significance actually have more than a one in twenty chance of rejecting the null hypothesis when it is true) when there are few studies in the meta-analysis. They suggest a Monte-Carlo permutation test (Section 14.8) to control for this issue. A further problem is that there may be several candidate predictors that we wish to test by meta-regression in the same meta-analysis. This leads to further inflation of the false-positive error rate due to multiple testing (Section 9.2.5). As ever, we can protect against this problem by only testing a small number of pre-specified potential predictors. Higgins and Thompson (2004) extend their permutation test to allow for multiple testing.

12.5   Pooling tabular data

Sometimes meta-data are collected as tabular data. In particular, 2×2 tables, each identical in format to Table 3.1, are collected from each study. These data might arise from case–control studies, cohort studies, intervention studies (where the row labels in Table 3.1 should be altered to, say, 'active treatment' and 'placebo'), or some combination. Such meta-data may be analysed to produce pooled estimates and other quantities, just as in Section 12.3 in which we assumed that estimates and weights (e.g., standard errors, required for the IV weighting scheme) were directly available.

12.5.1   Inverse variance weighting

If we adopt IV weighting, all we need to do, in the presence of tabular meta-data, is to use the relevant formulae of earlier chapters to produce estimates and standard errors and then apply the methodology of Section 12.3.

Example 12.10 In Table 12.3, raw data were included (not used up to now), which are equivalent to 2×2 tables, for each study of risk factor (diabetes) exposure versus disease (CBV) outcome. Suppose we decide to calculate a pooled relative risk from these data. This requires repeated use of (3.2) to obtain the relative risk estimates (used to calculate log relative risks) and (3.5) to obtain the standard errors of log relative risks. Armed with the set of estimates and their standard errors, we then simply apply the formulae of Section 12.3. In this case, we arrive at a fixed effect, IV weighted, pooled estimate (95% confidence interval) of 3.03 (2.42, 3.79). The corresponding random effects results are 2.97 (1.97, 4.46).

12.5.2   Mantel–Haenszel methods

An alternative to IV weighting is to adopt the Mantel–Haenszel (MH) methodology of Section 4.6. In this earlier section, we were concerned with pooling subtables defined by levels of a confounding variable. In the context of meta-analysis, we consider each subtable to represent a different study, and thus let 'study' take the role of 'level of the confounding variable' in the analyses of Chapter 4.

For fixed effect meta-analysis, we obtain pooled MH estimates of odds ratios from (4.10), and of relative risks from (4.15). This is equivalent to choosing weights in (12.1) as $b_i c_i / n_i$ and $c_i(a_i + b_i)/n_i$, respectively, using the notation of Table 4.12. Corresponding confidence intervals for these pooled estimates come from (4.14) for the pooled odds ratio and (4.18) for the pooled relative risk. We can use the Cochran–Mantel–Haenszel (CMH) test, (4.21), to test whether either of these pooled estimates is significantly different from unity. However, many meta-analysts use the simpler procedure of dividing the logarithm of the estimate by its estimated standard error, (4.11) or (4.16), and comparing against the standard normal distribution. This approach is consistent with (12.4) and gives similar p values to the CMH test in practice.

We can test for homogeneity by using the test for a common relative risk or odds ratio, (4.23) with (4.24) or (4.29), or by computing the Q statistic, (12.7), where the pooled estimate is the MH result. Meta-analysts generally take the latter approach but, again, these two approaches tend to give similar results in practice. When computing Q, we use IV weights, (12.5). Where necessary to improve the normality assumption, as before, we compute Q using estimates on the log scale.

For MH random effects meta-analysis, the usual approach taken is to follow exactly the same procedures as for IV weighting, that is, calculating the results of (12.15) to (12.17), but now with the MH version of Q. However, the statistical justification for this approach is problematic and thus the procedure is not recommended.

Example 12.11 To apply MH relative risk meta-analysis to the raw data in Table 12.3, we apply (4.15) to obtain the fixed effect pooled estimate, $\hat{\lambda}_{MH} = 2.91$. From (4.16), its standard error on the log scale is 0.112. Then, from (4.18), the 95% confidence interval for the fixed effect pooled estimate is

$$\exp(\log_e(2.91) \pm 1.96 \times 0.112) = (2.34, 3.62).$$

The continuity-corrected CMH test statistic, (4.21), is 93.8, which is highly significant, $p < 0.0001$. The alternative test statistic, (12.4), is $\log_e(2.91)/0.112 = 9.54$ ($p < 0.0001$). To compare this directly with CMH (which is computed using squared units), we must square it, giving 91.0 — not very different.

Next, we consider tests of homogeneity. The test for a common relative risk, (4.23), gives a test statistic of 22.5 ($p = 0.004$). The more often used 'Q approach' requires all the individual log relative risks and their standard errors. For example, for the Busselton Health Study, the log relative risk is derived by using (3.2) and taking logs; the result is 0.641. The corresponding standard error is, from (3.5), 0.2259. Then, from (12.5), the IV weight for Busselton is $1/(0.2259)^2 = 19.6$. Repeating these steps for all studies gives the MH Q statistic, from (12.7), as

$$Q_{MH} = \{(19.6)(0.641 - \log_e(2.91))^2 + \cdots\} = 21.1.$$

As expected, this is similar to the result of the test for a common relative risk. Notice that the only way that Q_{MH} differs from Q with IV weighting is that $\log_e(\hat{\lambda}_{MH})$, which in this case is $\log_e(2.91)$, replaces the IV pooled log relative risk in (12.7).

In most cases, the IV and MH approaches will give similar results and thus the choice of which to use is unimportant. For instance, the results of Example 12.10 and Example 12.11 are not dissimilar.

12.5.3   The Peto method

Another fixed effect method for pooling odds ratios from 2×2 tables is the **Peto** method (Peto *et al.*, 1977). Although this is often included as an option in meta-analysis software, it is not generally recommended because it can give biased estimates (Greenland and Salvan, 1990).

12.5.4   Dealing with zeros

When one of the cells in the 2×2 table for a particular study is zero, the methods described previously can break down due to division by zero. For instance, if there are no events amongst the group unexposed to the risk factor of interest, the c term in Table 3.1 is zero. Since the standard errors for both the log relative risk, (3.5), and log odds ratio, (3.10), include the term $1/c$, these will be incalculable and hence we cannot calculate the IV weights used in the derivation of Q.

A solution to the problem of zeros is to add a continuity correction (Section 3.5.3). The simplest approach is to add 0.5 to all cells of all studies that have a zero cell. Sweeting *et al.* (2004) suggest alternative continuity corrections.

Sometimes a study has zeros in cells of each exposure group. Typically this is where there are no events in either the exposed or unexposed group (or the treatment and control group in a clinical trial). Theoretically these 'double zero' studies can give no information about the relative risk (or odds ratio) overall and are usually left out of the pooling process, especially as it may be that some property of the study design or conduct led to no events of the index type having been identified.

12.5.5   *Advantages and disadvantages of using tabular data*

Although the approach to be used is usually determined by which meta-data are available, it is helpful to summarise the advantages and disadvantages of the tabular approach compared to the approach of Section 12.3, which requires collection of estimates and measures of variability. The tabular approach allows for a range of different estimates to be pooled; for example, we might calculate pooled odds ratios and relative risks from the same meta-data (except from case–control studies). As we have seen, we can also choose from a number of methods for pooling. Another advantage is that the tabular approach does not require the individual study investigators to have carried out statistical analyses on their data. This would be an important consideration if we have reason to believe that some such analyses would be missing or inadequate.

A disadvantage of the tabular method is that there is no mechanism to allow for censoring when dealing with follow-up data. Notice that the pooled relative risk estimates in Example 12.10 (3.03 and 2.97) are much less than the pooled hazard ratios (4.41 and 4.16) of Example 12.5. This is explained by the much higher degree of censoring amongst those with diabetes, caused by the greater propensity for this group to die from diseases other than that studied, CBV. Although acceptable for the sake of an example, in this case relative risks are not ideal as epidemiological measures. Thus, when the meta-analysis involves cohort or intervention studies, analysis of tabulated data may lead to bias. Similarly, analyses of tabulated data cannot take account of confounding variables. A further practical disadvantage is that whilst the other approach is general and thus easily extendable to situations beyond this book without further research, the tabular method requires knowledge of explicit formulae, special to each circumstance.

12.6   Individual participant data

Some meta-analysts go to the extreme of collecting the complete set of raw data on all variables of interest (including potential confounding variables and censoring information, where appropriate) from each study. Such data are called **individual participant** (or, sometimes, **patient**) **data** (IPD). A clear advantage of this method is that the meta-analyst can then analyse each dataset as she or he sees fit, making sure that a standard approach is used (for example, avoiding the problems of Section

12.3.11) and applying standard checks, such as range checks, to each dataset. The practical disadvantage is that study investigators are often much more reticent to share complete datasets and the time taken to compile the meta-data might well be considerably lengthened. Stewart and Clarke (1995) give a detailed discussion of IPD in the context of clinical trials, much of which is relevant to epidemiological settings. Blettner *et al.* (1999) discuss the role of IPD analyses within the general approach to meta-analysis in epidemiology.

If IPD are available, the meta-analyst has two choices when deciding how to analyse the meta-data. The first approach is to calculate estimates and standard errors from each study and then pool as in Section 12.3. The second approach is to join all the datasets into a single complete dataset and then compute estimates and confidence intervals, using some statistical method that allows for study differences. Both are used in practice. For instance, the 'estimate then pool' method (sometimes called the 'two-step' method) has been adopted by the Emerging Risk Factors Collaboration (ERFC) and the 'pool then estimate' method by the Prospective Studies Collaboration; both these collaborations are epidemiological IPD meta-analyses of cardiovascular disease and its risk factors.

The Asia Pacific Cohort Studies Collaboration (see Example 12.5) is a third IPD meta-analysis with similar aims to the ERFC and PSC, but a restricted geographical focus. As its primary method of analysis, it has adopted the 'pool then estimate' approach. Cox regression models are fitted to the combined dataset taking study as a strata variable, thus only assuming proportional hazards within study and not between studies (Section 11.8.5). This gives a fixed effect approach to dealing with study differences. Note that the data in Table 12.3 (used in several examples) were produced from the IPD and then used here to illustrate the 'estimate then pool' approach. In practice, for large meta-analyses, such as the three major collaborations mentioned here, the two approaches are unlikely to give importantly different answers (Thompson *et al.* 2010). Tudur Smith *et al.* (2005) consider both fixed effect and random effects methods with IPD.

12.7   Dealing with aspects of study quality

Descriptive reports of quality, as discussed in Section 12.2.2, are essential in systematic reviews. The question then arises whether aspects of study quality should be incorporated into the quantitative meta-analysis. The weighting schemes described up to now take account only of sampling variability. As we have seen in Section 12.3.1, the most commonly used (IV) weighting scheme gives greater influence (on the pooled summary) to studies with smaller variance. Although inverse variance depends also on the design and method of analysis used for the study, it is thought of as a measure of quantity, rather than quality, in meta-analysis. Such weighting takes no account of bias error or any of the other issues discussed in Section 12.2.2. Hence, for instance, a case–control study with a large sample size but a poorly selected hospital control group (see Section 6.4.2) would have more influence on the summary odds ratio than a marginally smaller study with an unbiased selection of controls. We thus run the risk of shrinking the confidence limits around the pooled estimate at the expense of moving it away from its true position.

To be able to take account of all aspects of quality in the pooling process, we need to give a quality score to each study. Section 12.2.2 gives some general guidance for constructing quality scores; reporting guidelines for the type of study being assessed take a more detailed, structured approach (see http://www.equator-network.org/). The most useful such guidelines in epidemiology are the STROBE guidelines (von Elm *et al.*, 2007). As discussed in Section 12.2.2, specialist input is required to enhance the generalist approach. An example of a quality scoring system is given by Berlin and Colditz (1990) in their meta-analysis of physical activity as a protective factor against coronary heart disease. As in this published meta-analysis, we can obtain the quality-adjusted pooled estimate by multiplying the quality score from the ith study by, say, the IV weight for the same study and take this product to be the weight, w_i, in the general formulae for the summary meta-analysis estimate and its standard error, (12.1) and (12.2).

In many situations, it may prove very difficult to assign quality scores. Even if it is possible for an individual, or group, to produce a scoring system, there is no guarantee that a similar scoring system would arise when another group considered the problem. Juni *et al.* (1999) show that different quality scales can lead to important differences in inferences. Another problem is that quality is really multidimensional, so by combining over components of quality, we lose information regarding probable sources of heterogeneity (Greenland, 1994).

Due to these problems, many meta-analyses restrict to descriptive or exploratory treatments of study quality. Quality scores, or ranks, could be used to order a forest plot (Section 12.4.1) or label an influence plot (Section 12.4.2) or be taken as the observations for the x variable in a meta-regression (Section 12.4.4). The latter approach lends itself to situations in which we can score at least some of several broad quality characteristics; then meta-regressions for each component of quality should be informative. This approach might be extended so that each quality component contributes an explanatory variable to the meta-regression, allowing variable selection methods (Section 9.7) to tease out the most influential aspects of quality.

12.8 Publication bias

As well as studying the quality of each individual study, we should consider the quality of the set of study estimates we have compiled. In particular, it is useful to consider whether these studies appear to make a consistent whole. A particular worry is that studies that generated small, nonsignificant results (often incorrectly called 'negative results' when they are really neutral), or results that go against the grain of perceived wisdom, will never have been written up or will have been rejected by the editors of journals. This phenomenon is known as **publication bias**. This is a real issue in meta-analysis. Easterbrook *et al.* (1991) describe a study of 285 health research projects approved by an ethics committee that could be traced to the stage of analysis. They showed that projects which generated statistically significant results ($p < 0.05$) were more likely (odds ratio and 95% confidence interval: 2.96 (1.68, 5.21)) to be published than those that failed to find significance. Although this, and similar, studies have prompted the editors of leading medical journals to make a concerted effort to accept submitted papers with neutral results in recent years, there can be little doubt that such research is less likely to see the light of day, largely because the findings are less exciting. In drug trials the issue is likely to be worse than in epidemiological studies, due to financial interests. Two striking examples of publication bias are given by Turner *et al.* (2008) and Eyding *et al.* (2010), both of which compared the results of published and unpublished antidepressant drug trials. Both found that the pooled evidence from published data far overstated the efficacy of the drugs studied, compared to the unpublished data.

12.8.1   The funnel plot

If we selected an unbiased sample of similar studies (say, a collection of cohort studies) of varying size and calculated a similar estimate (say, an age-adjusted odds ratio) from each, we would expect to find that the estimates from our smaller studies were relatively widely dispersed and that the estimates from larger studies were less dispersed, either side of the overall pooled estimate. This is an expectation based upon ideas of sampling variability: the larger the sample is, the less the uncertainty. Thus, if we plotted size of estimate against size of study, we would expect to see a funnel shape produced, if the studies have overall consistency. The resulting plot is thus called a **funnel plot**. In fact, in order to allow for other factors (principally, study design) that affect sampling variability in general situations, it is more usual to plot the reciprocal of the standard error on the x axis of the funnel plot (as in Figure 12.5) or to use a reverse scale for its standard error (as in Figure 12.7). This is, of course, consistent with the approach to measuring precision taken throughout this chapter.

Figure 12.5(a) is a funnel plot in which there is no indication of publication bias because the plot is reasonably symmetrical. Contrast this with Figure 12.5(b), in which there is clearly skewness. This plot is what we expect to see when negative and small, nonsignificant, positive results are omitted due to publication bias. In fact, Figure 12.5(b) was based upon the same simulated data as the other plot, but with the five negative (log odds ratio below zero) and the smallest positive study removed. As we would expect, the pooled log odds ratio (indicated on the graph) increased when these smallest six individual log odds ratios were removed. Thus, if it had happened that the corresponding six studies were not published, the meta-analysis would have found an upwardly biased summary odds ratio.

As with any graphical technique, the funnel plot has the disadvantage of leading to subjective decision making. Several objective tests for deciding whether publication bias has occurred have been suggested, including methods based upon regressions from radial (Egger *et al.*, 1997) and funnel plots (Duval and Tweedie, 2000; Macaskill *et al.*, 2001).

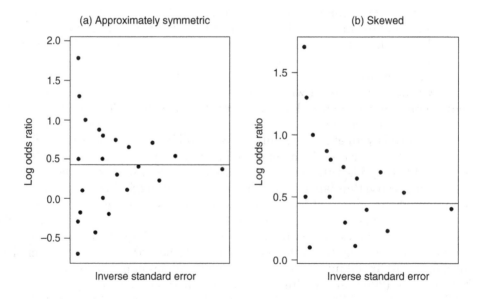

Figure 12.5. Funnel plots for simulated data from a collection of cohort studies showing age-adjusted log odds ratios and their inverse standard error. Each plot includes a horizontal line at the fixed effect inverse variance weighted pooled estimate of the log odds ratio for the data plotted.

Another problem with the funnel plot is that when few studies are available, as is often the case in meta-analysis in practice, there will likely be too few data points to enable identification of an underlying pattern.

12.8.2   Consequences of publication bias

If studies with 'unlikely' results have been omitted, the pooled estimate, or its standard error, may be biased. Thus, if the general expectation is that a certain factor increases the chance of disease, omitting studies that found it to be protective (because they were never published) would lead to an overestimate of the effect (as in Figure 12.5). In situations in which only significant results, in either direction, have been published, we would expect to see a 'hole' in the funnel plot near the zero estimate. This would lead to an upward bias in the width of the confidence interval for the pooled meta-analysis estimate but may well not cause bias in the estimate.

In practice, the degree of such biases is often not important. In many situations, the only studies lost due to publication bias are small and the pooled estimate obtained is then likely to be close to what would have been found if all studies had been included in the meta-analysis. For instance, in Figure 12.5, the pooled estimate when the six studies have been removed (Figure 12.5(b)) is only slightly bigger than when all 23 studies are included (Figure 12.5(a)). The log odds ratio changed from 0.4291 with 23 studies to 0.4520 with 17 studies; the corresponding odds ratios are 1.54 and 1.57. This is because the small studies that have been excluded due to publication bias are those that would have received small weights, and thus contributed minimally to the pooled estimate, had there not been publication bias. This is particularly true under fixed effect analyses; random effects weights will be more evenly distributed. Even so, in the real-life example of publication bias provided by Example 12.12 the random effects estimate and confidence interval, before and after correction for publication bias, are not greatly different.

Another situation in which publication bias often turns out to be unimportant is when the underlying true effect is large, because then results that fail to find significance, or go the 'wrong way' are unlikely. For instance, when comparing heavy smokers with people who have never smoked for lung cancer outcomes, the relative risk, is so high (over 30 in Example 1.2) that even small epidemiological studies are likely to find significant positive results.

12.8.3   Correcting for publication bias

Several methods are available to correct for publication bias, of which the **trim and fill** method of Duval and Tweedie (2000) is the easiest to understand amongst methods with statistical appeal. The method is easily applied through the METATRIM command in Stata. The idea is to identify the asymmetry in the funnel plot; trim those studies that cause this asymmetry (e.g., those studies in the top left portion of Figure 12.5(b)); calculate the pooled estimate for the remaining studies and then fill in the funnel plot by replacing the trimmed points and adding their mirror images about this pooled estimate. The final pooled results come from analyses using all the true estimates and the simulated mirror images.

Example 12.12 Huxley *et al.* (2005) carried out a systematic review of the association between diabetes and pancreatic cancer. Their data are available from the web site for this book. Figure 12.6 summarises the results they found from cohort studies (with the outcome metric taken to be the approximate relative risk) using random effects meta-analysis with IV weighting. Notice the inclusion of columns to convey information on the confounding variables that were accounted for in each study and the study weights, and (at the foot of the plot) specification of the zones within which

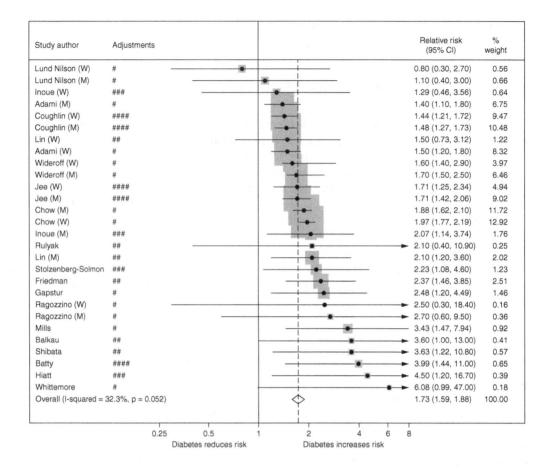

Study author	Adjustments	Relative risk (95% CI)	% weight
Lund Nilson (W)	#	0.80 (0.30, 2.70)	0.56
Lund Nilson (M)	#	1.10 (0.40, 3.00)	0.66
Inoue (W)	###	1.29 (0.46, 3.56)	0.64
Adami (M)	#	1.40 (1.10, 1.80)	6.75
Coughlin (W)	####	1.44 (1.21, 1.72)	9.47
Coughlin (M)	####	1.48 (1.27, 1.73)	10.48
Lin (W)	##	1.50 (0.73, 3.12)	1.22
Adami (W)	#	1.50 (1.20, 1.80)	8.32
Wideroff (W)	#	1.60 (1.40, 2.90)	3.97
Wideroff (M)	#	1.70 (1.50, 2.50)	6.46
Jee (W)	####	1.71 (1.25, 2.34)	4.94
Jee (M)	####	1.71 (1.42, 2.06)	9.02
Chow (M)	#	1.88 (1.62, 2.10)	11.72
Chow (W)	#	1.97 (1.77, 2.19)	12.92
Inoue (M)	###	2.07 (1.14, 3.74)	1.76
Rulyak	##	2.10 (0.40, 10.90)	0.25
Lin (M)	##	2.10 (1.20, 3.60)	2.02
Stolzenberg-Solmon	###	2.23 (1.08, 4.60)	1.23
Friedman	##	2.37 (1.46, 3.85)	2.51
Gapstur	#	2.48 (1.20, 4.49)	1.46
Ragozzino (W)	#	2.50 (0.30, 18.40)	0.16
Ragozzino (M)	#	2.70 (0.60, 9.50)	0.36
Mills	#	3.43 (1.47, 7.94)	0.92
Balkau	##	3.60 (1.00, 13.00)	0.41
Shibata	##	3.63 (1.22, 10.80)	0.57
Batty	####	3.99 (1.44, 11.00)	0.65
Hiatt	###	4.50 (1.20, 16.70)	0.39
Whittemore	#	6.08 (0.99, 47.00)	0.18
Overall (I-squared = 32.3%, p = 0.052)		1.73 (1.59, 1.88)	100.00

Diabetes reduces risk — Diabetes increases risk
(0.25 0.5 1 2 4 6 8)

Figure 12.6. Forest plot for Example 12.12, produced by METAN in Stata. Data from Huxley *et al.* (2005). (M) and (W) refer to men and women, respectively. Adjustments made were: # age and sex; ## age, sex and smoking or social class; ### age, sex, smoking and social class; #### age, sex, smoking, social class and diet. The p value shown is for the Q test of heterogeneity.

diabetes either decreases or increases risk. In this forest plot, light shading is used to show the boxes around the point estimates because solid shading (as used in Figure 12.2) masks the actual location of the estimate and the confidence interval, due to overlapping boxes.

The studies in the plot have been ordered by the size of their relative risk. Careful inspection will show that relatively few studies with estimates to the left of the pooled estimate (1.73) have wide confidence limits (i.e., they are not generally small studies). This is plainly seen from the funnel plot (Figure 12.7), produced by the METAFUNNEL routine in Stata; apparently there is publication bias, with missing studies, compared to what is expected, in the lower left portion of the plot (i.e., small studies with relatively low relative risks (less than one) are likely to have been missed).

METAFUNNEL produces a funnel plot which differs from Figure 12.5 in four ways. First, the axes have been turned through ninety degrees, so that the effect (the relative risk, here) now labels the x axis. Second, this axis is drawn on a log scale, but labeled for the raw scale. Third, instead of showing the inverse standard error, METAFUNNEL shows the standard error on a reverse scale (which has the same visual outcome). Finally, it includes a 'pseudo 95% confidence interval': for each value of the standard error (of the log relative risk), SE, this interval goes from the fixed effect pooled estimate (of log relative risk) to ± 1.96SE.

Figure 12.8 shows the results of a trim and fill analysis produced by METATRIM in Stata. Six simulated studies have been filled in: see the open circles. These are the mirror images, about the updated fixed effect pooled estimate, of the six studies with the largest relative risks in Figure 12.6. Published reports of meta analyses will often include a figure similar

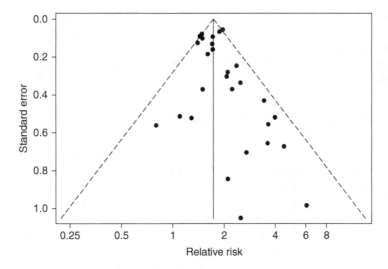

Figure 12.7. Funnel plot corresponding to Figure 12.6. The standard error is for the log relative risk. The vertical line is plotted at the fixed effect estimate and the dashed lines indicate the extremes of the pseudo 95% confidence intervals.

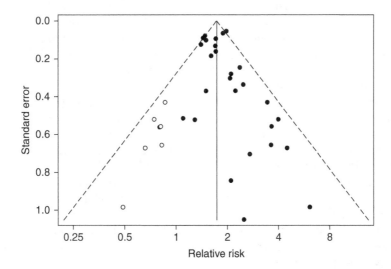

Figure 12.8. Filled-in funnel plot corresponding to Figure 12.7. The filled-in 'quasi-studies' are indicated by open circles (one of which overlaps with the solid circle from a real study). The vertical line is plotted at the updated fixed effect estimate (which is only slightly less than the original).

to Figure 12.7, but not Figure 12.8 which is included here purely as an aid to understanding the methodology. METATRIM reports the updated random effects estimate (with 95% confidence interval) of the relative risk of pancreatic cancer, diabetes versus not, after accounting for publication bias, to be 1.69 (1.55, 1.85).

12.8.4   Other causes of asymmetry in funnel plots

It is important to recognise that asymmetry in the funnel plot may arise from sources other than publication bias. Asymmetry may, alternatively, be due to differences in study design and analysis. As in other plots, such differences may stand out if colour coding (or similar) is used to show different aspects of design and analysis, such as degrees of adjustment for confounding. Egger *et al.* (1997) give a list of potential causes of asymmetry in funnel plots from meta-analyses of clinical trials, most of which have more universal application.

12.9 Advantages and limitations of meta-analysis

In concluding this chapter, it is appropriate to record that not everyone is content to apply meta-analysis in epidemiological research. The most often quoted complaint is that many (perhaps all) of the individual studies are biased and yet the pooling process seems to lend an element of authority, and spurious precision, to the summary result (Shapiro, 1994; Egger *et al.,* 1998). For instance, a certain epidemiological association might have been studied in many case–control studies, each of which is subject to (unknown) selection bias, which leads to overestimation of the odds ratio. Meta-analysis of all the studies thus arrives at an artificially inflated pooled estimate that, nevertheless, has tight confidence limits because of the great volume of information used. The comprehensive nature of the research and the limited sampling error suggest that the pooled estimate may receive wide acceptance.

As the foregoing has shown, meta-analysis is far more than a pooling procedure. In particular, systematic review and exploration of heterogeneity are crucial components that provide important information to the epidemiological researcher. For instance, when an epidemiological association differs by region of the world — perhaps because of genetic or cultural differences — this may not be seen without a forest plot. When several study designs have been used, the very fact that different designs give different results (when they do) gives clues to the aetiology and shows where the study design has likely failed, potentially leading to avoidance of the problem in future. Even in the extreme situation of the last paragraph, without structured sifting of the total evidence base, it would be impossible to determine that only case–control studies have been carried out on the topic of interest, suggesting a gap in current research.

Thus, without pooling, meta-analysis is a sensible approach for an epidemiologist as she or he seeks to understand the underlying nature of the association of interest. When pooling is included, some care is required to acknowledge the problem of possible bias, particularly when all the studies are similar in design. As stressed earlier, when study designs differ, it is important to consider pooled estimates from different study designs separately, at least as a sensitivity analysis.

The final justification for use of meta-analysis in epidemiology is its utility in putting new results in context. When a new study has its final result, it is natural to want to compare this with what was found before. Meta-analysis supplies the tools to do this in the most comprehensive and systematic way, perhaps leading to discussion of how novelties in the current design may have led to different outcomes and, if appropriate, to computation of the current best quantitative evidence on the association of interest after updating the pooled estimate of (say) relative risk.

Exercises

12.1   There is interest in the possibility that smoking by expectant mothers causes brain tumours in their children. Conduct a systematic review of the literature on this association, including a data extraction table.

Huncharek *et al.* (2002) report a review of such literature in which they identified 12 studies with quantitative measures of the association between maternal smoking and childhood brain tumours. Details are given in the following table. Make sure that all 12 studies are included in your review.

Study author	Type of study[a]	Odds ratio	95% Confidence limits	
			Lower	Upper
Bunin	population	1.0	0.6	1.7
Cordier	population	1.6	0.7	3.5
Filippini	population	1.6	0.7	3.6
Gold	population	1.08	0.80	1.45
Howe	hospital	1.42	0.70	3.00
Hu	hospital	1.20	0.45	3.23
John	population	0.8	0.3	2.2
Kuijten	population	1.0	0.6	1.7
McCredie	population	0.9	0.5	1.8
Norman	population	0.98	0.72	1.3
Pershagen	cohort	0.96	0.59	1.56
Stjernfeldt	population	0.93	0.50	1.74

[a] Case–control with source of controls as stated, except for Pershagen.

12.2 Using the preceding table,
  (i) Produce a forest plot with the 12 studies shown in order of decreasing width of confidence interval.
  (ii) Calculate the pooled odds ratio, assuming a fixed effect, and the corresponding 95% confidence interval. Add these results to the forest plot as a summary diamond.
  (iii) Calculate the Q test for homogeneity and test its significance.
  (iv) Calculate the I^2 statistic.
  (v) Why would random effects analysis be unnecessary here?
  (vi) Produce an influence plot. Which studies have great influence on the pooled estimate and heterogeneity?
  (vii) Is there any evidence that the odds ratio derived might vary according to the design of the study? What implications would this have?
  (viii) Does the evidence from this table suggest that maternal smoking is a risk factor for childhood brain tumours?
12.3 Although Exercise 12.2 (vii) required sensitivity analyses taking account of type of study, the systematic review carried out for Exercise 12.1 might have identified other factors that affect study quality. If so, carry out further sensitivity analyses, such as omitting any study with potential bias due to nonresponse. If your review identified any further studies with a quantitative measure of the association between maternal smoking and childhood brain tumours, you should add these to the meta-analysis and produce an updated summary odds ratio.
12.4 Table C.13 (see Appendix C) contains data extracted from a review of passive smoking and lung cancer (Boffetta, 2002). All studies identified in this review are included except one which was reported with inconsistent results.
  (i) Produce a forest plot with the studies grouped by type of study.
  (ii) Calculate the pooled relative risk, assuming a fixed effect, and the corresponding 95% confidence interval.

(iii) Calculate the Q test for homogeneity and test its significance.

(iv) Calculate the I^2 statistic, together with its 95% confidence interval.

(v) Calculate the pooled relative risk, assuming random effects, and the corresponding 95% confidence interval.

(vi) Decide whether you prefer to assume fixed or random effects and thus add the appropriate pooled result to the forest plot.

(vii) Produce an influence plot. Which studies contribute large amounts to the Q statistic?

(viii) One study is especially influential because it has both the greatest (fixed and random effects) weight and contributes the greatest portion to the homogeneity test statistic. Identify this study, remove it and repeat part (ii) to part (v). Draw conclusions. Replace the study temporarily deleted before undertaking the remaining questions.

(ix) One concern with the overall pooling of the studies is that different study designs are generally more reliable than others. Investigate the possibility that results differ by study design by calculating separate pooled random effects relative risks by study type. Also draw an influence plot with study type distinguished through using different plotting symbols or colours. What do you conclude?

(x) Draw a bubble plot, showing year of study on the x axis. Do the log relative risks seem to vary with year?

(xi) Carry out a fixed effect meta-regression using year of study as the explanatory variable. Test the significance of the slope and interpret the result.

(xii) Draw a funnel plot. Is there evidence of possible publication bias? If so, in what way does this appear to have occurred?

12.5 Bachrach *et al.* (2003) conducted a systematic review of breastfeeding and the risk of hospitalisation for respiratory disease in infancy. Seven cohort studies were identified; the following table shows the number hospitalised for respiratory disease and the total number of infants, amongst those breast-fed and those not.

| Study | Breastfed | | Not breastfed | |
author	Hospitalised	Total	Hospitalised	Total
Ball	2	323	3	155
Beaudry	0	49	27	346
Fergusson	1	196	10	226
Hoey	1	41	4	107
Howie	1	90	18	246
Nafstad	38	1376	5	27
Oddy	32	1126	10	217

(i) Calculate relative risks, breastfed against not breastfed, for all these studies (use a continuity correction: add 0.5 to all values in the second study). Also calculate the corresponding 95% confidence intervals. Put them into a forest plot.

(ii) Calculate the pooled relative risk, assuming a fixed effect model and using inverse variance weighting, and the corresponding 95% confidence interval.

(iii) Carry out the corresponding test of homogeneity.

(iv) Calculate the pooled relative risk (and 95% confidence interval), assuming random effects and using inverse variance weighting.

(v) Do the answers to (ii)–(iv) seem to agree with the visual evidence in the forest plot of (i)?

(vi) Repeat (ii)–(iv) for the odds ratio.

(vii) Calculate the pooled relative risk (and 95% confidence interval), assuming fixed effect Mantel–Haenszel weighting.

(viii) Carry out the corresponding test of homogeneity.

(ix) Calculate the negative square root of the Cochran–Mantel–Haenszel test statistic. Compare this with the test statistics calculated by dividing the logarithms of the Mantel–Haenszel estimates of the fixed effect pooled relative risk and odds ratio by their respective standard errors. Why would you expect these three results to be similar?

(x) Compute the test statistic given in Section 4.8 for the test of a common relative risk across the studies (i.e., no interaction between the study and breastfeeding). Compare to the result of (iii).

(xi) Repeat (x) for the test of a common odds ratio, and compare to the homogeneity test in (vi).

(xii) Do the results of the analyses of these meta-data seem to be sensitive to the analytical methods chosen?

12.6 The results of a review of retrospective cohort studies investigating the association between taking naproxen, a nonsteroidal anti-inflammatory drug (NSAID), and the risk of myocardial infarction (MI) are shown below. In each study, naproxen users are compared to patients who took no NSAIDs; each measure of comparative risk reported was interpreted as the relative risk. In most of the ten studies, data were derived from a large medical database, such as general practitioner records and the MEDICAID system in the US. When studies with overlapping data were identified, only one of the studies was included.

| | | 95% confidence limits | |
Study author	Relative risk	Lower	Upper
Ray, Jan. 2002	0.95	0.82	1.09
Watson	0.61	0.39	0.94
Solomon	0.84	0.72	0.98
Ray, Oct. 2002	0.93	0.82	1.06
Mamdani	1	0.6	1.7
Kimmel	0.48	0.28	0.82
Graham	1.14	1	1.3
Levesque	1.17	0.75	1.84
Johnsen	1.5	0.99	2.29
Hippisley-Cox	1.27	1.01	1.6

(i) Draw a forest plot.

(ii) Discuss the main features of these meta-data.

(iii) Draw a funnel plot.

(iv) Is there any suggestion of publication bias?

CHAPTER 13

Risk scores and clinical decision rules

13.1 Introduction

Preceding chapters in this book have presented the essential theory underlying quantitative epidemiology. In the main, the methodology developed has had the goals of identifying whether a putative risk factor is truly associated with the disease in question, or which of a set of candidate risk factors have such an association, and determining the magnitude of such associations. In this chapter we shall consider how epidemiological data might be used to produce clinical algorithms to determine just who should be considered eligible for intervention aimed at preventing future disease events.

13.1.1 Individual and population level interventions

Policies developed from epidemiological results may be designed for application at the individual or population level. These are often contrasted as clinical and public health interventions, respectively. Often the appropriate level depends upon the nature of the intervention that is envisaged.

Examples of population level interventions include salt (i.e., sodium) reduction in processed foods, fluoride in drinking water, distribution of free mosquito nets and compulsory vehicle seat-belt legislation. In the main, it is relatively straightforward to estimate the expected effects of such interventions using the methods explained in earlier chapters, provided suitable data are available. For instance, Bibbins–Domingo *et al.* (2010) projected the effects on coronary heart disease (CHD) events in the US of each of a 1-, 2- and 3-gram reduction in dietary salt using (amongst other things) the results of a meta-analysis of the relationship between salt reduction and change in systolic blood pressure (SBP), distributions of risk factors from the US National Health and Nutrition Examination Survey, hazard ratios relating SBP and CHD from the Framingham Heart Study and published national CHD incidence rates. As in this example, we can think of a population intervention as seeking to move the entire distribution of the risk factor to the left, assuming a single continuous risk factor with a normal distribution (at least, after transformation), for which lower values are 'better' (see Figure 13.1).

Most medical treatments could not, sensibly, be allocated at a population level, because of undesirable side effects and the prohibitive cost. Intervention should then be at the individual level. For instance, strong analgesics, such as heroin or morphine, might well be prescribed for patients who are at high risk of pain, for example after an operation, but there would be no question of distributing such drugs to every citizen merely because all of us are prone to occasional accidents that might cause us pain. As in this example, individual level interventions seek to identify, and subsequently treat (more generally, to intervene — for example, through dietary advice) those at high risk of the disease, as exemplified in Figure 13.2.

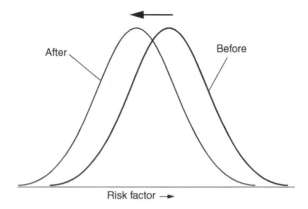

Figure 13.1. Schematic diagram of a population level intervention, showing the risk factor distribution before and after the intervention (and assuming a single risk factor is involved).

An example where monetary cost is the over-riding factor, when deciding whether to intervene universally or just in high-risk groups, is where a decision has to be made about the provision of mosquito nets. These are likely to be of some benefit to virtually everybody living in a country such as Zimbabwe, but the chance of contracting malaria will be relatively low in urban areas at high altitude, such as Harare (the capital city). Unless funds are essentially unlimited, it is unlikely that a programme of free mosquito net distribution would include all of Zimbabwe. In general, the expected benefits have to outweigh the expected costs for the intervention to include individuals at low or moderate risk, and, in general, undesirable side effects would have to be included in the cost side of this comparison.

Another example of the issues involved comes from the suggestion that a combination pill should be freely distributed to the entire population above a certain age, regardless of their level of risk for CHD (Wald and Law, 2003). Such a pill (a 'polypill') would, at least, include compounds to reduce blood pressure and cholesterol. If such a polypill can be produced sufficiently cheaply, the anticipated medical benefits are likely to outweigh the costs, including the detrimental effects of inappropriate use (for example, an increase in falls due to new hypotension) that will inevitably occur in a small percentage of the population. This is primarily because the polypill should prevent many CHD events in the group of people that have moderate risk. This group, whose members would not

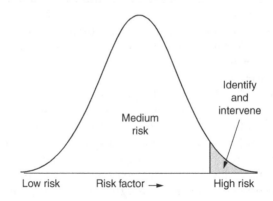

Figure 13.2. Schematic diagram of the scope of an individual level intervention (assuming a single risk factor is involved).

routinely be identified as candidates for medical treatment, contains the vast majority of the population at large (consider the large central portion of Figure 13.2) and consequently most CHD events will occur in this group.

13.1.2   Scope of this chapter

Individual level interventions will be the assumed policy tool for the remainder of this chapter. These are especially challenging because many diseases are multi-factorial and hence we must decide how to assess risk, and the expected consequences of interventions, based on data for several risk factors. However, this is an important challenge to face in modern medical research since, as technology develops in such fields as genomics and proteomics, individual level decision-making and consequent treatment, or **personalised medicine**, is set to become more common.

As stated in the introduction, we shall consider the development of an algorithm, known as a **risk algorithm**, **risk score** or **risk engine**, for determining the level of *future* risk for individuals. Thus the data required will be prospective, and we shall speak of the risk factors used in the risk algorithm as **prognostic variables**. An immediate issue is how long should we 'wait' for disease to develop? That is, do we want to have an algorithm for risk within the next 6 months; the next 5 years; etc.? Different time horizons have been used in published risk scores, most often related more to the availability of the data rather than to clinical utility. To give just one example, most cardiovascular risk scores predict 10-year risk, but it has been argued that this is too long a time horizon for potential sufferers to relate to with sufficient concern to cause them to change unhealthy habits (Wells *et al.*, 2010). Others argue that lifetime risk is most important. For obvious reasons, prognosis is usually considered only for people who currently are free of the disease in question (as in the worked examples given in this chapter). However, in certain situations it can make sense to apply the same ideas to recurrent cases of disease.

Notice that much of the methodology developed in this chapter may also be used for disease prevalence; the exceptions are the methods devised to deal with censored data. For example, Muntner *et al.* (2011) describe an algorithm for determining who is most likely to have albuminuria using only variables that can be self-reported by the general public, such as age, race and smoking status, so that the algorithm may be administered online. This was constructed from a cross-sectional study. In these situations we would call the variables involved in the risk algorithm **diagnostic variables**. Cross-sectional data are easier to deal with than prospective data, and some of what follows builds upon the relatively simple situation of decision making when using cross-sectional data described in Section 2.10.

An applied summary of much of the material covered by this chapter is given in the pair of papers by Moons *et al.* (2012a and 2012b). What is not included in either this chapter or these summary papers is the economic side of clinical decision making. As we have already seen, this is almost inevitably part of the decision-making process in real life. Assuming that the cost of an intervention can be quantified, per person to whom it is applied, it is quite simple to calculate the cost per expected event saved when intervening above a certain threshold of risk. Going beyond such a simple economic evaluation is beyond our current scope.

As usual in this book, the development of the subject will begin by considering the simple case of a single risk factor. Given that the practical outcome of the clinical decision rule will be whether or not to intervene for any specific individual, in both this and multivariable situations, a secondary question will be how to determine the threshold for high risk.

13.2   Association and prognosis

Suppose that there is a single risk factor from which we wish to develop a clinical decision rule. In earlier chapters we have already seen how to determine whether a risk factor is related to the risk of the index disease. For example, in Example 10.14 we concluded that systolic blood pressure (SBP) has an effect on CHD, with and without also taking account of cholesterol, because the likelihood ratio (deviance) tests were significant at the 5% level. However, when statistical tests were introduced in Section 2.5.1, the significance level was defined as the chance of type I error: the probability of rejecting the null hypothesis (of no effect) when it is really true. Subsequently, in Section 8.2, type II error was defined as the probability of failing to reject the null hypothesis when it is really false. A clinical decision rule must take account of both types of error, since a rule that correctly identifies the high-risk people who are going to develop the disease is unlikely to be of practical use as a screening tool, for deciding who should receive treatment, if the rule also identifies a large proportion of people who will not get the disease to be at high risk, and thus apparently suitable for intervention. Certainly, a prognostic variable must have a strong association with the disease of interest, but (as we shall see later) a strong association does not necessarily infer utility in prognosis.

One further general contrast with measures of association may be made. When we conclude that one variable predicts another because the statistical model using the first variable (the explanatory variable) to model the second variable (the outcome variable) gives a better fit than the corresponding model without it, we do not necessarily mean that the explanatory variable must precede the outcome variable in time. In general, all we mean is that we have a better idea what the value of the outcome variable will be for a new subject when we know the value of the explanatory variable for that subject than when we do not (see Section 9.1). Prognostic (explanatory) variables, by contrast, must have utility in forecasting future outcomes.

For a continuous risk factor to be a useful prognostic variable it must have a threshold which gives acceptable ratings for both types of error. Furthermore, it will be more useful than a competing variable if it shows superior ratings across its range. For a binary variable, such as family history of disease (yes/no), there is no question of choice in threshold levels. Categorical variables fall in-between, as they allow a limited number of high-risk thresholds (e.g., current smoking alone or current and former smoking together). For multiple risk factors (discussed in Section 13.3.2), their joint prognosis is encapsulated in a risk score constructed as a mathematical function of the individual variables (which can be both quantitative and qualitative). The high-risk threshold is then defined for the score rather than the individual variables.

Example 13.1 Fibrinogen is a clotting factor which stops us from bleeding to death following severe cuts. But when clotting occurs in the wrong place, a heart attack or stroke may result. Fibrinogen has, thus, long been identified as a potential risk factor for cardiovascular disease (CVD). Does it have any role in identifying the minority of healthy persons (currently free of CVD) who would most benefit from preventive treatment for CVD?

To answer this question we should first see whether fibrinogen is a predictor of CVD risk. An excellent way of doing this would be through a published meta-analysis. To produce a complete example here, we will look only at results from the Scottish database used routinely through much of this book. In fact, we shall look at the combined data from the Scottish Heart Health Study (SHHS) and MONICA study, called the Scottish Heart Health Extended Cohort (SHHEC) study, with a median of 19.2 years follow-up (Woodward *et al.*, 2009). These data include around 13000 men and women who, at baseline, were aged 30 years or

Table 13.1. Summary statistics and tests for fibrinogen in the SHHEC study. Multiple adjustment is for age, systolic blood pressure, total cholesterol and smoking.

Sex	CVD during follow-up?	n	Mean (g/l)	Median (g/l)	p value after adjustment for None	Age	Multiple
Men	No	4875	2.71	2.60	<0.0001	<0.0001	0.04
	Yes	1634	2.87	2.74			
Women	No	5559	2.82	2.71	<0.001	<0.001	0.02
	Yes	992	3.04	2.92			

more, were free of CVD and had fibrinogen measured. The data are available from the web site for this book (see Appendix A).

One simple way of checking whether fibrinogen predicts CVD is to compare the mean fibrinogen at baseline between those who subsequently went on to get CVD and those who did not. Table 13.1 shows the results from general linear models comparing these groups. Since fibrinogen is right-skewed, log transformations were used before testing to compare the means. The results show that those who developed CVD have a tendency to have started the study with higher values of fibrinogen. Adjustment for multiple classical CVD risk factors attenuates the significance, but still leaves fibrinogen a significant predictor, for both sexes, at the usual 5% level.

A more illuminating analysis, dealing with the issues of dose–response and censoring, is obtained from fitting Cox models to the SHHEC data. Figure 13.3 shows the (unadjusted) hazard ratios by tenth of fibrinogen for women (a similar pattern is found for men). This suggests that, on the log scale, there is a linear relationship between fibrinogen and the risk of CVD, so that the summary estimates of Table 13.2 are meaningful: for women, an extra 1 g/l of fibrinogen confers an additional 17% risk of CVD, after allowing for classical risk factors.

According to the epidemiological and statistical criteria we have used in this book we can safely conclude that fibrinogen predicts CVD. Indeed, there is a reasonable case to conclude that elevated fibrinogen is likely to be a cause of CVD since all the relevant Bradford-Hill principles are satisfied

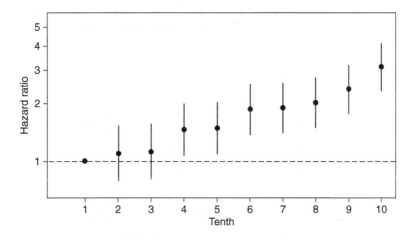

Figure 13.3. Cardiovascular disease hazard ratios (95% confidence intervals) by tenth of fibrinogen for women in the SHHEC study. The first tenth is the reference group. The vertical axis uses a logarithmic scale.

Table 13.2. Cardiovascular disease hazard ratios (95% confidence intervals) for a one unit (g/l) increase in fibrinogen in the SHHEC study. Multiple adjustment is for age, systolic blood pressure, total cholesterol and smoking (sample sizes vary due to missing values). All p values for fibrinogen are <0.0001.

| | Adjustment | | |
	None	Age	Multiple
Men	1.28 (1.22, 1.34)	1.20 (1.14, 1.27)	1.14 (1.08, 1.21)
Women	1.36 (1.28, 1.44)	1.24 (1.16, 1.33)	1.17 (1.09, 1.25)

(see Section 1.6.3). That is, there is a strong association between fibrinogen and CVD; the value of fibrinogen was obtained before CVD was diagnosed; there is a plausible biological explanation for the association; the association has been found in a large meta-analysis (Fibrinogen Studies Collaboration, 2005); there is a dose–response association; and the association persists after adjustment for the leading CVD risk factors (furthermore, Woodward *et al.* (2009) show a residual effect of fibrinogen after further adjustments to those included here). But does this necessarily mean that fibrinogen is useful as a prognostic variable?

13.2.1   The concept of discrimination

To answer the last question of Example 13.1, we will, first, consider the general issue. Figure 13.4 shows a potential situation where the variable under consideration has, as in Example 13.1, a higher mean in the group with the disease. Here we introduce the concept of **discrimination**: how well the risk factor separates the distributions of those with and without the disease. The distributions of the two groups are almost completely separate in Figure 13.4, meaning that the disease is well discriminated by the risk factor. Contrast this with Figure 13.5, where the mean is still higher (we can assume it is significantly so) in the disease positive group than the disease negative group, but the distributions have a large overlap, and hence discrimination is poor. As in Figure 13.1 and Figure 13.2, normal distributions are assumed here, for simplicity.

We could also look at the degree of overlap using boxplots: Figure 13.6 does this, separately by sex, for Example 13.1 (showing only the middle 98% of the distributions to simplify the interpretation — note that the skewness is apparent even without the

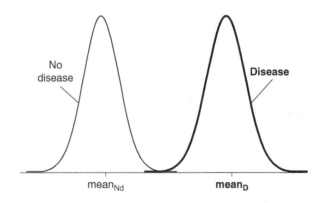

Figure 13.4. Schematic diagram of the distribution of a risk factor with good discrimination, shown separately for those with and without the disease of interest. The D suffix and bold type/lines denote the group with the disease; the Nd suffix denotes the group with no disease.

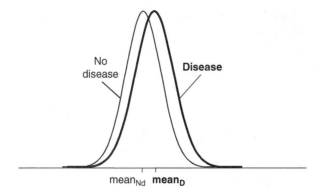

Figure 13.5. Schematic diagram of the distribution of a risk factor with poor discrimination, shown separately for those with and without the disease of interest. Conventions as in Figure 13.4.

extreme values). From Figure 13.6 it is very obvious that the values of fibrinogen at baseline overlap considerably for those who did, and did not, go on to develop CVD. That is, it appears that fibrinogen does not discriminate CVD at all well. In Section 13.4 we shall see how to quantify discrimination.

13.2.2   Risk factor thresholds

Since CVD is a multi-factorial disease, it is really quite unreasonable to expect anything like the separation for fibrinogen in Figure 13.6 that is implied by Figure 13.4, which would be more typical for a disease which has only one predictor. Also, Figure 13.6 relates to the risk factor itself, rather than to the clinical decision rule which we really want to evaluate in the current context. If we are to use a single risk factor in a clinical algorithm, where we either decide to intervene or not, we need to define a threshold (cut-point) at or above which the risk factor is high enough (assuming that risk increases with the risk factor) to justify intervention.

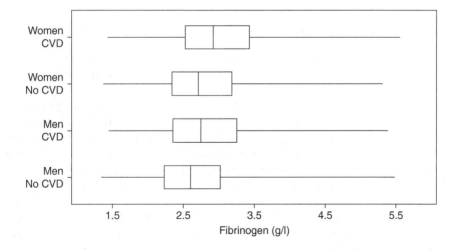

Figure 13.6. Boxplot for fibrinogen by sex and incident CVD in the SHHEC study. The whiskers go to the 1st and 99th percentiles.

Table 13.3. Probabilities arising when applying decision rules.[a]

Test result	True disease status	
	Positive	Negative
Positive	True +ve Sensitivity Power	False +ve Type I error (p value)
Negative	False −ve Type II error	True −ve Specificity

[a] This corresponds with Table 2.21 and Table 3.1 which arose in related contexts. All probabilities are specific to columns (i.e., the true disease status): e.g., the probability of a false negative is the number with a negative test result amongst those who are truly positive. Thus all the probabilities in a column are the complement of those in the other row of the same column: e.g., the probability of a true positive is one minus the probability of a false negative.

We now need to decide how to evaluate the performance of the test based on any specific threshold. The materials for doing this have already been introduced in the context of diagnostic tests (Section 2.10); the most basic of these are sensitivity and specificity. Example 13.2 applies these principles. To facilitate interpretation of these basic ideas, the analogy with hypothesis tests (discussed in Section 8.2) is presented in Table 13.3.

Example 13.2 Returning to Example 13.1, Table 13.4 shows the distribution of CVD cases during the first 10 years of follow-up according to tenth of fibrinogen at baseline, for women. Again, we see the general dose–response effect, this time by examining the percentages in parentheses. Suppose that we choose the 9th decile (i.e., the 90% percentile) of 3.85 g/l as the intervention threshold.

Using this threshold, how accurate is our decision rule? This is answered by Table 13.5, which has been structured to look like Table 2.21. From (2.37),

$$\text{Sensitivity} = 77/404 = 0.19.$$
$$\text{Specificity} = 5567/6147 = 0.91.$$

The proposed clinical decision rule is thus quite satisfactory for picking out non-cases but not for identifying cases (those who will go on to develop CVD within 10 years).

In fact, the conclusion of Example 13.2 was predictable because of the high degree of overlap seen in Figure 13.6. To see this in general terms, consider Figure 13.7 and Figure 13.8, which reproduce Figure 13.5 but add probabilities below and above a threshold, T, placed far to the right of the centre of the distribution of the risk factor (fibrinogen, in the example). T (the 90th percentile in the example) is the border between a positive (at or above the threshold) and a negative (below the threshold) test decision. Figure 13.7 shows the probabilities (areas within appropriate ranges of the curves) which correspond to false negative conclusions (where the decision rule predicts no disease — the risk factor takes a value below the threshold — but the person really did develop the disease) and false positive conclusions (where the decision rule predicts disease — value at or above the threshold — when the person really did not develop the disease). Figure 13.8 conveys the same message, but the converse probabilities are

Table 13.4. Incident CVD over 10 years follow-up by tenth of fibrinogen for women in the SHHEC study. The tenths vary somewhat in size due to clustering at the deciles.

	Tenth (maximum value; g/l)										Total
	1st (2.01)	2nd (2.25)	3rd (2.43)	4th (2.59)	5th (2.74)	6th (2.91)	7th (3.10)	8th (3.37)	9th (3.85)	10th (11.32)	
CVD	23 (3.5%)	27 (4.1%)	26 (4.0%)	30 (4.5%)	38 (5.7%)	44 (7.0%)	43 (6.5%)	41 (6.3%)	55 (8.4%)	77 (11.7%)	404 (6.2%)
No CVD	631	631	617	643	626	588	617	615	599	580	6147
Total	654	658	643	673	664	632	660	656	654	657	6551

Table 13.5. Results of a clinical decision rule which identifies those in the highest 10% of the distribution of fibrinogen as predicted CVD cases in the next 10 years, for women in the SHHEC study.

In 90th percentile for fibrinogen?	True CVD outcome		
	Positive	Negative	Total
Positive	77	580	657
Negative	327	5567	5894
Total	404	6147	6551

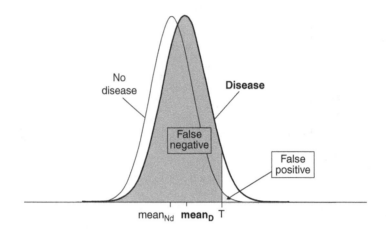

Figure 13.7. Schematic diagram of the probabilities of false positives and negatives. The D suffix and bold type/lines denote the group with the disease; the Nd suffix denotes the group with no disease. T denotes the clinical decision threshold for the risk factor.

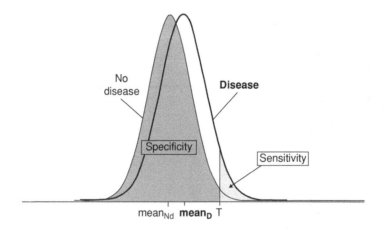

Figure 13.8. Schematic diagram of sensitivity and specificity. Conventions as in Figure 13.7 (which shows the complementary probabilities).

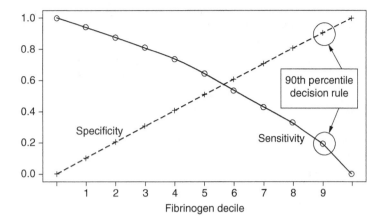

Figure 13.9. Sensitivity and specificity against the threshold (deciles or extreme values) used to distinguish 10-year CVD from not, for women in the SHHEC study. The threshold used in Example 13.2 is highlighted. The unlabelled ticks at the extreme ends of the horizontal scale denote the extreme values. Note that the horizontal axis is not scaled to the fibrinogen distribution.

shown. With the distributions of those with and without disease overlapping as much as in Figure 13.8, for a risk factor positively related to the disease, any high threshold value is clearly sure to give poor sensitivity. Since it would be hard to imagine choosing anything other than a high decision threshold for a risk factor that is positively related to the disease in question, this is important to bear in mind when assessing clinical decision rules in practice.

For further insight, Figure 13.9 shows the sensitivities and specificities for separate clinical decision rules based on each specific decile for the fibrinogen data. This was constructed from the data in Table 13.4. To understand this plot, imagine Figure 13.8 representing the fibrinogen problem (after log transforming fibrinogen) and consider where the threshold (T) would come for any specific decile. If we take the decision threshold to lie at the first decile (10th percentile), this places T off to the far left, giving a large area to represent sensitivity and a small area to represent specificity. As we have already seen, the opposite is true when we take the 9th decile (90th percentile). This explains why specificity rises and sensitivity falls as the threshold increases. At the two extremes, either all or none of the area of both curves is to the right. At the left extreme, the threshold is the lowest value of fibrinogen and then all future cases are identified (sensitivity = 1) but no one is classed as a future non-case, so specificity must be zero. The converse is true at the right extreme, when the threshold corresponds to the largest value of fibrinogen.

Rather than choosing an extreme value of the risk factor, we could fix the decision threshold using (2.40); that is, by finding the value of the risk factor where the sum (or weighted sum) of sensitivity and specificity is maximised. In Figure 13.9 this is the 5th decile. However, this approach is generally unworkable in practical clinical decision making, since (as in this example) it tends to identify a substantial portion of the population for treatment — far more than can be afforded.

13.2.3   Risk thresholds

In practice, a threshold is usually picked according to the predicted level of risk, rather than by selecting a particular value of the risk factor (or risk factor combination). For example, we might decide that someone with a chance of 10%, or more, of developing the disease in the next 10 years should be offered treatment, perhaps because denial of treatment to someone at this level of risk would be unacceptable. Changing to such risk thresholds makes no difference to the concepts discussed already, but does immediately suggest problems with using observed data. For instance, we can see from Table 13.4 that the chance of CHD within 10 years is about 12% for those in the top 10% of fibrinogen values, and that all other tenths have below 10% risk, but it is not possible to isolate the group with exactly 10% risk from this table. Furthermore, as evidenced by Table 13.4 (where the risk in succeeding tenths does not increase monotonically), sampling variation adds random error to the operation. Risk thresholds are, thus, better derived from mathematical models, which smooth the data: see Section 13.3.4.

13.2.4   Odds ratios and discrimination

In many of the preceding chapters in this book the odds ratio, or a similar measure of relative risk, has been the primary index of association between a risk factor and the disease in question. The essential problem with this approach, when we come to issues of personalised medicine, is that this is a one-dimensional index which merely establishes the degree of association. As we have already seen, if we are to assess the consequences of clinical interventions, we must consider the chances of making the wrong decision in the false negative situation, as well as the false positive situation that is considered in standard hypothesis testing using p values.

Here we shall consider the relationship between the odds ratio, ψ, and the sensitivity, s, and specificity, p. The odds ratio is chosen here both for convenience and because it may be computed from case–control studies, as well as from other types of epidemiological design — the material in this section is equally applicable to retrospective and cross-sectional (diagnostic) studies.

From (2.37) and (3.9) we can show that

$$\psi = \left(\frac{s}{1-s}\right)\left(\frac{p}{1-p}\right). \tag{13.1}$$

This relationship has been used repeatedly to produce Table 13.6, which shows how the odds ratio changes as sensitivity and specificity are varied from 0.1 to 0.9. For simplicity, this table only considers odds ratios of one or more (values below one would appear above the diagonal). What is very striking here is how large ψ has to be before we have reasonably adequate values of sensitivity and specificity. Even with ψ around 9, we see that we will miss:

- 50% of true positives and 10% of true negatives, or
- 50% of true negatives and 10% of true positives, or
- 20% of true positives and 30% of true negatives, or
- 20% of true negatives and 30% of true positives, or
- similar combinations not covered by the table.

It appears that we need an odds ratio of at least 16 to obtain even moderately good decision criteria.

Table 13.6. The odds ratios (≥ 1) which correspond to various combinations of sensitivity and specificity.

Sensitivity	Specificity								
	0.1	0.2	0.3	0.4	0.5	0.6	0.7	0.8	0.9
0.1									1
0.2								1	2.2
0.3							1	1.7	3.9
0.4						1	1.6	2.7	6.0
0.5					1	1.5	2.3	4.0	9.0
0.6				1	1.5	2.2	3.5	6.0	13.5
0.7			1	1.6	2.3	3.5	5.4	9.3	21.0
0.8		1	1.7	2.7	4.0	6.0	9.3	16.0	36.0
0.9	1	2.2	3.9	6.0	9.0	13.5	21.0	36.0	81.0

Looking at the issue in another way, we shall now consider what the disease-specific curves (in the style of Figure 13.4 and Figure 13.5) would look like (assuming a normal distribution) when the odds ratio takes a value which would conventionally be considered large.

In practical epidemiology, with a continuous risk factor, we generally divide the risk factor into groups and compare each other group to the pre-defined reference group. Often the groups chosen are fifths and the lowest is taken as the reference (e.g., as in Example 10.11). Should the odds ratio comparing the extreme fifths (highest versus lowest) be 4 (or more) we would likely conclude that the risk factor appears to be an important predictor (a significant hypothesis test would strengthen this conclusion). This is approximately the case, for instance, when comparing cholesterol fifths in the real-life data from Table 10.14: see Table 13.7 which isolates the extreme fifths from this earlier table. When the odds ratio comparing the extreme fifths is 4, it may be shown that the mean values of the disease and non-disease groups will be separated by about $0.5s$, where s is the standard deviation of the risk factor (assumed equal in each group). In deriving this, it was assumed that the overall quintiles are approximately the same as the quintiles in the non-diseased sub-group, which is reasonable if the disease is fairly rare. Example 13.3 illustrates the degree of separation of disease curves that can be expected when the odds ratio is 4. This clearly shows that a substantial odds ratio does not guarantee good discrimination. Indeed, an odds ratio of around 17 is required to separate the curves by one standard deviation, whilst we only get a separation of $2s$ or more when $\psi > 300$.

Table 13.7. Comparison of extreme fifths for cholesterol, extracted from Table 10.14. The odds ratio (highest versus lowest fifth) is $(65 \times 810)/(18 \times 722) = 4.05$.

Cholesterol fifth	True CVD outcome		Total
	Positive	Negative	
Highest	65	722	787
Lowest	18	810	828
Total	83	1532	1615

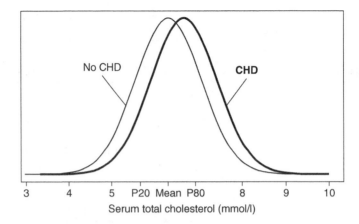

Figure 13.10. Distribution of cholesterol amongst those with and without CHD when the odds ratio comparing extreme fifths is 4. P20, mean and P80 are, respectively, the 20th percentile, mean and 80th percentile in the CHD-free group. The mean and standard deviation in the CHD-free group were estimated from Table 2.12, and a normal distribution was assumed.

Example 13.3 In Section 2.6 we found that cholesterol (in a small, but real-life, dataset) was approximately normally distributed with mean 6.287 and standard deviation (SD) 0.757 mmol/l. We shall assume that people without CHD have cholesterol values following this distribution, whilst people with CHD have cholesterol values with the same standard deviation, but a higher mean. Suppose that, when we divide people up into the fifths of the non-CHD group (approximately the same as the overall fifths for all people) we find that the odds ratio comparing the top to bottom fifth is 4. What do the disease-specific curves then look like?

To answer this we need, first, to find the mean in the diseased group. Assuming the approximate result given in this section, this is $6.287 + 0.5 \times 0.787 = 6.680$. Then we can construct the form of each of the two normal distributions using the NORM.DIST function in Excel for each value of cholesterol within whatever range we are interested in. Figure 13.10 was constructed this way. The high percentage of overlap between the curves is clear: cholesterol by itself is unlikely to be a good discriminator of CHD.

Here we have only looked at the case of a binary comparison to produce the odds ratio. Pepe *et al.* (2004) consider the case of a continuously varying risk factor and draw similar conclusions. Cook (2008) considers the multivariable case.

13.3   Risk scores from statistical models

13.3.1   *Logistic regression*

As already discussed in Section 13.2.3, the method of tabulating risk according to arbitrary ordinal groups (as in Table 13.4), and then picking a decision threshold which identifies the group at sufficiently high risk for intervention, is limited in practical utility and generalisability. A regression modelling approach, using raw data, is preferable for deriving clinical decision rules, and this method will be used from here on. Many different models can be used, but the simplest is logistic regression, which will be described here. This model is most appropriate within the situation of a fixed cohort (see Section 5.2.1) since it cannot deal satisfactorily with censoring; if this is an important issue a survival model should be used instead (see Section 13.3.3).

Example 13.4 A logistic regression model was fitted to the raw data, available on the web site for this book, on fibrinogen and the binary outcome variable recording whether or not CVD occurred during 10 years of follow-up for women in the SHHEC study. Based on these data, and past literature, a linear relationship between fibrinogen and the log of the odds ratio for CVD was assumed.

PROC LOGISTIC in SAS returned coefficients of −3.8063 and 0.3645 for the intercept and slope for fibrinogen, respectively. The fitted model is thus

$$\text{log\^it} = -3.8063 + 0.3645 \times \text{fibrinogen}. \tag{13.2}$$

We can use (10.8) to turn this into an equation for predicted risk,

$$\hat{p} = \{1 + \exp(-(-3.8063 + 0.3645 \times \text{fibrinogen}))\}^{-1} \tag{13.3}$$

For example, when fibrinogen is 5 g/l, (13.3) gives:

$$\hat{p} = 1/\{1 + \exp(3.8063 - 0.3645 \times 5)\} = 0.12.$$

From (13.3), Figure 13.11 was produced. This shows the predicted values corresponding to each observed value of fibrinogen, as well as the fitted curve.

(13.3) is our first example of a risk score. The scale upon which a risk score is expressed may either be as in Figure 13.11 (a proportion), in which case scores must range between 0 and 1, or as a percentage (i.e., multiply by 100), in which case they range between 0 and 100. As discussed in Section 13.1.2, all risk scores have an element of time (10 years in the example), which should always be made clear.

Although, for simplicity, we shall only consider linear models for risk scores in this chapter, non-linear associations should also be considered in practice. Just as for standard regression problems, it may be that a non-linear, or a spline, model leads to more accurate prognosis. For instance, a risk score based on log(fibrinogen) might have better properties than one, such as (13.3), based on fibrinogen itself.

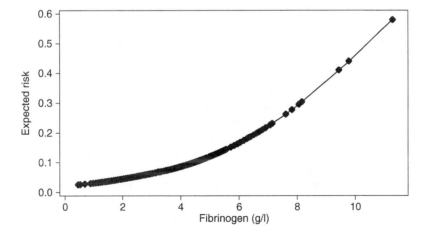

Figure 13.11. Expected risk of CVD within 10 years according to value of fibrinogen for women in the SHHEC study. Dots show the expected risk corresponding to observed values of fibrinogen (observed values cluster considerably).

13.3.2   *Multiple variable risk scores*

The approach of Example 13.4 is generalised to deal with several potential prognostic variables simultaneously by fitting a multiple logistic regression model. The right-hand side of the logistic regression equation then has several x values:

$$\text{log\^{i}t} = b_0 + b_1 x_1 + b_2 x_2 + b_3 x_3 + \ldots\ldots$$

As with a single risk factor, the equation for a risk score involving several variables then comes from (10.8):

$$\hat{p} = \left\{ 1 + \exp(-\text{log\^{i}t}) \right\}^{-1}.$$

Given many potential prognostic variables, the question arises about how the variables should be selected. The usual way in which multiple variable risk scores are constructed is to start with a set of risk factors considered, by expert opinion, to be the important predictors of the index disease. Most risk scores are developed from existing cohort studies, in which case any variables that were not collected at baseline must inevitably be left out of the model, unless they can now be derived from administrative databases or stored biological materials (such as frozen blood samples). If this means excluding key risk factors, this might lead to searching for an alternative developmental dataset or abandoning the project entirely. Otherwise, we might continue by developing a parsimonious set of independent (in the sense of being significant after cross-adjustment) predictive factors, using the methods described in Chapter 10 or Chapter 11. Parsimony in predicting association is certainly not the only possible criterion for our final selection although, for pragmatic reasons, it may be a reasonable first step. We may, for example, wish to see whether adding extra variables, beyond those independently predictive, improves discrimination, whilst the costs of measuring the variables may also be an important consideration. Interaction terms should certainly be considered in this process.

Assuming that the disease in question has many risk factors, multivariable risk scores provide a convenient way of expressing the joint effects of several risk factors, leading to an efficient clinical decision rule. For instance, blood pressure lowering medication is often prescribed to reduce the risk of CHD. A naïve approach to allocating such treatment would be to only give it to those with hypertension (high blood pressure, at levels above nationally defined norms). However, many (if not, most) of the people at high risk of CHD have sub-optimal, but moderate, levels of blood pressure, falling below the level of hypertension. They may be at high risk because they smoke and have high levels of cholesterol; these factors add risk on top of the moderate contribution from their blood pressure. Such people would also benefit from blood pressure reduction, conceivably more than others who are hypertensive but have no other coronary risk factors. A decision rule based upon a risk score which measures the totality of (absolute) risk is likely to allocate blood pressure lowering treatment more effectively than the naïve approach.

Example 13.5 In Example 10.15 we considered the best logistic regression model for future coronary heart disease (CHD) for men initially free of CHD, using the data given on the web site for this book (originating from Example 10.12). Although various models were considered in Example 10.15, here we shall take that model with the variables that were found to be significant

($p < 0.05$) predictors in cross-adjusted models: total cholesterol, systolic blood pressure and smoking status.

In Example 13.4 we derived 10-year risk, and we might like to estimate 10-year risk here also. However, in Section 5.2.3 it was stated that the maximum elapsed time (baseline to end of follow-up) was only 9.1 years in the study data used for the current example. Thus we could only consider evaluating up to 9.1 years' risk here. However, even this is too large a number, because the participants who started after the first wave of recruitment inevitably had less than 9.1 years potential follow-up, and so estimation of 9.1-year risk is bound to be biased downwards. In fact, it is only risk over elapsed periods of less than or equal to the minimum potential follow-up (i.e., the time between the final recruitment and end of follow-up) that may be estimated without bias in a logistic regression model. In our case, this is 6.2 years (see Section 5.2.3). In practice, we would prefer to choose a round number of years for our time horizon, such as 5 years, since this is more interpretable. Since the data on the web site include total follow-up time, we can easily censor all follow-up at 5 years by reclassifying any CHD event post 5 years as a non-event before running the logistic regression model. The data give time in days; allowing for leap years, we shall take 5 years as 1827 days.

The three-variable prognostic model turns out to be:

$$\hat{\text{logit}} = -9.1372 + 0.3391(\text{TOTCHOL}) + 0.0208(\text{SYSTOL})$$
$$+ 0.4016(\text{ex}) + 0.7089(\text{current})$$

where TOTCHOL denotes total cholesterol, SYSTOL is systolic blood pressure and 'ex' = 1 only for ex-smokers and 'current' = 1 only for current smokers. The predicted 5-year CHD risk scores then come from (10.8):

$$\hat{p} = \{1 + \exp(9.1372 - 0.3391(\text{TOTCHOL}) - 0.0208(\text{SYSTOL})$$
$$- 0.4016(\text{ex}) - 0.7089(\text{current}))\}^{-1}.$$

13.3.3 Cox regression

Risk scores developed from survival data, allowing for censoring, are most commonly derived from Cox regression models. Although other survival models, particularly the Weibull, have been used in practice, this is the only such model that will be considered here. As we have seen in Section 11.5 and Section 11.6, a Cox proportional hazards model produces an expression for the log hazard ratio $\log_e \hat{\phi}$, of an event, given a risk factor set $\{x\}$, of the form (11.30):

$$\log_e \hat{\phi} = b_1 x_1 + b_2 x_2 + b_3 x_3 + \ldots$$

Compared to logistic models, this lacks an intercept term with which to 'anchor down' estimates of risk. This anchor is commonly taken as the estimated survival probability when all the variables in the model, $\{x\}$, attain their mean values, although this is a broad approximation and so other methods might be considered (see Nieto and Coresh, 1996). This estimated survival probability, often called the **baseline survivor function** (where 'baseline' refers to the chosen values for $\{x\}$, rather than time) is evaluated at time t, where t is the length of time over which we wish to make prognostic assertions (e.g., 10 years). We will represent the baseline survival probability up to time t for subjects who have mean values for all the risk variables as $S(t, \bar{x})$. The BASELINE command in SAS PROC PHREG automatically produces $S(t, \bar{x})$, and PREDICT used after STCOX in Stata also produces it, provided the variables entered into the Cox model are each centred at their mean (see Section 11.5.3).

An estimate of the risk of disease during t years for any combination of values for the prediction variables, $\{x\}$, may be shown to be:

$$\hat{p} = 1 - S(t, \bar{x})^z \qquad (13.4)$$

where

$$z = \exp(w) \quad \text{and} \quad w = \sum_i b_i x_i - \sum_i b_i \bar{x}_i.$$

Thus (13.4) is a risk score from a Cox model.

Note that another way of writing the last equation is:

$$w = \sum b_1(x_1 - \bar{x}_1) + b_2(x_2 - \bar{x}_2) + b_3(x_3 - \bar{x}_3) + \dots$$

which illustrates that the predicted risk for someone with any specific values of the risk factors, $\{x\}$, takes into account how far her or his specific combination differs from the baseline (mean) combination.

Example 13.6 The fibrinogen data of Example 13.4 arose from a cohort study where some follow-ups were censored. Hence a Cox model is likely to be a suitable one to analyse these data; indeed, more suitable than the logistic model, used in Example 13.4, which cannot allow for censoring. We shall, as before, compute 10-year risks; since most women in this large study were observed for at least 10 years the survival probability at 10 years should be reliable.

Fitting a Cox model to the female fibrinogen data available from the web site for this book (Appendix A) gives the fitted model:

$$\log_e \hat{\phi} = 0.30671 \times \text{fibrinogen}.$$

The mean level of fibrinogen is 2.8578546 g/l. The estimate of 10-year (or 3652 days, allowing for leap years) survival when fibrinogen = 2.8578546, $S(10, 2.8578546)$, was found from PROC PHREG in SAS to be 0.93916, the cumulative risk of survival at the time of the last event recorded up to and including day 3652. Then, using (13.4), the predicted risk is:

$$\hat{p} = 1 - 0.93916^z,$$

where $z = \exp(0.30671x - 0.30671 \times 2.8578546) = \exp(0.30671x - 0.97653)$.

For example, a woman whose fibrinogen level is 2 g/l has $z = \exp(0.30671 \times 2 - 0.97653) = 0.76865$, and thus a predicted 10-year risk of $\hat{p} = 1 - 0.93916^{0.76865} = 0.04711$.

Example 13.7 The data used in Example 13.5 also derive from a cohort study: see Example 11.10. The Cox model relating CHD to total cholesterol, systolic blood pressure and smoking, using PROC PHREG in SAS applied to the data available from the web site for this book, is:

$$\log_e \hat{\phi} = 0.29483(\text{TOTCHOL}) + 0.02186(\text{SYSTOL}) + 0.32380(\text{ex})$$

$$+ 0.65894(\text{current}), \qquad (13.5)$$

where the variable names are as in Example 13.5.

Table 13.8. Computation table for Example 13.7.

Variable	b	Mean	Product
Total cholesterol (mmol/l)	0.29483	6.35832	1.87462
Systolic blood pressure (mmHg)	0.02186	133.223	2.91226
Ex-smoking	0.32380	0.25537	0.08269
Current smoking	0.65894	0.52038	0.34290
Total			5.21247

The mean values of the three risk factors (one of which has two constituent dummy variables) are easily found (e.g., using PROC MEANS in SAS) and are shown in Table 13.8. Here the estimated beta coefficients are shown again, and the cross-product of each of these with their respective means is included to demonstrate how w is computed. For the two binary variables, i.e., the dummy variables, the means are the proportion of men who are, respectively, ex-smokers and current smokers in the entire sample.

As in Example 13.5, we will choose to predict CHD outcomes over 5 years: i.e., $t = 5$ years (or 1827 days) in (13.4). From SAS PROC PHREG, the estimated probability of survival (free of CHD) for 5 years, $S(5, \bar{x})$, in the (mean) baseline group is 0.97648. Using (13.4), the equation for the predicted risk is thus:

$$\hat{p} = 1 - 0.97648^{\exp(0.29483(\text{TOTCHOL}) + 0.02186(\text{SYSTOL}) + 0.32380(\text{ex}) + 0.65894(\text{current}) - 5.21247)}. \qquad (13.6)$$

13.3.4   Risk thresholds

In Section 13.2.3 the idea of a risk threshold was introduced. Here we shall construct and evaluate a risk threshold from a risk score using, as an example, (13.3). For instance, suppose it is felt that we should give anti-CVD medication, such as statins, whenever the chance of a CVD event in the next 10 years is 10% or more. To determine the threshold, we turn around (13.3) to make the fibrinogen value appear on the left side of the equation. Solving that, when the estimated risk is 0.1, gives a fibrinogen value of 4.42 g/l. Thus our rule is to give statins to every woman with a fibrinogen value of 4.42 g/l or more.

Having generated such a rule, it is reasonable to want to know the likely ramifications. Sensitivity and specificity result from the usual 2×2 table: Table 13.9. These turn out to be 7 and 96%, respectively. As expected from the earlier discussion, a decision rule based on fibrinogen alone has poor sensitivity but good — indeed, excellent — specificity.

Table 13.9. Clinical decision rule for anti-CVD intervention based on a risk threshold of 10%: women in SHHEC.

Test	True CVD outcome		Total
	Positive	Negative	
Positive (i.e., fibrinogen ≥ 4.42; i.e., predicted risk ≥ 0.1)	30 (7%)	224	254
Negative	374	5923 (96%)	6297
Total	404	6147	6551

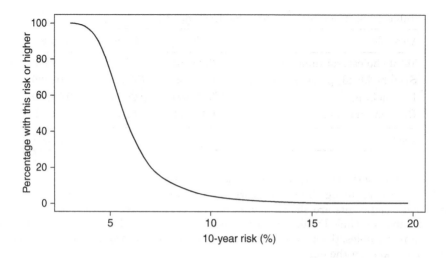

Figure 13.12. Inverse ogive for the risk score produced from the SHHEC data for women.

In clinical practice, a critical statistic is the proportion that would be expected to be treated when the decision rule is used in the general population. Under the assumption that the sample used is a fair representation of the population at large, this is estimated from Table 13.9 to be 254/6551 = 0.0388. Thus we expect to treat 3.88% (about 4%) of the population of women aged 30+ years who are currently free of CVD. To turn this into expected numbers we need other data. Given that 6.91% of women (with fibrinogen measurements) in SHHEC had baseline CVD and the population of Scottish women aged 30 years or more is about 1.76 million (from official data in 2009), this means that we would expect to be treating about 64 thousand women without CVD on the basis of the clinical decision rule. Presumably, the estimated 122 thousand with prevalent CVD would be treated as well.

It can be informative to illustrate the distribution of risk scores using an ogive (see Section 2.6.6) or, better still, an inverse ogive which plots the risk on the horizontal axis and the percentage at or above each risk value on the vertical axis. This is shown, for the female fibrinogen data, in Figure 13.12; since there are few women with risk scores below 3% or above 20%, the horizontal axis has been foreshortened. Although this plot has been drawn from a risk score based on a single risk factor, exactly the same methodology can be used for multiple risk factors, as are more commonly met in practice.

An inverse ogive allows us to see the expected consequences, in proportionate terms, of choosing different decision thresholds. In Figure 13.12, draw a line up from 10% risk to the plot and then across to the vertical axis to see (at least approximately) the result of 3.88% that was given above. We also see, for instance, that adopting a risk threshold of 5% would mean treating around three-quarters of all women without pre-existing CVD. If required, a second vertical scale showing the number in the general population corresponding to each percentage could be drawn on the right side of the plot.

13.3.5   Multiple thresholds

Although the clinical decision rule itself is often based upon a single threshold, there are situations where several thresholds may be required. For example, a national policy might involve doing nothing for people at low risk, giving lifestyle advice to people at moderate risk and giving drug therapy to people at high risk, thus requiring two thresholds. Furthermore, the level of advice or therapy might be varied according to position within a risk group.

13.4   Quantifying discrimination

We have already seen that sensitivity and specificity are key elements of discrimination. In Section 2.10.1 the receiver operating characteristic (ROC) plot was introduced as a way of summarizing sensitivity and specificity in diagnostic testing. As already discussed, prognostic and diagnostic testing procedures are methodologically the same, up to a point, so it is natural to consider ROC plots for clinical decision making.

A ROC plot for the risk score (13.3) is shown as Figure 13.13. In such plots, using all the raw data, every person in the database donates a point to the plot, unless there are duplicates (i.e., two or more people with the same fibrinogen level, in our example), in which case each distinct *value* donates a point. Note that a drawback with the ROC plot is that it does not allow any particular data value (for fibrinogen, in our example) to be identified.

We could also draw a ROC plot for the 'decile model' defined by Table 13.4. This would have just 11 points, one for each decile and one for each of the two extreme values. This would show a stepped pattern, roughly following the same essential overall shape as the continuous model does in Figure 13.13. For example, the point corresponding to the 90th percentile threshold, with sensitivity = 0.19 and specificity = 0.91 (i.e., 1 − specificity = 0.09) can roughly be seen to lie on the plot shown in Figure 13.13.

Figure 13.13 adds the plots we would see should we have a perfectly discriminating test; and should we have a test with no discrimination. The ROC plots for these extreme situations were mentioned in Section 2.10.1, but now we can use Figure 13.4, Figure 13.5 and Figure 13.8 to understand why they arise. When the two distributions, disease positive and negative, have no overlap (a situation close to, but more extreme than, Figure 13.4), if we adopt a clinical decision threshold at the far left of the scale, the specificity will be zero but the sensitivity will be at its maximum, i.e., 1 (we can see this by analogy to Figure 13.8). Moving the threshold progressively

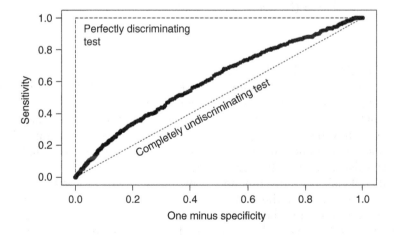

Figure 13.13. ROC plot for the fibrinogen risk score for women in the SHHEC study. Theoretical best and worst test results are also shown, for comparison. Individual values have been plotted — often these are 'smoothed out', as in Figure 13.15.

to the right, but keeping to the left of the entire 'disease curve' makes the specificity decrease (and thus 1 − specificity must increase) but the sensitivity will remain at 1. Once we reach the mid-point between the 'no disease' and 'disease' curves, the specificity and sensitivity will both be 1. From there on, as we move the threshold to the right, the specificity stays the same but the sensitivity decreases progressively, until it reaches 0 at the extreme right. The result is the corner-shaped plot in Figure 13.13, which is drawn right to left and then top to bottom as the threshold increases. At the other extreme, the two curves overlap completely, in which case the sensitivity must always equal the complement of the specificity, i.e., sensitivity = 1 − specificity, giving the diagonal line on Figure 13.13.

13.4.1   The area under the curve

It is clear that the fibrinogen risk score has non-zero discrimination, but the points are much closer to the theoretical situation of no discrimination than to that of perfect discrimination. We need a measure of discrimination to be able to compare our score to the theoretical extremes and, when this situation arises, to other risk scores.

The ROC plot shows how the probability of a true positive (vertical axis) relates to the probability of a false positive (horizontal axis): see Table 13.3. Obviously we would like the former to exceed the latter as much as possible — that is, the area under the curve (the **AUC**) transcribed by the plot should be as large as possible. The AUC is by far the most popular index of discrimination. The AUC for a test with perfect discrimination is 1, and the AUC for a test with no discrimination (where the probabilities of true positives and false negatives are equal) is 0.5. In practice, the AUC must lie between these extremes of 0.5 and 1 (if it were less than 0.5 we would simply reverse the decisions made at each threshold to get a better test).

Since the AUC has an unusual scale (0.5 to 1), a more easily interpretable measure of discrimination is **Somers' rank correlation coefficient** (Somers, 1962). In general situations, D is an alternative to the Spearman rank correlation coefficient, introduced in Section 9.3.2, and is the measure of correlation that corresponds to the Wilcoxon test (see Section 2.8.2 and later comments in this section). In the current situation it can be shown (Newson, 2001) that

$$D = 2c - 1, \qquad\qquad (13.7)$$

where c is the AUC. Notice that, as we would expect from a correlation, D lies between −1 and +1 and, furthermore, it takes the value 0 for no discrimination, which is analogous to the situation of 'no correlation'.

Using theory relevant to Somers' D statistic, a rather different definition of the population AUC may be derived: given a random pair of subjects, one of whom will develop the disease and one who will not, the AUC is the probability that the one who will develop the disease has the higher risk score. Equivalently, the AUC is the probability that the predicted risk is higher amongst someone who will be a future case compared to a non-case. For this reason, the AUC is sometimes known as the concordance statistic, or **c-statistic**. The agreement between the two approaches to defining the AUC can be proven using probability theory, but a couple of artificial examples (Examples 13.7 and 13.8) will suffice for our purposes. In practice, we will generally use statistical packages which draw the ROC and estimate the AUC and its 95% confidence interval, such as PROC LOGISTIC in SAS and the ROCTAB routine in Stata.

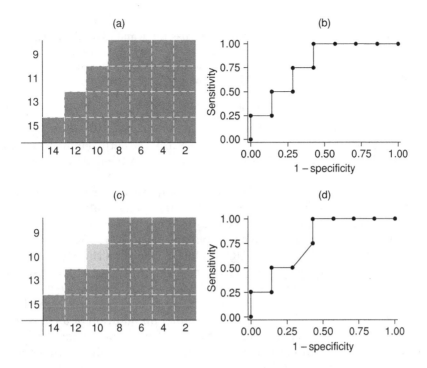

Figure 13.14. Demonstration of the agreement between two definitions of the AUC.

Example 13.8 Suppose the risk score has eleven outcomes in a sample of individuals, four of whom go on to develop the disease of interest. The baseline values of the risk score, X, are 2, 4, 6, 8, 10, 12 and 14 in the disease-free group and 9, 11, 13 and 15 in the disease group.

Panel (a) of Figure 13.14 tabulates the distribution of X amongst those who get the disease against the distribution of X amongst those who do not. In the cross-tabulation of pairs of values from these two distributions, a solid box is shown when the value which comes from the disease distribution is higher and an empty box when the value which comes from the no disease distribution is higher. So, for instance, the pair (14, 9) in the top left of panel (a) has an empty cell because 14 (from the no disease group) is higher than 9 (from the disease group). If we then count the number of filled cells and divide by the total number of cells, we get the probability that, in a randomly chosen pair of subjects with one from each group, the member of the pair from the disease group is the one with the highest value. This is 22/28 = 0.7857, and gives the solid area of the cross-table as a proportion of the whole.

Panel (b) of the same figure shows the ROC for this example, produced by ROCTAB in Stata. This procedure also gave the AUC (95% confidence interval) as 0.7857 (0.49710, 1.00000). Since the ROC plot is the same as the outline of the solid region in the accompanying table, the agreement between the two areas computed is not surprising. This demonstrates the probabilistic interpretation of the AUC.

There is one snag with using the approach illustrated by Example 13.8: when the pair of values gives a tie we have to make a corresponding allowance in our definition. We do this by redefining the AUC from pairs (as before, one from each group defined by disease status) as the probability that the value in the disease group has the higher score plus one half the probability that the scores are equal. Example 13.9 shows that this works accordingly. In theory, a tie is impossible; in practice it is common because risk factor values are inevitably rounded. The practitioner will find the theoretical definition most interpretable, and we will accordingly ignore the issue of ties following Example 13.9.

Example 13.9 Take the last example again, but now suppose that the outcome of 11 in the disease group is replaced by 10. The corresponding cross-table and ROC plot are given as panels (c) and (d), respectively, in Figure 13.14. In the cross-table the cell where the tie, (10, 10), occurs has only been filled with light colour, depicting no superiority or inferiority of the value from the disease distribution. The redefined AUC, by the pairing method, is

$$21/28 + 0.5 \times (1/28) = 0.7679.$$

This agrees with the AUC given in a ROCTAB analysis from Stata which gave an AUC (95% confidence interval) of 0.7679 (0.46814, 1.00000). Clearly the outline in panel (c) would look the same as the ROC if we choose to depict a tie by the area of a one-half block, suitably drawn.

Another way of thinking of the AUC is as a comparison of ranks: the ranks of the scores (or predicted risks) amongst those who do, and do not, suffer the disease during follow-up. In Section 2.8.2 we considered a test based on comparing two sets of ranks, the Wilcoxon test, which was noted to be equivalent to the Mann–Whitney test. Hanley and McNeill (1982) showed that the AUC can be derived from the Mann–Whitney test statistic, thus consolidating the interpretation of the AUC as a comparison of ranks. Notice that this highlights a weakness of the AUC statistic. Just as we noted in Section 2.8.2, using ranks alone is wasteful of information. In this case, the actual scores are not used in deriving the AUC, so that (for example) an addition of a constant to each risk score would produce the same AUC. This is not an issue for measuring discrimination — it just means that both curves get shifted to the right by an equal amount, if we think in terms of Figure 13.3, etc. It will, however, be important when we consider other aspects of risk scores.

The AUC for the fibrinogen risk score, (13.3), with 95% confidence interval, was found, from ROCTAB, to be 0.6069 (0.5784, 0.6354). We interpret this as saying that, if we were to select a woman who will go on to get CVD, and another who will not, the chance that the risk score will be highest in the woman who will get CVD is 0.6069. Equivalently, the chance that a woman who will get CVD in the next 10 years has a higher value of fibrinogen than one who will not is 61%.

To decide whether this makes fibrinogen a useful discriminator of CVD requires some knowledge of past research. In practice, AUCs above 0.85 are rare when the disease in question is multi-factorial. For example, the 2008 version of the most commonly used CVD risk score, from the Framingham Heart Study, has AUCs of 0.763 in men and 0.793 in women (D'Agostino et al., 2008). Diamond (1992) shows that, under some idealised conditions, the AUC cannot exceed 0.83. Hence the practical range of the AUC (beginning at 0.5) is narrow, leading to small differences in AUCs between risk scores even when we have good reason to believe that they differ importantly in discriminative utility. Hence, the use of four or five decimals is not unreasonable when expressing the AUC. As well, this has led to seeking alternative ways of quantifying discrimination (see Section 13.4.4, Section 13.4.5 and Section 13.9).

Thus we should conclude that fibrinogen discriminates poorly, even though Example 13.1 concluded that there is a good case for concluding that fibrinogen is a cause of CVD. Fibrinogen is a predictor of CVD, but it seems not to be, by itself, a useful prognostic variable. Given the multi-factorial nature of CVD prediction, this is not a surprising result; a risk score with several variables, such as the Framingham score, will likely be required to achieve good discrimination. Note that the present conclusion does not rule out fibrinogen's utility in adding importantly to the discrimination given by other prognostic variables (see Section 13.4.2 and Section 13.9).

Although some authors may express the result for the fibrinogen-based risk score by saying that the risk score is about 61% successful, this is misleading since a randomly allocated score would, correspondingly, give 50% success. The Somers' *D* statistic, from (13.7), of 0.2138 is a more reasonable index of success. This may be interpreted, in a randomly chosen pair of women, only one of whom will get CVD, as the difference between the probability that the score is highest in the woman who will get CVD in the next 10 years and the probability that the score is highest in the woman who will not. This is sometimes said to be the difference between the probabilities of concordance and discordance.

13.4.2 Comparing AUCs

We can use ROC curves and AUCs to compare the discrimination of two risk scores constructed from the same dataset. Most often this is used to see whether a new variable adds discrimination to variables that are already well established as prognostic variables. For example, Woodward *et al.* (2009) considered whether fibrinogen adds discrimination to the set of variables used in the Framingham Heart Study CVD risk score — it added a significant ($p < 0.05$) amount for women, but not men. When an additional variable is used in a risk score in clinical applications there will usually be cost implications. In this situation, a one-sided test of equality against the alternative hypothesis that the new score has a higher AUC might be more appropriate than the usual two-sided alternative.

Stata and SAS commands for ROC curves are listed in Section 2.10.1. AUCs from different risk scores, derived from the same dataset, can be compared quantitatively using the ROCCONTRAST subcommand to PROC LOGISTIC in SAS or ROCCOMP in Stata, as well as other software. See De Long *et al.* (1988) for a theoretical exposition.

Example 13.10 The model used in Example 13.5 excluded body mass index (BMI). This was left out of the risk score because it failed to be significant in the presence of total cholesterol (TOTCHOL), systolic blood pressure (SYSTOL) and smoking status in Example 10.15. However, in that example we saw that BMI was only marginally non-significant, and thus it was included in the final regression equation there. Thus it seems reasonable to test whether a revised risk score, including BMI, has better discrimination than the score without it.

The new logistic model, when BMI is included, is:

$$\hat{\text{logit}} = -9.7186 + 0.3301(\text{TOTCHOL}) + 0.0266(\text{BMI})$$
$$+ 0.0203(\text{SYSTOL}) + 0.4000(\text{ex}) + 0.7258(\text{current}).$$

Figure 13.15 has the ROCs with and without (as in Example 13.5) BMI. Although the plot with BMI tends to lie just above that without, there is little 'daylight' between the two plots, and no systematic superiority of the enlarged score across the range of specificities. To give further insight, Figure 13.15 also includes the ROC curve for the prognostic model with systolic blood pressure alone:

$$\hat{\text{logit}} = -6.6447 + 0.0226(\text{SYSTOL}).$$

This is clearly much worse than the three-variable prognostic model of Example 13.5 since, for virtually every value of (one minus) specificity, the corresponding sensitivity is lower. These findings are consistent with the model building process in Example 10.15.

A formal comparison of the AUCs is shown in Output 13.1. Here the ROCCOMP procedure has been used twice, comparing each of the other two scores, in turn, against the three-variable score from Example 13.5. As anticipated, there is a significant difference between the score only involving systolic blood pressure and the reference ($p = 0.0003$) but not between the BMI-enriched score and the reference ($p = 0.37$). Note that a two-sided test is reported by ROCCOMP. If our alternative hypothesis is (for example) that BMI increases discrimination (AUC) then we should halve the p value in Output 13.1.

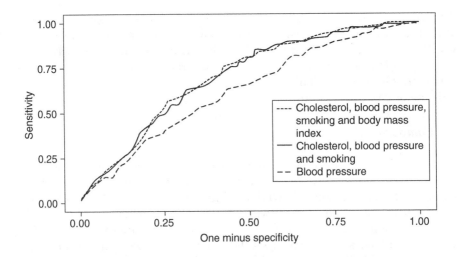

Figure 13.15. ROC curves for three risk scores constructed from SHHS data in Example 13.11.

Note that the AUC for the three-variable model is 0.6977. This would be interpreted as the probability that a man who will get CHD within the next 5 years has a higher risk score than a man who will not. Using BMI as an additional predictor makes little difference to this probability, but taking away cholesterol and smoking makes a considerable difference.

Cook (2008) notes that the change in the AUC on adding a new predictor to a risk score depends on the strength of the risk factors in the original risk score, as well as the strength of the new predictor and the correlation between the two. She demonstrates that, even if the new risk predictor has an independent effect to the original risk score, it will need to have an unusually large effect (for example, as measured by its odds ratio) to

Output 13.1 Stata ROCCOMP results comparing (i) the risk score involving only systolic blood pressure ('single') and the score involving systolic blood pressure, total cholesterol and smoking ('multi') and (ii) comparing the latter with the score involving the same three variables plus BMI ('multiplus').

(i) Single versus multi

	Obs	ROC Area	Std. Err.	—Asymptotic Normal— [95% Conf. Interval]	
multi	4049	0.6977	0.0222	0.65419	0.74124
single	4049	0.6255	0.0254	0.57558	0.67532

Ho: area(multi) = area(single)
chi2(1) =   13.04   Prob>chi2 = 0.0003

(ii) Multi versus multiplus

	Obs	ROC Area	Std. Err.	—Asymptotic Normal— [95% Conf. Interval]	
multi	4049	0.6977	0.0222	0.65419	0.74124
multiplus	4049	0.7006	0.0218	0.65781	0.74345

Ho: area(multi) = area(multiplus)
chi2(1) =   0.83   Prob>chi2 = 0.3633

have any discernible effect on the ROC curve and AUC when the original risk score is a strong predictor. This complements the discussion of Section 13.2.4.

Discrimination is only one component of prognostic utility, as we shall consider subsequently. Thus, whilst it is useful to consider whether adding a certain selection of risk factors improves discrimination, it would be dangerous to base variable selection upon questions of discrimination alone. Furthermore, statistical considerations are only part of the story when deciding whether a variable 'adds' to prediction. For instance, a variable which is very expensive to measure may not have sufficient additional discrimination to be worth taking account of. The cost of screening the entire population, so as to be able to find their risk score with the added variable, may just not be worth the extra precision. In this case a two-step procedure may be useful, where the additional variable is only measured whenever the clinical decision rule derived from the basic risk score is inconclusive.

13.4.3 Survival data

Since sensitivity and specificity are, for any given threshold, defined in terms of the classic two-by-two table (exemplified by Table 13.3) it is clear that they cannot allow for censoring. Yet often censoring is present in the prospective data that are used to develop risk scores. With this in mind, Harrell et al. (1982) defined a generalised c statistic as the probability that, in two randomly chosen subjects, at least one of whom will have an event during the observation period, the person with the lower risk score will survive the longest. Equivalently, it is the probability that the predicted risk is higher amongst someone who will survive for a shorter length of time. Once follow-up is complete, this is estimated by selecting all possible pairs of subjects, rejecting any selection where both are still event-free at end of follow-up. Any pair in which the person with the lowest risk score survived longer without experiencing an event is given a score of one, and any pair with tied event times is given a score of 0.5. Else the score is zero. Harrell's c statistic is the sum of the scores divided by the number of pairs not discarded. This may be obtained in Stata from using the ESTAT CONCORDANCE post-estimation command after using the Cox regression command (STCOX), which itself follows an STSET command to set up the survival time data. This does not provide a confidence interval, but such can be obtained from the user-defined SOMERSD command (Newson, 2011) or from the methods described in Pencina and D'Agostino (2004): see the corresponding Stata and SAS programs provided on the web site for this book.

Using these programs on the fibrinogen data, Harrell's c statistic was found to be 0.6002, with a 95% confidence interval of (0.5822, 0.6182). In computing this result all survival times were used; if we are only interested in (say) 10-year risk we should cap the time over which events are accrued at 10 years. Pencina and D'Agostino allow this explicitly in their equations; otherwise, events after 10 years can be treated as non-events. With such a cap, Harrell's c statistic (and confidence interval) becomes 0.6059 (0.5782, 0.6337). This estimate is similar to the AUC, suitable for fixed cohorts, for 10-year risk of 0.6069 reported in Section 13.4.1.

The SOMERSD command can also be used to compare c statistics. Again, this could be done using all survival times or with events capped — say, at 5 years. Using the multi and multiplus models of Example 13.10, but produced from a Cox model (the multi model is given by (13.6)), Harrell's c statistics (with 95% confidence intervals), from SOMERSD, for discrimination of 5-year risk of CHD are 0.6956 (0.6528, 0.7384), when systolic blood pressure, cholesterol and smoking are the predictors and 0.6985 (0.6564, 0.7407) when BMI is added to the predictors. The difference in c statistics is 0.002981 (−0.003039,

0.009002), so that BMI does not add significantly to discrimination (the p value for a test of the null hypothesis of a difference in c statistics of zero is 0.33). These are similar results to the equivalent computations for a fixed cohort in Example 13.10.

Other types of c statistics that allow for censoring have been suggested: see Uno *et al.* (2011) and Chambless *et al.* (2011) for discussions.

13.4.4   The standardised mean effect size

An alternative approach to using c statistics is to measure the distance between the means of the risk factor distributions for those who do, and those who do not, go on to have an event. This is easily understood from Figure 13.4: if the means are relatively close then separation, and thus discrimination, is relatively poor. However, it is also clear that if the spread of each curve in Figure 13.4 is relatively narrow (i.e., the distributions are tight) then, for fixed positions of the two means, the amount of overlap, and thus discrimination, will be relatively poor. Hence the appropriate measure of discrimination should correct the distance between the means for the underlying variability in the risk factors. Assuming that variability can be appropriately measured by the standard deviation (SD) a sensible index of discrimination is

$$(\bar{x}_1 - \bar{x}_2)/\,\mathrm{SD}, \tag{13.8}$$

where $\bar{x}_1$ is the mean of those in group 1 (in risk scoring, those with the disease) and $\bar{x}_2$ is the mean in group 2 (those without disease), assuming that the former is larger than the latter. Such a statistic is called a **standardised mean effect size** (SMES), a special case of an **effect size**: in general, a quantification of the strength of a process. Dividing the difference in means by the SD makes (13.8) unit-free, which allows direct comparison between different applications. Figure 13.16 was drawn from Figure 13.4 to illustrate how the SMES relates to the risk factor distributions.

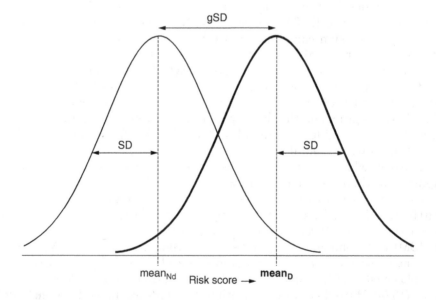

Figure 13.16. Schematic representation of the standardised mean effect size, represented by Hedge's g statistic, when the risk score is normally distributed with a common standard deviation (SD), in the diseased (D) and non-diseased (Nd) groups.

There are currently three popular forms of the SMES based on (13.8), which only differ in the way SD is defined. All can be obtained from the ESIZE routine in Stata. Hedges's g statistic takes SD as the pooled standard deviation, s_p^2, as given by (2.16). Cohen's d statistic is not uniquely defined, but is usually taken with SD the same as for g, except that the divisor for the SD lacks subtraction of 2. Hence, d can be found from g using

$$d = g\sqrt{\frac{n_1 + n_2}{n_1 + n_2 - 2}},$$

where, as usual, the n's are the sample sizes in the two groups (diseased and not, in risk scoring). The third option is to take SD as the sample standard deviation in the comparison group, such as the control group in a clinical trial or the no disease group in the situation of this chapter. This is called Glass's Δ. The g and d statistics implicitly assume that the two groups being compared have equal variance. Even if this is not true, the methodology is defensible, in an averaging sense, although most researchers would then prefer to use Δ. The Δ statistic is most useful when several groups are to be compared to a single standard, such as grades of disease (by time or severity) versus no disease. In most practical situations in risk scoring, there is little to choose between the three methods.

We shall continue by assuming that g is to be used. Hedges and Olkin (1985) showed that a large sample approximation to the variance of g is

$$\mathrm{var}(g) = \frac{n_1 + n_2}{n_1 n_2} + \frac{h^2}{2(n_1 + n_2)}$$

where

$$h = \left(1 - \frac{3}{4(n_1 + n_2) - 9}\right)g. \tag{13.9}$$

If we are prepared to assume that g has an approximate normal distribution, the 95% confidence interval for g is

$$g \pm 1.96\sqrt{\mathrm{var}(g)}. \tag{13.10}$$

In general, the SMES is useful in applications where we wish to compare, or summarise, the effects of the same risk factor between data measured on different scales, such as in meta-analysis (see Section 12.3.9). It can also be useful when we want to compare the effects of different risk factors on the same disease and when the measurements recorded for comparison are not familiar to a general audience. For example, in a clinical trial educating children about healthy lifestyle choices where the outcome measure is a subjective score (in the range 0–100) of the children's knowledge of healthy behaviours, the SMES might be used to compare the intervention and control groups in a standardised way. Due to their universal application and unit-free measurement, some have suggested that effect sizes, in general, might be used as an alternative to the significance testing paradigm that forms the basis of much of the scientific method in medicine and elsewhere. Their advantage over significance testing is their lack of dependence on the sample size (see Section 3.5.5).

Table 13.10. Standardised mean effect sizes (95% confidence intervals) for three scores of 5-year risk for CHD, each computed from two statistical models: SHHS data for men.

Variables in model	Logistic model	Cox model
SBP	0.4771 (0.2906, 0.6636)	0.4770 (0.2905, 0.6635)
SBP, total cholesterol and smoking	0.6936 (0.5068, 0.8805)	0.6927 (0.5059, 0.8796)
SBP, total cholesterol, smoking and BMI	0.6983 (0.5114, 0.8851)	0.6953 (0.5085, 0.8821)

However, a drawback with the SMES is that the use of the means and the SD implicitly assumes that these are sensible measures of average and spread (see Section 2.6). This is unlikely to be so for risk scores derived from logistic and Cox models, which tend to be skewed. As usual, we may be able to get round this problem by taking a transformation. In the current application, it is usual to define the SMES for the linear predictor (see Section 10.3), which is the estimated logit for logistic regression and the log hazard ratio for Cox regression.

Example 13.11 For the female fibrinogen data available on the web site for this book, (13.2) defines the logits. The mean (standard deviation) of these logits in the non-diseased ($n = 6147$) and diseased ($n = 404$) groups are -2.7771 (0.2929) and -2.6619 (0.3139), respectively. From (13.8), using (2.16) to obtain the (pooled) SD of 0.2942, the SMES, $g = 0.3915$. Hence the prognostic model involving only fibrinogen separates those with and without CVD by just under 40% of a standard deviation. From (13.9), $h = 0.39145$ and var(g) = 0.00265. Using (13.10), the approximate 95% confidence interval for g is thus (0.2906, 0.4924).

Example 13.12 For the SHHS data available on the web site for this book, as used to derive logistic risk scores in Example 13.5 and Example 13.10, the SMESs (using linear predictors) for the three logistic prognostic models investigated earlier are given in Table 13.10. In agreement with the findings in Example 13.10, adding BMI to the reference risk model (that in the middle line of Table 13.10) adds little to discrimination, as measured here by the SMES, but restricting to systolic blood pressure reduces discrimination substantially.

In Example 13.7 a Cox risk score was derived from the same data. The corresponding SMESs are also shown in Table 13.10. As expected, due to the low rate of censoring in these data, results from logistic and Cox models are similar.

It will not always be possible to find a transformation that makes the risk score approximately symmetric within both the disease and no disease groups. Indeed, the fibrinogen logits, (13.2), show some skewness (as we can see from Figure 13.6, since, in each case, the logit is simply a linear transformation of the fibrinogen values), although far less than the fibrinogen risk scores, (13.3), which are highly skewed. Experience suggests that this may rarely be an issue with multi-factor risk scores. For instance, for the multivariable Cox model used in Example 13.7, the log hazard ratios, (13.5), have a distribution with no important skew. In general, when a transformation to induce symmetry is not available, we could bootstrap the SMES (Section 14.2). Alternatively, an obvious modification of (13.8) is to take the standardised effect size for medians,

$$(Q_{21} - Q_{22})/(Q_3 - Q_1), \tag{13.11}$$

where Q denotes a quartile and Q_{2i} is the second quartile (median) in the ith group ($i = 1$ or 2). As with means, there is a question about which group to use to get the first and third quartiles in the denominator, whilst the skewness makes it unlikely that the inter-quartile range will be equal in the two groups. In risk scoring the 'disease negative' group will very likely be the largest and so it seems more reasonable to use its interquartile range in (13.11).

When the two risk score distributions are normal with equal variance, (13.11) will give an answer that is (13.8) divided by 1.349. This is so because, under normality, the mean and median are the same and the interquartile range is 1.349 times the standard deviation. We can see this approximately from Table A.2, and exactly from Excel's NORM.S.INV function, which gives $P(Z < 0.6745) = 0.75$ and $P(Z < -0.6745) = 0.25$, where Z is a standard normal variable. Thus the distance between the quartiles is $0.6745 - (-0.6745) = 1.349$ for a standard normal, which has a standard deviation of 1, by definition. For this reason, and due to the pivotal position of the normal distribution in statistical theory, (13.11) is often multiplied by 1.349 to give the normalised standardised median effect size,

$$e = 1.349(Q_{21} - Q_{22})/(Q_3 - Q_1).$$

For the fibrinogen logits, this gives

$$e = \frac{1.349 \times (-2.7162 - (-2.8114))}{-2.6376 - (-2.9548)} = 0.4049,$$

which is very close to the result for g (of 0.3915) found in Example 13.11.

A general approach to the SMES, allowing for variation in sampling distributions, is given by Kelly (2005). However, for the remainder of this section we shall assume that the data from the two groups being compared have normal distributions with equal variance. This assumption allows for easily understandable pictorial representations of the SMES (see Figure 13.17) and also allows some simple summary statistics to be calculated from the SMES, which help in interpretation. Furthermore, some simple relationships can then be found between the SMES and other measures introduced earlier in this chapter.

Under the normality assumption, the SMES may be used to estimate the chance that a randomly chosen individual from one group (say, group 1) has a higher value

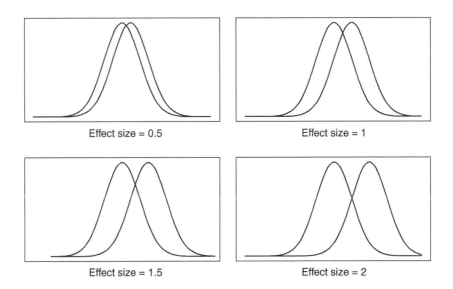

Figure 13.17. Two normal distributions with equal variance when the standardised mean effect size (shortened to 'effect size' on the figure) linking them varies from 0.5 to 2.

than the population mean of group 2. This estimate is $P(Z < g)$, where Z is a standard normal random variable, which can be read directly from Table B.1. For example, a SMES of 0.5 means that the proportion of people in the disease group that has a higher value than the average in the non-diseased group is 0.6915. Another useful derived estimate, in the special case of equally dispersed normal distributions, is the chance that a randomly chosen individual from group 1 will have a higher value than a randomly chosen individual from group 2. This is $P(Z < g/\sqrt{2})$. When the SMES is 0.5 this is 0.6382. This also suggests that the AUC may be approximated by $P(Z < g/\sqrt{2})$. For instance, in the fibrinogen example we have seen that $g = 0.3915$, whence $P(Z < g/\sqrt{2}) = P(Z < 0.2768) = 0.6090$. In Section 13.4.1 we found the AUC to be 0.6069, which is very similar. Using this normal model, the standarised effect sizes of 0.5, 1, 1.5 and 2 illustrated in Figure 13.17 are translated to AUCs of 0.64, 0.76, 0.86 and 0.92, respectively. According to practical considerations discussed in Section 13.4.1, an effect size of 1.5 or more would thus suggest good discrimination of a multifactorial disease.

Royston and Altman (2010) discuss the relationship between g and the AUC, under the normality assumption, in more detail.

We will now return briefly to the situation of using the risk score to make the clinical decision of whether or not a person is likely to develop the disease in question. Under the normal model with common variance, g can be related to the threshold, T, and the sensitivity, s, and specificity, p, in the context of Figure 13.8. For a standard normal variable Z, it can be shown that

$$p = P\left(Z < \frac{T - \mu_{Nd}}{SD}\right) \qquad (13.12)$$

and

$$s = P\left(Z < g - \frac{T - \mu_{Nd}}{SD}\right). \qquad (13.13)$$

Substituting the sample mean and standard deviation for the no disease group into these equations enables the appropriate decision threshold, T, and the SMES, g, to be derived from any given s and p, at least for the theoretical model assumed. For example, suppose that a given risk score has a mean of 20 with a standard deviation of 2 amongst those with no disease. Using (13.12), to obtain a specificity of 0.9 we must choose the cut-off for identifying people as disease positive to satisfy

$$0.9 = P\left(Z < \frac{T - 20}{2}\right).$$

From Table B.2 we can see that $(T - 20)/2$ is, therefore, 1.2816. Hence the threshold should be set at 22.5632. Having established this, we might now want to know what the sensitivity will be when, for example, the SMES is 1.4. Using (13.13), this is given by

$$s = P\left(Z < 1.4 - \frac{22.5632 - 20}{2}\right) = P(Z < 0.1184) = 0.5471,$$

which is little better than chance. The latter value was found exactly from Excel; Table B.1 gives an approximation.

Using (13.1), or approximately from Table 13.6, we can also use (13.12) and (13.13) to relate the SMES and threshold to the odds ratio for a clinical decision rule. With the threshold set at 1.2816 standard deviations above the mean of the non-diseased group, to obtain a SMES of 1.4 requires an odds ratio of 10.9.

Finally, one drawback of the SMES for risk scoring that arises in special circumstances should be noted. Risk scores are sometimes derived from clinical trials, by treating the trial data as we would an observational study. However, the trial may have less variability in its risk scores than would a corresponding observational study (involving the same risk factors) just because the trial has inclusion and exclusion criteria which restrict the type of person that is included (see Section 7.2.1). Assuming that the difference in means is estimated without bias, this will lead to an overestimate of the SMES in general populations. This problem is less important for the AUC as it only depends upon the rank ordering in the disease and disease-free groups.

13.4.5   Other measures of discrimination

Several other approaches for measuring discrimination have been suggested. Two will be mentioned here, although their details and computational implications are beyond the scope of this book. First, Rom and Hwang (1996) estimated the degree by which the 'no disease' and 'disease' distributions overlap. When the distributions cross only once, the overlap will increase as the SMES decreases, as is clear from Figure 13.16. When they have normal distributions with equal variance, they must cross at $g(\mathrm{SD})/2$ where SD is the common standard deviation, as in Figure 13.16. The probability of overlap is then $P(Z < -g/2)$ where Z is a standard normal variable; this is a special case of the Rom and Hwang measure of discrimination. Second, some measures of discrimination (such as the D statistic of Royston and Sauerbrei, 2004) are based upon the separation of the individual Kaplan–Meier curves. Unlike Rom and Hwang's measure, these indices take account of censoring.

13.5   Calibration

Calibration measures the agreement between the predicted and observed risks. If the risk algorithm underlying the clinical decision rule is to be robust, it clearly needs to be able to separate future cases from non-cases, so discrimination is of paramount importance; but this cannot be the only consideration. For example, consider two risk scores, score one having all its predictions exactly 0.1 higher than score two. In terms of discrimination, these scores are equal, since they separate future cases and non-cases by the same amount. Suppose that clinicians require that all people with anticipated risk greater than, say, 20% (i.e., 0.2) in the next 10 years should be treated. Score one will clearly identify more people for treatment, so that its practical impact is far different from score two. Similarly, a test that assigns probabilities of 0.4 to all future cases and 0.2 to all non-cases must surely be considered inferior to a more emphatic score that assigns probabilities of 0.99 and 0.01, yet these would not differ in their c statistic (which is one in this extreme example). In general, we would naturally prefer to use the score with predicted risks as near as possible to actual risks. Discrimination does not address this issue.

We can identify (at least) four kinds of calibration. Most extreme would be **perfect calibration** in which the predicted risks from the score are exactly the same as the true risks (otherwise called absolute risks or probabilities). Since each individual's true risk, evaluated at the study's end, must either be one (they get the disease) or zero (they don't), this would be achieved only when the score correctly assigns each person to her or his true future disease state. This might occur when an easily identifiable genetic abnormality is the sole precursor of a certain disease, but is generally highly unlikely. Instead, we might find that the observed and predicted risks are not significantly different, which will mean there is **overall calibration**: see Section 13.5.1. Next, we might examine **mean calibration**, which occurs when the mean of the predicted risks equals the mean of the observed risks (i.e. the disease incidence): see Section 13.5.2. In practice, many researchers only consider **grouped calibration** (usually just called 'calibration') where observed and predicted mean risks are compared within a set of mutually exclusive and exhaustive subgroups. This is most usefully done by choosing groups according to predicted risk, using ordinal groups obtained from ranking the entire set of risk scores for the cohort: see Section 13.5.3. Mean calibration and overall calibration can be viewed as extreme versions of grouped calibration (using the minimum and the maximum number of groups, respectively), which are too crude for most uses.

In general, there is no one overall test for calibration, just as there is no one overall definition. In practice, descriptive plots, such as those introduced in Section 13.5.4, generally offer the best information on what we intuitively recognise as 'agreement'. Certainly, all assessments of calibration should include such a plot. The tests described in what follows may help in deciding whether a risk score lacks calibration, but it would be dangerous to rely upon these as the sole source of evaluation.

13.5.1   Overall calibration

The null hypothesis in the test for overall calibration is that the true and predicted risks are all equal. This may be tested by comparing

$$\frac{\Sigma(y_i - p_i)(1 - 2p_i)}{\sqrt{\Sigma(1 - 2p_i)^2 p_i(1 - p_i)}} \tag{13.14}$$

with the upper tail of the standard normal distribution (Spiegelhalter, 1986). Here y is the observed outcome ($y = 0$ for no disease and $y = 1$ for disease) and p_i is the risk score for the ith person. The summations are over all subjects. As always, both the observed outcomes and predicted risks are evaluated over the same time interval, such as 10 years.

For the fibrinogen-based 10-year CVD risk score, (13.3), the result of (13.14) is 0.09. Clearly this is not significant at any reasonable significance level, so there is no lack of overall calibration. See Section 13.7 for more examples using Speigelhalter's test.

13.5.2   Mean calibration

If the data arise from a fixed cohort (or if censoring, although present, is ignored) then the observed risk, r, is calculated as the number of positive outcomes over t years, where t is the interval over which risk has been predicted, divided by the number of subjects in the study. The estimated standard error of r, $\widehat{se}(r)$, is given by (3.3). If censoring is allowed for, the observed risk is the Kaplan–Meier (KM) estimate of risk at t years, and its standard error is the corresponding KM estimate. Either way, an approximate test of the null hypothesis that the observed risk equals the mean predicted risk, $\bar{p}$, is to compare

$$\frac{r - \bar{p}}{\widehat{se}(r)} \qquad (13.15)$$

with the standard normal distribution.

For example, the mean predicted score for the fibrinogen-only based CVD score in Example 13.4 is obtained as the mean result of (13.3) across all 6551 women. This turns out to be 0.0616796. Correspondingly, from Table 13.4, the observed risk (ignoring censoring) is $404/6551 = 0.0616700$. Clearly these are so similar that we can immediately conclude no evidence of lack of mean calibration. A similar finding comes from testing mean calibration for the SHHS multivariable CHD score of Example 13.7. Both observed (KM) risk and mean predicted risk (using (13.6)) are 0.0284 to four decimal places. In fact, such equality as seen in these examples can be expected when mean calibration is tested on the same data from which the risk score was derived. Hence it is only meaningful to test for mean calibration when a score is tested in a different study population to that from which it was derived (Section 13.10).

13.5.3 Grouped calibration

As already discussed, it is most effective to test for calibration by dividing the predicted risks into ordinal groups and comparing observed and expected values within these groups. This gives a clear picture of how well the risk score behaves across all levels of risk. Most often, 10 ordinal groups are used. Values other than 10 may also be used: it will be sensible to use fewer groups when the total number of events is relatively small.

The Hosmer–Lemeshow (HL) test (Section 10.7.2) is often applied to test for grouped calibration. The HL test statistic is

$$\sum \frac{n_i (r_i - \bar{p}_i)^2}{\bar{p}_i (1 - \bar{p}_i)}, \qquad (13.16)$$

where r_i is the observed (true) risk of disease in the ith group and $\bar{p}_i$ is the mean predicted probability in the ith group; i ranges from 1 to ℓ, the number of groups ($\ell = 10$ when tenths are used). If the cohort is closed (i.e., no censoring) then r_i is calculated as the number of events divided by the number at risk in the ith group, and the test statistic is to be compared against chi-square on $\ell - 2$ degrees of freedom. If censoring is allowed for (typically when a Cox model was used to generate the risk score), KM estimates of observed risk, r, should be used rather than relative frequencies, and the test statistic should be compared to chi-square on $\ell - 1$ d.f. (D'Agostino et al., 2008).

It should be noted that the HL test has shortcomings, as discussed (amongst others) by Hosmer et al. (1997). Various alternatives have been suggested; Kuss (2001) describes several of these, and presents a SAS macro to implement them. However, (13.16) is widely used in current practice.

Example 13.13 To investigate calibration by tenths for the fibrinogen data used in earlier examples, the 6551 predicted risks, calculated in Example 13.4 as (13.3), need to be ranked and then split into 10 groups, each of about 655 women (as close as clustering around the deciles, and rounding, will permit): see Table 13.11. Within each tenth, the predicted risk is calculated as the mean risk score for that tenth. In parallel, the observed risk is calculated

Table 13.11. Calculations required in Example 13.13 for the HL test statistic using a logistic risk score.

Tenth of predicted risk	Maximum value	Mean predicted risk ($\bar{p}$)	Number with CVD in 10 years	No. at risk	Observed risk (r)	Difference ($r - \bar{p}$)	Component of (13.16)
1	0.04427	0.0401665	23	654	0.0351682	−0.0049983	0.423802
2	0.04823	0.0463951	27	658	0.0410334	−0.0053617	0.427548
3	0.05117	0.0496492	26	643	0.0404355	−0.0092137	1.156876
4	0.05407	0.0525586	30	673	0.0445765	−0.0079821	0.861094
5	0.05712	0.0555252	38	664	0.0572289	0.0017037	0.036752
6	0.06030	0.0586200	44	632	0.0696203	0.0110003	1.385835
7	0.06462	0.0623053	43	660	0.0651515	0.0028462	0.091515
8	0.07083	0.0674428	41	656	0.0625000	−0.0049428	0.254823
9	0.08325	0.0758906	55	654	0.0840979	0.0082073	0.628149
10	0.57958	0.1081535	77	657	0.1171994	0.0090459	0.557362
						Total	5.823757

Table 13.12. Calculations required in Example 13.14 for the HL test statistic using a Cox regression risk score.

Tenth of predicted risk	Mean predicted risk $(\bar{p})$	No. at risk	Observed risk (r)	Difference $(r - \bar{p})$	Component of (13.16)
1	0.0088142	404	0.00501	−0.00380	0.66922
2	0.0126888	405	0.00753	−0.00516	0.86036
3	0.0154418	405	0.0124	−0.00304	0.24648
4	0.0182010	405	0.0100	−0.00820	1.52430
5	0.0212337	405	0.0225	0.00127	0.03125
6	0.0248029	405	0.0321	0.00730	0.89158
7	0.0288603	405	0.0351	0.00624	0.56260
8	0.0346800	405	0.0451	0.01042	1.31353
9	0.0437601	405	0.0597	0.01594	2.45913
10	0.0757065	405	0.0548	−0.02091	2.52973
				Total	11.08818

simply as the number of events divided by the number at risk in that tenth. The HL test statistic then comes from (13.16). Table 13.11 shows all the calculations required, by tenth. The HL statistic, 5.82 (to two decimal places) is to be compared to chi-square on $10 - 2 = 8$ d.f. Table B.3 shows us that this test is not significant at any conventional level of significance; the precise p value is 0.67. There is no evidence of lack of calibration for this risk score.

HL tests for fixed cohorts can be obtained directly from packages such as SAS and Stata. For example, as described in Section 10.7.2, PROC LOGISTIC in SAS gives the HL statistic as a by-product of fitting a logistic regression model. Although SAS uses a different expression for the HL statistic to that given in (13.16), the result is the same. When a proprietary computer package is applied to the fibrinogen data provided on the web site to this book, a slightly different result to that given in Example 13.13 may be produced simply because the clustering of fibrinogen values (which was noted in Table 13.4) means that the tenths of predicted risk are not unique for these data.

Example 13.14 In Example 13.7 a 5-year multivariable CHD risk score was derived from a Cox model as (13.6). Applying this formula repeatedly gave the predicted risks for all 4049 men, which were then averaged within each of their tenths. PROC LIFETEST was used, in SAS, to find the KM estimate of the observed risk of surviving for 5 years (1827 days, allowing for leap years) in each tenth of the predicted risks. Results appear in Table 13.12: the p value for the HL test is 0.27 and there is thus no evidence of lack of calibration.

Another test for calibration, although only applicable in fixed cohorts, appears in Section 13.6.2.

13.5.4 Calibration plots

As already discussed, a sensible graph will often provide the best insight into how well a risk score calibrates with the observed data. In many publications on risk

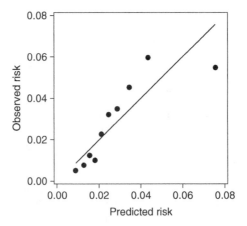

Figure 13.18. Calibration plot for Example 13.14. Observed against mean predicted risk is plotted for each tenth of predicted risk.

scores, the mean predicted risk within each risk group (usually the tenths — often, confusingly, called the deciles) is plotted alongside the observed risk in the same group so as to produce the format of a grouped bar chart (see Section 2.4). However, scatterplots are more useful for understanding (lack of) calibration; two types of calibration scatterplot will be illustrated here.

First, a graph of observed against predicted (expected) risk; Figure 13.18 shows such a plot for Example 13.14. For a well-calibrated score, the points will cluster around the diagonal line included on this plot. A score that is uniformly poorly calibrated will have its points either all above the line (showing that it underestimates risk) or all below the line (showing that it overestimates risk). Figure 13.18 suggests that calibration is good except amongst those at highest risk of CHD.

Second, a graph of observed divided by predicted risk against the predicted risk; Figure 13.19 shows such a plot for Example 13.14. Note that here the tenth of risk,

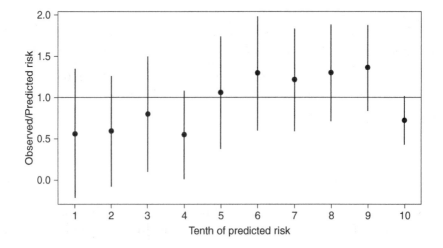

Figure 13.19. Alternative calibration plot for Example 13.14, including 95% confidence limits. Predicted risks are mean values within their tenths.

rather than the actual mean predicted risk in that tenth, has been plotted on the horizontal axis. This hides the fact that the final tenth is well separated from the rest; sometimes it may be useful to draw readers' attention to such skewness. In this type of plot, a well-calibrated score will have its points clustering around a horizontal line placed at unity on the vertical scale. A score that always underestimates risk will have points above the line and one that overestimates will have points below the line. If the proportionate degree of bias up or down is constant, the points will lie on a line parallel to the horizontal.

In Figure 13.19 confidence intervals have been added for the observed/predicted ratio. These emphasize the lack of calibration at high risk for the current risk score — the 95% confidence limit barely includes the point of equality (observed/predicted = 1). The confidence intervals were derived by finding confidence intervals for the observed risk and then dividing the lower and upper confidence limits by the predicted risk, within each tenth. Standard errors for the observed risk were taken from the output from PROC LIFETEST in SAS and the corresponding confidence limits were then found using (5.5). In the situation where censoring is not an issue (i.e., as assumed in Example 13.13) we would use (3.4) to find the confidence limits for the observed risk.

13.6   Recalibration

If a risk score is poorly calibrated one of a number of 'fixes' can be tried to improve the situation. A generic term for such processes is **recalibration**. This operation is often used to 'correct' a score that was generated in one population so it can be used with greater accuracy in a new population. In the situation where risk predictions are being updated so as to be contemporary, the new population would be the original population considered at a later date.

13.6.1   Recalibration of the mean

The simplest type of recalibration is **mean recalibration**. If the true overall risk is r and the mean predicted risk (from the risk score) is $\bar{p}$, then recalibration of the mean is achieved by multiplying all risk scores by $r/\bar{p}$. Whilst this obviously guarantees perfect mean calibration, it may not produce an acceptable calibration plot, although it will often improve it. For instance, Figure 13.20 plots the risk scores for the Framingham CVD risk score applied to all women in the SHHEC study in Scotland. The overall 10-year risk of CVD in SHHEC women is 0.0626 and the mean Framingham score for SHHEC women is 0.0966. Thus the mean recalibrated score was obtained, for each person, by multiplying their Framingham scores by 0.0626/0.0966 = 0.648033. The resulting scores are also plotted on Figure 13.20. There is clearly a great improvement in the calibration plot: indeed, the recalibrated score shows excellent calibration across the tenths.

13.6.2   Recalibration of scores in a fixed cohort

The first type of calibration scatterplot presented here suggests another way of testing calibration, due to Cox (1958). Consider fitting a line through the dots, for example on Figure 13.20. If the score predicts well the fitted line should have a slope of one and should intersect the vertical axis at zero. If the cohort is closed (i.e., no censoring) then, as explained in Section 10.3, the line can be fitted using a logistic regression model. Since the outcome from such a model is a logit, the logical approach is to predict

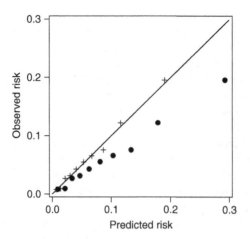

Figure 13.20. Calibration plot for the Framingham 10-year CVD risk score (dots) and the mean recalibrated Framingham score (crosses), applied to Scottish women. Observed against mean predicted risk is plotted for each tenth of predicted risk.

the observed logits from the predicted logits. Using subscripts O and P for observed and predicted, respectively, this means fitting the model

$$\text{logit}_O = \alpha + \beta \, \text{logit}_P. \tag{13.17}$$

Cox's calibration test is a test of $\alpha = 0$, given that β is fixed to be unity; expressed another way, this is a test of a zero intercept when the slope is one. In the context of a calibration plot, this emphasizes that calibration is a measure of the 'correct size' of the predictions, rather than their distribution. In practical terms, we need, first, to compute the predicted logits from the risk score, recalling that $\text{logit} = \log(p/(1 - p))$, where p is the predicted risk. Then we fit the model which regresses the observed logits against a null model (containing only an intercept) with the predicted logits as an offset (Section 11.10.1).

Example 13.15 Suppose that we want to apply the fibrinogen CVD risk score (13.3), created from data on Scottish women, to Scottish men. Although this is an artificial example, it has the benefit of having a ready interpretation (also the data are available on the web site for this book: see Appendix A). It is well known that the risk of CVD is higher for men than for women, so we would expect the 'female risk score', (13.3), to underestimate the risk for men, which is indeed what the pattern of dots (all above the diagonal) in Figure 13.21 suggests. Using SAS, predicted logits were calculated from the risk score (note that (13.2) gives a direct equation for these logits) and declared as an offset in PROC GENMOD. The fitted null (intercept-only) model was $\text{log}\hat{\text{it}}_0 = 0.7369$, and the test for a zero intercept was highly significant ($p < 0.0001$). Hence there is evidence of poor calibration for the female risk score when applied to men — just as we would expect.

Should Cox's test be applied in the cohort from which a logistic regression model-based score was produced, the result is certain to be perfect; that is, the intercept will be zero and the slope unity. So the test is only applicable when either an existing score is used in a new (closed) study population (as in Example 13.15), or when the score was derived in a study population by a method other than logistic regression, and is now to be calibrated within the same (closed) study population (for instance, where the scores are subjective probabilities expressed by a forecaster).

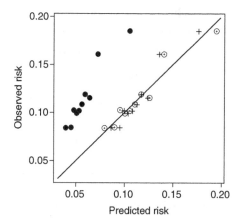

Figure 13.21. Calibration plot for the fibrinogen-only logistic regression risk score for women (dots), the intercept recalibrated logistic risk score (crosses) and the logistic recalibrated risk score (circles around points), when applied to men. Observed against mean predicted risk is plotted for each tenth of predicted risk.

Should Cox's test show poor calibration, we can use the same construct to recalibrate the logistic intercept. This will be called **intercept recalibration**. This proceeds by fitting (as in Example 13.15) the model

$$\text{logit}_O = \alpha + \text{logit}_P. \tag{13.18}$$

The recalibrated logit, logit_R, is then

$$\hat{\text{logit}}_R = a + \text{logit}_P$$

where a is the estimated value of α from the logistic model with an offset. The recalibrated risk score then comes from converting the new logits to predicted risks using (10.8). The result is a rescaling of the risk score which will make the overall observed and mean predicted (after recalibration) risks equal — that is, this is one way of achieving mean recalibration.

Intercept recalibration merely shifts the predicted probabilities up (when a is positive) or down (when a is negative). If this is not successful, we can consider 'tilting' the original predicted probabilities as well. To do this, we fit (13.17) and then take the recalibrated logit as

$$\hat{\text{logit}}_R = a + b\,\text{logit}_P,$$

where a and b are the estimated intercept and slope, respectively. This is generally called **logistic recalibration** or **Cox recalibration**. As with intercept recalibration, this forces the mean predicted risk to equal the overall observed risk; it should also achieve better grouped calibration.

Example 13.16 As we saw in Example 13.15, fitting (13.18) to the fibrinogen data for men gave recalibrated logits which are 0.7369 bigger than the predicted logits from the original (female) score. Hence the recalibrated scores, using (10.8), are

$$\{1 + \exp(-\hat{\text{logit}}_R)\}^{-1} = \{1 + \exp(-(\hat{\text{logit}}_P + 0.7369))\}^{-1}.$$

From (13.2), $\hat{\text{logit}}_P = -3.8063 + 0.3645 \times$ fibrinogen. Hence the intercept recalibrated score (predicted 10-year CVD risk for any value of fibrinogen) is

$$\{1 + \exp(-(-3.0694 + 0.3645 \times \text{fibrinogen}))\}^{-1}.$$

For example, when fibrinogen is 5 g/l, this gives

$$p = 1/\{1 + \exp(3.0694 - 0.3645 \times 5)\} = 0.22,$$

which may be compared with the prediction of 0.12 using the original score (see Example 13.4). As desired, this recalibration, of a CVD score from a female to a male population, has caused the score to increase.

On the other hand, when (13.17) is applied to the same data, the fitted model is

$$\hat{\text{logit}}_O = 0.1649 + 0.7915 \times \text{logit}_P.$$

From this, logistic recalibrated logits are:

$$\hat{\text{logit}}_R = 0.1649 + 0.7915 \times (-3.8063 + 0.3645 \times \text{fibrinogen})$$

$$= -2.84779 + 0.288502 \times \text{fibrinogen}.$$

The recalibrated risk score is then, from (10.8),

$$\{1 + \exp(-\hat{\text{logit}}_R)\}^{-1} = 1/\{1 + \exp(2.84779 - 0.288502 \times \text{fibrinogen})\}.$$

For example, when fibrinogen is 5 g/l, the logistic recalibrated predicted risk is 0.20.

The mean predicted risk for the original score is 0.0595. The corresponding results for both the intercept and logistic recalibrated scores are 0.1158, the same as for the true overall risk (since 754/6509 men in SHHEC had incident CVD within 10 years).

The two recalibrated risks scores are shown on Figure 13.21. Both are clearly considerably superior to the original score, as they are closer to the diagonal line and show no systematic pattern of variation around this diagonal. A slight advantage, in terms of approximate fit to the diagonal reference line, appears for the logistic recalibrated score. Calibration is excellent in the low and middle ranges of predicted risks with the recalibrated scores, but not ideal in the upper 20%. Any improvement would likely require fitting extra prognostic variables. The HL test of lack of fit (see Section 13.5.3) is highly significant ($p < 0.0001$) for the original score but not for the intercept recalibrated ($p = 0.67$) or the logistic recalibrated ($p = 0.85$) scores. Mean recalibration (see Section 13.6.1), although not shown here, gave very similar results to intercept recalibration.

13.6.3   Recalibration of parameters from a Cox model

When the original score was calculated from a Cox regression model, recalibration may be undertaken by updating the baseline survival probability in concert with updating the mean. Whereas the original t-year risk score, (13.4), is

$$\hat{p} = 1 - S(t, \overline{x})^{\exp(\Sigma b_i x_i - \Sigma b_i \overline{x}_i)},$$

where $\overline{x}_i$ is the mean for the ith variable in the original dataset, the recalibrated risk score is

$$\hat{p} = 1 - S'(t, \overline{x}')^{\exp\left(\Sigma b_i x_i - \Sigma b_i \overline{x}_i'\right)}, \tag{13.19}$$

where S' and $\overline{x}_i'$ are, respectively, the survival probability and mean for the ith variable in the new population. This recalibration technique does not generally produce perfect mean calibration, unlike the earlier recalibration methods we have seen.

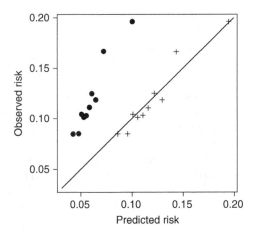

Figure 13.22. Calibration plot for the fibrinogen-only Cox regression risk score for women (dots) and the recalibrated risk score (crosses), when applied to men. Observed against mean predicted risk is plotted for each tenth of predicted risk.

Example 13.17 In Example 13.6 the female risk score from a Cox model, using fibrinogen as the single prognostic variable, was found to be $\hat{p} = 1 - 0.93916\,{}^{\exp(0.30671x - 0.97653)}$, where x is the value of fibrinogen. For this score applied to the male data for fibrinogen (available on the web site for this book) the resultant calibration plot is shown by the dots on Figure 13.22. Clearly this is poorly calibrated; to provide a quantitative result, the HL test was applied, using (13.16). As Figure 13.22 suggests it should be, this was highly significant ($p < 0.0001$). Note that Example 13.16 has already pointed towards this conclusion.

In the male data the mean value of fibrinogen is 2.75219 g/l (slightly lower than for women) and the probability of CVD-free survival for 10 years for men with this mean value for fibrinogen was estimated to be 0.88266 (much lower than for women). Taking these two parameters for $\bar{x}'$ and $S'(t, \bar{x}')$, respectively, in (13.19) gives the recalibrated score, $\hat{p} = 1 - 0.88266\,{}^{\exp(0.30671x - 0.30671 \times 2.75219)}$. The recalibrated plot is shown with crosses on Figure 13.22. This is much better calibrated than the original score, with no systematic variation around the diagonal. The HL test had a p value of 0.83: no evidence of lack of calibration.

The overall observed (KM) 10-year risk is 0.1192. The mean predicted risk for the original score is 0.0609 and for the recalibrated score is 0.1205.

13.6.4 Recalibration and discrimination

Although the rank ordering of risk for people with particular risk factor profiles is likely to be reasonably homogeneous across time and location, 'background' risk is much more likely to be heterogeneous. This is related to issues with pooling relative risks and risk differences, discussed in Section 12.3.8. We are dealing with prospective accumulation of results in this chapter, and the results of a risk scoring exercise must necessarily use data collected over several years in the past. Hence it may be unreasonable to expect calibration, as opposed to discrimination, to be good even for a risk score derived in the same place (e.g., country) as the one for which we currently want reliable risk scores. As we have seen, there are several simple ways to update a risk score to improve calibration. Unfortunately there are no such easy fixes for a poorly discriminating score. None of the methods of recalibration described here will change the rank ordering of the predicted risks. Importantly, this means that recalibration has no effect on discrimination. As an example, using the datasets available for this book, we can show that the AUC (95% confidence interval) for all three scores shown on Figure 13.21 is 0.578 (0.556, 0.600).

If we want to improve discrimination we need to consider making changes to the linear predictor, $\sum bx$, which underlies the statistical models. We might pool new data with old data to update the regression (b) coefficients, using meta-analysis; we might change the form of some of the prognostic (x) variables, for instance, by taking logarithms; and we might add new prognostic variables by refitting the statistical model with an expanded set of explanatory variables. Of course, such changes may also affect calibration.

Although it is clearly clinically useful to obtain, and communicate, accurate risk predictions, in some situations calibration may be a moot point. For example if a health authority can only afford to treat, say, a million people then, in a sense, it does not matter what the risk of the millionth person in risk order is: all that is necessary is to rank people correctly, which is the realm of discrimination.

These considerations lead to a conclusion that the ability to discriminate well is a more important property of a risk score than is good calibration.

13.7 The accuracy of predictions

We have seen how to quantify the two most important features of a risk score, discrimination and calibration. It can also be useful to evaluate the overall fit of a prediction model to observed data using a single index. This can be done by extending the concept of the r^2 statistic, as described in Section 9.3.1. Mittlböck and Schemper (1996) and Schemper and Stare (1996) show how this can be done for binary and survival data, respectively. Here we shall consider a simple method, due to the meteorologist Glenn Brier, which evaluates the mean square error of prediction.

13.7.1 The Brier score

The **Brier score** (Brier, 1950) is the average of the squared differences between the observed and predicted risks:

$$\frac{1}{n}\sum_{i=1}^{n}(y_i - p_i)^2,$$

where, as in (13.14), y is the observed outcome ($y = 0$ for no disease and $y = 1$ for disease), for example over a ten-year period of observation, p is the risk score and i refers to the ith person out of n (the total number of subjects). In essence, the Brier score measures the average error in the predictions. As with other applications in statistics, such as in the definition of the standard deviation (Section 2.6.3), the squaring operation is required to ensure that the effects of positive and negative errors do not get cancelled out. Note that the word 'score' in 'Brier score' refers to an index of error, rather than the predicted chance of an individual developing disease, as in 'risk score', and that the smaller the Brier score is, the better the score. It must lie between 0 and 1, but the effective practical range for useful Brier scores is from 0 to 0.25, since a Brier score of 0.25 can be obtained by guessing each forecast as exactly one half (see score S_5 in Table 13.13 for an example).

To understand the relationships between discrimination, calibration and the Brier score, Table 13.13 presents a range of hypothetical risk scores for a population of size 24, of whom 6 (25%) get the disease, and 18 do not, during observation. Score S_1 gives

Table 13.13. Illustrative risk scores for a hypothetical population of size 24. y is the true outcome (1 = disease; 0 = no disease) and S_i is the set of predicted probabilities for the ith forecast. Note that the overall risk, r, is $6/24 = 0.25$.

y	S_1	S_2	S_3	S_4	S_5	S_6	S_7	S_8	S_9	S_{10}	S_{11}
1	1.00	0.00	1.00	0.00	0.50	0.25	0.90	0.60	0.50	0.70	0.95
1	1.00	0.00	1.00	0.00	0.50	0.25	0.90	0.60	0.45	0.65	0.70
1	1.00	0.00	1.00	0.00	0.50	0.25	0.90	0.60	0.40	0.60	0.50
1	1.00	0.00	1.00	0.00	0.50	0.25	0.90	0.60	0.35	0.50	0.40
1	1.00	0.00	1.00	0.00	0.50	0.25	0.90	0.60	0.30	0.40	0.30
1	1.00	0.00	1.00	0.00	0.50	0.25	0.90	0.60	0.25	0.30	0.10
0	1.00	0.00	0.00	1.00	0.50	0.25	0.10	0.40	0.31	0.51	0.80
0	1.00	0.00	0.00	1.00	0.50	0.25	0.10	0.40	0.26	0.41	0.40
0	1.00	0.00	0.00	1.00	0.50	0.25	0.10	0.40	0.20	0.31	0.30
0	1.00	0.00	0.00	1.00	0.50	0.25	0.10	0.40	0.10	0.10	0.25
0	1.00	0.00	0.00	1.00	0.50	0.25	0.10	0.40	0.10	0.10	0.20
0	1.00	0.00	0.00	1.00	0.50	0.25	0.10	0.40	0.10	0.10	0.18
0	1.00	0.00	0.00	1.00	0.50	0.25	0.10	0.40	0.10	0.10	0.16
0	1.00	0.00	0.00	1.00	0.50	0.25	0.10	0.40	0.10	0.10	0.16
0	1.00	0.00	0.00	1.00	0.50	0.25	0.10	0.40	0.10	0.10	0.15
0	1.00	0.00	0.00	1.00	0.50	0.25	0.10	0.40	0.10	0.10	0.14
0	1.00	0.00	0.00	1.00	0.50	0.25	0.10	0.40	0.10	0.10	0.14
0	1.00	0.00	0.00	1.00	0.50	0.25	0.10	0.40	0.10	0.10	0.12
0	1.00	0.00	0.00	1.00	0.50	0.25	0.10	0.40	0.10	0.10	0.12
0	1.00	0.00	0.00	1.00	0.50	0.25	0.10	0.40	0.10	0.10	0.10
0	1.00	0.00	0.00	1.00	0.50	0.25	0.10	0.40	0.10	0.10	0.10
0	1.00	0.00	0.00	1.00	0.50	0.25	0.10	0.40	0.10	0.10	0.05
0	1.00	0.00	0.00	1.00	0.50	0.25	0.10	0.40	0.10	0.10	0.05
0	1.00	0.00	0.00	1.00	0.50	0.25	0.10	0.40	0.10	0.10	0.01
$\bar{p}$	1.00	0.00	0.25	0.75	0.50	0.25	0.30	0.45	0.19	0.25	0.27
$r - \bar{p}$	**-0.75**	**0.25**	0.00	**-0.50**	**-0.25**	0.00	-0.05	**-0.20**	0.06	0.00	-0.02
Spieg						0	-1.63	-4.00	-0.51	-1.33	-0.09
AUC	0.5	0.5	1	0	0.5	0.5	1	1	0.97	0.94	0.81
Brier	0.75	0.25	0.00	1.00	0.25	0.19	0.01	0.16	0.11	0.09	0.13

Notes: $\bar{p}$ = mean risk score; $r - \bar{p}$ is the difference between the true overall risk (0.25) and the mean predicted risk ($p < 0.05$ in bold, using (13.15)); Spieg = Spiegelhalter's test statistic (here, this test must be non-significant each time, since no results are positive; else use (13.14)).

everyone a predicted risk of 1; that is, everyone is forecast to suffer the disease. S_2 forecasts that everyone will fail to get the disease, S_3 gets the forecast right every time and S_4 gets it wrong every time. None of these risk algorithms have any practical relevance, but it is instructive to see their results. Each of S_1 and S_2 naturally has zero discrimination (AUC = 0.5), but the Brier scores for S_1 and S_2 are quite different: because more people are really disease negative, S_2 gets a lower (better) score than S_1. Score S_3 has perfect discrimination (AUC = 1) and a perfect Brier score (zero); S_4 has perfect negative discrimination (AUC = 0) and the worst possible Brier score (unity). In terms of mean calibration (i.e. the absolute value of $r - \bar{p}$): S_3 is (once again) perfect; just as with the Brier score, S_2 does better than S_1; S_4 has poor calibration, although (opposite to the Brier score) it does better than S_1.

Scores S_5 and S_6 each give a constant score to everyone and so, like S_1 and S_2, they have no discrimination. S_5 gives everyone the score of 0.5, which might be chosen by a forecaster with no knowledge of the application, and S_6 gives everyone a score equal to the overall prevalence (in practice, this would be an estimate, perhaps informed by recent data). In terms of discrimination, S_5 and S_6 are no different from each other or S_1 and S_2, but calibration is necessarily at its best when all the scores are 0.25. The Brier score is also better for S_6 than S_5.

Scores S_7 and S_8 directly illustrate the ordinal nature of the AUC, and its limitation as an overall index of prediction. In both cases, discrimination is perfect yet calibration and the Brier score are much better for S_7, since it separates the cases and non-cases more extremely. Going from S_9 to S_{10} or S_9 to S_6, discrimination worsens and calibration improves, yet the Brier score gets better in the first comparison and worse in the other. This shows that comparisons of Brier scores can be informative even when differences in discrimination and calibration are already known.

S_{10} has perfect mean calibration, at least to 16 decimal places, so that this score has equivalent calibration (in the restricted sense used here) to S_6, despite their very different scoring patterns and completely different AUCs. Finally, S_{11} represents a 'reasonable' scoring pattern in that the average score is similar to the prevalence, few in the no disease group were given a relatively high score and few in the disease group were given a relatively low score. The Brier score here is 0.13. However, real-life scores often do appreciably better. For instance, when the Framingham CVD risk score was applied to men and women in the Scottish Heart Health Extended Cohort Study, the Brier scores were 0.097 and 0.057, respectively.

The Brier score may be decomposed in several ways, so as to express it in terms of additive components of various aspects of model fit and the distribution of the scores. This helps in understanding how calibration (for example) can improve as the Brier score worsens. One such decomposition gives rise to Spiegelhalter's test for overall calibration, (13.14). Results for this test are included in Table 13.13; examination of (13.14) will show that this test is undefined in the unrealistic situations when all the score components are 0, 1 or 0.5 or when they are all 0 or 1, since then the denominator becomes zero.

In Stata, the BRIER command produces both the Brier score and the result of Spiegelhalter's test.

13.7.2   Comparison of Brier scores

Redelmeier et al. (1991) devised a test to compare two Brier scores when each has overall calibration, taken to mean that Speigelhalter's test is not significant at the 5% level. Defining p_{1i} to be the score given to the ith individual using the first scoring system, p_{2i} to be the corresponding score for the same individual using the second scoring system and (as usual) y_i to be the true disease status (1 for disease, 0 for no disease) for this individual, Redelmeier's test statistic is

$$\frac{\sum (p_{1i} - p_{2i})(p_{1i} + p_{2i} - 2y_i)}{\sqrt{\sum (p_{1i} - p_{2i})^2 (p_{1i} + p_{2i})(2 - p_{1i} - p_{2i})}}.$$

For the last three scores (S_9–S_{11}) in Table 13.13, the Brier scores are 0.11, 0.09 and 0.13, respectively. Redelmeier test statistics (p values) are: S_9 versus S_{10}, 1.17 ($p = 0.24$); S_{10} versus S_{11}, 2.17 ($p = 0.03$); and S_9 versus S_{11}, 0.62 ($p = 0.54$). Thus, only the Brier scores of S_{10} and S_{11} (not surprisingly, those that are furthest apart) are significantly different. Interestingly, the corresponding AUCs are not significantly different ($p = 0.18$), using ROCCOMP in STATA. Note that the usual issues of significance tests apply here, including multiple testing (see Section 9.2.5). Another method of comparing two scores in terms of overall prediction is given in Section 13.9.

13.8 Assessing an extraneous prognostic variable

In some situations a risk score, derived by others, is already in use for clinical decision making, but the question arises as to whether a variable excluded from that risk score should also be considered when making clinical decisions. As an example, the Framingham risk score for CVD has been used for several years in many parts of the world. Socio-economic status (SES) is widely accepted as a risk factor for CVD, in that those in relatively deprived circumstances generally have higher risk, even after allowing for the effect of classical CVD risk factors (an example, using housing tenure as a measure of SES, appeared in earlier chapters). Yet the Framingham score, currently in use, omits SES. When this score is used to allocate treatment (so as to target those most at risk) does this bias against underprivileged people?

In such cases it will not usually be possible to see whether the new variable 'adds' to the score using standard methods (Section 13.4.2 and Section 13.9) because the data used to generate the original score are not available or because the new variable was not recorded (and cannot now be measured) in the study population from which the original data were derived. However, if a similar dataset, including all the variables of the existing risk score plus the variable to be tested, is available, calibration plots can be used to check whether there is a systematic pattern in the comparison of observed and predicted risks — existence of such a pattern suggests that the new variable is important in prognosis. This is similar to the ideas behind residual analyses described in Section 9.8, whilst the mechanics of the process are identical to those in Section 13.5.4.

Tunstall–Pedoe and Woodward (2006) carried out such analyses to see whether SES would improve risk prediction, above that achieved by the Framingham score for CHD, in Scotland. Figure 13.23 shows their results, using data from the Scottish Heart Health Extended Cohort Study. For each subject, the Framingham score (predicted 10-year risk) was computed using a published formula and social deprivation was scored using Census data on the general affluence of the neighbourhood where the subject lived (see Example 10.45 for details). Subjects were then allocated to groups defined by the quintiles of this SES measure. Within each group, the mean Framingham CHD score (predicted risk) was compared with the observed (KM) risk of CHD.

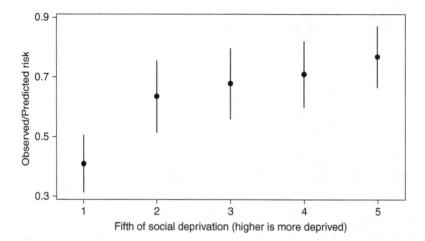

Figure 13.23. Ratios of observed to mean predicted coronary risks from the Framingham score, by fifths of social deprivation in Scotland. Note that the Framingham CHD score is used here, in contrast to the Framingham CVD score used in Figure 13.20.

The first thing to notice in Figure 13.23 is that all the observed/predicted ratios are below one, which indicates that the Framingham score is poorly calibrated to the Scottish environment (it overestimates risk). Second, there is an obvious trend in the summary ratios: the relative amount of overestimation is greatest in the 20% most socially advantaged (1st fifth) and progressively decreases as social advantage decreases. The ratio is approximately twice as high in the most deprived 20% as in the least deprived 20%. As the source paper points out, this means that when the standard Framingham score is applied for deciding treatment in Scotland (as was the norm, prior to this study), the most socially deprived would receive proportionately half the treatment in relation to their prospective disease burden of that given to the least deprived.

13.9   Reclassification

A common issue in determining appropriate clinical decision rules is whether the addition of a new variable to an existing score improves the prediction of the outcome in question. In Section 13.8 we saw how we might identify this issue in the case where the new variable is available only in a different dataset from the one used to generate the original risk score. In this section we consider the case where the new variable is available within the same dataset. For example, suppose a standard risk algorithm is used to identify those at high risk for end-stage kidney disease. A novel biomarker, which can be assayed from blood samples — stored in freezers at baseline — is now identified as having a strong association with this condition. Should the risk algorithm be updated to include the biomarker?

One approach to such a question would be to compare discrimination with and without the biomarker (see Section 13.4.2), but discrimination is not the only issue to consider. Another possibility would be to use Redelmeier's test (of Section 13.7.2), but this is only valid in restricted circumstances. Instead we shall return to fundamental issues of prediction, and develop indices concerned with how much better we classify who will and will not get the outcome of interest.

13.9.1 The integrated discrimination improvement from a fixed cohort

Consider a fixed cohort, where there is no censoring to account for. As discussed in Section 2.10 and Section 13.2.2, the two principal measures of the performance of a binary prediction are the sensitivity and specificity. In Section 13.2.2 we saw how these move in opposite directions as the threshold for deciding who is 'test positive' increases. A reasonable measure of how well a test based on a risk score classifies future disease status is thus the Youden index (Section 2.10.1), the average, or sum, of sensitivity and (1 − specificity), averaged over all thresholds — i.e., all observed values of the risk score. Hence a reasonable comparison of the overall performance of one risk score (call it 'new') and another (call it 'base') is the difference between their averaged (or 'integrated') Youden indices. Pencina *et al.* (2008) call this the **integrated discrimination improvement (IDI)**. When testing the addition of a biomarker, we would take the base score to be that derived from the original model, which comprises all the standard, established risk factors, and the new score to be that derived from the model with the standard risk factors plus the biomarker. In general, any two risk models can be compared using the same method.

For a fixed cohort an alternative definition of the IDI, suggested by Pencina *et al.* (2008), is more intuitive, easier to implement, and a basis for defining another type of index of reclassification (Section 13.9.2). Consider how well, on average, the new risk score (e.g., with the biomarker) outperforms the original score. To do this we have to consider subjects that did go on to get the index disease, and those that did not, separately. Amongst only those who did get the disease, the best risk score is one that gives a 'perfect' score of one to everyone. In practice this will not occur, but it suggests that a score that is, on average, nearer to one will be better than one that is further from one; that is, for those who are disease positive, a new score is better than the old score if it has the higher mean. We can measure the average degree of superiority of the new (extended) score over the base (original) score as $\bar{p}_{N+} - \bar{p}_{B+}$, where the two p's represent the observed values of the risk score amongst those positive for the disease (hence the + subscripts) for the base ('B') and new ('N') scores. We can test for no improvement (when adding the new prognostic variable) amongst those with the disease by comparing

$$\frac{\bar{p}_{N+} - \bar{p}_{B+}}{\mathrm{SE}(p_{N+} - p_{B+})} \tag{13.20}$$

to the standard normal (SE is the standard error). We can evaluate (13.20) by finding the differences between the two scores (new and base) within subjects and then use a computer procedure (for example, PROC MEANS in SAS or the SUMMARIZE command in Stata) to find the mean and SE of these differences, thus producing the numerator and denominator of (13.20) (noting that a mean of differences is the same as a difference of means). An approximate 95% confidence interval comes from

$$(\bar{p}_{N+} - \bar{p}_{B+}) \pm 1.96 \times \mathrm{SE}(p_{N+} - p_{B+}).$$

Conversely, for those who did not go on to get the disease, the new score is better if its mean is lower than that of the base score. Thus, for the 'no disease' group, the average degree of superiority of the new score over the base score is $\bar{p}_{B-} - \bar{p}_{N-}$, where the p's with negative subscripts represent the observed values of the two risk scores amongst those without the disease. An associated test and confidence interval for subjects with no disease follows, using the same steps as for those with the disease.

Taking all subjects together, and assuming that a misclassification is equally important in either direction, the net degree of superiority of the extended risk score over the original is thus

$$(\bar{p}_{N+} - \bar{p}_{B+}) + (\bar{p}_{B-} - \bar{p}_{N-})$$

or

$$(\bar{p}_{N+} - \bar{p}_{B+}) - (\bar{p}_{N-} - \bar{p}_{B-}). \tag{13.21}$$

A simple interpretation of the IDI, in this sense, is as the mean of the differences between the two scores for those who are disease positive minus the same difference for those who are disease negative.

An approximate test for a zero improvement in risk scoring, when moving from the base to the new score, is given by comparing

$$\frac{(\bar{p}_{N+} - \bar{p}_{B+}) - (\bar{p}_{N-} - \bar{p}_{B-})}{\sqrt{[\text{SE}(p_{N+} - p_{B+})]^2 + [\text{SE}(p_{N-} - p_{B-})]^2}} \tag{13.22}$$

with the standard normal distribution. An approximate 95% confidence interval for the IDI is

$$(\bar{p}_{N+} - \bar{p}_{B+}) - (\bar{p}_{N-} - \bar{p}_{B-}) \pm 1.96 \sqrt{[\text{SE}(p_{N+} - p_{B+})]^2 + [\text{SE}(p_{N-} - p_{B-})]^2}. \tag{13.23}$$

Both the test and confidence interval for the IDI, and its two components, depend upon an assumption of (at least approximate) normality. Kerr *et al.* (2011) suggest that this assumption is not always reasonable, in which case the two-sided test is too conservative (biased towards not finding significance) but a one-sided test is too liberal. Since the question at issue here is whether adding a new variable *improves* classification, a one-sided test may be more appropriate than the usual two-sided test (as was noted for comparing AUCs in Section 13.4.2). However, although introduced as a comparison of an original score with an extended score (where the extensions can involve any number of 'new' risk factors), (13.20)–(13.23) can equally well compare two scores which differ entirely. All that is necessary is that the two scores can be computed for the same people. Two-sided tests are then most natural.

Example 13.18 Consider the three risk scores (single with systolic blood pressure only, multi which adds total cholesterol and smoking and multiplus which adds body mass index) of Example 13.10. The mean risk scores and the SEs of the within-subject differences for single versus multi and multi versus multiplus, by CHD group, were computed from PROC MEANS in SAS, and are shown in Table 13.14.

For those with CHD, when the multi score is used instead of the single risk factor score the mean score is improved by $0.041468 - 0.034472 = 0.006996$. For those without CHD, the improvement is -0.000086. Overall, the improvement is $0.006996 + (-0.000086) = 0.00691$, the IDI. To test the null hypothesis that multi is no better at classifying future CHD than single, we use (13.22) which gives

$$\frac{(0.041468 - 0.034472) - (0.027870 - 0.027784)}{\sqrt{0.002023^2 + 0.000256^2}} = 3.39.$$

Table 13.14. Summary statistics for three risk scores in Example 13.18.

	CHD	No CHD
Means		
single	0.034472	0.027784
multi	0.041468	0.027870
multiplus	0.041430	0.027832
Standard errors		
multi versus single	0.002023	0.000256
multiplus versus multi	0.000399	0.000047

This has a one-sided p value of 0.0004, so we can conclude that taking account of total cholesterol and smoking does give improved prediction of CHD compared with merely using systolic blood pressure as a prognostic variable. From (13.23), the approximate 95% confidence interval for the IDI is $0.00691 \pm 1.96 \times 0.002039$, i.e., (0.00291, 0.01091).

Similarly, the test statistic for comparing multiplus with multi is –0.0007 (one-sided $p = 0.50$). BMI does not improve prediction once the other three variables are appropriately accounted for. The IDI is minus zero to several decimal places with a 95% confidence interval of (–0.00079, 0.000786).

Note that the conclusions in Example 13.18 are much the same as in Example 13.10. However, in general, there is no reason why conclusions from comparing AUCs should agree with those from comparing classification, as is demonstrated by Pencina *et al.* (2008). Also, closer consideration of Table 13.14 shows that, of all the scores, whilst multi performs best for correctly classifying CHD, it is worst for classifying lack of CHD (since, in both cases, it has the highest score). If, for some reason, we wanted to give a greater weight to correctly classifying no CHD, then single or multiplus could turn out to be the best for our purpose.

Two drawbacks with the IDI are that its value is typically very small (as in Example 13.18) and it has no easy clinical interpretation. As a consequence, it may be more informative to estimate the **relative integrated discrimination improvement** (RIDI). This is derived by reordering (13.21) into the equivalent form,

$$(\bar{p}_{N+} - \bar{p}_{N-}) - (\bar{p}_{B+} - \bar{p}_{B-}).$$

In this form, we see that the IDI is the difference between a contrast of scores amongst positive and negative disease outcomes using the new score, and the same contrast using the base score. From this, the RIDI for the new score relative to the base score is logically defined as

$$\frac{(\bar{p}_{N+} - \bar{p}_{N-}) - (\bar{p}_{B+} - \bar{p}_{B-})}{(\bar{p}_{B+} - \bar{p}_{B-})};$$

i.e.,

$$\text{RIDI} = \frac{\text{IDI}}{(\bar{p}_{B+} - \bar{p}_{B-})}. \tag{13.24}$$

For Example 13.18, comparing multi to single, (13.24) becomes

$$\text{RIDI} = \frac{0.00691}{(0.034472 - 0.027784)} = 1.033.$$

Thus, taking appropriate additional account of total cholesterol and smoking, having already accounted for systolic blood pressure, improves classification of CHD by 103% in this study population. A confidence interval for the RIDI can be obtained from bootstrapping (see Chapter 14).

13.9.2   The net reclassification improvement from a fixed cohort

A variation on the second (mean-based) interpretation of the IDI in fixed cohorts is the **net reclassification improvement** (NRI), in which the net direction of change is accounted for, rather than the mean magnitude of change. That is, we count how many people had higher scores under the new risk algorithm, compared with the base (call this $n_{\uparrow+}$ in the group with an event and $n_{\uparrow-}$ in the group without an event) and how many had lower scores (call these $n_{\downarrow+}$ and $n_{\downarrow-}$, respectively). As discussed in deriving (13.21) for the IDI, having a higher score is good (the new score is better) when that person really does have the disease during follow-up and is bad (the new score is worse) when that person does not have the disease. So as to allow for the differential frequencies of events and non-events (the latter is usually much more common in cohort studies), the estimated net beneficial value of the new (extended) score, compared with the base (original) score, is then defined as a comparison of relative numbers, or probabilities, of movements up and down. That is,

$$\widehat{\text{NRI}} = (\hat{p}_{\uparrow+} - \hat{p}_{\downarrow+}) - (\hat{p}_{\uparrow-} - \hat{p}_{\downarrow-}), \tag{13.25}$$

where $\hat{p}$ is the observed probability of the movement denoted by its suffices, i.e., $\hat{p}_{\uparrow+} = n_{\uparrow+}/n_+$, where n_+ is the number who are disease positive (that is, they suffer the disease during follow-up), etc. Notice that (13.25) is analogous to (13.21); qualitative changes have now replaced quantitative changes.

The estimated standard error of the NRI can be obtained as

$$\widehat{\text{SE}} = \sqrt{\frac{n_{\uparrow+} + n_{\downarrow+}}{n_+^2} - \frac{(n_{\uparrow+} - n_{\downarrow+})^2}{n_+^3} + \frac{n_{\uparrow-} + n_{\downarrow-}}{n_-^2} - \frac{(n_{\uparrow-} - n_{\downarrow-})^2}{n_-^3}}, \tag{13.26}$$

whence the approximate 95% CI is $\widehat{\text{NRI}} \pm 1.96 \times \widehat{\text{SE}}$. A test for a net improvement of zero in correctly diagnosed counts (i.e., the null hypothesis of a zero NRI) is given by comparing $\widehat{\text{NRI}}/\sqrt{D}$ with the standard normal distribution, where

$$D = \frac{n_{\uparrow+} + n_{\downarrow+}}{n_+^2} + \frac{n_{\uparrow-} + n_{\downarrow-}}{n_-^2}. \tag{13.27}$$

Example 13.19 Consider the evaluation of the multi risk score relative to the single risk score of Example 13.18 using the NRI method. Table 13.15 shows the number of people whose score

Table 13.15. Number with increased scores, comparing multi to single in Example 13.19.

Movement	CHD	No CHD
Decreased	39 (34.21%)	2372 (60.28%)
Increased	75 (65.79%)	1563 (39.72%)
Total	114	3935

has decreased and the number whose score has increased when the single score is replaced by the multi score. No one had the same score by both methods.

From (13.25), the NRI is estimated as $0.6579 - 0.3421 - (0.3972 - 0.6028) = 0.5214$. From (13.26), the estimated SE of the NRI is

$$\sqrt{\frac{75+39}{114^2} - \frac{(75-39)^2}{114^3} + \frac{1563+2372}{3935^2} - \frac{(1563-2372)^2}{3935^3}} = 0.0902,$$

giving a 95% confidence interval of $0.5214 \pm 1.96 \times 0.0902$ or $(0.3445, 0.6982)$. To test the null hypothesis that the NRI is zero we compute D from (13.27). Since no subject has a tied score in this example, (13.27) simplifies to the sum of reciprocals of the marginal sample sizes, i.e., $(1/114) + (1/3935)$. From this, the test statistic for a zero NRI is 5.4879. Compared to the standard normal this is highly significant, $p < 0.0001$. Hence multi has improved the classification of CHD events compared to single; that is, smoking and cholesterol provide additional prognostic value over and above systolic blood pressure.

In some situations, a clinically meaningful risk threshold exists and this can be used to produce a targeted form of the NRI, which uses risk thresholds. For example, it may be that national policies are to treat, with pharmaceuticals, everyone who has a 10-year risk of the index disease of more than 20%. Then it would be important to see whether adding a new biomarker to the clinical risk algorithm improves the classification of risk above and below the 0.2 threshold. We can handle this problem using (13.25)–(13.27) provided we define each $\hat{p}$ to be the probability of moving into or out of the group with probability of disease > 0.2. Sometimes more than one threshold is defined, in which case each $\hat{p}$ is a probability of moving into either a higher or a lower risk category, as the following example (with two thresholds) illustrates.

Example 13.20 Suppose that guidelines suggest giving lifestyle and dietary advice to anyone with a 5-year coronary risk of more than 5%, and treating anyone with a risk of more than 10% with statins. General practitioners (GPs) then need a risk algorithm that correctly identifies whether a patient, currently free of CHD, falls into the risk groups: < 0.05, 0.05–0.1 and > 0.1. Is it sufficient for GPs to base their decisions on when to intervene appropriately on a measurement of systolic blood pressure alone, or should they also take into account the patient's cholesterol level and smoking habit?

This is a problem that can be addressed using the SHHS data used in the last two examples, comparing the single (systolic blood pressure only) and multi (adding cholesterol and smoking) scores. Table 13.16 shows the cross-classification of subjects according to the two risk scores, by CHD status on follow-up. Here the relevant thresholds have been used to group subjects by each score. The cells with entries in bold type include subjects who have moved to a more appropriate risk group, and those in italics have moved to a less appropriate risk group, when changing to an evaluation using the multi, rather than the single, risk score.

Table 13.16. Reclassification of subjects using pre-defined risk thresholds in Example 13.20.

| | Risk using multi score | | | | | |
| Risk using single score | CHD (n = 114) | | | No CHD (n = 3935) | | |
	<0.05	0.05-0.1	≥0.1	<0.05	0.05-0.1	≥0.1
<0.05	87	11	2	3437	254	17
0.05–0.1	4	5	1	97	91	25
≥0.1	0	1	3	1	3	10

From Table 13.16,

$$n_{\uparrow+} = 11 + 2 + 1 = 14, \ n_{\uparrow-} = 254 + 17 + 25 = 296,$$
$$n_{\downarrow+} = 4 + 0 + 1 = 5, \ n_{\downarrow-} = 97 + 1 + 3 = 101.$$

Hence, $\hat{p}_{\uparrow+}$ = 14/114 = 0.1228; $\hat{p}_{\downarrow+}$ = 5/114 = 0.0439; $\hat{p}_{\uparrow-}$ = 296/3935 = 0.0752; $\hat{p}_{\downarrow-}$ = 101/3935 = 0.0257. From (13.25), the estimated NRI is thus 0.0294, with 95% confidence interval, using (13.26), of (–0.0448, 0.1036). Using (13.27), the test statistic for a zero value of the NRI is 0.7621 (one-sided p = 0.22). Taking the thresholds proposed, there is no evidence that coronary risk is better classified by making extra use of cholesterol and smoking.

The threshold-based NRI of Example 13.20 is much smaller than the threshold-free (or continuous) NRI of Example 13.19. As a consequence, the negative conclusion of Example 13.20 is at odds with the conclusion of Example 13.19, as well as with earlier examples where the single and multi risk scores were compared across the entire range of risk (Examples 13.10 and 13.18). Which conclusion is reasonable to draw depends upon the practical use of the risk score. The threshold-free NRI is clearly more objective than the threshold-based NRI, since it does not depend upon the choice of thresholds. On the other hand, it treats each part of the range of risk equally and this may not be acceptable to the clinician, especially when treatment guidelines relating to level of risk are well established. In particular, we may not be concerned about relatively inaccurate prediction at extreme levels of risk, but feel that it is crucial to identify those falling above fixed risk thresholds accurately; in this case, Example 13.20 would give the key result. Since, in general, the value of the NRI depends on whether or not thresholds are employed and, when they are used, the actual thresholds chosen, it is important to specify how thresholds were used in any presentation of NRI analyses.

Just as for the IDI, the NRI from a fixed cohort can usefully be split into net reclassification indices for events and for non-events:

$$\widehat{\text{NDI}}_+ = (\hat{p}_{\uparrow+} - \hat{p}_{\downarrow+}) \quad \text{and} \quad \widehat{\text{NDI}}_- = (\hat{p}_{\downarrow-} - \hat{p}_{\uparrow-}),$$

whence $\widehat{\text{NDI}}$ = $\widehat{\text{NDI}}_+$ + $\widehat{\text{NDI}}_-$. This result can be seen from simple manipulation of (13.25). Such a split is suggested by the pair of reclassification tables presented as Table 13.16. In Example 13.20 the NRI for CHD events is 0.1228 – 0.0439 = 0.0789 and for non-events is 0.0257 – 0.0752 = –0.0496. Hence the extended score, adding cholesterol and smoking, does better for those who go on to have a coronary event; the effect of changing to the extended score is to correctly reclassify 8% of events. However, the extended score does worse than the base score for those who will not get a coronary: its effect is to correctly reclassify –5% of non-events. Assuming that equal importance is given to correctly reclassifying events and non-events, as in the standard definition of the NRI, the net effect is sometimes loosely interpreted by saying that classification is improved by $8 + (-5) = 3\%$ (corresponding to the value of 0.0294 in Example 13.20). If required, tests and confidence intervals for the individual components come from using only terms with either $+$ or $-$ suffices in (13.26) and (13.27).

13.9.3 The integrated discrimination improvement from a variable cohort

We turn, now, to the situation of a variable cohort where censoring is to be accounted for and thus risk scores may be generated from a Cox, rather than a logistic, regression model. In this situation, using the results of Chambless *et al.* (2011), the average Youden index for a risk score, Z, is

$$\bar{Y}_Z = \frac{\text{Var}\,(r_Z)}{S(t)(1 - S(t))},$$

where t is the follow-up time at which risk is to evaluated, $S(t)$ is the observed survival at time t and $\text{Var}(r_Z)$ is the variance of the risk score Z (which expresses risks at time t). $S(t)$ can be estimated by the KM method and the variance term is just the straightforward variance of the risk scores on all subjects. Then, using the fundamental definition of IDI as the difference in Youden indices between the new ('N') and the base ('B') score, the IDI that allows for censoring, IDI_c is defined as

$$\text{IDI}_c = \bar{Y}_N - \bar{Y}_B = \frac{\text{Var}\,(r_N) - \text{Var}\,(r_B)}{S(t)(1 - S(t))}. \tag{13.28}$$

Example 13.21 Taking the problem of Example 13.18 again, but now allowing for censoring, the three risk scores were compared in pairwise fashion, as before, but using the risk scores for 5 years (1827 days) from Cox models. The three risk scores are:

single $= 1 - 0.97415^{\exp(0.02357(\text{SYSTOL}) - 3.14007)}$,
multi $= 1 - 0.97648^{\exp(0.29483(\text{TOTCHOL}) + 0.02186(\text{SYSTOL}) + 0.32380(\text{ex}) + 0.65894(\text{current}) - 5.21247)}$,
multiplus $= 1 - 0.97669^{\exp(0.03676(\text{BMI}) + 0.28277(\text{TOTCHOL}) + 0.02118(\text{SYSTOL}) + 0.31873(\text{ex}) + 0.67913(\text{current}) - 6.00921)}$,

where (as before) SYSTOL is systolic blood pressure, TOTCHOL is total cholesterol, BMI is body mass index and 'ex' and 'current' are dummy variables for ex-smoking and current smoking, respectively. Note that the multi risk score was defined earlier as (13.6).

For every member of the study population, utilizing the data on this book's web site, each of the three risk scores were computed and the variances derived using PROC MEANS in SAS. The values were: $\text{Var}(r_{\text{single}}) = 0.000229945$; $\text{Var}(r_{\text{multi}}) = 0.000438829$; and $\text{Var}(r_{\text{multiplus}}) = 0.000452747$. The KM estimate of survival to 5 years is 0.9716 from PROC LIFEREG in SAS. Hence the IDI_c for adding total cholesterol and smoking to systolic blood pressure (i.e., multi versus single) is, from (13.28),

$$\text{IDI}_c = \frac{0.0043889 - 0.000229945}{0.9716(1 - 0.9716)} = 0.0076.$$

Similarly, the IDI_c comparing multiplus and multi (i.e., adding BMI to the others) is 0.0005. Both are similar to the equivalent values found from risk scores based on logistic models in Example 13.18.

There is no simple equation for the confidence interval of IDI_c. In this situation we might use bootstrapping (see Chapter 14). For example, using a SAS program available on the web site for this book, the 95% confidence interval for IDI_c (multi versus single) was found using a rudimentary bootstrap routine to be (0.0054, 0.0102). The relative IDI for a variable cohort is

$$\mathrm{RIDI}_c = \frac{\mathrm{IDI}}{\bar{Y}_B} = \frac{\mathrm{Var}(r_N) - \mathrm{Var}(r_B)}{\mathrm{Var}(r_B)}.$$

The relative IDI for the survival data–based comparison of the multi and simple risk scores is 0.908, so the relative improvement in classification is about 91%. A bootstrap 95% confidence interval for this, derived from the same SAS program as above, is (0.631, 1.229).

13.9.4   The net reclassification improvement from a variable cohort

Pencina *et al.* (2011) define a variation on the basic NRI for use in the presence of censoring. To derive this, (13.25) needs to be written in an equivalent (but more complex) form,

$$\widehat{\mathrm{NDI}}_c = \frac{\hat{p}_{+\uparrow}\hat{p}_\uparrow - \hat{p}_{+\downarrow}\hat{p}_\downarrow}{\hat{p}_+} + \frac{(1 - \hat{p}_{+\downarrow})\hat{p}_\downarrow - (1 - \hat{p}_{+\uparrow})\hat{p}_\uparrow}{1 - \hat{p}_+}. \tag{13.29}$$

Here $\hat{p}$ are observed probabilities, as before. However, whereas in (13.25) $\hat{p}_{\uparrow+}$ represents the observed probability of upward movement (across thresholds or overall) amongst those positive for disease within a fixed period of time, say t years, in (13.29) $\hat{p}_{+\uparrow}$ represents the observed probability of contracting the disease within t years amongst those who have a higher score using the new score compared to the old (an upwards movement). Also, $\hat{p}_+$ is the observed overall probability of an event within t years. So as to account for censoring, all the $\hat{p}$ terms for events in (13.29), i.e., $\hat{p}_{+\uparrow}$, $\hat{p}_{+\downarrow}$ and $\hat{p}_+$, will be derived from KM estimation. We can use (13.29) with or without imposing thresholds, and we can have as many thresholds as we wish. A 95% confidence interval for the NRI_c may be estimated by bootstrapping: the same SAS program as used in Section 13.9.3 might be used to obtain such a confidence interval (but see Section 14.3 for ways of improving bootstrap estimates).

As with the logistic case, it is insightful to give the estimated NRI_c for events and non-events separately. From first principles (see Pencina *et al.*, 2011), these are, respectively, the left and right portions of the equation for the overall estimated NRI_c, (13.29).

Example 13.22 Consider, now, the problems of Example 13.19 and Example 13.20 in the situation of a variable cohort; that is, now taking account of the censoring in the SHHS data that was ignored previously. The two risk scores to be compared, multi and simple, derived from Cox models, are expressed in Example 13.21.

First consider NRI_c with no threshold. To use (13.29), first, we should compute the number of people who have been given a higher score (i.e. reclassified upwards), and those given a lower score (reclassified downwards), using multi compared to simple. These are 1657 and 2392, respectively (no one had the same score). Since there are 4049 men in the sample, $\hat{p}_\uparrow = 1657/4049 = 0.4092$ and $\hat{p}_\downarrow = 2392/4092 = 0.5908$. Next, we find KM estimates of a CHD event within 5 years for (i) everyone, $\hat{p}_+$ (ii) those reclassified upwards, $\hat{p}_{+\uparrow}$ (iii) those reclassified downwards, $\hat{p}_{+\downarrow}$. From PROC LIFETEST in SAS these were (i) 0.0284, (ii) 0.0464, (iii) 0.0160. Substituting into (13.29) gives

$$\mathrm{NRI}_c = \frac{0.0464 \times 0.4092 - 0.0160 \times 0.5908}{0.0284}$$
$$+ \frac{(1 - 0.0160) \times 0.5908 - (1 - 0.0464) \times 0.4092}{(1 - 0.0284)}$$
$$= 0.335 + 0.197 = 0.531$$

(after rounding).

This answer is similar to that found in Example 13.19 when a logistic model was used. Note that 33.5% of those having events, and 19.7% not having events, are correctly reclassified when using the multi score compared to the single score.

Next, consider the NRI with thresholds at 5 and 10%, as in Example 13.20. In this case, Table 13.17 (Overall portion) shows the reclassification table. From this, the number reclassified upwards and downwards are, respectively, 112 and 272, giving $\hat{p}_\uparrow = 0.0672$ and $\hat{p}_\downarrow = 0.0277$. From SAS PROC LIFETEST, KM estimates for the probability of an event within 5 years are 0.0284 overall (as when no thresholds are used), 0.0482 for those moving upwards and 0.0536 for those moving downwards. From (13.29), $\mathrm{NRI}_c = 0.062 + (-0.039) = 0.023$. This is similar to the NRI found in Example 13.20 when a logistic model was used. The first of the two components of NRI_c is the proportion of all men with an event who are correctly reclassified when the multi score is used rather than the single score; i.e., 6.2% of events are correctly reclassified. Similarly, from the second component, −3.9% of non-events are correctly reclassified. As when logistic regression is used, ignoring censoring, the multiple-variable score does better than the single-variable score only for those who have an event. Table 13.17 also shows separate sub-tables for events and non-events. Notice that these are for events and non-events over the entire follow-up, which varies for each subject, unlike Table 13.16 which shows events within 5 years only. This emphasises the difference between fixed and variable cohorts. We cannot tabulate, correctly, events/non-events at 5 years because those censored within 5 years have unknown event times. This means that the reclassification table cannot be used to compute the NRI, unlike the situation with a fixed cohort.

Table 13.17. Reclassification of subjects using pre-defined risk thresholds in Example 13.22.

Risk using single score	Risk using multi score		
	< 0.05	0.05–0.1	≥ 0.1
Overall ($n = 4049$)			
< 0.05	3522	240	8
0.05–0.1	104	124	24
≥ 0.1	2	6	19
CHD ($n = 196$)			
< 0.05	145	21	2
0.05–0.1	8	10	3
≥ 0.1	0	3	4
No CHD ($n = 3853$)			
< 0.05	3377	219	6
0.05–0.1	96	114	21
≥ 0.1	2	3	15

13.9.5   Software

Software to perform reclassification is scarce, but emerging, at the time of writing. For example, Kennedy and Pencina (2010) describe a SAS macro for use in fixed cohorts; this and a similar program for variable cohorts (utilised in Section 13.9.3) are available on the web site for this book. This web site also has Stata programs with similar utility.

13.10 Validation

In the main, up to now we have only considered the worth of a risk algorithm, such as its calibration and discrimination, within the data from which it was derived. Since the risk score is conceived as a tool for use in clinical decision making amongst future subjects, this begs the question of its worth in a wider setting. We must expect a risk score to perform better within the data from which it was derived than it would elsewhere, because the statistical model from which the score was constructed was that which fitted the data in an optimal fashion. So the measures of calibration, discrimination and reclassification, derived within the data used to construct the score, are too optimistic for general use.

There are two general approaches to overcoming this self-testing bias: internal and external validation. **Internal validation** is where the original dataset is sampled so as to provide both development and testing subsets. A simple way of doing this is to split the data into two, perhaps taking a random sample of 2/3 of the data in which to develop the risk score and using the remaining 1/3 as the testing (validation) sample. All the material of preceding sections of this chapter can be used directly. However, this makes inefficient use of the data available to derive the risk score: the proportion of the data put aside for use in testing could have been used to improve estimation (which is why, in practice, the percentage used for testing is generally less than 50%). Cross-validation is repeated data splitting where, for example, 10 random subsamples of equal size are defined. The prognostic model is developed on the entirety of nine subsamples and tested on the remaining subsample. Repeating this so that each of the 10 subsamples is, in turn, the validation sample, gives 10-fold cross-validation. Measures of discrimination, etc. can be averaged over the 10 operations. Intuitively this is better than a single data split since it protects against chance differences in the single validation sample.

Harrell *et al.* (1996) suggest that the best internal validation comes from bootstrapping (see Chapter 14), which uses all the available data to derive the risk score. A large number (at least 200) of bootstrap samples should be generated, in each of which a risk score is generated and then assessed (e.g., for discrimination) on both the bootstrap sample and on the original dataset. In principle, all the steps used to generate the score, including variable selection, should be repeated for each bootstrap sample. The mean (over all bootstrap samples) difference between the two measures (e.g., the AUC) quantifies the degree of optimism in the measures (e.g. of discrimination) derived using self-testing on the original dataset. For example, Marchioli *et al.* (2001) derived a risk score for death, within 4 years, after a myocardial infarction. From a basic analysis, quantifying discrimination within the dataset used to develop their risk score, they reported that the score had an AUC of 0.774 for men and 0.786 for women. From 200 bootstrap replications, they found that the mean difference between the AUCs in the bootstrap and original samples was 0.006 for men and 0.027 for women. Thus they concluded that the AUCs, adjusted for optimism, were 0.768 for men and 0.759 for women.

Unfortunately, experience suggests that internal validation underestimates the bias inherent in self-testing when the risk score is used in other populations; for an example see Bleeker *et al.* (2003). Hence, **external validation** is preferable whenever a second, independent cohort is available. External validation can then be performed using the methods described earlier in this chapter, without alteration. The second cohort should have available data with the same prognostic variables, measured in the same way, and the same outcome of interest reported as in the data from the development cohort. Otherwise differences may be due to practical issues rather than over-optimism. For example, in Example 13.5 and elsewhere in this chapter, a risk score for CHD was developed from a Scottish cohort study. A cohort from elsewhere may use a different definition for CHD, involving broader criteria, such as including deaths due to heart failure. Although it may well be reasonable to assume that the risk factors act in the same way for CHD with and without heart failure, it would be expected that the average predicted risk would be higher, all else being equal, in the testing cohort than in the development cohort. Thus calibration tests would be compromised. Furthermore, thresholds used in NRI calculations would require appropriate modification when moving from the development to the testing cohort. Another issue to consider is whether subjects in the testing cohort have been observed for a sufficiently long length of time. For instance, if the risk score to be validated is for disease within 10 years, ideally everyone in the testing cohort should have been entered into the cohort at least 10 years before the date of termination of follow-up. Otherwise, in the case of a fixed cohort (with logistic modelling), we are likely to discover that the score appears to over-estimate 10-year risk even when the score is truly well calibrated within the minimum elapsed time. With Cox models, incomplete follow-up for some will mean that, although the estimated 10-year risk (in the example) may well be unbiased, it will be relatively poorly estimated — the fewer the number who had an elapsed time of 10 years, the greater the sampling error.

Sometimes the testing cohort can be a new cohort within the same setting as the original (development) cohort; for example, Aekplakorn *et al.* (2006) derived a risk score for incident diabetes from an occupational cohort and examined its performance within a second cohort whose subjects were different people employed in the same company, but recruited 13 years after the original cohort. Such external validation is relatively easy for a research team that has ready access to both datasets. It does, however, raise the question of whether the two datasets ought to be combined to improve estimation of the risk model, in much the same way as was discussed for split samples, above. More importantly, when the testing sample is much like the development sample we can only really claim to have performed validation in a specific type of population, such as company employees in the diabetes example. An illustration of a broadly different testing sample is given by Kengne *et al.* (2010) who tested the Framingham CVD risk score, developed in a general population within the US, in a cohort of patients with diabetes, but without CVD, drawn from 20 countries excluding the US. They found that, on average, the Framingham score overestimated risk by a factor of two. As discussed in Section 13.6.4, when external validation fails, often the problem lies with calibration, rather than discrimination, since 'background' risks tend to vary. This can often be fixed by recalibration (see Section 13.6), as was the case for Kengne *et al.* (2010).

13.11 Presentation of risk scores

Once the final risk score has been formulated and approved for use, we need to decide how to present it for convenient use in clinical decision making. An ideal approach is to encapsulate the algorithm into a web-based 'calculator'. Figure 13.24 is an example,

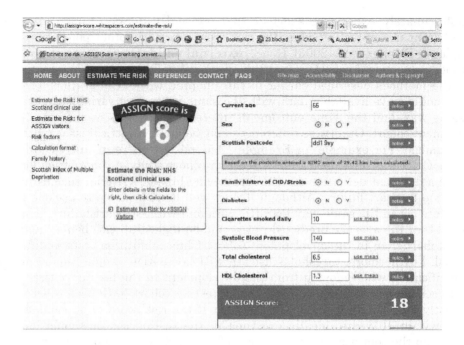

Figure 13.24. On-line risk calculator for the ASSIGN CVD risk score. A user has filled in responses on the right side and the calculator has returned the score (18% chance of a CVD event within the next 10 years) at the bottom, on the right side. Note that the ASSIGN calculator has also returned a 'social deprivation' score of 29.42 based on the postcode (zipcode) that the subject has entered: see Example 10.45.

being a screen dump from the web site for the ASSIGN cardiovascular risk score (http://www.assign-score.com). This score was derived from the Scottish database used in Example 13.1 and in many other places in this book. Such automatic scoring systems are sometimes consolidated within general practitioners' routine information systems, so that a risk score may be immediately viewed during a consultation with a patient, and stored electronically for future comparisons. Similarly, 'apps' can provide instant risk scores from mobile cellular telephones.

For ease of reference and for purposes of education, risk maps (heat maps) or charts can be useful. These are diagrams that allow an approximate risk to be obtained by eye; generally colours are used to indicate grades of risk. An example of a score that is similar to ASSIGN is the European SCORE project, whose risk charts are available from http://www.escardio.org/communities/EACPR/toolbox/health-profes-sionals/Pages/SCORE-Risk-Charts.aspx).

13.11.1 Point scoring

All of the above approaches to risk scoring have the disadvantage that they do not easily show the importance of one risk factor relative to another. This can be remedied by adopting a point scoring algorithm. This allocates points to each level of each risk factor in the risk algorithm, for example being aged 50–59 years old might give one 3 risk points, and having diabetes might give one 2 risk points. Points are summed and then converted to an approximate risk score using a standard look-up table. Assuming integer scores are used, this gives a very simple arithmetic procedure which anyone can use in the absence of an electronic aid.

In Section 10.3, the concept of a linear predictor was introduced. The point scoring approach uses the fact that all standard risk scores are ultimately a transformation of the linear predictor $\Sigma b_i x_i$ where $\{b_i\}$ are the regression parameters (the estimated beta coefficients) and $\{x_i\}$ are the prognostic variables (e.g., age, sex, smoking, etc.) in the risk score. By simple algebra and approximation, each $\Sigma b_i x_i$ combination is made into an integer, leaving the user to do the summation and then look up the risk corresponding to whatever total is obtained. Before formalising the approach, we first shall explore the methodology through three artificial examples.

Example 13.23 Suppose that our risk score has just two binary variables, sex and smoking. A logistic regression model has been fitted and the resulting logit is:

$$-5.6 + 2.5 \times \text{sex} + 1.3 \times \text{smoking}, \tag{13.30}$$

where sex = 1 for men and 0 for women, and smoking = 1 for smokers and 0 for non-smokers. We can think of sex as being the first risk factor (with symbol x_1) and smoking (x_2) as the second. Then the $b \times x$ 'regression units' are $b_1 x_1 = 2.5 \times 1 = 2.5$ for men and $2.5 \times 0 = 0$ for women, and $b_2 x_2 = 1.3 \times 1 = 1.3$ for smokers and $1.3 \times 0 = 0$ for non-smokers.

The first step in generating point scores is to choose a standard number of regression units to serve as a scaling factor; denote this as s. Suppose we choose this to be the regression units for smoking; then s is the bx product for smokers, which is 1.3. Hence we continue by dividing all other bx products by 1.3. The resulting scaled bx values are 2.5/1.3, 0, 1, 0 when taking terms in the same order as above. The final step is to round these values to the nearest integer: here the only term requiring rounding is 2.5/1.3 = 1.92, which is rounded up to 2. This gives points (for risk) of 2, 0, 1, 0 to male sex, female sex, smoking and non-smoking, respectively. Notice that this shows that being male confers about twice the risk as does smoking.

Having obtained these points for each personal trait, we need to consider what the estimated risk will consequently be for every possible combination of traits. In this simple example there are only four possible combinations: female non-smokers (with 0 points), female smokers (with 1 point), male non-smokers (with 2 points) and male smokers (with 3 points). Before we deal with these point totals, consider how to estimate the arithmetically exact risks. This is done using (10.8),

$$\left\{ 1 + \exp\left(-\left(b_0 + \sum_{i=1}^{k} b_i x_i \right) \right) \right\}^{-1},$$

where b_0 is the intercept, which is -5.6 in (13.30), and k predictors are involved (in this example $k = 2$). For example, for male non-smokers the arithmetically exact risk is, from using (10.8) in combination with (13.30),

$$\{1 + \exp(-(-5.6 + 2.5 \times 1 + 1.3 \times 0))\}^{-1} = 0.0431.$$

The equivalent calculation using point totals replaces the Σbx component with the point total, after scaling back up by the number of standard regression units. If we call the point total P, then the approximate risk is

$$\{1 + \exp(-(b_0 + Ps))\}^{-1}.$$

For male non-smokers, where the point total is 2, the approximate risk is thus:

$$\{1 + \exp(-(-5.6 + 2 \times 1.3))\}^{-1} = 0.0474.$$

Table 13.18 shows all the exact and approximate (point scoring) results. Results for women are the same using the two methods, of necessity since Σbx and Ps are the same for female

Table 13.18. Exact and point scoring estimates of risk for Example 13.23.

	Exact method					Point scoring method			
	x_1	b_1	x_2	b_2	$\Sigma b_i x_i$	Risk	Sex pts.	Smoke pts.	Total pts. (P)	Risk
Female, non-smoker	0	2.1	0	1.3	0	0.0037	0	0	0	0.0037
Female, smoker	0	2.1	1	1.3	1.3	0.0134	0	1	1	0.0134
Male, non-smoker	1	2.1	0	1.3	1.8	0.0431	2	0	2	0.0474
Male, smoker	1	2.1	1	1.3	3.1	0.1419	2	1	3	0.1545

non-smokers and smokers, but the point scoring system slightly over-estimates the risk amongst men, since the male regression units were rounded up in the determination of points. Some error is inevitable in point scoring; the magnitude of error will generally decrease as more risk factors are added to the prognostic model.

Example 13.24 The last example only had binary variables. Now we consider a hypothetical case where there is one binary variable, sex, and a categorical variable, age, which was divided, before model fitting, into four ordinal 10-year age groups. Suppose, this time, that a Cox model was fitted to the data and produced the estimates shown in Table 13.19. Note that the reference groups are females and those aged 40–49 years. Since a Cox model was used, by reference to (13.4), we shall need to know the mean values of each risk factor in order to derive the risks. Age can be represented as a set of four dummy variables (see Section 9.2.6). The mean of the dummy variable for each age group is the proportion of people in that specific age group. Similarly, the mean for sex is the proportion of men. In Table 13.19 these proportions are shown, although the base levels have been omitted as they will not contribute to further calculations (these base levels will also be omitted from computer output when the Cox model is fitted). To use (13.4) we also need to know the cumulative survival, over whatever time period (say, 12 years) we wish to use in our clinical decision rule, for an 'average' person. Suppose that the KM estimate of survival to 12 years for someone with the mean values of each prognostic variable, $S(12, \bar{x})$, in the dataset is 0.98.

For the purpose of illustration, we shall start by estimating risks using the arithmetically exact method. The risk is, from (13.4),

$$1 - S(12, \bar{x})^z$$

where

$$z = \exp(w) \quad \text{and} \quad w = \sum_i b_i x_i - \sum_i b_i \bar{x}_i.$$

From Table 13.19, $\sum_i b_i \bar{x}_i = 0.7 \times 0.25 + 2.1 \times 0.25 + 3.1 \times 0.20 + 1.8 \times 0.48 = 2.184$.

For example, for a 50- to 59-year-old man,

$$z = \exp(0.7 \times 1 + 1.8 \times 1 - 2.184) = \exp(0.316) = 1.37163,$$

and hence the estimated risk is

$$\hat{p} = 1 - 0.98^{1.37163} = 0.0273.$$

Notice that all the x values in the calculation of w will be 1 or 0 when the fitted terms in the model are all dummy variables. Besides the x values corresponding to the index person (in the

Table 13.19. Fitted estimates from a Cox model and the proportion in each risk group for Example 13.24.

Term	Estimated beta coefficient (b)	Proportion in sample
Age 50–59 years	0.7	0.25
Age 60–69 years	2.1	0.25
Age 70–79 years	3.1	0.20
Male sex	1.8	0.48

Table 13.20. Exact 12-year predicted risks in Example 13.24.

Sex	Age (yrs)	Σbx	w	0.98^w	Risk
Female	40–49	0	−2.184	0.997728	0.0023
Female	50–59	0.7	−1.484	0.995430	0.0046
Female	60–69	2.1	−0.084	0.981596	0.0184
Female	70–79	3.1	0.916	0.950761	0.0492
Male	40–49	1.8	−0.384	0.986334	0.0137
Male	50–59	2.5	0.316	0.972670	0.0273
Male	60–69	3.9	1.716	0.893712	0.1063
Male	70–79	4.9	2.716	0.736785	0.2632

specific example, those for age 50–59 years and the male sex), all other terms in Σbx will correspond to x values of zero and thus can make no contribution to w. Continuing in this way gives all the exact predicted risks in Table 13.20; we shall use this to make comparisons with the point scoring method subsequently.

To make a points algorithm here we will arbitrarily choose the number of regression units for male sex to have unit size. That is, we shall scale the results by dividing by the product of b and x for male sex before rounding. Sex must thus confer 0 points for women and 1 for men. For age, 40–49 years has 0 points, since it is the reference group. For age 50–59 we compute, from Table 13.19, 0.7/1.8 = 0.3888 and round to the nearest integer, which is zero. Continuing in this way gives points to successive age groups of 0, 0, 1 and 2. In the point totalling approach, the effect of being male and of being aged 60–69 years is thus the same. Bearing in mind the approximate nature of the methodology, this should be interpreted as the impact, on 12-year risk, of being male being roughly equal to that of being aged 60–69 years. Finally we can now see that the points allocated to the six possible types of person listed in Table 13.20, in order, must be 0, 0, 1, 2, 1, 1, 2 and 3 (see the first few columns of Table 13.21).

We now have the points system worked out, but for this to be useful we need a look-up table of corresponding risks (which will be approximations to the exact predicted values). To get any single approximate risk we need to consider how, within the limits of rounding, we can convert total points back to an approximation for $\Sigma b_i x_i$ and substitute into (13.4). As in Example 13.23, this requires us to multiply the point total by the scaling factor we used (the raw regression units for male sex, 1.8) and use this in place of Σbx in the calculations. Otherwise, we proceed as for the exact risks. For example, for a man aged 50–59 years, the point total is 1 and s is 1.8 and so Σbx is approximated by 1.8. The approximate risk is thus:

$$1 - S(12, \bar{x})^z \text{ where } z = \exp(1.8 - v) \text{ and } v = \sum_i b_i \bar{x}_i.$$

We already know that $S(12, \bar{x}) = 0.98$ and $v = 2.184$. Thus $z = \exp(1.8 - 2.184) = 0.6811$, and the approximate risk is $1 - 0.98^{0.6811} = 0.0137$. Table 13.21 shows the complete set of approximate risks for each possible type of person. Naturally the risks are the same for any combination of age and sex values that share a common point total. In practice, the look-up table would only be provided in terms of total points, rather than for each type of person (see Table 13.24 and Table 13.25 for examples).

It is clear from Example 13.24 that some risks can be poorly estimated using a points system, whilst the true differences in risk between types of person are sometimes lost. As noted before, such problems are less likely when several prognostic factors are involved, rather than the two risk factors in this example.

Table 13.21. Approximate 12-year risks using a points system in Example 13.24.

Sex	Age (yrs)	Sex points	Age points	Total points	Est(Σbx)[a]	w	0.98^w	Risk
Female	40–49	0	0	0	0	−2.184	0.997728	0.0023
Female	50–59	0	0	0	0	−2.184	0.997728	0.0023
Female	60–69	0	1	1	1.8	−0.384	0.986334	0.0137
Female	70–79	0	2	2	3.6	1.416	0.920124	0.0799
Male	40–49	1	0	1	1.8	−0.384	0.986334	0.0137
Male	50–59	1	0	1	1.8	−0.384	0.986334	0.0137
Male	60–69	1	1	2	3.6	1.416	0.920124	0.0799
Male	70–79	1	2	3	5.4	3.216	0.604341	0.3957

[a] Est(Σbx) is the estimated sum of regression units (denoted by Ps when using the notation of Example 13.23).

Table 13.22. Fitted estimates from a Cox model and means for
Example 13.25.

Term	Estimated beta coefficient (b)	Mean in sample
Age (per year)	0.107	54.63
Male sex	1.8	0.48

Example 13.25 Sometimes a continuous variable is left in its continuous form in the risk score
and yet we would like to allocate points according to standard intervals or according to groups
that are considered importantly clinically distinct. For example, suppose that the model of the
last example was fitted, instead, with age as a continuous risk factor (i.e., assuming a log linear
increase in the hazard with age). The table of estimates and means corresponding to Table
13.19 is Table 13.22. The estimated beta coefficient for age is the log hazard ratio for a unit
(i.e., 1 year) increase in age. The mean age in the sample replaces the mean for the dummy
variables representing age (i.e., the proportions) in Table 13.19.

Supposing that 10-year age groups are to be used for point scoring, we proceed by constructing artificial regression units for each 10-year group. First, we pick a reference group; 40–49
years seems a reasonable choice (as in the last example). The centre of this can be approximated
by the mid-range, 45 years, and we will assume this as the value of concentration of the risk
inherent to this group. If we then take similar mid-ranges to represent the risk concentration
for the other three groups, that is, 55, 65 and 75 years, we want the regression units for each
of the other three groups, relative to the zero units that will now be fixed in the 40–49 year
group, to be those for an increase of 10, 20 and 30 years of age. From Table 13.22 we can see
that the beta coefficients for such increases will be predicted to be 0.107×10 for the 50–59
year group, 0.017×20 for the 60–69 year group and 0.107×30 for the 70–79 year group.
Finally, to get the points for each term, as before, we choose a suitable standard for the
regression units. In many cases, age is a strong risk factor and it can be helpful to phrase the
risk contributions from other factors in terms of easily-understood age equivalents. Here we
shall take the regression units for 5 years of age as the standard (that is, everything else will
be expressed in risk units of ageing 5 years). From Table 13.22, this requires dividing each
regression unit by $5 \times 0.107 = 0.535$. Results appear in Table 13.23; for instance, being male
is approximately equivalent to $3 \times 5 = 15$ extra years of age, in terms of risk. Note that the
reference groups have been included in this table to help understanding, although they will
make no contribution to the individual point scores.

Table 13.23. Points system derived from the Cox model in Example 13.25.

Term	Value of concentration (c)	Estimated beta coeff. (b)*	$c -$ reference (d)	$(b) \times (d)$	Points**
Age 40–49	45 (reference)	0.107	0	0	0
Age 50–59	55	0.107	10	1.07	2
Age 60–69	65	0.107	20	2.14	4
Age 70–79	75	0.107	30	3.21	6
Female sex	0 (reference)	0	0	0	0
Male sex	1	1	1	1.8	3

* From Table 13.22.
** Previous column divided by the scaling factor, 0.535, rounded to the nearest integer.

Table 13.24. Points converted to
approximate 12-year risk for
Example 13.25.

Points	Risk
0	0.0049
2	0.0142
3	0.0241
4	0.0407
5	0.0685
6	0.1142
7	0.1870
9	0.4530

To interpret the point total for any individual we now need to derive a look-up table for (approximate) risk. To do this, as in Example 13.24, we use (13.4) but with Σbx replaced by its approximation. In this case, we not only have to back-multiply the point total by 0.535 but also to add back the contribution, to the sum of cross-products, Σbx, of the reference group (centred on 45 years) that we arbitrarily constructed (for age). Suppose that 12-year predictions are to be made, and that the 'average' 12-year survival is 0.968. The approximate risk corresponding to a point total of P is thus:

$$1 - 0.968^z \text{ where } z = \exp(0.535 \times P + 0.107 \times 45 - v) \text{ and, as before, } v = \sum_i b_i \bar{x}_i.$$

From Table 13.22,

$$v = 0.107 \times 54.63 + 1.8 \times 0.48 = 6.70941.$$

Thus,

$$z = \exp(0.535 \times P + 4.815 - 6.70941).$$

For example, a 53-year-old man would get a points score of $2 + 3 = 5$. Hence, for him,

$$z = \exp(0.535 \times 5 + 4.815 - 6.70941) = 2.18276.$$

The approximate 12-year risk for this man is thus $1 - 0.968^{2.18276} = 0.0685$. Table 13.24 shows the complete set of approximate risks for each possible point total.

As in the other examples in this section, it is of interest to compare these approximate risks to the exact predictions from the model. For a 53-year-old man, (13.4) gives the arithmetically exact risk as

$$1 - 0.968^{\exp(0.107 \times 53 + 1.8 \times 1 - 6.70941)} = 0.0673.$$

The approximate answer (0.0685) is very close to this.

To provide a general approach to that used in the last three examples, it is necessary to consider how the logistic and Cox models utilise the linear predictor, $L = \sum_i b_i x_i$. To give a general account here, L will be taken to exclude the intercept term, b_0, for logistic regression models (Cox models do not have an intercept). Using (10.8), as discussed in Section 13.3.1, and (13.4), as discussed in Section 13.3.3, the predicted risks under the logistic and Cox models are, respectively,

$$\{1 + \exp(-(b_0 + L))\}^{-1}$$

and

$$1 - S(t,\overline{x})^{\exp(L - \Sigma b\overline{x})} .$$

As our three examples have shown, the point scoring system approximates L by a function of the appropriate point total. Whilst deriving points for each personal trait (e.g., male sex) is straightforward, the back-calculation to convert point totals into (approximate) risk predictions is relatively complex. Following the applied logic of the examples, a general recipe for deriving approximate risks is to replace L by its approximation,

$$\tilde{L} = sP + \sum_{j=1}^{m} b_j c_j, \tag{13.31}$$

in the appropriate risk formula, such as those above based on (10.8) and (13.4). Here, s is the scaling factor, P is the point total, m is the number of continuous variables that have been converted to categories (in Example 13.25, $m = 1$) and c_j is the value of concentration of risk in the reference group for the jth of these variables (in Example 13.25 there was a single c, for age, of 45 years). Although this chapter is restricted to logistic and Cox models, (13.31) can be used with other regression models, such as Poisson and Weibull models, that involve linear predictors, should these be suitable models for the study data.

We shall complete this account by constructing a point scoring algorithm for the real data used in Example 13.7.

Example 13.26 In Example 13.7 the fitted model, (13.6), was:

$$\hat{p} = 1 - 0.97648^{\exp(0.29483\,(\text{TOTOCHOL}) + 0.02186(\text{ SYSTOL}) + 0.32380(\text{ex}) + 0.65894(\text{current}) - 5.21247)}.$$

Note that a Cox regression model was employed to estimate the hazard ratios for CHD and that total cholesterol (TOTCHOL) and systolic blood pressure (SYSTOL) were fitted as continuous variables and smoking status was fitted using dummy variables with never smoking as the reference group. Suppose that we wish to have a risk algorithm with grouped continuous variables; then the first question is how to group blood pressure and cholesterol. A good choice would be to use national guidelines: US national guidelines (at the time of writing) suggest the groupings (with textural interpretation) given in Table 13.25. Within each of these groups we need to decide upon the value of concentration of risk, c. As in the situations met in Section 3.6.2 and Section10.7.5, here we shall assume that the median in each group is a reasonable representation of c. Using the data supplied with the web site for this book (attributed to Example 10.12 in Appendix A), the medians corresponding to the first seven rows of Table 13.25 are 113, 129, 147 and 169 mmHg, and 4.79, 5.77 and 7.00 mmol/l. Next, we need to choose the reference groups for each variable. We shall take those with the lowest blood pressure, lowest cholesterol and those who never smoked, respectively. Finally, we must decide what to use as the standard measure of risk; i.e., the standard number of regression units, s. We will take the regression units for a 5 mmHg increase in systolic blood pressure as the scaling factor; i.e., $s = 5 \times 0.02186 = 0.1093$.

This time, all the working calculations have been suppressed and Table 13.25 only shows the results that would be used in practice, should the risk scoring model of Example 13.7 be accepted for clinical use in this simplified form. We see that, for example, being in the pre-hypertensive stage, having borderline high cholesterol and being an ex-smoker all confer the same risk, at least in approximate terms.

Table 13.25. Point scoring algorithm for Example 13.26.

Risk factor	Category	Range	Points
Systolic blood pressure (mmHg)	Normal	<120	0
	Pre-hypertension	120–139	3
	Hypertension stage I	140–159	7
	Hypertension stage II	160+	11
Serum total cholesterol (mmol/l)*	Desirable	<5.17	0
	Borderline high	5.17–6.20	3
	High	>6.20	6
Smoking	Never smoked		0
	Ex-smoker		3
	Current smoker		6

* Converted from mg/ml (in the US guidelines) using the division factor of 38.67.

To use the information in Table 13.25 in clinical decision making, we need to compute the approximate risks for all possible point totals. Expressed in terms of the linear predictor, L, (13.4) gives the risk as

$$\hat{p} = 1 - 0.97648^{\exp(L - 5.21247)}.$$

This is then used to compute the approximate risks using (13.31), which here has the form

$$\tilde{L} = 0.1093 \times P + 0.02186 \times 113 + 0.29483 \times 4.79$$
$$= 0.1093 \times P + 3.8824157$$

for any point total, P. For example, when $P = 7$, $\tilde{L} = 4.647516$ and the approximate risk is $1 - 0.97648^{0.568386} = 0.0134$. Figure 13.25 gives a complete package for the risk scoring process, suitable for use in practice, which combines the key information from Table 13.25 and the 'look up' table of predicted risks. Notice that the risks have been converted to percentages, to make the presentation, and interpretation, easier.

For an example of the use of Figure 13.25, suppose that a General Practitioner (GP) is consulted by a man who is an ex-smoker with a SBP of 150 mmHg and a TC of 6.1 mmol/l. The GP could use Figure 13.25 to get her patient's point total of 13 and then find the corresponding predicted risk of 2.57% (or 0.0257). She, thus, might tell the patient that his chance of getting a heart attack in the next 5 years is roughly two and a half percent.

For our own satisfaction, and to check that the approximation procedure is robust, it is helpful, as in other examples, to compare the approximate and arithmetically exact predictions. For instance, using (13.4) gives a prediction of 0.0275 for the patient mentioned above. In this case, the approximate and exact predictions are not importantly different.

Evidently, the process of setting up the point scoring scheme can be quite tedious, but then the resultant risk algorithm is extremely easy to use. A second, and more important disadvantage is quite obvious — the results are approximations. We may prefer an exact method, for instance using a web-based calculator. A further drawback arises when a continuous variable is grouped, as in the last two examples, since alternative choices of grouping thresholds, reference group and scaling factor can give different estimates of risk for the same person. Further details of the methodology, and other examples, are given by Sullivan et al. (2004).

Step 1

Systolic blood pressure (mmHg)	Points
<120	0
120–139	3
140–159	7
160+	11

Step 2

Total cholesterol (mmol/l)	Points
<5.17	0
5.17–6.20	3
>6.20	6

Step 3

Smoking	Points
Never	0
Previously	3
Currently	6

Step 4

Sum up points from steps 1 to 3

Step 5

Look up predicted 5-year

% risk of CHD in the table

Point total	Risk (%)
0	0.63
3	0.87
6	1.21
7	1.34
9	1.67
10	1.86
11	2.07
12	2.31
13	2.57
14	2.87
15	3.19
16	3.55
17	3.96
19	4.90
20	5.45
23	7.48

Figure 13.25. Risk scoring algorithm for Example 13.26.

13.12 Impact studies

A clinical decision rule is an important vehicle for the translation of epidemiological research into clinical practice. However, for widespread adoption, not only does the underlying risk score have to have satisfactory statistical qualities, of which the most crucial is validated evidence of good discrimination, but the rule has to be demonstrated to be useful in practice.

To this end, **impact studies** are necessary, where the utility of a decision rule is tested in real life (as described in Moons *et al.*, 2012a). This might simply involve testing physicians' acceptance of a risk score for use during patient contacts, the ease of capturing information on certain risk factors included in the score during clinic appointments or the ability of existing health care computer systems to deal with the information required, and the result returned, by the risk score. However, such studies are limited because they lack a control group. The cluster randomised trial design (see Section 7.4.2), where, for instance, health care centres are randomised to either apply the clinical decision rule to their patients or to continue with usual care, is particularly useful for an impact study. Usual care here would typically involve subjective assessments of risk based on the doctor's knowledge and experience. In this example, the cluster design is better because it 'isolates' doctors (and other health care providers) and patients using the two separate protocols. This lessens the chance of 'contamination' of those allocated to control (usual care), compared to a standard randomised controlled trial in which patients are randomised. Contamination might occur through a learning effect of experience with the risk score amongst doctors who have patients allocated to both protocols, or by contact between patients in the same health centre who are allocated to different protocols. The end-points analysed could include both between-patient variables, such as change in health status and satisfaction with care, and between-doctor variables, such as a comparison of objective (from the risk score) and subjective (usual care) predictions of patients' outcomes.

Exercises

(These exercises require the use of a computer package with appropriate procedures.)

13.1 The web site for this book contains data from the PROGRESS study (see Appendix A for details). PROGRESS was a clinical trial of blood pressure lowering following a stroke or transient ischaemic attack (MacMahon *et al.*, 2001). Fit logistic regression models to find the "best" model, using the Akaike Information Criterion (AIC), Bayesian Information Criterion (BIC) and -2 log likelihood statistics, to predict stroke from a selection of the explanatory variables age, body mass index, systolic blood pressure (SBP), diastolic blood pressure, sodium, creatinine and Barthel score. Consider the discrimination and calibration (with 10 groups, where possible) of the models you have chosen, and contrast the changes between models with the corresponding changes in the AIC and BIC.

13.2 One particular choice of "best" model in Exercise 13.1 would be that which only includes variables that are significant ($p < 0.05$) predictors in the presence of other variables. This should turn out to be the model with age, SBP, creatinine and Barthel score. Taking this as the base model, add each of the six pairwise interaction terms between age, SBP, creatinine and Barthel score, in turn. Show that the age*SBP interaction is the only one that is significant ($p < 0.05$) after adjustment for the four main effects above. The extended model will then be defined as age*SBP added to the base model.

    (i)   Evaluate the extended model for discrimination, through the area under the receiver operating characteristic curve (AUC), and test for (grouped) calibration. Compare these results, descriptively, with those for the other models you have fitted for this exercise.

    (ii) Write out the formula for the risk scores derived from both the extended model and the base model.

(iii) Draw ROC curves for the two risk scores on the same graph and comment upon them.

(iv) Test the null hypothesis that the AUCs for these two risk scores are equal, using a two-sided test.

(v) Compute the IDI and its 95% confidence interval, comparing the two risk scores. Test the null hypothesis that the IDI is zero.

(vi) Compute the RIDI.

(vii) Subjects in PROGRESS were followed for roughly 4 years, on average. Suppose that 4-year risks of 10% and 15% are thought to be meaningful clinical decision thresholds for recurrent stroke. Grouping according to these risk thresholds, cross-tabulate the base score against the extended score, separately for stoke cases and non-cases.

(viii) From this table, find how many cases were correctly, and how many were incorrectly, reclassified when moving from the base score to the extended score. Find corresponding numbers for the non-cases. Covert these numbers to net proportions correctly reclassified; add them together to get the NRI.

(ix) Compute the 95% confidence interval for the NRI. Test the null hypothesis that the NRI is zero, and the equivalent tests for null reclassification of cases and non-cases.

(x) Compute the continuous (threshold-free) NRI and its 95% confidence interval. Test the null hypothesis that the continuous NRI is zero.

(xi) What is the net percentage of cases of stroke, and the net percentage of non-cases, that was correctly reclassified when moving from the base score to the extended score, using the criteria of the continuous NRI? Test, in turn, that each of these percentages is zero.

(xii) Which risk score is most appropriate for clinical use: the base or the extended? Why?

13.3 The age*Barthel score interaction should have been found to be almost significant ($0.05 < p < 0.06$) in Exercise 13.2. Add this term to the chosen model (of Exercise 13.2) and consequently see if it improves fit in any important way, including:

(i) Make informal comparisons of the AIC and BIC metrics.

(ii) Write down the AUC, and its corresponding 95% confidence interval, for risk scores derived from each of the two models: the base, without age*Barthel, and the new, with age*Barthel. Test the null hypothesis that the AUCs are equal.

(iii) Compute Brier scores for both risk scores.

(iv) Compute Spiegelhalter tests of overall calibration for the risk scores produced from each of the two models.

(v) Compute Redelmeier's test of equal Brier scores.

(vi) Compute the IDI and 95% confidence interval comparing the two scores. Test the null hypothesis of zero improvement in risk scoring.

(vii) Compute the NRI, using the risk thresholds of Exercise 13.2, and 95% confidence interval. Test the null hypotheses of zero NRI.

(viii) Compute the continuous (threshold-free) NRI and 95% confidence interval. Test the null hypotheses of zero continuous NRI.

(ix) Decide whether the new risk score is better than the base.

13.4 Fit any further models that you think should be considered before settling upon a risk score. Assuming this leads to taking the model of Exercise 13.2 (four main effects plus one interaction) as the chosen model for the risk score:

(i) Draw the calibration plot using tenths of predicted risk.

(ii) Test for mean calibration.

(iii) Draw boxplots for the risk score amongst those with and without a stroke event during follow-up.

(iv) Estimate discrimination through the standardised mean effect size. Compute the g statistic and its 95% confidence interval, applied to the logits of the risk score. Compare this result for g with those for the risk scores evaluated in Section 13.4.4. Does the degree of discrimination suggested by g agree with that of the c statistic found in Exercise 13.2?

13.5 For the lung cancer data of Exercise 11.10 we found the best Cox model to be that with education and tumour status.

(i) Write down the risk score for death within 6 months corresponding to this best Cox model.

(ii) Evaluate the discrimination of this risk score by finding the c-statistic (taking account of censoring) and its 95% confidence interval.

(iii) Find the g statistic and its 95% confidence interval.

(iv) Compare the observed risk of death within 6 months and the mean predicted risk according to the risk score.

(v) Divide the predicted risks into four ordinal groups of (as near as possible) equal size. Tabulate the observed and predicted 6-month risks across these four groups and test the calibration of the risk score through use of the Hosmer–Lemeshow test.

(vi) Carry out Spiegelhalter's test of overall calibration.

(vii) Compute the Brier score for this risk score.

(viii) Construct a point scoring system, taking the risk due to illiteracy as the scaling factor. Show the point allocation table and the risk 'look-up' table.

(ix) From the points system, how does the extra risk due to having a regional, rather than a local, tumour compare to the risk due to illiteracy?

(x) Compare the (approximate) risk distribution using the point system to the numerically exact risks from the Cox model.

(xi) Do you consider that this risk score (using the Cox model exactly or the point system) should be acceptable for clinical use?

13.6 The risk score for CHD used in Example 13.7, and elsewhere in this chapter, is unusual in practice, because it fails to include age which is a major determinant of coronary risk. The choice of the three prognostic variables total cholesterol (TOTCHOL), systolic blood pressure (SYSTOL) and smoking (ex- and current versus never) is based on the findings of Example 10.15. To investigate whether age should be included in the risk score from these data:

(i) Fit Cox models to the predictor set including age, TOTCHOL, SYSTOL and smoking, and write down the corresponding risk score for a CHD event within 5 years (1827 days).

(ii) Compute the IDI for survival data to compare the risk score (13.6) with that of (i), so as to quantify the degree of appropriate reclassification achieved by adding age to the existing 'best' risk score for these data. Since measuring age has no real practical issues, two-sided tests may reasonably be used here.

(iii) Do the same as in (ii) but for the NRI with no threshold, and then with the thresholds of 0.05 and 0.1 (as used in Example 13.20). In each case, also state the percentage of CHD events and the percentage of non-events correctly reclassified.

(iv) Repeat (i)–(iii) for the model and risk score which has the variables age, TOTCHOL and SYSTOL, to compare, again, with (13.6).

(v)   What do you conclude?

(vi) Regardless of your conclusion in (v), construct a points scoring system for the risk score with age, TOTCHOL, SYSTOL and smoking. Divide age into four 5-year groups, defining the first group as the reference; otherwise use the groups defined by Table 13.25. Assume that the points of concentration of risk are the mid-points (42.5 years, etc.) for age, and as in Example 13.26 otherwise. Take the additional risk incurred from 5 extra years of age as the scaling factor.

(vii) To check your point scores, compute and compare the true and approximate (point score) risks of coronary disease within 5 years for a 53-year-old man who is an ex-smoker with a SBP of 150 mmHg and a cholesterol level of 6.1 mmol/l. Why are both results higher than that evaluated for the same person in Exercise 13.26?

13.7 A research team publishes a risk score which uses age, systolic blood pressure (SBP), smoking (current versus non-current) and physical activity (inactive versus some activity) to predict CHD within 4 years amongst people currently fee of CHD. Their risk score (i.e., the predicted risk of CHD within 4 years), for men, is:

$$1/\{1+\exp(8.5 - 0.04(\text{age}) - 0.02(\text{SBP}) - 0.44(\text{smoke}) - 0.09(\text{PA}))\},$$

where age is in years, SBP is in mmHg, smoke is 1 if currently smoking and 0 otherwise, and PA is 1 if physically active and 0 otherwise.

(i)   By producing a calibration plot and carrying out a Hosmer–Lemeshow (HL) test with 10 groups, decide whether this score is well calibrated for use in the SHHS data which was utilised in Exercise 13.6.

(ii) Carry out Cox's test for lack of calibration.

(iii) Recalibrate the score using intercept recalibration, writing down the revised risk score. Carry out the HL test.

(iv) Recalibrate the score using logistic recalibration, writing down the revised risk score. Carry out the HL test.

(v)   Plot the original, intercept recalibrated and logistic recalibrated scores on the same calibration plot.

(vi) Which of the three scores best calibrates?

(vii) Recalibrate the score using mean recalibration. Tabulate this, using the same 10 groups as for the HL tests above, together with the intercept recalibration, and thus demonstrate their similarity.

13.8 Suppose that another research team, using a different database, produces a similar score to that in Exercise 13.7 but with different coefficients:

$$1/\{1+\exp(7.3 - 0.02(\text{age}) - 0.17(\text{SBP}) - 0.37(\text{smoke}) - 0.06(\text{PA}))\}.$$

(i)   Using the SHHS data again, produce a calibration plot for this score, together with the intercept recalibrated and logistic recalibrated scores.

(ii) Carry out HL tests for all three scores.

(iii) Which score of the three best calibrates?

CHAPTER 14

Computer-intensive methods

14.1   Rationale

The results of any epidemiological study are limited both by the data that are available and, on the face of it, the existence of a mathematical approach to solving the problem that the data are desired to address. In this final chapter of the book we shall consider three approaches to generating 'quasi-data' that use the observed data to construct data that could have been found under similar conditions. This approach offers relief from the mathematical constraints of classical statistics and allows for an extended range of inferences. In each case this is achieved through exploitation of the immense computational power and speed of modern computers. These three approaches are:

- The bootstrap, which is ideally suited for problems of estimation – precisely, expressions of confidence intervals (CIs). This is covered in Section 14.2 to Section 14.7.
- Permutation tests, which involve a non-parametric approach to hypothesis testing. This is covered in Section 14.8.
- Multiple imputation, which is a powerful method for dealing with missing values. The main issues involved with missing values are introduced in Section 14.9; some simple methods for imputation are described in Section 14.10; multiple imputation is the topic of Section 14.11 and Section 14.12; and concluding comments appear in Section 14.13.

Although this is our current scope, it is appropriate to mention that several other computer-intensive methods are also used in epidemiological research. Also, what qualifies as 'computer-intensive' is sure to vary with time. Indeed, some of the methods met in earlier chapters, such as generalised linear and Cox regression models, would not be of practical use without the aid of a computer. The expression seems to have been coined by Bradley Efron, the inventor of the bootstrap (Efron, 1979), and this is where we will start.

14.2   The bootstrap

In this book, whenever estimates are given, the corresponding CI — or, sometimes just the standard error (SE) — is routinely given. This is essential to express the amount of uncertainty we have in our sample-based estimate. In the vast majority of cases, the formulae presented in this book, and elsewhere, depend upon an assumption regarding applicability of the normal distribution, from the simple case of estimating the mean of a continuous variable in Section 2.7.2 to estimating CIs for regression parameters in Chapter 9 to Chapter 11. In real life, *nothing* follows a normal distribution exactly.

Thus, whilst experience, backed up by the Central Limit Theorem (see Section 2.7), has shown that the normal is a robust approximation when the sample size is large, we are left to wonder whether the normal assumption really is reasonable (even after transformation) in any particular case. Furthermore, even when an estimate for a specific parameter is easily obtained, sometimes there is no reliable theoretical formula for the corresponding CI, typically because of lack of a closed formula for the variance of the estimator. Examples include the median, the ratio of two means and the difference between the means of two highly skewed variables (see Section 2.8). Such problems can be solved by using **bootstrap resampling.**

Bootstrapping is one of a number of techniques that come under the general heading of **resampling methods.** The basic idea of resampling methods is to use the single set of sample data that has been collected to create a set of like samples from which the summary statistic of interest can be computed. As the name suggests, this is achieved by resampling within the observed, true, sample. In bootstrapping, this is achieved by randomly sampling with replacement within the sample data so as to achieve a new sample of the same size as the original. Sampling with replacement is essential because the more intuitive style of sampling — that is, without replacing chosen items — will only shuffle the observed data into a different order with no subsequent change in summary statistics, such as the mean or the median. (Re)sampling is done many times (typically thousands); each time the mean value of the summary statistic is found and the consequent set of results gives a basis for estimating the variability of this summary statistic, and consequently a CI. Recall that the Central Limit Theorem invokes ideas of repeat sampling which is untenable in practice (if we could sample extra people, we would simply make our inferences using the larger set of observed data). Bootstrap resampling is a surrogate for such true repeat sampling.

For example, take the sample of data given in Table 2.10, which has $n = 50$. To draw a bootstrap sample we could take 50 identical balls and write unique identifiers on each ball, to represent each of the 50 people in the observed dataset. We would then put the balls in a container and start the sampling process by drawing one ball out at random. This ball is then replaced into the container and is thus a potential draw when the second ball is chosen. Continuing in this way, 50 balls are drawn in sequence; each time the number drawn is recorded and the corresponding ball is replaced into the container. Interpreting the numbers as unique identifiers for subjects, the result is a sample in which we can expect that some people are included more than once and thus, conversely, some people are not included at all. Figure 14.1 illustrates the selection of a set of 10 000 bootstrap samples from Table 2.10. Of course, in real life we are not going to draw balls 10 000 times; instead, we will get a computer to do the work for us. Sophisticated statistical computer packages, such as Stata, have built-in bootstrap commands whilst others, such as Excel and SAS, have the basic programming capabilities to allow the user to draw her or his own bootstrap samples.

The underlying assumption in a bootstrap process is that each bootstrap sample is a valid representation of a sample (of the index size; 50 in the example) that could have been taken from the parent population. The replacement process implicitly assumes that each person in the observed data represents a certain type of person in the population at large; since there are conceivably several people of any one type in the population, a random sample should have the possibility of including more than one of each type. Bootstrapping thus represents the repeated sampling artifact that is the basis of statistical inference, for example the interpretation of CIs, as introduced in Section 2.5.2. Thus, it gives an alternative to the classical methods for estimation which are based on normal distributions, or distributions, such as the t distribution, that are derived from it.

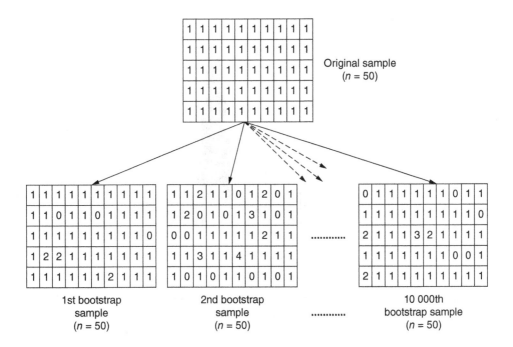

Figure 14.1. Schematic diagram of bootstrap sampling 10 000 times; each cell represents a person with an enumeration of the number of times she or he is included.

In what follows we shall assume that bootstrap samples of the same size as the original population will be drawn; in general, this is not necessary, although it is usual practice.

14.2.1 Bootstrap distributions

Having done bootstrap sampling, we can find the estimates of whatever statistic is of interest (e.g., the mean, median, coefficient of skewness, etc.) from every resample and examine them so as to understand how this statistic is likely to vary if the parent population, from which the observed sample data were taken, could itself be resampled.

Take the data of Table 2.10, and suppose we wish to make inferences about the mean serum total cholesterol. Table 2.12 shows us that the observed mean cholesterol from these data is 6.287 mmol/l. This is our best estimate of the mean for all Scots (the parent population), assuming these are the only data available. Bootstrapping cannot improve on this as the best estimate, but bootstrapping has other important uses. Under the schema of Figure 14.1, the 50 values of cholesterol were resampled 10 000 times; each time the mean of the resample was found. Figure 14.2 shows a histogram for this bootstrap sample of 10 000 means. Here a histogram of the observed data (Figure 2.9 shows the same data, but using broader class limits) is laid over the bootstrap histogram to illustrate that the bootstrap sample distribution of means clusters more tightly than the distribution of the raw data. This is what we expect, since means de-emphasize outliers in data. As explained in Section 2.6.4, the standard deviation (SD) of the mean is the SE and may be calculated as $s/\sqrt{n}$, where s is the SD of the raw data (the spread of the distribution shown with hashed lines in Figure 14.2). Hence, from basic theory, we know that the spread of the sample means is drawn in by a factor of $1/\sqrt{n}$, which is 0.1414 in this case.

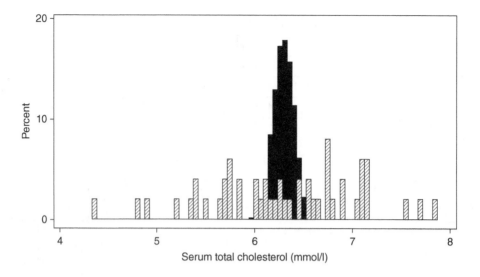

Figure 14.2. The distributions of the values of total cholesterol in the original data of Table 2.10 (hashed bars) and of the means of 10 000 bootstrap resamples from the original cholesterol data (solid bars).

It appears that the centres of the bootstrap and observed distributions are close. We can easily see how close they are by finding the sample mean of the bootstrap distribution: this might be achieved by saving the bootstrap distribution (of means) and using the appropriate command in a computer package to obtain its mean (e.g., the AVERAGE function in Excel). In the bootstrap distribution of size 10 000 created here it was 6.287 mmol/l, exactly the same as for the observed data (to three decimals). We conclude that the bootstrap mean is unbiased for the observed statistic.

Finally, we see that the bootstrap distribution is reasonably close to a normal shape, being fairly symmetric either side of a peak. Figure 14.3 and Figure 14.4 give further evidence for near-normality of the bootstrap distribution of cholesterol means.

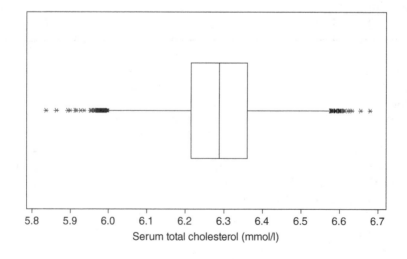

Figure 14.3. Boxplot for the bootstrap sample of 10 000 cholesterol means.

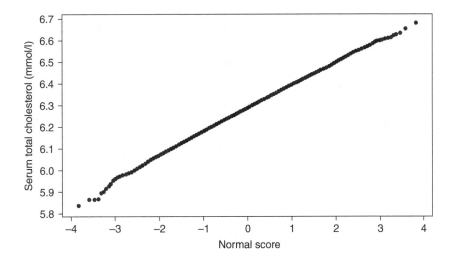

Figure 14.4. Normal plot for the bootstrap sample of 10 000 cholesterol means.

This bootstrapping exercise has justified our use of the normal distribution (or, rather, the t distribution derived from it) to estimate the 95% CI for cholesterol in Chapter 2. That is, it suggests that the sample of size 50 was big enough for near-normality of the distribution of sample means to be achieved in this case. All the same, we can see, perhaps most obviously from Figure 14.4 (where the straight line 'wobbles' in the extremes), that the bootstrap distribution is not exactly normal. Should it be that very precise estimation of the CI is essential, we might still wish to consider bootstrap CIs which do not necessarily require normal distributions, as we shall see.

The top left panel of Figure 14.5 shows the distribution of bootstrap cholesterol means again, but now on a narrower scale. From this, the approximate normality of the means is, again, clear. The other panels in the top row of Figure 14.5 show the corresponding bootstrap distributions for alcohol and cotinine for the data from Table 2.10. Both of these also have shapes that are very much closer to a normal curve than the raw data (see the histogram for alcohol given as Figure 2.10, and the boxplot for cotinine shown in Figure 2.8). The same is true for the other quantitative variables presented in Tables 2.10 and 2.12, which are not shown here to save space. This is as expected from the Central Limit Theorem — and with larger sample sizes the approximation should be better still. Whether the approximation to normality is good enough for the inferences required is still in question, although the histograms for mean alcohol and mean cotinine suggest that, despite worries expressed in Section 2.7 due to skewness of the observed data, use of t distributions will not give wholly inaccurate results.

Of course, the mean is not the only summary statistic that we may wish to estimate. With other statistics we may not be able to rely upon so-called asymptotic (extremely large sample) theoretical results, such as the Central Limit Theorem, to assure us of approximate normality (or, indeed, any other distribution) 'as long as the sample is large enough'. In general, the bootstrap distribution approximates the distribution of sample statistics; that is, the (theoretical) distribution of statistics from repeated samples. The bottom row of Figure 14.5 shows the distributions of the inter-quartile ranges (IQRs) of cholesterol, alcohol and cotinine from the same 10 000 bootstrap resamples as before. None of these approximate the normal shape anything like as

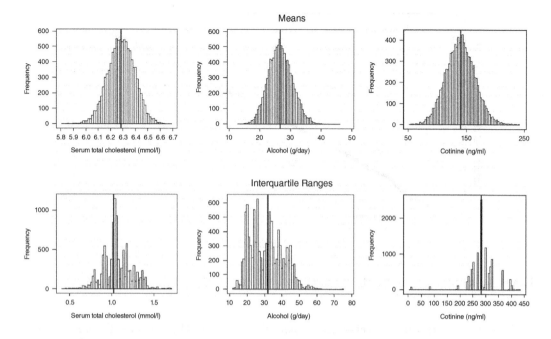

Figure 14.5. Results of 10 000 bootstrap samples of the data in Table 2.10. The top panels show the distributions of the means of the bootstrap samples and the bottom panels show the distributions of the inter-quartile ranges (IQRs). The vertical lines are placed at the observed values of the corresponding statistic (mean or IQR) in the original data (i.e., as shown in Table 2.12).

closely as the corresponding distributions for means. The implications of this are discussed in Section 14.3.1.

14.3   Bootstrap confidence intervals

A number of methods are available for producing bootstrap CIs: see Efron (1987); Efron and Tibshirani (1993); Carpenter and Bithell (2000) and Davison and Hinkley (2006). Here we shall look at four approaches: the first two are intuitive methods and the last has theoretically optimal features. All four are readily available from Stata.

First, we shall need some notation. Suppose that we select b bootstrap samples. From each sample we then compute the required summary statistic of interest (e.g., the mean, median, coefficient of skewness, etc.); call the result from the ith bootstrap sample $\tilde{\theta}_i$. From (2.8), we define the mean of the bootstrap statistics to be

$$\bar{x}_{\text{boot}} = \frac{1}{b}\sum_{1}^{b}\tilde{\theta}_i \,.\tag{14.1}$$

Now define the **bootstrap bias** as

$$\text{Bias} = \bar{x}_{\text{boot}} - \hat{\theta},\tag{14.2}$$

where $\hat{\theta}$ is the point estimate found from the observed data, which is to be derived by standard formulae — as appear throughout this book, for various parameters —

or directly from a computer package. The bootstrap bias is thus the amount by which the bootstrap mean over-estimates the point estimate.

Next, we define the **bootstrap standard error** to be the SD of the bootstrap distribution of the statistic of interest. From (2.10) this is computed as

$$\mathrm{SE}_{\mathrm{boot}}(\hat{\theta}) = \sqrt{\frac{1}{b-1}\sum_{1}^{b}(\tilde{\theta}_i - \bar{x}_{\mathrm{boot}})^2}. \tag{14.3}$$

If our goal is, for example, to find a bootstrap CI for the mean, $\tilde{\theta}_i$ is the mean in (re)sample i and $\bar{x}_{\mathrm{boot}}$ is the mean of the b means. To take one other example, if our goal is to find a bootstrap CI for the IQR, $\tilde{\theta}_i$ is now the IQR in (re)sample i and $\bar{x}_{\mathrm{boot}}$ is the mean of the b IQRs. Whatever the goal, (14.1) and (14.3) can easily be applied by saving the bootstrap distribution of the index statistic and using computer commands (e.g., PROC MEANS in SAS or SUMMARIZE in Stata) which produce means and standard deviations.

14.3.1 Bootstrap normal intervals

If the bootstrap results of the statistic of interest in any practical situation have a symmetric distribution, then $\mathrm{SE}_{\mathrm{boot}}(\hat{\theta})$ should be a good estimate of the SE of the point estimate of that statistic. If the bootstrap distribution looks approximately normal, and the bias is small, then a reasonable estimate of the 95% confidence interval (95% CI) will be the bootstrap normal 95% CI,

$$\hat{\theta} \pm 1.96 \times \mathrm{SE}_{\mathrm{boot}}(\hat{\theta}), \tag{14.4}$$

where 1.96, as always, derives from the normal distribution (e.g., see Table B.2). Notice that a bootstrap normal CI will always be symmetric about the observed sample estimate.

Example 14.1 Return to the problem of estimating a 95% CI for the mean cholesterol from the data of Table 2.10, using the 10 000 bootstrap samples derived earlier. In this case, $\hat{\theta}$ is the sample mean of cholesterol, which is 6.287, to three decimal places. As we have seen in Section 14.2, the distribution of means of the 10 000 bootstrap samples looks close to the normal and there is no difference between the bootstrap and observed means for cholesterol, so there is no bias (at least to three decimal places). Hence we are justified in using (14.4). The bootstrap SE can be computed from (14.3) applied to the bootstrap sampling distribution. This gave an answer of 0.108 for the bootstrap samples drawn; this is strikingly close to the SE of cholesterol (0.107) in the observed data — see Table 2.12. Plugged into (14.4) this gives a 95% CI of $6.287 \pm 1.96 \times 0.108 = (6.075, 6.499)$. In Section 2.7.2 the theoretical 95% CI from the observed data was given as (6.07, 6.50); when showing three places of decimals, this is (6.071, 6.502). Clearly the normal bootstrap approach gives virtually the same result as the theoretical method.

Table 14.1 includes bootstrap normal 95% CIs for all the six statistics illustrated by Figure 14.5, as well as further bootstrap CIs yet to be described. First, we consider the means. The similarity of the results for mean cholesterol, using observed data and using the normal bootstrap, was not surprising because the original sample data followed a normal distribution quite closely (see Figure 2.5, Figure 2.9, Figure 2.11 and Figure 2.14). What about the other variables in Table 2.10? For brevity, here only two other variables from this table are analysed. These are two variables for which

Table 14.1. Results of 10 000 bootstrap samples of Table 2.10: 95% confidence intervals.

Method	Means			Interquartile ranges		
	Cholesterol (mmol/l)	Alcohol (g/day)	Cotinine (ng/ml)	Cholesterol (mmol/l)	Alcohol (g/day)	Cotinine (ng/ml)
Observed	6.29	26.8	139.5	1.03	32.1	284
	(6.07, 6.50)	(18.9, 34.7)	(89.0, 190.0)			
Normal	(6.07, 6.50)	(19.2, 34.3)	(91.1, 187.8)	(0.72, 1.34)	(13.8, 50.4)	(185, 382)
Percentile	(6.07, 6.50)	(19.5, 34.7)	(92.4, 188.7)	(0.76, 1.39)	(17.2, 49.0)	(189, 395)
BC	(6.07, 6.50)	(19.9, 36.2)	(92.9, 189.1)	(0.75, 1.38)	(18.2, 51.7)	(233, 404)
BCa	(6.07, 6.49)	(20.3, 35.8)	(94.6, 191.1)	(0.77, 1.39)	(18.6, 54.0)	(233, 404)

Notes: Point and interval estimates from the observed data are also given, in italics, above the main table. These were found using the original data in Table 2.10 (see also Table 2.12) and assuming a *t* distribution (i.e., no bootstrapping). BC = bias corrected; BCa = bias corrected and accelerated.

the observed data showed obvious skew: alcohol (see Figure 2.6, Figure 2.10 and Figure 2.15) and cotinine (see Figure 2.8); neither could thus be said to be approximately normally distributed. The top line of Figure 14.5 includes histograms of the bootstrap sampling distributions for the means of alcohol and cotinine — as already discussed, both are suggestive of a fair approximation to a normal distribution for the distribution of means. Boxplots and normal plots, omitted here, are similarly suggestive of a reasonable approximation to normality for alcohol and cotinine bootstrap means. Not surprisingly, then, the observed and normal bootstrap results, for both alcohol and continine, are similar. This emphasises the robustness of the normal model for means that is used so frequently in statistical theory.

Now consider the problem of finding a bootstrap normal 95% CI for the IQR. Since there is no theoretical expression for the CI of an IQR, there is no way of obtaining a 95% CI from the observed data, unlike the case of a mean (under appropriate conditions), and hence the gaps in Table 14.1. On the face of it, bootstrapping presents a neat way of overcoming the absence of a plug-in formula. However, can we reasonably use (14.4) in this situation? The bottom line of Figure 14.5 suggests not: the bootstrap distributions for IQRs of cholesterol, alcohol and cotinine do not approximate to a normal distribution. Hence bootstrap normal CIs are not likely to be reliable here, and another approach is needed.

14.3.2   Bootstrap percentile intervals

To get round the problem of non-normal bootstrap distributions, percentile intervals may be useful. The percentile method of estimating bootstrap 95% CIs uses the whole distribution of bootstrap summary statistics, rather than just the standard deviations of such (as is the case with the normal bootstrap method). The basic idea is very simple: rank the bootstrap statistics and take the 95% confidence limits as the values 2.5% and 97.5% of the way along the ordered results; i.e., take the 2.5th and 97.5th percentiles of the bootstrap distribution. The result is a range in which the middle 95% of the bootstrap summary statistics should lie. Unlike normal bootstrap intervals, percentile intervals may be asymmetric around the point estimate.

Bootstrap percentile intervals have the advantage over normal intervals that they make no assumption about the way the bootstrap summaries are spread. In particular, they are preferable when the bootstrap distribution is skewed, such as is the case for the IQR of alcohol in Figure 14.5. Equality of the normal and percentile approaches can be seen as a mutual justification of each method. If they are importantly different, the percentile method may be preferred; however, each of the other two approaches yet to be described has more attractive theoretical properties than the percentile approach.

Example 14.2 As already discussed, Figure 14.5 suggests that the bootstrap distribution for the IQR of alcohol is not normal. This is further emphasised by Figure 14.6 and Figure 14.7. So, bootstrap normal CIs are unlikely to be accurate. Instead, we might use a percentile CI. To obtain the percentile 95% CI we take the summary estimates from the 10 000 bootstrap samples (that is, the data used to create Figure 14.6 and Figure 14.7) and place them in rank order.

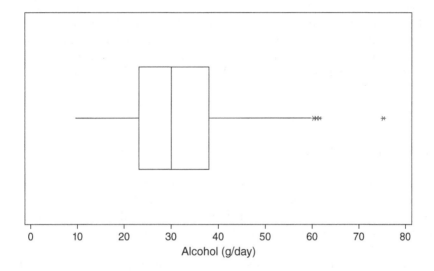

Figure 14.6. Boxplot for the bootstrap sample of 10 000 alcohol inter-quartile ranges.

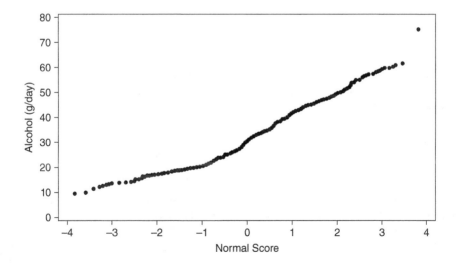

Figure 14.7. Normal plot for the bootstrap sample of 10 000 alcohol inter-quartile ranges.

Then we find the position of the 2.5th percentile: $(2.5/100) \times 10\ 000 = 250$. Using the rule expressed in Section 2.6.2, the 2.5th percentile is then the mean of the 250th and 251st values in rank order. Since there are only 50 values in the sample dataset, inevitably there are many repetitions within the 10 000 bootstrap estimates of the IQR, and it thus happens that the 250th and 251st values are both 17.2. Thus the lower limit of the CI is 17.2. The upper limit is, similarly, the mean of the 9750th and 9751st values. These were 49.0 and 49.1 and thus the upper limit is 49.05. Hence the 95% bootstrap percentile 95% CI is (17.2, 49.05). Recall, from Table 2.12, that the observed IQR from our original sample of size 50 is 32.1 g. As in all situations, this is our point estimate around which the interval is expressed, i.e., the sample IQR is our realisation of $\hat{\theta}$ in this example. Notice that the percentile 95% CI is skewed with a smaller lower side than upper side. Looking at Table 14.1, we see that the bootstrap percentile 95% CI for the alcohol IQR is narrower than the normal interval, being drawn in at both ends, but more especially at the lower end.

Bootstrap percentile 95% CIs from all the distributions shown in Figure 14.5 are given in Table 14.1. The CIs can be seen to be the same (to the given level of accuracy) for the normal and percentile approaches for the cholesterol mean, and virtually so for the alcohol mean. All the rest show clear differences; the difference for the IQR of alcohol is likely to be the most important for practical purposes.

14.3.3   Bootstrap bias-corrected intervals

The bootstrap bias-corrected (BC) interval is derived by a simple extension of the idea behind the percentile interval. If the bootstrap mean $\bar{x}_{boot}$ differs from the sample estimate, $\hat{\theta}$, in any important way then it seems sensible to shift the percentile evaluations accordingly so as to appropriately reposition the interval. If the bootstrap mean lies below the observed sample statistic, then we would wish to shift the interval upwards; if above, we want it to move downwards.

Since the percentile approach requires identification of the rank positions in the bootstrap sample, this upwards or downwards shift is achieved by recomputing these positions according to the proportion of bootstrap estimates that are below the observed point estimate. This is achieved by assuming a convenient normal model for the repositioning process. Explicitly, let

$$p_{boot} = P(x_{boot} \leq \hat{\theta}), \tag{14.5}$$

where P denotes a probability, which is estimated by the proportion in the bootstrap distribution below the point estimate in the observed data, and x_{boot} represents a random bootstrap estimate. Then let

$$z_0 = Z^{-1}(p_{boot}), \tag{14.6}$$

where Z^{-1} is the inverse standard normal function, sometimes called the **probit** function (e.g., $Z^{-1}(0.8159) = 0.9$ from Table B.1). We will refer to z_0 as the **bias correction**. Next, let

$$y_{95\%L} = z_0 + Z^{-1}(0.025) \tag{14.7}$$

and

$$y_{95\%U} = z_0 + Z^{-1}(0.975). \tag{14.8}$$

Then the BC 95% confidence limits are defined as (L, U) where the position of L is at the percentile defined by

$$Y_{95\%L} = 100 \times Z(z_0 + y_{95\%L}) \tag{14.9}$$

and the position of U is at the percentile defined by

$$Y_{95\%U} = 100 \times Z(z_0 + y_{95\%U}), \tag{14.10}$$

and Z is the standard normal function (e.g., Z(0.9) = 0.8159).

In essence, all this does is to modify the percentiles required according to information about the difference between the central point around which the bootstrap means cluster and the estimate from the observed data.

Consider the special case where the bootstrap means are equally likely to lie either side of the observed statistic: this is termed as being **median unbiased.** Then, by definition, (14.5) becomes

$$P(x_{boot} \leq \hat{\theta}) = 0.5.$$

This gives a value of z_0 of 0. Then $y_{95\%L} = Z^{-1}(0.025)$ and $Y_{95\%L} = 100 \times Z(y_{95\%L}) = 2.5$. Similarly $Y_{95\%U} = 97.5$. That is, under median unbiasedness, the positions are (rightly) unchanged, compared with the percentile bootstrap approach.

Example 14.3 For the 10 000 bootstrap sample estimates of the IQR of alcohol used in Example 14.2, the bootstrap mean was 30.81, which is slightly less than the observed IQR of 32.10. Hence the bootstrap bias is −1.29. Furthermore, 5559 of the 10 000 were less than or equal to the observed IQR and hence, in (14.5), p_{boot} is estimated as 0.5559 and consequently (14.6) gives $z_0 = Z^{-1}(0.5559)$. The easiest way to evaluate this may be to use the NORM.S.INV function in Excel, which gave a result of 0.14058.

To obtain the lower 95% confidence limit, (14.7) gives

$$y_{95\%L} = 0.14058 + Z^{-1}(0.025) = 0.14058 + (-1.95996) = -1.81938.$$

Notice that 1.95996 is a more accurate version of the familiar 5% two-sided critical value from a normal distribution, 1.96. This leads to, from (14.9),

$$Y_{95\%L} = 100 \times Z(0.14058 + (-1.81938)) = 4.6596.$$

Thus we need to extract the 4.6596th percentile of the bootstrap distribution. Since there are 10 000 estimates in that distribution, we need the 466th value in rank order. In the bootstrap distribution that was generated, this value is 18.2. Similarly, to obtain the upper 95% confidence limit, (14.8) and (14.10) give:

$$y_{95\%U} = 0.14058 + Z^{-1}(0.975) = 0.14058 + 1.95996 = 2.10055;$$

$$Y_{95\%U} = 100 \times Z(0.14058 + 2.10055) = 98.7491.$$

Thus we need the 9875th value in rank order, which turns out to be 51.7. Thus the BC 95% CI is (18.2, 51.7). This is slightly wider than the percentile interval, with both ends of the interval having been pushed upwards to account for the bias (see Table 14.1).

14.3.4 Bootstrap bias-corrected and accelerated intervals

Unfortunately, the BC method does not always have the correct coverage for a 95% CI, in the sense that the estimates from 2.5% of samples can be expected to fall below, and 2.5% to fall above, the BC 95% CI. This may be due to the normal assumption used in its calculation. Efron (1987) suggested a generalised version of the normal assumption used in the BC method, leading to the bias-corrected and accelerated (BCa) interval. The theoretical details are beyond the scope of this book, but the main concept behind moving from BC to BCa is to use an additional correction for skewness, as well as the bias correction, z_0, to further perturbate the percentile method. This extra correction involves use of the skewness correction, more often called the **acceleration coefficient,** a. The name 'acceleration coefficient' is used because this parameter measures the rate of change of the bootstrap SE with respect to the value of the parameter being estimated.

The acceleration coefficient is usually computed using **jackknife** methodology. This is another resampling technique which can sometimes be used instead of, or even in preference to, the bootstrap (see Shao and Tu, 1995). Like the bootstrap, it can be used to estimate the SE of a sample statistic. In its simplest, and most commonly used, form it generates multiple versions of the data by generating repeated samples, with each resample missing out a unique different observation. Given a sample of size n, this process continues until n resampled datasets, each of size $n - 1$, are obtained. Each individual in the observed dataset is represented in all but one of the resamples. Notice that, unlike the bootstrap, a unique set of resamples is obtained using this basic version of the jackknife.

The acceleration statistic is computed as

$$a = \frac{\Sigma(\bar{x}_{\text{jack}} - \ddot{\theta}_j)^3}{6\left\{\Sigma(\bar{x}_{\text{jack}} - \ddot{\theta}_j)^2\right\}^{1.5}}, \tag{14.11}$$

where both sums run from 1 to n; $\ddot{\theta}_j$ is the summary statistic of interest (e.g., the median) in the jth jackknife sample; and $\bar{x}_{\text{jack}}$ is the mean of the n jackknife estimates. Then, by analogy with (14.7) and (14.8), we calculate

$$y_{95\%L} = \frac{z_0 + Z^{-1}(0.025)}{1 - a\{z_0 + Z^{-1}(0.025)\}} \tag{14.12}$$

and

$$y_{95\%U} = \frac{z_0 + Z^{-1}(0.975)}{1 - a\{z_0 + Z^{-1}(0.975)\}}. \tag{14.13}$$

We finish by using (14.9) and (14.10) to obtain the positions of the BCa 95% confidence limits within the bootstrap sample.

Example 14.4 Suppose we wish to find the BCa 95% CI for the IQR of alcohol from Table 2.10 (where $n = 50$). To use (14.11) to compute the acceleration coefficient for the IQR of alcohol we need to find such IQRs from all jackknife samples, each with one of the 50 excluded. The first jackknife sample has the first sample member excluded. Without loss of generality, take this first person to be the one whose data fills the first row of Table 2.10 — as in the data stored on the web site for this book. This person has an alcohol consumption of 5.4 g; for the remaining 49 people the 1st quartile is 7.2 and the 3rd quartile is 38.3, giving a IQR of $\ddot{\theta}_1 = 31.1$ (recall that the IQR for all 50 is 32.1). Continuing in this way, we get all 50 values of $\ddot{\theta}_{.i}$. The mean of all these, $\bar{x}_{\text{jack}} = 29.968$. The sum of the squares of the deviations between each jackknife estimate and the mean of all is 459.6488 and the sum of the cubes is 1440.768, whence, from (14.11),

$$a = \frac{1440.768}{6\left\{\sqrt{459.6488}\right\}^3} = 0.024367.$$

So far, bootstrapping has not been used. To proceed, we will use the 10 000 bootstrap samples already exploited in the last two examples. For this bootstrap evaluation we know, from Example 14.3, that the bias correction, $z_0 = 0.14058$. Hence (14.12) becomes

$$y_{95\%L} = \frac{0.14058 + Z^{-1}(0.025)}{1 - 0.024367 \times \{0.14058 + Z^{-1}(0.025)\}} = \frac{0.14058 + (-1.95996)}{1 - 0.024367 \times \{0.14058 + (-1.95996)\}} = -1.74215.$$

Then, using (14.9),

$$Y_{95\%L} = 100 \times Z(0.14058 + (-1.74215)) = 5.4626.$$

Hence we need the 547th value in the ordered bootstrap data, which is 18.6. Similarly, from (14.13) and (14.10),

$$y_{95\%U} = \frac{0.14058 + Z^{-1}(0.975)}{1 - 0.024367 \times \{0.14058 + Z^{-1}(0.975)\}} = \frac{0.14058 + 1.95996}{1 - 0.024367 \times \{0.14058 + 1.95996\}} = 2.213854;$$

$$Y_{95\%U} = 100 \times Z(0.14058 + 2.213854) = 99.0725.$$

Hence we need the 9908th value in the ordered bootstrap data, which is 54.0. Hence the BCa 95% CI is (18.6, 54.0). This is slightly more asymmetric than the BC interval (see Table 14.1).

14.3.5   Overview of the worked example

Now that all four bootstrap methods have been introduced, it is useful to compare them with reference to our observed dataset using Table 14.1. This example includes situations where classical methods for CIs (of Chapter 2),

1. Should work well (for mean cholesterol)
2. Might not work well (for mean alcohol and cotinine)
3. Do not exist (for IQRs)

In the case of making inferences about mean cholesterol, it is clear that bootstrapping is not necessary. In the cases of mean alcohol and cotinine, classical methods (i.e., based on Student's t distribution) work reasonably well, but produce a CI which is too symmetric. For IQRs, bootstrapping gives us new inferences, not available from classical theory. Within the sets of bootstrap CIs, there is no regular pattern of differences, but the case of alcohol shows that each method can give somewhat different results. Whether these differences have any clinical significance is another matter, but these results show that we should now consider which bootstrap method to use in any given situation.

14.3.6   Choice of bootstrap interval

The BCa approach is generally recognised to be the most reliable of the four methods described here. However, the price to pay for this superiority is a good deal more computation, and thus a greater demand for computer resources and more time required to get an answer. Furthermore, it requires more replications than the others to achieve convergence to a stable solution. Unlike the other three methods, which can be used in all situations, the BCa approach does not always work, even when employing packages such as SAS or Stata. Hence, sometimes another approach is necessary. Of the other three methods described here, the BC method would then be the method of choice, albeit with the worry that skewness may not have been sufficiently accounted for. Carpenter and Bithell (2000) describe some other methods that may be considered, giving a guide to which to use in particular situations, whilst the ABC method of DiCiccio and Efron (1992) may also be worth considering when resources are limited. The normal and percentile methods are simple, and thus useful for introducing concepts, but they are unsuitable when there is bias or skewness; hence they cannot be recommended in general situations.

14.4   Practical issues when bootstrapping

14.4.1   Software

Bootstrapping is only feasible because of the power of modern computers. Bootstrap analyses can now be achieved using any of the leading proprietary statistical software packages. However, this often requires the user to be proficient at writing computer code. One exception is Stata, which allows many of its standard methods, such as a regression analysis, to be performed using bootstrap resampling by the simple use of a BOOTSTRAP prefix to the standard command. Bootstrapping of a simple arithmetic manipulation of the results that are automatically stored by a standard command is also easy to achieve, again by an extension of the standard command. For example, the IQR requires computation of $Q3 - Q1$, where the Qs are the quartiles, before bootstrapping. Thus many results shown in this chapter were obtained using an extended version of Stata's SUMMARIZE command. More complex pre-bootstrapping manipulation of estimates from Stata commands or descriptive statistics, such as smoothed lines from scatterplots, require programming in Stata. Examples of all three approaches within Stata are included in the code provided on the web site for this book.

When using SAS, the %JACKKNIFE, %BOOT and %BOOTCI macros are all relevant to the current issue, the latter being the most useful. These may be downloaded from http://support.sas.com/kb/24/982.html. Alternatively, some authors have posted bootstrap algorithms to do specific analyses in SAS, such as finding bootstrap CIs for the kappa coefficient (Vierkant, 1997). A SAS macro to compute bootstrap CIs for any statistic that is returned by PROC MEANS is available from the web site for this book (ascribed to Examples 14.1 to 14.4).

Due to the benefits of using Stata, all the bootstrap results presented in this chapter were produced from that package.

14.4.2   How many replications should be used?

Just as with any random process, bootstrapping will generally produce more stable estimates with larger numbers. So far, all examples have used 10 000 bootstrap replications. Is this enough, or is it too many? In general, we would wish to use the number of replications that just gives a stable solution, but this number will not be known in advance of bootstrapping.

Consider Table 14.2 which, once again, shows bootstrap results from the data in Table 2.10 for the six problems posed in Table 14.1, but now uses eight possible values for the number of replications used, b. Here only three methods of obtaining bootstrap CIs are shown for brevity: normal, percentile and BCa. The BCa approach is the most complex, so it is not surprising that there is a general tendency for greater variation in confidence limits with increasing values of b when this method is used. For estimating confidence limits for mean cholesterol (the variable with a sample distribution closest to the normal) $b = 50$ is ample, except for the BCa method where a value of b closer to 100 appears to be needed. For mean alcohol, except for the normal method, $b = 100$ does not appear to be enough and for mean cotinine, $b = 5000$ does not seem excessive. For estimating CIs for IQRs, $b = 50$ seems enough for cholesterol for all but the normal method, which seems to need around 100 to get a reasonably stable estimate. For alcohol, 1000, 5000 and even 50 000 replications might be required for normal, percentile and BCa, respectively. For cotinine, the corresponding values seem to be around 5000, 500 and 1000.

Although the values in Table 14.2 are never wildly different, there is obviously considerable variation in where the process 'settles down', even for the relatively simple scenario analysed here. We can expect the play of chance to have more impact in a more complex situation. This, and the clear issue that what degree of error is acceptable depends upon the practical situation, means that it is difficult to give precise advice regarding the most appropriate value for b. Experienced practitioners suggest that at least 1000 to 2000 replications should be used, whilst Poi (2004) describes Stata commands to determine b according to the prescribed acceptable degree of error. The results in Table 14.2 were obtained from using Stata on a standard household laptop of 2005 vintage. None of the analyses took more than two minutes, even with $b = 100 000$, so it does not seem excessive to have used $b = 10 000$ in Table 14.1. However, as already acknowledged, the problems considered so far have been simple and the sample size is small. Depending upon the forbearance of the user and the importance of getting an accurate result for the CI, it is worth considering using a value of b that is greater than those generally recommended as sufficient. Stata takes $b = 50$ by default, but this would be dangerous to use in anything other than when testing code.

For simplification, the values of b considered here are always round numbers ending in at least one zero. However, it can save computer time to, instead, choose b to be an odd number, such as 999 or 1999. This is because of the way percentiles are estimated. Consider the method for estimating quantiles (a more general word for percentiles) expressed in Section 2.6.2, which is the one adopted by Stata. Whenever the rank position of the percentile required is an integer, the calculation involves averaging two numbers, whereas when the rank position is a fraction, no arithmetic is required — the percentile is taken to be one of the numbers in the bootstrap sample — thus saving time. For example, when $b = 1000$ the percentile method for estimating the 95% CI first requires identification of the 2.5th percentile. According to the method of Section 2.6.2, this will be the average of the 25th and 26th highest values in the 1000. Similarly, the required 97.5th percentile is the average of the 975th and 976th highest values. Thus two arithmetic operations are required to obtain the CI.

Table 14.2. Results of b bootstrap samples from Table 2.10: 95% confidence intervals.

b	Means			Interquartile ranges		
	Cholesterol (mmol/l)	Alcohol (g/day)	Cotinine (ng/ml)	Cholesterol (mmol/l)	Alcohol (g/day)	Cotinine (ng/ml)
	6.29	*26.8*	*139.5*	*1.03*	*32.1*	*284*
	(6.07, 6.50)	*(18.8, 34.6)*	*(89.0, 190.0)*			
	Normal bootstrap confidence intervals					
50	(6.08, 6.49)	(18.6, 35.0)	(85.8, 193.1)	(0.74, 1.32)	(13.9, 50.3)	(188, 380)
100	(6.08, 6.49)	(19.2, 34.3)	(89.4, 189.6)	(0.72, 1.34)	(15.1, 49.1)	(184, 384)
500	(6.08, 6.49)	(19.3, 34.2)	(93.4, 185.5)	(0.73, 1.33)	(14.1, 50.1)	(192, 376)
1000	(6.08, 6.49)	(19.1, 34.4)	(92.1, 186.8)	(0.72, 1.34)	(13.8, 50.4)	(191, 377)
5000	(6.08, 6.49)	(19.1, 34.5)	(91.0, 187.9)	(0.72, 1.34)	(13.6, 50.6)	(188, 380)
10 000	(6.08, 6.49)	(19.1, 34.4)	(90.7, 188.3)	(0.71, 1.35)	(13.8, 50.4)	(187, 381)
50 000	(6.08, 6.49)	(19.1, 34.4)	(90.6, 188.4)	(0.71, 1.35)	(13.6, 50.6)	(187, 381)
100 000	(6.08, 6.49)	(19.1, 34.4)	(90.6, 188.4)	(0.71, 1.35)	(13.6, 50.6)	(186, 382)
	Percentile bootstrap confidence intervals					
50	(6.07, 6.49)	(18.4, 35.6)	(95.7, 191.2)	(0.77, 1.38)	(16.6, 47.3)	(230, 404)
100	(6.08, 6.49)	(18.1, 33.0)	(92.5, 190.9)	(0.77, 1.39)	(16.6, 47.3)	(189, 403)
500	(6.09, 6.50)	(19.3, 34.6)	(93.8, 186.3)	(0.77, 1.38)	(17.0, 48.4)	(189, 395)
1000	(6.09, 6.50)	(19.3, 34.8)	(94.2, 188.8)	(0.76, 1.39)	(17.2, 48.5)	(189, 395)
5000	(6.08, 6.49)	(19.5, 34.8)	(92.6, 189.6)	(0.76, 1.39)	(17.4, 49.2)	(189, 395)
10 000	(6.08, 6.49)	(19.5, 34.8)	(92.6, 190.1)	(0.76, 1.39)	(17.4, 49.2)	(189, 395)
50 000	(6.08, 6.49)	(19.5, 34.8)	(91.9, 189.6)	(0.76, 1.39)	(17.2, 49.2)	(189, 395)
100 000	(6.08, 6.49)	(19.5, 34.7)	(91.9, 189.4)	(0.76, 1.39)	(17.2, 49.2)	(189, 395)
	Bias-corrected and accelerated (BCa) bootstrap confidence intervals					
50	(6.11, 6.51)	(22.6, 36.5)	(95.7, 201.8)	(0.78, 1.39)	(21.2, 56.8)	(245, 407)
100	(6.08, 6.49)	(21.6, 36.5)	(95.7, 191.2)	(0.77, 1.39)	(20.0, 56.8)	(233, 407)
500	(6.07, 6.47)	(20.4, 36.0)	(96.1, 190.0)	(0.77, 1.39)	(18.8, 56.0)	(244, 404)
1000	(6.06, 6.48)	(20.1, 35.8)	(96.8, 191.2)	(0.76, 1.39)	(18.6, 56.0)	(233, 405)
5000	(6.07, 6.48)	(20.1, 35.8)	(94.6, 191.2)	(0.76, 1.39)	(18.6, 54.8)	(233, 404)
10 000	(6.07, 6.49)	(20.1, 35.7)	(94.9, 192.5)	(0.76, 1.39)	(18.6, 54.8)	(233, 404)
50 000	(6.08, 6.49)	(20.2, 35.8)	(93.8, 191.7)	(0.76, 1.39)	(18.2, 54.0)	(233, 404)
100 000	(6.07, 6.49)	(20.2, 35.7)	(94.2, 192.2)	(0.77, 1.39)	(18.2, 54.0)	(233, 404)

Notes: Point and interval estimates from the observed data are also given, in italics, above the main table. The same random seed (Section 14.4.3) was used each time, and this was different from the random seed used to produce Table 14.1.

When $b = 999$ the percentile 'positions' will be $999 \times (2.5/100) = 24.975$ and $999 \times (97.5/1000) = 94.025$, which are not integers, and thus the 25th and 975th values in rank order are used for the CI with no arithmetic being necessary. A further advantage of taking b to be a number such as 999 can arise in bootstrap hypothesis testing (see Boos, 2003).

14.4.3 Sensible strategies

Bootstrapping is applied by using random numbers, such as those in Table B.6 or, more likely, according to an algorithm 'hidden' within the software package. These numbers are used to select the bootstrap samples. As discussed in Section 7.7 we need to start a random number sequence off at a random starting point of our choice, often called the **random seed,** or just the **seed.** Software such as SAS and Stata, unless asked to do otherwise, will pick a random seed for themselves — generally one that varies with the time on the computer's clock. This is sensible, since it ensures that the software does not give the same results every time, which clearly runs contrary to the very concept of random sampling. However, it is usually better to choose a random seed ourselves, to make sure that the same random sequence can be reproduced at a future time, both so as to be able to reproduce past results and so that the performance of different bootstrap methods can be compared fairly. Any number is acceptable within the range allowed by the package; for example, in Stata the range allowed is any integer between 1 and $2^{31} - 1$.

Another useful tip when developing bootstrap methods is to start small and simple. That is, choose a low value of b, even a value below ten, and omit the more time-consuming BCa method, in the first tries of any new set of bootstrap commands. It may also be sensible to start with a cut-down version of the original sample dataset. Otherwise a lot of time may be wasted in developing operational code. Sometimes bootstrap runs can take hours. Once results are obtained that seem useful, they should be saved immediately. There is nothing more annoying than having to rerun a long exercise just because the original output has been accidently, or automatically, deleted or overwritten.

A more technical issue arises when a researcher writes her or his own bootstrap routine from scratch. The researcher has a decision to make: should the routine generate each bootstrap sample, and then the summary estimate from it, in turn; or should it generate all the bootstrap samples at once and then carry out the estimation process simultaneously (i.e., using a single executed command) on the combined mega-sample? In general, the first method is easier to think through and write out, but the second may be more efficient. For example, Barker (2005) gives a simple example where the first method took almost three minutes to do the same task as took the second method only one second to achieve, in SAS.

14.5   Further examples of bootstrapping

In this section a set of examples of the use of bootstrap CIs are presented, based on examples introduced in earlier chapters. Corresponding Stata DO files are available from the web site for this book.

Example 14.5 Consider the data from 61 developing countries given in Table 9.8. In Example 9.6 a regression line was fitted to predict the log of the number of decayed, missing or filled teeth (LDMFT) from the sugar consumption, per country. We will use bootstrapping to see whether the CI computed using the classical methods of Section 9.3.1 seems to accurately describe the uncertainty in the estimate of the slope in this case.

Output 14.1 shows (i) the results obtained from running the regression on the observed data (i.e., as used to produce Table 9.10) and (ii) the results obtained from repeating the REGRESS procedure in 2000 bootstrap samples in Stata (see the web site for this book for the code used). In the current situation we are only interested in the lines of output relating to sugar — the explanatory variable. Using more decimal places than would be usual in a practical situation, classical methods estimate that LDMFT will increase by 0.0213944 for an extra kg/person/year of sugar, with a 95% CI of (0.0120054, 0.0307834).

For the bootstrap results, two tables are presented; these required two commands in Stata. First, the basic BOOTSTRAP command (in conjunction with the REGRESS command) produced results from the normal bootstrap method. This includes estimates of the intercept (denoted '_cons') and slope (here denoted 'sugar') from the observed data. The SE now is (as indicated by Stata) for the bootstrap sample; that is, the SE for the slope is the SD of the distribution of 2000 estimates of slope, as computed by (14.3) when $b = 2000$ and $\tilde{\theta}_i$ is the estimate of slope in the ith bootstrap sample. The z column contains Wald test statistics using the bootstrap SEs (i.e., for the slope: $0.0213944/0.0046639 = 4.59$) and similarly the 95% CI for the slope is $0.0213944 \pm 1.96 \times 0.0046639 = (0.012253, 0.030535)$.

The second table of bootstrap results are the 'post-estimation' (ESTAT) results produced by Stata, showing all four bootstrap methods described in this chapter (note that the BCa method is only applied when explicitly asked for when running the bootstrap command in Stata). In the first column we see the estimates from the observed data, once again. The second column shows the bias, computed using (14.2), for the slope and intercept. In the third column we see (as in the first table) the bootstrap SE. The lower and upper limits of the four 95% CIs appear in the last two columns.

Stata was asked to store the 2000 bootstrap results, thus creating a file of size 2000 by 2. Here we are only interested in the 2000 results for the slope, which seemed to have a distribution close to a normal distribution upon plotting. We can use this file to obtain the results in the second bootstrap table for ourselves. The bootstrap SE for the slope comes from using the SUMMARIZE command in Stata applied to the saved 2000 bootstrap results. Here, this gave the standard deviation of the 2000 slopes as 0.0046639, as in Output 14.1. We can find the bootstrap bias from the 2000 bootstrap results, using the SUMMARIZE command to obtain the bootstrap mean and subtracting the observed estimate, 0.0213944, from this. As seen in Example 14.3 and Example 14.4, percentile and BC intervals can be obtained from the saved 2000 bootstrap results, after sorting them in ascending order and using the rule for computing quantiles expressed in Section 2.6.2. For example, consider the percentile 95% confidence limits. These are the 2.5th and 97.5th percentiles of the distribution of bootstrap sample slopes. To obtain these we first compute $(2.5/100) \times 2000 = 50$. As this is a whole number, we take the mean of the 50th and 51st values in rank order. With the 2000 bootstrap samples taken here, these were 0.01231061 and 0.0124008. The 2.5th percentile is thus the mean of these, 0.012356, as given (with one extra decimal place) in Output 14.1 as the lower 95% confidence limit for the percentile method. A similar calculation for the upper limit requires averaging the 1950th and 1951st slopes in rank order.

The main finding from these analyses is that the original (observed) results seem robust. The distribution of the bootstrap samples is near to normal and none of the bootstrap CIs is very different from the CI for the sample data. Bias is small and the two SEs are almost the same. The small, unimportant, differences found are:

- The normal bootstrap CI is slightly narrower than the observed CI, explained by the bootstrap SE being marginally smaller than the original sample-based estimate, plus the use of Student's t distribution in the calculation of the latter (t on 59 degrees of freedom is 2.001, which exceeds 1.96).
- The percentile CI shifts the lower limit up and the upper limit down, compared with the normal CI, and so is slightly narrower; also, it is slightly 'heavier' on the lower side of the point estimate.
- The BC and BCa CIs are similar, both wider than the percentile CI and with the weight shifted to the upper side.

Output 14.1. Stata REGRESS results for Example 14.5.

(i) Using REGRESS on the observed data

```
   Source  |      SS       df       MS              Number of obs =      61
-----------+----------------------------           F(  1,    59) =   20.79
    Model  | 7.59333811    1  7.59333811           Prob > F      = 0.0000
 Residual  | 21.5490868   59   .365238759          R-squared     = 0.2606
-----------+----------------------------           Adj R-squared = 0.2480
    Total  | 29.1424249   60   .485707082          Root MSE      = .60435
```

```
    ldmft  |      Coef.  Std. Err.    t    P>|t|   [95% Conf. Interval]
-----------+----------------------------------------------------------------
    sugar  |    .0213944   .0046922   4.56  0.000    .0120054    .0307834
    _cons  |    .0955066   .138912    0.69  0.494   -.1824557    .3734689
```

(ii) Using REGRESS with bootstrap resampling

Linear regression

```
                                             Number of obs =      61
                                             Replications   =    2000
                                             Wald chi2(1)   =   21.04
                                             Prob > chi2    = 0.0000
                                             R-squared      = 0.2606
                                             Adj R-squared  = 0.2480
                                             Root MSE       = 0.6043
```

```
           |  Observed   Bootstrap                  Normal-based
    ldmft  |     Coef.   Std. Err.    z    P>|z|   [95% Conf. Interval]
-----------+----------------------------------------------------------------
    sugar  |   .0213944   .0046639   4.59  0.000    .0122534    .0305354
    _cons  |   .0955066   .1463349   0.65  0.514   -.1913045    .3823177
```

Linear regression

```
                                             Number of obs   =      61
                                             Replications    =    2000
```

```
           |  Observed              Bootstrap
    ldmft  |     Coef.      Bias     Std.Err.    [95% Conf. Interval]
-----------+----------------------------------------------------------------
    sugar  |  .02139441  -.0000193  .00466387    .0122534   .0305354   (N)
           |                                     .0123557   .0302137   (P)
           |                                     .0127621   .0307046   (BC)
           |                                     .0128035   .0307169  (BCa)
    _cons  |   .0955066   .0017721  .14633488   -.1913045   .3823177   (N)
           |                                    -.1842951   .3833357   (P)
           |                                    -.1843598   .3832871   (BC)
           |                                    -.1903026   .3756871  (BCa)
```

(N) normal confidence interval
(P) percentile confidence interval
(BC) bias-corrected confidence interval
(BCa) bias-corrected and accelerated confidence interval

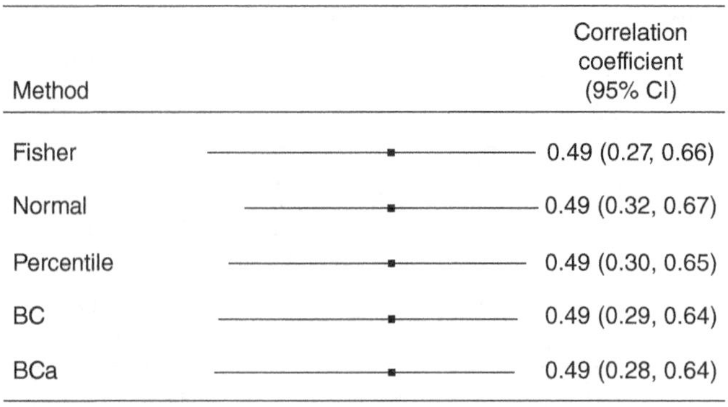

Method		Correlation coefficient (95% CI)
Fisher	—————————•—————	0.49 (0.27, 0.66)
Normal	—————————•—————	0.49 (0.32, 0.67)
Percentile	—————————•—————	0.49 (0.30, 0.65)
BC	—————————•—————	0.49 (0.29, 0.64)
BCa	—————————•—————	0.49 (0.28, 0.64)

Figure 14.8. Correlation coefficient with Fisher and bootstrap confidence intervals for Example 14.6.

Example 14.6 The sugar-caries data may also be used to illustrate the ascertainment of a CI for the Pearson correlation coefficient. In Section 9.3.2 the correlation was found to be 0.49, but the issue of finding a CI around this estimate was left unaddressed. Although a simple formula for such a CI, attributed to Sir Ronald Fisher, has been available for many years, this requires an unusual transformation and a subsequent approximation to normality which may be in question. Indeed, Stata's CORRELATE command (the basic Stata command for correlation) does not produce a CI. It is thus of interest to obtain a 95% CI using bootstrapping.

The easiest way to apply bootstrapping to this problem in Stata is to bootstrap the REGRESS command, as in Example 14.5, but now making use of the Stata's storage of the r^2 statistic, this being the square of Pearson's correlation coefficient. Figure 14.8 shows the results obtained from this bootstrapping; in this case the bias was a negligible 0.0003376, and hence bias correction made little difference. For comparison, the results from using Fisher's method, applied using PROC CORR in SAS, are included in the figure. Although Fisher's method appears to be too conservative and we would do best to use the BCa CI due to its better theoretical properties, there are no big differences between these CIs.

Example 14.7 The regression paradigm can also be exploited to address another common problem through bootstrapping. As we saw in Section 2.7.3, the task of comparing two means can be tackled through simple formulae, but only if a normal distribution can be assumed for the difference between the means. In Section 2.8.1 an example was cited (for the alcohol data in Table 2.10) where such an assumption is in doubt and a transformation, which works well for a single mean, is not very useful for a difference between means. Here we shall apply bootstrapping to this problem using most of the variables from Table 2.10 — to conserve space, diastolic blood pressure (which is highly correlated with systolic blood pressure) is not considered. The two groups to be compared will be those with and without CHD.

Regression can be used in this context by defining the outcome variable as (for example) alcohol and the explanatory variable as CHD. In fact, since CHD is coded 1 for yes and 2 for no in Table 2.10, a new variable CHD2 = 2 − CHD was defined, and used as the explanatory variable, so that the differences between (for example) alcohol were computed for those with CHD minus those without CHD, rather than vice-versa. The regression model fitted is then

$$y = b_0 + b_1 x,$$

where $x = 1$ for CHD and 0 for no CHD. The fitted values (i.e., estimated means) for CHD and no CHD are thus b_0 and, $b_0 + b_1$, respectively, and hence the difference of the means is estimated by b_1

In Stata, the bootstrap procedure then follows much as in Example 14.5. As in that example, simple Stata code will give bootstrap results for the required parameter — the estimated beta coefficient for CHD2 — as well as the intercept. Table 14.3 shows results of the difference in means for each of the six variables considered.

Table 14.3. Results from 2000 bootstrap samples of differences between means: Example 14.7.

	Total cholesterol (mmol/l)	Systolic BP (mmHg)	Alcohol (g/day)	Cigarettes (per day)	Carbon monoxide (ppm)	Cotinine (ng/ml)
Observed estimate	*0.5405*	*8.874*	*0.163*	*4.762*	*14.851*	*98.245*
Bias	−0.0015	−0.069	0.201	−0.076	−0.043	−0.722
Observed SE	*0.2492*	*4.757*	*9.573*	*4.243*	*4.689*	*59.480*
Bootstrap SE	0.2682	5.926	8.822	4.384	6.350	60.314
Observed 95% CI	*(0.0395, 1.0415)*	*(−0.690, 18.438)*	*(−19.09, 19.41)*	*(−3.769, 13.294)*	*(5.423, 24.278)*	*(−21.35, 217.84)*
Normal 95% CI	(0.0149, 1.0661)	(−2.741, 20.489)	(−17.13, 17.45)	(−3.830, 13.354)	(2.406, 27.296)	(−19.97, 216.46)
Percentile 95% CI	(−0.0169, 1.0599)	(−2.248, 21.092)	(−16.08, 18.70)	(−3.446, 13.607)	(2.480, 27.103)	(−21.51, 216.72)
BC 95% CI	(−0.0168, 1.0599)	(−1.610, 22.310)	(−15.87, 18.92)	(−2.996, 13.927)	(2.276, 26.930)	(−20.90, 217.73)
BCa 95% CI	(−0.0305, 1.0499)	(−0.993, 23.000)	(−14.64, 21.53)	(−2.800, 14.450)	(2.511, 27.329)	(−21.54, 216.52)

Notes: Mean for those with coronary heart disease less the mean for those without. BC = bias corrected; BCa = bias corrected and accelerated. BP = blood pressure. Sample-based (observed) results are in italics.

Alcohol is the only variable of the six where the bias is positive; also, as an absolute percentage of the estimate itself, bias is greatest for alcohol, at 1.2%. Alcohol is also the only variable for which the bootstrap SE is less than the observed SE, and consequently the only variable for which the normal bootstrap CI is narrower than that for the observed data. Cholesterol is the only variable for which the three CIs that allow for skewness are weighted towards the left of the estimate derived from the observed data; the CIs for carbon monoxide and cotinine show no lack of symmetry when skewness is allowed for. Interestingly, in every case it appears that bootstrapping was justified, even for cholesterol where Table 14.1 suggested no variation in results across different methodologies. The preferred BCa CI is noticeably different from the CI for the observed data (i.e., without bootstrapping) in every case. The BCa CI is also often quite dissimilar to the simple normal bootstrap CI; least so in the cases of carbon monoxide and cotinine, for which the extra resources spent on the BCa approach seem to have been unnecessary. As always, the statistical differences indicated here may not be considered important for practical purposes.

In Section 10.16 the binomial regression model was introduced as a way of estimating a CI for a risk, both with and without adjustment for confounding variables. This method was seen (Section 10.16.3) to run into difficulties in certain situations, unlike the logistic regression model which is more robust. In such cases a bootstrap approach to CI estimation, through logistic modelling, might be useful. The next example considers this for a simple (unadjusted) problem where the results can be compared with alternative methods.

Example 14.8 In Example 3.1 the risk of a cardiovascular death amongst smokers was estimated to be 0.02188, to five decimal places, in the EGAT study. What is a suitable 95% CI for this estimate?

In Example 3.1, the simple equations (3.3) and (3.4), and a normal approximation, were employed to produce a 95% CI. Another approach would be to assume that the number of cardiovascular deaths follows a binomial distribution, and use this directly. In Stata this was achieved using the CI command with a BINOMIAL option. In Example 10.38 the same problem was addressed using a binomial regression model. Now, a bootstrap evaluation of the 95% CI was obtained by running 2000 replications of a logistic model (via Stata's GLM command), employing (10.8) to get the risk from the log odds produced by GLM.

Results for the various 95% CIs are shown in Table 14.4. In this case the bootstrap bias was <0.0001, so bias correction was clearly unnecessary. We might assume that the exact binomial approach is the gold standard, since this is the most reasonable probability model for a risk. Comparing all else to this, we see that every method gives good answers. Another point of view

Table 14.4. Estimates of 95% confidence intervals for the risk of a cardiovascular death amongst smokers in the EGAT study: Example 14.8.

Data	Analysis method	Bootstrap method	95% confidence interval
Observed	Binomial		(0.0149, 0.0309)
Observed	Normal approximation		(0.0143, 0.0295)
Observed	Binomial regression		(0.0154, 0.0310)
Bootstrap	Logistic regression	Normal	(0.0141, 0.0297)
Bootstrap	Logistic regression	Percentile	(0.0144, 0.0300)
Bootstrap	Logistic regression	BC	(0.0147, 0.0300)
Bootstrap	Logistic regression	BCa	(0.0150, 0.0306)

Note: Two thousand bootstrap evaluations were summarised.

might be that the binomial model is in doubt, generally because of issues concerning under- or over-estimation of the variability (Section 10.7.1). Warning signs might be indications of systematic patterns in response, for example when smokers collude to lie about their habit, or problems seen when fitting models. In such situations, the BCa results might, rather, be taken as the gold standard.

In some situations it may be useful to compare regression coefficients that arise from fitting different models to the same data. For instance, we might want to compare the hazard ratios due to smoking for cancer and heart disease or the hazard ratios from Cox and Poisson models fitted to the same survival data. There is no simple way to obtain a CI for such a comparison, but such a problem is easily addressed using bootstrapping.

Example 14.9 In Chapter 11, Cox models were fitted to data from the Scottish Heart Health Study (SHHS) for the same problems that logistic regression models had previously been used for in Chapter 10. We saw that the odds ratios and hazard ratios were very similar. Although a survival approach, such as the Cox proportional hazards model, is preferable with these data, because it makes appropriate allowance for censoring, in the context of this book it is useful to see how much error is induced by ignoring censoring (precisely, assuming that those lost to follow-up have no event) in the relevant examples in Chapter 10.

For brevity, only one problem, and a single set of explanatory variables, will be considered here: the full model for the SHHS data, available from the web site for this book, ascribed to Example 10.12. The second column of Table 14.5 shows odds ratios for CHD in the observed (sample) data; these are the exponents of the log odds ratios listed in Table 10.6. The third column shows hazard ratios for CHD, which previously appeared in Output 11.4 (although here they were computed from Stata, with exactly the same results as those produced by SAS for Output 11.4). Table 14.5 then shows that the difference between the log hazard ratio and logit are small for all variables; correspondingly, each ratio of the hazard ratio to the odds ratio is close to unity. We can, of course, see these similarities from comparing Example 10.12 and Example 11.10.

Next, Table 14.5 shows the results of 2000 bootstrap evaluations. Bootstrapping was performed on the difference between the log hazard ratio and the logit. Since both the log hazard ratio and logit are known to have, approximately, a normal distribution their difference will also have an approximate normal distribution, and thus normal bootstrap results should be acceptable. Should BCa results be hard to obtain, this will be a useful result, although adoption of normal bootstrap results should still be justified, at least in part, by comparison with percentile and BC outcomes. In this case, BCa results were easily obtainable using the BOOTSTRAP command in Stata together with a simple bespoke Stata program. This program (available from the web site for this book) is easily adaptable to make comparisons between estimated beta coefficients in other situations. We can see from Table 14.5 that the bootstrap bias is always small, suggesting that bias correction will have little effect (which is as expected). More usefully, we can see that the 95% CIs for the difference, the metric on which bootstrap results were performed (results taken directly from Stata), are narrow. Correspondingly, the 95% CIs for the ratio (obtained by taking exponents of the results from Stata) are also narrow. Taking the Cox model as the gold standard, we might thus conclude that the error when using the logistic model is unlikely to be important in this example.

14.5.1 Complex bootstrap samples

All the foregoing examples have taken each bootstrap sample from the observed data as a whole. There are occasions when this is not sensible. For example, when the observed sample data were obtained from clustered or stratified sampling, we would wish to preserve the original structure in each bootstrap sample. Similarly, in a randomised controlled trial with two treatments allocated equally to subjects, it would make sense to have each bootstrap sample with the same number of subjects in each treatment arm, rather than allowing some bootstrap samples to have disproportionate numbers on one or other treatment. Then we will need to draw separate samples with replacement from each treatment group on each bootstrap replication. This is easily

Table 14.5. Observed and BCa bootstrap (2000 replications) results for Example 14.9.

Variable	Observed results (sample data)				Bootstrap results		
	Odds ratio (95% CI)	Hazard ratio (95% CI)	Difference	Ratio	Bias for difference	95% CI for difference	95% CI for ratio
AGE	1.017 (0.990, 1.045)	1.018 (0.992, 1.045)	0.0009	1.001	-0.00002	(-0.0008, 0.0026)	(0.999, 1.003)
TOTCHOL	1.359 (1.209, 1.528)	1.331 (1.195, 1.483)	-0.0210	0.979	-0.00026	(-0.0414, -0.0099)	(0.959, 0.990)
BMI	1.043 (1.000, 1.087)	1.039 (0.998, 1.081)	-0.0036	0.996	-0.00022	(-0.0068, -0.0003)	(0.993, 1.000)
SYSTOL	1.021 (1.013, 1.028)	1.020 (1.013, 1.028)	-0.0003	1.000	-0.00003	(-0.0011, 0.0005)	(0.999, 1.000)
SMOKE2	1.381 (0.845, 2.256)	1.366 (0.847, 2.205)	-0.0104	0.990	-0.00058	(-0.0551, 0.0134)	(0.946, 1.014)
SMOKE3	2.074 (1.350, 3.187)	2.014 (1.325, 3.059)	-0.0297	0.971	-0.00132	(-0.0713, -0.0069)	(0.931, 0.993)
ACT2	0.827 (0.581, 1.176)	0.828 (0.590, 1.163)	0.0018	1.002	0.00029	(-0.0249, 0.0312)	(0.975, 1.032)
ACT3	0.904 (0.572, 1.428)	0.896 (0.577, 1.390)	-0.0087	0.991	0.00082	(-0.0452, 0.0323)	(0.956, 1.033)

Notes: Difference is log hazard ratio minus log odds ratio. Ratio is the hazard ratio divided by the odds ratio (i.e., the exponent of the difference). Details of variables are given in Table 10.16.

Table 14.6. Results from 2000 bootstrap samples of differences, active minus placebo, between delta means (also showing sample-based (observed) results in italics: Example 14.10.

	Nonverbal score	Verbal score
Observed estimate	*2.405*	*0.506*
Bias	−0.00776	−0.00005
Observed SE	*1.944*	*1.398*
Bootstrap SE	1.940	1.392
Observed 95% CI	*(−1.462, 6.272)*	*(−2.273, 3.286)*
Normal 95% CI	(−1.397, 6.207)	(−2.222, 3.235)
Percentile 95% CI	(−1.483, 6.255)	(−2.196, 3.310)
BC 95% CI	(−1.436, 6.279)	(−2.108, 3.364)
BCa 95% CI	(−1.429, 6.299)	(−2.161, 3.338)

Note: Sample-based (observed) results are in italics.

achieved in Stata using the STRATA option to the BOOTSTRAP command (the same command also has a CLUSTER option). This can be expected to produce narrower bootstrap CIs since the samples drawn, in total, will tend to be less variable than when choosing single bootstrap samples. In a case where the 'group' variable is not fixed to have any particular distribution in advance of data collection, such as in Example 14.7 where CHD status was not fixed by design to be as it was observed, the argument for stratification by bootstrapping is less strong and would require justification. Thus the bootstrap samples of size 50 used in Example 14.7 had varying numbers of members who were positive for CHD.

Example 14.10 The data of Table 7.1 are available on the web site for this book in 'long and thin form', with a variable denoting the treatment group. These data were downloaded to Stata and the REGRESS command used, just as in Example 14.7, but now including the STRATA option so that every bootstrap sample had 42 members with active treatment and 44 with placebo treatment. Results, both from the original sample and from bootstrap samples, for the two IQ test scores recorded in the trial, are shown in Table 14.6. In this example the bias from bootstrapping is small and the bootstrap and observed SEs are very similar. There are no important differences between straightforward analyses, based on t distributions, on the raw data and the bootstrap evaluations. Bootstrapping has thus justified the use of standard analyses with these data.

14.6   Bootstrap hypothesis testing

Although bootstrapping is generally applied so as to understand and quantify variability in estimates, it can also be used for tests of hypotheses. This may be done by forcing the null hypothesis to be true in the sample data and then bootstrapping the test statistic. The p value for the test is then estimated as the proportion of times the bootstrapped test statistic is at least as extreme as the observed value of the test statistic in the sample data (Efron and Tibshirani, 1993). Provided that we can see how to force the null hypothesis to be true, without simultaneously introducing bias, this is a simple procedure.

One instance where the null hypothesis can readily be imposed is the test for equality of two means: the two-sample t test. As stated in Section 2.7.3, when the variances are equal an exact procedure, at least when normality can be assumed, is available: the pooled t test. When the variances are unequal, only approximate solutions are available. Four main classes of approximate solutions include: (1) use (2.17) and an approximate degrees of freedom, as explained in Section 2.7.3; (2) use robust SEs (Section 9.11), which make no assumption of constant variance; (3) use bootstrapping; (4) use a permutation test. We will use (1) to (3) in the next example, and (4) in Example 14.12.

Example 14.11 Consider the data in Table 2.10 once again. In Example 2.10 the mean cholesterol was compared between those with and without CHD, assuming equal variances in each group — using a pooled t test. Suppose we were not prepared to accept the results of the F test given in Example 2.10, on the grounds that the sample was too small for such a test to have much power. Results of methods (1) and (2) from Stata appear as Output 14.2. Method (2) was applied by fitting a simple linear regression of cholesterol on CHD status, similar to Example 14.7 but asking the software employed to use robust SEs. Currently, Stata allows two choices for the approximate degrees of freedom approach (here Satterthwaite's method was used) and three choices for the type of robust SE (here the conservative 'HC3' robust option in Stata was used). Method (1) gave a p value of 0.0619, and (2) gave a similar p value of 0.058, for the test of equal means.

Output 14.2. Two-sample t test variants from Stata: Example 14.11.

(i) Two-sample t test with unequal variances

Group	Obs	Mean	Std.Err.	Std.Dev.	[95% Conf.	Interval]
1	11	6.708182	.2421751	.8032038	6.168582	7.247781
2	39	6.167692	.1135808	.709312	5.93776	6.397625
combined	50	6.2866	.1070505	.7569612	6.071474	6.501726
diff		.5404895	.2674871		−.0306748	1.111654

```
    diff = mean(1) - mean(2)                                    t =   2.0206
Ho: diff = 0                     Satterthwaite's degrees of freedom = 14.696
   Ha: diff < 0              Ha: diff != 0                   Ha: diff > 0
Pr(T < t) = 0.9690     Pr(|T| > |t|) = 0.0619       Pr(T > t) = 0.0310
```

(ii) Robust regression

```
Linear regression                              Number of obs =       50
                                               F(  1,    48) =     3.76
                                               Prob > F       =   0.0585
                                               R-squared      =   0.0893
                                               Root MSE       =   .72987
```

tc	Coef.	Robust HC3 Std. Err.	t	P>|t|	[95% Conf.	Interval]
chd	−.5404895	.2788436	−1.94	0.058	−1.101142	.020163
_cons	7.248671	.5208595	13.92	0.000	6.201413	8.29593

We will now use the t test in Output 14.2 as the basis for a bootstrap test. There the t statistic was 2.0206. So we need to bootstrap t statistics and find what proportion equals or exceeds 2.0206 in absolute value, assuming a two-sided test. First we need to transform the sample data so as to make the null hypothesis of equal means true in this sample. An easy way to do this is to subtract the subgroup-specific sample means from each member of the two subgroups. From Output 14.2 we see that this requires subtracting 6.708182 from each of the 11 subjects with CHD and 6.167692 from each of the 39 subjects without CHD. Call the new variable TC2 (for 'total cholesterol, version 2'). The mean of TC2 in each of the two groups is now zero and thus the null hypothesis is true in the revised sample. Importantly, subtracting a constant from each member of each subgroup leaves the subgroup-specific variances unchanged; only the mean has been changed, consistent with the restricted nature of the null hypothesis. Next, we bootstrap TC2 a large number of times. Since we certainly want the sample sizes within the two subgroups to be the same each time, to give a fair representation of repeated sampling, bootstrapping should be done within strata, as in Example 14.10. This procedure was followed in Stata with 2000 replications, using the program supplied on the web site for this book. The bootstrap distribution of 2000 test statistics was saved and the proportion of bootstrap test statistics with values greater than or equal to 2.0206 or less than or equal to –2.0206 was computed to be 0.0615. This is the bootstrap p value for this test. Clearly this is compatible with the results for both the non-bootstrap tests in Output 14.2 and thus they are all mutually demonstrated to be reasonable approaches to testing the equality of two means when variances are unequal.

As an aside, notice that the pooled t test result given in Example 2.10 was $p = 0.035$, meaning that we fail to reject the null hypothesis of equal means using the standard 5% threshold for decision making. The new methods employed in Example 14.11 would all draw the opposite conclusion: reject the null hypothesis. Whilst it is always valid to use a t test which does not assume equal variances, when it is reasonable to assume equal variances the resultant test with this assumption (i.e., the pooled t test) will always be more powerful. With large numbers, the differences are likely to be small.

14.7 Limitations of bootstrapping

Since the bootstrap depends upon random sampling, as we have seen, the results produced are not unique. Thus, whilst any question of inference has to deal with the fact that the sample is not a unique representation of the population at large, the bootstrap introduces a second stage of sampling variation and bias that we have not previously seen in this book. We can take more bootstrap samples and use a reliable bootstrapping procedure to protect against this new feature having an important effect on our results, but bootstrapping cannot rescue a researcher from a poor sample— such as one that is too small or is not representative. An implicit assumption made by bootstrap methodology is that the original, observed, data represents the entire population. Clearly a sample of size 50 to represent the Scottish population of several millions, as we have used in most of the previous examples in this chapter, is insufficient for this purpose: Table 2.10 is only used as a source of observed data here because it provides a tractable example.

Another obvious limitation is that some skill with writing computer code is essential to solve even simple bootstrap problems, unless we are familiar with Stata, or another package that has built-in bootstrap functionality. Even then, some problems will require custom-written code, as can be seen from the Stata bootstrap commands supplied on the web site for this book.

A more technical issue is that, since the bootstrap mimics the sampling distribution, we can only draw valid inferences from it if the bootstrap and sampling distributions of the estimator are the same. Conceptually this means that the (unknown) theoretical distribution function of the estimator, $\hat{\theta}$, which might have the normal shape of Figure 2.13, has to be well approximated by the histogram, such as those in Figure 14.5, drawn from the bootstrap evaluations of the estimator, $\bar{\theta}$. Simulation studies and experience show this to be a good assumption when the number of bootstrap replications, b, is large, whilst bias correction and acceleration (or other advanced bootstrap formulations, not covered in this book) can help reduce problems of mismatch. It is also crucial that bootstrap sampling follows the sampling process used to obtain the observed data (or the null hypothesis in testing), for instance when complex sampling is involved.

The basic introduction to bootstrapping given here has only scratched the surface of what is a very powerful and wide-reaching technique. In essence the idea behind it is very simple and its promise as a general method for obtaining CIs is beguiling. Furthermore, for experienced users of Stata, it is often very easy to apply by simply adding the term 'bootstrap' to syntax that is already familiar, such as Cox regression commands. However, not all bootstrap results are as good as others — we have seen some examples of this here, but approaches not covered in this chapter may be preferable in specific situations. Certainly, anyone reporting bootstrap results should specify exactly what she or he did; for example, stating b and the type of CI computed. Ideally, sensitivity of results to these criteria should also be explored. Finally, the methods given in earlier chapters are generally robust when samples are large, so that bootstrapping may not be necessary. For instance, the CI and test for a difference between two means using a normal approximation works well in many real-life situations, even when the distributions show skewness. Where necessary, transformations to near-normality work well in many single-sample problems.

Other variations to the basic bootstrap approach considered here include allowing the size of each bootstrap (re)sample to vary and the **parametric bootstrap,** where samples are taken from a fitted model for the data. Details of the strengths and limitations of bootstrap methodology, and further examples of practical uses of bootstrapping, are given in two seminal textbooks: Efron and Tibshirani (1993) and Davison and Hinkley (2006). Carpenter and Bithell (2000), Efron and Gong (1983) and Manly (2007) are further useful references. For the practitioner, the case study of bootstrapping in health economics by Walters and Campbell (2004) is recommended reading.

14.8   Permutation tests

Permutation tests, or **exact tests,** consider all possible outcomes of the test statistic associated with any hypothesis test, given the observed numbers, and take the p value to be the proportion of such outcomes that are at least as extreme as that observed. We have already seen an example of such a test in Section 3.5.4: Fisher's exact test for 2×2 tables. The concept of a permutation test will now be introduced through some hypothetical data concerning levels of creatinine (μmol/l) collected from two women and three men with severe alcoholic hepatitis — women: 0.65 and 0.85; men: 0.80, 0.95 and 1.00. To create a permutation distribution, we have to decide:

1. What is the null hypothesis we wish to test?
2. What is the alternative hypothesis we wish to test against the null?
3. What test statistic shall we use to perform our test?

All these are fundamental issues when constructing hypothesis tests, even if their meaning is sometimes overlooked when the same type of test has been used routinely in the past. In our simple example, the most usual null hypothesis would be that the

Table 14.7. All possible permutations and the permutation distribution for hypothetical creatinine data (µmol/l)

1st value	2nd value	3rd value	4th value	5th value	Female mean	Male mean	Absolute difference[a]
0.65	*0.85*	*0.8*	*0.95*	*1*			
WOMEN	*WOMEN*	*MEN*	*MEN*	*MEN*	*0.75*	*0.92*	**0.17**
WOMEN	MEN	WOMEN	MEN	MEN	0.73	0.93	**0.21**
WOMEN	MEN	MEN	WOMEN	MEN	0.80	0.88	0.08
WOMEN	MEN	MEN	MEN	WOMEN	0.83	0.87	0.04
MEN	WOMEN	WOMEN	MEN	MEN	0.83	0.87	0.04
MEN	WOMEN	MEN	WOMEN	MEN	0.90	0.82	0.08
MEN	WOMEN	MEN	MEN	WOMEN	0.93	0.80	0.13
MEN	MEN	WOMEN	WOMEN	MEN	0.88	0.83	0.04
MEN	MEN	WOMEN	MEN	WOMEN	0.90	0.82	0.08
MEN	MEN	MEN	WOMEN	WOMEN	0.98	0.77	**0.21**

Notes: The values in italics are those observed. Values of the test statistic (absolute difference in means) in bold are greater than or equal to the observed value.

[a] Female mean minus male mean, with sign ignored.

two (female and male) means are equal; the most usual alternative would be the two-sided alternative of unequal means; and the test statistic might be the difference between the means. Notice that this test statistic makes no assumption about a distribution (such as the normal) and so gives a non-parametric test. The idea of the permutation test, for a two-sample problem, is that under the null hypothesis of no effect (no difference in the mean creatinine for women and men, in the example), the data items assigned by nature to one group might equally well have been any of the data items observed. In our example, under the null hypothesis, any two of the five creatinine values would be just as likely to be found for the women as are any other two values. The permutation test thus proceeds by considering all possible permutations of the labels 'women' and 'men', keeping the outcomes (i.e., of creatinine) intact. Since there are two women and three men, from probability theory there are 5!/(3!2!) ways of allocating two items to women (and thus three to men). See Section 3.5.4 for a definition of the ! operator. Table 14.7 shows all possible permutations, with the observed permutation in italics.

In this simple example, the p value is easily seen to be 3/10 = 0.3. Since this is >0.05, we fail to reject the null hypothesis of no difference between the means at the usual 5% level of significance.

14.8.1   Monte Carlo permutation tests

So far, no Monte Carlo (MC) random sampling methods have been used in permutation tests, but real-life problems in epidemiology rarely (if ever) have sample sizes as small as five. The number of possible permutations rapidly rises with the sample size. Consider the problem met in Example 14.11 where $n = 50$ (still very small compared with typical epidemiological sample sizes), divided by CHD status into groups of size 11 and 39. In this case, the number of possible permutations is 50!/(11!39!) = 37 353 738 800. If some of the observed values of the explanatory variable were the same then this would be reduced somewhat, but even then the number would be so big that it may be impractical to consider all permutations.

Output 14.3. Stata results from a MC permutation test corresponding to Table 14.7.

T	T(obs)	c	n	p=c/n	SE(p)	[95% Conf. Interval]	
diff	.1666667	2946	10000	0.2946	0.0046	.2856761	.3036436

```
Note: confidence interval is with respect to p=c/n.
Note: c = #{|T| >= |T(obs)|}
```

Hence MC methods are used to sample the permutations and then create a permutation distribution of the values of the test statistic from them, against which to test the observed test statistic, much as in the complete permutation example above. In MC permutation tests, sometimes called **randomisation tests**, it is generally reasonable to use a large number of permutations, to protect against chance outlier results, since there are no time-consuming ancillary computations as, for example, required by the bootstrap BCa method. Certainly in the examples considered in this section, there was considerable difference between p values obtained after 100 and 10 000 permutations. Furthermore, it would be reasonable to use an extremely large number of permutations if the p values being produced are close to a pre-defined decision threshold, such as $p = 0.05$.

MC permutation tests can be programmed into any statistical package, although we shall only view results produced by Stata, which has a convenient PERMUTE command to achieve such tests. To begin with, the hypothetical data shown in Table 14.7 were read into Stata and the MC permutation test was run with 10 000 permutations. The key results from Stata appear as Output 14.3. The p value is shown as $p = c/n$, where c is the number of permutations for which the 'permuted' value of the test statistic, denoted 'T', is greater than or equal to the observed value, denoted 'T(obs)' and n is the total number of permutations performed. The answer returned is 0.2946, a very close approximation to the known true value of 0.3. Of course, this is a rather artificial example, not least because we already know the true answer.

As further examples, MC permutation tests were run for the two problems addressed in Output 14.2. Again using 10 000 permutations, the PERMUTE command in Stata gave a p value of 0.0614 for the t test with variance computed using (2.17), compared with the 0.062 found from looking up the value of the t statistic for the observed data in tables — which is, effectively, what Stata did to produce the p value in Output 14.2 (i). Similarly, the permutation form of the robust regression procedure gave a p value of 0.0621 after 10 000 permutations, similar to the 0.058 reported in Output 14.2 (ii). Once again, the Stata commands that produced these results are supplied on this book's web site.

If we can now accept that MC permutation works, at least approximately, when a large number of permutations are used, then we can use it to verify approximations made in common statistical procedures. For example, a Wilcoxon test was applied to the same data used above (on cholesterol and CHD status), to be compared with the result given in Example 2.12. As explained in Section 2.8.2, the p value from the Wilcoxon test is generally obtained from a normal approximation, using (2.23). In Stata, (2.23) was repeatedly evaluated when the CHD yes/no labels were permuted 10 000 times and the resultant p value was 0.0498. This is close to the Wilcoxon normal approximation p value of 0.048 reported in Example 2.12, and thus the normal approximation seems robust. This is important, because the sample size in this example, 50, is not large, and it is thus reasonable to ask whether it is large enough for the normal approximation used in Example 2.12 to be acceptable.

Finally, we consider using MC permutation tests to perform a test for which no reliable closed formula exists: a test for the equality of two medians. Yet again, we will take the cholesterol and CHD data. A Stata program to perform 10 000 MC permutations of the difference between the median TC for those with and without CHD returned a p value of 0.0469, so we can conclude that there is evidence of a difference. Notice that this is (again) close to the Wilcoxon test statistic for the same problem, 0.048, stated above. See Section 2.8.2 for comments on why the Wilcoxon test may sometimes be considered a test of equality of means or medians.

14.8.2   Limitations

As with bootstrapping, permutation tests require insight into the structure of the observed data and an ability to write computer code, although familiarity with Stata makes the latter much less of a drawback. The MC version, also like the bootstrap, is subject to sampling variation. There are two other major drawbacks with permutation tests. First, it is not always possible to permute labels: an obvious instance is a one-sample test. More broadly, it may not be possible to conceive how to formulate the permutation process to replicate the conditions of the real-life data, such as when a complex sampling design was used. Second, an inherent assumption in the permutation procedure is that the distributions involved are the same (although the central points may differ). That is, in the first example used here, we must assume that the shape and spread of the two distributions of male and female creatinine are the same. Hence when we compare means between groups using a permutation test we are necessarily assuming that that the variances for each group are the same. Thus the permutation test, in this context, has the same limitation as does the pooled t test. However, the permutation test makes no assumption of the actual form of distribution, unlike the t test which assumes a normal distribution, or at least the t distribution, a small-sample variant of the normal. When the normal is a good model, the two approaches should give similar results. Thus whilst the pooled t test of Example 2.10, using (2.16), had a p value of 0.035, using an MC permutation pooled t test with 10 000 permutations the p value was, as expected, very similar at 0.0355.

Provided that we are content to make an assumption of a common distribution, the permutation test is liable to be preferred to the bootstrap in two-sample tests similar to those described here. However, in general the bootstrap approach to hypothesis testing is a more flexible approach, and is likely to be the method of choice whenever standard (typically normal-based) methods are not available or are in doubt (typically due to small samples). For a thorough description of permutation tests, and a comparison with bootstrap procedures, see Good (2005), Good (2006) or the more technical brief account by Janssen and Pauls (2003).

14.9   Missing values

The final sections of this chapter consider another situation where Monte Carlo methods, harnessing the power of modern computing, can effectively address long-standing common problems in the analysis of data. This is how to deal with the vexing issue of missing data items; that is, variables that are incompletely enumerated.

Table 14.8 gives a very simple example where there are three variables (besides the identification code) in the dataset, one of which, systolic blood pressure (SBP),

Table 14.8. Hypothetical dataset with missing values
for systolic blood pressure.

Subject number	Sex	Age (years)	Systolic blood pressure (mmHg)
1	Male	50	163.5
2	Male	41	126.4
3	Male	52	150.7
4	Male	58	190.4
5	Male	56	172.2
6	Male	45	
7	Male	42	136.3
8	Male	48	146.8
9	Male	57	162.5
10	Male	56	161.0
11	Male	55	148.7
12	Male	58	163.6
13	Female	57	
14	Female	44	140.6
15	Female	56	
16	Female	45	118.7
17	Female	48	
18	Female	50	104.6
19	Female	59	131.5
20	Female	55	126.9

Note: These data may be downloaded (see Appendix A).

has missing values for subjects 6, 13, 15 and 17 — the other two variables are complete. Missing values can arise for many reasons, such as refusal or inability to answer a question, lost information or failed assays due to contamination of blood samples. More precisely, we will define a missing value to be something that should be included in the database, but is absent. This extended definition clarifies that values that are absent of necessity are not included. For example, the question 'At what age did you start smoking?' is not answerable if the subject has never smoked.

Missing value imputation is the process of 'filling in' the missing values with plausible answers. In the remainder of this chapter we shall look at various ways of doing this, with discussion of the comparative strengths of different methods. However, at the outset it should be understood that the best way of coping with missing values comes at the data collection phase, rather than during data analysis. That is — avoid them. No post-collection missing value 'fix' can be as good as not having any missing values in the first instance. Of course the larger the sample size, and the greater the number of variables collected, the more likely it is to have something missing, and it may be unreasonable to suppose that every piece of information will be obtained in a large epidemiological study. Good practice in data collection, such as the use of pre-tested, comprehendible questionnaires, or making adequate allowance for wastage when extracting blood volumes, can reduce the problem. When missing values are unavoidable, they should at least be missing at random (as will be formally explained) to allow reliable imputation. This requires making appropriate decisions in designing the study and its protocol, and care in data collection.

14.9.1   Dealing with missing values

At the outset of any data analysis, it is essential to be sure that missing values are correctly identified to the chosen computer package. Many erroneous results have been produced from epidemiological studies because of errors in identifying missing values; getting this right may well be more important than choosing the best modelling strategy for the data. The first step to avoiding problems is to understand how the computer package deals with missing values.

Example 14.12 The data of Table 14.8 were read into Excel, and the SUM function was used to sum the numbers in the SBP column. The answer returned was 2344.4. Dividing this by the number of observations in the dataset (20) gave the answer of 117.2. On the face of it, these operations should give the same answer as when using the AVERAGE function applied to the same data cells. However, the latter gives the answer 146.5. Why do they differ?

The answer is that the blank cells in the SBP column of the spreadsheet are treated as zeros by the basic SUM function, but as missing values by the AVERAGE function, and indeed other statistical functions in Excel. It is not hard to see how such discrepancies could easily lead to erroneous inferences if not recognised and accounted for, especially in large datasets where such mismatches may be hard to spot. Although Excel is not ideal for statistical analyses, it is extremely useful for many everyday tasks in epidemiology, during which the presence of missing values may cause issues which will later compromise formal analyses.

SAS and Stata recognise a period (i.e., a full stop) as a missing value. However, not all packages use this convention; for instance MINITAB uses an asterisk (i.e., *), and thus reading data from package to package has to be done with care to make sure the missing value codes come over correctly; possibly they may need recoding. Data collected on questionnaires often use a much different number than would be obtained in real data, such as 999.999, to represent missing values. In addition, it is often useful to use another, clearly not real, value (such as 888.888) to represent items that could not possibly be answered by the respondent (as discussed already, these are not formally defined as missing values in this exposition). Before using the computer package for analysis, these special values need recoding to the package's default code for missing values or, if the package allows (e.g., SPSS will do so), should be declared as a special missing value code. As well as the period, Stata has a further 26 missing value codes, .a, .b, ..., .z, that can be used to denote different kinds of missing values, if desired.

When missing values are used in computations, commercial packages will *generally* miss out the complete observation when the operation involved makes sense, as where Excel's AVERAGE function was used in Example 14.12. When it would not be possible to get a sensible answer by deleting the observation, the package will *generally* simply generate a missing answer. For instance, suppose we ask SAS to add variable X to variable Y to get the new variable to be called Z; and suppose that X or Y is missing for observation 564. The value of Z for observation 564 will then also be missing. The word 'generally' in this paragraph is a note of caution!

In the vast majority of cases, all the above is quite straightforward and causes no difficulties to the user. However, many errors in the handling of epidemiological data arise through incorrect assignment of missing values during recoding or grouping operations, such as dividing a continuous variable into ordinal groups. Such errors occur because the missing values, although coded as (for example) a period, are actually stored as numbers. Both SAS and Stata store missing values as extremely large positive numbers; SPSS stores them as a large negative number. To see why this can cause a problem, we will take SAS as an example.

Example 14.13 Many studies have found SBP to have a positive association with the risk of renal disease. Imagine that data, similar to Table 14.8 but expanded to a more realistic size of several thousand, were collected at baseline and subjects followed up for several years to observe incident renal disease. Perhaps a few hundred subjects had missing values of SBP at baseline. A standard epidemiological analysis would be to divide SBP into (say) four ordinal groups and compare the log hazard ratios for renal disease across these groups, in order to investigate the potential dose–response relationship. Suppose thresholds of 120, 140 and 160 mmHg were used to do this division. The following code would make the new variable, SBP4, coded as 1–4 for the four ordinal groups, from the original variable SBP (containing the raw SBP data) in SAS.

```
SBP4 = 1 ;
IF SBP > 120 THEN SBP4 = 2 ;
IF SBP > 140 THEN SBP4 = 3 ;
IF SBP > 160 THEN SBP4 = 4 ;
```

Even someone who has never used SAS should understand the logic of this code (the semi-colons denote the ends of lines of commands). Following running this code, a Cox regression model was run by the researchers and the hazard ratios produced, in group order, were 1, 1.46, 1.80 and 1.78, with narrow CIs. The researchers were disappointed in these results since they have apparently failed to show the expected strong linearity of the association, due to the downturn in the highest group.

Subsequently a member of the research group reran the code. She additionally ran an analysis of SBP as a continuous variable; i.e., using SBP in the Cox model, rather than the categorical variable SBP4. She noticed that the degrees of freedom for the categorical analysis were much higher than for the continuous analysis. Very soon, she realised that this was because the missing values were automatically excluded by SAS when SBP was the explanatory variable, but not when SBP4 was the explanatory variable. What had happened was that those with missing values, stored as high values in SAS, were treated as >160 and thus included in group 4 of SBP4. Those with missing SBP values were roughly representative of people with an average risk, lower than the risk amongst those who truly had high recorded SBP values. Thus they attenuated the risk in group 4. Adding the following extra line of code,

```
IF SBP = . THEN SBP4 = . ;
```

removed the missing values from the ordinal analysis and changed the hazard ratio for the fourth versus first group to 2.35 — now following the upward progression of the other hazard ratios.

Exactly the same problem could occur with other computer packages and, leaving aside variations in syntax, the same solution would have solved it. The same problem would also be found if, instead of constructing a single variable (SBP4), with codes for the four groups, three dummy variables for SBP group had been defined and fitted. Then all three dummy variables would have to be defined to have missing values whenever SBP is missing.

The only way to be confident with handling missing data is to read the description of the computer routine being used. This is reasonably easy for a specific type of analysis, but not for general data manipulation. Online searches should be useful in this regard, although trials using simple hypothetical data will often suffice. As in Example 14.13, it is most advisable to check all the basic numbers in computer output to ensure that they are as expected.

14.9.2   Types of missingness

Rubin (1976) laid out the basis of modern methods to deal with missing values. His textbook (Rubin, 1987) contains far more detail, and rigour, than can be fit within the confines of this general textbook. Other textbooks worth consulting, for a comprehensive understanding of the subject, include Little and Rubin (2002) and Molenberghs and Kenward (2007). Less theoretical accounts of the subject are given in Allison (2001) and McKnight *et al.* (2007). Useful resources may be found at www.missingdata.org.uk.

Rubin distinguished two types of random processes that might lead to missingness. First, values could be missing **completely at random (MCAR)**: the probability of a certain value being missing does not depend on the true (unknown) value or on the value of any of the other variables in the dataset. Take the example of a study of married people which included a question on the number of sexual partners before marriage. It is conceivable that relatively old women will be more likely to refuse to answer this question than others; if this were so, then this question would not be MCAR. When, as in this example, a certain systematic mechanism for MCAR is suspected, it can be tested using the available dataset. For another example, take a study of vitamin D levels and colorectal cancer. Suppose we suspected that vitamin D (derived from blood serum samples) was less likely to be obtained from a certain ethnic group, perhaps because of religious beliefs. Then we could compare the proportion of people with missing values in the index group and in the remaining subjects; if there is an important difference then MCAR is unlikely to be true. Although the hypothetical data of Table 14.8 are far too limited for any reliable analyses, we can use these data for a simple illustration of the testing process. The proportion of men with missing SBP values is $1/12 = 0.08$, whilst the proportion of women is $3/8 = 0.375$, which is suggestive of a real difference. With a larger sample we might use a CI and a hypothesis test for the difference to guide our decision regarding whether to reject the MCAR assumption. We might want to test for dependence across both age and sex, perhaps by splitting the data categorically into four groups by both younger/older age and sex. We might also use logistic regression to test whether missingness depends upon either, or both, age and sex.

The second type of random missing value mechanism is where the probability of a value being missing is unrelated to its true (unknown) value only after controlling for — i.e., taking account of — other variables. Values are then said to be **missing at random (MAR).** For example, if the chance of SBP being missing depends upon the sex of the individual concerned, but the chance of any one woman having a missing SBP result is the same as that for any other woman, and similarly for men, then SBP is MAR. It may be useful to think of this as SBP being MCAR within the sex groups — overall SBP is MAR but within sex it is MCAR.

Roughly speaking, MCAR is the process of total randomness of missingness, and MAR is randomness only within the levels of what may be called the **conditioning variables.** In this sense, MCAR is a special type of MAR with one stratum. If MCAR is not tenable, MAR is a very attractive alternative, since we should (given suitable data on the conditioning variables) be able to make use of the randomness within levels of the conditioning variable(s) to make plausible estimates for the missing values. Most of the rest of this chapter looks at ways of doing this.

Unfortunately, there is no simple test for MAR, unlike that for MCAR. However, the test suggested above for MCAR really is only testing whether MAR is more reasonable than MCAR, because we can only test for observed conditioning variables. Since the true value of that missing can never be known, there is no test that can absolutely rule in MCAR, just as there is no test that can absolutely rule in MAR. Hence we can never be absolutely sure that we have controlled to such a degree that the residual missing value mechanism is purely random. All we can reasonably do is to condition on all available variables with a known, hypothesised or plausibly important association with the variable that has missing values (this is discussed in more detail in Section 14.11.3). In our SBP example, SBP is associated with age as well as sex (in Table 14.8 values of SBP tend to be higher, within sex groups, at older age; Figure 14.9 illustrates this relationship for men), so that SBP is not MAR after only allowing for sex. We might take as a working hypothesis that it is MAR after conditioning on both sex and age, but we cannot prove it.

Sometimes a variable may be MAR by design. An example of this is the third US National Health and Nutrition Examination Survey wherein cystatin-C (a marker of renal disease) was measured, amongst those aged 12–59 years, in a random sample plus all individuals with high serum creatinine (>1.2 mg/dl in men and >1.0 mg/dl in women). Cystatin-C is then MAR in that it is randomly missing within those without high creatinine and missing with a probability of zero amongst those with high creatinine. Here, creatinine is the conditioning variable.

Sometimes a value is **not missing at random (NMAR)**, in either sense. In this situation the observed data are not sufficient to make reliable imputations: the process that generated the missingness needs to be known, or at least assumed, and the missing value mechanism is then **non-ignorable.** We will see various methods that lend themselves to MAR or MCAR mechanisms, the best of which should be reasonably robust to most types of non-ignorable missingness, but direct allowance for a non-ignorable mechanism is beyond our scope: see Rubin (1987). One particular type of missing value process that is certainly non-ignorable, and cannot be satisfactorily coped with by the methods described here, is where values at the end of a follow-up study are missing due to death, such as in a cohort study wherein computerised axial tomography (CAT) scanning is used to compare the progression of atherosclerosis between subjects with and without diabetes. We could certainly use methods described here to estimate missing values of CAT parameters after death, but their meaning would be moot given that the very disease we are studying could have led to the death. In these situations it may be sensible to include a composite endpoint, such as a change in the key CAT measure above a certain threshold or death (see also Section 11.9.1).

14.9.3   Complete case analyses

One way to deal with missing values is to just ignore them, giving a so-called **complete case** (or **casewise deletion** or **listwise deletion**) analysis. We treat the data as if the subjects with missing data were not there. This is, by far, the most commonly used method in medical research, largely because it is so simple to apply. Analysing the data of Table 14.8 according to the methods of Chapter 2, the complete case analysis ($n = 16$) of mean SBP gives an answer of 146.53 mmHg with a SE of 5.53, giving a 95% CI of (134.80, 158.25).

What are the costs of this simplicity? If the data are MCAR, then the observed data is a random subsample of the whole sample. Hence any estimates derived from it will be unbiased estimates of corresponding quantities in the sample. Assuming that the sample is, itself, a random sample of the parent population of overall interest, the results will be unbiased in the general sense and complete case analysis is a valid approach. However, the sampling variability will be larger than if there were no missing data, so that CIs will be wider and power reduced, compared with the non-missing situation. Even if missingness is sparse for any specific variable, missingness can accumulate to cause a considerable loss of power when fitting regression models with several confounding variables.

Inferences from a complete case analysis are, by definition, only valid for the type of person who does not have missing values. If the data are only MAR, inferences from a complete case analysis will be biased (except in special circumstances, as explained by Allison, 2001). Suppose respondents in a survey have missing data more often when they are sick — then the complete case analysis will include relatively fewer sick people than there are in the population at large. Hence estimates of mean values and proportions from a complete case analysis will be biased against sick people; corresponding hypothesis tests will be similarly compromised. Seldom will this be unimportant bias in epidemiological studies of general populations. Now consider a variable that is more likely to be missing for women, such as SBP in Table 14.8. If, as well, the values of that variable tend to be lower (or higher) amongst women than amongst men, then the complete case estimate of the mean will be higher (or lower) than it should be. The mean SBP for women and men are 124.46 and 156.55 mmHg, respectively, so that women tend to have lower values of SBP in our example. The results of the complete data analysis are thus biased upwards; i.e., the value of 146.53 mmHg is really too high to be representative of the sample, and thus (by implication) the study population.

In reports of epidemiological investigations it is common to have a set of analyses in which a dependent variable is regressed upon a putative predictor variable controlling for different, often accumulating, sets of potential confounding factors. Table 4.8 gives a simple example. In this situation, the series of complete case analyses will generally be based upon different sets of observations (and, thus, different sample sizes) because the distribution of missingness varies across the variables. Leaving aside the concern that any one complete case analysis may be biased, the regression coefficient for the variable of interest, and especially its SE and corresponding p value, will not then be directly comparable between adjustment sets. The latter problem can be overcome by restricting all analyses to those people without missing data for any of the analyses: a **complete dataset analysis.** However, this can lead to a dramatic reduction in sample size even when rates of missingness are low for each individual variable, throwing away much data that could be used to give more reliable specific estimates.

To give an example of the contrasting use of complete case and complete dataset analyses, consider the way SAS deals with correlations through PROC CORR, its flagship correlation procedure. Using PROC CORR with (say) three variables, each with missing values, produces a set of three correlation coefficients: for the correlations between the first two variables, the last two variables and the first and the third variables. Each is produced using the reduced sample with non-missing observations for both the variables whose correlation has been measured, so that the sample sizes used will generally vary. This is a complete case analysis; since variables are considered in pairs here, this is sometimes called **pairwise deletion.** However, if PROC CORR is used to obtain partial correlation coefficients, the results produced for the three correlation coefficients are all based on the same sample; that is, without missing values for any of the variables to be correlated (or to be used in adjustment). So this is a complete dataset analysis. This confirms the message of Section 14.9.1: care is required when dealing with missing values in computer packages. To be fair to SAS, the log file does state that only complete data are used when the partial correlation option, PARTIAL, is invoked.

Since a complete case analysis has relatively low power and may introduce bias, this method of analysis cannot be recommended on statistical grounds in general situations. If missingness is rare or very common, then a complete case analysis may be justified on the grounds that nothing else can be expected to do much better (see Section 14.13); otherwise it can only be justified on the grounds of simplicity. All the datasets used (up to now) in this book were set up for complete dataset analyses by removing anyone with missing values. This was purely to avoid complexity, and this condition will be removed from here on.

14.10 Naïve imputation methods

Missing values are clearly a nuisance when summarising data in reports and comparing different methodologies, such as different levels of adjustment for confounding. If for no other reason than having a single, easily referable, value for n, a complete data matrix would be preferable. Consequently, some simple methods for filling in missing values have been suggested, and are sometimes used in epidemiological research. The most common ones are described here; none of them are recommended, so our coverage will be brief. In subsequent sections, methods with more attractive theoretical properties will be described. Unlike the methods described in this section, the methods we shall explore later fully exploit the power of modern computing.

14.10.1 Mean imputation

In **mean imputation** (or **marginal mean imputation**), each missing value is filled in by the overall mean. Thus for the data in Table 14.8 we would replace each of the four missing values by the mean SBP of the 16 true observations, 146.53. Arithmetically, the estimate of the mean after mean imputation must always be the same as the observed mean for the true data; in our example, the estimate of SBP is the same as in the complete case analysis, 146.53. This is an advantageous feature if the data are MCAR, but explicitly not in other situations, since then the missing data mechanism is not an 'average' process. More important is the effect that the mean imputation method has on the estimate of variability, or uncertainty, of point estimates. As we saw in Section 14.9.3, the SE of the 16 true SBP values is 5.53, but after mean imputation the corresponding SE for the filled-in data with $n = 20$ is only 4.39. In most statistical operations one method is better than another if it reduces the uncertainty of the estimate, but in this case the reduction is unrealistic. Consider that every time we add an extra quasi-observation to the dataset, with its presumed value taken to be the mean of the observed data, the sum of squared deviations about the mean will be unchanged but the SE will inevitably go down (see the definition of the SE of the mean in Section 2.6.4). That is, since the SE measures the precision of the estimate of the mean, the mean is apparently more reliably estimated as more quasi-data (set equal to the observed mean) are added. Taken to a ridiculous length, if mean imputation were acceptable practice then it would be advantageous to add, *ad infinitum*, people to the study of Table 14.8 from whom we deliberately fail to measure SBP, perhaps just by extracting age and sex from taxation or electoral records. In reality, although we should strive to obtain more precise estimates by appropriate treatment of missing values, there must always be a price to pay in uncertainty, in estimates and the results of hypothesis tests, for the values being missing.

In summary, even if the data are MCAR, mean imputation provides a downward-biased estimate of variability, and thus artificially tight CIs; a complete case analysis is preferable. If the data are not MCAR, it has no rational scientific basis.

14.10.2 Conditional mean and regression imputation

Instead of using the overall mean as the 'filler' for missing values, the idea behind **conditional mean imputation** is to take the mean only over all people with the same, or similar, characteristics as the person with missing values. This is a more plausible value to use as a substitute for the unknown quantity, and is clearly a more suitable approach than mean imputation if the data are MAR — provided the appropriate conditioning variable(s) are used.

In the data of Table 14.8, using conditional mean imputation by sex, the missing value for subject 6 is filled in with the observed mean for men of 156.55, and the missing values for subjects 13, 15 and 17 are filled in with the observed mean for women of 124.46. The estimate of the overall mean is then 143.72 with a SE of 4.80. Note that this SE is not much bigger than that (4.39) found using mean imputation and much smaller than that (5.53) for the observed data: the problem of inappropriately reduced variation has not been resolved. Of course, the estimated subgroup means, after this filling-in process, must be equal to those in the observed data; i.e., when a complete case analysis is used in each stratum. Thus conditional mean imputation on the data of Table 14.8 gives an estimated mean for women of 124.46, and for men of 156.55, exactly as expected. However, once again, the SEs for both estimates (3.64 and 4.81, respectively) are unrealistically low compared with the equivalent values (6.10 and 5.27) from a complete case analysis.

In fact the above analysis has not properly conditioned for the MAR mechanism because (as we have already noted) SBP appears to rise with age, as well as being higher for men compared with women, from the data in Table 14.8 (as well as the relevant past literature). That is, even if we make an imputation specifically for a man, the imputation should logically take account of our knowledge (or, at least, expectation) that the true value we are imputing is likely to be greater if the man is relatively old.

If the conditioning variable is continuous, as is the case for age in Table 14.8, a regression analysis could be run to predict the missing values: we shall call this **regression imputation.**

Example 14.14 Figure 14.9 shows the observed values, and the fitted simple linear regression line that predicts SBP from age, for the twelve male subjects in Table 14.8. There is just one man for whom we know his age, 45 years, but not his SBP value. The dashed line shows the zone of uncertainty for this missing value (in general these range from minus to plus infinity). The open circle is where we would be placing the imputation if we used the method of mean

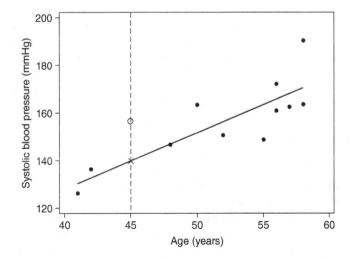

Figure 14.9. Missing value imputation by regression imputation for the male data from Table 14.8.

imputation, i.e., at 156.55 mmHg, the observed mean SBP for men. This is clearly not a sensible choice. The cross shows the predicted value at age 45 according to the fitted regression line, which comes at a SBP value of 139.8758, which is the imputation from regression imputation. Intuitively, this is a better choice.

When there are several conditioning variables, multiple regression can be used. For example, a general linear model for SBP was fitted to the complete data of Table 14.8 with age (continuous) and sex (coded as 1 = male; 2 = female). The fitted equation was

$$SBP = 100.1421 + 1.6518(age) - 29.63184(sex). \qquad (14.14)$$

For subject 6, the fill-in value from (14.14) is $100.1421 + 1.6518 \times 45 - 29.63184 \times 1 = 144.84$ mmHg. Similarly, subjects 13, 15 and 17 get fill-in values of 135.03, 133.38 and 120.17, respectively. With these imputations, the SBP data now have a mean of 143.89, which is the estimated mean after regression imputation based on age and sex. Assuming that the missing values occur randomly after controlling for both sex and age, but not after controlling for sex alone, this is a better estimate (because it is then unbiased) than that obtained from conditioning on sex alone (found earlier). However, the SE (4.65) associated with this estimate, once again, is lower than seems realistic.

Regression imputation can give rise to filled-in values that are impossible in real life. The classic example is a negative value, or lower confidence limit, which (for example) can arise when the intercept for a fitted regression line with a positive slope is positive but close to zero. A further issue with the conditional mean/regression method of imputation is that the correlation(s) between the variable that has been filled in and the conditioning variable(s) will be artificially inflated. Depending upon the aims of the investigation, this can lead to biased inferences. In summary, conditional mean/regression imputation has an advantage over mean imputation when the data are MAR, but is still far from ideal.

14.10.3 *Hot deck imputation and predictive mean matching*

In **hot deck imputation** a 'donor' with similar characteristics to the person having a missing value on a variable is selected from people with observed values for that variable. The missing value is then filled in with the donor's value. In essence, the idea behind hot decking is similar to that for conditional mean imputation, the difference being that now a single value is chosen from amongst the set of 'like people' who contributed data for computation of the mean in the former method. One simple, and effective, method of drawing the donor is to create a set of cross-classifications for each of the set of chosen characteristics for matching (transforming continuous variables into categorical variables) and choosing the donor at random within the index cross-class. For instance, to hot deck the data in Table 14.8 by sex and age groups, we might construct cross-classification by sex and two age groups, < 50 years and 50+ years (the sparseness of these artificial data does not suggest finer groupings). Subject 4 is a male aged 45 years, so to find his donor we would sample from amongst the three men aged below 50 years with SBP values: subjects 2, 7 and 8. Using simple random sampling, suppose we choose subject 2: the fill-in value for subject 4 is hence 126.4 mmHg. The cross-classification set of like subjects from which we draw the actual donor is called the **donor pool** or the **nearest neighbour set.**

One obvious disadvantage of hot decking is that it assumes categorical predictor variables. Little (1988) proposed a similar technique to hot decking, called **predictive mean matching (PMM).** In the simplest form of this method, a regression model is used to predict the variable with missing values from other variables. For each subject with a missing value, the donor is chosen to be the subject with a predicted value of her or his own that is closest to the prediction for the subject with the missing value. Rather than just taking the closest match, sometimes a choice is made at random from a set of close matches, i.e., using a donor pool. This pool can be of any size, although a large pool can clearly lead to poor matches and hence a pool of fewer than five subjects may be preferable in PMM. See Andridge and Little (2010) for a discussion of metrics of 'closeness' and a more general approach to hot decking/PMM in practice.

Hot deck/PMM imputation is commonly used to deal with missing values in large-scale government surveys. One advantage it has, compared with conditional mean/regression imputation, is that it will always give a realistic imputation, i.e., the imputation will necessarily be within the practically achievable range, and of the same degree of accuracy, as the observed values. Generally speaking, we can expect hot deck/PMM imputation to give better estimates than complete case analysis when the data are MCAR, and often (depending upon the methods of donor selection and analysis) when the data are MAR. Andridge and Little (2010) show that the best results are expected when the combination of values defining the cross-classification cells are associated both with the chance of non-response and the outcome (e.g., SBP in our example).

However, once again, the undesirable feature of this method of imputation is its underestimation of the variability of estimates. To reduce this problem, Rubin (1987) suggested a method for estimating the set of missing values together in a hot deck imputation. Suppose there are N_{obs} observed values of a variable and N_{miss} missing values, in the donor pool. Then we should randomly sample, with replacement, N_{obs} values from amongst the N_{obs}. From the results, we take a second random sample with replacement of size N_{miss} from amongst the N_{obs} and fill in the missing values with these. We repeat for all donor pools. Having the two sampling operations puts back more of the unknown variation due to missing values compared to basic PMM. See Section 14.11.6 for another variation on basic PMM.

14.10.4 Longitudinal data

When data are longitudinal, missing values often occur; for example, because some respondents drop out after a certain time. In such cases it makes sense to use information on the same variable taken from the same individual at other times: typically, but not necessarily, in the past. A common strategy is to impute each missing value as the last value that was taken from the same person. This imputation method is called 'last observation carried forward' or LOCF. For instance, if we have recorded urinary creatinine on five occasions in the past, but the respondent fails to attend at the clinic when the sixth creatinine measurement is due to be taken, LOCF imputes the missing sixth creatinine value as the fifth value. If that respondent fails to attend at all future clinics, then all these missing creatinine values will also be imputed as the value recorded at the fifth visit.

LOCF has similar advantages and disadvantages to all the other naïve methods of imputation: it is very simple to use, but it underestimates variability, leading to over-optimistic test results, and can lead to bias, such as where drop-out is more common amongst certain types of people (e.g., those in the intervention group in a randomised controlled trial). See Gadbury et al. (2003) and Cook et al. (2004) for more detailed comments.

When it satisfies the aims of the analysis, a better approach than LOCF is to use generalised estimating equations (see Section 9.11 and Section 10.15), as these have general time structures that deal directly with gaps in the time sequence. However, Li *et al.* (2006) show that a principled multiple imputation method that deals with longitudinal data (Section 14.12.6) has statistical advantages over a repeated measure regression approach.

14.11 Univariate multiple imputation

In this section, we shall consider problems where there are potentially several variables involved in analyses but only one has missing values: this will lead to a **univariate imputation.** Section 14.12 will consider the more complex case wherein more than one variable has missing values. We shall assume that data are MAR, here and in Section 14.12. We shall approach both topics using **multiple imputation (MI),** a MC process involving repeated imputation of each missing value and then averaging over imputations. This general method will first be introduced in the context of the normal regression model, extending the naïve method of regression imputation.

14.11.1 Multiple imputation by regression

Consider, again, Example 14.14. The cross on Figure 14.9 seems a reasonable starting point for our imputation, but (as already discussed) we need to bring in the uncertainties of the estimation process to obtain a valid imputation procedure. Recall that the estimates, or predicted values, from a fitted regression line are subject to random error (Section 9.3.1). We can use MC methods to make a random draw of sampling error, assuming a known error distribution, such as the normal distribution. Such a draw gives us an error-enriched imputed value for the corresponding missing value (the example being discussed only has one missing value; in general there may be many) and subsequently the estimated value of the mean or whatever other summary statistic we wish to estimate. To start the random process (across the set of missing values), we should use a random seed for random number generation. This might be generated by the computer package but, as in bootstrap and permutation problems, it is better to pick a number, at random, that can be re-employed later, should results need to be reproduced or extended. This number should be changed every time a new problem is started (Section 14.4.3). MI routines in commercial software packages, such as PROC MI in SAS and MI IMPUTE REGRESSION in Stata, provide convenient tools to produce such random draws.

Example 14.15 The MI IMPUTE REGRESSION command in Stata was used to make a single imputation of SBP for subject 6 in Table 14.8 accounting for the linear association with age, using only the 12 data items for men. The resulting imputation for subject 6, for the random seed used, was 139.8143 mmHg. This is very slightly below the naïve regression estimate, found in Example 14.14, of 139.8758; that is, when allowing for imperfect estimation in a single imputation, by chance, the imputation has been located just below the fitted regression line, along the dashed line of uncertainty in Figure 14.9. Using this imputed value, the estimated mean SBP ($n = 12$) is 155.16 (SE = 5.01); this is slightly lower than the sample value (using the 11 male observations) of 156.55 (SE = 5.27).

Although adding this random error gives some comfort that the imputation process is more honest than before in accounting for uncertainty, it does not address the fundamental problem of adding appropriate variability into the estimation process following imputation. A clever way of doing this is to add the random error repeatedly; i.e., make several draws for each missing value. This gives MI: each missing value will be imputed several times. From each completed imputation set we can estimate whatever summary statistic is of interest. We then can produce a summary, overall, estimate as a mean of the individual estimates.

Example 14.16 In Example 14.15 only one imputation was extracted. To take a more reasonable account of uncertainty, four further imputations were extracted using MI IMPUTE REGRESSION. The five imputations obtained (including the first, already seen in Example 14.15) were:

139.8143, 137.7417, 125.4214, 153.3632 and 138.739.

We might imagine plotting these five on the line of uncertainty in Figure 14.9. Each result may be thought of as adding random error (positive or negative) to the 'central' naïve regression estimate of 139.8758. Each of these five separate results was substituted for the missing value in Table 14.8 (amongst men only), in turn. The five resulting means (each for $n = 12$) were:

155.1595, 154.9868, 153.9601, 156.2886 and 155.0699.

The mean of these five individual estimates is 155.09 mmHg, our MI estimate of the mean SBP amongst men, allowing for the influence of age. Stata's MI ESTIMATE command gave the same result — see the program supplied on the web site for this book, and reported that the associated SE was 5.16 (see Section 14.11.4 for details of how to compute this SE by hand).

14.11.2 The three-step process in MI

In general, MI involves filling in data several times and thus a set of quasi-datasets, all of size n (the number of people in the study), are produced. These quasi-datasets are routinely called **imputed datasets,** although they are actually composed of a fixed portion — the observed data — and a varying portion — the filled-in values. In MI, each individual imputation is considered a random draw from the probability distribution of the unknown true value corresponding to the missing value; thus the imputed datasets are not 'made-up' data, but samples of what could have been observed without missingness. Under this scenario, it is reasonable to think of making inferences using each imputed dataset and averaging results to obtain the final estimate, such as the mean or a regression coefficient.

As we shall see, by repeating the imputation process, additional variability is given to the final estimate, thus making appropriate allowance for uncertainty, unlike when naïve methods are used. Furthermore, bias can be avoided by appropriate conditioning, Even when the data are NMAR, MI can generally be expected to improve on a complete case analysis and the naïve methods of imputation (see Shafer, 1997).

We shall use M to denote the number of imputations performed (meaning, the number of imputed datasets produced) and m to denote the number of any specific imputation (where $m = 1, 2, \ldots, M$). As implied above, the general three-step process of MI is:

1. Produce M imputed datasets;
2. Estimate the quantity required in each of the M imputed datasets;
3. Pool the M estimates into a single final estimate.

As we shall see, the only complex part of this is step one: formulating a good imputation process, to be used M times. The second step, producing the final estimate, is straightforward as it treats each imputed dataset as if it were a real dataset (e.g., to get an adjusted odds ratio we can use multiple logistic regression, just as in Chapter 10); we just have to do the simple things M times. As Shafer (1997) says, multiple imputation works by "solving an incomplete-data problem by repeatedly solving the complete-data version". The third step merely involves simple arithmetic.

Different computer packages may implement these three steps in different ways. SAS users can carry out step 1 using PROC MI, step 2 using non-MI procedures (such as PROC GLM or PROC PHREG) and step 3 using PROC MIANALYZE. Stata users can use the suite of commands with an MI prefix: MI IMPUTE carries out step 1 and MI ESTIMATE carries out both steps 2 and 3. Some other MI commands in Stata are referred to later: see also the programs on the web site for this book.

One of the attractive things about this stepped approach is that the principal investigators of a study can use skilled personnel, and their own insight into the missing value mechanisms, to produce the best possible M imputed datasets, storing the results for future use by both themselves and less well-informed secondary users of the data. Rubin (1987) gives theoretical insight into what makes for a good imputation (a 'proper imputation', in his terminology), but for our purposes a good imputation is one that produces an unbiased estimate, taking account of all sources of variability, and that lends itself to use by the process for step 3 (see Section 14.11.4). In this book we shall not delve into the complexities of how to generate the imputations. Such material is covered in specialist textbooks, such as those cited earlier. Rather, some basic advice is provided as to how to produce good imputations and the currently most popular methods of MI in epidemiology are described.

14.11.3 Imputer's and analyst's models

As with naïve imputation methods, the MI procedure uses other variables to impute missing values for an index variable under an assumption of MAR; for example in Section 14.11.1 we used age to impute missing values for SBP. To do this we had to decide upon the statistical model that was most reasonable to represent the association between SBP and age in the observed data: a simple linear regression model, based upon a normal distribution, was used in Section 14.11.1. In general, the imputation process requires the formulation of a model; this is often called the **imputer's model.** This model should include all variables:

1. With missing values;
2. Upon which missingness may depend;
3. Which are highly correlated with the variables that have missing data;
4. Which are to be subsequently used in estimation (typically via regression models).

Criterion 1 is quite obvious; in the current setting we are assuming that only one variable will have missingness, but in general there could be many.

Criterion 2 explicitly shows that we will be assuming that the data are MAR after conditioning on these variables, just as in the naïve approaches described earlier.

Criterion 3 requires the inclusion of other variables which, although not part of the aims of an investigation (i.e., not in the analyst's model — explained below), may be expected to be good predictors of missing values for at least one of the variables which are of interest (and have missing data). Example 14.18, Example 14.20 and Example 14.22 all include use of such 'ancillary' prediction variables. In some situations, the investigators of a study might make use of variables in imputations that are not made available for secondary users. These might be confidential data, such as income or self-reports of sexual proclivities which are correlated with at least one of the variables to be imputed.

Criterion 4 requires inclusion, in the imputer's model, of *every* variable in whatever model (often called the **analyst's model**) will be used to make inferences following imputation. This should include any interactions and transformations included in the analyst's model. For any explanatory variables in the analyst's model that have been omitted from the imputation model, the regression coefficient (i.e., the slope or estimated beta coefficient) will be biased towards zero. Notice that sometimes the aims of an investigation will require several statistical models to be fitted to make all the required inferences, in which case the total number of variables to be included in the imputer's model may be large.

The imputer's model should always include the outcome (dependent) variable. This may seem odd, but if we consider the imputation process separately from the inferential process it should be apparent that the outcome variable has no special place in imputation. Although Figure 14.9 looks like the kind of regression analysis that might be performed in an epidemiological investigation, if age were missing for some individuals, and the missing value mechanism made it a sensible thing to do, we could perfectly well impute age from SBP values, rather than the other way around. It is only at the second step of MI that the variables are assigned special meanings due to the inferential process envisaged, as generally determined by our understanding, or belief, in the causal relationships between variables. Furthermore, we want the imputed values, of the variables with missing data, to have the same relationship with the outcome variable as do the observed values of the same variables. This may not be so unless the dependent variable is used in the imputer's model.

If a survival model, such as Cox's proportional hazards model, is to be used to draw inferences, both the outcome variable (or, equivalently, the censoring indicator) and a second variable with information on the survival time should be included in the imputer's model. This second variable might be the censoring time (as used by Barzi and Woodward, 2004), or its logarithm. White and Royston (2009) suggest that a better choice for this second variable is the Nelson–Aalen estimate of the cumulative baseline hazard function (Section 11.3.4), although in practice any advantage seems to be negligible.

14.11.4   Rubin's equations

Once we have all the M imputed datasets, thus completing step 1 of Section 14.11.2, we use standard methods, as given earlier in this book for most common situations in epidemiology, to carry out step 2. The result will be M estimates and corresponding variances. As discussed already, these estimates will most often be means or regression parameters. The method, due to Donald Rubin, for combining these estimates, and their variances, so as to make practical inferences (step 3) is described here: for details, see Rubin (1987).

Suppose we wish to estimate a quantity θ. Let the M imputed estimates of this be $\hat{\theta}_1, \hat{\theta}_2, \hat{\theta}_3, \ldots, \hat{\theta}_M$. Then the obvious summary estimate, to use as our best estimate of the quantity in question, is the mean of all these,

$$\bar{\theta} = \frac{1}{M} \sum_{m=1}^{M} \hat{\theta}_m, \tag{14.15}$$

the estimated value of θ after allowing for missing values.

As ever, we should quantify the variability associated with this estimate. Similar to meta-analysis (Chapter 12), this variability consists of two parts: within- and between-imputations. Within-imputation variance is akin to the variance we find in observed data; it decreases with increasing sample size. Between-imputation variance decreases as the number of missing values decreases and, to a limited extent, as the number of imputations, M, increases (Section 14.11.8). A relatively large between-imputation variance means there is considerable heterogeneity in the individually imputed estimates; in this situation the overall variance (i.e., the degree of uncertainty in the estimate) can be large even when the sample size is large.

If $\hat{w}_i$ is the estimated SE of $\hat{\theta}_i$ then the (average) within-imputation variance is

$$\overline{W} = \frac{1}{M} \sum_{m=1}^{M} \hat{w}_m^2 \; ; \tag{14.16}$$

the between-imputation variance is

$$B = \frac{1}{M-1} \sum_{m=1}^{M} (\hat{\theta}_m - \overline{\theta})^2 ; \tag{14.17}$$

and the SE of $\overline{\theta}$ is

$$s = \sqrt{\overline{W} + \frac{M+1}{M} B} \, . \tag{14.18}$$

If there were no missing data (contributing to the estimation of θ), then B would be equal to zero and the estimated total variation, s^2, would be $\overline{W}$. Thus the additional variation in the estimation of θ due to missing values is $s^2 - \overline{W}$ and the relative increase in variance (i.e., uncertainty about the value of θ) due to missingness is

$$r = \frac{\dfrac{M+1}{M} B}{\overline{W}} = \frac{(M+1)B}{M\overline{W}} \, . \tag{14.19}$$

A 95% CI for θ is given by

$$\overline{\theta} \pm t_R s, \tag{14.20}$$

where t_R is Student's t distribution on R degrees of freedom, evaluated at the 5% level. For large samples, R is taken to be

$$R = (M-1)\left(\frac{r+1}{r}\right)^2 . \tag{14.21}$$

Notice that R depends upon both M and r, but not the sample size of the observed data. This can lead to situations where the degrees of freedom are larger than those for the complete case analysis, which is inappropriate. To avoid this problem, Stata makes an automatic correction to R when the sample size is small. Since the formula used is quite complex, it is not included here; see Barnard and Rubin (1999) and Marchenko and Reiter (2009) for details.

Finally, the fraction of lost information about θ due to missing values is computed as

$$\hat{\lambda} = \frac{2 + (R+3)r}{(R+3)(r+1)}.$$ (14.22)

See Schafer (1997) for a derivation of $\hat{\lambda}$. This statistic, like r, can be used to understand the effect of missingness on the uncertainty of estimation. It tells us how much of the statistical information about the parameter of interest has been lost due to missing data, taking account of the missingness in all variables in the dataset that have contributed to the estimation of θ.

Example 14.17 Generalising upon Example 14.16, we shall now use MI to impute SBP from both age and sex using the data from Table 14.8. MI IMPUTE REGRESSION in Stata was used again, but now using age and sex in the imputer's model and taking all the 20 subjects together. The results, and corresponding summary statistics from standard formulae, are included in Table 14.9. Notice that each of the five imputations gives different results. Mean values range between 139.875 and 144.624; each of these is smaller than the value from a complete case analysis. This is to be expected because three women, but only one man, have had their missing SBP values imputed (and women tend to have lower values of SBP). Although the estimates derived from the imputed datasets are useful in order to understand, and evaluate, the imputation process, to the practitioner the interesting results are the combined estimates and SEs. To get the combined MI estimate we use (14.15); that is, we find the mean of the five estimates: in this case, the mean of the five means. This is 142.950 mmHg, our MI estimate of the mean SBP. Next, we apply (14.16) to find the within-imputation variance. This is

$$\overline{W} = \frac{1}{5}(5.42^2 + 4.93^2 + 4.52^2 + 5.20^2 + 4.81^2) = 24.87.$$

Note that a few extra decimal places have been used in intermediate calculations than are shown here. From (14.17), the between-imputation variance is

$$B = \frac{1}{4}((139.87 - 142.95)^2 + (143.98 - 142.95)^2 + (144.62 - 142.95)^2 + (141.85 - 142.95)^2$$
$$+ (144.42 - 142.95)^2) = 4.17.$$

From these we see that the within-imputation variance much exceeds the between-imputation variance. The estimated SE of our estimate of the mean SBP then comes from (14.18) as

$$\sqrt{24.87 + \frac{6}{5} \times 4.17} = \sqrt{29.87} = 5.47.$$

Next, using (14.19), $r = 0.2010$, and hence the percentage increase in the variance of our estimate of the mean SBP due to the three missing values is 20%. All of these results can be obtained directly from the MI ESTIMATE command in Stata or PROC MI in SAS, as well as from other statistical software.

Table 14.9. Results from observed data (as in Table 14.8, shown in italics) and from five imputations ('Imps'): Example 14.17.

Subject number	Sex	Age (yrs)	Systolic blood pressure (mmHg)					
			Observed	Imp1	Imp2	Imp3	Imp4	Imp5
1	*Male*	*50*	*163.5*	163.5	163.5	163.5	163.5	163.5
2	*Male*	*41*	*126.4*	126.4	126.4	126.4	126.4	126.4
3	*Male*	*52*	*150.7*	150.7	150.7	150.7	150.7	150.7
4	*Male*	*58*	*190.4*	190.4	190.4	190.4	190.4	190.4
5	*Male*	*56*	*172.2*	172.2	172.2	172.2	172.2	172.2
6	*Male*	*45*		127.5482	154.2816	140.1439	139.1031	137.1012
7	*Male*	*42*	*136.3*	136.3	136.3	136.3	136.3	136.3
8	*Male*	*48*	*146.8*	146.8	146.8	146.8	146.8	146.8
9	*Male*	*57*	*162.5*	162.5	162.5	162.5	162.5	162.5
10	*Male*	*56*	*161.0*	161.0	161.0	161.0	161.0	161.0
11	*Male*	*55*	*148.7*	148.7	148.7	148.7	148.7	148.7
12	*Male*	*58*	*163.6*	163.6	163.6	163.6	163.6	163.6
13	*Female*	*57*		109.927	145.1663	140.3396	126.1301	150.4562
14	*Female*	*44*	*140.6*	140.6	140.6	140.6	140.6	140.6
15	*Female*	*56*		105.0237	130.8897	140.181	94.26609	147.9549
16	*Female*	*45*	*118.7*	118.7	118.7	118.7	118.7	118.7
17	*Female*	*48*		110.5982	104.8428	127.419	133.1865	108.4016
18	*Female*	*50*	*104.6*	104.6	104.6	104.6	104.6	104.6
19	*Female*	*59*	*131.5*	131.5	131.5	131.5	131.5	131.5
20	*Female*	*55*	*126.9*	126.9	126.9	126.9	126.9	126.9
		Mean	*146.525*	139.875	143.979	144.624	141.854	144.416
		SE	*5.529613*	5.420848	4.934473	4.516167	5.201727	4.814755

The remaining relevant equations supplied in this section, (14.20) — (14.22), rely upon a large sample assumption, which is clearly not valid here since the total n is only 20. Nevertheless, for completeness, these equations were used with the current data. From (14.21),

$$R = 4 \times \left(\frac{1.2010}{0.2010} \right)^2 = 142.79.$$

A 95% CI for the mean SBP then comes from (14.20) as $142.950 \pm t_{142.79} \times 5.47$. From Excel, the 5% critical value of t with 142.79 degrees of freedom is 1.9768. Hence the 95% CI for mean SBP is (132.14, 153.75). This is wide, reflecting the small size of the sample ($n = 20$) rather more than the effect of the missing values. Finally, (14.22) gives

$$\hat{\lambda} = \frac{2 + 145.79 \times 0.2010}{145.79 \times 1.2010} = 0.179.$$

For these data, MI ESTIMATE in Stata automatically uses the small sample versions of (14.20) – (14.22), producing the answers for the 95% CI and λ of (131.15, 154.75) and 0.198, respectively: see Output 14.4. These results are theoretically preferable. So we conclude that about 20% of the information about the estimated mean level of SBP is lost due to missing data.

Output 14.4. Extract from Stata MI IMPUTE REGRESSION, followed by MI ESTIMATE: Example 14.17. Here RVI is the relative variance increase (r) and FMI is the fraction of missing (i.e., lost) information due to missingness ($\hat{\lambda}$). Relative efficiency is defined in Section 14.11.8.

Variance information

| | Imputation variance | | | | | Relative |
	Within	Between	Total	RVI	FMI	efficiency
_cons	24.874	4.16677	29.8742	.201018	.198128	.961885

Multiple-imputation estimates		Imputations	=	5
Linear regression		Number of obs	=	20
		Average RVI	=	0.2010
		Largest FMI	=	0.1981
		Complete DF	=	19
		DF: min	=	13.07
		avg	=	13.07
DF adjustment: Small sample		max	=	13.07

sbp	Coef.	Std. Err.	t	P>|t|	[95% Conf. Interval]	
_cons	142.9496	5.465727	26.15	0.000	131.1477	154.7516

The problem of estimating the mean value of SBP using the hypothetical data of Table 14.8 was chosen as a simple example to illustrate key concepts in imputation. The remaining examples will illustrate how to estimate regression parameters, accounting for missingness. Although this may seem a more difficult task, the results obtained from MI ESTIMATE in Stata for Example 14.16 and Example 14.17 came from using an empty analyst's regression model to get the imputed mean SBP, so we have already seen imputation used for a regression parameter: the intercept term. In this sense, a mean is just a simple case of a regression parameter.

Before leaving the problem of estimating the SBP mean, consider Table 14.10 which compiles the various estimates produced. The sample size of the hypothetical data used is so small that chance has a greater role to play, in the relative sizes of means and SEs, than would normally be the case in epidemiology. Also, to some extent, the results are specific to the particular methodology used in earlier computations; for instance, our example of conditional mean imputation only conditioned on sex. Nevertheless, it is useful to summarise our findings. The most noticeable thing is that the mean value is somewhat smaller for the three methods that allow for age and/or sex than for those that do not. As these data are clearly not MCAR (e.g., see Figure 14.9), the bias in the complete case and mean imputation estimates is not surprising. Apart from MI, all the imputation methods produce an unrealistically small SE. MI has a lower SE than the complete case analysis, but only marginally so — it has added a reasonable amount of uncertainty due to missing value imputation, compared with the naïve regression approach, but not so much as to have no gain in precision compared with the complete case analysis, which ignored subjects with missing values.

Table 14.10. Summary of previous results from analyses of the data in Table 14.8, with comments.

Method	Mean (standard error)	Limitations
Complete case	146.53 (5.53)	Ignores apparent associations of SBP with age and sex
Mean imputation	146.53 (4.39)	As above; also artificially inflates precision
Conditional mean imputation (on sex)	143.72 (4.80)	Ignores association with age; artificially inflates precision
Regression imputation	143.89 (4.65)	Artificially inflates precision; assumes a normal model
Multiple imputation (using normal regression)	142.95 (5.47)	Subject to random variation; assumes a normal model

As we have seen, compared with other methods considered here, MI is to be recommended on two criteria: reducing bias and making a realistic estimate of uncertainty. However, it is not without limitations. As Table 14.10 states, MI is limited in not giving a unique answer (different random number seeds will give different results) and it has assumed a normal distribution. We cannot remove the first limitation, although having more imputations might help stability (Section 14.11.8). The second limitation probably is not too much of a problem here since SBP is reasonably normally distributed — Section 14.11.6, Section 14.11.7 and Section 14.12.5 describe ways of avoiding this limitation. Furthermore, notice that although MI will very often reduce the overall variability compared with a complete case analysis, as in Table 14.10, it can lead to an increase in the overall variability of the final estimate, compared with a complete case analysis. This often happens when missingness is common (see Section 14.13), in which case the estimate of uncertainty is, not surprisingly, large. This is a limitation of the data, rather than the method of MI.

14.11.5   Imputation diagnostics

Whenever imputations are derived, it is worthwhile checking them to see whether they seem reasonable, in relation to the observed data and the perceived underlying mechanism of missingness (Abayomi et al., 2008). In Table 14.9 we went the whole way and looked at each imputed set in its entirety; clearly this would be impractical with a large dataset or when there are many imputations. Instead, summary analyses, such as means, minimum and maximum values and plots (typically, histograms or kernel density plots) of distributions are often used. Such summaries are compared between the filled-in values in one, or perhaps a few, imputations and the equivalent summary from the observed data. It is not so useful to compare summaries of a complete imputed set (containing both the observed and filled-in values — such as a mean from an 'Imp' column in Table 14.9), with the equivalent complete case summary statistic (e.g., the mean for the observed data in Table 14.9), since the portion of observed data will often far outweigh the imputed data and thus all imputed means (for example) will inevitably be similar to the complete case mean. Notice that the summary statistics being compared do not *have* to be close because we are allowing the data to be MAR, rather than MCAR. But it would be unlikely that the distributions would differ substantially, without us knowing a good reason why they should. Outliers in the distribution of imputations tend to be particularly useful for suggesting problems in the imputation process.

Notice that the imputed values in Table 14.9 have more decimals than do the reported observed values. This is to be expected because of the regression process behind the imputations. Sometimes rounding is enforced to ensure that imputed values have the same level of accuracy as observed values. Although this can introduce bias (Horton *et al.*, 2003) it can be attractive for the sake of plausibility, especially when the multiply imputed datasets are distributed to end users.

14.11.6 Skewed continuous data

When the variable with missing values is continuous with a skewed distribution, the assumption of a normal distribution in the imputer's model may well not be viable. In cases where the observed mean is close to zero, but the variable can never possibly take values less than zero, an obvious problem is that some imputations may be negative — exactly as for naïve regression imputation (Section 14.10.2). This may cause bias in the final results, such as a downwardly biased mean. We can avoid this problem using MI by PMM (Section 14.10.3). Although this is by no means the only situation when PMM imputation can be used, it is one situation where it is often the best choice.

Example 14.18 The web site for this book gives access to a dataset extracted from the SHHEC data (see Example 13.1), containing records on age, sex and cotinine at baseline from 5388 men and women, without CVD, living in north Glasgow. These subjects were followed for up to almost 24 years, and the dataset also includes a binary variable (coded 0/1 for no death/death) and another variable recording the follow-up time (in days) per subject. Suppose that the research question is, 'What is the association between cotinine level and the risk of premature death?' From past experience we expect this association to be non-linear, and we also wish to make adjustments for age and sex. Accordingly, the model to be fitted to the data is

$$\log_e \hat{\phi} = b_1 x_1 + b_2 x_2 + b_3 x_3 + b_4 x_3^2,$$

where ϕ is the hazard for death, x_1 is age (in years) x_2 is sex (coded appropriately) and x_3 is cotinine. This book's web site also gives access to two Stata programs that were used to analyse these data using MI, as will now be explained.

Inspection of the data shows that 858 (16%) of the cotinine values are missing. We should use the remaining variables in the (analyst's) model to impute these. Two other variables collected from the same people are strongly related to cotinine and should be used to improve the imputation — that is, make it more likely that the MAR assumption is realised. These are carbon monoxide in expired air (CO) and self-reported cigarette status (see Section 2.8.1 and Example 2.16). In real life these two variables had a small number of missing values; in the extracted data, to make an example of univariate imputation, subjects with missing values of CO or self-declared smoking status were excluded. The imputer's model thus will contain, as predictors: age, sex, death during follow-up (yes/no), the Nelson–Aalen estimate of the cumulative baseline hazard, CO and smoking status (current smoker/not).

In the first attempt at imputation, a normal regression model was assumed for the imputer's model and applied, with five imputations, using Stata's MI IMPUTE REGRESSION command (as in Example 14.17). The method appeared to work well; when the analyst's model was fitted, using MI ESTIMATE, the values for b_1, b_2, b_3 and b_4 were all similar to those in the complete case analysis (shown in Output 14.5), but with slightly smaller SEs. However, inspection of the five imputed datasets showed that each contained negative values, which are physically impossible. It seems unreasonable to allow such imputations to influence the final results. Consequently, in preference, PMM imputation was used — applied using MI IMPUTE PMM in Stata — using sets of three nearest neighbours. Again, five imputations were run. Results appear in Output 14.5.

Output 14.5. Stata results from a complete case analysis and from PMM imputation:
Example 14.18. *Note*: COT is cotinine and COTSQ is its square.

(i) Complete case analysis

_t	Coef.	Std. Err.	z	P>|z|	[95% Conf. Interval]	
age	.1000601	.0032803	30.50	0.000	.0936309	.1064894
sex	-.4870172	.0645327	-7.55	0.000	-.613499	-.3605354
cot	.0039384	.0004759	8.28	0.000	.0030057	.0048711
cotsq	-3.08e-06	9.55e-07	-3.22	0.001	-4.95e-06	-1.20e-06

(ii) PMM

_t	Coef.	Std.Err.	t	P>|t|	[95% Conf. Interval]	
age	.0989626	.0030334	32.62	0.000	.0930163	.1049089
sex	-.4160689	.0581495	-7.16	0.000	-.5300399	-.3020979
cot	.004483	.0004505	9.95	0.000	.0035992	.0053667
cotsq	-3.98e-06	9.14e-07	-4.35	0.000	-5.77e-06	-2.18e-06

Output 14.6. More Stata results from the PPM analysis of Example 14.18.

| | Imputation variance | | | | | Relative |
	Within	Between	Total	RVI	FMI	efficiency
age	9.0e-06	1.8e-07	9.2e-06	.023933	.02364	.995294
sex	.003377	3.2e-06	.003381	.001144	.001143	.999771
cot	1.9e-07	8.7e-09	2.0e-07	.054433	.052884	.989534
cotsq	7.8e-13	4.4e-14	8.4e-13	.068092	.065648	.987041

Comparing the regression parameters in the complete case and PMM imputation analyses, the values are similar, suggesting that the complete case analysis does not have substantial bias. All four SEs are somewhat smaller in the PMM analysis, by almost 10% in the case of sex, once the 858 subjects with missing cotinine were 'put back'. Hence the PMM analysis has additional power.

For completeness, the table of variance information from the PMM imputation is shown as Output 14.6. Unlike Example 14.17 (where the sample size was small), here Stata recognised that the large sample version of degrees of freedom and fraction of missing information was applicable; i.e., (14.21) and (14.22).

A related, principled method of imputation deserves mention at this juncture: an MI generalisation of the hot deck procedure. This is easily implemented using the HOTDECK command which may be downloaded to Stata, but has limited applicability and appears to have been little used in epidemiology.

14.11.7 Other types of variables

When the variable to be imputed has a binary form, a sensible imputation model to use is the logistic regression model (see Chapter 10). In Stata this is implemented using the MI IMPUTE LOGIT command. Similarly, when the single variable with missing values is categorical with multiple categories the MI IMPUTE MLOGIT command is applicable, and when these categories are ordered the MI IMPUTE OLOGIT command is applicable. Stata also allows for other special types of imputer's models, such as a Poisson regression model which is handled through MI IMPUTE POISSON. All of these procedures are applied similarly to the way MI IMPUTE REGRESSION is used for the normal regression model.

14.11.8 How many imputations?

In the examples so far, five imputations were used because this is the number recommended by several authors. Such a small number of imputations are often judged to be acceptable because of another result due to Rubin (1987). He showed that the relative efficiency of using M imputations, compared with the maximum theoretical number of imputations of infinity, is $M/(M + \lambda)$. Even when the fraction of missing information, λ, is as much as one half, the relative efficiency when $M = 5$ is 0.91; i.e., this is 91% efficient. In Example 14.17, with five imputations, the relative efficiency can be seen from Output 14.4 as 0.961885; i.e., about 96%. Similarly, in Example 14.18 all four relative efficiencies were above 98.7% (see Output 14.6).

Even so, averaging processes, such as the one involved in (14.15), are intuitively more reliable when the number of items averaged over is higher, whilst modern computing power should be able to handle many imputations in a reasonable amount of time for all but the largest datasets. Thus it seems worth investigating whether $M > 5$ may be worthwhile.

Example 14.19 We shall now look at results from rerunning Example 14.18 using the same $M = 5$ several times with different random seeds, and also trying $M = 20$. As in other instances in this chapter, this gives insight into how the random element of the estimation process works. To make things simple, only the regression coefficient for cotinine from the analyst's model will be shown (multiplied up, for easier reading). Results from using MI IMPUTE PMM, followed by MI ESTIMATE to apply Rubin's equations, in Stata are shown in Table 14.11. In each half of the table ten random results have been ordered by the size of the relative efficiency, to make results easier to interpret.

First, notice how all the results vary with the (unspecified) random seed used; this is because each random draw will, except in unusual circumstances, give different imputation sets and thus different associated variances. We can be unlucky and end up with a relatively poor relative efficiency. By comparing to the observed results in Output 14.5, we can see that the only time the SE in the MI analysis is greater than that in the complete case analysis is when the relative efficiency is below 97%. Second, comparing the two halves of the table, we can see that the variation in all three results (estimate, SE and relative efficiency) is considerably less when $M = 20$ than when $M = 5$. Finally, when $M = 20$ the relative efficiency never falls below 99%.

Table 14.11 underlines the fact that a MI estimate is not a definitive answer: just as with bootstrap methodology, the result will change when different random numbers are used. This is the price to be paid for missing data; MI cannot remove

Table 14.11. Results for the cotinine regression slope from PMM imputation using twenty different random seeds: Example 14.19.

	$M = 5$			$M = 20$	
Estimate[a]	SE[b]	Relative efficiency (%)	Estimate[a]	SE[b]	Relative efficiency (%)
44.778	5051	94.47	44.078	4727	99.17
44.532	4877	95.54	45.399	4734	99.26
45.993	4703	97.02	44.889	4637	99.32
44.206	4614	97.96	44.993	4628	99.38
44.397	4578	98.20	45.231	4678	99.40
43.873	4558	98.39	45.884	4688	99.41
45.359	4511	98.57	45.408	4635	99.44
45.356	4513	98.78	45.527	4638	99.47
45.260	4400	99.46	45.358	4608	99.51
45.315	4423	99.72	44.697	4499	99.65

Notes: Ten results were generated using five imputations and another ten using twenty imputations. M is the number of imputations; SE is the standard error.

Results multiplied by [a] ten thousand and [b] ten million (divide by these multipliers to compare with Output 14.5).

all the uncertainty incurred by missingness. Whilst a restricted evaluation, such as Example 14.19, cannot give a complete picture even for PMM imputation, let alone the general case, it does suggest that something may be gained by taking more than five imputations. In Example 14.18 we found a relative efficiency, with five imputations, for the cotinine regression parameter of 98.95%. That was a great result, and gave us some considerable confidence that MI, with $M = 5$, had worked well. We should be less sanguine having seen Table 14.11; it seems that we were moderately lucky to get such a high relative efficiency. With $M = 20$, it appears that we can have considerably more confidence in any one specific run.

Moving to the general case, as in other situations in this chapter, it is not possible to give a definitive answer as to how many imputations should be used: see Graham *et al.* (2007) for a thorough discussion of this topic. What is large enough depends on many factors, such as the complete case sample size, the degree of missingness and the computing power available. As Example 14.19 suggests, examination of Rubin's statistics concerning the impact of missingness allows an informed decision as to whether enough have been used after a particular choice of M. One popular approach is to take M to be larger than the percentage of missing information; when several variables with missing values are involved, as would be most typical, we would take the maximum percentage of missing information over all the parameters of interest. In Example 14.17 the percentage missing is 100×0.198, suggesting that twenty or more imputations are needed to get reliable results. In Example 14.18 the percentage of missing information is 6.56%, suggesting that M should exceed 6; but unfortunately Example 14.19 suggests that a value of M of around 7 may be too small for comfort. Taking account of all known issues and results, if resources allow, it seems sensible to use a value for M of at least twenty. Sensitivity analyses, similar to Example 14.19, are always worthwhile, even if just using the same value of M to test reproducibility.

Another practical consideration arises when the imputations are designed for use by multiple users. A large epidemiological study is likely to be used for several purposes and, rather than impute values each time, it may be possible to create M versions of the data, each with separately imputed data, such as the five sets shown in Table 14.9, which can cover a multitude of purposes (recall that all variables to be used in making future inferences from the data should have been included in the original imputation model). It may be that these M datasets will be distributed to users as well as, or instead of, the observed data. In this situation it may not be practically feasible to consider even moderately large values of M, due to limitations of transfer or computational speed, or restricted storage capacity, at least for some of the potential users.

14.12 Multivariate multiple imputation

In general, a dataset may have many variables with missing values. To make good imputations we should use a **multivariate analysis,** by which is meant the analysis of all variables within a single platform. Three methods for dealing with missingness in several variables will be described in this section: monotone imputation, which assumes that missingness has a hierarchical structure; data augmentation, which assumes the data have a multivariate normal distribution; and chained imputation, which makes no assumptions about the distributions of either missingness or the variables observed. Rubin's equations apply to multivariate MI without change from the univariate situation.

Before starting on a multivariate imputation it is useful to examine the pattern of missingness across the variables. This examination should encompass both item-specific rates of missingness and the relationships between missingness amongst the variables. Knowledge of the structure of missingness can sometimes be exploited to cut down the work, or to obtain better imputations. For example, if a small percentage of values are missing on a certain variable in a large study it may well make sense to simply exclude such people, since the bias and loss of power caused by the missingness are unlikely to be important (Section 14.13). When missingness in one variable is seen to depend upon missingness in other variables, the pattern of missingness may suggest causal hypotheses for missingness which inform our judgment of how best to impute. The Stata commands with the prefix MI MISSTABLE exhibit the patterns of missingness in the dataset: for an example, see Output 14.7. Similarly, SAS PROC MI automatically produces details of missingness: for an example, see Output 14.8.

14.12.1 Monotone imputation

One specific pattern of missingness is easily dealt with: **monotone missingness.** This pertains whenever the variables can be ordered such that each element of every successive variable is missing whenever the same element in the preceding variable is missing. Figure 14.10 gives a schematic example. A practical example would be a longitudinal study where, once a subject drops out, her or his data are missing forever after.

Special techniques are available for data with monotone missingness (see Schafer, 1997): for example, as part of the PROC MI procedure in SAS and with the MI IMPUTE MONTONE routine in Stata. These techniques, which have a direct solution, should be faster than other procedures in multivariate MI, which use an iterative approach to a solution. The drawback with the monotone approach is that it is rarely applicable in epidemiology, because missingness is unlikely to be as well behaved as in Figure 14.10.

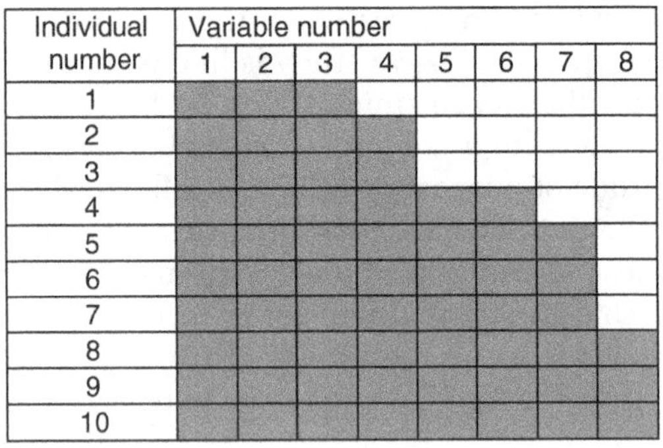

Individual	Variable number							
number	1	2	3	4	5	6	7	8
1								
2								
3								
4								
5								
6								
7								
8								
9								
10								

Figure 14.10. Schematic representation of a specific monotone missingness pattern. Filled cells represent observed data; empty cells represent missing data.

Hence, this topic will not be further developed here. However, in some cases, the pattern of missingness may be almost monotone — for example, where certain few people in a longitudinal study have missing values, additional to those due to drop-out, at various clinic visits during follow-up. In such cases a hybrid technique, due to Li (1988), may be worthwhile. This is easy to implement in standard software: for example, using the IMPUTE=MONOTONE option to the MCMC statement in SAS PROC MI. Once again, see Schafer (1997) for details.

14.12.2 Data augmentation

Data augmentation (DA) is, essentially, a generalisation of the univariate MI regression procedure of Section 14.11.1; a key feature is that it assumes all the variables involved in the imputer's model have a normal distribution. Unlike a multiple regression model, in a multivariate regression model no variable is granted the special status of 'the' outcome variable, i.e., that to be predicted from the others. A key reference for DA is the seminal textbook by Schafer (1997); a succinct account of the method appears in Schafer and Olsen (1998). Amongst other software, PROC MI in SAS and the MI IMPUTE MVN command in Stata apply DA.

DA deals with all the variables in the imputer's model, many of which may have missing values, together. It is applied iteratively such that, at each iteration, the current estimates of missing values are included in the complete data, thus producing an updated regression model each time before the current set of predicted fill-in values are randomly selected. As described in detail by Shafer (1997), and succinctly by Alison (2002), this to-and-fro-ing between random draws of the regression parameters (which depend on the latest imputations of the missing data) and random draws of the missing values (which depend on the latest estimates of the regression parameters) should eventually settle down to producing random draws of the missing values which are independent of the last regression parameters estimated and thus, by extension, the starting values for the iterative procedure. The simulated chain of iterations, each one depending upon the last, is called a **Monte Carlo Markov Chain.**

The settling down process depends upon, amongst other things, the starting values that are used for the regression parameters in the imputation series. A good way of starting is to use the **Expectation-Maximization (EM) procedure,** which is a deterministic (i.e., non-random) version of the DA procedure; this is yet another way of estimating missing values, this time using maximum likelihood methods.

Since this method fails to deal with the uncertainty behind missing values it is generally not as good as DA, but it is still useful for obtaining starting values for the latter process. We should also be careful to use several iterations, to ensure that the iterative process has gone far enough to have lost its dependence on previous iterations, tracing back to the starting values. The question of how many is enough is impossible to answer definitely; it depends on data-specific issues, such as the percentage of data that is missing, as well as methodological issues, such as the starting values for iterations. As with other methods described in this chapter, the larger the number of iterations the more confident we can be of success, but practical considerations must also come into play. If the EM procedure has first been run, this gives a rough guide to the number of iterations required for DA. A reasonable, if liberal, target would be to use twice as many iterations in DA as were required for convergence in EM.

We start the iterative process with a random seed. Due to the dependence of one iteration on the next, it is sensible to have a **burn-in period;** that is, to throw away the first sequence of iterations produced by DA and then draw the imputation. Typically the first 100–200 iterations are used as the burn-in period. Since we require M imputations, each imputation can be based on separate sequences of iterations, each with a burn-in period. More commonly, a single chain is produced; after throwing away the burn-in period, an interval of (typically) around 100 iterations is left between draws of the imputations, so as to create a good degree of independence. Figure 14.11 illustrates an iterative process with three imputations (i.e., $M = 3$), a burn-in of 200 iterations and 99 iterations discarded between draws of the imputation sets. Following the notation used by Stata, the burn-in period is counted up from −200 to −1 in Figure 14.11.

Since the DA process is estimating the distribution for the missing values, there is no formal test to see when the process has converged, because there is no single number towards which the process should be heading. Instead we might check to see whether the process is drifting by plotting key parameters (such as the mean of each variable to be imputed) against the iteration number: this is called a **trace plot.** If the trace plot shows, in the right side of the plot (i.e., after the burn-in period has

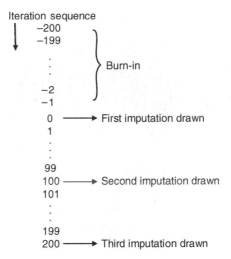

Figure 14.11. Schematic diagram of a data augmentation process with three imputations. A burn-in of 200 iterations is used and every 100th iteration thereafter is taken as an imputation.

elapsed), a zig-zag pattern around a constant flat trend, then convergence seems likely. In some situations there can be so many parameters that need checking this way that, instead of looking at single parameters, only a linear combination of all the mean and variance parameters is examined on a trace plot. The linear combination routinely used is that which can be expected, under certain conditions, to have the slowest convergence, called the **worst linear function** (Shafer, 1997).

We should also examine the correlations of key parameters, or the worst linear function, with preceding estimates of the same parameter, for instance the correlation of a mean value now with a mean value several score iterations in the past. In general, such correlations between a variable at different points in time are called **autocorrelations**. Again, examination is often done using a plot: this time of autocorrelation against the lag (the number of iterations between evaluations), called an **autocorrelation plot**. The autocorrelation plot should not show any large spikes in the right-hand side of the plot; 95% CIs for expected values under the null hypothesis of zero autocorrelation are often included in the plot to enable judgement of what is 'large'.

Examples of trace and autocorrelation plots, produced by SAS and derived within Example 14.20, are given as Figure 14.12 and Figure 14.13. These illustrate a case where convergence appears to be achieved, a condition known as **stationarity**. See Schafer and Olsen (1998) for examples where convergence has failed; Section 14.12.4 discusses what to do in this situation.

Although DA has a sound theoretical underpinning, it clearly suffers from the practical disadvantage of assuming that all data are normally distributed. Shafer (1997) and others argue that the DA approach still works well in practice when the data are non-normal. However, to make the variables used fit the assumptions better, certain manipulations are often done when DA is used with overtly non-normal data. With skewed data a transformation to approximate normality is often employed; typically a log transformation. This will often be helpful in avoiding impractical

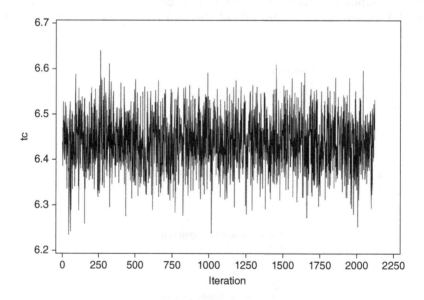

Figure 14.12. A trace plot for mean total cholesterol (tc) for Example 14.20, produced by PROC MI in SAS.

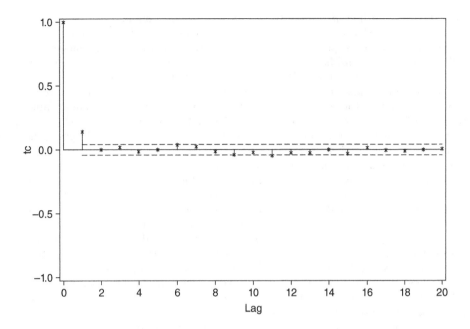

Figure 14.13. A correlogram for mean total cholesterol (tc) for Example 14.20, produced by PROC MI in SAS.

negative imputations (Section 14.11.6). A disadvantage of this method is that the form of the variable in the imputer's and analyst's models may then be different, which can lead to bias. When random draws are outside the practically acceptable range, we may wish to reject them and resample — this is another way of avoiding impractical negative values. See von Hippel (2012) for a general discussion of how to deal with skewed variables when a normal model is assumed in imputation. Even binary data are sometimes included in DA. Although not necessary, fractional imputations are then often replaced by 0 or 1 — whichever is nearest. Bernaards *et al.* (2007) demonstrate that this generally works well in practice.

Example 14.20 The web site for this book includes the dataset, for a restricted number of variables and only for women aged 30 years or more without cardiovascular disease (CVD) at baseline, from the Edinburgh MONICA study ($n = 663$). In this study, with an average follow-up of well over 20 years, we shall consider the problem of predicting the hazard ratio, from Cox regression, for incident coronary heart disease (CHD) amongst women from five classic CHD risk factors: age, systolic blood pressure (SBP), total cholesterol (TC), body mass index (BMI) and smoking status (current cigarette smoker/not). We shall assume that all these risk factors, except smoking, have a linear relationship with the log hazard of CHD.

Of the explanatory variables in the Cox model, age, SBP and BMI are all complete; TC has 122 (18%) of its values missing; and smoking status has 5 (<1%) missing (see Output 14.7). So the main issue, for current purposes, will be how to handle the missing values for TC. The set of variables available for use includes two other blood lipid variables, HDL-cholesterol and triglycerides, both of which would be expected to have a strong association with TC, and thus be useful variables in the imputation model. A further variable that was available and that we might expect to be related to TC will be included in the imputation model: dietary cholesterol (which is missing for only six subjects). This was computed from a food frequency questionnaire, taking account of average portion sizes and using national data on nutrient distributions in foodstuffs (Bolton–Smith *et al.*, 1991). In fact, the bivariate, complete case, Spearman correlations between TC and HDL-cholesterol, triglycerides and dietary cholesterol are 0.29, 0.41 and 0.11, respectively. Based on past experience, of the covariates in the Cox model to be fitted, age, SBP and BMI would all be expected to have an association with TC: here the Spearman correlations are 0.49, 0.31 and 0.20. We would also expect TC at baseline to be related to CHD on follow-up: here the mean TC is 6.3 mmol/l for those who did not go on to have a coronary event and 7.2 mmol/l for those who did. In contrast, the mean TC for nonsmokers and smokers showed little difference in these data (6.3 and 6.7 mmol/l, respectively).

The imputer's model should include all the variables likely to be good predictors of the missing data items plus all the variables in the analyst's model. In practice, there may be other variables available, such as dietary saturated fat and use of statins, that should be considered, but we shall assume otherwise. The analyst's model will thus consist of age, SBP, TC, BMI, smoking status (the variable SMOKER, coded as one for smokers and zero otherwise), CHD status (yes/no), days to censoring, HDL-cholesterol, triglycerides and dietary cholesterol. However, since triglycerides is heavily skewed, this was log-transformed to make the assumption of normality more reasonable. Amongst the five variables with missing values, a minimum acceptable value of zero for imputations was imposed (i.e., values <0 were discarded) for all but the log of triglycerides (which is theoretically boundless), whilst SMOKER was also forced to have a maximum imputed value of 1 and was also rounded to whole numbers (i.e., it was made to have imputed values of 0 or 1). Imputed values for TC, HDL-cholesterol and dietary cholesterol were rounded as in the observed dataset, but as log(triglycerides) is a derived variable it was not rounded. Notice that taking logs of triglycerides also avoids the problem of imputing many negative values for triglycerides in its raw form (since this variable has a large variance and a low mean), which would lead to many rejected imputations and slow down the computer routine greatly.

SAS PROC MI was used to do the primary analyses, with Stata used to perform a similar parallel analysis but without the truncation and rounding referred to above and using the Nelson–Aalen estimate of the cumulative baseline hazard function, instead of days to censoring, in the imputer's model: results were similar. Both used 20 imputations. Programs are available from the web site for this book. Although the log transformation of triglycerides can be done within PROC MI, which will then back-transform for the imputation sets, here triglycerides was transformed before calling the procedure. In what follows, LTRIGS is the log of triglycerides (other labels are obvious).

The first step was to look at the patterns of missingness, some of which have already been commented upon. Output 14.7 shows results from MI MISSTABLE SUMMARIZE in Stata: notice that both TRIGS and LTRIGS are included. As discussed in Section 14.9.1, Stata has two types of missing value, a standard (or 'system') missing value, denoted by a period, and several special (or 'user-defined') values. The former is stored as a large number, but the latter are stored as even larger numbers. Hence the results for '>.' in Output 14.7 refer to the special missing values, of which there are none here. The results for '<.' are the smaller numbers that constitute the observed data. Output 14.8 shows the clustered patterns of missingness, as produced by PROC MI in SAS (MI MISSTABLE PATTERNS in Stata gives similar results). There are 10 different types of missing value distributions; about 21% of subjects had at least one missing value, most (116) of whom had all three blood lipid variables missing.

The simple descriptive analysis clearly shows that, although, theoretically, HDL-cholesterol and triglycerides should be useful variables in the imputer's model for TC, in this specific example they have no useful role. This illustrates the importance of understanding the nature of missingness in a practical situation; in this case, TC, HDL-cholesterol and triglycerides are all measured from blood samples, and thus when one is missing the others are likely to be missing also. Although clearly not the case here, missingness from blood samples is sometimes monotonic (Section 14.12.1), due to incomplete samples. For example, TC might have been measured first, on everyone who provided a sample, and the other two measured only when enough residual blood is available. In our example, we would be justified, at this stage, to omit HDL-cholesterol and triglycerides from the imputer's model. Nevertheless, for the sake of a simple, and substantive, example, we shall continue with the model that was originally formulated.

Output 14.7. Summary statistics from MI MISSTABLE SUMMARIZE in Stata for Example 14.20.

Variable	Obs=.	Obs>.	Obs<.	Obs<. Unique values	Min	Max
cholest	6		657	>500	51.1	928.7
hdlc	132		531	247	.548	3.157
trigs	123		540	330	.374	6.774
tc	122		541	397	3.43	11.44
smoker	5		658	2	0	1
ltrigs	123		540	330	-.9834995	1.913092

Output 14.8. Missing value patterns identified by PROC MI in SAS for Example 14.20.

Group	sbp	age	bmi	chdevent	dayschd	cholest	ltrigs	hdlc	tc	smoker	Freq	Percent
1	X	X	X	X	X	X	X	X	X	X	523	78.88
2	X	X	X	X	X	X	X	X	X	.	3	0.45
3	X	X	X	X	X	X	X	X	.	X	1	0.15
4	X	X	X	X	X	X	X	.	X	X	10	1.51
5	X	X	X	X	X	X	.	X	X	X	1	0.15
6	X	X	X	X	X	X	.	.	X	X	1	0.15
7	X	X	X	X	X	X	.	.	.	X	116	17.50
8	X	X	X	X	X	X	.	.	.	.	2	0.30
9	X	X	X	X	X	.	X	X	X	X	3	0.45
10	X	X	X	X	X	.	.	.	.	X	3	0.45

Notes: X denotes that the variable was observed; cholest is dietary cholesterol; dayschd is censoring time (time to CHD event, withdrawal or end of study).

Imputations were run with default parameters for PROC MI, except for the specific restrictions on values taken by imputations already mentioned. The trace and autocorrelation plots for TC (Figure 14.12 and Figure 14.13) did not suggest any problems. The imputed and observed values had similar means and overall distributions (e.g., see Figure 14.14 from the Stata analyses).

The desired Cox model, relating the hazard of a CHD event to age, SBP, TC, BMI and smoking, was fitted, using PROC PHREG, for all twenty imputed datasets, and the results were pooled using PROC MIANALYZE. Results are shown in Output 14.9; with twenty imputations DA has more than 99% efficiency for all the regression coefficients. About 20% of the information regarding TC has been lost due to missing values; as would be expected, all other variables show a small (below 2%) loss of information.

The estimated relationship between CHD and the five predictors after MI via DA is:

$$\log_e \hat{\phi} = 0.090054 \,(\text{age}) + 0.048375 \,(\text{SBP10}) + 0.073609 \,(\text{BMI}) + 0.430740 \,(\text{SMOKER}) + 0.213616 \,(\text{TC}),$$

where ϕ is the hazard for CHD and SBP10 is SBP divided by 10 (so as to avoid a small estimated beta coefficient).

Table 14.12 shows the hazard ratios for each component of this fitted model (i.e., the exponents of each term). These estimate the hazard ratio for a unit increase in each variable, adjusting

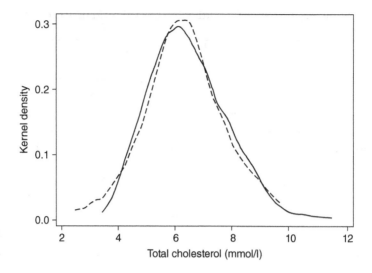

Figure 14.14. Kernel density plots for total cholesterol showing observed data (solid line) and imputed values from the first imputation made (dashed line): Example 14.20. This graph was produced by using DA in Stata with the MI IMPUTE MVN command.

for all the others (for SBP a unit is now a 10 mmHg increase, and for SMOKER, smokers are compared with non-smokers). For comparative purposes, the equivalent hazard ratios for the complete case analysis (i.e. omitting anyone with a missing value for any of the variables in the Cox model) are shown. Quite clearly, accounting appropriately for the missing values has had only minor effects on the estimates: the biggest changes are for smoking and TC, but even then there is only a change in the second decimal place. For every variable, the 95% CI is narrower after the imputation, so that the results from imputations have less random error. Another way to see this would be to compare the SEs from Output 14.9 with the SEs obtained from a complete case analysis. Yet another way is by noting the more extreme p values in the MI results compared with the complete case results; indeed, smoking has almost reached the conventional threshold of 5% significance after MI, whereas it is nowhere near any conventional significance threshold when only the observed data are used. So it appears that the complete case analysis was unbiased but relatively underpowered.

Table 14.12. Hazard ratios for CHD before and after multiple imputation: Example 14.20.

Variable (units)	Complete case ($n = 538$)		Multiple imputation ($n = 663$)	
	Estimate (95% CI)	p	Estimate (95% CI)	p
Age (years)	1.094 (1.053, 1.137)	<0.0001	1.094 (1.059, 1.130)	<0.0001
Systolic blood pressure (10 mmHg)	1.047 (0.933, 1.175)	0.44	1.050 (0.950, 1.159)	0.34
Body mass index (kg/m²)	1.077 (1.011, 1.147)	0.02	1.076 (1.023, 1.132)	0.004
Current smoking	1.520 (0.888, 2.601)	0.13	1.538 (0.975, 2.428)	0.06
Serum total cholesterol (mmol/l)	1.247 (1.021, 1.522)	0.03	1.238 (1.024, 1.497)	0.03

Output 14.9. SAS PROC MIANALYZE results for Example 14.20.

	Variance Information							
		Variance				Relative Increase in Variance	Fraction Missing Information	Relative Efficiency
Parameter		Between	Within	Total	DF			
age		0.000003068	0.000273	0.000276	139493	0.011809	0.011685	0.999416
sbp10		0.000037006	0.002522	0.002561	82528	0.015407	0.015197	0.999241
bmi		0.000006732	0.000659	0.000666	168598	0.010730	0.010627	0.999469
smoker		0.000564	0.053643	0.054235	159498	0.011035	0.010927	0.999454
tc		0.001736	0.007532	0.009355	500.61	0.241952	0.198014	0.990196

	Parameter Estimates									
Parameter	Estimate	Std Error	95% Confidence Limits		DF	Minimum	Maximum	Theta0	t for H0: Parameter=Theta0	Pr > |t|
age	0.090054	0.016615	0.05749	0.122619	139493	0.086783	0.093370	0	5.42	<.0001
sbp10	0.048375	0.050605	−0.05081	0.147559	82528	0.033565	0.058435	0	0.96	0.3391
bmi	0.073609	0.025804	0.02303	0.124184	168598	0.068645	0.077926	0	2.85	0.0043
smoker	0.430740	0.232884	−0.02571	0.887187	159498	0.360853	0.464848	0	1.85	0.0644
tc	0.213616	0.096719	0.02359	0.403641	500.61	0.137439	0.293466	0	2.21	0.0277

In the last example, it seems a reasonable assumption that TC can be considered to be missing at random once the known values of age, SBP, BMI, HDL-cholesterol, triglycerides, dietary cholesterol and CHD are taken into account, i.e., TC is MAR, conditional on these variables. However, this would not be a reasonable assumption if other variables, not available to us, controlled the missingness; nor would it be reasonable if we could not assume TC to be MAR even when the other lipid variables are also missing. All the same, even if we suspect it is not MAR we might well conclude that continuing to use DA, or some other form of multivariate MI, is better than to use the other analytic methods available to us, such as a complete case analysis, because of the strong associations between several of the variables in the imputation model and TC.

14.12.3 Categorical variables

Categorical variables with several levels may also be handled through DA. To achieve this, they should be represented using dummy variables in the imputer's model. As we have seen in previous chapters, this requires $\ell - 1$ dummy variables for a variable with ℓ levels. With such a representation, we will have $\ell - 1$ imputed values and will need to decide whether to assign 0's or 1's in some rational fashion. Effectively this means deciding which of the ℓ levels is most likely, at the current imputation. Allison (2002) suggests computing one minus the sum of the $\ell - 1$ imputed values to represent the imputed value for the reference category, and then taking the current imputed category to be that with the highest value (ties might be reconciled at random). For example, consider the categorical variable 'smoking status' with outcomes for never, ex- and current smoking. Two dummy variables, EX and CURRENT, are defined as EX = 1 for ex-smokers and 0 otherwise; CURRENT = 1 for current smokers and 0 otherwise. The reference category is thus never-smokers. Suppose three imputations are extracted from a DA, with results as in Table 14.13. In the first imputation, the imputer's model gives values of 0.2 for EX and also 0.2 for CURRENT. To use these to obtain an imputed category, we see which of the results for EX, CURRENT and one minus their sum (taken to represent never smokers) has the highest value. Clearly this is $1 - 0.2 - 0.2 = 0.6$. Hence we decide that this imputation is 'never smoker' and thus EX = 0 and CURRENT = 0. The other two imputations in the table are handled similarly.

14.12.4 What to do when DA fails

DA has broad application, attractive theoretical properties and is easy to apply using standard software. As with other imputation schemes, DA may fail to provide

Table 14.13. Hypothetical results for three imputations of smoking status from a multivariate normal model.

Imputation	Results from imputer's model			Assigned imputations	
	EX	CURRENT	1 − EX − CURRENT	EX	CURRENT
1	0.2	0.2	0.6	0	0
2	0.8	−0.1	0.3	1	0
3	0.5	0.6	−0.1	0	1

unbiased results if used inappropriately, even when the data are MAR. This may be because the imputer's model has excluded terms, typically interactions or non-linear relationships, which are included in the analyst's model. The solution to this is obvious, but it may be difficult to make any changes once the imputed datasets have already been produced and distributed. Another example of bias is when stationarity has not been achieved. Increasing the burn-in period or the number of iterations between imputations may solve this problem, but does not always do so. The cause of failure may be a very high rate of missingness in one or more variables, which is beyond the rescue of available techniques. Another may be the incorrect specification of the imputation model, such as where several binary variables with substantial amounts of missingness are modelled using the multivariate normal (see Section 14.12.5 for a possible solution to this problem).

On occasion, a DA implementation can fail to provide any answer at all, due to computational problems. This most often occurs when the number of variables is not several times smaller than the number of observations, or when a set of variables within the imputer's model has high **multicollinearity,** which means that a linear combination of the variables can be constructed such that its sum is zero, or approximately so. Essentially this is high correlation between clusters of variables. In such situations it can be very useful to get the imputation process going by taking less notice of the covariances than would routinely be done, when starting with only the observed data as a guide to the imputation process. This can be done, using standard software, by using a **ridge prior** (see Schafer, 1997). This starts the imputation process, for example an EM algorithm, using a covariance matrix that is a weighted average of that suggested by the observed data and a covariance matrix with zeros for all the covariances. We can make the ridge prior closer or further from the 'observed' form by varying the weight — in the absence of any other information, a weight of 0.5 may be reasonable. This has no effect on the starting values for means or variances, but acts to stabilise the DA process, allowing reliable results to be obtained when they otherwise could not be, due to numerical problems. In general, ridge priors may be expected to decrease variance at the cost of increased bias. Since multicollinearity is more likely when more variables are employed, it is not sensible to simply throw all possible variables into the imputer's model, without consideration of their utility.

One clear case of multicollinearity that should be avoided is having a sum of variables in the imputer's model together with the constituent variables. For instance, we should not include the SF-36 quality of life total score as well as all the components of this score. Either the components or their summary should be included; generally the former is better when there are few components, but the latter may be better when there are many components and missingness tends to cluster within the components (see Graham, 2009).

14.12.5 Chained equations

As we have seen, the approach to MI through DA has one big drawback: its assumption of the multivariate normal distribution. In epidemiology it is common to have datasets with many variables and it is unlikely that all will have near-normal distributions, even after transformation. Even small datasets frequently have binary or categorical variables, whilst issues concerning restricted ranges of imputations, and imputations that are only necessary within a subset of subjects (such as imputing number of cigarettes smoked per day, which would only be necessary for smokers) do not fit comfortably within the multivariate normal paradigm. Despite findings that DA generally works well in practice, its theoretical underpinning and the simplicity of its consistent approach, it is attractive to have a flexible procedure that, in principle, handles all kinds of distributions and restrictions on imputations. Here a procedure known as **MI by chained equations** (abbreviated to MICE, or sometimes just ICE) is described. This is also known as **regression switching, sequential multiple imputation** and **fully conditional specification**.

Taken simply, MICE fits a sequence of univariate imputations wherein each variable with missing values has these values imputed from some (or all) of the others, in turn. The beauty of this approach is that each variable can be imputed exactly as we wish to, provided we have the right computing tools. For example, if the variable is binary we might impute it from logistic regression; if it is a count we might impute it using Poisson regression; if it has a restricted range we might impute it using truncated regression. The entire process works similarly to DA, being iterative and based upon simulation. Full details are given by Raghunathan *et al.* (2001) and van Buuren (2007). White *et al.* (2011) provide a useful summary of how the method should be used, and sound advice for MI in general.

Example 14.21 To explain MICE, consider an example with four variables, X1, X2, X3, and X4, of which all but X4 have missing values. The MICE procedure is illustrated by Figure 14.15. As with DA, we have to start the process of MICE somewhere; we might start by imputing each missing value as the mean of the variable concerned. That is, each missing value of X1 is imputed by the mean of X1 amongst the observed data on X1, etc. This is simply assuming a so-called 'uninformative prior'. Then we develop a regression model using X1 as the dependent variable, only using observed data for X1 (ignoring the current imputations for X1). This regression model (which is an early-stage imputer's model) might have all the other variables as explanatory variables (in which case all the current imputations for X2 and X3 would be included, as well as all the observed data for X2, X3 and X4). If X1 is approximately normally distributed then this should be a normal linear regression imputation model with three explanatory variables. We use this prediction model to update the imputations for X1. Next, we run an imputer's model to predict the observed values for X2 from the observed and currently imputed values for X1 and X3, plus X4. Again, if X2 has a near-normal distribution a normal linear regression would be used, but if the distribution is approximately binomial a logistic regression would be more appropriate, etc. We use this prediction model to update the imputations for X2. Finally, we impute X3 using the currently imputed values and observed values for X1 and X2, plus X4, using all cases in the database where X3 is non-missing. This completes the first iteration of the process. We cycle round again, starting now with the first stage updated imputations for X1, X2 and X3. After the desired number of iterations (i.e., the burn-in period) we take the updated imputations at that point as the first imputation set. We continue iterating until we draw the Mth imputation set, as when using DA, with several iterations between imputation draws.

A choice to be made during imputation is how to order the variables: generally the best method will be to enter them in ascending order of missingess; i.e., the most complete variable should come first (i.e., taking the place of X1 in Example 14.14). Notice that it is not necessary that all other variables be considered as predictors at each stage, although that is what was done in Example 14.21. If there are very many variables in the dataset it may be necessary to be selective in choosing the predictors for any one variable, to avoid computational problems or excessive time in imputations. Of course, we still have to adhere to the rules that all variables in the analyst's model be included in the imputation process and that the missingness should be MAR (i.e., all important predictors in the imputation process are included in the set to be used).

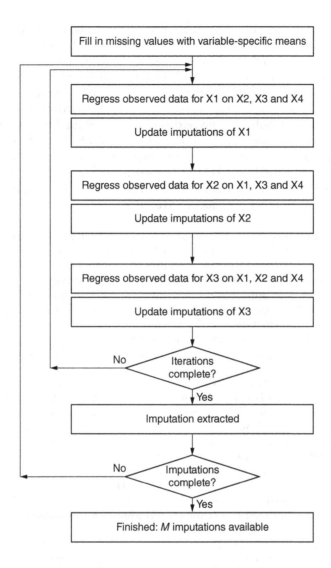

Figure 14.15. Example of MICE for Example 14.21 wherein there are three variables with missing values (X1, X2 and X3) and one variable with no missing values (X4). The regression imputation models at each stage can, in principle, be of any type.

Unlike DA, MICE does not have a strong theoretical justification, although research is ongoing. Its popularity for imputation lies more in its proven utility in applications (e.g., see He *et al.* (2010) and Stuart *et al.*, 2009) and in simulation studies (e.g., Lee and Carlin (2010) and Marshall *et al.*, 2010). The major drawback with MICE is that the conditional imputation models used (i.e., where one variable is imputed conditioning on others) may not be mutually consistent, and consequently the imputations may not be reliable. As with DA, it is a good idea to run some diagnostics, to check the compatibility between the imputations and the observed data, and sensitivity analyses, to assess how consistent the imputations are, using, for example, different random seeds or possibly different orders of imputing variables.

MICE can be applied in standard statistical software, such as SAS, SPSS and Stata, whilst the MICE package is available for users of R. SAS uses the IVEware programs, which are also available as a stand-alone package from http://www.isr.umich.edu/src/smp/ive/. Version 12 of Stata introduced the MI IMPUTE CHAINED routine; the user-defined ICE routine, which uses the same imputation methods but has different functionality, pre-dates this routine (from version 9 onwards). MI IMPUTE CHAINED is an attractive tool for MI as it utilises not only the myriad features of Stata but also Stata's efficient univariate MI procedures, such as MI IMPUTE REGRESS. Since Stata embeds MICE within the general MI framework, the transition across methods is relatively easy to make. By default, MI IMPUTE CHAINED uses all other variables as missing value predictors for each variable and introduces the variables into the chain in increasing order of missingness, although other options are available.

Example 14.22 In Example 14.20 the binary variable SMOKER was treated as normally distributed when the multivariate normal-based DA process was run. A more appropriate approach may be to use MICE, predicting missing values for SMOKER using a logistic regression equation. However, as only five values of SMOKER are missing, this is unlikely to make much difference. Instead, to provide a meaningful contrast in methods, suppose that we wish to consider hypercholesterolaemia as a risk factor, represented by the new variable HC which takes a value of one if total cholesterol is 6.5 mmol/l or greater, and a value of zero if cholesterol is below 6.5 mmol/l (whilst preserving missingness). Similar to before, suppose that our ultimate aim is to fit the Cox model predicting the hazard for CHD from HC together with age, SBP, BMI and smoking.

Using Stata, the estimated beta coefficients from the Cox model were found from the observed data only, after imputation by DA and after imputation by MICE, assuming a logistic regression analyst's model for HC. In the chained imputation, missing values for SMOKER were also predicted from a logistic model but dietary cholesterol, HDL-cholesterol and log(triglycerides) were assumed to have normal distributions. The same random seed was used for each of the two MI analyses, and each used twenty imputations. Results for HC are shown in Table 14.14 (note that these are on the log scale, unlike Table 14.12). There is a suggestion of a slight overestimation of the effect of high cholesterol on CHD using the observed data (before the missing values are accounted for). Both the MI methods give a lower SE than in the observed data, suggesting some additional power for the MI approach. As suggested by the literature, the results for the DA and MICE approaches are similar.

The chained MI results in Table 14.14 were obtained using the default burn-in of 10 imputations in MI IMPUTE CHAINED. To check whether this was enough, concerning ourselves only with the variable (HC), with several missing values in the analyst's model, a set of 200 iterations was run and the trace plot for the proportion hypercholesterolaemic (i.e., the mean of HC) was produced: Figure 14.16. Since this suggests regular fluctuation and no evidence of a drift, it seems that there is stationarity and no advantage would be gained from increasing the burn-in. Finally, when the twenty individual imputation sets were examined, the majority (17) of the twenty filled-in subsets had a higher proportion of subjects with hypercholesterolaemia than the 0.447 in the observed data.

Table 14.14. Adjusted Cox regression coefficients for hypercholesterolaemia: results from Stata for Example 14.22.

Method	Estimate	SE	95% confidence interval	p
Complete case ($n = 538$)	0.611898	0.305647	(0.01284, 1.21096)	0.045
Data augmentation ($n = 663$)	0.589245	0.277949	(0.04320, 1.13529)	0.034
Chained equations ($n = 663$)	0.607292	0.287063	(0.04352, 1.17106)	0.035

Note: The STCOX, MI ESTIMATE MVN and MI ESTIMATE CHAINED procedures were used for successive rows.

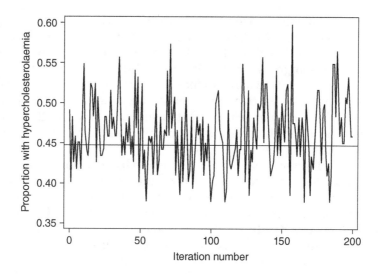

Figure 14.16. Trace plot for the proportion hypercholesterolaemic: Example 14.22. The reference line is drawn at the proportion in the observed dataset (0.447).

14.12.6 Longitudinal data

When data are longitudinal, multivariate MI can be used by expressing the data such that each subject has a single record which has the results (or missing values) for every repeated variable labelled, and treated, as different variables. For example, if creatinine is measured from urine taken at each of ten scheduled clinic visits for 5000 people in a randomised controlled trial, then the database might consist of 5000 lines, each of which includes (as well as other variables):

identification code; randomised treatment; age at baseline; sex; cr-1; cr-2; ... ; cr-9; cr-10,

where cr-j is the creatinine at visit j (for j = 1 to 10). We could then impute cr-j using, for example, an imputer's model which includes (as well as other variables):

treatment; age; sex; cr-1; cr-2; ... ; cr-$(j - 1)$.

Notice that, regardless of the usual advantages of MI, this improves greatly upon LOCF (see Section 14.10.4) since it makes use of all previous information from the index subject, not just the last recorded, and uses both baseline data and information on relationships from other subjects. Imputations that weight according to time since each particular recording was made, or which use subsequent recordings, are also possible to implement.

A case study of the use of multivariate MI techniques in nutritional epidemiology with longitudinal data, including a comparison of methods, is given by Barzi *et al.* (2006). Nevalainen *et al.* (2009) extend the basic methodology within the same applied context.

14.13 When is it worth imputing?

As the foregoing sections of this chapter have demonstrated, when appropriately conducted, imputation has real benefits in terms of reducing bias and improving power, as compared with a complete case analysis. As we have seen, when imputation is worthwhile, MI is likely to be the best method to use. However, if missingness is rare, the benefits may be outweighed by the additional complexity of a procedure such as multivariate MI. If missingness is common, the additional uncertainty introduced by estimation of the missing values may produce estimates with a higher total error than for a complete case analysis. In this sense, total error is often measured by the **mean square error** (bias squared plus variance), the sum of systematic and random error, or its square root. So when there are few or many missing values, it is likely that a complete case analysis is a reasonable choice.

Since the impact of imputation methodology also depends upon the form of the data, the pattern of missingness and the aims of the analysis, it is not possible to state any general rule as to what degree of missingness must be present to make imputation worthwhile. Furthermore, few investigators have used real-life data to look at this issue. An exception is Barzi and Woodward (2004), who compared several imputation procedures, including MI, and complete case analysis, as applied to 28 different epidemiological studies. They concluded that there was not much to choose between the methods when missingness was below about 10%. When missingness exceeded 60%, no imputation method worked well. The simulation study of Marshall *et al.* (2010) came to similar conclusions.

Exercises

These exercises require the use of a computer package with appropriate procedures.

14.1   Consider the oats challenge data ($n = 10$) of Exercise 2.5. Calculate the after minus before differences. Generate 9999 bootstrap samples and save the bootstrap distribution of the 9999 mean differences. Use the latter only to obtain the results following (most of which can be obtained directly using the BOOTSTRAP command in Stata, and from other software).
   (i)   Draw a histogram. Does this look to be near-normally distributed?
   (ii)   Find the bootstrap mean, standard error and bias.
   (iii) Compute the bootstrap normal 90% confidence interval for the mean difference.
   (iv)   Compute the bootstrap percentile 90% confidence interval for the mean difference.
   (v)   Find p_{boot} and the bias correction.
   (vi)   Compute the BC 90% confidence interval for the mean difference.
   (vii) Identify the ten jackknife samples (each with a different observed value deleted) of size nine. Find the mean difference in each sample.
   (viii) Find the acceleration statistic.
   (ix)   Compute the BCa 90% confidence interval for the mean difference.
   (x)   Compare the four bootstrap intervals with one another, and to the answer found using the observed data in Exercise 2.5 (ii).
14.2   The web site for this book (see Appendix A) contains data, provided by Professor B. C. Neal, on the salt (i.e., sodium) content of all 7017 unique food items that were identified during surveys of supermarkets in Australia in 2008. Also provided is a coded variable denoting whether or not any particular food product was covered by the Australian Division of World Action on Salt and Health (AWASH)'s 'Drop the Salt!' program. Products made by a company are covered by AWASH if they had committed to a program of reducing salt. An

interesting feature of these data is that they are severely skewed and yet the large sample size may be sufficient to allow a normal approximation to the distribution of the mean salt to be reasonable.

(i)   Draw a histogram of the data. Note the skewness.

(ii) Create a bootstrap distribution of 2000 mean salt values and draw its histogram. Does this approximate a normal distribution?

(iii) Find a suitable bootstrap 95% confidence interval for the mean salt and compare this with a 95% confidence interval obtained from standard methods, assuming a t distribution, from the observed data on salt.

(iv) To gain further insight into how large a sample size is required before the distribution of means is likely to approximate a normal distribution with highly skewed data, sample r results from each hundredth of the salt distribution, where r varies from trial to trial. For example, when $r = 1$ we could simply take the 99 percentiles plus the maximum value. Each sample will then be smaller than the actual observed sample, but with similar skew. For each value of r you decide to use, repeat the steps of (i)–(iii).

(v)   Now consider a comparison of the average salt content of those food items covered and not covered by AWASH. Find a 95% confidence interval for the difference between the mean salt content of foods not covered and foods covered by AWASH. First, from standard methods applied to the observed data; and second, from bootstrapping, using at least the normal and percentile methods, each with a large number of replications. Draw a histogram of the bootstrap means and compare this to the normal distribution. For a further descriptive test of approximate normality, produce a normal plot for the bootstrap distribution. Draw conclusions.

14.3   Adiposity (excess weight) is known to be related, probably causally, to high blood pressure. What is not well characterised is whether the relationship is stronger for body mass index (BMI) or waist circumference (WC) and for systolic or diastolic blood pressure (SBP or DBP). This can be explored by comparing the slopes of regression lines for SBP on BMI, DBP on BMI, SBP on WC and DBP on WC. To make a fair comparison, all four variables should be standardised to have the same variance and, because age is related to all four, regressions should be adjusted for age. A dataset available on the web site for this book contains data on the necessary variables for women in the third north Glasgow MONICA study. Find the relative slopes for the regression models taking the SBP-BMI slope as the reference (slope = 1). Use an appropriate bootstrap method to find corresponding 95% confidence intervals. Summarise your findings.

14.4   In the ADVANCE trial, 11 140 patients with type 2 diabetes were randomised to undergo either standard glucose control or intensive glucose control over a median of five years follow-up. Using Cox models, the hazard ratio for the primary (composite) outcome of a major macro- or micro-vascular event, intensive compared to standard control, was reported as 0.90 with a 95% confidence interval of 0.82 to 0.98 (see Patel *et al.*, 2008). The basic data from ADVANCE needed to compute these statistics is available from the web site for this book (see Appendix A).

(i)   Check that the published results are correct.

(ii) The confidence interval for the hazard ratio depends upon a normal assumption (on the log scale). By using an appropriately large number of replications, use bootstrapping (stratified by treatment) to check whether this assumption seems reasonable.

(iii) One alternative model that could be fitted to these data is the logistic (which ignores censoring and thus is not as good as the Cox model). The odds ratio (with confidence limits) should be a reasonable approximation to the hazard ratio since follow-up is fairly complete in ADVANCE. Fit a logistic model and see how good the approximation is.

(iv) As with the Cox model, the confidence interval from the logistic model relies upon a normal approximation. Use bootstrapping to assess whether this is a reasonable assumption in this case.

(v) Similar to (iii), fit a binomial model (with log link) to the ADVANCE data.

(vi) Similar to (iv), bootstrap the binomial.

(vii) Compare and contrast the observed and bootstrap results for all three models.

14.5 The web site for this book contains another set of data from ADVANCE, this time for the 9304 subjects in ADVANCE with a glycated haemoglobin (HbA1c) level of 8% or below. In Zoungas *et al.* (2012) this dataset was employed to estimate the value of HbA1c at which the hazard for death was least. This was achieved by fitting a Cox model for the log hazard ratio for death using a quadratic function in HbA1c. In general, for a quadratic model,

$$\text{log hazard ratio} = bx + cx^2.$$

The minimum will occur when $x = -b/(2c)$. In the ADVANCE problem, HbA1c takes the place of x and b and c are the estimated beta coefficients for HbA1c and its square, respectively.

(i) Fit the quadratic Cox model, and plot it. By eye, estimate where the curve achieves its minimum. Use the equation in x above to estimate the level of HbA1c where this minimum occurs.

(ii) There is no standard formula for the confidence interval for such a minimum risk threshold. Use bootstrapping to obtain a 95% confidence interval.

(iii) Consider the clinical implications of these results.

14.6 Consider the problem of Exercise 14.2 (v) anew. Suppose we wish to test whether the food products covered by AWASH have different levels of salt than those not covered. Given such a problem, a standard approach would be to run a two-sample t test. However, virtually any simple descriptive analyses (such as the histogram suggested in Exercise 14.2 (i)) will show the extreme skew in these data and, in such cases, it is common practice in medical research to run the t test after a logarithmic transformation.

(i) Run a preliminary test of equality of variances, and then run the appropriate two-sample t test of equality between the mean levels of salt amongst products covered and not covered by AWASH.

(ii) Repeat the two steps in (i), but for the logarithm of salt.

(iii) Assuming the usual 5% threshold for statistical significance, what do you conclude from these two t tests?

(iv) Find the p value for the test of equal means by bootstrapping.

(v) Find the p value for the test of equal means by using a Monte Carlo permutation test.

(vi) Another possible approach to this problem would be to run a two-sample Wilcoxon test. Run this test and report the p value.

(vii) Yet another approach would be to test the difference between the medians, rather than the means. Do this using a Monte Carlo permutation test. Report the p value.

(viii) Draw a conclusion: is there evidence that products covered by AWASH have different levels of salt to those not covered?

14.7 The following table shows a small artificial dataset with three missing values:

Subject number	Age (years)	Sex	Vitamin D (ng/ml)
1	47	Male	1.8
2	76	Male	23.6
3	52	Male	2.2
4	59	Male	
5	43	Female	3.1
6	39	Female	4.7
7	45	Male	
8	60	Male	12.4
9	57	Female	44.2
10	38	Female	
11	63	Female	3.0
12	61	Male	8.5
13	36	Male	57.6

(i) Carry out a complete case analysis to find the mean value of vitamin D overall, and by sex. Also compute the associated standard error of the mean.

(ii) Impute the missing values of vitamin D by mean imputation. Use these filled-in values to estimate the mean vitamin D with corresponding standard error.

(iii) Impute the missing values of vitamin D by conditional mean imputation, conditioning on sex. Use these filled-in values to estimate the mean vitamin D, overall and by sex, with corresponding standard error.

(iv) Impute the missing values for vitamin D by regression imputation, regressing on sex and age. Write down the regression equation used and the three imputed values obtained. Use these to estimate the mean vitamin D with corresponding standard error.

(v) Suppose hot deck imputation is to be used with strata defined by sex and age (<50 years and 50+ years). What are the possible forms of the imputed data? Taking one of these, estimate the mean vitamin D with corresponding standard error.

(vi) Summarise the various answers obtained here in a table, with comments on the disadvantages of each of the methods used.

14.8 Data augmentation, involving all the variables available, was used to generate five imputations for the data in Exercise 14.7. The results obtained according to imputation ("Imp") number for those with missing vitamin D values were:

Subject	Imp 1	Imp 2	Imp 3	Imp 4	Imp 5
4	3.0	30.6	10.7	10.8	15.1
7	36.9	36.2	39.1	28.8	23.9
10	24.0	58.0	30.0	27.8	11.7

Use Rubin's equations to find:

(i)   The estimated mean vitamin D.

(ii)   The within-imputation variance.

(iii)   The between-imputation variance.

(iv)   The standard error of the mean vitamin D.

(v)   The percentage increase in the variance of the estimate of the mean vitamin D due to the three missing values.

(vi)   A 95% confidence interval for mean vitamin D (using (14.21) to obtain R).

(vii)   The percentage of information on vitamin D that is lost due to missingness.

(viii) The relative efficiency of using five imputations.

14.9   Carry out multiple imputation by data augmentation on the data of Exercise 14.7 from first principles. Use five imputations. Compare your answers with those given in Exercise 14.8. Use trace and autocorrelation plots to check whether the imputation process seems to have worked acceptably.

14.10   Repeat the process in Exercise 14.9, keeping all the conditions the same except for varying the random number seed and the number of imputations used, M. Let M take the values 5, 20, 100, 1 000, 10 000 and 100 000. Repeat the use of each M five times. Each time, report the mean and standard error of vitamin D (i.e., produce results five times for each value of M). Discuss your findings.

14.11   Suppose the goal of our research is to estimate how vitamin D depends upon age, having adjusted for sex and having used multiple imputation to take account of missing values, and the only information available is that given in these exercises and your solutions to them. How could you do this, using only a simple calculator or basic Excel? Hence, or otherwise, estimate the sex-adjusted rate of decrease in vitamin D with increasing age. Comment on how far this result might be useful, assuming the data of Exercise 14.7 are real. How much of a limitation, to practical utility of the estimated slope, is the missing values?

14.12   Take the Scottish Heart Health Study data first introduced in Example 10.12 (available on the web site for this book).

(i)   Fit a Cox model to predict the hazard of coronary heart disease from serum total cholesterol, systolic blood pressure and smoking. Confirm that the fitted model is as specified in Example 13.7.

(ii)   Set the level of systolic blood pressure to missing for the first 200 subjects in the dataset. Set the levels of total cholesterol to missing for the next 200 subjects; the level of smoking to missing for the next 200 subjects; and the level of activity to missing for the next 200 subjects. This gives a revised dataset which includes 800 subjects with a single missing value. Fit the same Cox model as in (i) to this new dataset.

(iii)   Impute the missing values by any principled method of choice and compare the results to those in (i) and (ii). Discuss whether any differences seen were as expected.

14.13   This book's web site contains data from the Fletcher Challenge Study (MacMahon et al., 1995), as included in the Asia Pacific Cohort Studies Collaboration. Suppose the research goal is to estimate the effect of blood glucose on the odds of a premature death, adjusting for age and sex. Since most past studies have analysed the logarithm of glucose, rather than glucose itself (due to its skewness), find the odds of death for a one unit increase in log glucose, adjusting for age and sex:

(i)   Using a complete case analysis.
(ii) Using 25 imputations from multiple imputation by chained equations. The imputer's model is to include all variables in the regression model plus body mass index (BMI) and history of a doctor diagnosis of diabetes — both of which were strongly related to the level of glucose in past studies. Two variables have missing values: log glucose and BMI. Both should be imputed using normal regression.
(iii) Contrast your results.
(iv) Examine the sensitivity of your results by repeating (ii) using different random seeds, using different numbers of imputations and using different methods of imputation (predictive mean matching and data augmentation are obvious alternatives).

Materials available on the web site for this book

The catalogue page for this book is:

http://www.crcpress.com/product/isbn/9781439839706.

The items listed in this appendix, as well as any updates to the text, are available from the Downloads & Updates tab on this catalogue page.

In addition, a solutions manual is available from the publisher for lecturers adopting the book for a course. They should contact orders@taylorandfrancis.com to request the solutions manual or to request an evaluation copy of this book. Evaluation copies may also be requested by completing the form at:

www.crcpress.com/textbooks/evaluation/9781439839706.

A.1   SAS programs

These are named according to the example to which they first refer in the text. The set includes all the SAS programs used to produce outputs included in the text.

A.2   Stata programs

These are also labelled by the example to which they refer. Again, all Stata programs used to produce outputs in the text are included.

A.3   Sample size spreadsheet (authors: L.M.A. Francis and M. Woodward)

This is an Excel spreadsheet which should be self-explanatory to use.

A.4   Floating absolute risks macros (author: A. Palmer)

This is a bundle of SAS macros with embedded annotation to explain how to use them.

A.5   SAS and Stata programs for the integrated discrimination improvement and net reclassification improvement (authors: M. Pencina, K. Kennedy and Y. Sang)

This is a set of programs that deal with both fixed and variable cohorts. Note that the bootstrap methods used for survival data are rudimentary.

A.6   SAS program for a c-statistic from survival data
         (author: M. Pencina)

A.7   Datasets

The following lists the datasets on the web site that are used in the text. In each case, the place where the dataset first appears in the text is indicated (many are used in subsequent places) and the order of the variables listed is as in the dataset. The list is split into data that derive (at least in their first appearance) in examples, tables or exercises. All the datasets have been constructed in free format (i.e., with spaces between the variables). Data generally appear as on the source database from which they were taken; in some instances the observations have several more decimal places than the accuracy of their measurement justifies. See Appendix C for full listings of additional, small datasets used in exercises.

AWASH = Australian Division of World Action on Salt and Health; BMI = body mass index; CHD = coronary heart disease; CVD = cardiovascular disease; DBP = diastolic blood pressure; HDL = high density lipoprotein; SBP = systolic blood pressure.

Point of origin	Variables (outcomes)
Examples	
2.13	Fibrinogen by prothrombin time (g/l); fibrinogen by the von Clauss method (g/l).
5.9	Age (years); tenure (1 = owner–occupier; 2 = renter); CHD (0 = no; 1 = yes); survival time (days).
9.8	Diet (1 = omnivores; 2 = vegetarians; 3 = vegans); cholesterol (mmol/l); sex (1 = male; 2 = female).
9.12	Serum HDL-cholesterol (mmol/l); age (years); alcohol (units/week); dietary cholesterol (mg/day); fibre (g/day).
9.16	Fibrinogen (g/l); age (years); *H. pylori* status (0 = no; 1 = yes).
9.19	Table 2.15 in long form.
9.20	Table 7.5 in long form.
9.21	Subject identification number (arbitrary); week number; group (C = control; R = reduced salt); acceptability score; flavour score; change detected (0 = no; 1 = yes). A period (full stop) denotes a missing value.
10.10	Age (years); death (0 = no; 1 = yes).
10.12	Age (years); cholesterol (mmol/l); BMI (kg/m^2); SBP (mmHg); smoking (1 = never; 2 = ex; 3 = current); activity (1 = active; 2 = average; 3 = inactive); CHD (0 = no; 1 = yes); survival time (days).
10.23	Sex (1 = male; 2 = female); Bortner score; Bortner quarter; CHD (0 = no; 1 = yes); survival time (days).
10.26	Estimated glomerular filtration rate (ml/min/1.73 m^2); stroke (0 = no; 1 = yes)
10.39	Table 4.6 in generic form.
10.45	Age (years); deprivation score; smoker (0 = no; 1 = yes); heavy drinker (0 = no; 1 = yes); cancer (0 = no; 1 = yes).
11.8	Cholesterol fifth; SBP fifth; CHD event (0 = no; 1 = yes); survival time (days).
11.20	Smoker (0 = no; 1 = yes); age (years); time to event (days); event (0 = no event; 1 = CVD; 2 = death from a non-CVD cause).
12.13	First author (with sex code); level of adjustment (hash notation); estimate; lower 95% confidence limit; upper 95% confidence limit.
13.1	Sex (1 = male, 2 = female); fibrinogen (g/l); CVD within 10 years (0 = no; 1 = yes); CVD during follow-up (0 = no; 1 = yes); survival time (days).
14.8	Table 3.1 in generic form.

Point of origin	Variables (outcomes)
14.18	Age (years); sex (1 = male; 2 = female); carbon monoxide in expired air (ppm); smoker (0 = no; 1 =yes); cotinine (ng/ml); survival time (days); death (0 = no; 1 = yes). A period denotes a missing value.
14.20	SBP (mmHg); age (years); BMI (kg/m^2); CHD (0 = no; 1 = yes); survival time (days); dietary cholesterol (mg/day); serum HDL-cholesterol (mmol/l); serum triglycerides (mmol/l); serum total cholesterol (mmol/l); smoker (0 = no; 1 = yes). A period denotes a missing value.

Tables

2.10	As in the table.
4.9	Age group (1 to 8 in rank order); number of events; population; deprivation group (1 to 4 in rank order).
5.14	Age group (1 to 6 in rank order); tenure (1 = owner–occupier; 2 = renter); number of events; person-years.
7.1	As in the table except for treatment (1 = placebo; 2 = active).
9.1	Diet (1 = omnivores; 2 = vegetarians; 3 = vegans); cholesterol (mmol/l).
9.8	Type of country (1 = industrialised; 2 = developing); sugar (kg/head/year); DMFT score.
9.11	Diet (1 = omnivores; 2 = vegetarians; 3 = vegans); cholesterol (mmol/l); sex (1 = male; 2 = female).
9.15	As in the table.
10.4	Age (years); death (0 = no; 1 = yes); number of subjects.
10.14	SBP fifth; cholesterol fifth; CHD (0 = no; 1 = yes); number of subjects.
10.42	As in the table.
11.1	Time (weeks); cellularity (1 = low; 2 = high).
14.8	As in table except for sex (1 = male; 2 = female). A period denotes a missing value.

Exercises

2.2	Survival time (days); censored (0 = no; 1 = yes); sex (1 = male; 2 = female); age (years); education (1 = literate; 2 = illiterate); religion (1 = Hindu; 2 = Christian; 3 = Muslim); marital status (1 = single; 2 = separated/divorced; 3 = married); type of tumour (1 = local; 2 = regional; 3 = advanced).
2.4	Age (years); alcohol group (1 = nondrinker; 2 = occasional drinker (zero consumption in the past week); 3 = mild; 4 = medium; 5 = heavy); protein C (iu/dl); protein S (%pool).
6.12	Matched set (arbitrary number); case–control status (0 = control; 1 = case); hormone replacement therapy use (0 = not a current user; 1 = current user); BMI (kg/m^2). An asterisk denotes a missing value.
10.19	Propensity score; matched set (arbitrary number); current smoker (0 = no; 1 = yes); age (years); total cholesterol (mmol/l); BMI (kg/m^2); SBP (mmHg).
13.1	Age (years); BMI (kg/m^2); SBP (mmHg); DBP (mmHg); sodium (mmol/l); creatinine (μmol/l); Barthel score; stroke (0 = no; 1 = yes).
14.2	AWASH code (1 = covered; 2 = not covered); sodium (mg/100g).
14.3	Age (years); BMI (kg/m^2); waist circumference (cm); DBP (mmHg); SBP (mmHg).
14.4	Treatment (0 = standard care; 1 = intensive care); primary outcome event (0 = no event; 1 = event); survival time (days).
14.5	Glycated haemoglobin (%); death (0 = no; 1 = yes); survival time (days).
14.13	Death (0 = no; 1 = yes); age (years); sex (0 = male; 1 = female); glucose (mmol/l); BMI (kg/m^2); previous doctor diagnosis of diabetes (0 = no; 1 = yes).

APPENDIX B

Statistical tables

TABLE B.1. The standard normal distribution.

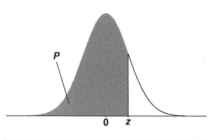

The normal distribution with mean 0 and standard deviation 1 is tabulated below. For each value z, the quantity given is the proportion P of the distribution less than z. For a normal distribution, with mean μ and variance σ^2, the proportion of the distribution less than some value, x, is obtained by calculating $z = (x - \mu)/\sigma$ and reading off the proportion corresponding to this value of z.

z	P	z	P	z	P	z	P	z	P	z	P
−4.00	0.00003	−2.05	0.0202	−1.00	0.1587	0.00	0.5000	1.05	0.8531	2.10	0.9821
−3.50	0.00023	−2.00	.0228	−0.95	.1711	0.05	.5199	1.10	.8643	2.15	.9842
−3.00	0.0013	−1.95	.0256	−0.90	.1841	0.10	.5398	1.15	.8749	2.20	.9861
−2.95	0.0016	−1.90	0.0287	−0.85	0.1977	0.15	0.5596	1.20	0.8849	2.25	0.9878
−2.90	.0019	−1.85	.0322	−0.80	.2119	0.20	.5793	1.25	.8944	2.30	.9893
−2.85	.0022	−1.80	.0359	−0.75	.2266	0.25	.5987	1.30	.9032	2.35	.9906
−2.80	0.0026	−1.75	0.0401	−0.70	0.2420	0.30	0.6179	1.35	0.9115	2.40	0.9918
−2.75	.0030	−1.70	.0446	−0.65	.2578	0.35	.6368	1.40	.9192	2.45	.9929
−2.70	.0035	−1.65	.0495	−0.60	.2743	0.40	.6554	1.45	.9265	2.50	.9938
−2.65	0.0040	−1.60	0.0548	−0.55	0.2912	0.45	0.6736	1.50	0.9332	2.55	0.9946
−2.60	.0047	−1.55	.0606	−0.50	.3085	0.50	.6915	1.55	.9394	2.60	.9953
−2.55	.0054	−1.50	.0668	−0.45	.3264	0.55	.7088	1.60	.9452	2.65	.9960
−2.50	0.0062	−1.45	0.0735	−0.40	0.3446	0.60	0.7257	1.65	0.9505	2.70	0.9965
−2.45	.0071	−1.40	.0808	−0.35	.3632	0.65	.7422	1.70	.9554	2.75	.9970
−2.40	.0082	−1.35	.0885	−0.30	.3821	0.70	.7580	1.75	.9599	2.80	.9974
−2.35	0.0094	−1.30	0.0968	−0.25	0.4013	0.75	0.7734	1.80	0.9641	2.85	0.9978
−2.30	.0107	−1.25	.1056	−0.20	.4207	0.80	.7881	1.85	.9678	2.90	.9981
−2.25	.0122	−1.20	.1151	−0.15	.4404	0.85	.8023	1.90	.9713	2.95	.9984
−2.20	0.0139	−1.15	0.1251	−0.10	0.4602	0.90	0.8159	1.95	0.9744	3.00	0.9987
−2.15	.0158	−1.10	.1357	−0.05	.4801	0.95	.8289	2.00	.9772	3.50	.99977
−2.10	.0179	−1.05	.1469	0.00	.5000	1.00	.8413	2.05	.9798	4.00	.99997

Table B.2. Critical values for the standard normal distribution.

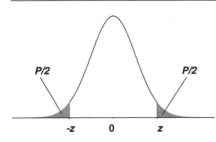

This table gives (two-sided) critical values for the standard normal distribution. These are the values of z for which a given percentage, P, of the standard normal distribution lies outside the range from $-z$ to $+z$.

P	z
90	0.1257
80	0.2533
70	0.3853
60	0.5244
50	0.6745
40	0.8416
30	1.0364
20	1.2816
15	1.4395
10	1.6449
5	1.9600
2	2.3263
1	2.5758
0.2	3.0902
0.1	3.2905
0.02	3.7190
0.01	3.8906

TABLE B.3. Critical values for the chi-square distribution.

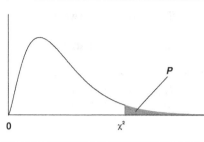

This table gives (one-sided) critical values for the chi-square distribution on v degrees of freedom. These are the values of χ^2 for which a given percentage, P, of the chi-square distribution is greater than χ^2.

P	97.5	95	50	10	5	2.5	1	0.1
$v = 1$	0.000982	0.00393	0.45	2.71	3.84	5.02	6.64	10.8
2	0.0506	0.103	1.39	4.61	5.99	7.38	9.21	13.8
3	0.216	0.352	2.37	6.25	7.81	9.35	11.3	16.3
4	0.484	0.711	3.36	7.78	9.49	11.1	13.3	18.5
5	0.831	1.15	4.35	9.24	11.1	12.8	15.1	20.5
6	1.24	1.64	5.35	10.6	12.6	14.5	16.8	22.5
7	1.69	2.17	6.35	12.0	14.1	16.0	18.5	24.3
8	2.18	2.73	7.34	13.4	15.5	17.5	20.1	26.1
9	2.70	3.33	8.34	14.7	16.9	19.0	21.7	27.9
10	3.25	3.94	9.34	16.0	18.3	20.5	23.2	29.6
11	3.82	4.57	10.3	17.3	19.7	21.9	24.7	31.3
12	4.40	5.23	11.3	18.5	21.0	23.3	26.2	32.9
13	5.01	5.89	12.3	19.8	22.4	24.7	27.7	34.5
14	5.63	6.57	13.3	21.1	23.7	26.1	29.1	36.1
15	6.26	7.26	14.3	22.3	25.0	27.5	30.6	37.7
16	6.91	7.96	15.3	23.5	26.3	28.8	32.0	39.3
17	7.56	8.67	16.3	24.8	27.6	30.2	33.4	40.8
18	8.23	9.39	17.3	26.0	28.9	31.5	34.8	42.3
19	8.91	10.1	18.3	27.2	30.1	32.9	36.2	43.8
20	9.59	10.9	19.3	28.4	31.4	34.2	37.6	45.3
22	11.0	12.3	21.3	30.8	33.9	36.8	40.3	48.3
24	12.4	13.9	23.3	33.2	36.4	39.4	43.0	51.2
26	13.8	15.4	25.3	35.6	38.9	41.9	45.6	54.1
28	15.3	16.9	27.3	37.9	41.3	44.5	48.3	56.9
30	16.8	18.5	29.3	40.3	43.8	47.0	50.9	59.7
35	20.6	22.5	34.3	46.1	49.8	53.2	57.3	66.6
40	24.4	26.5	39.3	51.8	55.8	59.3	63.7	73.4
45	28.4	30.6	44.3	57.5	61.7	65.4	70.0	80.1
50	32.4	34.8	49.3	63.2	67.5	71.4	76.2	86.7
55	36.4	39.0	54.3	68.8	73.3	77.4	82.3	93.2
60	40.5	43.2	59.3	74.4	79.1	83.3	88.4	99.7

Table B.4. Critical values for Student's t distribution.

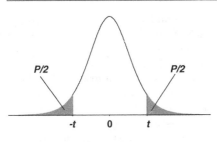

This table gives (two-sided) critical values for the t distribution on υ degrees of freedom. These are the values of t for which a given percentage, P, of the t distribution lies outside the range $-t$ to $+t$. As the number of degrees of freedom increases, the distribution becomes closer to the standard normal distribution.

P	50	20	10	5	2	1	0.2	0.1
$\upsilon = 1$	1.00	3.08	6.31	12.7	31.8	63.7	318	637
2	0.82	1.89	2.92	4.30	6.96	9.92	22.3	31.6
3	0.76	1.64	2.35	3.18	4.54	5.84	10.2	12.9
4	0.74	1.53	2.13	2.78	3.75	4.60	7.17	8.61
5	0.73	1.48	2.02	2.57	3.36	4.03	5.89	6.87
6	0.72	1.44	1.94	2.45	3.14	3.71	5.21	5.96
7	0.71	1.42	1.89	2.36	3.00	3.50	4.79	5.41
8	0.71	1.40	1.86	2.31	2.90	3.36	4.50	5.04
9	0.70	1.38	1.83	2.26	2.82	3.25	4.30	4.78
10	0.70	1.37	1.81	2.23	2.76	3.17	4.14	4.59
11	0.70	1.36	1.80	2.20	2.72	3.11	4.03	4.44
12	0.70	1.36	1.78	2.18	2.68	3.05	3.93	4.32
13	0.69	1.35	1.77	2.16	2.65	3.01	3.85	4.22
14	0.69	1.35	1.76	2.14	2.62	2.98	3.79	4.14
15	0.69	1.34	1.75	2.13	2.60	2.95	3.73	4.07
16	0.69	1.34	1.75	2.12	2.58	2.92	3.69	4.01
17	0.69	1.33	1.74	2.11	2.57	2.90	3.65	3.96
18	0.69	1.33	1.73	2.10	2.55	2.88	3.61	3.92
19	0.69	1.33	1.73	2.09	2.54	2.86	3.58	3.88
20	0.69	1.32	1.72	2.09	2.53	2.85	3.55	3.85
22	0.69	1.32	1.72	2.07	2.51	2.82	3.51	3.79
24	0.68	1.32	1.71	2.06	2.49	2.80	3.47	3.75
26	0.68	1.32	1.71	2.06	2.48	2.78	3.44	3.71
28	0.68	1.31	1.70	2.05	2.47	2.76	3.41	3.67
30	0.68	1.31	1.70	2.04	2.46	2.75	3.39	3.65
35	0.68	1.31	1.69	2.03	2.44	2.72	3.34	3.59
40	0.68	1.30	1.68	2.02	2.42	2.70	3.31	3.55
45	0.68	1.30	1.68	2.01	2.41	2.69	3.28	3.52
50	0.68	1.30	1.68	2.01	2.40	2.68	3.26	3.50
55	0.68	1.30	1.67	2.00	2.40	2.67	3.25	3.48
60	0.68	1.30	1.67	2.00	2.39	2.66	3.23	3.46
∞	0.67	1.28	1.64	1.96	2.33	2.58	3.09	3.29

Table B.5. Critical values for the F distribution.

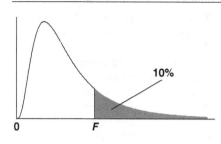

These tables give (one-sided) critical values of the F distribution. In each subtable, the percentage of the F distribution in the title is above the tabulated F value. The F distribution arises from the ratio of two independent estimates of variance; v_1 and v_2 are (respectively) the degrees of freedom of the estimates in the numerator and denominator.

(a) 10% critical values for the F distribution

v_1	1	2	3	4	5	6	7	8	10	12	24
$v_2 = 2$	8.53	9.00	9.16	9.24	9.29	9.33	9.35	9.37	9.39	9.41	9.45
3	5.54	5.46	5.39	5.34	5.31	5.28	5.27	5.25	5.23	5.22	5.18
4	4.54	4.32	4.19	4.11	4.05	4.01	3.98	3.95	3.92	3.90	3.83
5	4.06	3.78	3.62	3.52	3.45	3.40	3.37	3.34	3.30	3.27	3.19
6	3.78	3.46	3.29	3.18	3.11	3.05	3.01	2.98	2.94	2.90	2.82
7	3.59	3.26	3.07	2.96	2.88	2.83	2.78	2.75	2.70	2.67	2.58
8	3.46	3.11	2.92	2.81	2.73	2.67	2.62	2.59	2.54	2.50	2.40
9	3.36	3.01	2.81	2.69	2.61	2.55	2.51	2.47	2.42	2.38	2.28
10	3.28	2.92	2.73	2.61	2.52	2.46	2.41	2.38	2.32	2.28	2.18
11	3.23	2.86	2.66	2.54	2.45	2.39	2.34	2.30	2.25	2.21	2.10
12	3.18	2.81	2.61	2.48	2.39	2.33	2.28	2.24	2.19	2.15	2.04
13	3.14	2.76	2.56	2.43	2.35	2.28	2.23	2.20	2.14	2.10	1.98
14	3.10	2.73	2.52	2.39	2.31	2.24	2.19	2.15	2.10	2.05	1.94
15	3.07	2.70	2.49	2.36	2.27	2.21	2.16	2.12	2.06	2.02	1.90
16	3.05	2.67	2.46	2.33	2.24	2.18	2.13	2.09	2.03	1.99	1.87
17	3.03	2.64	2.44	2.31	2.22	2.15	2.10	2.06	2.00	1.96	1.84
18	3.01	2.62	2.42	2.29	2.20	2.13	2.08	2.04	1.98	1.93	1.81
19	2.99	2.61	2.40	2.27	2.18	2.11	2.06	2.02	1.96	1.91	1.79
20	2.97	2.59	2.38	2.25	2.16	2.09	2.04	2.00	1.94	1.89	1.77
22	2.95	2.56	2.35	2.22	2.13	2.06	2.01	1.97	1.90	1.86	1.73
24	2.93	2.54	2.33	2.19	2.10	2.04	1.98	1.94	1.88	1.83	1.70
26	2.91	2.52	2.31	2.17	2.08	2.01	1.96	1.92	1.86	1.81	1.68
28	2.89	2.50	2.29	2.16	2.06	2.00	1.94	1.90	1.84	1.79	1.66
30	2.88	2.49	2.28	2.14	2.05	1.98	1.93	1.88	1.82	1.77	1.64
35	2.85	2.46	2.25	2.11	2.02	1.95	1.90	1.85	1.79	1.74	1.60
40	2.84	2.44	2.23	2.09	2.00	1.93	1.87	1.83	1.76	1.71	1.57
45	2.82	2.42	2.21	2.07	1.98	1.91	1.85	1.81	1.74	1.70	1.55
50	2.81	2.41	2.20	2.06	1.97	1.90	1.84	1.80	1.73	1.68	1.54
55	2.80	2.40	2.19	2.05	1.95	1.88	1.83	1.78	1.72	1.67	1.52
60	2.79	2.39	2.18	2.04	1.95	1.87	1.82	1.77	1.71	1.66	1.51

Table B.5. (continued). Critical values for the F distribution.

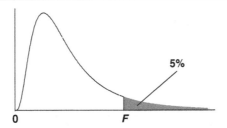

0   F

(b) 5% critical values for the F distribution

v_1	1	2	3	4	5	6	7	8	10	12	24
$v_2 = 2$	18.5	19.0	19.2	19.2	19.3	19.3	19.4	19.4	19.4	19.4	19.5
3	10.1	9.55	9.28	9.12	9.01	8.94	8.89	8.85	8.79	8.74	8.64
4	7.71	6.94	6.59	6.39	6.26	6.16	6.09	6.04	5.96	5.91	5.77
5	6.61	5.79	5.41	5.19	5.05	4.95	4.88	4.82	4.74	4.68	4.53
6	5.99	5.14	4.76	4.53	4.39	4.28	4.21	4.15	4.06	4.00	3.84
7	5.59	4.74	4.35	4.12	3.97	3.87	3.79	3.73	3.64	3.57	3.41
8	5.32	4.46	4.07	3.84	3.69	3.58	3.50	3.44	3.35	3.28	3.12
9	5.12	4.26	3.86	3.63	3.48	3.37	3.29	3.23	3.14	3.07	2.90
10	4.96	4.10	3.71	3.48	3.33	3.22	3.14	3.07	2.98	2.91	2.74
11	4.84	3.98	3.59	3.36	3.20	3.09	3.01	2.95	2.85	2.79	2.61
12	4.75	3.89	3.49	3.26	3.11	3.00	2.91	2.85	2.75	2.69	2.51
13	4.67	3.81	3.41	3.18	3.03	2.92	2.83	2.77	2.67	2.60	2.42
14	4.60	3.74	3.34	3.11	2.96	2.85	2.76	2.70	2.60	2.53	2.35
15	4.54	3.68	3.29	3.06	2.90	2.79	2.71	2.64	2.54	2.48	2.29
16	4.49	3.63	3.24	3.01	2.85	2.74	2.66	2.59	2.49	2.42	2.24
17	4.45	3.59	3.20	2.96	2.81	2.70	2.61	2.55	2.45	2.38	2.19
18	4.41	3.55	3.16	2.93	2.77	2.66	2.58	2.51	2.41	2.34	2.15
19	4.38	3.52	3.13	2.90	2.74	2.63	2.54	2.48	2.38	2.31	2.11
20	4.35	3.49	3.10	2.87	2.71	2.60	2.51	2.45	2.35	2.28	2.08
22	4.30	3.44	3.05	2.82	2.66	2.55	2.46	2.40	2.30	2.23	2.03
24	4.26	3.40	3.01	2.78	2.62	2.51	2.42	2.36	2.25	2.18	1.98
26	4.23	3.37	2.98	2.74	2.59	2.47	2.39	2.32	2.22	2.15	1.95
28	4.20	3.34	2.95	2.71	2.56	2.45	2.36	2.29	2.19	2.12	1.91
30	4.17	3.32	2.92	2.69	2.53	2.42	2.33	2.27	2.16	2.09	1.89
35	4.12	3.27	2.87	2.64	2.49	2.37	2.29	2.22	2.11	2.04	1.83
40	4.08	3.23	2.84	2.61	2.45	2.34	2.25	2.18	2.08	2.00	1.79
45	4.06	3.20	2.81	2.58	2.42	2.31	2.22	2.15	2.05	1.97	1.76
50	4.03	3.18	2.79	2.56	2.40	2.29	2.20	2.13	2.03	1.95	1.74
55	4.02	3.16	2.77	2.54	2.38	2.27	2.18	2.11	2.01	1.93	1.72
60	4.00	3.15	2.76	2.53	2.37	2.25	2.17	2.10	1.99	1.92	1.70

Table B.5. (continued). Critical values for the F distribution.

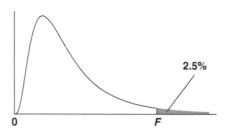

(c) 2.5% critical values for the F distribution

v_1	1	2	3	4	5	6	7	8	10	12	24
$v_2 = 2$	38.5	39.0	39.2	39.3	39.3	39.3	39.4	39.4	39.4	39.4	39.5
3	17.4	16.0	15.4	15.1	14.9	14.7	14.6	14.5	14.4	14.3	14.1
4	12.2	10.7	9.98	9.60	9.36	9.20	9.07	8.98	8.84	8.75	8.51
5	10.0	8.43	7.76	7.39	7.15	6.98	6.85	6.76	6.62	6.52	6.28
6	8.81	7.26	6.60	6.23	5.99	5.82	5.70	5.60	5.46	5.37	5.12
7	8.07	6.54	5.89	5.52	5.29	5.12	4.99	4.90	4.76	4.67	4.41
8	7.57	6.06	5.42	5.05	4.82	4.65	4.53	4.43	4.30	4.20	3.95
9	7.21	5.71	5.08	4.72	4.48	4.32	4.20	4.10	3.96	3.87	3.61
10	6.94	5.46	4.83	4.47	4.24	4.07	3.95	3.85	3.72	3.62	3.37
11	6.72	5.26	4.63	4.28	4.04	3.88	3.76	3.66	3.53	3.43	3.17
12	6.55	5.10	4.47	4.12	3.89	3.73	3.61	3.51	3.37	3.28	3.02
13	6.41	4.97	4.35	4.00	3.77	3.60	3.48	3.39	3.25	3.15	2.89
14	6.30	4.86	4.24	3.89	3.66	3.50	3.38	3.29	3.15	3.05	2.79
15	6.20	4.77	4.15	3.80	3.58	3.41	3.29	3.20	3.06	2.96	2.70
16	6.12	4.69	4.08	3.73	3.50	3.34	3.22	3.12	2.99	2.89	2.63
17	6.04	4.62	4.01	3.66	3.44	3.28	3.16	3.06	2.92	2.82	2.56
18	5.98	4.56	3.95	3.61	3.38	3.22	3.10	3.01	2.87	2.77	2.50
19	5.92	4.51	3.90	3.56	3.33	3.17	3.05	2.96	2.82	2.72	2.45
20	5.87	4.46	3.86	3.51	3.29	3.13	3.01	2.91	2.77	2.68	2.41
22	5.79	4.38	3.78	3.44	3.22	3.05	2.93	2.84	2.70	2.60	2.33
24	5.72	4.32	3.72	3.38	3.15	2.99	2.87	2.78	2.64	2.54	2.27
26	5.66	4.27	3.67	3.33	3.10	2.94	2.82	2.73	2.59	2.49	2.22
28	5.61	4.22	3.63	3.29	3.06	2.90	2.78	2.69	2.55	2.45	2.17
30	5.57	4.18	3.59	3.25	3.03	2.87	2.75	2.65	2.51	2.41	2.14
35	5.48	4.11	3.52	3.18	2.96	2.80	2.68	2.58	2.44	2.34	2.06
40	5.42	4.05	3.46	3.13	2.90	2.74	2.62	2.53	2.39	2.29	2.01
45	5.38	4.01	3.42	3.09	2.86	2.70	2.58	2.49	2.35	2.25	1.96
50	5.34	3.97	3.39	3.05	2.83	2.67	2.55	2.46	2.32	2.22	1.93
55	5.31	3.95	3.36	3.03	2.81	2.65	2.53	2.43	2.29	2.19	1.90
60	5.29	3.93	3.34	3.01	2.79	2.63	2.51	2.41	2.27	2.17	1.88

Table B.5. (continued). Critical values for the F distribution.

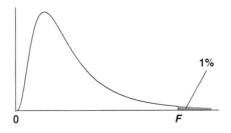

(d) 1% critical values for the F distribution

v_1	1	2	3	4	5	6	7	8	10	12	24
$v_2 = 2$	98.5	99.0	99.2	99.3	99.3	99.3	99.4	99.4	99.4	99.4	99.5
3	34.1	30.8	29.5	28.7	28.2	27.9	27.7	27.5	27.2	27.1	26.6
4	21.2	18.0	16.7	16.0	15.5	15.2	15.0	14.8	14.6	14.4	13.9
5	16.3	13.3	12.1	11.4	11.0	10.7	10.5	10.3	10.1	9.89	9.47
6	13.8	10.9	9.78	9.15	8.75	8.47	8.26	8.10	7.87	7.72	7.31
7	12.3	9.55	8.45	7.85	7.46	7.19	6.99	6.84	6.62	6.47	6.07
8	11.3	8.65	7.59	7.01	6.63	6.37	6.18	6.03	5.81	5.67	5.28
9	10.6	8.02	6.99	6.42	6.06	5.80	5.61	5.47	5.26	5.11	4.73
10	10.0	7.56	6.55	5.99	5.64	5.39	5.20	5.06	4.85	4.71	4.33
11	9.65	7.21	6.22	5.67	5.32	5.07	4.89	4.74	4.54	4.40	4.02
12	9.33	6.93	5.95	5.41	5.06	4.82	4.64	4.50	4.30	4.16	3.78
13	9.07	6.70	5.74	5.21	4.86	4.62	4.44	4.30	4.10	3.96	3.59
14	8.86	6.51	5.56	5.04	4.69	4.46	4.28	4.14	3.94	3.80	3.43
15	8.68	6.36	5.42	4.89	4.56	4.32	4.14	4.00	3.80	3.67	3.29
16	8.53	6.23	5.29	4.77	4.44	4.20	4.03	3.89	3.69	3.55	3.18
17	8.40	6.11	5.18	4.67	4.34	4.10	3.93	3.79	3.59	3.46	3.08
18	8.29	6.01	5.09	4.58	4.25	4.01	3.84	3.71	3.51	3.37	3.00
19	8.18	5.93	5.01	4.50	4.17	3.94	3.77	3.63	3.43	3.30	2.92
20	8.10	5.85	4.94	4.43	4.10	3.87	3.70	3.56	3.37	3.23	2.86
22	7.95	5.72	4.82	4.31	3.99	3.76	3.59	3.45	3.26	3.12	2.75
24	7.82	5.61	4.72	4.22	3.90	3.67	3.50	3.36	3.17	3.03	2.66
26	7.72	5.53	4.64	4.14	3.82	3.59	3.42	3.29	3.09	2.96	2.58
28	7.64	5.45	4.57	4.07	3.75	3.53	3.36	3.23	3.03	2.90	2.52
30	7.56	5.39	4.51	4.02	3.70	3.47	3.30	3.17	2.98	2.84	2.47
35	7.42	5.27	4.40	3.91	3.59	3.37	3.20	3.07	2.88	2.74	2.36
40	7.31	5.18	4.31	3.83	3.51	3.29	3.12	2.99	2.80	2.66	2.29
45	7.23	5.11	4.25	3.77	3.45	3.23	3.07	2.94	2.74	2.61	2.23
50	7.17	5.06	4.20	3.72	3.41	3.19	3.02	2.89	2.70	2.56	2.18
55	7.12	5.01	4.16	3.68	3.37	3.15	2.98	2.85	2.66	2.53	2.15
60	7.08	4.98	4.13	3.65	3.34	3.12	2.95	2.82	2.63	2.50	2.12

Table B.5. (continued). Critical values for the F distribution.

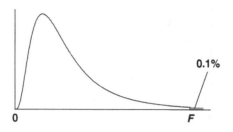

(e) 0.1% critical values for the F distribution

v_1	1	2	3	4	5	6	7	8	10	12	24
$v_2 = 2$	998.5	999.0	999.2	999.3	999.3	999.3	999.4	999.4	999.4	999.4	999.5
3	167.0	148.5	141.1	137.1	134.6	132.9	131.6	130.6	129.3	128.3	125.9
4	74.1	61.3	56.2	53.4	51.7	50.5	49.7	49.0	48.1	47.4	45.8
5	47.2	37.1	33.2	31.1	29.8	28.8	28.2	27.7	26.9	26.4	25.1
6	35.5	27.0	23.7	21.9	20.8	20.0	19.5	19.0	18.4	18.0	16.9
7	29.3	21.7	18.8	17.2	16.2	15.5	15.0	14.6	14.1	13.7	12.7
8	25.4	18.5	15.8	14.4	13.5	12.9	12.4	12.1	11.5	11.2	10.3
9	22.9	16.4	13.9	12.6	11.7	11.1	10.7	10.4	9.89	9.57	8.72
10	21.0	14.9	12.6	11.3	10.5	9.93	9.52	9.20	8.75	8.45	7.64
11	19.7	13.8	11.6	10.4	9.58	9.05	8.66	8.35	7.92	7.63	6.85
12	18.6	13.0	10.8	9.63	8.89	8.38	8.00	7.71	7.29	7.00	6.25
13	17.8	12.3	10.2	9.07	8.35	7.86	7.49	7.21	6.80	6.52	5.78
14	17.1	11.8	9.73	8.62	7.92	7.44	7.08	6.80	6.40	6.13	5.41
15	16.6	11.3	9.34	8.25	7.57	7.09	6.74	6.47	6.08	5.81	5.10
16	16.1	11.0	9.01	7.94	7.27	6.80	6.46	6.19	5.81	5.55	4.85
17	15.7	10.7	8.73	7.68	7.02	6.56	6.22	5.96	5.58	5.32	4.63
18	15.4	10.4	8.49	7.46	6.81	6.35	6.02	5.76	5.39	5.13	4.45
19	15.1	10.2	8.28	7.27	6.62	6.18	5.85	5.59	5.22	4.97	4.29
20	14.8	9.95	8.10	7.10	6.46	6.02	5.69	5.44	5.08	4.82	4.15
22	14.4	9.61	7.80	6.81	6.19	5.76	5.44	5.19	4.83	4.58	3.92
24	14.0	9.34	7.55	6.59	5.98	5.55	5.23	4.99	4.64	4.39	3.74
26	13.7	9.12	7.36	6.41	5.80	5.38	5.07	4.83	4.48	4.24	3.59
28	13.5	8.93	7.19	6.25	5.66	5.24	4.93	4.69	4.35	4.11	3.46
30	13.3	8.77	7.05	6.12	5.53	5.12	4.82	4.58	4.24	4.00	3.36
35	12.9	8.47	6.79	5.88	5.30	4.89	4.59	4.36	4.03	3.79	3.16
40	12.6	8.25	6.59	5.70	5.13	4.73	4.44	4.21	3.87	3.64	3.01
45	12.4	8.09	6.45	5.56	5.00	4.61	4.32	4.09	3.76	3.53	2.90
50	12.2	7.96	6.34	5.46	4.90	4.51	4.22	4.00	3.67	3.44	2.82
55	12.1	7.85	6.25	5.38	4.82	4.43	4.15	3.92	3.60	3.37	2.75
60	12.0	7.77	6.17	5.31	4.76	4.37	4.09	3.86	3.54	3.32	2.69

Table B.6. Random numbers.

In generating this table, the digits 0 to 9 were equally likely to occur in each place.

14	72	60	92	72	97	83	00	02	77	28	11	37	33
78	02	65	38	92	90	07	13	11	95	58	88	64	55
77	10	41	31	90	76	35	00	25	78	80	18	77	32
85	21	57	89	27	08	70	32	14	58	81	83	41	55
75	05	14	19	00	64	53	01	50	80	01	88	74	21
57	19	77	98	74	82	07	22	42	89	12	37	16	56
59	59	47	98	07	41	38	12	06	09	19	80	44	13
76	96	73	88	44	25	72	27	21	90	22	76	69	67
96	90	76	82	74	19	81	28	61	91	95	02	47	31
63	61	36	80	48	50	26	71	16	08	25	65	91	75
65	02	65	25	45	97	17	84	12	19	59	27	79	18
37	16	64	00	80	06	62	11	62	88	59	54	12	53
58	29	55	59	57	73	78	43	28	99	91	77	93	89
79	68	43	00	06	63	26	10	26	83	94	48	25	31
87	92	56	91	74	30	83	39	85	99	11	73	34	98
96	86	39	03	67	35	64	09	62	36	46	86	54	13
72	20	60	14	48	08	36	92	58	99	15	30	47	87
67	61	97	37	73	55	47	97	25	65	67	67	41	35
25	09	03	43	83	82	60	26	81	96	51	05	77	72
72	14	78	75	39	54	75	77	55	59	71	73	15	56
59	93	34	37	34	27	07	66	15	63	14	50	74	29
21	48	85	56	91	43	50	71	58	96	14	31	55	61
96	32	49	79	42	71	79	69	52	39	45	04	49	91
16	85	53	65	11	36	08	14	86	60	40	18	51	15
64	28	96	90	23	12	98	92	28	94	57	41	99	11
60	54	36	51	15	63	83	42	63	08	01	89	18	53
42	86	68	06	36	25	82	26	85	49	76	15	90	13
00	49	62	15	53	32	31	28	38	88	14	97	80	33
26	64	87	61	67	53	23	68	51	98	60	59	02	33
02	95	21	53	34	23	10	82	82	82	48	71	02	39
65	47	77	14	75	30	32	81	10	83	03	97	24	37
28	55	15	36	46	33	06	22	29	23	81	14	20	91
59	75	78	49	51	02	20	17	02	30	32	78	44	79
87	54	57	69	63	31	61	25	92	31	16	44	02	10
94	53	87	97	15	23	08	71	26	06	25	87	48	97
79	43	75	93	39	10	18	51	28	17	65	43	22	06
48	38	71	77	53	37	80	13	60	63	59	75	89	73
98	30	59	32	90	05	86	12	83	70	50	30	25	65
85	80	16	77	35	74	09	32	06	30	91	55	92	33
87	03	96	27	05	59	64	25	33	07	03	08	55	58

Table B.7. Sample size requirements for testing the value of a single mean or the difference between two means.

The table gives requirements for testing a single mean with a one-sided test directly. For two-sided tests, use the column corresponding to half the required significance level. For tests of the difference between two means, the total sample size (for the two groups combined) is obtained by multiplying the requirement given below by 4 if the two sample sizes are equal or by $(r + 1)^2/r$ if the ratio of the first to the second is $r : 1$ (assuming equal variances).
Note that S = difference/standard deviation.

	5% Significance		2.5% Significance		1% Significance		0.5% Significance		0.1% Significance		0.05% Significance	
S	90% Power	95% Power	90% Power	95% Power	90% Power	95% Power	90% Power	95% Power	90% Power	95% Power	90% Power	95% Power
0.01	85 639	108 222	105 075	129 948	130 170	157 705	148 794	178 142	191 125	224 211	209 040	243 580
0.02	21 410	27 056	26 269	32 487	32 543	39 427	37 199	44 536	47 782	56 053	52 260	60 895
0.03	9 516	12 025	11 675	14 439	14 464	17 523	16 533	19 794	21 237	24 913	23 227	27 065
0.04	5 353	6 764	6 568	8 122	8 136	9 857	9 300	11 134	11 946	14 014	13 065	15 224
0.05	3 426	4 329	4 203	5 198	5 207	6 309	5 952	7 126	7 645	8 969	8 362	9 744
0.06	2 379	3 007	2 919	3 610	3 616	4 381	4 134	4 949	5 310	6 229	5 807	6 767
0.07	1 748	2 209	2 145	2 652	2 657	3 219	3 037	3 636	3 901	4 576	4 267	4 972
0.08	1 339	1 691	1 642	2 031	2 034	2 465	2 325	2 784	2 987	3 504	3 267	3 806
0.09	1 058	1 337	1 298	1 605	1 608	1 947	1 837	2 200	2 360	2 769	2 581	3 008
0.10	857	1 083	1 051	1 300	1 302	1 578	1 488	1 782	1 912	2 243	2 091	2 436
0.15	381	481	467	578	579	701	662	792	850	997	930	1 083
0.20	215	271	263	325	326	395	372	446	478	561	523	609
0.25	138	174	169	208	209	253	239	286	306	359	335	390
0.30	96	121	117	145	145	176	166	198	213	250	233	271
0.35	70	89	86	107	107	129	122	146	157	184	171	199
0.40	54	68	66	82	82	99	93	112	120	141	131	153
0.45	43	54	52	65	65	78	74	88	95	111	104	121
0.50	35	44	43	52	53	64	60	72	77	90	84	98
0.55	29	36	35	43	44	53	50	59	64	75	70	81

0.60	24	31	30	37	37	44	42	50	54	63	59	68
0.65	21	26	25	31	31	38	36	43	46	54	50	58
0.70	18	23	22	27	27	33	31	37	40	46	43	50
0.75	16	20	19	24	24	29	27	32	34	40	38	44
0.80	14	17	17	21	21	25	24	28	30	36	33	39
0.85	12	15	15	18	19	22	21	25	27	32	29	34
0.90	11	14	13	17	17	20	19	22	24	28	26	31
0.95	10	12	12	15	15	18	17	20	22	25	24	27
1.00	9	11	11	13	14	16	15	18	20	23	21	25
2.00	3	3	3	4	4	4	4	5	5	6	6	7

Table B.8. Sample size requirements for testing the value of a single proportion.

These tables give requirements for a one-sided test directly. For two-sided tests, use the table corresponding to half the required significance level. Note that π_0 is the hypothesised proportion (under H_0) and d is the difference to be tested.

(a) 5% significance, 90% power

d	π_0										
	0.01	0.10	0.20	0.30	0.40	0.50	0.60	0.70	0.80	0.90	0.95
0.01	1 178	8 001	13 923	18 130	20 625	21 406	20 475	17 830	13 473	7 400	3 717
0.02	366	2 070	3 534	4 567	5 172	5 349	5 097	4 417	3 308	1 769	833
0.03	192	950	1 593	2 045	2 305	2 376	2 255	1 944	1 443	748	322
0.04	123	551	908	1 158	1 300	1 335	1 262	1 083	795	398	148
0.05	88	362	589	746	834	853	804	686	498	239	
0.06	67	258	414	521	580	591	555	471	338	155	
0.07	54	194	308	385	427	434	405	342	242	104	
0.08	44	152	238	296	327	331	308	258	181	71	
0.09	38	123	190	235	259	261	242	201	139	48	
0.10	32	102	156	191	210	211	195	161	109		
0.15	18	49	72	87	93	92	83	66	40		
0.20	12	30	42	49	52	50	44	33			
0.25	9	20	27	31	33	31	26	18			
0.30	7	14	19	22	22	20	16				
0.35	5	11	14	16	16	14	10				
0.40	4	9	11	12	11	10					
0.45	4	7	8	9	8	6					
0.50	3	6	7	7	6						

Table B.8 (continued). Sample size requirements for testing the value of a single proportion (one-sided test).

(b) 5% significance, 95% power

d	0.01	0.10	0.20	0.30	0.40	π_0 0.50	0.60	0.70	0.80	0.90	0.95
0.01	1 552	10 163	17 634	22 938	26 076	27 051	25 860	22 505	16 984	9 297	4 636
0.02	494	2 642	4 485	5 784	6 542	6 759	6 434	5 568	4 160	2 208	1 022
0.03	263	1 218	2 026	2 592	2 917	3 001	2 845	2 448	1 809	927	386
0.04	171	708	1 157	1 469	1 645	1 686	1 591	1 361	994	489	171
0.05	123	468	751	947	1 056	1 077	1 012	860	621	291	
0.06	95	334	529	662	735	747	698	590	420	185	
0.07	76	253	394	489	541	547	509	427	300	123	
0.08	63	198	305	377	414	418	387	322	223	82	
0.09	54	161	244	299	328	329	303	251	170	54	
0.10	47	133	200	244	266	266	244	200	133		
0.15	27	65	93	110	118	115	103	80	46		
0.20	18	39	54	63	65	63	54	39			
0.25	13	27	35	40	41	38	32	20			
0.30	10	19	25	28	28	25	19				
0.35	8	15	18	20	19	17	12				
0.40	6	11	14	15	14	11					
0.45	5	9	11	11	10	7					
0.50	4	7	8	8	7						

Table B.8 (continued). Sample size requirements for testing the value of a single proportion (one-sided test).

(c) 2.5% significance, 90% power

d	π_0										
	0.01	0.10	0.20	0.30	0.40	0.50	0.60	0.70	0.80	0.90	0.95
0.01	1 402	9 781	17 056	22 228	25 297	26 265	25 131	21 895	16 557	9 116	4 601
0.02	428	2 523	4 323	5 595	6 342	6 563	6 259	5 429	4 073	2 189	1 043
0.03	222	1 154	1 946	2 503	2 826	2 915	2 770	2 392	1 780	931	409
0.04	141	667	1 108	1 417	1 593	1 638	1 552	1 333	983	498	193
0.05	100	438	718	912	1 022	1 047	988	845	617	301	
0.06	76	311	504	637	711	726	683	581	420	196	
0.07	61	234	374	470	523	532	499	422	302	133	
0.08	50	183	289	362	401	407	380	320	226	93	
0.09	42	147	231	287	317	321	298	249	174	64	
0.10	36	122	189	233	257	259	240	200	137		
0.15	20	59	87	105	114	113	103	82	51		
0.20	13	35	50	60	64	62	55	42			
0.25	10	24	33	38	40	38	33	23			
0.30	7	17	23	26	27	25	21				
0.35	6	13	17	19	19	17	13				
0.40	5	10	13	14	14	12					
0.45	4	8	10	11	10	8					
0.50	3	6	8	8	8						

Table B.8 (continued). Sample size requirements for testing the value of a single proportion (one-sided test).

(d) 2.5% significance, 95% power

d	π_0										
	0.01	0.10	0.20	0.30	0.40	0.50	0.60	0.70	0.80	0.90	0.95
0.01	1 809	12 159	21 140	27 520	31 300	32 481	31 063	27 046	20 428	11 209	5 618
0.02	566	3 151	5 369	6 935	7 851	8 116	7 732	6 698	5 013	2 675	1 253
0.03	298	1 447	2 422	3 105	3 499	3 604	3 420	2 947	2 184	1 129	481
0.04	192	840	1 382	1 759	1 973	2 025	1 914	1 640	1 203	599	219
0.05	138	553	896	1 133	1 266	1 294	1 218	1 038	753	359	
0.06	105	395	630	792	881	897	841	712	510	231	
0.07	84	297	468	585	648	658	614	517	365	154	
0.08	70	233	363	450	497	502	467	390	272	105	
0.09	59	188	290	357	393	396	366	304	209	70	
0.10	51	156	237	291	318	319	294	243	164		
0.15	29	76	110	131	141	139	125	99	59		
0.20	19	46	64	75	78	76	66	49			
0.25	14	31	42	48	49	46	39	26			
0.30	11	22	29	33	33	30	24				
0.35	8	17	21	24	23	21	15				
0.40	7	13	16	18	17	14					
0.45	6	10	13	13	12	9					
0.50	5	8	10	10	9	9					

Table B.9. Total sample size requirements (for the two groups combined) for testing the ratio of two proportions (relative risk) with equal numbers in each group.

These tables give requirements for a one-sided test directly. For two-sided tests, use the table corresponding to half the required significance level. Note that π is the proportion for the reference group (the denominator) and λ is the relative risk to be tested.

(a) 5% significance, 90% power

μ	π								
	0.001	0.005	0.010	0.050	0.100	0.150	0.200	0.500	0.900
0.10	23 244	4 636	2 310	448	216	138	100	30	8
0.20	32 090	6 398	3 188	618	298	190	136	40	10
0.30	45 406	9 052	4 508	874	418	268	192	56	14
0.40	66 554	13 268	6 606	1 278	612	390	278	78	18
0.50	102 678	20 466	10 190	1 968	940	598	426	118	26
0.60	171 126	34 104	16 976	3 274	1 562	990	706	192	38
0.70	323 228	64 410	32 058	6 176	2 940	1 862	1 322	352	62
0.80	770 020	153 422	76 348	14 688	6 980	4 412	3 128	814	126
0.90	3 251 102	647 690	322 264	61 924	29 380	18 534	13 110	3 346	450
1.10	3 593 120	715 666	355 984	68 240	32 272	20 282	14 288	3 496	292
1.20	941 030	187 410	93 208	17 846	8 426	5 286	3 716	890	
1.30	437 234	87 068	43 298	8 280	3 904	2 444	1 714	402	
1.40	256 630	51 098	25 406	4 854	2 284	1 428	1 000	228	
1.50	171 082	34 062	16 934	3 232	1 518	948	662	148	
1.60	123 556	24 596	12 226	2 330	1 094	680	474	104	
1.80	74 842	14 896	7 402	1 408	658	408	284	58	
2.00	51 318	10 212	5 074	962	448	278	192		
3.00	17 102	3 400	1 688	316	146	88	60		
4.00	9 498	1 886	934	174	78	46	30		
5.00	6 410	1 272	630	116	52	30			
10.00	2 318	458	226	40					
20.00	992	194	94						

Table B.9 (continued). Total sample size requirements (for the two groups combined) for testing the ratio of two proportions (relative risk) with equal numbers in each group (one-sided test).

(b) 5% significance, 95% power

μ	0.001	0.005	0.010	0.050	0.100	0.150	0.200	0.500	0.900
0.10	29 372	5 856	2 918	5 66	272	174	126	36	10
0.20	40 552	8 086	4 026	780	374	240	172	50	12
0.30	57 378	11 438	5 696	1 102	528	336	240	68	16
0.40	84 102	16 764	8 346	1 612	772	490	350	98	20
0.50	129 754	25 860	12 874	2 484	1 186	754	536	146	30
0.60	216 250	43 094	21 450	4 136	1 970	1 250	888	238	44
0.70	408 460	81 390	40 506	7 800	3 712	2 348	1 666	440	74
0.80	973 072	193 874	96 476	18 556	8 816	5 568	3 946	1 024	154
0.90	4 108 420	818 476	407 234	78 240	37 116	23 408	16 554	4 216	556
1.10	4 540 658	904 406	449 874	86 248	40 796	25 644	18 068	4 432	384
1.20	1 189 190	236 838	117 794	22 560	10 656	6 688	4 704	1 132	
1.30	552 540	110 034	54 720	10 470	4 938	3 094	2 172	512	
1.40	324 310	64 576	32 110	6 138	2 890	1 808	1 266	292	
1.50	216 202	43 046	21 402	4 086	1 922	1 200	840	190	
1.60	156 142	31 086	15 454	2 948	1 384	864	602	132	
1.80	94 582	18 826	9 356	1 782	834	518	360	76	
2.00	64 852	12 906	6 414	1 218	570	352	244		
3.00	21 612	4 298	2 132	402	184	112	76		
4.00	12 004	2 384	1 182	220	100	60	40		
5.00	8 102	1 608	796	146	66	38			
10.00	2 930	580	286	50					
20.00	1 252	246	120						

Table B.9 (continued). Total sample size requirements (for the two groups combined) for testing the ratio of two proportions (relative risk) with equal numbers in each group (one-sided test).

(c) 2.5% significance, 90% power

μ	π 0.001	0.005	0.010	0.050	0.100	0.150	0.200	0.500	0.900
0.10	28 518	5 688	2 834	550	266	170	122	38	10
0.20	39 374	7 852	3 912	760	366	234	168	50	14
0.30	55 710	11 108	5 532	1 072	514	328	236	68	18
0.40	81 658	16 278	8 106	1 568	752	478	342	98	24
0.50	125 984	25 112	12 502	2 416	1 154	734	524	146	32
0.60	209 964	41 846	20 832	4 020	1 918	1 218	866	236	48
0.70	396 588	79 030	39 334	7 578	3 610	2 286	1 624	434	78
0.80	944 780	188 246	93 680	18 026	8 570	5 416	3 840	1 004	160
0.90	3 988 950	794 694	395 412	75 986	36 058	22 748	16 092	4 114	560
1.10	4 408 574	878 078	436 766	83 716	39 586	24 876	17 520	4 280	350
1.20	1 154 592	229 938	114 356	21 892	10 334	6 480	4 554	1 086	
1.30	536 462	106 824	53 120	10 156	4 786	2 996	2 100	488	
1.40	314 870	62 692	31 170	5 952	2 800	1 750	1 224	278	
1.50	209 908	41 788	20 774	3 962	1 860	1 160	810	178	
1.60	151 596	30 176	15 000	2 858	1 340	834	580	124	
1.80	91 826	18 274	9 080	1 726	806	500	346	70	
2.00	62 964	12 528	6 224	1 180	550	340	234		
3.00	20 982	4 170	2 068	388	178	108	72		
4.00	11 654	2 314	1 146	212	96	56	36		
5.00	7 864	1 560	772	142	62	36			
10.00	2 844	562	276	48					
20.00	1 216	238	114						

Table B.9 (continued). Total sample size requirements (for the two groups combined) for testing the ratio of two proportions (relative risk) with equal numbers in each group (one-sided test).

(d) 2.5% significance, 95% power

μ	0.001	0.005	0.010	0.050	0.100	0.150	0.200	0.500	0.900
0.10	35 268	7 034	3 504	680	328	210	150	44	12
0.20	48 694	9 708	4 836	938	450	288	206	60	16
0.30	68 896	13 736	6 840	1 324	634	404	290	82	20
0.40	100 986	20 130	10 024	1 938	928	590	422	118	26
0.50	155 802	31 054	15 460	2 984	1 426	906	646	178	36
0.60	259 664	51 748	25 758	4 968	2 368	1 502	1 068	288	54
0.70	490 462	97 732	48 642	9 368	4 460	2 822	2 004	532	92
0.80	1 168 420	232 800	115 848	22 286	10 590	6 692	4 742	1 234	190
0.90	4 933 188	982 796	488 996	93 958	44 578	28 118	19 888	5 072	678
1.10	5 452 174	1 085 950	540 172	103 550	48 972	30 780	21 684	5 310	450
1.20	1 427 912	284 378	141 436	27 082	12 788	8 024	5 640	1 352	
1.30	663 456	132 118	65 700	12 566	5 924	3 710	2 604	610	
1.40	389 410	77 538	38 552	7 366	3 468	2 168	1 518	348	
1.50	259 600	51 684	25 696	4 904	2 304	1 438	1 004	224	
1.60	187 484	37 322	18 552	3 536	1 660	1 034	720	156	
1.80	113 566	22 604	11 232	2 136	1 000	620	430	88	
2.00	77 870	15 496	7 698	1 462	682	422	292		
3.00	25 950	5 158	2 560	480	220	134	90		
4.00	14 414	2 862	1 418	264	118	70	46		
5.00	9 726	1 930	956	176	78	46			
10.00	3 518	694	342	60					
20.00	1 504	294	142						

Table B.10. Total sample size requirements (for the two groups combined) for unmatched case–control studies with equal numbers of cases and controls.

These tables give requirements for a one-sided test directly. For two-sided tests, use the table corresponding to half the required significance level. Note that P is the prevalence of the risk factor in the entire population and λ is the approximate relative risk to be tested.

(a) 5% significance, 90% power

					P				
μ	0.010	0.050	0.100	0.200	0.300	0.400	0.500	0.700	0.900
0.10	2 318	456	224	108	70	50	40	30	38
0.20	3 206	638	316	158	104	80	66	56	88
0.30	4 546	912	458	232	160	124	106	98	176
0.40	6 676	1 348	684	356	248	200	176	172	330
0.50	10 318	2 098	1 074	566	404	332	296	306	616
0.60	17 220	3 522	1 816	974	706	588	536	576	1 206
0.70	32 570	6 698	3 476	1 890	1 390	1 174	1 088	1 206	2 612
0.80	77 686	16 052	8 382	4 614	3 438	2 944	2 764	3 146	7 012
0.90	328 374	68 156	35 786	19 922	15 020	13 006	12 354	14 400	32 892
1.10	363 666	76 090	40 352	22 918	17 630	15 574	15 096	18 316	43 550
1.20	95 332	20 020	10 664	6 112	4 744	4 228	4 134	5 102	12 340
1.30	44 334	9 342	4 998	2 888	2 260	2 032	2 002	2 510	6 166
1.40	26 044	5 506	2 958	1 722	1 358	1 230	1 222	1 554	3 870
1.50	17 376	3 684	1 986	1 166	926	846	846	1 090	2 748
1.60	12 558	2 672	1 446	854	684	628	632	826	2 106
1.80	7 618	1 630	888	532	432	400	408	546	1 420
2.00	5 230	1 124	616	374	306	288	296	404	1 074
3.00	1 754	386	218	138	120	118	126	184	522
4.00	978	220	126	84	74	76	84	130	380
5.00	664	150	88	60	56	58	66	104	316
10.00	244	60	38	30	30	34	40	70	224
20.00	108	30	20	18	20	24	30	56	190

Table B.10 (continued). Total sample size requirements (for the two groups combined) for unmatched case–control studies with equal numbers of cases and controls (one-sided test).

(b) 5% significance, 95% power

μ	P								
	0.010	0.050	0.100	0.200	0.300	0.400	0.500	0.700	0.900
0.10	2 928	576	282	136	86	64	50	36	46
0.20	4 052	804	400	198	132	100	82	70	110
0.30	5 744	1 152	578	294	200	156	134	124	220
0.40	8 436	1 704	864	448	314	252	220	218	414
0.50	13 036	2 650	1 356	716	510	418	374	386	778
0.60	21 760	4 450	2 294	1 230	892	742	678	726	1 524
0.70	41 158	8 462	4 392	2 386	1 756	1 484	1 374	1 522	3 300
0.80	98 172	20 284	10 590	5 828	4 344	3 718	3 492	3 974	8 858
0.90	414 966	86 130	45 222	25 174	18 980	16 434	15 612	18 196	41 566
1.10	459 566	96 154	50 994	28 962	22 278	19 682	19 076	23 144	55 034
1.20	120 472	25 298	13 476	7 722	5 994	5 342	5 222	6 448	15 592
1.30	56 024	11 804	6 316	3 650	2 856	2 566	2 530	3 172	7 790
1.40	32 910	6 956	3 736	2 176	1 716	1 554	1 544	1 964	4 890
1.50	21 958	4 656	2 510	1 472	1 170	1 066	1 066	1 376	3 472
1.60	15 870	3 374	1 826	1 080	864	792	798	1 042	2 660
1.80	9 626	2 058	1 122	672	544	506	516	688	1 794
2.00	6 610	1 420	778	472	386	364	374	510	1 356
3.00	2 214	486	274	174	150	148	158	232	658
4.00	1 236	276	158	104	94	94	104	162	480
5.00	838	190	110	76	70	72	82	132	400
10.00	308	74	46	36	36	40	50	86	282
20.00	136	36	26	22	24	30	38	70	238

Table B.10 (continued). Total sample size requirements (for the two groups combined) for unmatched case–control studies with equal numbers of cases and controls (one-sided test).

(c) 2.5% significance, 90% power

μ	0.010	0.050	0.100	0.200	0.300	0.400	0.500	0.700	0.900
0.10	2 844	560	274	132	86	62	48	36	46
0.20	3 934	782	390	194	128	98	80	68	108
0.30	5 578	1 120	562	286	196	154	132	122	216
0.40	8 192	1 656	840	436	306	246	216	212	404
0.50	12 658	2 574	1 318	696	496	406	364	376	756
0.60	21 128	4 322	2 228	1 194	866	722	658	706	1 480
0.70	39 962	8 218	4 264	2 318	1 706	1 442	1 336	1 480	3 206
0.80	95 318	19 696	10 284	5 660	4 220	3 612	3 390	3 860	8 602
0.90	402 898	83 626	43 908	24 442	18 430	15 958	15 160	17 668	40 358
1.10	446 202	93 358	49 512	28 120	21 632	19 110	18 522	22 472	53 434
1.20	116 970	24 562	13 086	7 500	5 820	5 188	5 072	6 260	15 140
1.30	54 396	11 462	6 132	3 544	2 774	2 492	2 456	3 080	7 564
1.40	31 954	6 756	3 628	2 114	1 668	1 510	1 500	1 908	4 750
1.50	21 320	4 522	2 438	1 432	1 138	1 038	1 038	1 338	3 372
1.60	15 410	3 278	1 774	1 048	840	770	776	1 012	2 584
1.80	9 348	2 000	1 090	652	530	492	502	670	1 744
2.00	6 418	1 380	756	460	376	354	364	496	1 318
3.00	2 152	472	266	170	146	144	154	226	640
4.00	1 200	268	154	104	92	94	104	158	466
5.00	814	186	108	74	68	72	80	128	390
10.00	300	74	46	36	36	40	48	86	274
20.00	134	36	26	22	26	30	38	70	232

Table B.10 (continued). Total sample size requirements (for the two groups combined) for unmatched case–control studies with equal numbers of cases and controls (one-sided test).

(d) 2.5% significance, 95% power

μ	0.010	0.050	0.100	0.200	0.300	0.400	0.500	0.700	0.900
0.10	3 516	692	338	162	104	76	60	44	56
0.20	4 864	966	480	238	158	120	98	84	134
0.30	6 898	1 382	694	352	242	188	162	150	266
0.40	10 130	2 046	1 038	538	376	302	266	262	498
0.50	15 654	3 182	1 628	860	614	502	450	464	936
0.60	26 130	5 344	2 754	1 476	1 072	892	814	874	1 830
0.70	49 420	10 162	5 274	2 866	2 110	1 782	1 652	1 828	3 964
0.80	117 880	24 358	12 716	7 000	5 218	4 466	4 192	4 772	10 638
0.90	498 270	103 420	54 300	30 228	22 790	19 734	18 746	21 850	49 910
1.10	551 824	115 458	61 230	34 776	26 752	23 632	22 904	27 790	66 082
1.20	144 656	30 376	16 182	9 274	7 198	6 414	6 272	7 742	18 724
1.30	67 272	14 174	7 584	4 382	3 430	3 082	3 038	3 808	9 354
1.40	39 518	8 354	4 486	2 614	2 062	1 866	1 854	2 358	5 874
1.50	26 366	5 590	3 014	1 768	1 406	1 282	1 282	1 652	4 170
1.60	19 056	4 052	2 192	1 296	1 036	952	958	1 252	3 194
1.80	11 560	2 472	1 346	806	654	608	618	826	2 156
2.00	7 936	1 706	936	566	464	436	450	614	1 628
3.00	2 660	584	328	210	180	176	190	280	790
4.00	1 484	332	190	126	112	114	126	196	576
5.00	1 006	228	134	92	84	88	98	158	480
10.00	370	90	56	44	44	50	60	104	338
20.00	164	44	30	28	29	35	45	84	286

Table B.11.   Critical values for Pearson's correlation
coefficient.

The table shows the smallest value of the correlation coefficient that is significant at the particular significance
level. These are to be used in two-sided significance tests
where the null hypothesis is that the correlation is zero.

Sample size	Significance level			
	10%	5%	1%	0.1%
3	0.9877	0.9969	0.9999	0.9999
4	0.900	0.950	0.990	0.999
5	0.805	0.878	0.959	0.991
6	0.729	0.811	0.917	0.974
7	0.669	0.754	0.875	0.951
8	0.621	0.707	0.834	0.925
9	0.582	0.666	0.798	0.898
10	0.549	0.632	0.765	0.872
11	0.521	0.602	0.735	0.847
12	0.497	0.576	0.708	0.823
13	0.476	0.553	0.684	0.801
14	0.457	0.532	0.661	0.780
15	0.441	0.514	0.641	0.760
16	0.426	0.497	0.623	0.742
17	0.412	0.482	0.606	0.725
18	0.400	0.468	0.590	0.708
19	0.389	0.456	0.575	0.693
20	0.378	0.444	0.561	0.679
21	0.369	0.433	0.549	0.665
22	0.360	0.423	0.537	0.652
27	0.323	0.381	0.487	0.597
32	0.296	0.349	0.449	0.554
42	0.257	0.304	0.393	0.490
52	0.231	0.273	0.354	0.443
62	0.211	0.250	0.325	0.408
82	0.183	0.217	0.283	0.357
102	0.164	0.195	0.254	0.321

APPENDIX C

Additional datasets for exercises

Table C.1. Summary data from the complete third Glasgow MONICA survey.

This table gives summary results, analysed in more detail by Woodward et al. (1997), from the same survey that was used in Exercise 2.4, but now using the complete dataset. The variables tabulated are sex, 10-year age group, factor IX status (high = above sex-specific median; low = below) by prevalent cardiovascular disease (CVD) status.

Factor IX status	Age group (years)												
	25–34		35–44		45–54		55–64		65–74		Total	
	CVD	No CVD	CVD	No CVD	CVD	No CVD	CVD	No CVD	CVD	No CVD	CVD	No CVD
Males												
Low	6	75	12	56	24	40	35	39	34	33	111	243
High	4	20	15	56	29	52	36	54	38	52	122	234
Total	10	95	27	112	53	92	71	93	72	85	233	477
Females												
Low	18	69	21	87	21	62	19	37	27	24	106	279
High	11	32	11	34	36	58	39	59	57	62	154	245
Total	29	101	32	121	57	120	58	96	84	86	260	524

Table C.2. Brain metastases data.

The following table shows survival times for 17 consecutive patients with brain metastases from lung tumours who were treated with hyperthermia plus nitrosoureas, as reported by Pontiggia *et al.* (1995).

Age (years)	Prior treatment	Outcome	Survival time (months)
69	No	Death	20
52	Yes	Drop-out	13
62	No	Drop-out	19
49	No	Death	12
60	Yes	Death	5
61	Yes	Death	23
61	Yes	Death	5
60	No	Other cause	12
56	No	Death	2
59	No	Death	28
64	Yes	Death	12
51	No	Death	7
67	No	Death	16
62	No	Death	12
45	No	Death	5
62	No	Alive	11
39	Yes	Alive	8

Note: 'Other cause' means a non-tumour-related death. All other deaths are due to tumours.

Table C.3. Smelter workers data.

Breslow and Day (1994) give the following data from the Montana smelter workers study. These data are for men employed prior to 1925, showing the number of deaths and man-years (PYs) of low and high arsenic exposure within age groups and calendar periods. Low exposure means less than 1 year, and high exposure means 15 or more years, of work in areas which are known to have a considerable amount of arsenic trioxide in their atmosphere. The study concluded in September 1977.

Age group (years)	Exposure	Calendar period							
		1938–1949		1950–1959		1960–1969		1970–1977	
		Deaths	PYs	Deaths	PYs	Deaths	PYs	Deaths	PYs
40–49	High	0	337.29	0	121.00				
	Low	2	3075.27	0	936.75				
50–59	High	4	626.72	3	349.53	1	142.33		
	Low	2	2849.76	3	2195.59	3	747.77		
60–69	High	9	672.09	7	441.10	3	244.82	1	100.64
	Low	2	2085.43	7	1675.91	10	1501.73	1	440.21
70–79	High	1	277.25	2	268.27	1	197.20	2	92.75
	Low	3	833.61	6	973.32	6	1027.12	6	674.44

Table C.4. Cerebral palsy data.

In a randomised controlled single-blind parallel group study, lumbo-sacral selective posterior rhizotomy (SPR) followed by intensive physiotherapy was compared with physiotherapy alone in improving motor function in children with diplegic cerebral palsy (Steinbok *et al.*, 1997). The following table shows the gross motor function measure before and after therapy (lasting for 9 months) for each subject.

SPR + physiotherapy group		Physiotherapy group	
Before	After	Before	After
81.7	89.7	70.3	74.0
48.1	58.2	39.9	52.9
69.2	87.0	82.0	89.7
87.7	92.4	65.3	62.8
43.1	66.6	62.4	69.6
67.8	75.0	82.2	85.7
59.9	63.6	52.5	61.6
42.2	53.3	62.5	65.6
72.4	86.5	65.0	69.2
43.9	59.5	70.4	75.2
48.8	52.5	58.3	63.5
81.7	90.6	48.5	55.6
44.9	67.8	33.0	35.7
58.7	65.2	86.0	89.1

Table C.5. Norwegian Multicentre Study data.

In the Norwegian Multicentre Study, survivors of acute myocardial infarction were randomly allocated to Blocadren or placebo (Hwang and Rodda, 1992). The following table shows the number at risk at the start of each month and the number of deaths within that month, over 34 months of study.

Month	Blocadren		Placebo	
	At risk	Deaths	At risk	Deaths
1	945	19	939	31
2	926	10	908	9
3	916	7	899	4
4	909	3	895	10
5	906	5	885	7
6	901	6	878	10
7	895	5	868	10
8	890	2	858	3
9	888	5	855	7
10	883	2	848	4
11	881	3	844	6
12	878	5	838	5
13	873	1	833	6
14	836	0	801	2
15	806	5	764	5
16	767	5	737	3
17	722	0	702	3
18	672	0	649	4
19	631	0	599	1
20	592	2	558	3
21	542	2	523	2
22	507	1	483	1
23	463	2	442	1
24	419	0	393	3
25	375	1	352	2
26	337	0	315	1
27	295	0	278	2
28	267	2	242	2
29	237	2	207	0
30	197	2	172	2
31	145	1	126	0
32	100	0	81	3
33	50	0	39	0
34	12	0	7	0

Source: Reprinted from Peace, K.E., Ed. (1992, p. 222), *Biopharmaceutical Sequential Statistical Applications*. Statistics, Textbooks and Monographs, vol. 128. Courtesy of Marcel Dekker Inc., New York.

Table C.6. Rheumatoid arthritis data.

In the rheumatoid arthritis cross-over study of Hill *et al.* (1990), carried out at Leeds General Infirmary (UK) and described in Example 7.7, subjects were asked to record how many paracetamol tablets they took, to alleviate pain, over each of their 2-week treatment periods. These results follow.

Ibuprofen–Aspergesic group		Aspergesic–ibuprofen group	
Period 1	Period 2	Period 1	Period 2
2.400	2.133	2.462	0.857
2.667	0.400	1.429	5.846
1.571	1.571	0.000	3.429
4.142	4.571	0.286	0.400
0.733	1.429	0.143	0.286
3.000	1.142	7.571	6.714
2.667	3.067	0.000	0.000
0.000	0.000	0.000	0.000
1.571	0.000	1.538	0.615
1.857	2.857	6.143	7.143
0.000	0.000	2.933	3.143
5.385	5.571	0.000	0.000
0.000	6.923	0.857	0.923
3.000	2.000	1.140	1.710
0.000	2.267		

Table C.7. Data from a sequential intervention study.

For definitions of variables, see Exercise 7.8.

Observation	m	n	S	T
1	0	1	0	0
2	1	1	1	0
3	1	2	1	0
4	2	2	1	0
5	2	3	1	0
6	2	4	1	0
7	2	5	1	1
8	3	5	2	1
9	4	5	3	2
10	4	6	3	2
11	4	7	3	2
12	4	8	3	2
13	5	8	4	2
14	6	8	4	2
15	6	9	4	2
16	6	10	4	2
17	6	11	4	3
18	6	12	4	3
19	6	13	4	3
20	7	13	5	3
21	8	13	5	3
22	8	14	5	3
23	9	14	6	3
24	10	14	7	3
25	11	14	8	3
26	12	14	9	3
27	12	15	9	4
28	12	16	9	4
29	13	16	10	4
30	14	16	11	4

Source: Reprinted from Peace, K.E., Ed. (1992, p. 195), *Biopharmaceutical Sequential Statistical Applications*. Statistics, Textbooks and Monographs, vol. 128. Courtesy of Marcel Dekker Inc., New York.

Table C.8. Epilepsy data.

Braathan *et al.* (1997) give data for 19 children with epilepsy who participated in a prospective study concerning
the duration of treatment with carbamazepine. These children were selected for entry to a further study. Selected
variables follow: the BO test is the Bruininks–Oseretsky
test of motor proficiency.

Child Number	Diagnosis	Duration of treatment (years)	BO test (μmol/l)
1	PS	1	22
2	GTCS	3	21
3	GTCS	3	32
4	PS	1	17
5	BECT	1	27
6	GTCS	1	30
7	PS	3	37
8	GTCS	1	19
9	GTCS	1	18
10	GTCS	3	21
11	PS	1	26
12	BECT	3	29
13	GTCS	1	23
14	PS	3	33
15	PS	3	10
16	BECT	3	27
17	GTCS	3	26
18	GTCS	3	27
19	GTCS	1	23

Notes: PS = partial seizures; GTCS = generalised
tonic–clonic seizures; BECT = benign partial epilepsy with
centro-temporal spikes.

Table C.9. Ozone exposure data.

When humans are exposed to high levels of ozone, reversible
changes in lung function occur. The following data show
part of an investigation by Ying *et al.* (1990), who exposed
13 nonsmoking men to 0.4 ppm ozone. This shows lung
function (FEV_1) before and after exposure, together with
age, height and weight.

Subject number	Age (yr)	Height (cm)	Weight (kg)	FEV_1 Before	FEV_1 After
1	22	170	68	4.52	3.92
2	22	178	73	5.21	4.14
3	26	163	61	3.10	2.27
4	31	188	89	4.25	3.16
5	27	170	72	3.19	2.81
6	30	173	66	4.24	2.23
7	28	185	73	4.41	4.29
8	27	185	76	4.30	4.20
9	22	188	75	4.76	3.50
10	24	190	91	4.38	2.71
11	23	178	57	4.49	3.19
12	18	180	66	4.66	4.17
13	26	185	68	5.08	5.13

Table C.10. Anorexia data.

Ben–Tovim *et al.* (1979) report a case-control study to test the hypothesis that anorexic people tend to overestimate their true waist measurements. Eight anorexic women were identified from a hospital in-patient unit and compared with eleven nonanorexic adolescent schoolgirls. The outcome variable used to compare cases and controls was the body perception index,

$$\text{BPI} = 100 \times \frac{\text{perceived waist width}}{\text{true waist width}}.$$

The following data were collected.

Subject	Waist width (cm)		
number	True	Perceived	BPI
Cases			
1	22.6	29.5	130.5
2	19.2	30.6	159.6
3	21.9	31.1	142.0
4	23.4	28.1	119.9
5	22.9	32.7	143.0
6	19.1	37.1	194.0
7	21.4	32.9	153.7
8	28.3	33.5	118.2
Controls			
9	24.9	32.9	132.3
10	16.6	27.9	168.1
11	22.0	28.7	130.5
12	22.2	34.1	153.6
13	21.4	33.9	158.4
14	19.1	39.3	206.0
15	18.2	36.9	202.7
16	21.4	31.4	146.5
17	17.6	40.4	229.5
18	20.0	34.6	172.8
19	24.3	31.8	130.9

Table C.11. UK population data.

The following data show the size of
the UK population at successive 10-
year population censuses.

Census year	Population size (thousands)
1801	11 944
1811	13 368
1821	15 472
1831	17 835
1841	20 183
1851	22 259
1861	24 525
1871	27 431
1881	31 015
1891	34 264
1901	38 237
1911	42 182
1921	44 227
1931	46 338
1951	50 525
1961	52 609
1971	55 515
1981	55 776
1991	57 801

Table C.12. Nasal cancer data.

Breslow and Day (1994) give data on nasal sinus cancer mortality amongst Welsh nickel refinery workers, as reproduced below. Column 1 has age when first employed (1 = <20; 2 = 20 to 27.4; 3 = 27.5 to 34.9; 4 = 35.0 to 54.4 years). Column 2 has year of first employment (1 = 1902 to 1909; 2 = 1910 to 1914; 3 = 1915 to 1919; 4 = 1920 to 1924). Column 3 has duration of exposure to nickel compounds (1 = 0.0; 2 = 0.5 to 4.0; 3 = 4.5 to 8.0; 4 = 8.5 to 12.0; 5 = 12.5 or more years). Column 4 has the number of deaths and column 5 has the number of person-years. The five columns of data have been further split into three segments.

1	1	2	0	19406	2	2	2	1	528066	3	3	2	2	169654
1	1	3	0	70000	2	2	3	4	497481	3	3	3	1	111962
1	1	4	0	52836	2	2	4	2	279542	3	3	4	0	55060
1	1	5	0	33209	2	2	5	2	97982	3	3	5	1	840
1	2	1	0	2166	2	3	1	0	82886	3	4	1	0	679445
1	2	2	1	175294	2	3	2	0	253653	3	4	2	0	686531
1	2	3	0	179501	2	3	3	0	206343	3	4	3	1	458838
1	2	4	1	121217	2	3	4	2	111541	3	4	4	1	183701
1	2	5	0	77877	2	3	5	0	45434	3	4	5	0	42665
1	3	1	0	71400	2	4	1	0	1021139	4	1	2	0	14773
1	3	2	0	267774	2	4	2	1	1088072	4	1	3	0	36570
1	3	3	0	267714	2	4	3	0	869314	4	1	4	0	17290
1	3	4	0	210773	2	4	4	3	585779	4	2	1	0	3176
1	3	5	0	157445	2	4	5	0	250398	4	2	2	2	164801
1	4	1	0	279472	3	1	2	3	116939	4	2	3	5	56130
1	4	2	0	344109	3	1	3	1	262567	4	2	4	0	7258
1	4	3	0	315170	3	1	4	1	151760	4	3	1	0	34540
1	4	4	0	267320	3	1	5	1	32238	4	3	2	2	124253
1	4	5	0	176503	3	2	1	0	3824	4	3	3	1	68881
2	1	2	1	174418	3	2	2	3	330710	4	3	4	0	4382
2	1	3	2	521768	3	2	3	2	265273	4	4	1	1	354720
2	1	4	0	304922	3	2	4	3	90851	4	4	2	3	319077
2	1	5	2	142282	3	2	5	0	19540	4	4	3	0	141845
2	2	1	0	3831	3	3	1	0	49453	4	4	4	0	17203

Table C.13. Studies of lung cancer and passive exposure to smoking by the spouse.

Summary results of a review of passive smoking and lung cancer carried out by Boffetta (2002) are given below.

Study author	Year	Type of study[a]	Sex group	Relative risk[b] (95% conf. interval)	
Akiba	1986	C–C, population controls	females	1.5	(1.0, 2.5)
Akiba	1986	C–C, population controls	males	1.8	(0.5, 5.6)
Boffetta	1998	C–C, mixed controls	females	1.09	(0.85, 1.40)
Boffetta	1998	C–C, mixed controls	males	1.55	(0.82, 2.94)
Boffetta	1999	C–C, hospital controls	females	1.0	(0.5, 1.8)
Brownson	1992	C–C, population controls	females	1.1	(0.8, 1.3)
Buffler	1984	C–C, population controls	females	0.78	(0.34, 1.81)
Buffler	1984	C–C, population controls	males	0.52	(0.14, 1.74)
Butler	1988	cohort	females	2.02	(0.48, 8.56)
Cardenas	1997	cohort	females	1.2	(0.8, 1.6)
Cardenas	1997	cohort	males	1.1	(0.6, 1.8)
Chan	1982	C–C, hospital controls	females	0.75	(0.43, 1.30)
Correa	1983	C–C, hospital controls	females	2.07	(0.82, 5.20)
Correa	1983	C–C, hospital controls	males	2.0	(0.4, 10)
Fontham	1994	C–C, population controls	females	1.29	(1.04, 1.60)
Gao	1987	C–C, hospital controls	females	0.9	(0.6, 1.4)
Garfinkel	1985	C–C, hospital controls	females	1.22	(0.97, 1.71)
Garfinkel	1981	cohort	females	1.17	(0.94, 1.44)
Geng	1988	C–C, hospital controls	females	2.16	(1.08, 4.29)
Hirayama	1984	cohort	females	1.45	(1.02, 2.08)
Hirayama	1984	cohort	males	2.25	(1.06, 4.76)
Hole	1989	cohort	females	2.41	(0.45, 12.8)
Humble	1987	C–C, population controls	females	2.6	(1.2, 5.6)
Inoue	1988	C–C, hospital controls	females	2.55	(0.74, 8.78)
Janerich	1990	C–C, population controls	both	0.93	(0.55, 1.57)
Jee	1999	cohort	females	1.9	(1.0, 3.5)
Kabat	1984	C–C, hospital controls	females	0.9	(0.4, 2.1)
Kabat	1984	C–C, hospital controls	males	1.3	(0.3, 4.9)
Kabat	1995	C–C, hospital controls	females	0.95	(0.53, 1.67)
Kabat	1995	C–C, hospital controls	males	1.13	(0.53, 2.45)
Kalandidi	1990	C–C, hospital controls	females	2.11	(1.09, 4.08)
Ko	1997	C–C, hospital controls	females	1.3	(0.7, 2.5)
Koo	1987	C–C, population controls	females	1.64	(0.87, 3.09)
Lam	1985	C–C, population controls	females	2.01	(1.09, 3.72)
Lam	1987	C–C, hospital controls	females	1.65	(1.16, 2.35)
Lee	1986	C–C, hospital controls	females	1.0	(0.37, 2.71)
Lee	1986	C–C, hospital controls	males	1.3	(0.38, 4.39)
Lee	2000	C–C, hospital controls	females	2.2	(1.5, 3.3)
Liu	1991	C–C, population controls	females	0.77	(0.30, 1.96)
Liu	1993	C–C, hospital controls	females	1.7	(0.7, 3.8)
Pershagen	1987	C–C, population controls	females	1.2	(0.7, 2.1)
Rapiti	1999	C–C, hospital controls	both	1.1	(0.5, 2.6)

Table C.13 (continued). Studies of lung cancer and passive exposure to smoking by the spouse.

Study author	Year	Type of study[a]	Sex group	Relative risk[b] (95% conf. interval)	
Shen	1998	C–C, population controls	females	1.63	(0.68, 3.89)
Shimizu	1988	C–C, hospital controls	females	1.08	(0.64, 1.82)
Sobue	1990	C–C, hospital controls	females	1.13	(0.78, 1.63)
Stockwell	1992	C–C, population controls	females	1.6	(0.8, 3.0)
Sun	1996	C–C, hospital controls	females	1.16	(0.80, 1.69)
Svensson	1989	C–C, population controls	females	1.26	(0.57, 2.81)
Trichopoulos	1983	C–C, hospital controls	females	2.1	(1.2, 3.6)
Wang	1996	C–C, population controls	females	1.11	(0.65, 1.88)
Wang	2000	C–C, population controls	females	1.03	(0.6, 1.7)
Wang	2000	C–C, population controls	males	0.56	(0.2, 1.4)
Wu	1985	C–C, population controls	females	1.2	(0.5, 3.3)
Wu–Williams	1990	C–C, population controls	females	0.7	(0.6, 0.9)
Zaridze	1998	C–C, hospital controls	females	1.53	(1.06, 2.21)
Zhong	1999	C–C, population controls	females	1.1	(0.8, 1.5)
Zhou	2000	C–C, population controls	females	0.94	(0.45, 1.97)

[a] C–C = case–control study.
[b] Approximated from an odds ratio where necessary.

References

Abayomi, K., Gelman, A. and Levy, M. (2008) Diagnostics for multivariate imputations. *J. R. Statist. Soc.*, **57**, 273–291.

Aekplakorn, W., Bunnag, P., Woodward, M. *et al.* (2006) A risk score for predicting incident diabetes in the Thai population. *Diabetes Care,* **29**, 1872–1877.

Agresti, A. (1996) *Introduction to Categorical Data Analysis.* John Wiley & Sons, New York.

Agresti, A. and Min, Y. (2004) Effects and non-effects of paired identical observations in comparing proportions with binary matched-pairs data. *Statist. Med.*, **23**, 65–75.

Akaike, H. (1974) A new look at statistical model identification. *IEEE Trans. Automatic Control*, **19**, 716–723.

Allison, P.D. (1995) *Survival Analysis Using the SAS System, A Practical Guide.* SAS Institute Inc., Cary, NC.

Allison, P.D. (2001) *Missing Data.* Sage University Press, Thousand Oaks, CA.

Altman, D.G. (1985) Comparability of randomized groups. *Statistician*, **34**, 125–136.

Altman, D.G. (1991) *Practical Statistics for Medical Research.* Chapman & Hall, London.

Altman, D.G. (1998) Confidence intervals for the number needed to treat. *BMJ*, **317**, 1309–1312.

Altman, D.G. and Andersen, P.K. (1999) Calculating the number needed to treat for trials where the outcome is time to an event. *BMJ*, **319**, 1492–1495.

Altman, D.G. and De Stavola, B.L. (1994) Practical problems in fitting a proportional hazards model to data with updated measurements of the covariates. *Statist. Med.*, **13**, 301–341.

Altman, D.G., Machin, D., Bryant T.N. and Gardner, M.J. (Eds.) (2000) *Statistics with Confidence: Confidence Intervals and Statistical Guidelines.* BMJ Books, London.

Andersen, P.K. and Gill, R.D. (1982) Cox's regression model for counting processes: a large sample study. *Ann. Statist.*, **10**, 1100–1120.

Anderson, P., Bartlett C., Cook, G. and Woodward, M. (1985) Legionnaires disease in Reading — possible association with a cooling tower. *Comm. Med.*, **7**, 202–207.

Andridge, R.R. and Little, R.J.A. (2010) A review of hot deck imputation for survey non-response. *Int. Statist. Rev.,* **78**, 40–64.

Arbogast, P.G. (2010) Performance of floating absolute risks. *Int. J. Epidemiol.*, **162**, 487–490.

Armitage, P. (1955) Tests for linear trends in proportions and frequencies. *Biometrics*, **11**, 375–386.

Armitage, P., Berry, G. and Matthews, J.N.S. (2001) *Statistical Methods in Medical Research*, 4th ed. Blackwell, Oxford.

Armstrong, B.G. and Sloan, M. (1989) Ordinal regression models for epidemiologic data. *Am. J. Epidemiol.*, **129**, 191–204.

Ashton, J. (Ed.) (1994) *The Epidemiological Imagination.* Open University Press, Buckingham.

Asia Pacific Cohort Studies Collaboration (2003a) Cholesterol, coronary heart disease and stroke in the Asia–Pacific region. *Int. J. Epidemiol.*, **32**, 563–572.

Asia Pacific Cohort Studies Collaboration (2003b) The effects of diabetes on the risks of major cardiovascular diseases and death in the Asia–Pacific region. *Diabetes Care*, **26**, 360–366.

Austin, P.C. (2007) Propensity-score matching in the cardiovascular surgery literature from 2004 to 2006: a systematic review and suggestions for improvement. *J. Thorac. Cardiovasc. Surg.*, **134**, 1128–1135.

Austin, P.C. (2008) A critical appraisal of propensity-score matching in the medical literature between 1996 and 2003. *Statist. Med.*, **27**, 2037–2049.

Austin, P.C. (2009) Balance diagnostics for comparing the distribution of baseline covariates between treatment groups in propensity-score matched samples. *Statist. Med.*, **28**, 3083–3107.

Austin, P.C. (2010) Statistical criteria for selecting the optimal number of untreated subjects matched to each treated subject when using many-to-one matching on the propensity score. *Am. J. Epidemiol.*, **172**, 1092–1097.

Austin, P.C. (2011) Optimal caliper widths for propensity-score matching when estimating differences in means and differences in proportions in observational studies. *Pharmaceut. Statist.*, **10**, 150–161.

Austin, P.C. and Mamdani, M.M. (2006) A comparison of propensity score methods: a case-study estimating the effectiveness of post-AMI statin use. *Statist. Med.*, **25**, 2084–2106.

Autier, P., Dore, J.-F., Lejeune, F.J. *et al.* (1996) Sun protection in childhood or early adolescence and reduction of melanoma risk in adults: an EORTC case-control study in Germany, Belgium and France. *J. Epidemiol. Biostatist.*, **1**, 51–57.

Bachrach, V.R.G., Schwarz, E. and Bachrach, L.R. (2003) Breastfeeding and the risk of hospitalisation for respiratory disease in infancy. *Arch. Pediatr. Adolesc. Med.*, **157**, 237–243.

Badger, G.D., Nursten, J., Williams, P. and Woodward, M. (1999) *Systematic Review of the International Literature on Mentally Disordered Offending*. NHS Centre for Reviews and Dissemination Report 15, University of York.

Bakoyannis, G. and Touloumi, G. (2012) Practical methods for competing risks data: a review. *Stat. Methods Med. Res.*, **21**, 257–272.

Barbash, G.I., White, H.D., Modam, M. *et al.* (1993) Significance of smoking in patients receiving thrombolytic therapy for acute myocardial infarction. *Circulation*, **87**, 53–58.

Barker, N. (2005) A practical introduction to the bootstrap using the SAS system. http://www.lexjansen.com/phuse/2005/pk/pk02.pdf.

Barker, N., Hews, R.J., Huitson, A. and Poloniecki, J. (1982) The two period cross-over trial. *BIAS*, **9**, 67–116.

Barlow, W.E., Ichikawa, L., Rosner, D. and Izumi, S. (1999) Analysis of case-cohort designs. *J. Clin. Epidemiol.*, **52**, 1165–1172.

Barnard, J. and Rubin, D.B. (1999) Small-sample degrees of freedom with multiple imputation. *Biometrika*, **86**, 948–955.

Barzi, F. and Woodward, M. (2004) Imputations of missing values in practice: results from imputations of serum cholesterol in 28 cohort studies. *Am. J. Epidemiol.*, **160**, 34–45.

Barzi, F., Woodward, M., Marfisi, R.M. *et al.* (2003) Mediterranean diet and all-causes mortality after myocardial infarction: results from the GISSI-Prevenzione trial. *Eur. J. Clin. Nutr.* **57**, 604–611.

Basnayake, S., De Silva, S.V., Miller, P.C. and Rogers, S. (1983) A comparison of Norinyl and Brevicon in 3 sites in Sri Lanka. *Contraception*, **27**, 453–464.

Bates, D.M. and Watts, D.G. (1988) *Non-linear Regression Analysis and Its Applications*. John Wiley & Sons, New York.

Belsley, D.A., Kuh, E. and Welsch, R.E. (1980) *Regression Diagnostics: Identifying Influential Data and Sources of Collinearity*. John Wiley & Sons, New York.

Bender, R. and Blettner, M. (2002) Calculating the 'number needed to be exposed' with adjustment for confounding variables in epidemiological studies. *J. Clin. Epidemiol.*, **55**, 525–530.

Benichou, J. (1991) Methods of adjustment for estimating the attributable risk in case-control studies: a review. *Statist. Med.*, **10**, 1753–1773.

Benichou, J. (2001) A review of adjusted estimators of attributable risk. *Stat. Methods Med. Res.*, **10**, 195–216.

Benichou, J. and Gail, M.H. (1990) Variance calculations and confidence intervals for estimates of the attributable risk based on logistic models. *Biometrics*, **46**, 991–1003.

Ben–Tovim, D., Whitehead, J. and Crisp, A.H. (1979) A controlled study of the perception of body width in anorexia nervosa. *J. Psychosomatic Res.*, **23**, 267–272.

Berkey, C.S., Hoaglin, D.C., Mosteller, F. and Colditz, G.A. (1995) A random-effects regression model for meta-analysis. *Statist. Med.*, **14**, 395–411.

Berlin, J.W. and Colditz, G.A. (1990) A meta-analysis of physical activity in the prevention of coronary heart disease. *Am. J. Epidemiol.*, **132**, 612–628.

Bernaards, C.A., Belin, T.R. and Schafer, J.L. (2007) Robustness of a multivariate normal approximation for imputation of incomplete binary data. *Statist. Med.*, **26**, 1368–1382.

Berry, D.A. (2011) Adaptive clinical trials in oncology. *Nature Rev.* **9**, 199–207.

Berry, G. (1983) The analysis of mortality by the subject-years method. *Biometrics*, **39**, 173–184.

Bibbins-Domingo, K., Chertow, G.M., Coxson, P.G. *et al* (2010) Projected effect of dietary salt reductions on future cardiovascular disease. *New England J. Med.*, **362**, 590–599.

Biesheuvel, C.J., Vergouwea, Y., Steyerberg, E.W., Grobbee, D.E. and Moons, K.G.M. (2008) Polytomous logistic regression analysis could be applied more often in diagnostic research. *J. Clin. Epidemiol.*, **61**, 125–134.

Birkes, D. and Dodge, Y. (1993) *Alternative Methods of Regression.* John Wiley & Sons, New York.

Bland, J.M. and Altman, D.G. (1986) Statistical methods for assessing agreement between two methods of clinical measurement. *Lancet*, **i**, 307–310.

Bland, J.M. and Altman, D.G. (1987) Statistics notes: Cronbach's alpha. *BMJ*, **314**, 572.

Bland, J.M. and Altman, D.G. (1994) Statistics notes: some examples of regression towards the mean. *BMJ*, **309**, 780.

Bland, M. (2000) *An Introduction to Medical Statistics*, 3rd ed. Oxford University Press, Oxford.

Bleeker, S.E., Moll, H.A., Steyerberg, E.W., *et al.* (2003) External validation is necessary in prediction research: a clinical example. *J. Clin. Epidemiol.*, **56**, 826–832.

Blettner, M., Sauerbrei, W., Schlehofer, B., Scheuchenpflug, T. and Friedenreich, C. (1999) Traditional reviews, meta-analysis and pooled analyses in epidemiology. *Int. J. Epidemiol.*, **28**, 1–9.

Boffetta, P. (2002) Involuntary smoking and lung cancer. *Scand. J. Work Environ. Health*, **28** Suppl. 2, 30–40.

Bolton–Smith, C., Smith, W.C.S., Woodward, M. and Tunstall–Pedoe, H. (1991) Nutrient intakes of different social-class groups: results from the Scottish Heart Health Study. *Br. J. Nutr.*, **65**, 321–335.

Bolton–Smith, C. and Woodward, M. (1995) Intrinsic, non-milk extrinsic and milk sugar consumption by Scottish adults. *J. Human Nutr. Dietetics*, **8**, 35–49.

Bolton–Smith, C. and Woodward, M. (1997) Trends in energy intake and body mass index across smoking habit groups for men. *Proc. Nutr. Soc.*, **56**, 66A.

Bolton–Smith, C., Woodward, M., Smith, W.C.S. and Tunstall–Pedoe, H. (1991) Dietary and nondietary predictors of serum total and HDL-cholesterol in men and women: results from the Scottish Heart Health Study. *Int. J. Epidemiol.*, **20**, 95–104.

Boos, D.D. (2003) Introduction to the bootstrap world. *Statist. Sci.*, **2**, 168–174.

Borenstein, M., Hedges, L.V., Higgins, J.P.T. and Rothstein, H.R. (2009) *Introduction to Meta-Analysis.* Wiley, Chichester.

Bortner, K.W. (1969) A short rating scale as a potential measure of pattern A behaviour. *J. Chronic Dis.*, **22**, 87–91.

Box, G.E.P. and Cox, D.R. (1964) An analysis of transformations. *J. R. Statist. Soc. B*, **26**, 211–252.

Boyce, T.G., Koo, D., Swerdlow, D.L. *et al.* (1996) Recurrent outbreaks of *Salmonella* enteritidis infections in a Texas restaurant: phage type 4 arrives in the United States. *Epidemiol. Infect.*, **117**, 29–34.

Boyle, P., Maisonneuve, P. and Doré, J.F. (1995) Epidemiology of malignant melanoma. *Br. Med. Bull.*, **51**, 523–547.

Braathan, G., von Bahr, L. and Theorell, K. (1997) Motor inpairments in children with epilepsy treated with carbamazepine. *Acta Paediatr.*, **86**, 372–376.

Breslow, N.E. (1984) Elementary methods of cohort analysis. *Int. J. Epidemiol.*, **13**, 112–115.

Breslow, N.E. and Day, N.E. (1993) *Statistical Methods in Cancer Research. Volume I — The Analysis of Case–Control Studies.* Oxford University Press, New York.

Breslow, N.E. and Day, N.E. (1994) *Statistical Methods in Cancer Research. Volume II —The Design and Analysis of Cohort Studies.* Oxford University Press, New York.

Breslow, N.E., Day, N.E., Halvorsen, K.T., Prentice, R.L. and Sabai, C. (1978) Estimation of multiple relative risk functions in matched case–control studies. *Am. J. Epidemiol.*, **108**, 299–307.

Breslow, N.E., Lumley, T., Ballantyne, C.M., Chambless, L.E. and Kulich, M. (2009) Using the whole cohort in the analysis of case-cohort data. *Am. J. Epidemiol.*, **169**, 1398–1405.

Bretz, F., Koenig, F., Brannath, W., Glimm, E. and Posch, M. (2009) Adaptive designs for confirmatory clinical trials. *Statist. Med.*, **28**, 1181–1217.

Brier, G.W. (1950) Verification of forecasts expressed in terms of probability. *Monthly Weather Rev.*, **78**, 1–3.

Bristol, D.R. (1989) Sample sizes for constructing confidence intervals and testing hypotheses. *Statist. Med.*, **8**, 803–811

Brown, H. and Prescott, R. (2006) *Applied Mixed Models in Medicine.* 2nd ed. John Wiley & Sons, Chichester.

Buck, C., Llopis, A., Nájera, E. and Terris, M. (Eds.) (1988) *The Challenge of Epidemiology. Issues and Selected Readings.* World Health Organization, Washington, DC.

Calle, E.E., Mervis, C.A., Wingo, P.A., Thun, M.J., Rodriguez, C. and Heath, C.W. (1995) Spontaneous abortion and risk of fatal breast cancer in a prospective cohort of United States women. *Cancer Causes Control*, **6**, 460–468.

Campbell, I. (2007) Chi-squared and Fisher–Irwin tests of two-by-two tables with small sample recommendations. *Statist. Med.*, **26**, 3661–3675.

Campbell, M., Grimshaw, J. and Steen, N. (2000) Sample size calculations for cluster ran-domised trials. *J. Health Serv. Res. Policy*, **5**, 12–16.

Campbell, M.J., Machin, D. and Walters, S.J. (2007) *Medical Statistics. A Textbook for the Medical Sciences*, 4th ed. John Wiley & Sons, Chichester.

Campbell, M.K., Feuer, E.J. and Wun, L.-M. (1994) Cohort-specific risks of developing breast cancer to age 85 in Connecticut. *Epidemiology*, **5**, 290–296.

Campbell, M.K., Mollison, J. and Grimshaw, J.M. (2001) Cluster trials in implementation research: estimation of intracluster correlation coefficients and sample size. *Statist. Med.*, **20**, 391–399.

Carpenter, J. and Bithell, J. (2000) Bootstrap confidence intervals: when, which, what? A practical guide for medical statisticians. *Statist. Med.*, **19**, 1141–1164.

Carroll, R.J., Ruppert, D., Stefanski, L.A. and Crainiceanu, C.M. (2006) *Measurement Error in Nonlinear Models.* 2nd ed. Chapman & Hall/CRC Press, Boca Raton, FL.

Casagrande, J.T., Pike, M.C. and Smith, P.G. (1978) The power function of the exact test for comparing two binomial distributions. *Appl. Statist.*, **27**, 176–180.

Chambless, L.E., Cummiskey, C.P. and Cui, G. (2011) Several methods to assess improvement in risk prediction models: extension to survival analysis. *Statist. Med.*, **30**, 22–38.

Chan, A.-W., Tetzlaff, J.M., Altman, D.G. *et al.* (2013) SPIRIT 2013 statement: defining standard protocol items for clinical trials. *Annals Int. Med.,* **158**, 200–207.

Chatterjee, S. and Price, B. (2000) *Regression Analysis by Example*, 3rd ed. John Wiley & Sons, New York.

Choudhury, J.B. (2002). Non-parametric confidence interval estimation for competing risks analysis: application to contraceptive data. *Statist. Med.*, **21**, 1129–1144.

Clarke, G.M. and Cooke, D. (2004) *A Basic Course in Statistics*, 5th ed. Arnold, London.

Clarke, G.M. and Kempson, R.E. (1997) *Introduction to the Design and Analysis of Experiments.* Arnold, London.

Clarke, R., Shipley, M., Lewington, S. *et al.* (1999) Underestimation of risk associations due to regression dilution in long-term follow-up of prospective studies. *Am. J. Epidemiol.*, **150**, 341–353.

Clayton, D. and Cuzick, J. (1985) Multivariate generalizations of the proportional hazards model (with discussion). *J. R. Statist. Soc. A,* **148**, 82–117.

Clayton, D. and Hills, M. (1993) *Statistical Models in Epidemiology.* Oxford University Press, Oxford.

Clayton, D. and Schifflers, E. (1987a) Models for temporal variation in cancer rates. I: Age–period and age–cohort models. *Statist. Med.*, **6**, 449–468.

Clayton, D. and Schifflers, E. (1987b) Models for temporal variation in cancer rates. II: Age–period–cohort models. *Statist. Med.*, **6**, 469–481.

Cleveland, W. S. (1979) Robust locally weighted regression and smoothing scatterplots. *J. Am. Statist. Assoc.*, **74**, 829–836.

Cochran, W.G. (1977) *Sampling Techniques*, 3rd ed. John Wiley & Sons, New York.

Cochrane, A.L., St. Leger, A.S. and Moore, F. (1978) Health service 'input' and mortality 'output' in developed countries. *J. Epidemiol. Comm. Health*, **32**, 200–205.

Cohen, J. (1968) Weighted kappa: nomial scale agreement with provision for scaled disagreement or partial credit. *Psychol. Bull.*, **70**, 213–220.

Cole, P. and McMahon, B. (1971) Attributable risk percent in case-control studies. *Br. J. Prev. Soc. Med.*, **25**, 242–244.

Collett, D. (2002) *Modelling Binary Data*, 2nd ed. Chapman & Hall, London.

Collett, D. (2003) *Modelling Survival Data in Medical Research*, 2nd ed. Chapman & Hall, London.

Conover, W.J. (1999) *Practical Nonparametric Statistics*, 3rd ed. John Wiley & Sons, New York.

Cook, N.R. (2008) Statistical evaluation of prognostic versus diagnostic models: beyond the ROC curve. *Clin. Chem.*, **54**, 17–23.

Cook, R.J, Zeng, L. and Yi, G.Y. (2004) Marginal analysis of incomplete longitudinal binary data: a cautionary note on LOCF imputation. *Biometrics*, **60**, 820–828.

Cornfield, J. (1956) A statistical problem arising from retrospective studies, in *Proceedings of the Third Berkeley Symposium on Mathematical Statistics and Probability* (Ed. J. Newman). University of California Press, Berkeley.

Coughlin, S.S., Benichou, J. and Weed, D.L. (1994) Attributable risk estimation in case–control studies. *Epidemiol. Rev.*, **16**, 51–64.

Cox, D.R. (1958) Two further applications of a model for binary regression. *Biometrika*, **45**, 562–565.

Cox, D.R. (1972) Regression models and life tables (with discussion). *J. R. Statist. Soc. B*, **74**, 187–220.

Cox, D.R. and Oakes, D. (1984) *Analysis of Survival Data*. Chapman & Hall, London.

Crombie, I.K., Todman, J., McNeill, G., Florey, C. du V., Menzies, I. and Kennedy, R.A. (1990) Effect of vitamin and mineral supplementation on verbal and nonverbal reasoning of schoolchildren. *Lancet*, **335**, 744–747.

Crowther, C.A., Verkuyl, D.A.A., Neilson, J.P., Bannerman, C. and Ashurst, H.M. (1990) The effects of hospitalization for rest on fetal growth, neonatal morbidity and length of gestation in twin pregnancy. *Br. J. Obstet. Gynae.*, **97**, 872–877.

Crowther, M.J., Abrams, K.R. and Lambert, P.C. (2012) Flexible parametric joint modelling of longitudinal and survival data. *Statist. Med.*, **31**, 4456–4471.

Cui, J. (2007) QIC program and model selection in GEE analyses. *Stata J.*, **7**, 209–220.

Cumming, R.G. and Le Couteur, D.G. (2003) Benzodiazepines and risk of hip fractures in older people: a review of the evidence. *CNS Drugs*, **17**, 825–837.

D'Agostino, R.B. Sr., Vasan, R.S., Pencina, M.J. *et al.* (2008) General cardiovascular risk profile for use in primary care: the Framingham Heart Study. *Circulation*, **117**, 743–753.

Dahabreh, I.J., Sheldrick, R.C., Paulus, J.K. *et al.* (2012) Do observational studies using propensity score methods agree with randomized trials? A systematic comparison of studies on acute coronary syndromes. *Eur. Heart J.*, **33**, 1893–1901.

Daly, E., Vessey, M.P., Hawkins, M.M., Carson, J.L., Gough, P. and Marsh, S. (1996) Risk of venous thromboembolism in users of hormone replacement therapy. *Lancet*, **348**, 977–980.

Davison, A.C. and Hinkley, D.V. (2006) *Bootstrap Methods and Their Application*. Cambridge University Press, Cambridge.

Day, N.E., Byar, D.P. and Green, S.B. (1980) Overadjustment in case–control studies. *Am. J. Epidemiol.*, **112**, 696–706.

de Boor, C. (1978) *A Practical Guide to Splines*. New York, Springer-Verlag.

DeLong, E.R., DeLong, D.M. and Clarke-Pearson D.L. (1988) Comparing the areas under two or more correlated receiver operating characteristic curves: a nonparametric approach. *Biometrics*, **44**, 837–845.

DeMets, D.L. and Lan, K.K. (1994) Interim analysis: the alpha spending function approach. *Statist. Med.*, **13**, 1341–1352.

DerSimonian, R. and Laird, N. (1986) Meta-analysis in clinical trials. *Control. Clin. Trials*, **7**, 177–188.

Diamond, G.A. (1992) What price perfection? Calibration and discrimination of clinical prediction models. *J. Clin. Epidemiol.*, **45**, 85–89.

DiCiccio, T. and Efron, B. (1992) More accurate confidence intervals in exponential families. *Biometrika*, **79**, 231–245.

Dickersin, K. (2002) Systematic reviews in epidemiology: why are we so far behind? *Int. J. Epidemiol.*, **31**, 6–12.

Diggle, P.J., Heagerty, P., Liang, K.-Y. and Zeger, S.L. (2002) *Analysis of Longitudinal Data.* 2nd ed. Oxford University Press, New York.

Ditchburn, R.K. and Ditchburn, J.S. (1990) A study of microscopical and chemical tests for the rapid diagnosis of urinary tract infections in general practice. *Br. J. Gen. Practice.*, **40**, 406–408.

Dobson, A.J., Kuulasmaa, K. and Eberle, E. (1991) Confidence intervals for weighted sums of Poisson parameters. *Statist. Med.*, **10**, 457–462.

Doll, R. and Hill, A.B. (1950) Smoking and carcinoma of the lung. Preliminary report. *BMJ*, ii, 739–748.

Doll, R. and Hill, A.B. (1952) A study of the aetiology of carcinoma of the lung. *BMJ*, ii, 1271–1286.

Doll, R. and Hill, A.B. (1964) Mortality in relation to smoking: ten years' observations of British doctors. *BMJ*, i, 1399–1410, 1460–1467.

Doll, R. and Peto, R. (1976) Mortality in relation to smoking: 20 years' observations on male British doctors. *BMJ*, ii, 1525–1536.

Doll, R., Peto, R., Boreham, J. and Sutherland, I. (2004) Mortality in relation to smoking: 50 years' observations on male British doctors. *BMJ,* **328**, 1519–1527.

Doll, R., Peto, R., Wheatley, K., Gray, R. and Sutherland, I. (1994) Mortality in relation to smoking: 40 years' observations on male British doctors. *BMJ*, **309**, 901–911.

Donner, A. and Klar, N. (2000) *Design and Analysis of Cluster Randomisation Trials in Health Research.* Oxford University Press, New York.

Donner, A. and Li, K.Y.R. (1990) The relationship between chi-square statistics from matched and unmatched analyses. *J. Clin. Epidemiol.*, **43**, 827–831.

Dorman, P.J., Slattery, J., Farrell, B. *et al.* (1997) A randomised comparison of the EuroQol and Short Form-36 after stroke. *BMJ*, **315**, 461.

Draper, N.R. and Smith, H. (1998) *Applied Regression Analysis*, 3rd ed. John Wiley & Sons, New York.

Drews, C.D., Kraus, J.F. and Greenland, S. (1990) Recall bias in a case–control study of sudden infant death syndrome. *Int. J. Epidemiol.*, **19**, 405–411.

Du Mond, C. (1992) An application of the sequential probability ratio test to an unblinded clinical trial of ganciclovir versus no treatment in the prevention of CMV pneumonia following bone marrow transplantation, in *Biopharmaceutical Sequential Statistical Applications* (Ed. K.E. Peace), Statistics, Textbooks and Monographs Vol. 128. Marcel Dekker, New York.

Duffy, J.C. (1995) Alcohol consumption and all-causes mortality. *Int. J. Epidemiol.*, **24**, 100–105.

Durkheim, E. (1951) *Suicide: A Study in Sociology.* Free Press, New York.

Duval, S. and Tweedie, R. (2000) Trim and fill: a simple funnel plot based method of testing and adjusting for publication bias in meta-analysis. *Biometrics*, **56**, 455–463.

Easterbrook, P.J., Berlin, J.A., Gopalan, R. and Matthews, D.R. (1991) Publication bias in clinical research. *Lancet*, **337**, 867–872.

Easton, D.F., Peto, J. and Babiker, A.G.A.G. (1991) Floating absolute risk: an alternative to relative risk in survival and case–control analysis avoiding an arbitrary reference group. *Statist. Med.*, **10**, 1025–1035.

Efron, B. (1979) Bootstrap methods: another look at the jackknife. *Annals Statist.*, **7**, 1–26.

Efron, B. (1987) Better bootstrap confidence intervals. *JAMA*, **82**, 171–185.

Efron, B. and Gong, G. (1983) A leisurely look at the bootstrap, the jackknife, and cross-validation. *Am. Statistician*, **37**, 36–48.

Efron, B. and Tibshirani, R.J. (1993) *An Introduction to the Bootstrap.* Chapman & Hall, New York.

Egger, M., Schneider, M. and Smith, G.D. (1998) Spurious precision? Meta-analysis of observational studies. *BMJ*, **316**, 140–144.

Egger, M., Smith, G.D., Schneider, M. and Minder, C. (1997) Bias in meta-analysis detected by a simple, graphical test. *BMJ*, **315**, 629–634.

Elbourne, D.R., Altman, D.G., Higgins, J.P.T., Curtin, F., Worthington, H.V. and Vail, A. (2002) Meta-analysis involving cross-over trials: methodological issues. *Int. J. Epidemiol.*, **31**, 140–149.

Ernster, V.L. (1994) Nested case-control studies. *Prev. Med.*, **23**, 587–590.

Eyding, D., Lelgemann, M., Grouven, U. *et al.* (2010) Reboxetine for acute treatment of major depression: systematic review and meta-analysis of published and unpublished placebo and selective serotonin reuptake inhibitor controlled trials. *BMJ*, **341**, c4737. doi: 10.1136/bmj.c4737.

Feinstein, A.R., Walter, S.D. and Horwitz, R.I. (1986) An analysis of Berkson's bias in case–control studies. *J. Chronic Dis.*, **39**, 495–504.

Fibrinogen Studies Collaboration (2005) Plasma fibrinogen level and the risk of major cardiovascular diseases and nonvascular mortality: an individual participant meta-analysis. *JAMA*, **294**, 1799–1809.

Fihn, S.D., Boyko, E.J., Normand, E.H. *et al.* (1996) Association between use of spermicidecoated condoms and *Escherichia coli* urinary tract infection in young women. *Am. J. Epidemiol.*, **144**, 512–520.

Fine, J.P. and Gray, R.J. (1999) A proportional hazards model for the subdistribution of a competing risk. *J. Am. Statist. Assoc.*, **94**, 496–509.

Fisher, R.A. and Yates, F. (1963) *Statistical Tables for Biological, Agricultural and Medical Research,* 6th ed. Oliver and Boyd, Edinburgh.

Flanders, W.D., DeSimonian, R. and Freedman, D.S. (1992) Interpretation of linear regression models that include transformations or interaction terms. *Ann. Epidemiol.*, **2**, 735–744.

Flanders, W.D. and Rhodes, P.H. (1987) Large sample confidence intervals for regression standardized risks, risk ratios, and risk differences. *J. Chron. Dis.*, **40**, 697–704.

Fleiss, J.L. (1993) The statistical basis of meta-analysis. *Statist. Methods Med. Res.*, **2**, 121–145.

Fleiss, J.L. and Levin, B. (1988) Sample size determination in studies with matched pairs. *J. Clin. Epidemiol.*, **41**, 727–730.

Fleiss, J.L., Levin, B. and Paik, M.C. (2003) *Statistical Methods for Rates and Proportions*, 3rd ed. John Wiley & Sons, New York.

Fleming, T.R. and Harrington, D.P. (1991) *Counting Processes and Survival Analysis*. John Wiley & Sons, New York.

Forster, D.P., Newens, A.J., Kay, D.W.K. and Edwardson, J.A. (1995) Risk factors in clinically diagnosed presenile dementia of the Alzheimer type: a case–control study in northern England. *J. Epidemiol. Comm. Health*, **49**, 253–258.

Fransen, M., Woodward, M., Norton, R., Robinson, E., Butler, J. and Campbell, A.J. (2002) Excess mortality or institutionalisation following hip fracture: men are at greater risk than women. *J. Am. Geriatr. Soc.*, **50**, 685–690.

Freedman, D., Pisani, R. and Purves, R. (1997) *Statistics*, 3rd ed. Norton, New York.

Freedman, L.S. (1982) Tables of the number of patients required in clinical trials using the logrank test. *Statist. Med.*, **1**, 121–130.

Freiman, J.A., Chalmer, T.C., Smith, H. and Kuebler, R.R. (1978) The importance of beta, the type II error and sample size in the design and interpretation of the randomized control trial. *N. Engl. J. Med.*, **299**, 690–694.

Frost, C. and Thompson, G. (2000) Correcting for regression dilution bias: comparison of methods for a single predictor variable. *J. R. Statist. Soc. A*, **163**, 173–189.

Gadbury, G.L., Coffey, C.S. and Allison, D.B. (2003) Modern statistical methods for handling missing repeated measurements in obesity trial data: beyond LOCF. *Obesity Rev.*, **4**, 175–184.

Galbraith, R.F. (1988) A note on graphical presentation of estimated odds ratios from several clinical trials. *Statist. Med.*, **7**, 889–894.

Ganna, A., Reilly, M., de Faire, U., Pedersen, N., Magnusson, P. and Ingelsson, E. (2012) Risk prediction measures for case–cohort and nested case–control designs: an application to cardiovascular disease. *Am. J. Epidemiol,* **175**, 715–724.

Gart, J.J. (1969) An exact test for comparing matched proportions in crossover designs. *Biometrika*, **56**, 75–80.

Gault, L.V., Shultz, M. and Davies, K.J. (2002) Variations in Medical Subject Headings (MeSH) mapping: from the natural language of patron terms to the controlled vocabulary of mapped lists. *J. Med. Libr. Assoc.*, **90**, 173–180.

Gefeller, O. (1992) Comparison of adjusted attributable risk estimators. *Statist. Med.*, **11**, 2083–2091.

Gillespie, B.W., Halpern, M.T. and Warner, K.E. (1994) Patterns of lung cancer risk in exsmokers, in *Case Studies in Biometry* (Eds. N. Lange *et al.*), John Wiley & Sons, New York.

Girgis, S., Neal, B., Prescott, J. *et al.* (2003) A one-quarter reduction of the salt content of bread can be made without detection. *Eur. J. Clin. Nutr.*, **57**, 616–620.

Good, P.I. (2005) *Permutation, Parametric, and Bootstrap Tests of Hypotheses*. 3rd ed. Springer, New York.

Good, P.I. (2006) *Resampling Methods: A Practical Guide to Data Analysis*, 3rd ed. Birkhauser, Boston.

Gore, S.M. and Altman, D.G. (1982) *Statistics in Practice*. British Medical Association, London.

Graham, J.W. (2009) Missing data analysis: making it work in the real world. *Ann. Rev. Psych.*, **60**, 549–576.

Graham, J.W., Olchowski, A.E. and Gilreath, T.D. (2007) How many imputations are really needed? Some practical clarifications of multiple imputation theory. *Prev. Sci.*, **8**, 206–213.

Gray, R. (1988). A class of K-sample tests for comparing the cumulative incidence of a competing risk. *Annals Statist.*, **16**, 1141–1154.

Greenland, S. (1989) Modeling and variable selection in epidemiologic analysis. *Am. J. Epidemiol.*, **79**, 340–349.

Greenland, S. (1994) A critical look at some popular meta-analytic methods (with discussion). *Am. J. Epidemiol.*, **140**, 290–302.

Greenland, S. (2004) Estimating standardized parameters from generalized linear models. *Statist. Med.*, **10**, 1069–1074.

Greenland, S. and Longnecker, M.P. (1992) Methods for trend estimation from summarized dose response data, with applications to meta-analysis. *Am. J. Epidemiol.*, **135**, 1301–1309.

Greenland, S., Michels, K.B., Robins, J.M., Poole, C. and Willett, W.C. (1999). Presenting statistical uncertainty in trends and dose–response relations. *Am. J. Epidemiol.*, **149**, 1077–1086, plus Letters on pages 393–394 of same journal (2000).

Greenland, S. and Robins, J.M. (1985) Estimation of a common effect parameter from sparse follow-up data. *Biometrics*, **41**, 55–68.

Greenland, S. and Salvan, A. (1990) Bias in the one-step method for pooling study results. *Statist. Med.*, **9**, 247–252.

Greenwood, M. (1926) *Reports on Public Health and Medical Subjects*. No. 33, Appendix 1. HMSO, London.

Guo, S. and Fraser, M.W. (2010). *Propensity Score Analysis: Statistical Methods and Applications*. Sage, Thousand Oaks, CA.

Haneuse, S., Schildcrout, J. and Gillen, D. (2012) A two-stage strategy to accommodate general patterns of confounding in the design of observational studies. *Biostatistics*, **13**, 274–288.

Hanley, J.A. and McNeil, B.J. (1982) The meaning and use of the area under a receiver operating characteristic (ROC) curve. *Radiology*, **143**, 29–36.

Hardin, J.W. and Hilbe, J.M. (2013) *Generalized Estimating Equations*, 2nd ed. CRC Press, Boca Raton, FL.

Härdle, W. (1990) *Applied Nonparametric Regression*. Cambridge University Press, Cambridge.

Harrell, F.E. Jr. (2001) *Regression Modeling Strategies*. Springer-Verlag, New York.

Harrell, F.E. Jr., Califf, R.M., Pryor, D.B., Lee, K.L. and Rosati, R.A. (1982) Evaluating the yield of medical tests. *JAMA*, **247**, 2543–2546.

Harrell, F.E. Jr., Lee, K.L. and Mark, D.B. (1996) Multivariable prognostic models: issues in developing models, evaluating assumptions and adequacy, and measuring and reducing errors. *Statist. Med.*, **15**, 361–387.

Hastie, T.J., Botha, J.L. and Schnitzler, C.M. (1989) Regression with an ordered categorical response. *Statist. Med.*, **8**, 785–794.

Hastie, T., Tibshirani, R. and Friedman, J. (2001) *The Elements of Statistical Learning.* Springer-Verlag, New York.

He, Y., Zaslavsky, A.M., Landrum, M.B., Harrington, D.P. and Catalano, P. (2010) Multiple imputation in a large-scale complex survey: a practical guide. *Statist. Methods Med. Res.*, **19**, 653–670.

Hedges, L.V. and Olkin, I. (1985) *Statistical Methods for Meta-Analysis.* Academic Press, London.

Heinrich, J., Balleisen, L., Schulte, H., Assmann, G. and van de Loo, J. (1994) Fibrinogen and factor VII in the prediction of coronary risk. Results from the PROCAM study in healthy men. *Arterioscler. Thromb.*, **14**, 54–59.

Higgins, J.P.T. and Thompson, S.G. (2002) Quantifying heterogeneity in a meta-analysis. *Statist. Med.*, **21**, 1539–1558.

Higgins, J.P.T. and Thompson, S.G. (2004) Controlling the risk of spurious findings from meta-regression. *Statist. Med.* **23**, 1663–1682.

Higgins, J.P.T., Thompson, S.G., Deeks, J.J. and Altman, D.G. (2003) Measuring inconsistency in meta-analyses. *BMJ*, **327**, 557–560.

Hill, J., Bird, H.A., Fenn, G.C., Lee, C.E., Woodward, M. and Wright, V. (1990) A double-blind crossover study to compare lysine acetyl salicylate (Aspergesic) with ibuprofen in the treatment of rheumatoid arthritis. *J. Clin. Pharm. Therapeutics*, **15**, 205–211.

Hills, M. and Armitage, P. (1979) The two-period cross-over clinical trial. *Br. J. Clin. Pharm.*, **8**, 7–20.

Horton, N.J., Lipsitz, S.R. and Parzen, M. (2003) A potential for bias when rounding in multiple imputation. *Am. Statist.*, **57**, 229–232.

Horwitz, R.I. and Feinstein, A.R. (1978) Methodologic standards and contradictory results in case–control research. *Am. J. Med.*, **66**, 556–564.

Hosmer, D.W., Hosmer, T., Le Cessie, S. and Lemeshow, S. (1997) A comparison of goodness-of-fit tests for the logistic regression model. *Statist. Med.*, **16**, 965–980.

Hosmer, D.W. and Lemeshow, S. (2000) *Applied Logistic Regression*, 2nd ed. John Wiley & Sons, New York.

Hsieh, F.Y. (1989) Sample size tables for logistic regression. *Statist. Med.*, **8**, 795–802.

Hsieh, F.Y., Bloch, D.A. and Larsen, M.D. (1998) A simple method of sample size calculation for linear and logistic regression. *Statist. Med.*, **17**, 1623–1634.

Hsieh, F.Y. and Lavori, P.W. (2000) Sample-size calculations for the Cox proportional hazards regression model with nonbinary covariates. *Control. Clin. Trials*, **21**, 552–560.

Huncharek, M., Kupelnick, B. and Klassen, H. (2002) Maternal smoking during pregnancy and the risk of childhood brain tumours: a meta-analysis of 6566 subjects from twelve epidemiological studies. *J. Neuro-Oncol.*, **57**, 51–57.

Hussey, M.A. and Hughes, J.P. (2007) Design and analysis of stepped wedge cluster randomized trials. *Contemp. Clin. Trials*, 28, 182–191.

Huxley, R., Moghaddam, A., Berrington de Gonzalez, A., Barzi, F. and Woodward, M. (2005) Type-II diabetes and pancreatic cancer: a meta-analysis of 36 studies. *Br. J. Cancer*, **92**, 2076–2083.

Hwang, I.K. and Rodda, B.E. (1992) Interim analysis in the Norwegian Multicenter Study, in *Biopharmaceutical Sequential Statistical Applications* (Ed. K.E. Peace), Statistics, Textbooks and Monographs Vol. 128. Marcel Dekker, New York.

Iman, R.L., Quade, D. and Alexander, D.A. (1975) Exact probability levels for the Kruskal–Wallis test. *Selected Tables Math. Statist.*, **3**, 329–384.

Infante–Rivard, C., Mur, P., Armstrong, B., Alvarez–Dardet, C. and Bolumar, F. (1991) Acute lymphoblastic leukaemia among Spanish children and mothers' occupation: a case–control study. *J. Epidemiol. Comm. Health*, **45**, 11–15.

Irwig, L., Macaskill, P., Glasziou, P. and Fahey, M. (1995) Meta-analytic methods for diagnostic test accuracy. *J. Clin. Epidemiol.*, **48**, 119–130.

Janssen, A. and Pauls, T. (2003) How do bootstrap and permutation tests work? *Annals Statist.*, **31**, 768–806.

Jenicek, M. (2003) *Foundations of Evidence-Based Medicine.* CRC Press, Boca Raton, FL.

Jennison, C.J. and Turnbull, B.W. (1990) Statistical approaches to interim monitoring of medical trials: a review and commentary. *Statist. Sci.*, **5**, 299–317.

Johansson, I., Tidehag, P., Lundberg, V. and Hallmans, G. (1994) Dental status, diet and cardiovascular risk factors in middle-aged people in northern Sweden. *Comm. Dent. Oral Epidemiol.*, **22**, 431–436.

Jones, B. and Kenward, M.G. (2003) *Design and Analysis of Cross-Over Trials*, 2nd ed. Chapman & Hall, London.

Julious, S.A. (2004) Sample sizes for clinical trials with normal data. *Statist. Med.*, **23**, 1921–1986.

Julious, S.A. and Campbell, M.J. (2012) Sample sizes for parallel group clinical trials with binary data. *Statist. Med.*, **31**, 2904–2936.

Juni, P., Witschi, A., Bloch, R. and Egger, M. (1999) The hazards of scoring the quality of clinical trials for meta-analysis. *JAMA*, **282**, 1054–1060.

Kahn, H.A. and Sempos, C.T. (1989) *Statistical Methods in Epidemiology*. Oxford University Press, New York.

Kalbfleisch, J.D. and Prentice, R.L. (2002) *The Statistical Analysis of Failure Time Data*, 2nd ed. John Wiley & Sons, New York.

Kaplan, E.L. and Meier, P. (1958) Nonparametric estimation from incomplete observations. *J. Am. Statist. Assoc.*, **53**, 457–481.

Karkavelas, G., Mavropoulou, S., Fountzilas, G. *et al.* (1995) Correlation of proliferating cell nuclear antigen assessment, histologic parameters and age with survival in patients with glioblastoma multiforme. *Anticancer Res.*, **15**, 531–536.

Katz, D., Baptista, J., Azen, S.P. and Pike, M.C. (1978) Obtaining confidence intervals for the risk ratio in cohort studies. *Biometrics*, **34**, 469–474.

Kaufman, D.W., Helmrich, S.P., Rosenberg, L., Miettinen, O.S. and Shapiro, S. (1983) Nicotine and carbon monoxide content of cigarette smoke and the risk of myocardial infarction in young men. *N. Engl. J. Med.*, **308**, 409–413.

Kauhanen, J., Kaplan, G.A., Goldberg, D.E. and Salonen, J.K. (1997) Beer binging and mortality: results from the Kuopio ischaemic heart disease risk factor study, a prospective population based study. *BMJ*, **315**, 846–851.

Kay, R. (1984) Goodness of fit methods for the proportional hazards regression model: a review. *Rev. Épidémiol. Santé Publique*, **32**, 185–198.

Kelly, K. (2005) The effects of nonnormal distributions on confidence intervals around the standardized mean difference: bootstrap and parametric confidence intervals. *Educ. Psychol. Meas.*, **65**, 51–69.

Kengne, A., Patel, A., Colagiuri, S. *et al.* (2010) The Framingham and UK Prospective Diabetes Study (UKPDS) risk equations do not reliably estimate the probability of cardiovascular events in a large ethnically diverse sample of patients with diabetes: the Action in Diabetes and Vascular Disease: Preterax and Diamicron-MR Controlled Evaluation (ADVANCE) Study. *Diabetologia*, **53**, 821–831.

Kennedy, K.F. and Pencina, M.J. (2010). A SAS macro for computing added predictive ability of new markers predicting a dichotomous outcome. Paper SDA-07 in *Proceedings of the Seventeenth Annual South East SAS Users Group Conference,* Savannah, GA.

Kerr, K.F., McClelland, R.L., Brown, E.R. and Lumley, T. (2011). Evaluating the incremental value of new biomarkers with integrated discrimination improvement. *Am. J. Epidemiol.*, **174**, 364–374.

Kiechl, S., Willeit, J., Poewe, W. *et al.* (1996) Insulin sensitivity and regular alcohol consumption: large, prospective, cross-sectional population study (Bruneck Study). *BMJ*, **313**, 1040–1044.

Kim, M., Munter, P., Sharma, S. *et al.* (2013). Assessing patient-reported outcomes and preferences for same-day discharge after percutaneous coronary intervention: results from a pilot randomized, controlled trial. *Circ. Cardiovasc. Qual. Outcomes,* **6**, 186–192.

Kitange, H.M., Machibya, H., Black, J. *et al.* (1996) Outlook for survivors of childhood in sub-Saharan Africa — adult mortality in Tanzania. *BMJ*, **312**, 216–220.

Kleinbaum, D.G., Kupper, L.L. and Morgenstern, H. (1982) *Epidemiologic Research: Principles and Quantitative Methods*. Van Nostrand Reinhold, New York.

Kramer, O.S. and Shapiro, S. (1984) Scientific challenges in the application of randomized trials. *JAMA,* **252**, 2739–2745.

Kupper, L.L., Karon, J.M., Kleinbaum, D.G., Morgenstern, H. and Lewis, D.K. (1981) Matching in epidemiologic studies: validity and efficiency considerations. *Biometrics,* **37**, 271–291.

Kupper, L.L., Janis, J.M., Karmous, A. and Greenberg, B.G. (1985) Statistical age–period–cohort analysis: a review and critique. *J. Chronic Dis.,* **38**, 811–830.

Kushi, L.H., Fee, R.M., Sellers, T.A., Zheng, W. and Folsom, A.R. (1996) Intake of vitamins A, C and E and postmenopausal breast cancer. The Iowa Women's Health Study. *Am. J. Epidemiol.,* **144**, 165–174.

Kuss, O. (2001) A SAS/IML-Macro for Goodness-of-Fit Testing in Logistic Regression Models with Sparse Data. Paper 265–26 in *Proceedings of the 26th Annual SAS Users Group International Conference,* CD-Rom Version.

Kvålseth, T.O. (1985) Cautionary note about R^2. *Am. Statistician,* **39**, 279–285.

Langholz, B. and Clayton, D. (1994) Sampling strategies in nested case–control studies. *Environ. Health Perspect.,* **102** Suppl. 8, 47–51.

Langholz, B. and Thomas, D.C. (1990) Nested case-control and case–cohort methods of sampling from a cohort: a critical comparison. *Am. J. Epidemiol.,* **131**, 169–176.

Le, C.T. and Zelterman, D. (1992) Goodness of fit tests for proportional hazards regression models. *Biom. J.,* **5**, 557–566.

Lee, K.J. and Carlin, J.B. (2010) Multiple imputation for missing data: fully conditional specification versus multivariate normal imputation. *Am. J. Epidemiol.,* **171**, 624–632.

Lee, P.N. (2001) Lung cancer and type of cigarette smoked. *Inhalation Toxicol.,* **13**, 951–976.

Leung, H.M. and Kupper, L.L. (1981) Comparisons of confidence intervals for attributable risk. *Biometrics,* **37**, 293–302.

Li, K.H. (1988) Imputation using Markov chains. *J. Statist. Comp. Simulation,* **30**, 57–79.

Li, X., Mehrotra, D.V. and Barnard, J. (2006) Analysis of incomplete longitudinal binary data using multiple imputation. *Statist. Med.,* **25**, 2107–2124.

Liddell, F.D.K. (1980) Simplified exact analysis of case-referent studies: matched pairs; dichotomous exposure. *J. Epidemiol. Comm. Health,* **37**, 82–84.

Liddell, F.D.K., McDonald, J.C. and Thomas, D.C. (1977) Methods of cohort analysis: appraisal by application to asbestos mining. *J. R. Statist. Soc. A,* **140**, 469–491.

Lilienfeld, D.E. and Stolley, P.D. (1994) *Foundations of Epidemiology,* 3rd ed. Oxford University Press, New York.

Lin, G., So, Y. and Johnston, G. (2012) Analyzing survival data with competing risks using SAS software. SAS Global Forum paper 344-2012, Orlando, FL.

Lin, J.-T., Wang, L.-Y., Wang, J.-T., Wang, T.-H., Yang, C.-S. and Chen, C.-J. (1995) A nested case–control study on the association between *Helicobacter pylori* infection and gastric cancer risk in a cohort of 9775 men in Taiwan. *Anticancer Res.,* **15**, 603–606.

Little, R.J.A. (1988) Missing data in large surveys. *J. Business Econ. Statist.,* 6, 287–301.

Little, R.J.A. and Rubin, D.B. (2002) *Statistical Analysis with Missing Data,* 2nd ed. John Wiley & Sons, Hoboken, NJ.

Lopez, A.D., Mathers, C.D., Ezzati, M., Jamison, D.T. and Murray, C.J. (Eds.) (2006) *Global Burden of Disease and Risk Factors.* Oxford University Press, New York.

Lowe, G.D.O., Rumley, A., Woodward, M. *et al.* (1997) Epidemiology of coagulation factors, inhibitors and activation markers: The Third Glasgow MONICA Survey. I Illustrative reference ranges by age, sex and hormone use. *Br. J. Haematology,* **97**, 775–784.

Macaskill, P., Walter, S.D., and Irwig, L. (2001) A comparison of methods to detect publication bias in meta-analysis. *Statist. Med.,* **20**, 641–654.

Machin, D., Campbell, M.J., Tan, S.-B. and Tan, S.-H. (2009) *Sample Size Tables for Clinical Studies,* 3rd ed. Wiley–Blackwell, Chichester.

Maclure, M. and Greenland, S. (1992) Tests for trend and dose response: misinterpretations and alternatives. *Am. J. Epidemiol.,* **135**, 96–104.

Maclure, M. and Mittleman, M.A. (2000) Should we use a case-crossover design? *Annu. Rev. Public Health,* **21**, 193–221.

MacMahon, B. and Trichopoulos, D. (1996) *Epidemiology. Principles and Methods,* 2nd ed. Lippincott–Raven, Hagerstown, MD.

MacMahon, S., Neal, B., Tzourio, C. *et al.* (2001) Randomised trial of a perindopril-based blood-pressure-lowering regimen among 6105 individuals with previous stroke or transient ischaemic attack. *Lancet*, **358**, 1033–1041.

MacMahon, S., Norton, R., Jackson, R. *et al.* (1995). Fletcher Challenge-University of Auckland Heart and Health Study: design and baseline findings. *N.Z. Med. J.*, **108**, 499–502.

MacMahon, S., Peto, R., Cutler, J. *et al.* (1990) Blood pressure, stroke and coronary heart disease. Part 1, prolonged differences in blood pressure: prospective observational studies corrected for the regression dilution bias. *Lancet*, **335**, 765–774.

Manly, B.F.J. (2007) *Randomization, Bootstrap and Monte Carlo Methods in Biology*, 3rd ed. Chapman & Hall/CRC Press, Boca Raton, FL.

Marchenko, Y.V. and Reiter, J. P. (2009) Improved degrees of freedom for multivariate significance tests obtained from multiply imputed, small-sample data. *Stata J.*, **9**, 388–397.

Marchioli, R., Avanzini, F., Barzi, F. *et al.* (2001) Assessment of absolute risk of death after myocardial infarction by use of multiple-risk-factor assessment equations: GISSI-Prevenzione mortality risk chart. *Eur. Heart J.*, **22**, 2085–2103.

Marshall, A., Altman, D.G. and Holder, R.L. (2010) Comparison of imputation methods for handling missing covariate data when fitting a Cox proportional hazards model: a resampling study. *BMC Med. Res. Method.*, **10**: 112.

Matsushita, K., van der Velde, M., Astor, B.C. *et al.* (2010) Association of estimated glomerular filtration rate and albuminuria with all-cause and cardiovascular mortality: a collaborative meta-analysis of general population cohorts. *Lancet*, **375**, 2073–2081.

McCullagh, P. (1980) Regression models for ordinal data (with discussion). *J. R. Statist. Soc. B*, **42**, 109–142.

McCullagh, P. and Nelder, J.A. (1989) *Generalized Linear Models*, 2nd ed. Chapman & Hall, London.

McDonagh, T.A., Woodward, M., Morrison, C.E. *et al.* (1997) *Helicobacter pylori* infection and coronary heart disease in the North Glasgow MONICA population. *Eur. Heart J.*, **18**, 1257–1260.

McEvoy, S.P., Stevenson, M.R., McCartt, A.T. *et al.* (2005) Role of mobile phones in motor vehicle crashes resulting in hospital attendance: a case-crossover study. *BMJ*, **331**, 428–432.

McKinlay, S.M. (1977) Pair matching — a reappraisal of a popular technique. *Biometrics*, **33**, 725–735.

McKinney, P.A., Alexander, F.E., Nicholson, C., Cartwright, R.A. and Carrette, J. (1991) Mothers' reports of childhood vaccinations and infections and their concordance with general practitioner records. *J. Public Health Med.*, **13**, 13–22.

McKnight, P.E., McKnight, K.M., Sidani, S. and Figueredo, A.J. (2007). *Missing Data: A Gentle Introduction*. Guilford Press, New York.

McLoone, P. (1994) *Carstairs Scores for Scottish Postcode Sectors from the 1991 Census*. Public Health Research Unit, University of Glasgow, Glasgow.

McMahon, J., Parnell, W.R. and Spears, G.F.S. (1993) Diet and dental caries in preschool children. *Eur. J. Clin. Nutr.*, **47**, 794–802.

McNeil, D. (1996) *Epidemiological Research Methods*. John Wiley & Sons, Chichester.

Mahoney, F.I. and Barthel, D.W. (1965) Functional evaluation: the Barthel Index. *Md. State Med. J.*, **14**, 61–65.

Mantel, N. and Greenhouse, S.W. (1968) What is the continuity correction? *Am. Statistician*, **22**, 27–30.

Mantel, N. and Haenszel, W. (1959) Statistical aspects of the analysis of data from retrospective studies. *J. Natl. Cancer Inst.*, **22**, 719–748.

Mason, D., Birmingham, L. and Grubin, D. (1997) Substance use in remand prisoners: a consecutive case study. *BMJ*, **315**, 18–21.

Mawson, A.R., Blundo, J.J., Clemmer, D.I., Jacobs, K.W., Ktsanes, V.K. and Rice, J.C. (1996) Sensation-seeking, criminality and spinal cord injury: a case-control study. *Am. J. Epidemiol.*, **144**, 463–472.

Mehta, C., Gao, P., Bhatt, D.L., Harrington, R.A., Skerjanec, S. and Ware, J.H. (2009) Optimizing trial design: sequential, adaptive, and enrichment strategies. *Circulation*, **119**, 597–605.

Mehta, C.R., Patel, N.R. and Gray, R. (1985) Computing an exact confidence interval for the common odds ratio in several 2 × 2 contingency tables. *J. Am. Statist. Assoc.*, **80**, 969–973.

Mezzetti, M., Ferraroni, M., Decarli, A., La Vecchia, C. and Benichou, J. (1996) Software for attributable risk and confidence interval estimation in case-control studies. *Computers Biomed. Res.*, **29**, 63–75.

Miao, L.M. (1977) Gastric freezing: an example of the evaluation of a medical therapy by randomized clinical trials, in *Costs, Risks and Benefits of Surgery*. (Eds. J.P. Bunker, B.A. Barnes and F. Mosteller). Oxford University Press, New York.

Miettinen, O.S. (1970) Estimation of relative risk from individually matched series. *Biometrics*, **26**, 75–86.

Miettenen, O.S. and Cook, E.F. (1981) Confounding: essence and detection. *Am. J. Epidemiol.*, **114**, 593–603.

Miller, C.T., Neutel, C.I., Nair, R.C., Marrett, L.D., Last, J.M. and Collins, W.E. (1978) Relative importance of risk factors in bladder carcinogenesis. *J. Chronic Dis.*, **31**, 51–56.

Millns, H., Woodward, M. and Bolton–Smith, C. (1995) Is it necessary to transform nutrient variables prior to statistical analysis? *Am. J. Epidemiol.*, **141**, 251–262.

Mittlböck, M. and Schemper, M. (1996) Explained variation for logistic regression. *Statist. Med.*, **15**, 1987–1997.

Mittleman, M.A., Maclure, M. and Robins, J.M. (1995) Control sampling strategies for case-crossover studies: an assessment of relative efficiency. *Am. J. Epidemiol.*, **142**, 91–98.

Moher, D., Liberati, A., Tetzlaff, J. and Altman, D.G. (2009) Preferred reporting items for systematic reviews and meta-analyses: the PRISMA statement. *PLoS Med.*, **21**, 6: e1000097. doi: 10.1371/journal.pmed.1000097.

Molenberghs, G. and Kenward, M.G. (2007). *Missing Data in Clinical Studies*. John Wiley & Sons, Chichester.

Montgomery, D.C. and Peck, E.A. (2012) *Introduction to Linear Regression Analysis*, 5th ed. John Wiley & Sons, New York.

Mood, A.M., Graybill, F.A. and Boes, D.C. (1974) *Introduction to the Theory of Statistics*, 3rd ed. McGraw–Hill, Tokyo.

Moons, K.G., Kengne, A.P., Grobbee, D.E., *et al.* (2012a) Risk prediction models: II. External validation, model updating, and impact assessment. *Heart*, **98**, 691–698.

Moons, K.G., Kengne, A.P., Woodward, M. *et al.* (2012b) Risk prediction models: I. Development, internal validation, and assessing the incremental value of a new (bio)marker. *Heart*, **98**, 683–690.

Morgenstern, H. (1982) Uses of ecologic analysis in epidemiologic research. *Am. J. Public Health*, **72**, 1336–1344.

Moritz, D.J., Kelsey, J.L. and Grisso, J.A. (1997) Hospital controls versus community controls: differences in influences regarding risk factors for hip fracture. *Am. J. Epidemiol.*, **145**, 653–660.

Morrison, A.S. (1992) Risk factors for surgery for prostatic hypertrophy. *Am. J. Epidemiol.*, **135**, 974–980.

Morrison, C., Woodward, M., Leslie, W. and Tunstall–Pedoe, H. (1997) Effect of socioeconomic group on incidence of, management of, and survival after myocardial infarction and coronary death: analysis of community coronary event register. *BMJ*, **314**, 541–546.

Morton, V. and Torgerson, D.J. (2003) Effect of regression to the mean on decision making in health care. *BMJ*, **326**, 1083–1084.

Moser, C.A. and Kalton, G. (1971) *Survey Methods in Social Investigation,* 2nd ed. Heinemann, London.

Moss, A.J., Jackson Hall, W., Cannon, D.S. *et al.* (1996) Improved survival with an implanted defibrillator in patients with coronary disease at high risk for ventricular arrhythmia. *N. Engl. J. Med.*, **335**, 1933–1940.

Müller, R. and Büttner, P. (1994) A critical discussion of intraclass correlation coefficients. *Statist. Med.*, **13**, 2465–2476.

Muntner, P., Woodward, M., Carson, A.P. *et al.* (2011) Development and validation of a self-assessment tool for albuminuria: results from the REasons for Geographic And Racial Differences in Stroke (REGARDS) Study. *Am. J. Kidney Dis.*, **58**, 196–205.

National Cancer Institute (1997) *Changes in Cigarette-Related Disease Risks and Their Implication for Prevention and Control.* Smoking and Tobacco Control Monograph 8. National Institutes of Health, Bethesda, MD.

National Cancer Institute (2001) *Risks Associated with Smoking Cigarettes with Low Machine-measured Yields of Tar and Nicotine.* National Institutes of Health, Bethesda, MD.

Nevalainen, J., Kenward, M.G. and Virtanen, S.V (2009) Missing values in longitudinal dietary data: A multiple imputation approach based on a fully conditional specification *Statist. Med.,* **28**, 3657–3669.

Newson, R. (2000) sg151: B-splines and splines parameterized by their values at reference points on the X-axis. *Stata Tech. Bull.,* 57, 20–27.

Newson, R. (2001) Parameters behind "non-parametric" statistics: Kendall's τ_a, Somers' D and median differences. *Stata J.,* **1**, 1–20.

Newson, R.B. (2011) Comparing the predictive power of survival models using Harrell's c or Somers' D. *Stata J.,* **10**, 339–358.

Nieto, F.J. and Coresh, J. (1996) Adjusting survival curves for confounders: a review and a new method. *Am. J. Epidemiol.,* **143**, 1059–1068.

Office of Population Censuses and Surveys (1980) *Classification of Occupations, 1980.* HMSO, London.

Ohkubo, T., Chapman, N., Neal, B., Woodward, M., Omae, T. and Chalmers, J. (2004) Effects of an angiotensin converting enzyme inhibitor-based regimen on pneumonia risk. *Am. J. Respiratory Critical Care Med.,* **169**, 1041–1045.

Ornish, D., Brown, S.E., Scherwitz, L.W. *et al.* (1990) Can lifestyle changes reverse coronary heart disease? The Lifestyle Heart Trial. *Lancet,* **336**, 129–133.

Pan, W. (2001) Akaike's information criterion in generalized estimating equations. *Biometrics,* **57**, 120–125.

Parmar, M.K.B. and Machin, D. (2006) *Survival Analysis. A Practical Approach,* 2nd ed. John Wiley & Sons, Chichester.

Parsonnet, J. (1995) The incidence of *Helicobacter pylori* infection. *Aliment. Pharmacol. Ther.,* **9**, Suppl. 2, 45–51.

Parsons, L.S. (2001) Reducing bias in a propensity score matched-pair sample using greedy matching techniques. SUGI-26 paper 214-26, Long Beach, CA.

Passaro, K.T., Little, R.E., Savitz, D.A. and Noss J. (1996) The effect of maternal drinking before conception and in early pregnancy on infant birth-weight. *Epidemiology,* **7**, 377–383.

Patel, A., MacMahon, S., Chalmers, J. *et al.* (2008) Intensive blood glucose control and vascular outcomes in patients with type 2 diabetes. *New Engl. J. Med.,* **358**, 2560–2572.

Patel, P., Mendall, M.A., Carrington, D. *et al.* (1995) Association of *Helicobacter pylori* and *Chlamydia pneumoniae* infections with coronary heart disease and cardiovascular risk factors. *BMJ,* **311**, 711–714.

Paul, C., Skegg, D.C.G., Spears, G.F.S. and Kaldor, J.M. (1986) Oral contraceptives and breast cancer: a national study. *BMJ,* **293**, 723–726.

Peace, K.E. (Ed.) (1992) *Biopharmaceutical Sequential Statistical Applications.* Statistics, Textbooks and Monographs, Vol. 128. Marcel Dekker, New York.

Peace, L.R. (1985) A time correlation between cigarette smoking and lung cancer. *Statistician,* **34**, 371–381.

Pearl, R. (1929) Cancer and tuberculosis. *Am. J. Hyg.,* **9**, 97–159.

Pearson, M., Spencer, S. and McKenna, M. (1991) Patterns of uptake and problems presented at Well Women clinics in Liverpool. *J. Public Health Med.,* **13**, 42–47.

Pencina, M.J. and D'Agostino, R.B. (2004) Overall c as a measure of discrimination in survival analysis: model specific population value and confidence interval estimation. *Statist. Med.,* **23**, 2109–2123.

Pencina, M.J., D'Agostino, R.B. Sr. and D'Agostino, R.B. Jr. (2008) Evaluating the added predictive ability of a new marker: from area under the ROC curve to reclassification and beyond. *Statist. Med.,* **27**, 157–172.

Pencina, M.J., D'Agostino, R.B. Sr. and Steyerber, E.W. (2011) Extensions of net reclassification improvement calculations to measure usefulness of new biomarkers. *Statist. Med.*, **30**, 11–21.

Pepe, M.S., Janes, H., Longton, G., Leisenring, W. and Newcomb, P. (2004) Limitations of the odds ratio in gauging the performance of a diagnostic, prognostic, or screening marker. *Am. J. Epidemiol.*, **159**: 882–890.

Petersen, M.R. and Deddens, J.A. (2008) A comparison of two methods for estimating prevalence ratios. *BMC Med. Res. Methodology*, 8: 9. doi:10.1186/1471-2288-8-9.

Peterson, B. (1990) Re: ordinal regression models for epidemiologic data. *Am. J. Epidemiol.*, **131**, 745–746.

Peto, R., Pike, M.C., Armitage, P. *et al.* (1977) Design and analysis of randomized clinical trials requiring prolonged observation of each patient. II. Analysis and examples. *Br. J. Cancer*, **35**, 1–39.

Piaggio, G., Elbourne, D.R., Pocock, S.J., Evans, S.J. and Altman, D.G. (2012). Reporting of noninferiority and equivalence randomized trials: extension of the CONSORT 2010 statement. *JAMA*, **308**, 2594–2604.

Phillips, A.N. and Davey Smith, G. (1992) Bias in relative odds estimation owing to imprecise measurement of correlated exposures. *Statist. Med.*, **11**, 953–961.

Piantadosi, S. (2005) *Clinical Trials: A Methodologic Perspective,* 2nd ed. John Wiley & Sons, New York.

Pike, M.C. and Morrow, R.H. (1970) Statistical analysis of patient-control studies in epidemiology. Factor under investigation an all-or-none variable. *Br. J. Prev. Soc. Med.*, **24**, 42–44.

Pike, M.C., Morrow, R.H., Kisuule, A. and Mafigiri, J. (1970) Burkitt's lymphoma and sickle cell trait. *Br. J. Prev. Soc. Med.*, **24**, 39–41.

Pocock, S.J. (1979) Allocation of patients to treatment in clinical trials. *Biometrics*, **35**, 183–197.

Pocock, S.J. (1983) *Clinical Trials: A Practical Approach.* John Wiley & Sons, Chichester.

Poi, B.P. (2004) From the help desk: some bootstrapping techniques. *Stata J.*, **4**, 312–328.

Pollard, A.H., Yusuf, F. and Pollard, G.N. (1990) *Demographic Techniques*, 3rd ed. Pergamon, Sydney.

Pontiggia, P., Curto, F., Rotella, G., Sabato, A., Rizzo, S. and Butti, G. (1995) Hyperthermia in the treatment of brain metastates from lung cancer. Experience in 17 cases. *Anticancer Res.*, **15**, 597–602.

Poole, C. (1986) Exposure opportunity in case–control studies. *Am. J. Epidemiol.*, **123**, 352–358.

Poole, C. (2010) On the origin of risk relativism. *Epidemiology*, **21**, 3–9.

Porta, M. (Ed.) (2008) *A Dictionary of Epidemiology,* 5th ed. Oxford University Press, New York.

Pounder, R.E. and Ng, D. (1995) The prevalence of *Helicobacter pylori* infection in different countries. *Aliment. Pharmacol. Ther.*, **9**, Suppl. 2, 33–39.

Prescott, R.J. (1981) The comparison of success rates in cross-over trials in the presence of an order effect. *J. R. Statist. Soc. C*, **30**, 9–15.

Putter, H., Fiocco, M. and Geskus, R.B. (2007) Tutorial in biostatistics: competing risks and multi-state models. *Statist. Med.*, **26**, 2389–2430.

Raghunathan, T.W., Lepkowksi, J.M., Van Hoewyk, J. and Solenbeger, P. (2001) A multivariate technique for multiply imputing missing values using a sequence of regression models. *Survey Methodol.*, **27**, 85–95.

Rawnsley, K. (1991) The National Counselling Service for Sick Doctors. *Proc. R. Coll. Physicians Edinburgh*, **21**, 4–7.

Reading, R., Harvey, I. and Mclean, M. (2000) Cluster randomised trials in maternal and child health: implications for power and sample size. *Arch. Dis. Child.*, **82**, 79–83.

Redelmeier, D.A., Bloch D.A. and Hickam, D.H. (1991) Assessing predictive accuracy: how to compare Brier scores. *J. Clin. Epidemiol.*, **44**, 1141–1146.

Robins, J.M., Gail, M.H. and Lubin, J.H. (1986a) More on 'biased selection of controls for case-control analyses of cohort studies'. *Biometrics*, **42**, 293–299.

Robins, J., Greenland, S. and Breslow, N.E. (1986b) A general estimator for the variance of the Mantel–Haenszel odds ratio. *Am. J. Epidemiol.*, **124**, 719–723.

Rodrigues, L.C., Gill, O.N. and Smith, P.G. (1991) BCG vaccination in the first year of life protects children of Indian subcontinent ethnic origin against tuberculosis in England. *J. Epidemiol. Comm. Health*, **45**, 78–80.

Rom, D.M. and Hwang, E. (1996) Testing for individual and population equivalence based on the proportion of similar responses. *Statist. Med.*, **15**, 1489–1505.

Rose, G.A., McCartney, P. and Reid, D.D. (1977) Self-administration of questionnaire on chest pain and intermittent claudication. *Br. J. Prev. Soc. Med.*, **31**, 42–48.

Rosenbaum, P.R. and Rubin, D.B. (1983) The central role of the propensity score in observational studies for causal effects. *Biometrika*, 70, 41–55.

Rosenberger, W.F. and Lachin, J.M. (2002) *Randomization in Clinical Trials: Theory and Practice*. John Wiley & Sons, New York.

Rosner, B. (2010) *Fundamentals of Biostatistics*, 7th ed. Brooks/Cole, Boston.

Rosner, B., Spiegelman, D. and Willett, W.C. (1990) Correction of logistic regression relative risk estimates and confidence intervals for measurement error: the case of multiple covariates measured with error. *Am. J. Epidemiol.*, **132**: 734–745.

Rothman, K.J. and Boice, J.D. (1979) *Epidemiological Analysis with a Programmable Calculator*, NIH Publications 79–1649. U.S. Government Printing Office, Washington, DC.

Rothman, K.J. and Greenland, S. (1998) *Modern Epidemiology*, 2nd ed. Lippincott–Raven, Philadelphia, PA.

Roumie, C.L., Hung, A.M., Greevy, R.A. *et al.* (2012). Comparative effectiveness of sulfonylurea and metformin monotherapy on cardiovascular events in type 2 diabetes mellitus: a cohort study. *Ann. Intern. Med.*, **157**, 601–610.

Royston, P. and Altman, D.G. (1994) Regression using fractional polynomials of continuous covariates: parsimonious parametric modelling. *Appl. Statist.*, **43**, 429–467.

Royston, P. and Altman, D.G. (2010) Visualizing and assessing discrimination in the logistic regression model. *Statist. Med.*, **29**, 2508–2520.

Royston, P. and Sauerbrei, W. (2004) A new measure of prognostic separation in survival data. *Statist. Med.*, **23**, 723–748.

Rubin, D.B. (1976) Inference and missing data. *Biometrika*, **63**, 581–592.

Rubin, D.B. (1987) *Multiple Imputation for Nonresponse in Surveys*. John Wiley & Sons, New York.

Rumley, A., Woodward, M., Hoffmeister, A., Koenig, W. and Lowe, G.D. (2003) Comparison of plasma fibrinogen by Clauss, prothrombin time-derived, and immunonephelometric assays in a general population: implications for risk stratification by thirds of fibrinogen. *Blood Coagul. Fibrinolysis*, **14**, 197–201.

Ruth, K.J. and Neaton, J.D. (1991) Evaluation of two biochemical markers of tobacco exposure. *Prev. Med.*, **20**, 574–589.

Sackett, D.L. (1979) Bias in analytic research. *J. Chronic Dis.*, **32**, 51–63.

Saetta, J.P., March, S., Gaunt, M.E. and Quinton, D.N. (1991) Gastric emptying procedures in the self-poisoned patient: are we forcing gastric content beyond the pylorus? *J. R. Soc. Med.*, **84**, 274–276.

Satterthwaite, F.E. (1946) An approximate distribution of estimates of variance components. *Biometrics Bull.*, **2**, 110–114.

Sayal, K., Draper, E.S., Fraser, R., Barrow, M., Davey Smith, G. and Gray, R. (2013) Light drinking in pregnancy and mid-childhood mental health and learning outcomes. *Arch. Dis. Child.*, **98**, 107–111.

Schafer, J.L. (1997) *Analysis of Incomplete Multivariate Data*. Chapman & Hall, London.

Schafer, J.L. and Olsen, M.K. (1998) Multiple imputation for multivariate missing-data problems: a data analyst's perspective. *Multivariate Behavioral Res.*, **33**, 545–571.

Scheaffer, R.L., Mendenhall, W. and Ott, R.L. (1995) *Elementary Survey Sampling*, 5th ed. Duxbury, Belmont, CA.

Schemper, M. and Stare, J. (1996) Explained variation in survival analysis. *Statist. Med.*, **15**, 1999–2012.

Schlesselman, J.J. (1974) Sample size requirements in cohort and case–control studies of disease. *Am. J. Epidemiol.*, **33**, 381–384.

Schlesselman, J.J. (1982) *Case–Control Studies: Design, Conduct and Analysis*. Oxford University Press, New York.

Schoenfeld, D.A. and Borenstein, M. (2005) Calculating the power or sample size for the logistic and proportional hazards models. *J. Statist. Comp. Simul.* **75**, 771–785.

Schonlau, M. (2005) Boosted Regression (Boosting): an introductory tutorial and a Stata plugin. *Stata J.*, **5**, 330–354.

Schwarz, G.E. (1978) Estimating the dimension of a model. *Annals Statist.*, **6**, 461–464.

Scott, A. and Wild, C. (1991) Transformations and R^2. *Am. Statistician*, **45**, 127–129.

Scragg, R., Mitchell, E.A., Taylor, B.J. *et al.* (1993) Bed sharing, smoking and alcohol in the sudden infant death syndrome. *BMJ*, **307**, 1312–1318.

Seber, G.A.F. and Wild, C.J. (2003) *Nonlinear Regression.* John Wiley & Sons, New York.

Senn, S. (2002) *Cross-Over Trials in Clinical Research*, 2nd ed. John Wiley & Sons, Chichester.

Shao, J. and Tu, D. (1995) *The Jackknife and Bootstrap.* Springer, New York.

Shaper, A.G., Wannamethee, G. and Walker, M. (1988) Alcohol and mortality in British men: explaining the U-shaped curve. *Lancet*, **ii**, 1267–1273.

Shapiro, S. (1994) Meta-analysis/Schmeta-analysis. *Am. J. Epidemiol*, **140**, 771–778.

Sheiner, L.B. and Rubin, D.B. (1995) Intention-to-treat analysis and the goals of clinical trials. *Clin. Pharmacol. Ther.*, **57**, 6–15.

Shewry, M.C., Smith, W.C.S., Woodward, M. and Tunstall–Pedoe, H. (1992) Variation in coronary risk factors by social status: results from the Scottish Heart Health Study. *Br. J. Gen. Practice*, **42**, 406–410.

Shryock, H.S., Siegel, J.S. and Stockwell, E.G. (1976) *The Methods and Materials of Demography,* condensed ed. Academic Press, New York.

Siemiatycki, J. (1989) Friendly control bias. *J. Clin. Epidemiol.*, **42**, 687–688.

Silverman, B.W. (1998) *Density Estimation for Statistics and Data Analysis.* Chapman & Hall/CRC Press, Boca Raton, FL.

Skov, T., Deddens, J., Petersen, M.R. and Endahl, L. (1998) Prevalence proportion ratios: estimation and hypothesis testing. *Int. J. Epidemiol.*, **27**, 91–95.

Smith, W.C.S., Crombie, I.K., Tavendale, R., Irving, I.M., Kenicer, M.B. and Tunstall–Pedoe, H. (1987) The Scottish Heart Health Study: objectives and development of methods. *Health Bull. (Edinburgh)*, **45**, 211–217.

Smith, W.C.S., Woodward, M. and Tunstall–Pedoe, H. (1991) Intermittent claudication in Scotland, in *Epidemiology of Peripheral Vascular Disease.* (Ed. F.G.R. Fowkes). Springer–Verlag, Berlin.

Snedecor, G.W. and Cochran, W.G. (1989) *Statistical Methods*, 8th ed. Iowa State University Press, Ames.

Somers, R.H. (1962) A new asymmetric measure of association for ordinal variables. *Am. Sociological Rev.*, **27**, 799–811.

Spiegelhalter, D.J. (1986) Probabilistic prediction in patient management and clinical trials. *Statist. Med.*, **5**, 421–433.

Srinivasan, U., Leonard, N., Jones, E. *et al.* (1996) Absence of oats toxicity in adult coeliac disease. *BMJ*, **313**, 1300–1301.

Sritara, P., Cheepudomwit, S., Chapman, N. *et al.* (2003) 12-year changes in vascular risk factors and their associations with mortality in a cohort of 3499 Thais. The Electricity Generating Authority of Thailand Study. *Int. J. Epidemiol.*, **32**, 461–468.

Steel, R.G.D. and Torrie, J.H. (1980) *Principles and Procedures of Statistics. A Biometrical Approach*, 2nd ed. McGraw–Hill, New York.

Steinbok, P., Reiner, A.M., Beauchamp, R., Armstrong, R.W. and Cochrane, D.D. (1997) A randomized controlled trial to compare selective posterior rhizotomy plus physiotherapy with physiotherapy alone in children with spastic diplegic cerebral palsy. *Develop. Med. Child. Neurol.*, **39**, 178–184.

Stephens, M.A. (1974) EDF statistics for goodness of fit and some comparisons. *J. Am. Statist. Assoc.*, **69**, 730–737.

Sterne, J. (Ed.) (2009) *Meta-Analysis: An Updated Collection from the Stata Journal.* Stata Press, College Station, TX.

Stewart, L.A. and Clarke, M.J. (1995) Practical methodology of meta-analyses (overviews) using updated individual patient data. *Statist. Med.*, **14**, 2057–2079.

Stolley, P.D. and Lasky, T. (1995) *Investigating Disease Patterns. The Science of Epidemiology.* W.H. Freeman, New York.

Storr, J., Barrell, E. and Lenny, W. (1987) Asthma in primary schools. *BMJ*, **295**, 251–252.

Stürmer, T., Joshi, M., Glynn, R.J., Avorn, J., Rothman, K.J. and Schneeweiss, S. (2006) A review of the application of propensity score methods yielded increasing use, advantages in specific settings, but not substantially different estimates compared with conventional multivariable methods. *J. Clin. Epidemiol.*, **59**, 437–447.

Strachan, D.P. (1988) Damp housing and childhood asthma: validation of reporting of symptoms. *BMJ*, **297**, 1223–1226.

Stroup, D.F., Berlin, J.A., Morton, S.C. *et al.* (2000) Meta-analysis of observational studies in epidemiology: a proposal for reporting. Meta-analysis of Observational Studies in Epidemiology (MOOSE) group. *J. Am. Med. Assoc.*, **283**, 2008–2012.

Stuart, E., Azur, M., Frangakis, C. and Leaf, P. (2009) Multiple imputation with large data sets: a case study of the children's mental health initiative. *Am. J. Epidemiol.*, **169**, 1133–1139.

Sullivan, L.M., Massaro, J.M. and D'Agostino, R.B. Sr. (2004) Presentation of multivariate data for clinical use: the Framingham Study risk score functions. *Statist. Med.*, **23**, 1631–1660.

Sutton, A.J., Abrams, K.R., Jones, D.R., Sheldon, T.A. and Song, F. (2000) *Methods for Meta-Analysis in Medical Research.* John Wiley & Sons, Chichester.

Swan, A.V. (1986) *GLIM 3.77 Introductory Guide.* Revision A. NAG, Oxford.

Sweeting, M.J., Sutton, A.J. and Lambert, P.C. (2004) What to add to nothing? Use and avoidance of continuity corrections in meta-analysis of sparse data. *Statist. Med.*, **23**, 1351–1375.

Sylvester, R.J., Machin, D. and Staquet, M.J. (1982) Cancer clinical trial protocols, in *Treatment of Cancer* (Ed. K.E. Halnan). Chapman & Hall, London.

Tarone, R.E. (1981) On summary estimations of relative risk. *J. Chronic Dis.*, **34**, 463–468.

Tetzchner, T., Sørensen, M., Jønsson, L., Lase, G. and Christiansen, J. (1997) Delivery and pudendal nerve function. *Acta Obstet. Gynecol. Scand.*, **76**, 324–331.

Tham, T.C.K., Collins, J.S.A., Molloy, C., Sloan, J.M., Banford, K.B. and Watson, R.G.P. (1996) Randomised controlled trial of ranitidine versus omeprazole in combination with antibiotics for eradication of *Helicobacter pylori. Ulster Med. J.*, **65**, 131–136.

Therneau, T.M. and Grambsch, P. (2000) *Modeling Survival Data: Extending the Cox Model.* Springer-Verlag, Berlin.

Thomas, D.C. and Greenland, S. (1983) The relative efficiencies of matched and independent sample designs for case–control studies. *J. Chronic Dis.*, **36**, 685–697.

Thomas, D.C. and Greenland, S. (1985) The efficiency of matching in case–control studies of risk factor interactions. *J. Chronic Dis.*, **38**, 569–574.

Thomas, D.G. (1975) Exact and asymptotic methods for the combination of 2×2 tables. *Comput. Biomed. Res.*, **8**, 423–426.

Thomas, L.H. (1992) Ischaemic heart disease and consumption of hydrogenated marine oils in England and Wales. *J. Epidemiol. Comm. Health*, **46**, 78–82.

Thompson, S.G. and Higgins, J.P.T. (2002) How should meta-regression analyses be interpreted? *Statist. Med.*, **21**, 1559–1573.

Thompson, S., Kaptoge, S., White, I., Wood, A., Perry, P. and Danesh, J. (2010) Statistical methods for the time-to-event analysis of individual participant data from multiple epidemiological studies. *Int. J. Epidemiol.*, **39**, 1345–1359.

Thompson, S.G. and Sharp, S. (1999) Explaining heterogeneity in meta-analysis: a comparison of methods. *Statist. Med.*, **18**, 2693–2708.

Thompson, W.D., Kelsey, J.L. and Walter, S.D. (1982) Cost and efficiency in the choice of matched and unmatched case-control study designs. *Am. J. Epidemiol.*, **116**, 840–851.

Tiku, M.L., Tan, W.Y. and Balakrishnan, N. (1986) *Robust Inference.* Marcel Dekker, New York.

Tudur Smith, C., Williamson, P.R. and Marson, A.G. Investigating heterogeneity in an individual patient data meta-analysis of time to event outcomes. *Statist. Med.*, **24**, 1307–1319.

Tunstall–Pedoe, H. (2003) *MONICA: Monograph and Multimedia Sourcebook.* World Health Organization, Geneva.

Tunstall–Pedoe, H., Smith, W.C.S., Crombie, I.K. and Tavendale, R. (1989) Coronary risk factor and lifestyle variation across Scotland: results from the Scottish Heart Health Study. *Scot. Med. J.*, **34**, 556–560.

Tunstall–Pedoe, H. and Woodward, M. (2006) By neglecting deprivation, cardiovascular risk scoring will exacerbate social gradients in disease. *Heart*, **92**, 307–310.

Tunstall–Pedoe, H., Woodward, M., Tavendale, R., A'Brook R. and McCluskey, M.K. (1997) Comparison of the prediction by 27 different factors of coronary heart disease and death in men and women of the Scottish Heart Health Study: cohort study. *BMJ*, **315**, 722–729.

Turner, E.H., Matthews, A.M., Linardatos, E., Tell, R.A. and Rosenthal, R. (2008) Selective publication of antidepressant trials and its influence on apparent efficacy. *N. Engl. J. Med.*, **358**, 252–260.

United Nations (1996) *Demographic Yearbook 1994*. United Nations, New York.

Uno, H., Cai, T., Pencina, M.J., D'Agostino, R.B. and Wei, L.J. (2011) On the c-statistics for evaluating overall adequacy of risk prediction procedures with censored survival data. *Statist. Med.*, **30**, 1105–1117.

Ury, H.K. (1975) Efficiency of case–control studies with multiple controls per case: continuous or dichotomous data. *Biometrics*, **31**, 643–649.

Valent, F., Brusaferro, S. and Barbone, F. (2001) A case-crossover study of sleep and childhood injury. *Pediatrics*, **107**, e23.

van Buuren, S. (2007) Multiple imputation of discrete and continuous data by fully conditional specification. *Statist. Methods Med. Res.*, **16**, 219–242.

Vierkant, R.A. (1997) A SAS macro for calculating bootstrapped confidence intervals about a kappa coefficient. http://www2.sas.com/proceedings/sugi22/STATS/PAPER295.PDF.

von Elm, E., Altman, D.G., Egger, M., Pocock, S.J., Gøtzsche, P.C. and Vandenbroucke, J.P. (2007) Strengthening the reporting of observational studies in epidemiology (STROBE) statement: guidelines for reporting observational studies. *Ann. Intern Med.*, **147**, 573–577.

von Hippel, P.T. (2013) Should a normal imputation model be modified to impute skewed variables? *Sociological Methods Res.*, **42**, 105–138.

Wacholder, S. (1991) Practical considerations in choosing between the case–cohort and nested case-control designs. *Epidemiology*, **2**, 155–158.

Wacholder, S. and Boivin, J.-F. (1987) External comparisons with the case–cohort design. *Am. J. Epidemiol.*, **126**, 1198–1209.

Wacholder, S. and Silverman, D.T. (1990) Re: 'Case-control studies using other diseases as controls: problems of excluding exposure-related diseases' (Letter). *Am. J. Epidemiol.*, **132**, 1017–1018.

Wacholder, S., McLaughlin, J.K., Silverman, D.T. and Mandel, J.S. (1992) Selection of controls in case–control studies. *Am. J. Epidemiol.*, **136**, 1019–1050.

Wald, N.J. and Law, M.R. (2003) A strategy to reduce cardiovascular disease by more than 80%. *BMJ*, **326**, 1419.

Walter, S.D. (1980a) Berkson's bias and its control in epidemiological studies. *J. Chronic Dis.*, **33**, 721–725.

Walter, S.D. (1980b) Matched case–control studies with a variable number of controls per case. *Appl. Statist.*, **29**, 172–179.

Wangensteen, O.H., Peter, E.T., Nicoloff, D.M., Walder, A.I., Sosin, H. and Bernstein, E.F. (1962) Achieving 'physiological gastrectomy' by gastric freezing. *JAMA*, **180**, 439–444.

Weiss, N. (2001) *Introductory Statistics*, 6th ed. Pearson Addison Wesley, Reading, MA.

Wells, S., Kerr, A., Eadie, S., Wiltshire, C. and Jackson, R. (2010) 'Your Heart Forecast': a new approach for describing and communicating cardiovascular risk? *Heart*, **96**, 708–713.

White, H. (1982) Maximum likelihood estimation of misspecified models. *Econometrica*, **50**, 1–25.

White, I.R. and Royston, P. (2009) Imputing missing covariate values for the Cox model. *Statist. Med.*, **28**, 1982–1998.

White, I.R., Royston, P. and Wood, A.M. (2011) Multiple imputation using chained equations: issues and guidance for practice. *Statist. Med.*, **30**, 377–399.

Whitehead, J. (1997) *The Design and Analysis of Sequential Clinical Trials*, 2nd ed. (rev.). John Wiley & Sons, Chichester.

Whittemore, A.S. (1983) Estimating attributable risk from case-control studies. *Am. J. Epidemiol.*, **117**, 76–85.

Williams, D.A. (1982) Extra-binomial variation in logistic linear models. *Appl. Statist.*, **31**, 144–148.

Williamson, E., Morley, R., Lucas, A. and Carpenter, J. (2012) Propensity scores: from naive enthusiasm to intuitive understanding. *Stat. Methods Med. Res.*, **21**, 273–293.

Williamson, P.R., Kolamunnage–Dona, R., Philipson, P. and Marson, A.G. (2008) Joint modelling of longitudinal and competing risks data. *Statist. Med.*, **27**, 6426–6438.

Wilson, D.C. and McClure, G. (1996) Babies born under 1000 g — perinatal outcome. *Ulster Med. J.*, **65**, 118–122.

Winn, D.M., Blot, W.J., McLaughlin, J.K. *et al.* (1991) Mouthwash use and oral conditions in the risk of oral and pharyngeal cancer. *Cancer Res.*, **51**, 3044–3047.

Wong, O. (1990) A cohort mortality study and a case-control study of workers potentially exposed to styrene in the reinforced-plastics and composites industry. *Br. J. Ind. Med.*, **47**, 753–762.

Woodward, M. (1992) Formulae for the calculation of sample size, power and minimum detectable relative risk in medical studies. *Statistician*, **41**, 185–196.

Woodward, M., Bolton–Smith, C. and Tunstall–Pedoe, H. (1994) Deficient health knowledge, diet and other lifestyles in smokers: is a multifactorial approach required? *Prev. Med.*, **23**, 354–361.

Woodward, M., Laurent, K. and Tunstall–Pedoe, H. (1995) An analysis of risk factors for prevalent coronary heart disease using the proportional odds model. *Statistician*, **44**, 69–80.

Woodward, M., Lowe, G.D.O., Campbell, D.J. *et al.* (2005) Associations of inflammatory and haemostatic variables with the risk of recurrent stroke. *Stroke*, **36**, 2143–2147.

Woodward, M., Lowe, G.D.O., Rumley, A. *et al.* (1997) Epidemiology of coagulation factors, inhibitors and activation markers: The Third Glasgow MONICA Survey. II. Relationships to cardiovascular risk factors and prevalent cardiovascular disease. *Br. J. Haematol.*, **97**, 785–797.

Woodward, M., Nursten, J., Williams, P. and Badger, G.D. (2000) Mental disorder and homicide: a review of epidemiological research. *Epidemiol. Psychiatr. Soc.*, **9**, 171–189.

Woodward, M., Shewry, M.C., Smith, W.C.S. and Tunstall–Pedoe, H. (1992) Social status and coronary heart disease: results from the Scottish Heart Health Study. *Prev. Med.*, **21**, 136–148.

Woodward, M. and Tunstall–Pedoe, H. (1992a) Biochemical evidence of persistent heavy smoking after a coronary diagnosis despite self-reported reduction. Analysis from the Scottish Heart Health Study. *Eur. Heart. J.*, **13**, 160–165.

Woodward, M. and Tunstall–Pedoe, H. (1992b) An iterative technique for identifying smoking deceivers with application to the Scottish Heart Health Study. *Prev. Med.*, **21**, 88–97.

Woodward, M., Tunstall-Pedoe, H., Rumley, A. and Lowe, G.D. (2009) Does fibrinogen add to prediction of cardiovascular disease? Results from the Scottish Heart Health Extended Cohort Study. *Br. J. Haematol.*, **146**, 442–446.

Woodward, M. and Walker, A.R.P. (1994) Sugar consumption and dental caries: evidence from 90 countries. *Br. Dent. J.*, **176**, 297–302.

Woolf, B. (1955) On estimating the relationship between blood group and disease. *Ann. Human Genet.*, **19**, 251–253.

World Health Organization (1995) *Physical Status: The Use and Interpretation of Anthropometry.* WHO Technical Report Series, 854. World Health Organization, Geneva.

Yanagwa, T., Fujii, Y. and Mastuoka, H. (1994) Generalized Mantel–Haenszel procedures for $2 \times J$ tables. *Environ. Health Perspect.*, **102** Suppl 8, 57–60.

Ying, R.L., Gross, K.B., Terzo, T.S. and Eschenbacher, W.L. (1990) Indomethacin does not inhibit the ozone-induced increase in bronchial responsiveness in human subjects. *Am. Rev. Respiratory Dis.*, **142**, 817–821.

Youden, W.J. (1950) Index for rating diagnostic tests. *Cancer*, **3**, 32–35.

Zhang, J., Savitz, D.A., Schwingl, P.J. and Cai, W.-W. (1992) A case–control study of paternal smoking and birth defects. *Int. J. Epidemiol.*, **21**, 273–278.

Zou, G. (2004) Modified Poisson regression approach to prospective studies with binary data. *Am. J. Epidemiol.*, **159**, 702–706.

Zoungas, S., Chalmers, J., Ninomiya, T. *et al.* (2012) Association of HbA_{1c} levels with vascular complications and death in patients with type 2 diabetes: evidence of glycaemic thresholds. *Diabetologia*, **55**, 636–643.

Zweig, M.H. and Campbell, G. (1993) Receiver-operating characteristic (ROC) plots: a fundamental evaluation tool in clinical medicine. *Clin. Chem.*, **39**, 561–577.

Index